	Hydroxyzine	Meperidine	Metoclopramide	Midazolam	Morphine	Nalbuphine	Pentazocine	Pentobarbital	Perphenazine	Prochlorperazine	Promazine	Promethazine	Ranitidine	Scopolamine	Secobarbital	Thiethylperazine
	C	C	C	C	C	C	C	C	C	C	C	C	C	C	I	
	C	C	C	C	C		C	I	C	C		C		C	I	C
	C	C	C	C	C		C	I	C	C	C	C	C	C	I	
								I							I	
	I	I	I		I	I	I	I	I	I	I	I		I	I	I
	I	C	C	I	C		C	I	C	I	I	I	C	C	I	
	C	C	C	C	C		C	I	C	C	C	C	C	C	I	
	C	C	C		C	C	C	I	C	C	C	C		C	I	
	C	C	C		C		C	I	C	C	C	C	C	C	I	
	C	C			C		I	I		C	C	C	C	C	I	
		I			I		I					I				
		C	C		C	C	C	I		C	C	C	I	C	I	
	C		C		I		C	I	C	C	C	C	C	C	I	
	C	C			C		C		C	C	C	C	C	C	I	
	C		C		C	C		I	I	I	C	C	I	C		C
	C	I	C				C	I	C	C	C	C	C	C	I	
	C							I		C		*	C	C	I	C
	C	C	C		C			I	C	C	C	C	C	C	I	
	I	I			I	I	I		I	I	I	I		C	I	
		C	C		C		C	I		C		C	C	C	I	I
	C	C	C		C	C	C	I	C		C	C	C	C	I	
	C	C	C		C		C	I		C		C		C	I	
	C	C	C		C	C	C	I	C	C	C		C	C	I	
		C	C	I	C	C	C		C	C		C		C		C
	C	C	C		C	C	C	C	C	C	C	C	C		I	
	I	I	I		I	I	I	I	I	I	I	I		I		I
						C			I				C		I	

Parenteral compatibility occurs when two or more drugs are successfully mixed without liquefaction, deliquescence, or precipitation.

Mosby's Drug Guide for Nurses

Fifth Edition

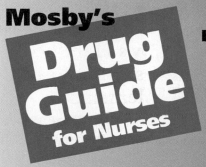

Linda Skidmore-Roth, RN, MSN, NP
Consultant
Littleton, Colorado
Formerly, Nursing Faculty
New Mexico State University
Las Cruces, New Mexico;
El Paso Community College
El Paso, Texas

Mosby's DrugSmart CD-ROM to accompany Mosby's Drug Guide for Nurses

with 190 *illustrations and* 2 *color inserts*

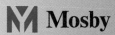

Mosby
An Affiliate of Elsevier Science
St. Louis London Philadelphia Sydney Toronto

Mosby
An Affiliate of Elsevier Science

11830 Westline Industrial Drive
St. Louis, Missouri 63146

MOSBY'S DRUG GUIDE FOR NURSES ISBN 0-323-01494-1

Notice

Pharmacology is an ever-changing field. Standard safety precautions must be followed, but as new research and clinical experience broaden our knowledge, changes in treatment and drug therapy may become necessary or appropriate. Readers are advised to check the most current product information provided by the manufacturer of each drug to be administered to verify the recommended dose, the method and duration of administration, and contraindications. It is the responsibility of the licensed health care provider, relying on experience and knowledge of the patient, to determine dosages and the best treatment for each individual patient. Neither the publisher nor the editor assumes any liability for any injury and/or damage to persons or property arising from this publication.

The Publisher

Previous editions copyrighted 1996, 1997, 1999, 2001

Vice President, Publishing Director: Sally Schrefer
Executive Editor, Nursing: Darlene Como
Senior Developmental Editor: Tamara A. Myers
Publishing Services Manager: Deborah L. Vogel
Design Manager: Bill Drone

GW/RDC

Printed in the United States of America

Last digit is the print number: 9 8 7 6 5 4 3 2 1

Consultants

Jean Krajicek Bartek, PhD, APRN
Associate Professor
University of Nebraska Medical Center
Colleges of Nursing and Medicine (Pharmacology)
Omaha, Nebraska

Rita Hanover Berdan, MS, RN, C
Nursing Faculty
St. Joseph's Hospital Health Center School of Nursing
Syracuse, New York

Barbara L. Cary, MSN, RN
Adjunct Faculty
University of Maine
Augusta, Maine

Tamara Conroy, RMA, CPT, SPN
Pittston, Pennsylvania

Henry B. Geiter, Jr, RN, C, CCRN
Vencor Hospital
St. Petersburg Junior College
St. Petersburg, Florida

F. James Grogan, PharmD
Executive Director
Grogan Communications
Swansea, Illinois

Jennifer L. Gudeman, PharmD
Product Surveillance Specialist
Corporate Product Monitoring
Mallinckrodt/Tyco Healthcare
St. Louis, Missouri

Scott Harrington, PharmD, RPh
Harrington Health Informatics
Tucson, Arizona

Phyllis Howard, RN, BSN
Associate Professor of Practical Nursing
Ashland Technical College
Ashland, Kentucky

Joan Ann Leach, RNC, MS, ME
Professor of Nursing
Capital Community College
Hartford, Connecticut

Mary Jo Mattocks, PhD, MN, BSN
Assistant Professor
Montana State University
Northern Great Falls Campus
Great Falls, Montana

Jennifer L. McQuade, PharmD
Medical Information Consultant
Douglasville, Georgia

Michelle M. Montpas, RN, MSN, OCN
CS Mott Community College
Flint, Michigan

Janet Rentfro, RN, ADN, ACLS
Medical Supervisor
Ascension Island
South Atlantic Ocean

Becky A. Ridenhour, PharmD
St. Louis College of Pharmacy
St. Louis, Missouri

Roberta Secrest, PharmD, PhD
Global Scientific Information and Communication
Eli Lilly and Company
Indianapolis, Indiana

Patricia R. Teasley, MSN, RN, CS
Central Texas College
Killeen, Texas

Brenda L. Thompson, PharmD
Assistant Professor
Pharmacy Practice Division
St. Louis College of Pharmacy
St. Louis, Missouri

Joyce S. Willens, PhD, RN
Assistant Professor
College of Nursing
Villanova University
Villanova, Pennsylvania

Preface

Mosby's Drug Guide for Nurses, 5th edition, is the most in-depth handbook available for nursing students and practicing nurses! Since its first publication in 1996, more than 100 U.S. and Canadian pharmacists and consultants have reviewed the book's content closely. Today, *Mosby's Drug Guide for Nurses* is more up-to-date than ever—with features that make it easy to find critical information fast!

NEW FACTS

This edition features over 2000 new drug facts, including:

- new drugs and new dosage information
- newly researched side effects and adverse reactions
- the latest precautions, interactions, and contraindications, including highlighted pediatric and geriatric considerations
- IV therapy updates
- revised nursing considerations
- updated patient/family teaching guidelines

NEW FEATURES

- Monographs for 118 "high-alert" medications are highlighted with a special monograph header in the A-to-Z section to remind you to use extra care in administering these drugs. Appendix C provides a complete list of "high-alert" drugs most capable of causing significant harm to patients.
- Appendix A, "Selected new drugs" provides detailed monographs for 24 drugs recently approved by the FDA. (See Table of Contents for complete list.) Included are monographs for:
  - frovatriptan (Frova) for treatment of migraines
  - bosentan (Tracleer) for treatment of pulmonary arterial hypertension
  - dutasteride (Duagen) for treatment of benign prostatic hyperplasia
  - valdecoxib (Bextra) for treatment of rheumatoid arthritis and osteoarthritis
- Appendix B, "Recent FDA drug approvals," lists generic/trade names and uses for 6 of the most recently approved drugs.
- DrugSmart CD-ROM offers a mini-database containing more than 35 common herbs, a complete dosages and calculations review program, and a dosing and lifespan pharmacology review.

ORGANIZATION

This handbook is organized into three main sections:

- Individual drug monographs (in alphabetical order by generic name)

- Drug categories
- Appendixes (identified by the wide blue thumb tabs on the edge)

and three smaller sections that provide additional valuable information for nursing students:

- Disorders Index (follows the Appendixes)
- Drug Identification Guide (full-color center insert)
- Photo Atlas of Drug Administration (full-color center insert)

The guiding principle behind this book is to provide fast, easy access to drug information and nursing considerations. Every detail—from the cover, binding, and paper to the typeface, two-color design, eye-catching icons, and appendixes—has been carefully chosen with the user in mind. Here's what you'll find in each section of the handbook:

Individual Drug Monographs

This book includes monographs for more than 4000 generic and trade name medications—those most commonly administered by students. Common trade names are given for all drugs regularly used in the United States and Canada, with drugs available only in Canada identified by a maple leaf icon (✱).

Each monograph provides the following information, whenever possible, for safe, effective administration of each drug:

High-alert status: Identifies drugs with the most potential to cause harm to patients, screened for easy identification.

Key drug status: Identifies drugs of special prominence within their functional class, often encountered by students during clinicals; denoted with a special icon (🔑).

Pronunciation: Helps the nurse master complex generic names.

Rx/OTC: Identifies prescription or over-the-counter drugs.

Functional and chemical classifications: Helps the nurse recognize similarities and differences among drugs in the same functional but different chemical classes.

Pregnancy category: FDA pregnancy categories A, B, C, D, or X are noted at the beginning of the monograph, as well as under Precautions or Contraindications depending on the FDA category. Appendix J provides a detailed explanation of each category.

Controlled substance schedule: Includes schedules for the United States (I, II, III, IV, V) and Canada (F, G).

Action: Describes pharmacologic properties concisely.

Therapeutic outcome: Details all possible results of medication use, denoted with a special icon (→).

Uses: Lists the conditions the drug is used to treat.

Investigational uses: Describes drug uses that may be encountered in practice but are not yet FDA-approved.

Dosage and routes: Lists all available and approved dosages and routes for adult, pediatric, and elderly patients.

"Pediatric" and "Geriatric" icons: Special icons (P and G) in the margins of theDosage and routes, Contraindications, and Precautions sections that denote lifespan content.

Available forms: Includes tablets, capsules, extended-release, injectables (**IV**, IM, SC), solutions, creams, ointments, lotions, gels, shampoos, elixirs, suspensions, suppositories, sprays, aerosols, and lozenges.

Adverse effects: Groups potential reactions by body system, with common side effects *italicized* and life-threatening reactions in **bold type** for emphasis.

Contraindications: Lists conditions under which the drug absolutely should not be given, including FDA pregnancy safety categories, D or X.

Precautions: Lists conditions that require special consideration when the drug is prescribed, including FDA pregnancy safety categories A, B, and C.

"Do not confuse" icon ( ): Denotes drug names that might easily be confused, within each appropriate monograph.

Pharmacokinetics/pharmacodynamics: Features a quick-reference chart of concise facts on pharmacokinetics (absorption, distribution, metabolism, excretion, half-life) and pharmacodynamics (onset, peak, duration).

Interactions: Includes confirmed drug, food, and herbal interactions, in alphabetical order by individual drug name, drug class name, or herbal product name.

"Herb-Drug Interaction" icon ( ): Highlights more than 400 potential interactions between herbal products and prescription or OTC drugs.

Lab test interferences: Identifies how the drug may affect lab test results.

Nursing considerations: Identifies key nursing considerations for each step of the nursing process: Assessment, Nursing Diagnoses (denoted with a special icon ✓), Implementation, Patient/Family Education, and Evaluation, including positive therapeutic outcomes. Instructions for giving drugs by various routes (e.g., **IV**, IM, SC, PO, topically, rectally) appear under Implementation, with route subheadings in bold.

Compatibilities: Lists syringe, Y-site, and additive compatibilities and incompatibilities. If no compatibilities are listed for a drug, the necessary compatibility testing has not been done and that compatibility information is unknown. To ensure safety, assume that the drug may not be mixed with other drugs unless specifically stated.

"Nursing Alert" icon (◆): Highlights situations in which the patient potentially could be at risk.

"Do Not Crush" icon (⃠): Denotes drugs that may not be administered in crushed form.

Treatment of overdose: Lists drugs and treatment for overdoses where appropriate.

Drug Categories

The Drug Categories section, following the individual drug monographs, provides general information about the various functional classes to promote learning about the similarities and differences among drugs in the same functional class. Summarizes action, uses, adverse effects, contraindications, precautions, pharmacokinetics, interactions, and nursing considerations for each functional class.

Appendixes

Selected new drugs: Includes comprehensive information on 24 key drugs approved by the FDA during the last 12 months.

Recent FDA drug approvals: Summarizes basic information, such as generic name, trade name and uses, for drugs so recently approved by the FDA that complete information was not yet available when this book went to press.

High-alert drugs: Lists the 118 drugs in *Mosby's Drug Guide for Nurses* that are considered high-alert because of their potential to cause significant harm to patients.

Ophthalmic, nasal, topical, and otic products: Provides monographs for more than 140 ophthalmic, otic, nasal, and topical products commonly used today, grouped by chemical drug class.

Combination products: Provides details on the forms and uses of more than 700 combination products.

Rarely used drugs: Provides concise monographs for 105 infrequently used drugs, including dosage and routes, uses, and contraindications.

Less frequently used antihistamines: Includes names, uses, doses, forms, interactions and contraindications.

Herbal products: Features basic usage information on more than 70 common herbs and natural supplements.

FDA pregnancy categories: Explains the 5 FDA pregnancy categories

Controlled substance chart: Covers both United States and Canadian drug schedules, with examples.

Commonly used abbreviations: Lists abbreviations alphabetically with their meanings.

IV drug/solution compatibility chart: Lists compatibilities for 52 **IV** drugs and solutions.

Nomogram for calculation of body surface area: Provides a quick, handy chart for calculating body surface area for patient drug calculations.

Disorders Index

This book includes both a general index and a disorders index, both of which are updated and expanded in this edition. Dovetailing with the content nursing students encounter in medical-surgical courses, the disorders index lists major disorders and major drugs used in their management. The page number for each drug listed follows.

Drug Identification Guide

Completely updated for the 5th edition, the Drug Identification Guide includes 160 full-color photos showing the top 60 prescribed drugs as tabulated in *Mosby's DrugConsult.* Photos are arranged alphabetically by generic name, with dosage strengths listed.

Photo Atlas of Drug Administration

This practical resource for students and practitioners lists standard precautions and provides 32 full-color illustrations depicting the physical landmarks and administration techniques used for **IV**, IM, SC, and ID drug delivery.

The following sources were consulted in the preparation of this edition:

Blumenthal M: *The complete German Commission E monographs: Therapeutic guide to herbal medicines,* Austin, 1998, American Botanical Council.

Clark JB, Queener SF, Karb VB: *Pharmacologic basis of nursing practice,* ed 6, St Louis, 2000, Mosby.

Drug information: Bethesda, American Hospital Formulary Service.

Facts and comparisons: St Louis, updated monthly.

Gahart BL: *Intravenous medications,* ed 18, St Louis, 2002, Mosby.

Goodman A and others: *Goodman and Gilman's the pharmacological basis of therapeutics,* ed 10, New York, 1998, Pergamon Press.

McKenry LM, Salerno E: *Mosby's pharmacology in nursing,* ed 21, St Louis, 2001, Mosby.

Mediphor Editorial Group: *Drug interaction facts,* Philadelphia, updated quarterly, JB Lippincott.

Review of natural products: Philadelphia, updated monthly, *Facts and Comparisons.*

Acknowledgments

I am indebted to the nursing and pharmacology consultants who reviewed the manuscript and galley pages, and I thank them for their thoughtful comments and encouragement. I would also like to thank Darlene Como and Tamara Myers, my editors, whose active encouragement and enthusiasm have made this book better than it might otherwise have been. I am likewise grateful to Deborah Vogel, Noelle Barrick, and Graphic World, Inc., for the coordination of the production process, and to Dana Knighten for assistance with development of the new edition.

Linda Skidmore-Roth

Contents

Drug Monographs New to This Edition (Appendix A)

alemtuzumab
almotriptan
anakinra
bosentan
cefditoren pivoxil
darbepoetin alfa
desloratadine
dexmethylphenidate
drotrecogin alfa
dutasteride
eprosartan mesylate/hydrochlorothiazide
ertapenem
esomeprazole
fondaparinux sodium
formoterol fumarate
frovatriptan
galantamine
imatinib
nesiritide
perflutren lipid microsphere
tenofovir disoproxil fumarate
valdecoxib
valganciclovir
zoledronic acid

abacavir (℞)

(aba-ka'veer)

Ziagen

Func. class.: Antiviral

Chem. class.: Nucleoside analog

Pregnancy category C

Action: A synthetic, nucleoside analog with inhibitory action against HIV. Inhibits replication of HIV by incorporating into cellular DNA by viral reverse transcriptase, thereby terminating the cellular DNA chain

➔ **Therapeutic Outcome:** Decreased symptoms of HIV

Uses: In combination with other antiretroviral agents for HIV-1 infection

Dosage and routes

Adult: PO 300 mg bid with other antiretrovirals

P ***Adolescents and children ≥3 mo:*** PO 8 mg/kg bid, max 300 mg bid with other antiretrovirals

Available forms: Tabs 300 mg; oral sol 20 mg/ml

Adverse effects

CNS: *Fever, headache, malaise, insomnia,* paresthesia

GI: *Nausea, vomiting, diarrhea, anorexia, cramps, abdominal pain, ↑ AST, ALT*

HEMA: **Granulocytopenia, anemia,** lymphopenia

INTEG: Rash, **fatal hypersensitivity reactions,** urticaria

META: **Lactic acidosis**

MISC: ↑ CPK

RESP: Dyspnea

Contraindications: Hypersensitivity

Precautions: Granulocyte count <1000/mm^3 or Hgb <9.5 g/dl, P pregnancy **C**, lactation, children, severe renal disease, severe hepatic function

Pharmacokinetics

Absorption	Well absorbed (PO)
Distribution	50% plasma protein binding
Metabolism	To inactive metabolite
Excretion	Kidneys, feces
Half-life	1½-2 hr

Pharmacodynamics

Unknown

Interactions

Individual drugs

Alcohol: ↑ abacavir levels

NURSING CONSIDERATIONS

Assessment

- Assess for lactic acidosis and severe hepatomegaly with steatosis
- ⚠ Assess for fatal hypersensitivity reactions: fever, rash, nausea, vomiting, diarrhea, abdominal discomfort; treatment should be discontinued and not restarted
- ⚠ Assess for pancreatitis: abdominal pain, nausea, vomiting, elevated liver enzymes; drug should be discontinued because condition can be fatal
- Monitor CBC, differential, platelet count qmo; withhold drug if WBC is <4000/mm^3 or platelet count is <75,000/mm^3; notify prescriber of results
- Monitor renal function studies; BUN, serum uric acid, urine CrCl before, during therapy; these may be elevated throughout treatment
- Monitor temp q4h, may indicate beginning infection
- Monitor liver function tests before, during therapy (bilirubin, AST, ALT, amylase, alkaline phosphatase prn or qmo)

Nursing diagnoses

- ✓ Infection, risk for (uses)
- ✓ Injury, risk for physical injury (adverse reactions)
- ✓ Knowledge deficit (teaching)

Implementation

PO route

- Give on empty stomach, q12h around the clock
- Give in combination with other antiretrovirals with food

Patient/family education

- Advise patient to report signs of infection: increased temp, sore throat, flu symptoms; to avoid crowds and those with known infections
- Instruct patient to report signs of anemia: fatigue, headache, faintness, shortness of breath, irritability
- Advise patient to report bleeding; avoid use of razors or commercial mouthwash
- Inform patient that drug is not a cure, but will control symptoms
- Inform patient that major toxicities may necessitate discontinuing drug
- Instruct patient to use contraception during treatment
- Caution patient to avoid OTC products or other medications without approval of prescriber
- Caution patient not to have any sexual contact without use of a condom, needles should not be shared, blood from infected individual should not come in contact with another's mucous membranes
- Give Medication Guide and Warning Card; discuss points on guide
- Advise patient to stop drug if skin rash, fever, cough, shortness of breath, GI symptoms occur, notify prescriber immediately; advise all health care providers that allergic reactions have occurred with this drug

Evaluation

Positive therapeutic outcome

- Decreased infection; symptoms of HIV

acarbose (℞)

(a-kar'bose)

Prandese ✤, Precose

Func. class.: Oral antidiabetic

Chem. class.: α-Glucosidase inhibitor

Pregnancy category B

Action: Delays the digestion of ingested carbohydrates, results in a smaller rise in blood glucose after meals; does not increase insulin production

Therapeutic Outcome: Decreased blood glucose levels in diabetes mellitus

Uses: Stable adult-onset diabetes mellitus (type II) NIDDM, alone or in combination with a sulfonylurea

Dosage and routes

Initial dose

Adult: PO 25 mg tid with first bite of meal

Maintenance dose

Adult: PO may be increased to 50-100 mg tid; dosage adjustment at 4-8 wk intervals

Adult <60 kg: PO not to exceed 100 mg tid

Available forms: Tabs 50, 100 mg

Adverse effects

GI: *Abdominal pain, diarrhea, flatulence, increased serum transaminase level*

Contraindications: Hypersensitivity, diabetic ketoacidosis, cirrhosis, inflammatory bowel disease, colonic ulceration, partial intestinal obstruction, chronic intestinal disease, serum creatinine >2 mg/dl

Precautions: Pregnancy **B,** renal disease, lactation, children, hepatic disease

Pharmacokinetics

Absorption	Unknown
Distribution	Unknown
Metabolism	GI tract
Excretion	Kidneys as intact drug
Half-life	Elimination 2 hr

Pharmacodynamics

Unknown

Interactions
Individual drugs
Insulin: ↑ hypoglycemia
Isoniazid: ↑ hypoglycemia
Nicotinic acid: ↑ hypoglycemia
Phenytoin: ↑ hypoglycemia
Thyroid: ↑ hypoglycemia
Drug classifications
Calcium channel blockers: ↑ hypoglycemia
Corticosteroids: ↑ hypoglycemia
Digestive enzymes: ↓ effect of acarbose
Diuretics: ↑ hypoglycemia
Estrogens: ↑ hypoglycemia
Intestinal absorbents: ↓ effect of acarbose
Oral contraceptives: ↑ hypoglycemia
Phenothiazines: ↑ hypoglycemia
Sulfonylureas: ↑ hypoglycemia
Sympathomimetics: ↑ hypoglycemia
Herb/drug
Alfalfa: possible ↑ hypoglycemia
Lab test interferences
↑ AST, bilirubin
↓ Calcium, vit B_6

NURSING CONSIDERATIONS
Assessment
- Assess for hypoglycemia, hyperglycemia; even though this drug does not cause hypoglycemia, if on a sulfonylurea or insulin, hypoglycemia may be additive; if hypoglycemia occurs, treat with glucose or if severe, **IV** dextrose or IM glucagon
- Monitor 1 hr postprandial for establishing effectiveness, then glycosylated Hgb q3 mo
- Monitor AST q3 mo × 1 yr, and periodically thereafter

Nursing diagnoses
- ✓ Nutrition altered, more than body requirements (uses)
- ✓ Nutrition altered, less than body requirements (adverse reactions)
- ✓ Knowledge deficit (teaching)
- ✓ Noncompliance (teaching)

Implementation
- Give tid with first bite of each meal
- Provide storage in tight container in cool environment

Patient/family education
- Teach patient the symptoms of hypoglycemia, hyperglycemia and what to do about each
- Instruct that medication must be taken as prescribed; explain consequences of discontinuing the medication abruptly
- Tell patient to avoid OTC medications, herbal products unless approved by prescriber
- Teach patient that diabetes is a life-long illness; drug will not cure condition
- Instruct patient to carry/wear ID as diabetic
- Teach patient that diet and exercise regimen must be followed

Evaluation
Positive therapeutic outcome
- Improved signs, symptoms of diabetes mellitus (decreased polyuria, polydipsia, polyphagia; clear sensorium, absence of dizziness, stable gait)

acebutolol (℞)
(a-se-byoo′ toe-lole)
Monitan ♣, Sectral
Func. class.: Antihypertensive
Chem. class.: Selective β_1-blocker; group II antidysrhythmic (II)
Pregnancy category B

Action: Competitively blocks stimulation of β-adrenergic receptors within vascular smooth muscle (decreases rate of SA node discharge, increases recovery time), slows conduction of AV node resulting in decreased heart rate (negative chronotropic effect), which decreases O_2 consumption in myocardium because of β_1-receptor antagonism, also decreases renin-aldosterone-angiotensin system at high doses, inhibits β_2-receptors in bronchial system (high doses)

Therapeutic Outcome: Decreased B/P, heart rate, AV conduction, control of dysrhythmias

Uses: Mild to moderate hypertension, sinus tachycardia, persistent atrial extrasystoles, tachydysrhythmias

Investigational uses: Prophylaxis of MI, treatment of angina pectoris, tremor, mitral valve prolapse, thyrotoxicosis, idiopathic hypertrophic subaortic stenosis

Dosage and routes

Hypertension

Adult: PO 400 mg qd or in 2 divided doses; may be increased to desired response; maintenance 200-1200 mg/qd in 2 divided doses

Ventricular dysrhythmia

Adult: PO 200 mg bid, may increase gradually; usual range 600-1200 mg daily; should be tapered over 2 wk before discontinuing

G ***Elderly:*** PO not to exceed 800 mg/qd

Renal dose

Creatinine clearance 25-50 ml/min, reduce dose by 50%; if <25 ml/min reduce dose by 75%

Available forms: Caps 200, 400 mg; tabs 100, 200, 400 mg ♣

Adverse effects

CNS: *Insomnia, fatigue, dizziness, mental changes,* memory loss, hallucinations, depression, lethargy, drowsiness, strange dreams, catatonia

CV: **Profound hypotension, bradycardia, CHF, cold extremities, postural hypotension, 2nd or 3rd degree heart block**

EENT: Sore throat; dry, burning eyes

ENDO: Increased hypoglycemic response to insulin

GI: *Nausea, diarrhea,* vomiting, **mesenteric arterial thrombosis, ischemic colitis**

GU: *Impotence*, decreased libido, dysuria, nocturia

HEMA: **Agranulocytosis, thrombocytopenia, purpura**

INTEG: Rash, fever, alopecia, dry skin

MS: Joint pain, cramping

RESP: **Bronchospasm**, dyspnea, wheezing, cough

Contraindications: Hypersensitivity to β-blockers, cardiogenic shock, heart block (2nd or 3rd degree), sinus bradycardia, CHF, cardiac failure

Precautions: Major surgery, pregnancy **B**, lactation, diabetes mellitus, renal disease, thyroid disease, COPD, asthma, well-compensated heart failure, aortic or mitral valve, hepatic disease

Pharmacokinetics

Absorption	Well
Distribution	Crosses placenta, minimal CNS
Metabolism	Liver to diacetolol
Excretion	Kidneys, unchanged
Half-life	8-13 hr diacetolol, 3-4 hr acebutolol

Pharmacodynamics

	PO (ANTIHYPERTENSIVE)	PO (ANTIDYSRHYTHMIAS)
Onset	1-1½ hr	1 hr
Peak	2-4 hr	4-6 hr
Duration	12-24 hr	8-10 hr

Interactions

Individual drugs

Alcohol: ↑ hypotension (large amounts)

Diltiazem: ↑ hypotension, bradycardia
Hydralazine: ↑ hypotension, bradycardia
Insulin: ↑ hypoglycemia
Prazosin: ↑ hypotension, bradycardia
Thyroid: ↓ effectiveness
Verapamil: ↑ myocardial depression

Drug classifications

Antidiabetics, oral: ↑ hypoglycemic effect
Antihypertensives: ↑ hypertension
Cardiac glycosides: ↑ bradycardia
Diuretics: ↑ hypotension, bradycardia
Nitrates: ↑ hypotension
NSAIDs: ↓ antihypertensive effect
Theophyllines: ↓ bronchodilatation

Herb/drug

Aloe: ↑ acebutolol effect
Buckthorn bark/berry: ↑ acebutolol effect
Cascara sagrada bark: ↑ acebutolol effect
Ephedra: ↑ dysrhythmia
Rhubarb root: ↑ acebutolol effect
Senna leaf/fruits: ↑ acebutolol effect

Lab test interferences

False positive: Antinuclear antibodies titer
Increased: Serum lipoprotein levels

NURSING CONSIDERATIONS

Assessment

- Monitor B/P during beginning treatment, periodically thereafter; pulse q4h; note rate, rhythm, quality; apical/radial pulse before administration; notify prescriber of any significant changes (pulse <50 bpm)
- Check for baselines in renal, liver function tests before therapy begins
- Assess for edema in feet, legs daily, monitor I&O, daily weight; check for jugular vein distention, rales bilaterally, dyspnea (CHF)
- Monitor skin turgor, dryness of mucous membranes for hydration status, especially elderly

Nursing diagnoses

- ✓ Cardiac output, decreased (side effects)
- ✓ Injury, risk for physical (side effects)
- ✓ Knowledge deficit (teaching)
- ✓ Noncompliance (teaching)

Implementation

- Given ac, hs; tablet may be crushed or swallowed whole; give with food to prevent GI upset; reduced dosage in renal dysfunction; check pulse before giving, hold dose and notify prescriber if pulse is <60 bpm
- Store protected from light, moisture; place in cool environment

Patient/family education

- Teach patient not to discontinue drug abruptly, severe cardiac reactions may occur, taper over 2 wk; may cause precipitate angina if stopped abruptly
- Teach patient not to use OTC products containing α-adrenergic stimulants (such as nasal decongestants, cold preparations); to avoid alcohol, smoking; to limit sodium intake as prescribed
- Teach patient how to take pulse and B/P at home, advise when to notify prescriber
- Instruct patient to comply with weight control, dietary adjustments, modified exercise program
- Tell patient to carry/wear ID to identify drug(s) that patient is taking, allergies; tell patient that drug controls symptoms but does not cure
- Caution patient to avoid hazardous activities if dizziness or drowsiness is present; that drug may cause sensitivity to cold
- Teach patient to report symptoms of CHF: difficult breathing, especially on exertion or when lying down, night cough, swelling of extremities or bradycardia, dizziness, confusion, depression, fever
- Teach patient to take drug as prescribed, not to double or skip doses; take any missed doses as soon

as remembered if several hours until next dose

- Advise patient to continue with required lifestyle changes (exercise, diet, weight loss, stress reduction)

Evaluation

Positive therapeutic outcome

- Decreased B/P in hypertension (after 1-2 wk)
- Absence of dysrhythmias

Treatment of overdose:

Lavage, **IV** atropine for bradycardia, **IV** theophylline for bronchospasm, digitalis, O_2, diuretic for cardiac failure, hemodialysis, **IV** glucose for hypoglycemia, **IV** diazepam (or phenytoin) for seizures

acetaminophen ⊶ (OTC)

(a-seat-a-mee′noe-fen)

Abenol ✤, Acephen, Aceta, Actimol, Aminofen, Apacet, APAP, Apo-Acetaminophen ✤, Arthritis Foundation Pain Reliever Aspirin-Free, Aspirin-Free Anacin, Aspirin-Free Pain Relief, Atasol ✤, Banesin, Children's Feverall, Dapa, Dapacin, Datril, Exdol ✤, FemEtts, Genapap, Genebs, Halenol, Liquiprin, Mapap, Maranox, Meda, Neopap, Oraphen-PD, Panadol, Redutemp, Robigesic ✤, Rounax ✤, Silapap, Tapanol, Tempra, Tylenol

Func. class.: Nonopioid analgesic

Chem. class.: Nonsalicylate, paraaminophenol derivative

Pregnancy category B

Action: May block pain impulses peripherally that occur in response to inhibition of prostaglandin synthesis; does not possess antiinflammatory properties; antipyretic action results from inhibition of prostaglandins in the CNS (hypothalamic heat-regulating center)

➔ **Therapeutic Outcome:** Decreased pain, fever

Uses: Mild to moderate pain or fever

Dosage and routes

P ***Adult and child >12 yr:*** PO/REC 325-650 mg q4h prn, max 4 g/day

P ***Child:*** PO 10-15 mg/kg q4h

P ***Child 6-12 yr:*** REC 325 mg q4-6h, max 2-6 g/day

P ***Child 3-6 yr:*** REC 125 mg q4-6h, max 720 mg/day

P ***Child 1-3 yr:*** REC 80 mg q4h

P ***Child 3-11 mo:*** REC 80 mg q6h

Available forms: REC supp 120, 125, 325, 600, 650 mg; chewable tabs 80, 160 mg; caps 500 mg; elix 120, 160, 325 mg/5 ml; liq 120, 160 mg/5 ml, 500 mg/15 ml; sol 100 mg/1 ml, 120 mg/2.5 ml; tabs 160, 325, 500, 650 mg; granules 80 mg/pkg or cup

Adverse effects

CNS: Stimulation, drowsiness

GI: Nausea, vomiting, abdominal pain; **hepatotoxicity, hepatic seizure (overdose)**

GU: **Renal failure** (high, prolonged doses)

HEMA: **Leukopenia, neutropenia, hemolytic anemia (long-term use), thrombocytopenia, pancytopenia**

INTEG: Rash, urticaria

SYST: **Hypersensitivity**

TOXICITY: **Cyanosis, anemia, neutropenia, jaundice, pancytopenia, CNS stimulation, delirium followed by vascular collapse, convulsions, coma, death**

Contraindications:

Hypersensitivity; intolerance to tartrazine (yellow dye #5), alcohol, table sugar, saccharin, depending on product

Precautions: Anemia, hepatic disease, renal disease, chronic alcoholism, pregnancy **B**, G elderly, lactation

Pharmacokinetics

Absorption	Well absorbed (PO), variable (REC)
Distribution	Widely distributed; crosses placenta in low concentrations
Metabolism	Liver 85%-95%; metabolites are toxic at high levels
Excretion	Kidneys—metabolites, breast milk
Half-life	3-4 hr

Pharmacodynamics

	PO	REC
Onset	½-1 hr	½-1 hr
Peak	1-3 hr	1-3 hr
Duration	3-4 hr	3-4 hr

Interactions

Individual drugs

Alcohol: ↑ hepatotoxicity, ↓ effect
Carbamazepine: ↓ effect, ↑ hepatotoxicity
Colestipol: ↓ absorption of acetaminophen
Cholestyramine: ↓ absorption of acetaminophen
Diflunisal: ↓ effect, ↑ hepatotoxicity
Isoniazid: ↓ effect, ↑ hepatotoxicity
Rifabutin: ↓ effect, ↑ hepatotoxicity
Rifampin: ↓ effect, ↑ hepatotoxicity
Sulfinpyrazone; ↓ effect, ↑ hepatotoxicity
Warfarin: Hypoprothrombinemia; long-term use, high doses of acetaminophen
Zidovudine: ↑ bone marrow suppression

Drug classifications

Barbiturates: ↓ effect, ↑ hepatotoxicity
Hydantoins: ↓ effect, ↑ hepatotoxicity
NSAIDs: ↑ renal adverse reactions
Salicylates: ↑ renal adverse reactions

Lab test interferences

Interference: Chemstrip G, Dextrostix, Visidex II, 5-HIAA

NURSING CONSIDERATIONS

Assessment

- Monitor liver function studies: AST, ALT, bilirubin, creatinine before therapy if long-term therapy is anticipated; may cause hepatic toxicity at doses >4 g/day with chronic use
- Monitor renal function studies: BUN, urine creatinine, occult blood; albumin indicates nephritis
- Monitor blood studies: CBC, protime if patient is on long-term therapy
- Check I&O ratio; decreasing output may indicate renal failure (long-term therapy)
- Assess for fever and pain: type of pain, location, intensity, duration, temperature, diaphoresis
- Assess for chronic poisoning: rapid, weak pulse; dyspnea; cold, clammy extremities; report immediately to prescriber
- Assess hepatotoxicity: dark urine, clay-colored stools, yellowing of skin and sclera; itching, abdominal pain, fever, diarrhea if patient is on long-term therapy
- Assess allergic reactions: rash, urticaria; if these occur, drug may have to be discontinued

Nursing diagnoses

- ☑ Pain (uses)
- ☑ Mobility, impaired physical mobility (uses)
- ☑ Injury, risk for (side effects)
- ☑ Knowledge deficit (teaching)

Implementation

- Administer to patient crushed or whole; chewable tabs may be chewed
- Give with food or milk to decrease gastric symptoms; give 30 min before or 2 hr after meals; absorption may be slowed

Patient/family education

- ❗ Teach patient not to exceed recommended dosage; acute poisoning with liver damage may result; acute toxicity includes symptoms of nausea, vomiting, and abdominal pain; prescriber should be notified immediately

• Tell patient to read label on other OTC drugs; many contain acetaminophen and may cause toxicity if taken concurrently
• Teach patient to recognize signs of chronic overdose: bleeding, bruising, malaise, fever, sore throat
• Inform patient that urine may become dark brown as a result of phenacetin (metabolite of acetaminophen)
• Tell patient to notify prescriber for pain or fever lasting more than 3 days

Evaluation

Positive therapeutic outcome
• Decreased pain
• Decreased fever

Treatment of overdose: Drug level q4h, gastric lavage, activated charcoal; administer oral acetylcysteine to prevent hepatic damage (*see acetylcysteine monograph,* p. 11)

acetazolamide (℞)

(a-set-a-zole′-a-mide)

Apo-Acetazolamide ♣, acetazolamide, Diamox, Diamox Sequels, Hydrazol

Func. class.: Diuretic carbonic anhydrase inhibitor; antiglaucoma agent, antiepileptic

Chem. class.: Sulfonamide derivative

Pregnancy category C

Action: Decreases the aqueous humor in the eye, which lowers intraocular pressure by the inhibition of carbonic anhydrase; also inhibits carbonic anhydrase activity in proximal renal tubules to decrease reabsorption of water, sodium, potassium, bicarbonate; decreases carbonic anhydrase in CNS, increasing seizure threshold; prevents uric acid or cysteine buildup in the renal system by the decrease in pH causing alkaline urine

➡ **Therapeutic Outcome:** Decreased intraocular pressure; control of seizures; prevention and treatment of acute mountain sickness; prevention of uric acid/cysteine renal stones; decreased edema in lung tissue and peripherally; decreased B/P

Uses: Open angle glaucoma, narrow angle glaucoma (preoperatively if surgery delayed), epilepsy (petit mal, grand mal, mixed), edema in CHF, drug-induced edema, acute mountain sickness

Investigational uses: Prevention of uric acid/cysteine renal stones, decrease CSF production in infants with hydrocephalus

Dosage and routes

Closed angle glaucoma

Adult: PO/IM/**IV** 250 mg q4h or 250 mg bid, to be used for short-term therapy or 500 mg ES bid

Open angle glaucoma

Adult: PO/IM/**IV** 250 mg-1g/day in divided doses for amounts over 250 mg or 500 mg SR bid

Edema in CHF

Adult: IM/**IV** 250-375 mg/day in AM

P ***Child:*** IM/**IV** 5 mg/kg/day in AM

Seizures

Adult: PO/IM/**IV** 8-30 mg/kg/day in 1-4 divided doses, usual range 375-1000 mg/day in divided doses tid or qid, or 300-900 mg/m^2/day, not to exceed 1.5 g/day

P ***Child:*** PO/IM/**IV** 8-30 mg/kg/day in divided doses tid or qid, or 300-900 mg/m^2/day, not to exceed 1 g/day

Mountain sickness

Adult: PO 250 mg q8-12h

Renal stones

Adult: PO 250 mg hs

P ***Infants with hydrocephalus***

Infant: **IV** 5 mg/kg/day q6h, may be increased up to 100 mg/kg/day if tolerated

Available forms: Tabs 125, 250 mg; caps ext rel 500 mg; inj 500 mg

Adverse effects

CNS: Drowsiness, paresthesia, anxiety, depression, headache, dizziness, confusion, stimulation, fatigue, **convulsions,** sedation, nervousness
EENT: Myopia, tinnitus
ENDO: Hyperglycemia, hypokalemia, hypocalcemia, hypomagnesemia, hyponatremia, hyperchloremia
GI: Nausea, vomiting, anorexia, constipation, diarrhea, melena, weight loss, **hepatic insufficiency,** taste alterations
GU: Frequency, hypokalemia, polyuria, **uremia,** glucosuria, hematuria, dysuria, crystalluria, renal calculi
HEMA: **Aplastic anemia, hemolytic anemia, leukopenia, agranulocytosis, thrombocytopenia, purpura, pancytopenia**
INTEG: Rash, pruritus, urticaria, fever, **Stevens-Johnson syndrome,** photosensitivity

Contraindications: Hypersensitivity to sulfonamides, severe renal disease, severe hepatic disease, electrolyte imbalances (hyponatremia, hypokalemia), hyperchloremic acidosis, Addison's disease, long-term use in narrow angle glaucoma

Precautions: Hypercalcemia, pregnancy **C**

Do Not Confuse:
acetazolamide/acetohexamide, Diamox/Dobutrex, Diamox/Trimox

Pharmacokinetics

Absorption	GI tract—65% if fasting, 75% with food); **IV**—complete
Distribution	Crosses placenta; widely distributed
Metabolism	None
Excretion	Kidneys, unchanged (80% within 24 hr); breast milk
Half-life	2½-5½ hr

Pharmacodynamics

	PO	PO–EXT REL	IV
Onset	1½ hr	2 hr	2 min
Peak	2-4 hr	3-6 hr	15 min
Duration	8-12 hr	18-24 hr	4-5 hr

Interactions

Individual drugs

Amphotericin B: ↑ hypokalemia
Aspirin: ↑ excretion of aspirin
Cyclosporine: ↑ toxicity
Diflunisal: ↑ side effects
Lithium: ↑ excretion of lithium
Methenamine: ↓ acetazolamide effect
Primidone: ↓ primidone level

Drug classifications

Amphetamines: ↑ action
Anticholinergics: ↑ anticholinergic action
Salicylates: ↑ toxicity

Lab test interferences

False positive: Urinary protein, 17-hydroxysteroids
Decreased: Thyroid iodine uptake

NURSING CONSIDERATIONS

Assessment

- Assess patient for tinnitus, hearing loss, ear pain; periodic testing of hearing is needed when high doses of this drug are given by **IV** route
- Monitor manifestations of hypokalemia: *RENAL:* acidic urine, reduced urine osmolality, nocturia, polyuria, polydipsia; *CARDIAC:* hypotension, broad T wave, U wave, ectopy, tachycardia, weak pulse; *NEURO:* muscle weakness, altered LOC, drowsiness, apathy, lethargy, confusion, depression; *GI:* anorexia, nausea, cramps, constipation, distention, paralytic ileus; *RESP:* hypoventilation, respiratory muscle weakness
- Monitor for CNS, GI, cardiovascular, integumentary, neurologic manifestations of hypocalcemia: *CNS:* personality changes, anxiety, disturbances, depression, psychosis, nausea, vomiting; *GI:* constipation, abdominal

pain from muscle spasm; *CV:* decreased contractility, decreased cardiac output, hypotension, lengthened ST segment, prolonged QT interval; *INTEG:* scaling eczema, alopecia, hyperpigmentation; *NEURO:* tetany, muscle twitching, cramping, grimacing, seizure, altered deep tendon reflexes, spasm

• Monitor for manifestations of hypomagnesemia: *CNS:* agitation; *NEURO:* muscle twitching, paresthesias, hyperactive reflexes, positive Babinski's reflex, dysphagia, nystagmus, seizures, tetany; *GI:* nausea, vomiting, diarrhea, anorexia, abdominal distention; *CARDIAC:* ectopy, tachycardia, broad, flat, or inverted T waves, depressed ST segment, prolonged QT, decreased cardiac output, hypotension

• Monitor for manifestations of hyponatremia: *CV:* increased B/P, cold, clammy skin, hypovolemia, or hypervolemia, vomiting, diarrhea, abdominal cramps; *NEURO:* lethargy, increased intracranial pressure, confusion, headache, seizures, coma, fatigue, tremors, hyperreflexia

• Monitor for manifestations of hyperchloremia: *NEURO:* weakness, lethargy, coma; *RESP:* deep, rapid breathing

• Assess fluid volume status: I&O ratio and record, count or weigh diapers as appropriate, distended neck veins, crackles in lung, color, quality and sp gr of urine, skin turgor, adequacy of pulses, moist mucous membranes, bilateral lung sounds, peripheral pitting edema; dehydration symptoms of decreasing output, thirst, hypotension, dry mouth, and mucous membranes should be reported

• Monitor electrolytes: potassium, sodium, calcium, magnesium; also include BUN, blood pH, ABGs, uric acid, CBC, blood sugar

• Assess B/P before and during therapy with patient lying, standing, and sitting as appropriate; orthostatic hypotension can occur rapidly

• Monitor blood, urine glucose in diabetic patients; glucose levels may be increased

• Assess for eye pain, change in vision when using drug for intraocular pressure

• Assess neurologic status when using drug for seizures

• Assess for decreased symptoms of acute mountain sickness: headache, nausea, vomiting, dizziness, fatigue, drowsiness, shortness of breath, insomnia

• Assess for cross-sensitivity between other sulfonamides and this drug

Nursing diagnoses

✓ Sensory-perceptual alterations: visual (uses)
✓ Fluid volume deficit (side effects)
✓ Fluid volume excess (uses)
✓ Knowledge deficit (teaching)

Implementation

• Give in AM to avoid interference with sleep

• Administer fluids 2-3 L/day to prevent renal calculi, unless contraindicated

• Potassium replacement if potassium level is <3.0 ml/dl

PO route

• Give with food, if nausea occurs, crush tabs and mix with sweet substance to counteract bitter taste; ES caps may be opened and sprinkled on food

⊘ • Do not crush or chew caps

IV **IV route**

• Do not use solution that is yellow or has a precipitate or crystals

IV*:* Dilute 500 mg of drug/5 ml or more sterile water for inj: use within 24 hr

Direct* IV:* Give over 1 min or more

Intermittent infusion: May be added to NS, D_5W, $D_{10}W$, 0.45% NaCl; give over 4-8 hr

Additive compatibilities: Cimetidine, ranitidine

Additive incompatibilities:
Multivitamins

Patient/family education

- Teach patient to take the medication early in the day to prevent nocturia
- Instruct patient to take with food or milk if GI symptoms of nausea and anorexia occur
- Teach patient to maintain a record of weight on a weekly basis and notify prescriber of weight loss of >5 lb
- Caution patient that this drug causes a loss of potassium, so food rich in potassium should be added to the diet; refer to a dietician for assistance in planning
- Advise patient to wear protective clothing and sunscreen in the sun to prevent photosensitivity
- Teach patient not to use alcohol or any OTC medications without prescriber's approval; serious drug reactions may occur
- Emphasize the need to contact prescriber immediately if muscle cramps, weakness, nausea, dizziness, or numbness occurs
- Teach patient to take own B/P and pulse and record
- Teach patient to continue taking medication even if feeling better; this drug controls symptoms but does not cure the condition
- Teach patient to see ophthalmologist periodically; glaucoma is a slow process
- Advise patient to ↑ fluids to 2-3 L/day if not contraindicated
- Instruct patient to report nausea, vertigo, rapid weight gain, change in stools

Evaluation

Positive therapeutic outcome

- Decreased intraocular pressure
- Decreased edema
- Decreased seizures
- Prevention of mountain sickness
- Prevention of uric acid/cysteine stones

Treatment of overdose:

Lavage if taken orally, monitor electrolytes, administer dextrose in saline, monitor hydration, CV, renal status

acetylcysteine (Rx)

(a-se-teel-sis'tay-een)
Mucomyst, Mucosil, Parvolex ✦
Func. class.: Mucolytic; antidote—acetaminophen
Chem. class.: Amino acid L-cysteine
Pregnancy category B

Action: Decreases viscosity of secretions in respiratory tract by breaking disulfide links of mucoproteins; increases hepatic glutathione, which is necessary to inactivate toxic metabolites in acetaminophen overdose

Therapeutic Outcome: Decreased hepatotoxicity from acetaminophen overdose (PO); decreased viscosity of mucus in respiratory disorders (inh)

Uses: Acetaminophen toxicity; bronchitis; pneumonia; cystic fibrosis; emphysema; atelectasis; tuberculosis; complications of thoracic surgery and cardiovascular surgery; diagnosis in bronchial lab tests

Investigational uses: Prevention of contrast media nephrotoxicity

Dosage and routes

Mucolytic

P ***Adult and child:*** INH 2-20 ml (10% sol) q1-4h prn, or 1-10 ml (20% sol)

Acetaminophen toxicity

P ***Adult and child:*** PO 140 mg/kg, then 70 mg/kg q4h × 17 doses to total 1330 mg/kg

Available forms: Sol 10%, 20%

Adverse effects

CNS: *Dizziness, drowsiness,* headache, fever, chills
CV: Hypotension

EENT: *Rhinorrhea,* tooth damage
GI: *Nausea,* stomatitis, constipation, vomiting, anorexia, **hepatotoxicity**
INTEG: Urticaria, rash, fever, clamminess
RESP: **Bronchospasm,** burning, **hemoptysis,** chest tightness

Contraindications: Hypersensitivity, increased intracranial pressure, status asthmaticus

Precautions: Hypothyroidism, Addison's disease, CNS depression, brain tumor, asthma, hepatic disease, renal disease, COPD, psychosis, alcoholism, convulsive disorders, lactation, pregnancy **B**

Pharmacokinetics

Absorption	Extensive (PO), locally (inh)
Distribution	Unknown
Metabolism	Liver
Excretion	Kidneys
Half-life	Unknown

Pharmacodynamics

	PO	INH
Onset	Unknown	1 min
Peak	Unknown	Unknown
Duration	Up to 4 hr	5-10 min

Interactions

Individual drugs

Activated charcoal: ↓ absorption of acetylcysteine
Iron, copper, rubber: Do not use with acetylcysteine

NURSING CONSIDERATIONS

Assessment

Mucolytic use

- Assess cough: type, frequency, character, including sputum
- Assess characteristics, rate, rhythm of respirations, increased dyspnea, sputum; discontinue if bronchospasm occurs; ABGs for increased CO_2 retention in asthma patients
- Monitor VS, cardiac status including checking for dysrhythmias, increased rate, palpitations

Antidotal use

- Assess liver function tests, acetaminophen levels, pro-time, glucose, electrolytes; inform prescriber if dose is vomited or vomiting is persistent; provide adequate hydration; decrease dosage in hepatic encephalopathy
- Assess for nausea, vomiting, rash; notify prescriber if these occur

Nursing diagnoses

- ✓ Injury, risk for physical (uses) (antidote)
- ✓ Impaired gas exchange (uses) (mucolytic)
- ✓ Airway clearance ineffective (uses) (mucolytic)
- ✓ Poisoning, risk for (uses) (antidote)
- ✓ Knowledge deficit (teaching)

Implementation

- G Give decreased dosage to elderly patients; their metabolism may be slowed; give gum, hard candy, frequent rinsing of mouth for dryness of oral cavity
- Use only if suction machine is available

PO route: *Antidotal use*

- Lavage, then give within 24 hr; give with cola or soft drink to disguise taste; can be given with H_2O through tubes; use within 1 hr

Inhalation route: *Mucolytic use*

- Use ac ½-1 hr for better absorption, to decrease nausea; only after patient clears airway by deep breathing, coughing
- Give by syringe 2-3 doses of 1-2 ml of 20% or 2-4 ml of 10% sol; 20% sol diluted with NS or water for injection; may give 10% sol undiluted
- Store in refrigerator: use within 96 hr of opening
- Provide assistance with inhaled dose: bronchodilator if bronchospasm occurs; wash face and rinse mouth after use to remove sticky feeling
- Use mechanical suction if cough

insufficient to remove excess bronchial secretions

Patient/family education

Mucolytic use

- Tell patient to avoid driving or other hazardous activities until patient is stabilized on this medication; avoid alcohol, other CNS depressants; will enhance sedating properties of this drug
- Teach patient that unpleasant odor will decrease after repeated use; that discoloration of solution after bottle is opened does not impair its effectiveness; avoid smoking, smoke-filled rooms, perfume, dust, environmental pollutants, cleaners

Evaluation

Positive therapeutic outcome

- Absence of purulent secretions when coughing (mucolytic use)
- Clear lung sounds bilaterally (mucolytic use)
- Absence of hepatic damage (acetaminophen toxicity)
- Decreasing blood toxicology (acetaminophen toxicity)

activated charcoal (OTC)

Actidose, Actidose-Aqua, Charco-Aid 2000, CharcoCaps, Liqu-Char,

Func. class.: Antiflatulent/antidote

Pregnancy category C

Action: Binds poisons, toxins, irritants; increases adsorption in GI tract; inactivates toxins and binds until excreted

Therapeutic Outcome: Prevention of toxicity and death resulting from absorption of drugs

Uses: Poisoning

Dosage and routes

Poisoning

P Children should not get more than 1 dose of products with sorbitol

P ***Adult and child:*** PO 5-10 × weight of substance ingested; minimum dosage 30 g/250 ml of water; may give 20-40g q6h for 1-2 days in severe poisoning

Available forms: Powder 15, 25, 30, 40, 120, 125, 240 g/container; oral susp 12.5 g/60 ml, 15 g/72 ml, 15 g/120 ml, 25 g/120 ml, 30 g/120 ml, 50 g/240 ml; ♣ 15 g/120 ml, 25 g/125 ml, 50 g/225 ml, 50 g/250 ml

Adverse effects

GI: Nausea, black stools, vomiting, constipation, diarrhea

Contraindications: Hypersensitivity to this drug, unconsciousness, semiconsciousness, poisoning of cyanide, mineral acids, alkalies

Precautions: Pregnancy **C**

Pharmacokinetics	
Absorption	None
Distribution	None
Metabolism	None
Excretion	Feces (unchanged)
Half-life	Unknown

Pharmacodynamics	
Onset	1 min
Peak	Unknown
Duration	4-12 hr

Interactions

Individual drugs

Acetylcysteine: ↓ effectiveness of both drugs

Ipecac: ↓ effectiveness of both drugs

Food/drug

Dairy products: ↓ effect of activated charcoal

NURSING CONSIDERATIONS

Assessment

- Assess neurologic status including LOC, pupil reactivity, cough reflex, gag reflex, and swallowing ability before administration; do not give if neurologic status is impaired; aspiration

may occur unless a protected airway is present
- Assess toxin, poison ingested, time of ingestion, and amount
- Monitor respiration, pulse, B/P to determine charcoal effectiveness if taken for barbiturate/narcotic poisoning

Nursing diagnoses
✓ Injury, risk for (uses)
✓ Poisoning, risk for (uses)
✓ Knowledge deficit (teaching)

Implementation
- Give after inducing vomiting unless vomiting contraindicated (i.e., cyanide or alkalies); mix with 8 oz of water or fruit juice to form thick syrup; do not use dairy products to mix charcoal; repeat dose if vomiting occurs soon after dose
- Space at least 2 hr before or after other drugs, or absorption will be decreased; use a laxative to promote elimination; constipation occurs often
- Give alone; do not administer with ipecac; if patient unable to swallow, dilute to a less thick sol; keep container tightly closed to prevent absorption of gases
- Give through a nasogastric tube if patient unable to swallow

Patient/family education
- Tell patient stools will be black
- Teach patient about overdose/poison prevention and about keeping poison control chart available

Evaluation
Positive therapeutic outcome
- Alert, PERL (poisoning)
- Absence of distention
- Absence of odor in wounds

acyclovir (Key Drug) (℞)
(ay-sye'kloe-ver)
Avirax (Can), Zovirax
Func. class.: Antiviral
Chem. class.: Acylic purine nucleoside analog
Pregnancy category B

See Appendix D for topical products

Action: Interferes with DNA synthesis by conversion to acyclovir triphosphate, causing decreased viral replication, time of lesional healing

Therapeutic Outcome: Decreased amount and time of healing of lesions

Uses: Mucocutaneous herpes simplex virus, herpes genitalis (HSV-1, HSV-2), herpes zoster; simple mucocutaneous herpes simplex in immunocompromised clients with initial herpes genitalis; herpes simplex encephalitis, cytomegalovirus, HSV after transplant

Dosage and routes
Renal dose
CrCl >50 ml/min dose q8h; CrCl 25-50 ml/min dose q12h; CrCl 10-25 ml/min dose q24h; CrCl 0-10 ml/min 50% of dose q24h

Herpes simplex
P ***Adult and child >12 yr:*** **IV** inf 5 mg/kg over 1 hr q8h × 5 days
P ***Child <12 yr:*** **IV** inf 250 mg/m^2 or 30 mg/kg/day divided q8h over 1 hr × 5 days

Genital herpes
Adult: PO 200 mg q4h 5 times a day while awake × 5 days to 6 mo depending on whether initial, recurrent, or chronic
P ***Adult and child:*** TOP apply to all lesions q3h while awake, 6 times a day × 1 wk

Herpes simplex encephalitis
P ***Child 3 mo-12 yr:*** **IV** 20 mg/kg q8h × 10 days

Child birth-3 mo: **IV** 10 mg/kg q8h × 10 days

Herpes zoster

Adult: PO 800 mg q4h while awake × 7-10 days; **IV** 5 mg/kg q8h

Varicella-zoster

Adult: PO 1000 mg q6h × 5 days or 600-800 mg q4h (5×/day while awake); **IV** 500 mg/m² q8h or 10 mg/kg q8h × 7 days

Chickenpox

Adult/child: PO 20 mg/kg qid × 5 days, max 800 mg/dose

P ***Child:*** PO 10-20 mg/kg (max 800 mg) qid × 5 days; **IV** 500 mg/m² q8h, or 10 mg/kg q8h × 7 days

Available forms: Caps 200 mg; tabs 400, 800 mg; inj **IV** 500 mg; top ointment 5% (50 mg/g); oral susp

Adverse effects

CNS: Tremors, confusion, lethargy, hallucinations, **convulsions,** *dizziness, headache,* encephalopathic changes

EENT: Gingival hyperplasia

GI: Nausea, vomiting, diarrhea, increased ALT, AST, abdominal pain, glossitis, colitis

GU: **Oliguria, proteinuria, hematuria,** vaginitis, moniliasis, **glomerulonephritis, acute renal failure,** changes in menses, polydipsia

INTEG: Rash, urticaria, pruritus, pain or phlebitis at **IV** site, unusual sweating, alopecia, stinging, burning, vulvitis

MS: Joint pain, leg pain, muscle cramps

Contraindications: Hypersensitivity

Precautions: Lactation, hepatic disease, renal disease, electrolyte imbalance, dehydration, pregnancy **B**

Pharmacokinetics

Absorption	Minimal (PO)
Distribution	Widely distributed, crosses placenta, CSF concentration 50% plasma
Metabolism	Liver, minimal
Excretion	Kidneys, 95% unchanged
Half-life	2.0-3.5 hr, increased in renal disease

Pharmacodynamics

	PO	IV	TOP
Onset	Unknown	Rapid	Unknown
Peak	1½-2½	Infusion's end	Unknown

Interactions

Individual drugs

Interferon: ↑ synergistic effect

Probenecid: ↑ neurotoxicity, nephrotoxicity

Zidovudine: ↑ CNS side effects

NURSING CONSIDERATIONS

Assessment

- Monitor for signs of infection, type of lesions, area of body covered, purulent drainage
- Check I&O ratio; report hematuria, oliguria, fatigue, weakness; may indicate nephrotoxicity; check for protein in urine during treatment
- Monitor any patient with compromised renal system, since drug is excreted slowly in poor renal system function; toxicity may occur rapidly
- Monitor liver studies: AST, ALT
- Monitor blood studies: WBC, RBC, Hct, Hgb, bleeding time; blood dyscrasias may occur; drug should be discontinued
- Monitor renal studies: urinalysis, protein, BUN, creatinine, CrCl; increased BUN, creatinine indicates renal failure and nephrotoxicity
- Obtain C&S before drug therapy; drug may be taken as soon as culture is taken; repeat C&S after treatment; determine the presence of other sexually transmitted diseases

• Monitor bowel pattern before, during treatment; if severe abdominal pain with bleeding occurs, drug should be discontinued
• Assess allergies before treatment, reaction of each medication; place allergies on chart in bright red letters; allergic reaction: burning, stinging, swelling, redness, rash, vulvitis, pruritus

Nursing diagnoses

✓ Infection, risk for (uses)
✓ Knowledge deficit (teaching)

Implementation

PO route

• Do not break, crush, or chew caps
• Give with food to lessen GI symptoms; may give without regard to meals with 8 oz of water
• Store at room temperature in dry place
• Shake suspension before use

Topical route

• Use finger cot or rubber glove to prevent further infection
• Enough medication to cover lesions completely
• After cleansing with soap and water before each application, dry well

IV route

• Provide increased fluids to 3 L/day to decrease crystalluria
• Give by int inf after reconstituting with 10 ml sterile water for injection/500 mg of drug (50 mg/ml); shake; dilute in 0.9% NaCl, LR, D_5W, D_5/0.25% NaCl, D_5/0.45% NaCl, D_5/0.9% NaCl (7 mg/ml); give over at least 1 hr (constant rate) by infusion pump to prevent nephrotoxicity; do not reconstitute with sol containing benzyl alcohol or parabens; check infusion site for redness, pain, induration; rotate sites
• Lower dosage in acute or chronic renal failure
• Store at room temperature for up to 12 hr after reconstitution; if refrigerated, sol may show a precipitate that clears at room temperature, yellow discoloration does not affect potency

Y-site compatibilities:

Allopurinol, amikacin, ampicillin, amphotericin B cholesteryl sulfate complex, cefamandole, cefazolin, cefonicid, cefoperazone, ceforanide, cefotaxime, cefoxitin, ceftazidime, ceftizoxime, ceftriaxone, cefuroxime, cephapirin, chloramphenicol, cimetidine, clindamycin, co-trimoxazole, dexamethasone sodium phosphate, dimenhydrinate, diphenhydramine, doxycycline, doxorubicin, erythromycin, famotidine, filgrastim, fluconazole, gallium, gentamicin, granisetron, heparin, hydrocortisone sodium succinate, hydromorphone, imipenem/cilastatin, lorazepam, magnesium sulfate, melphalan, methylprednisolone sodium succinate, metoclopramide, metronidazole, multivitamin infusion, nafcillin, oxacillin, paclitaxel, penicillin G potassium, pentobarbital, perphenazine, piperacillin, potassium chloride, propofol, ranitidine, remifentanil, sodium bicarbonate, tacrolimus, teniposide, tetracycline, theophylline, thiotepa, ticarcillin, tobramycin, trimethoprim-sulfamethoxazole, vancomycin, zidovudine

Y-site incompatibilities:

Dobutamine, dopamine, ondansetron, verapamil

Additive compatibilities:

Fluconazole

Additive incompatibilities:

Blood products, protein-containing solutions, dobutamine, dopamine

Patient/family education

Topical route

• Tell patient not to use in eyes; for use when there is no evidence of infection; apply with glove to prevent further infection
• Instruct patient to avoid use of OTC creams, ointments, lotions unless

directed by prescriber; may cause reinfection, delayed healing

- Teach patient to use asepsis (hand washing) before, after each application and avoid contact with eyes; to adhere strictly to prescribed regimen to maximize successful treatment outcome

PO route

- Teach patient that drug may be taken orally before infection occurs; that drug should be taken when itching or pain occurs, usually before eruptions; that partners need to be told that patient has herpes; they can become infected, so condoms must be worn to prevent reinfections; that drug does not cure infection, just controls symptoms and does not prevent infection to others
- Tell patient to report sore throat, fever, fatigue; may indicate superinfection; that drug must be taken in equal intervals around the clock to maintain blood levels for duration of therapy
- Tell patient to notify prescriber of side effects: bruising, bleeding, fatigue, malaise; may indicate blood dyscrasias
- Tell patient to seek dental care during treatment to prevent gingival hyperplasia
- Teach female patients with genital herpes to have regular Pap smears to prevent undetected cervical cancer
- Do not crush or chew caps

Evaluation

Positive therapeutic outcome

- Absence of itching, painful lesions
- Crusting and healed lesions

Treatment of overdose: Discontinue drug, hemodialysis, resuscitate if needed

HIGH ALERT

adenosine (℞)

(ah-den′oh-seen)

Adenocard, Adenoscan

Func. class.: Antidysrhythmic misc.

Chem. class.: Endogenous nucleoside

Pregnancy category C

Action: Slows conduction through AV node, can interrupt reentry pathways through AV node, and can restore normal sinus rhythm in patients with supraventricular tachycardia (SVT)

Therapeutic Outcome: Normal sinus rhythm in patients diagnosed with SVT

Uses: SVT, as a diagnostic aid to assess myocardial perfusion defects in CAD

Dosage and routes

Antidysrhythmic

Adult: **IV** bol 6 mg; if conversion to normal sinus rhythm does not occur within 1-2 min, give 12 mg by rapid **IV** bol; may repeat 12 mg dose again in 1-2 min

P ***Infants and children:*** 0.05 mg/kg; if not effective, increase dose by 0.05 mg/kg q2 min to a max of 0.25 mg/kg or 12 mg

Diagnostic use

Adult: **IV** 140 μg/kg/min × 6 min

Available forms: Inj 3 mg/ml (vial); 6 mg/2 ml (vial)

Adverse effects

CNS: Lightheadedness, dizziness, arm tingling, numbness, apprehension, blurred vision, headache

CV: Chest pain/pressure, **atrial tachydysrhythmias,** sweating, palpitations, hypotension, *facial flushing*

GI: Nausea, metallic taste, throat tightness, groin pressure

RESP: *Dyspnea, chest pressure,* hyperventilation

Contraindications: Hypersensitivity, 2nd- or 3rd-degree heart block, AV block, sick sinus syndrome, atrial flutter, atrial fibrillation

P G **Precautions:** Pregnancy **C**, lactation, children, asthma, elderly

Do Not Confuse:
Adenocard/adenosine

Pharmacokinetics

Absorption	Complete bioavailability
Distribution	Erythrocytes, cardiovascular endothelium
Metabolism	Liver, converted to inosine and adenosine monophosphate
Excretion	Kidneys
Half-life	10 sec

Pharmacodynamics

Onset	Rapid
Peak	Unknown
Duration	1-2 min

Interactions
Individual drugs
Caffeine: ↓ effects of adenosine
Carbamazepine: ↑ heart block
Digoxin: ↑ ventricular fibrillation
Dipyridamole: ↑ effects of adenosine
Theophylline: ↓ effects of adenosine
Smoking
↑ tachycardia
Herb/drug
Aloe: may ↑ adenosine effect
Angelica: may ↑ adenosine effect
Buckthorn bark/berry: may ↑ adenosine effect
Cascara sagrada bark: may ↑ adenosine effect
Rhubarb root: may ↑ adenosine effect
Senna leaf/fruits: may ↑ adenosine effect

NURSING CONSIDERATIONS
Assessment
- Monitor I&O ratio, electrolytes (potassium, sodium, chloride)
- Assess cardiopulmonary status: pulse, respiration, ECG intervals (PR, QRS, QT); check for transient dysrhythmias (PVCs, PACs, sinus tachycardia, AV block)
- Assess respiratory status: rate, rhythm, lung fields for rales, watch for respiratory depression; bilateral rales may occur in CHF patient; if increased respiration, increased pulse occurs, drug should be discontinued
- Assess CNS effects: dizziness, confusion, paresthesias; drug should be discontinued

Nursing diagnoses
- ✓ Cardiac output, decreased (uses)
- ✓ Impaired gas exchange (adverse reactions)
- ✓ Knowledge deficit (teaching)

Implementation
IV direct
- Give **IV** bol undiluted; give 6 mg or less by rapid inj; if using an **IV** line, use port near insertion site, flush with 0.9% NaCl (50 ml); warm to room temperature before giving

Continuous infusion
- Give 30-ml vial undiluted via peripheral vein

Solution compatibilities:
D_5LR, D_5W, LR, 0.9% NaCl
- Store at room temperature; sol should be clear; discard unused drug

Patient/family education
- Tell patient to report facial flushing, dizziness, sweating, palpitations, chest pain
- Instruct patient to rise from sitting or standing slowly to prevent orthostatic hypotension

Evaluation
Positive therapeutic outcome
- Normal sinus rhythm
- Diagnosis of perfusion defect

A

alatrofloxacin (℞)
(ah-lat-troh-floks'ah-sin)
Trovan IV

trovafloxacin (℞)
(troh-vah-floks'ah-sin)
Trovan

Func. class.: Antiinfective
Chem. class.: Fluoroquinolone

Pregnancy category C

Action: Interferes with conversion of intermediate DNA fragments into high-molecular-weight DNA in bacteria; DNA gyrase inhibitor

➔ **Therapeutic Outcome:** Bacterial action against the following: nosocomial pneumonia: *Escherichia coli, Pseudomonas aeruginosa, Haemophilus influenzae, Staphylococcus aureus;* community-acquired pneumonia: *Staphylococcus pneumoniae, Haemophilus influenzae, Staphylococcus aureus, Klebsiella pneumoniae, Mycoplasma pneumoniae, Mycoplasma catarrhalis, Legionella pneumophilia, Chlamydia pneumoniae*

Uses: Nosocomial pneumonia, community-acquired pneumonia, chronic bronchitis, acute sinusitis, complicated intraabdominal infections, gyn/pelvic infection, skin/skin structure infections, UTIs, chronic bacterial prostatitis, urethral gonorrhea in males, PID, cervicitis caused by susceptible organisms

Dosage and routes
Alatrofloxacin
Serious infections
Adult: **IV** 300 mg q24h
Other infections
Adult: **IV** 200 mg q24h
Perioperative prophylaxis
Adult: 200 mg ½-4 hr before surgery
Trovafloxacin
Gonorrhea
Adult: PO 100 mg as a single dose
Other infections
Adult: PO 100-200 mg q24h
Perioperative prophylaxis
Adult: PO 200 mg ½-4 hr before surgery

Available forms: Conc sol for inj 5 mg/ml (alatrofloxacin); tabs 100, 200 mg (trovafloxacin)

Adverse effects
CNS: Headache, *dizziness,* insomnia, anxiety, psychosis, **seizures**
GI: Nausea, flatulence, vomiting, diarrhea, abdominal pain, **pseudomembranous colitis**
GU: Vaginitis, crystalluria, ↑ BUN, creatinine
INTEG: Rash, pruritus, photosensitivity
HEMA: Anemia, **thrombocytopenia, leukopenia,** ↓ Hgb, Hct, ↑ platelets
MS: Arthralgia, myalgia
SYST: **Anaphylaxis, Stevens-Johnson syndrome**

Contraindications: Hypersensitivity to quinolones, seizure disorders, cerebral atherosclerosis, photosensitivity

Precautions: Pregnancy **C,** lactation, children

P

Pharmacokinetics

Absorption	Unknown
Distribution	Unknown
Metabolism	Liver
Excretion	Kidneys, unchanged
Half-life	Unknown

Pharmacodynamics

Onset	Unknown
Peak	Unknown
Duration	Unknown

Interactions
Individual drugs
Citric acid/sodium citrate: ↓ absorption
Cyclosporine: ↑ nephrotoxicity
Iron: ↓ absorption

Morphine IV: ↓ absorption of trovafloxacin
Sucralfate: ↓ absorption
Theophylline: ↑ theophylline level, ↑ toxicity
Warfarin: ↑ warfarin level
Drug classifications
Antacids with aluminum/ magnesium: ↓ absorption

NURSING CONSIDERATIONS
Assessment

- Assess for previous sensitivity reaction to fluoroquinolones
- Monitor for signs and symptoms of infection: characteristics of sputum, WBC >10,000/mm^3, fever; obtain baseline information before and during treatment
- Obtain C&S before beginning drug therapy to identify if correct treatment has been initiated
- Assess for allergic reactions: rash, urticaria, pruritus, chills, fever, joint pain; may occur a few days after therapy begins; epinephrine and resuscitation equipment should be available for anaphylactic reaction
- Assess bowel pattern qd; if severe diarrhea occurs, drug should be discontinued
- Assess for overgrowth of infection, perineal itching, fever, malaise, redness, pain, swelling, drainage, rash, diarrhea, change in cough, sputum
- Identify urine output; if decreasing, notify prescriber (may indicate nephrotoxicity); also check for increased BUN, creatinine
- Assess for CNS disorders; other fluoroquinolones cause seizures, stimulation
- Monitor blood studies: AST, ALT, CBC, Hct, bilirubin, LDH, alkaline phosphatase, Coombs' test monthly if patient is on long-term therapy
- Monitor electrolytes: potassium, sodium, chloride monthly if patient is on long-term therapy
- Assess for hepatotoxicity, use only for serious or life-threatening infection

Nursing diagnoses

- ✓ Infection, risk for (uses)
- ✓ Diarrhea (side effects)
- ✓ Injury, risk for (side effects)
- ✓ Knowledge deficit (teaching)
- ✓ Noncompliance (teaching)

Implementation
IV route

- Check for irritation, extravasation, phlebitis daily

Incompatibilities:
Do not use with magnesium in the same IV line

Solution compatibilities
D_5, ½% NaCl, D_5/0.2% NaCl, LR

Patient/family education

- Teach patient to report sore throat, bruising, bleeding, joint pain; may indicate blood dyscrasias (rare)
- Advise patient to avoid hazardous activities until response is known
- Advise patient to contact prescriber if vaginal itching, loose, foul-smelling stools, furry tongue occur, may indicate superinfection; report itching, rash, pruritus, urticaria
- Advise patient to rinse mouth frequently, use sugarless candy or gum for dry mouth
- Instruct patient to take all medication prescribed for the length of time ordered; drug must be taken around the clock to maintain blood levels; not to give medication to others; to avoid other medication unless approved by prescriber; not to use theophyllines, toxicity may occur
- Advise patient to notify prescriber of diarrhea with blood or pus, may indicate pseudomembranous colitis
- Advise patient to use sunscreen to prevent photosensitivity
- Teach patient that drug may be taken with or without food; separate sucralfate, antacids by ≥4 hr; to ↑ fluid intake to 2 L/day to prevent crystalluria

Evaluation

Positive therapeutic outcome

- Absence of signs/symptoms of infection (WBC <10,000/mm^3, temp WNL)
- Reported improvement in symptoms of infection

albumin, human (℞)

(al-byoo'min)

Albuminar 5%, Albutein 5%, Buminate 5%, Plasbumin 5%, Albuminar 25%, Albutein 25%, Buminate 25%, Plasbumin-25%

Func. class.: Blood derivative—volume expander

Chem. class.: Placental human plasma

Pregnancy category C

Action: Exerts colloidal oncotic pressure, which expands volume of circulating blood by pulling fluid from extravascular to intravascular spaces, and maintains cardiac output

➔ **Therapeutic Outcome:** Restoration of plasma volume by extravascular to intravascular fluid shift

Uses: Restores plasma volume in burns, hyperbilirubinemia, shock, hypoproteinemia, prevention of cerebral edema, cardiopulmonary bypass procedures, ARDS, hemorrhage; also replacement in nephrotic syndrome, hepatic failure

Dosage and routes

Burns

Adult: **IV** dose to maintain plasma albumin at 30-50 g/L, use 5% sol initially, then 25% sol after 24 hr

Shock

Adult: **IV** 500 ml of 5% sol q30 min, as needed

P ***Child:*** 0.5-1 g/kg/dose

Hypoproteinemia

Adult: **IV** 1000-2000 ml of 5% sol qd, not to exceed 5-10 ml/min or 25-100 g of 25% sol qd, not to exceed 3 ml/min, titrated to patient response

Hyperbilirubinemia/ erythroblastosis fetalis

P ***Infant:*** **IV** 1 g of 25% sol/kg before transfusion

Available forms: Inj 50, 250 mg/ml (5%, 25%)

Adverse effects

CNS: Fever, chills, flushing, headache

CV: **Fluid overload,** hypotension, erratic pulse, tachycardia

GI: Nausea, vomiting, increased salivation

INTEG: Rash, urticaria

RESP: Altered respirations, **pulmonary edema**

Contraindications: Hypersensitivity, CHF, severe anemia, renal insufficiency

Precautions: Decreased salt intake, decreased cardiac reserve, lack of albumin deficiency, hepatic disease, renal disease, pregnancy **C**

Pharmacokinetics	
Absorption	Complete bioavailability
Distribution	Intravascular spaces
Metabolism	Liver
Excretion	Unknown
Half-life	Unknown

Pharmacodynamics	
Onset	15-30 min
Peak	Unknown
Duration	Unknown

Interactions: None

Lab test interferences

↑ alkaline phosphatase

NURSING CONSIDERATIONS

Assessment

- Monitor blood studies: Hct, Hgb; if serum protein declines, dyspnea, hypoxemia can result; check for decreasing B/P, erratic pulse, respiration

• Monitor CVP: pulmonary wedge pressure will increase if overload occurs; I&O ratio: urinary output may decrease; CVP reading: distended neck veins indicate circulatory overload; shortness of breath, anxiety, insomnia, expiratory rales, frothy blood-tinged sputum, cough, cyanosis indicate pulmonary overload

• Assess for allergy: fever, rash, itching, chills, flushing, urticaria, nausea, vomiting, hypotension; requires discontinuation of infusion, use of new lot if therapy reinstituted; premedicate with diphenhydramine

Nursing diagnoses

- Fluid volume deficit (uses)
- Injury, risk for physical (uses)
- Fluid volume excess (adverse reactions)
- Knowledge deficit (teaching)

Implementation

• Check type of albumin; some are stored at room temperature, some need to be refrigerated; use only amber-colored sol without precipitate; solution should be clear

• Give **IV** slowly to prevent fluid overload; 5% may be given undiluted; 25% may be given diluted (D_5W, 0.9% NaCl) or undiluted; give over 4 hr, use infusion pump

• Provide adequate hydration before, during administration; whole blood may need to be given to prevent anemia; monitor hydration during treatment

Y-site compatibilities: Diltiazem, lorazepam

Solution compatibilities: LR, NaCl, Ringer's, D_5W, $D_{10}W$, $D_{2½}W$, dextrose/saline, dextran$_6$ D_5, dextran$_6$ NaCl 0.9%, dextrose/Ringer's, dextrose/LR

Patient/family education

• Explain use, reason for albumin; provide information on what to report to prescriber (hypersensitivity, fluid overload)

Evaluation

Positive therapeutic outcome

• Increased B/P, decreased edema (shock, burns)

• Increased serum albumin levels

• Increased plasma protein (hypoproteinemia)

albuterol (℞)

(al-byoo'ter-ole)

Airet, albuterol, Gen-Salbutamol ✱, Novo-Salmol ✱, Proventil, Salbutamol, Ventodisk, Ventolin, Volmax

Func. class.: Bronchodilator

Chem. class.: Adrenergic β_2-agonist, sympathomimetic, bronchodilator

Pregnancy category C

Action: Causes bronchodilatation by action on β_2 (pulmonary) receptors by increasing levels of cyclic adenosine monophosphate (cAMP), which relaxes smooth muscle; produces bronchodilatation; CNS, cardiac stimulation, increased diuresis, and increased gastric acid secretion; longer acting than isoproterenol

Therapeutic Outcome: Increased ability to breathe because of bronchodilatation

Uses: Prevention of exercise-induced asthma, acute bronchospasm, bronchitis, emphysema, bronchiectasis, reversible airway obstruction

Investigational uses: Hyperkalemia in dialysis patients

Dosage and routes

To prevent exercise-induced bronchospasm

Adult: INH (metered dose inhaler) 2 puffs 15 min before exercising

Other respiratory conditions

P ***Adult and child ≥12 yr:*** INH (metered dose inhaler) 2 puffs q4h; **PO** 2-4 mg tid-qid, not to exceed 8 mg; Volmax ext rel 8 mg q12h; Repetabs 4-8 mg q12h; Repetabs 4-8 mg q12h; NEB/IPPB 2.5 mg tid-qid

G ***Elderly:*** PO 2 mg tid-qid, may increase gradually to 8 mg tid-qid

P ***Child 2-12 yr:*** INH (metered dose inhaler) 0.1 mg/kg tid (max 2.5 mg tid-qid); NEB/IPPB 0.1-0.15 mg/kg/dose tid-qid or 1.25 mg tid-qid for child 10-15 kg or 2.5 mg tid-qid >15 kg

P ***Adult and child >4 yr:*** INH CAP (Rotahaler inhalation) 200 μg cap inhaled q4-6h; may use 15 min before exercise

Available forms: Aerosol 90, 100 μg/actuation; tabs 2, 4 mg; oral sol 2 mg/5 ml, ✤ ext rel 4, 8 mg; inh sol 0.83, 0.5, 1, 2.5 mg/ml; powder for inh (Rotacaps), 200, 400 μg; powder for inh (Ventodisk) 200, 400 μg; inh caps (Rotacaps) 200 μg; oral sol 2 mg/5 ml; 100 μg/spray, 80 inh/canister, 200 inh/canister

Adverse effects

CNS: *Tremors, anxiety,* insomnia, headache, dizziness, stimulation, *restlessness,* hallucinations, flushing, irritability

CV: *Palpitations, tachycardia, hypertension,* angina, hypotension, dysrhythmias

EENT: Dry nose, irritation of nose and throat

GI: *Heartburn, nausea, vomiting*

MISC: Flushing, sweating, anorexia, bad taste/smell changes

MS: Muscle cramps

RESP: Cough, wheezing, dyspnea, **bronchospasm,** dry throat

Contraindications: Hypersensitivity to sympathomimetics, tachydysrhythmias, severe cardiac disease, heart block

Precautions: Lactation, pregnancy **C,** cardiac disorders, hyperthyroidism, diabetes mellitus, hypertension, prostatic hypertrophy, narrow angle glaucoma, seizures, exercise-induced P bronchospasm (aero-sol) in children <12 yr

Do Not Confuse:
Ventolin/Vantin, Proventil/ Prinivil, albuterol/atenolol

Pharmacokinetics

Absorption	Well absorbed (PO)
Distribution	Unknown
Metabolism	Liver extensively, tissues
Excretion	Unknown, breast milk
Half-life	3-4 hr

Pharmacodynamics

	PO	PO–EXT REL	INH
Onset	½ hr	½ hr	5-15 min
Peak	2½ hr	2-3 hr	1-1½ hr
Duration	4-6 hr	12 hr	4-6 hr

Interactions
Drug classifications

β-Adrenergic blockers: Block therapeutic effect

Antidepressants, tricyclic: ↑ chance of hypertension, do not use together

Bronchodilators, aerosol: ↑ action of bronchodilator

Diuretics, potassium-losing: ↑ ECG changes/hypokalemia

MAOIs: ↑ chance of hypertensive crisis, do not use together

Oxytocics: Severe hypotension, do not use together

Sympathomimetics: ↑ adrenergic side effects

Xanthines: ↑ toxicity

NURSING CONSIDERATIONS
Assessment

- Assess respiratory function: vital capacity, forced expiratory volume, ABGs, lung sounds; heart rate, rhythm; B/P, sputum (baseline and during therapy)
- Determine that patient has not

received theophylline therapy before giving dose, to prevent additive effect; client's ability to self-medicate

- Monitor for evidence of allergic reactions; paradoxic bronchospasm; withhold dose; notify prescriber if bronchospasm occurs

Nursing diagnoses

- ✓ Airway clearance, ineffective (uses)
- ✓ Impaired gas exchange (uses)
- ✓ Knowledge deficit (teaching)

Implementation

PO route

- Give PO with meals to decrease P gastric irritation; oral sol for children (no alcohol, sugar)
- G In elderly patients, a spacing device is advised
- ⊘ Do not crush, break, or chew extended release tabs

Aerosol route

- Give after shaking metered dose inhaler; have patient exhale and place mouthpiece in mouth, inhale slowly, hold breath, remove inhaler, exhale slowly; allow at least 1 min between inhalations
- Store in light-resistant container; do not expose to temperatures over 86° F (30° C)

Nebulizer/IPPB

- Dilute 5 mg/ml sol/2.5 ml 0.9% NaCl for inhalation; other solutions do not require dilution for nebulizer O_2 flow or compressed air 6-10 L/min

Patient/family education

- Tell patient not to use OTC medications before consulting prescriber; excess stimulation may occur; instruct patient to use this medication before other medications and allow at least 5 min between each to prevent overstimulation; to limit caffeine products such as chocolate, coffee, tea, and cola
- Teach patient to use inhaler; review package insert with patient; to avoid getting aerosol in eyes or blurring may result; to wash inhaler in warm water and dry qd; to rinse mouth after using; to avoid smoking, smoke-filled rooms, persons with respiratory infections
- ! Teach patient that if paradoxic bronchospasm occurs to stop drug immediately and notify prescriber
- Instruct patient on administration of dose, not to use more than prescribed; serious side effects may occur; if taking PO regularly and dose is missed, take when remembered; space other doses on new time schedule; do not double doses
- G In elderly patients, a spacing device is advised

Evaluation

Positive therapeutic outcome

- Absence of dyspnea and wheezing after 1 hr
- Improved airway exchange
- Improved ABGs

Treatment of overdose:

Administer a β_1-adrenergic blocker

HIGH ALERT

aldesleukin (℞)

(al-dess-loo'kin)

interleukin-2, IL-2, Proleukin

Func. class.: Miscellaneous antineoplastics

Chem. class.: Interleukin-2, human recombinant, cytotine

Pregnancy category C

Action: Enhancement of lymphocyte mitogenesis and stimulation of IL-2–dependent cell lines; enhancement of lymphocyte cytotoxicity; induction of killer cell activity; induction of interferon-γ production; results in activation of cellular immunity and cytokines and inhibition of tumor growth

➡ **Therapeutic Outcome:** Prevention of rapid growth of malignant cells

Uses: Metastatic renal cell carcinoma in adults, phase II for HIV in combination with zidovudine, melanoma

Investigational uses: Kaposi's sarcoma given with zidovudine, metastatic melanoma given with cyclophosphamide, non-Hodgkin's lymphoma given with lymphokine-activated killer cells, AIDS (phase I) given with zidovudine

Dosage and routes

Adult: **IV** inf 600,000 IU/kg (0.037 mg/kg) over 15 min q8h × 14 doses; off 9 days; repeat schedule for another 14 doses, for a maximum of 28 doses/course

Available forms: Powder for inj 2.2 million IU/vial

Adverse effects

CNS: Mental status changes, dizziness, sensory dysfunction, syncope, motor dysfunction, fever, chills, headache, impaired memory, depression, sleep disturbances, hallucinations, rigors

CV: Hypotension, sinus tachycardia, dysrhythmias, bradycardia, PVCs, PACs, myocardial ischemia, **myocardial infarction, cardiac arrest,** capillary leak syndrome, **CVA**

EENT: Reversible visual changes

GI: Nausea, vomiting, *diarrhea,* stomatitis, anorexia, GI bleeding, dyspepsia, constipation, **intestinal perforation/ileus,** jaundice, ascites

GU: **Oliguria/anuria, proteinuria, hematuria,** dysuria, **renal failure**

HEMA: *Anemia,* **thrombocytopenia, leukopenia, coagulation disorders, leukocytosis, eosinophilia**

INTEG: Pruritus, *erythema, rash,* dry skin, **exfoliative dermatitis,** purpura, petechiae, urticaria

MS: Arthralgia, myalgia

RESP: Pulmonary congestion, dyspnea, **pulmonary edema, respiratory failure,** tachypnea, pleural effusion, wheezing, **apnea**

SYST: Infection

Contraindications: Hypersensitivity, abnormal thallium stress test or pulmonary function tests, organ allografts

Precautions: CNS metastases, bacterial infections, renal/hepatic, cardiac/pulmonary disease, pregnancy [P] **C,** lactation, children, anemia, thrombocytopenia

Do Not Confuse:
Proleukin/Prokine

Pharmacokinetics	
Absorption	Complete bioavailability
Distribution	Rapid extracellular, intravascular
Metabolism	Kidneys (convoluted tubules)
Excretion	Kidneys
Half-life	85 min

Pharmacodynamics	
Onset	4 wk
Duration	≤12 mo

Interactions

Individual drugs

Indomethacin: ↑ toxicity

Radiation: ↑ toxicity, bone marrow suppression

Drug classifications

Aminoglycosides: ↑ toxicity

Antihypertensives: ↑ hypotension

Antineoplastics: ↑ toxicity, bone marrow suppression

Glucocorticosteroids: ↓ tumor effectiveness

Psychotropics: Unpredictable reactions

Lab test interferences

↑ Bilirubin, ↑ BUN, ↑ serum creatinine, ↑ transaminase, ↑ alkaline phosphatase, ↑ hypomagnesemia, ↑ acidosis hypocalcemia, ↑ hypophosphatemia, ↑ hypokalemia, ↑ hyperuricemia, ↑ hypoalbuminemia, ↑ hypoproteinemia, ↑ hyponatremia, ↑ hyperkalemia, ↑ alkalosis (toxic effect of drug)

NURSING CONSIDERATIONS

Assessment

- Monitor CBC, differential, platelet count weekly; withhold drug if WBC is <2000/mm^3 or platelet count is <75,000/mm^3; notify prescriber of these results; transfusion of RBCs, platelets may be required
- Identify capillary leak syndrome (CLS), including a drop in mean arterial pressure (2-12 hr after initiating therapy); hypotension and hypoperfusion will occur; if B/P <90 mm Hg, monitor ECG, CVP in cardiac patients
- Monitor renal function studies: BUN, serum uric acid, urine CrCl, electrolytes before, during therapy; I&O ratio; report fall in urine output to <30 ml/hr
- Monitor temperature q4h; fever may indicate beginning infection
- Check liver function tests before, during therapy: bilirubin, AST, ALT, alkaline phosphatase, LDH as needed or monthly
- Monitor ECG; watch for ST-T wave changes, low QRS and T, possible dysrhythmias (sinus tachycardia, PVCs)
- Monitor baselines in pulmonary function; document FEV >2 L or ≥75% before therapy; check daily VS, pulse oximetry, dyspnea, rales, ABGs, watch for respiratory failure, intubate if necessary
- Obtain stress thallium study before therapy; document normal ejection fraction, unimpaired wall motion
- Assess for bleeding: hematuria, guaiac, bruising or petechiae, mucosa, or orifices q8h
- Assess for GI symptoms: frequency of stools, cramping
- Assess for acidosis, signs of dehydration: rapid respirations, poor skin turgor, decreased urine output, dry skin, restlessness, weakness
- Assess for cardiac status: B/P, pulse, character, rhythm, rate, ABGs, ECG
- Assess for infection: sore throat; antibiotics may be prescribed prophylactically

Nursing diagnoses

- ✓ Injury, risk for (adverse reactions)
- ✓ Body image disturbance (adverse reactions)
- ✓ Infection, risk for (adverse reactions)
- ✓ Knowledge deficit (teaching)

Implementation

IV intermittent infusion

- Give by intermittent **IV** inf after diluting 22 million IU (1.3 mg)/1.2 ml sterile (1.1 mg/ml) H_2O for inj at side of vial and swirl, do not shake; dilute dose with 50 ml D_5W and give over 15 min; use plastic bag; do not use an in-line filter; give through Y-tube or 3-way stopcock
- Give dopamine 1-5 kg/min before onset of hypotension; ↓ dose preserves kidney output
- Give hydrocortisone, dexamethasone, or sodium bicarbonate (1 mEq/1 ml) for extravasation, apply ice compresses
- Store in refrigerator any diluted drug; do not freeze; administer within 48 hr; bring to room temperature before infusing; discard unused portion

Y-site compatibilities:

Amikacin, **IV** fat emulsion, gentamicin, morphine, piperacillin, potassium chloride, ticarcillin, tobramycin, TPN #145, amphotericin B, calcium gluconate, diphenhydramine, dopamine, fluconazole, foscarnet, heparin, magnesium sulfate, metoclopramide, ondansetron, ranitidine, trimethoprim/sulfamethizole

Patient/family education

- Teach patient to avoid use of products containing aspirin or ibuprofen, razors, commercial mouthwash because bleeding may occur; to report symptoms of bleeding, hematuria, tarry stools
- Tell patient to report signs of

anemia: fatigue, headache, irritability, faintness, shortness of breath

• Tell patient to report any changes in breathing or coughing even several months after treatment

• Advise patient that contraception will be necessary during treatment; teratogenesis may occur

• Teach patient to report signs/symptoms of infection: fever, chills, sore throat; patient should avoid crowds or persons with known infections

• Advise patient to avoid alcohol, NSAIDs, salicylates; GI bleeding may occur

• Advise patient that visual problems may occur but are reversible

Evaluation

Positive therapeutic outcome

• Decreased spread of malignancy

alemtuzumab

See Appendix A, Selected New Drugs

alendronate (℞)

(al-en′droe-nate)

Fosamax

Func. class.: Bone-resorption inhibitor

Chem. class.: Biphosphonate

Pregnancy category C

Action: Absorbs calcium phosphate crystal in bone and may directly block dissolution of hydroxyapatite crystals of bone; inhibits bone resorption, apparently without inhibiting bone formation and mineralization

Therapeutic Outcome: Decreased symptoms of osteoporosis, Paget's disease

Uses: Osteoporosis in postmenopausal women, Paget's disease, prevention of osteoporosis, treatment of corticosteroid-induced osteoporosis in postmenopausal women not receiving estrogen, or in men

Dosage and routes

Osteoporosis in postmenopausal women

G ***Adult and elderly:*** PO 10 mg qd

Paget's disease

G ***Adult and elderly:*** PO 40 mg qd × 6 mo

Prevention of osteoporosis

Adult: PO 5 mg qd

Corticosteroid-induced osteoporosis

Adult: PO 10 mg qd

Available forms: Tabs 5, 10, 35, 40, 70 mg

Adverse effects

CNS: Headache

CV: Hypertension

GI: Abdominal pain, anorexia, constipation, nausea, vomiting, esophageal ulceration

GU: UTI, fluid overload

META: Anemia, hypokalemia, hypomagnesemia, hypophosphatemia

MS: Bone pain

Contraindications: Hypersensitivity to biphosphonates, hypocalcemia

P **Precautions:** Children, lactation, pregnancy **C**, CrCl <35 ml/min, esophageal disease, ulcers, gastritis

Pharmacokinetics	
Absorption	Unknown
Distribution	Mainly to bones
Metabolism	Unknown
Excretion	Via kidneys
Half-life	Unknown

Pharmacodynamics

Unknown

Interactions

Individual drugs

Ranitidine: ↑ alendronate effect

Drug classifications

Antacids: ↓ absorption

Calcium supplements: ↓ absorption
NSAIDs: ↑ GI reactions
Salicylates: ↑ GI reactions
Food/drug
Food: ↓ absorption

NURSING CONSIDERATIONS
Assessment
- Monitor renal studies and Ca, P, Mg, K; confirm osteoporosis with bone density test before use
- Assess for hypercalcemia: paresthesia, twitching, laryngospasm, Chvostek's, Trousseau's signs
- Monitor alkaline phosphatase; level of 2× upper limit of normal is indicated for Paget's disease

Implementation
- Give PO for 6 mo to be effective in Paget's disease; take with 8 oz of water 30 min ac
- Store in cool environment out of direct sunlight

Patient/family education
- Teach patient to remain upright for 30 min after dose to prevent esophageal irritation; if dose is missed, skip dose, do not double doses or take later in day
- Teach patient to take in AM, only before food, other meds, to take with 6-8 oz of water (not mineral water)
- To take calcium, vit D if instructed by provider
- To use weight-bearing exercise to increase bone density
- Teach patient to let provider know if pregnancy is planned or suspected or if nursing

Evaluation
Positive therapeutic outcome
- Increased bone mass, absence of fractures

alitretinoin (℞)
(al-ee-tret'i-noyn)
Panretin
Func. class.: Retinoid, 2nd generation
Pregnancy category D

Action: Controls cellular differentiation and proliferation of neoplastic and healthy cells by binding to retinoid receptors

➔ **Therapeutic Outcome:** Decreased size and number of lesions

Uses: Kaposi's sarcoma cutaneous lesions

Dosage and routes
Adult: TOP apply enough gel to cover lesions with a generous coating, allow to dry for 3-5 min before covering with clothing, do not apply near mucosal areas, apply as long as benefit occurs

Available forms: Top gel 0.1%

Adverse effects
INTEG: Rash, stinging, pain, warmth, redness, erythema, blistering, crusting, peeling, dermatitis

Contraindications: Hypersensitivity to retinoids, pregnancy **D**

Precautions: Lactation, eczema, sunburn, G elderly, cutaneous T-cell lymphoma

Pharmacokinetics	
Absorption	Small amounts
Distribution	Unknown
Metabolism	Unknown
Excretion	Kidneys
Half-life	Unknown

Pharmacodynamics
Unknown

Interactions
Individual drugs
DEET: Do not use around DEET (an insect repellant)

NURSING CONSIDERATIONS

Assessment

- Assess part of body involved, including time involved, what helps or aggravates condition, cysts, dryness, itching
- Assess for dermal toxicity that may start as erythema, then edema; drug may need to be discontinued and restarted

Nursing diagnoses

- ✓ Skin integrity, impaired (uses)
- ✓ Body image disturbances (uses)
- ✓ Knowledge deficit (teaching)

Implementation

- Apply bid initially to lesions, can be increased to tid-qid according to tolerance, discontinue for a few days if severe reactions occur
- Store at room temp
- Wash hands after application

Patient/family education

- Instruct patient to avoid application on normal skin, and to avoid getting cream in eyes, nose, other mucous membranes
- Advise patient to avoid sunlight, sunlamps or to use protective clothing or sunscreen to prevent burns
- Advise patient that treatment may cause warmth, stinging; dryness; peeling will occur
- Caution patient that drug does not cure condition; only relieves symptoms; that therapeutic results may be seen in 2-3 wk but may not be optimal until after 6 wk

Evaluation

Positive therapeutic outcome

- Decrease in size and number of lesions

allopurinol (℞)

(al-oh-pure'i-nole)

allopurinol, Aloprim, Apo-Allopurinol ✤, Lopurin, Purinol ✤, Zyloprim

Func. class.: Antigout drug

Chem. class.: Xanthine enzyme inhibitor

Pregnancy category C

Action: Inhibits the enzyme xanthine oxidase, reducing uric acid synthesis

➔ **Therapeutic Outcome:** Decreasing serum uric acid levels, decreasing joint pain

Uses: Chronic gout, hyperuricemia associated with malignancies, recurrent calcium oxalate calculi, Chagas disease, cutaneous/visceral leishmaniasis

Investigational uses: Stomatitis (mouthwash)

Dosage and routes

Increased uric acid levels in malignancies

Adult: **IV** inf 200-400 mg/m²/day, max 600 mg/day

Child: **IV** inf 200 mg/m²/day, initially

Gout/hyperuricemia

Adult: PO 200-600 mg qd depending on severity, not to exceed 800 mg/day

P ***Child 6-10 yr:*** 300 mg qd

P ***Child <6 yr:*** 150 mg qd

Impaired renal function

Adult, CrCl 30-40 ml/min: PO 200 mg qd

Adult, CrCl <20 ml/min: PO 100 mg qd

Recurrent calculi

Adult: PO 200-300 mg qd

Uric acid nephropathy prevention

P ***Adult and child >10 yr:*** PO 600-800 mg qd × 2-3 days

Stomatitis

Adult: Mouthwash dose varies, do not swallow mouthwash

Available forms: Tabs, scored, 100, 300 mg; powder for inj, lyophilized 500 mg

Adverse effects

CNS: *Headache,* drowsiness, neuritis, paresthesia

EENT: Retinopathy, cataracts, epistaxis

GI: ***Nausea, vomiting, anorexia, malaise,*** metallic taste, cramps, peptic ulcer, diarrhea, stomatitis

HEMA: **Agranulocytosis, thrombocytopenia, aplastic anemia, pancytopenia, leukopenia, bone marrow suppression, eosinophilia**

INTEG: Fever, chills, dermatitis, pruritus, purpura, erythema, ecchymosis, alopecia

MISC: Myopathy, arthralgia, hepatomegaly, **cholestatic jaundice, renal failure, exfoliative dermatitis**

Contraindications: Hypersensitivity

Precautions: Pregnancy **C**, lactation, renal disease, hepatic disease, P children

Do Not Confuse:
allopurinol/apresoline, Lopurin/Lupron

Pharmacokinetics

Absorption	80%
Distribution	Widely distributed
Metabolism	Liver to oxypurinol
Excretion	Kidneys
Half-life	2-3 hr, terminal 18-30 hr

Pharmacodynamics

	PO	IV
Onset	Unknown	Unknown
Peak	2-4 hr	Unknown
Duration	Unknown	Unknown

Interactions

Individual drugs

Ammonium chloride: ↑ kidney stone formation
Ampicillin: ↑ risk of rash
Azathioprine: ↑ action of azathioprine
Bacampicillin: ↑ risk of rash
Chlorpropamide: ↑ action of chlorpropamide
Cyclophosphamide: ↑ action of allopurinol
Mercaptopurine: ↑ action of mercaptopurine
Potassium/sodium phosphate: ↑ kidney stone formation
Theophylline: ↑ action of allopurinol
Vitamin C: ↑ kidney stone formation

Drug classifications

ACE inhibitors: ↑ action of ACE inhibitors
Aluminum salts: ↓ effects of allopurinol
Anticoagulants, oral: ↑ action of oral anticoagulants
Antineoplastics: ↑ bone marrow suppression
Diuretics, thiazide: ↑ allopurinol toxicity

NURSING CONSIDERATIONS

Assessment

- Assess for pain including location, characteristics, onset/duration, frequency, quality, intensity or severity of pain, precipitating factors
- Monitor uric acid levels q2 wk; normal uric acid levels are 6 mg/dl or less; check I&O ratio; increase fluids to 2 L/day to prevent stone formation, toxicity
- Monitor CBC, AST, BUN, creatinine before starting treatment, monthly; check blood glucose in diabetic patients receiving oral antidiabetic agents
- Monitor nutritional status: discourage organ meat, sardines, salmon, legumes, gravies (high-purine foods), alcohol

Nursing diagnoses

✓ Nutrition, more than body requirements (uses)
✓ Knowledge deficit (teaching)

Implementation

PO route

- Give with meals to prevent GI symptoms; crush and mix with food or fluids for patients with swallowing difficulties
- Give a few days before antineoplastic therapy if using for hyperuricemia associated with malignancy

IV Infusion

- Reconstitute 30-ml vial with 25 ml of sterile water for inj; dilute to desired conc with 0.9% NaCl for inj or D_5 for inj, begin inf within 10 hr

Solution incompatibilities: Amikacin, amphotericin B, carmustine, cefotaxime, chlorpromazine, cilastatin, cimetidine, clindamycin, cytarabine, dacarbazine, daunorubicin, diphenhydramine, doxorubicin, doxycycline, droperidol, floxuridine, gentamicin, haloperidol, hydroxyzine, idarubicin, imipenem, mechlorethamine, meperidine, metoclopramide, methylprednisolone, minocycline, nalbuphine, netilmicin, ondansetron, prochlorperazine, promethazine, sodium bicarbonate, streptozocin, tobramycin, vinorelbine

Patient/family education

- Tell patient to increase fluid intake to 2 L/day; to avoid taking large doses of vitamin C; kidney stone formation may occur; to maintain a diet enhancing urine alkalinity (e.g., milk, other dairy products); if taking for calcium oxalate stones, reduce dairy products, refined sugar, sodium, meat
- Tell patient to report skin rash, stomatitis, malaise, fever, aching; drug should be discontinued
- Advise patient to avoid hazardous activities if drowsiness or dizziness occurs; response may take several days to determine
- Tell patient to avoid alcohol, caffeine; these substances increase uric acid levels and decrease allopurinol levels
- Teach patient to report side effects and adverse reactions to prescriber, including rash, itching, nausea, vomiting

Evaluation

Positive therapeutic outcome

- Decreased pain in joints
- Decreased stone formation in kidney
- Decreased uric acid level to 6 mg/dl

almotriptan

See Appendix A, Selected New Drugs

alprazolam (℞)

(al-pray'zoe-lam)

Apo-Alpraz ✤, Novo-Alprazol ✤, Nu-Alpraz ✤, Xanax

Func. class.: Antianxiety/sedative/hypnotic

Chem. class.: Benzodiazepine

Pregnancy category D

Controlled substance schedule IV

Action: Depresses subcortical levels of CNS, including limbic system, reticular formation; potentiates GABA (γ-aminobutyric acid)

➡ **Therapeutic Outcome:** Decreased anxiety

Uses: Anxiety, panic disorders, anxiety with depressive symptoms

Investigational uses: Depression, social phobia, premenstrual syndrome, dysphoric disorders

Dosage and routes

Anxiety disorder

Adult: PO 0.25-0.5 mg tid, not to exceed 4 mg/day in divided doses

G ***Elderly:*** PO 0.125-0.25 mg bid; increase by 0.125 mg as needed

Panic disorder

Adult: PO 0.5 mg tid, max 10 mg/day; may ↑ q 3-4 days by 1 mg/day or less

Premenstrual dysphoric disorders

Adult: PO 0.25 mg bid-qid, starting on day 16-18 of menses, taper over 2-3 days when menses occurs

Social phobia

Adult: PO 2-8 mg/day

Hepatic dose

Reduce dose by 50%

Available forms: Tabs 0.25, 0.5, 1, 2 mg; oral sol 0.1, 1 mg/ml

Adverse effects

CNS: Dizziness, drowsiness, confusion, headache, anxiety, tremors, stimulation, fatigue, depression, insomnia, hallucinations

CV: Orthostatic hypotension, **ECG changes, tachycardia,** hypotension

EENT: Blurred vision, tinnitus, mydriasis

GI: Constipation, dry mouth, nausea, vomiting, anorexia, diarrhea

INTEG: Rash, dermatitis, itching

Contraindications: Hypersensitivity to benzodiazepines, narrow angle glaucoma, psychosis, pregnancy **D**, P child <18 yr

G **Precautions:** Elderly, debilitated, hepatic disease, renal disease

Do Not Confuse:
alprazolam/lorazepam, Xanax/Lanoxin, Xanax/Tylox, Xanax/Zantac

Pharmacokinetics

Absorption	Slow, complete
Distribution	Widely distributed; crosses placenta; crosses blood-brain barrier
Metabolism	Liver, to active metabolites
Excretion	Kidneys, breast milk
Half-life	12-15 hr

Pharmacodynamics

Onset	1 hr
Peak	1-2 hr
Duration	4-6 hr, therapeutic response 2-3 days

Interactions

Individual drugs

Alcohol: ↑ CNS depression
Cimetidine: ↑ action of alprazolam
Disulfiram: ↑ action of alprazolam
Erythromycin: ↑ action of alprazolam
Fluoxetine: ↑ action of alprazolam
Isoniazid: ↑ action of alprazolam
Ketoconazole: ↑ action of alprazolam
Levodopa: ↑ action of alprazolam
Metoprolol: ↑ action of alprazolam
Propoxyphene: ↑ action of alprazolam
Propranolol: ↑ action of alprazolam
Rifampin: ↓ action of alprazolam
Valproic acid: ↑ action of alprazolam

Drug classifications

Anticonvulsants: ↑ CNS depression
Antihistamines: ↑ CNS depression
Barbiturates: ↓ action of alprazolam
Oral contraceptives: ↑ action of alprazolam
Sedative/hypnotics: ↑ CNS depression
Xanthines: ↑ sedation

Food/drug

Grapefruit juice: ↑ drug level

Herb/drug

Kava: ↑ CNS depression

Lab test interferences

↑ AST/ALT, alkaline phosphatase; ↑ neutropenia

NURSING CONSIDERATIONS

Assessment

- Assess mental status: mood, sensorium, anxiety, affect, sleeping pattern, drowsiness, dizziness, especially G elderly; physical dependency, withdrawal symptoms: anxiety, panic attacks, agitation, convulsions, headache, nausea, vomiting, muscle pain, weakness; suicidal tendencies; indications of increasing tolerance and abuse; withdrawal seizures may occur after rapid decrease in dose or abrupt discontinuation; short duration of action makes it the drug of choice in G the elderly

- Monitor B/P (with patient lying, standing), pulse; if systolic B/P drops 20 mm Hg, hold drug, notify prescriber
- Monitor blood studies: CBC during long-term therapy; blood dycrasias have occurred rarely; decreased hematocrit, neutropenia may occur
- Monitor hepatic studies: AST, ALT, bilirubin, creatinine LDH, alkaline phosphatase, if on long-term treatment
- Monitor I&O; indicate renal dysfunction if on long-term treatment

Nursing diagnoses

✓ Anxiety (uses)
✓ Depression (uses)
✓ Injury, risk for (adverse reactions)
✓ Knowledge deficit (teaching)

Implementation

- Give with food or milk for GI symptoms; tab may be crushed, if patient is unable to swallow medication whole, and mixed with foods or fluids; may divide total daily dose into more times/day, if anxiety occurs between doses
- Give sugarless gum, hard candy, frequent sips of water for dry mouth

Patient/family education

- Tell patient that drug may be taken with food or fluids, and tabs may be crushed or swallowed whole
- Tell patient not to use for everyday stress or longer than 4 mo unless directed by prescriber; not to take more than prescribed amount; may be habit forming; not to double doses or skip doses; memory impairment is a sign of long-term use
- Tell patient to avoid OTC preparations unless approved by prescriber; alcohol and CNS depressants will increase CNS depression
- Tell patient to avoid driving, activities that require alertness, since drowsiness may occur; to avoid alcohol ingestion or other psychotropic medications; to rise slowly or G fainting may occur, especially elderly; that drowsiness may worsen at beginning of treatment
- Tell patient not to discontinue medication abruptly after long-term use; withdrawal symptoms include vomiting, cramping, tremors, seizures

Evaluation

Positive therapeutic outcome

- Decreased anxiety, restlessness, sleeplessness (short-term treatment only)

Treatment of overdose:

Lavage, VS, supportive care, flumazenil

HIGH ALERT

alteplase (℞)

(al-ti-plaze′)

Activase, Activase rt-PA ✱, Lysatec rt-PA ✱, Cathflo tissue plasminogin activator, t-PA

Func. class.: Thrombolytic enzyme
Chem. class.: Tissue plasminogen activator (TPA)

Pregnancy category C

Action: Produces fibrin conversion of plasminogen to plasmin; able to bind to fibrin, convert plasminogen in thrombus to plasmin, which leads to local fibrinolysis, limited systemic proteolysis

➡ **Therapeutic Outcome:** Lysis of thrombi in MI, pulmonary emboli (life threatening)

Uses: Lysis of obstructing thrombi associated with acute MI; conditions requiring thrombolysis, (e.g., PE, DVT, unclotting arteriovenous shunts), acute ischemic CVA

Investigational uses: Unstable angina, occluded catheters

Dosage and routes

Pulmonary embolism

Adult: **IV** 100 mg over 2 hr, then heparin

Acute ischemic stroke

Adult: **IV** 0.9 mg/kg, max 90 mg; give as inf over 1 hr, give 10% of dose

Standard infusion

Adult >65 kg: **IV** a total of 100 mg; 6-10 mg given **IV** bol over 1-2 min, 60 mg given over 1st hr, 20 mg given over 2nd hr, 20 mg given over 3rd hr

Adult <65 kg: **IV** 0.75 mg over 1st hr, 0.075-0.125 mg/kg given **IV** bol over first 1-2 min, 0.25 mg/kg over 2nd hr, 0.25 mg/kg over 3rd hr to a total dose of 1.25 mg/kg, max 100 mg total

Accelerated infusion

Adult: **IV** bol 15 mg; then 50 mg over ½ hr; 35 mg over 1 hr

Occluded catheters

Adult: 2 mg/2 ml infused in each port of dual lumen catheter; dwell time varies widely

Available forms: Powder for inj 20 mg (11.6 million IU/vial), 50 mg (29 million IU/vial), 100 mg (58 million IU/vial); 2 mg single-patient vial

Adverse effects

CV: **Sinus bradycardia, ventricular tachycardia, accelerated idioventricular rhythm**

INTEG: Urticaria, rash

SYST: **GI, GU, intracranial, retroperitoneal bleeding, surface bleeding, anaphylaxis**

Contraindications: Hypersensitivity, active internal bleeding, recent CVA, severe uncontrolled hypertension, intracranial/intraspinal surgery/trauma, aneurysm

Precautions: Pregnancy **C**, lactation, children

Pharmacokinetics	
Absorption	Complete
Distribution	Unknown
Metabolism	>80% liver
Excretion	Kidneys
Half-life	30 min

Pharmacodynamics	
Onset	Immediate
Peak	30-45 min
Duration	4 hr

Interactions

Individual drugs

Abciximab: ↑ bleeding
Aspirin: ↑ bleeding
Clopidogrel: ↑ bleeding
Dipyridamole: ↑ bleeding
Eptifibatide: ↑ bleeding
Heparin: ↑ bleeding
Plicamycin: ↑ bleeding
Ticlopidine: ↑ bleeding
Tirofiban: ↑ bleeding
Valproic acid: ↑ bleeding

Drug classifications

Anticoagulants, oral: ↑ bleeding
Cephalosporins, some: ↑ bleeding
NSAIDs: ↑ bleeding

Lab test interferences

↑ PT, ↑ APTT, ↑ TT

NURSING CONSIDERATIONS

Assessment

- Monitor VS q15 min, B/P, pulse, respirations (including peripheral), neurologic signs, temp at least q4h; temp >104° F (40° C) indicates internal bleeding; monitor rhythm closely; ventricular dysrhythmias may occur with hyperfusion; monitor heart, breath sounds, neurologic status, and peripheral pulses
- Assess for bleeding during 1st hr of treatment and 24 hr after procedure: hematuria, hematemesis, bleeding from mucous membranes, epistaxis,

ecchymosis, puncture sites; guaiac all body fluids and stools; obtain blood studies (Hct, platelets, PTT, PT, TT, APTT) before starting therapy; PT or APTT must be less than 2 times control before starting therapy; TT or PT q3-4h during treatment; obtain CPK—MB to identify drug effectiveness

- Assess hypersensitivity: fever, rash, facial swelling, dyspnea, itching, chills; mild reaction may be treated with antihistamines; report to prescriber
- Monitor ECG; on monitor, watch for segment changes, changes in rhythm: sinus bradycardia, ventricular tachycardia, accelerated idioventricular rhythm may occur due to reperfusion, cardiac enzymes, radionuclide myocardial scanning/coronary angiography

Nursing diagnoses

✓ Pain (uses)
✓ Tissue perfusion, altered (uses)
✓ Injury, risk for (adverse reactions)

Implementation

- Give after reconstituting with provided diluent; add appropriate amount of sterile water for injection (no preservatives); 20-mg vial/20 ml or 50-mg vial/50 ml (1 mg/ml); mix by slow inversion or dilute with 0.9% NaCl, D_5W to a concentration of 0.5 mg/ml further dilution; 1.5 to <0.5 mg/ml may result in precipitation of drug; use 18-gauge needle; flush line with NaCl after administration; use reconstituted **IV** sol within 8 hr or discard, within 6 hr of coronary occlusion for best results
- (!) Do not use 150 mg or more total dose; intracranial bleeding may occur
- Give heparin therapy after thrombolytic therapy is discontinued and when TT, ACT, and APTT less than 2 times control (about 3-4 hr)
- Avoid invasive procedures, inj, rec temp; apply pressure for 30 sec to minor bleeding sites; 30 min to sites of atrial puncture, followed by pressure dressing; inform prescriber if this does not attain hemostasis; apply pressure dressing
- Store powder at room temperature or refrigerate; protect from excessive light

Y-site compatibilities:
Lidocaine, metoprolol, propranolol

Y-site incompatibilities:
Dobutamine, dopamine, heparin, nitroglycerin

Additive compatibilities:
Lidocaine, morphine, nitroglycerin

Patient/family education

- Teach patient reason for alteplase, signs and symptoms of bleeding, allergic reactions, when to notify prescriber

Evaluation

Positive therapeutic outcome

- Lysis of pulmonary thrombi
- Adequate hemodynamic state
- Absence of congestive heart failure

altretamine (℞)

(al-tret'a-meen)

Hexalen, hexamethylmelamine, Hexastat ✦

Func. class.: Misc. antineoplastic
Chem. class.: *S*-Triazine derivative (formerly known as hexamethylmelamine)

Pregnancy category D

Action: Products of metabolism form covalent bonds with tissue macromolecules including DNA, which may be responsible for cytotoxicity; activity is not cell cycle phase specific

➔ **Therapeutic Outcome:** Prevention of rapid growth of malignant cells

Uses: Palliative treatment of recurrent, persistent ovarian cancer following first-line treatment with cisplatin or alkylating agent–based combination

Dosage and routes

Adult: PO 260 mg/m^2 day for 14 or 21 days in a 28-day cycle; give in 4 divided doses pc and hs

Available forms: Caps 50, 100 mg

Adverse effects

CNS: *Peripheral sensory neuropathy,* fatigue, **seizures,** mood disorders, disorders of consciousness, ataxia, dizziness, vertigo, Parkinson-like tremors

GI: *Nausea, anorexia, cramping, vomiting,* increased alkaline phosphatase, **hepatic toxicity**

GU: Increased BUN, serum creatinine

HEMA: **Leukopenia, thrombocytopenia, anemia**

INTEG: Rash, pruritus, alopecia, eczema

Contraindications: Hypersensitivity, severe bone marrow depression, severe neurologic toxicity, pregnancy **D**

P **Precautions:** Lactation, children

Pharmacokinetics

Absorption	Well absorbed
Distribution	Concentrated in liver, kidneys, small intestine
Metabolism	Liver (99%)
Excretion	Kidneys
Half-life	4½-10½ hr

Pharmacodynamics

Onset	Unknown
Peak	½-3 hr
Duration	Unknown

Interactions

Individual drugs

Cimetidine: ↑ toxicity

Radiation: ↑ toxicity

Drug classifications

Antineoplastics: ↑ bone marrow depression

Live virus vaccines: ↑ antibody reactions

MAOIs: ↑ orthostatic hypotension

NURSING CONSIDERATIONS

Assessment

- Monitor CBC, differential, platelet count weekly; withhold drug if WBC is <4000/mm^3 or platelet count is <75,000/mm^3; granulocytes <1000 mm^3, notify prescriber of results; nadir (leukopenia/thrombocytopenia) occurs in 1 mo; resolves in 6 wk
- Monitor renal function studies: BUN, serum uric acid, urine CrCl before, during therapy; I&O ratio; report fall in urine output of 30 ml/hr; monitor for decreased hyperuricemia
- Monitor for cold, fever, sore throat (may indicate beginning of infection)
- Assess for bleeding: hematuria, guaiac, bruising or petechiae, mucosa or orifices q8h; no rec temp; identify inflammation of mucosa, breaks in skin; use viscous lidocaine (Xylocaine) for oral pain
- Identify food preferences; list likes, dislikes
- Identify edema in feet, joint or stomach pain, shaking
- Assess neurologic status: paresthesia, numbness, tingling; pyridoxine may minimize neurologic reaction

Nursing diagnoses

- ✓ Injury, risk for (adverse reactions)
- ✓ Infection, risk for (adverse reactions)
- ✓ Knowledge deficit (teaching)

Implementation

- Give 1 hr before or 2 hr after meals to lessen nausea and vomiting or antacid before oral agent; give drug after evening meal, before bedtime; antiemetic 30-60 min before giving drug to prevent vomiting
- Give all medications PO, no rec temp, apply pressure to venipuncture sites for 10 min
- Store in tight container

Patient/family education

- Tell patient that contraceptive measures are recommended during therapy; teratogenic effects occur
- Teach patient to avoid use of products containing alcohol, aspirin, or

ibuprofen, razors, hard bristle toothbrush, and commercial mouthwash because bleeding may occur; to report symptoms of bleeding (hematuria, tarry stools)

- Tell patient to report signs of anemia (fatigue, headache, irritability, faintness, shortness of breath)
- Tell patient to report any changes in breathing or coughing even several months after treatment
- Tell patient that hair may be lost during treatment; a wig or hairpiece may make patient feel better; new hair may be different in color, texture
- Advise patient to avoid vaccinations during treatment; serious reactions may occur
- Advise patient to use contraception during and for 4 mo after treatment
- Teach patient to report signs/symptoms of infection: fever, chills, sore throat; patient should avoid crowds and persons with known infections; to report numbness in extremities

Evaluation

Positive therapeutic outcome

- Decreased size and spread of malignancy

aluminum hydroxide (OTC)

AlternaGEL, Alu-Cap, Alugel ✦, Aluminet, Aluminett, aluminum hydroxide, Alu-Tab, Amphojel, Basalgel, Basaljel, Dialume, Nephrox

Func. class.: Antacid, hypophosphatemic, antiulcer

Chem. class.: Aluminum product

Pregnancy category C

Action: Neutralizes gastric acidity, binds phosphates in GI tract; these phosphates are excreted

Uses: Peptic, gastric, duodenal ulcers; hyperphosphatemia in chronic renal failure; reflux esophagitis, hyperacidity, heartburn

Investigational uses: stress ulcer, GI bleeding

➔ **Therapeutic Outcome:** Decreased acidity, healing of ulcers; decreased phosphate levels in chronic renal failure

Dosage and routes

Adult: SUSP 5-10 ml 1 hr pc, hs; PO 600 mg 1 hr pc, hs, chewed with milk or water

GI bleeding

P ***Infant:*** PO 2-5 ml/dose q1-2h

P ***Child:*** PO 5-15 ml/dose q1-2h

Hyperphosphatemia in renal failure

Adult: SUSP 500 mg-2 g bid-qid

Available forms

Caps 475, 500 mg; tabs 300, 500, 600 mg; susp 450 mg/5 ml, 600 mg/5 ml; liq 320 mg/5 ml, 600 mg/5 ml, 675 mg/5 ml

Adverse effects

GI: *Constipation,* anorexia, **obstruction,** fecal impaction

META: *Hypophosphatemia,* hypercalciuria

Contraindications: Hypersensitivity to this drug or aluminum products, abdominal pain of unknown origin

G **Precautions:** Elderly, fluid restriction, decreased GI motility, GI obstruction, dehydration, renal disease, sodium-restricted diets, pregnancy **C**

Pharmacokinetics

Absorption	Not usually absorbed
Distribution	Widely distributed if absorbed; crosses placenta
Metabolism	Unknown
Excretion	Feces, kidneys (small amounts), breast milk
Half-life	Unknown

Pharmacodynamics	
Onset	20-40 min
Peak	½ hr
Duration	½-1½ hr

Interactions
Individual drugs
Allopurinol: ↓ allopurinol effect
Amphetamine: ↑ levels
Chlorpromazine: ↓ absorption
Ciprofloxacin: ↓ effectiveness
Diflunisal: ↓ diflunisal effect
Isoniazid: ↓ absorption
Mexiletine: ↑ levels
Quinidine: ↑ levels
Salicylate: ↓ levels
Tetracycline: ↓ absorption
Ticlopidine: ↓ ticlopidine effect
Drug classifications
Corticosteroids: ↓ corticosteroid effect
H_2 antagonists: ↓ corticosteroid effect
Thyroid hormones: ↓ thyroid effect

NURSING CONSIDERATIONS
Assessment
- Assess pain symptoms: location, duration, intensity, alleviating precipitating factors
- Monitor phosphate levels, since drug is bound in GI system; urinary pH, calcium, electrolytes; hypophosphatemia: anorexia, weakness, fatigue, bone pain, hyperreflexia
- Monitor constipation; increase bulk in diet if needed

Nursing diagnoses
✓ Pain, chronic (uses)
✓ Constipation (adverse reactions)
✓ Knowledge deficit (teaching)

Implementation
- Give laxatives or stool softeners if constipation occurs, especially elderly (G)
- Give after shaking liq; follow with water to facilitate passage
- Tab may be chewed if patient is unable to swallow; drink 8 oz of water after chewing; or by nasogastric tube if patient unable to swallow
- Give with 8 oz of water for hyperphosphatemia unless contraindicated
- Givc 1 hr before or after other medications to prevent poor absorption
- Give 15 ml 30 min pc and hs (esophagitis)
- May be given as prescribed q1-2h and given by gastric tube after diluting with water (peptic ulcer)

Patient/family education
- Instruct patient to increase fluids to 2000 ml/day unless contraindicated
- Instruct patient to avoid phosphate foods (most dairy products, eggs, fruits, carbonated beverages) during drug therapy; to add cheese, corn, pasta, plums, prunes, lentils after drug (hypophosphatemia)
- Instruct patient not to use for prolonged periods if serum phosphate is low or if on a low-sodium diet; CHF patients should check for sodium content and use sodium-reduced products
- Instruct patient that stools may appear white or speckled; constipation may result; to report black tarry stools, which indicate gastric bleeding
- Instruct patient to check with prescriber after 2 wk of self-prescribed antacid use; may be used for 4-6 wk after symptoms subside or as prescribed
- Instruct patient to separate other medications by 2 hr

Evaluation
Positive therapeutic outcome
- Absence of pain, decreased acidity
- Increased pH of gastric secretions
- Decreased phosphate levels

A

amifostine (℞)

(a-mi-foss'teen)

Ethyol

Func. class.: Cytoprotective agent for cisplatin

Pregnancy category C

Action: Binds and detoxifies damaging metabolites of cisplatin by converting this drug by alkaline phosphatasc in tissue to an active free thiol compound

➔ **Therapeutic Outcome:** Decreased toxic reaction from cisplatin

Uses: Used to reduce renal toxicity when cisplatin is given in ovarian cancer, reduces xerostomia in radiation therapy for head, neck cancer

Dosage and routes

Adult: **IV** 910 mg/m^2 qd, within ½ hr before chemotherapy, may reduce dose to 740 mg/m^2 if higher dose is poorly tolerated

Xerostomia

Adult: **IV** 200 mg/m^2 qd over 3 min as inf 15-30 min before radiation therapy

Available forms: Powder for inj 500 mg/vial with 500 mg mannitol

Adverse effects

CNS: Dizziness, somnolence

CV: Hypotension

EENT: Sneezing

GI: Nausea, vomiting, hiccups

INTEG: Flushing, feeling of warmth

MISC: Hypocalcemia, rash, chills

Contraindications: Hypersensitivity to mannitol, aminothiol; hypotension, dehydration, lactation

G P **Precautions:** Elderly, CV disease, pregnancy **C,** children

Pharmacokinetics

Absorption	Complete
Distribution	Unknown
Metabolism	To free thiol compound
Excretion	Unknown
Half-life	5-8 min

Pharmacodynamics

Unknown

Interactions

Drug classfications

Antihypertensives: ↑ hypotension

NURSING CONSIDERATIONS

Assessment

- Assess fluid status before administration; administer antiemetic before administration to prevent severe nausea and vomiting; also, dexamethasone 20 mg **IV** and a serotonin antagonist such as ondansetron, dolasetron, or granisetron
- Monitor calcium levels before and during treatment; calcium supplements may be given for low calcium levels
- Monitor blood pressure before and q5 min during infusion; if severe hypotension occurs, give **IV** 0.9% NaCl to expand fluid volume, place in Trendelenburg position

Nursing diagnoses

✓ Injury, risk for (uses)
✓ Knowledge deficit (teaching)

Implementation

- Give by **IV** intermittent inf after reconstituting with 9.5 ml of sterile 0.9% NaCl, further dilute with 0.9% NaCl to a concentration of 5-40 mg/ml, give at a rate over 15 min within ½ hr of chemotherapy

Y-site compatibilities: Amikacin, aminophylline, ampicillin, ampicillin/sulbactam, aztreonam, bleomycin, bumetanide, buprenorphine, butorphanol, calcium gluconate, carboplatin, carmustine, cefazolin, cefonicid, cefotaxime, cefotetan, cefoxitin, ceftazidime, ceftizoxime, ceftriaxone, cefuroxime, cimetidine, ciprofloxacin, clindamycin, cyclophosphamide, cytarabine, dacarbazine, dactinomycin, daunorubicin, dexamethasone, diphenhydramine, dobutamine, dopamine, doxorubicin, doxycycline, droperidol, enalaprilat, etoposide, famotidine, floxuridine, fluconazole, fludarabine, fluorouracil, furosemide, gallium, gentamicin, granisetron, haloperidol, heparin, hydrocortisone, hydromorphone, idarubicin, ifosfamide, imipenem-cilastatin, leucovorin, lorazepam, magnesium sulfate, mannitol, mechlorethamine, meperidine, mesna, methotrexate, methylprednisolone, metoclopramide, metronidazole, mezlocillin, mitomycin, mitoxantrone, morphine, nalbuphine, netilmicin, ondansetron, piperacillin, plicamycin, potassium chloride, promethazine, ranitidine, sodium bicarbonate, streptozocin, teniposide, thiotepa, ticarcillin, ticarcillin/clavulanate, tobramycin, trimethoprim-sulfamethoxazole, trimetrexate, vancomycin, vinblastine, vincristine, zidovudine

Additive incompatibilities: Do not mix with other drugs or solutions

Patient/family education

- Teach reason for medication and expected results, supine position during infusion
- Teach that side effects may cause severe nausea, vomiting, decreased B/P, chills, dizziness, somnolence, hiccups, sneezing

Evaluation

Positive therapeutic outcome

- Absence of renal damage

amikacin (℞)

(am-i-kay'sin)

amikacin sulfate, Amikin

Func. class.: Antibiotic

Chem. class.: Aminoglycoside

Pregnancy category D

Action: Interferes with protein synthesis in bacterial cell by binding to ribosomal subunit, which causes misreading of genetic code; inaccurate peptide sequence forms in protein chain, causing bacterial death

➔ **Therapeutic Outcome:** Bactericidal effects for the following organisms: *Pseudomonas aeruginosa, Escherichia coli, Enterobacter, Acinetobacter, Providencia, Citrobacter, Staphylococcus, Serratia, Proteus*

Uses: Severe systemic infections of CNS, respiratory, GI, urinary tract, bone, skin, soft tissues

Investigational uses: *Mycobacterium avium* complex (intrathecal or intraventricular) in combination; aerosolization

Dosage and routes

Severe systemic infections

P ***Adult and child:*** **IV** inf 15 mg/kg/day in 2-3 divided doses q8-12h in 100-200 ml D_5W over 30-60 min, not to exceed 1.5 g; decreased dosages are needed in poor renal function as determined by blood levels, renal function studies; IM 15 mg/kg/day in divided doses q8-12h; qd or extended internal dosing as an alternative dosing regimen

P ***Infants:*** **IV** 5 mg/kg q8h or 7.5 mg/kg q12h

P ***Neonates:*** IM/**IV** inf 10 mg/kg initially, then 7.5 mg/kg q12h in D_5W over 1-2 hr

P ***Premature neonates:*** **IV** 10 mg/kg initially, then 7.5 mg/kg q8-12h

A

Severe urinary tract infections
Adults: IM 250 mg bid
Adults with poor renal function: 5-7.5 mg/kg initially, then increased as determined by blood levels, renal function studies
Aerosolization
Adult: Aerosol varies widely, 250 mg q12h or 400 mg q8h

Available forms: Inj IM, **IV** 50, 250 mg/ml

Adverse effects

CNS: Confusion, depression, numbness, tremors, **convulsions,** muscle twitching, **neurotoxicity,** dizziness, vertigo, tinnitus
CV: Hypotension or hypertension, palpitations
EENT: Ototoxicity, deafness, visual disturbances
GI: *Nausea, vomiting, anorexia,* increased ALT, AST, bilirubin, hepatomegaly, **hepatic necrosis,** splenomegaly
GU: **Oliguria, hematuria, renal damage, azotemia, renal failure, nephrotoxicity**
HEMA: **Agranulocytosis, thrombocytopenia, leukopenia, eosinophilia, anemia**
INTEG: *Rash,* burning, urticaria, dermatitis, alopecia

Contraindications: Mild to moderate infections, hypersensitivity to aminoglycosides, pregnancy **D,** sulfites

P ***Precautions:*** Neonates, mild renal disease, myasthenia gravis, lactation, hearing deficits, Parkinson's disease, G elderly

Do Not Confuse:
Amikin/Amicar

Pharmacokinetics

Absorption	Well absorbed (IM), complete absorbed (**IV**)
Distribution	Widely distributed in extracellular fluids, poor in CSF; crosses placenta
Metabolism	Minimal; liver
Excretion	Mostly unchanged (79%) in kidneys, removed by hemodialysis
Half-life	2-3 hr, prolonged up to 7 hr in infants (P); increased in renal disease

Pharmacodynamics

	IM	IV
Onset	Rapid	Rapid
Peak	15-30 min	1-2 hr

Interactions

Individual drugs
Dimenhydrinate: ↑ masking of ototoxicity
Ethacrynic acid: ↑ masking of ototoxicity
Indomethacin: ↑ serum trough and peak

Drug classifications
Aminoglycosides: ↑ ototoxicity, neurotoxicity, nephrotoxicity
Anesthetics: ↑ neuromuscular blockade, respiratory depression
Cephalosporins: Inactivation of amikacin
Diuretics, loop: ↑ ototoxicity
Nondepolarizing neuromuscular blockers: ↑ neuromuscular blockade, respiratory depression
Penicillins: Inactivation of amikacin

Lab test interferences
↑ BUN, ↑ ALT, ↑ AST, ↑ bilirubin, ↑ LDH, ↑ alkaline phosphatase, ↑ creatinine
↓ Calcium, ↓ sodium, ↓ potassium, ↓ magnesium

NURSING CONSIDERATIONS

Assessment

- Assess patient for previous sensitivity reaction
- Assess patient for signs and symp-

toms of infection, including characteristics of wounds, sputum, urine, stool, WBC >10,000/mm^3, earache, temp; obtain baseline information before and during treatment
- Obtain C&S tests before beginning drug therapy to identify if correct treatment has been initiated
- Assess for allergic reactions: rash, urticaria, pruritus
- Identify urine output; if decreasing, notify prescriber (may indicate nephrotoxicity); also notify prescriber of increased BUN and creatinine, urine CrCl <80 ml/min; lower dosage should be given in renal impairment; urinalysis daily for protein, cells, casts, nephrotoxicity may be reversible if drug stopped at first sign
- Monitor blood studies: AST, ALT, CBC, Hct, bilirubin, LDH, alkaline phosphatase; Coombs' test monthly if patient is on long-term therapy
- Monitor electrolytes: potassium, sodium, chloride, magnesium monthly if patient is on long-term therapy
- Assess bowel pattern qd; if severe diarrhea occurs, drug should be discontinued
- Monitor for bleeding: ecchymosis, bleeding gums, hematuria, stool guaiac daily if on long-term therapy
- Assess for overgrowth of infection: perineal itching, fever, malaise, redness, pain, swelling, drainage, rash, diarrhea, change in cough, sputum
- Obtain weight before treatment; calculation of dosage is usually based on ideal body weight, but may be calculated on actual body weight
- Monitor VS during infusion, watch for hypotension, change in pulse
- Assess **IV** site for thrombophlebitis including pain, redness, swelling q30 min; change site if needed; apply warm compresses to discontinued site
- Obtain serum peak, drawn 30-60 min after **IV** infusion or 60 min after IM injection; trough level drawn just before next dose; 20-30 µg/ml, trough 4-8 µg/ml, blood level should be 2-4 times bacteriostatic level
- Urine pH if drug is used for UTI; urine should be kept alkaline
- ❗ Deafness by audiometric testing, ringing, roaring in ears, vertigo; assess hearing before, during, after treatment
- Dehydration: high sp gr, decrease in skin turgor, dry mucous membranes, dark urine
- Vestibular dysfunction: nausea, vomiting, dizziness, headache; drug should be discontinued if severe

Nursing diagnoses
- ✓ Infection, risk for (uses)
- ✓ Diarrhea (side effects)
- ✓ Knowledge deficit (teaching)
- ✓ Injury, risk for (side effects)

Implementation
IM route
- Give deeply in large muscle mass

IV route
- Dilute 500 mg of drug in 100-200 ml of **IV** D_5W, D_5NaCl, or 0.9% NaCl and give over ½-1 hr; flush after administration with D_5W or 0.9% NaCl

Syringe compatibilities:
Clindamycin, doxapram

Y-site compatibilities:
Acyclovir, amifostine, amiodarone, amsacrine, aztreonam, cisatracurium, cyclophosphamide, dexamethasone, diltiazem, enalamprilat, esmolol, filgrastim, fluconazole, fludarabine, foscarnet, furosemide, granisetron, idarubicin, IL-2, labetalol, lorazepam, magnesium sulfate, melphalan, midazolam, morphine, ondansetron, paclitaxel, perphenazine, remifentanil, sargramostim, teniposide, thiotepa, TPN #54, #61, #91, #203, #204, #212, vinorelbine, warfarin, zidovudine

Patient/family education
- Teach patient to report sore throat, bruising, bleeding, joint pain; may indicate blood dyscrasias (rare)
- Advise patient to contact prescriber if vaginal itching, loose foul-smelling

stools, furry tongue occur; may indicate superinfection
- Advise patient to report hypersensitivity: rash, itching, trouble breathing, facial edema and notify prescriber

Evaluation
Positive therapeutic outcome
- Absence of signs/symptoms of infection: WBC <10,000/mm^3, temp WNL; absence of red draining wounds; absence of earache
- Reported improvement in symptoms of infection

Treatment of overdose:
Withdraw drug; administer epinephrine, O_2, hemodialysis, exchange P transfusion in the newborn; monitor serum levels of drug; may give ticarcillin or carbenicillin

amiloride (℞)
(a-mill'oh-ride)
Amiloride HCl, Midamor
Func. class.: Potassium-sparing diuretic
Chem. class.: Pyrazine
Pregnancy category B

Action: Acts primarily on proximal distal tubule by inhibiting reabsorption of sodium and water and increasing potassium retention and conserving hydrogen ions

➡ **Therapeutic Outcome:** Diuretic and antihypertensive effect while retaining potassium

Uses: Diuretic-induced hypokalemia; used with other agents to treat edema, hypertension

Dosage and routes
Adult: PO 5 mg qd; may be increased to 10-20 mg qd if needed

Available forms: Tabs 5 mg

Adverse effects
CNS: *Headache,* dizziness, fatigue, weakness, paresthesias, tremor, depression, anxiety
CV: Orthostatic hypotension, dysrhythmias, angina
EENT: Loss of hearing, tinnitus, blurred vision, nasal congestion, increased intraocular pressure
ELECT: **Hyperkalemia**
GI: *Nausea, diarrhea,* dry mouth, *vomiting, anorexia,* cramps, constipation, abdominal pain, jaundice, bleeding
GU: *Polyuria,* dysuria, frequency, impotence
HEMA: **Aplastic anemia, neutropenia (rare)**
INTEG: *Rash, pruritus,* alopecia, urticaria
RESP: Cough, dyspnea, shortness of breath

Contraindications: Anuria, hypersensitivity, hyperkalemia, impaired renal function

Precautions: Dehydration, pregnancy **B,** diabetes, acidosis, lactation, hepatic disease

Pharmacokinetics
Absorption	Variable (10%-15%)
Distribution	Unknown
Metabolism	Unchanged in urine (50%) in feces (40%)
Excretion	Renal; breast milk
Half-life	6-9 hr

Pharmacodynamics
Onset	2 hr
Peak	6-10 hr
Duration	24 hr

Interactions
Individual drugs
Lithium: ↑ Lithium toxicity
Drug classifications
ACE inhibitors: ↑ hyperkalemia
Antihypertensives: ↑ action
Diuretics, potassium-sparing: ↑ hyperkalemia
NSAIDs: ↓ effectiveness of amiloride

Potassium products: ↑ hyperkalemia
Salt substitutes: ↑ hyperkalemia

Food/drug

Potassium foods: ↑ hyperkalemia

Lab test interferences

Interference: GTT

NURSING CONSIDERATIONS

Assessment

- Monitor manifestations of hyperkalemia: *MS:* fatigue, muscle weakness; *CARDIAC:* dysrhythmias, hypotension; *NEURO:* paresthesias, confusion; *RESP:* dyspnea
- Monitor for manifestations of hyponatremia: *CV:* increased B/P, cold, clammy skin, hypovolemia or hypervolemia; *GI:* anorexia, nausea, vomiting, diarrhea, abdominal cramps; *NEURO:* lethargy, increased ICP, confusion, headache, seizures, coma, fatigue, tremors, hyperreflexia
- Monitor for manifestations of hyperchloremia: *NEURO:* weakness, lethargy, coma; *RESP:* deep rapid breathing
- Assess fluid volume status: I&O ratios and record, weight, distended red veins, crackles in lung, color, quality and sp gr of urine, skin turgor, adequacy of pulses, moist mucous membranes, bilateral lung sounds, peripheral pitting edema; dehydration symptoms of decreasing output, thirst, hypotension, dry mouth and mucous membranes should be reported
- Monitor electrolytes: potassium, sodium, calcium, magnesium; also include BUN, ABGs, uric acid, CBC, blood sugar
- Assess B/P before and during therapy with patient lying, standing, and sitting as appropriate; orthostatic hypotension can occur rapidly

Nursing diagnoses

✓ Fluid volume deficit (side effects)
✓ Fluid volume excess (uses)
✓ Knowledge deficit (teaching)

Implementation

- Give in AM to avoid interference with sleep
- With food; if nausea occurs, absorption may be increased

Patient/family education

- Teach patient to take medication early in the day to prevent nocturia
- Instruct patient to take with food or milk if GI symptoms of nausea and anorexia occur
- Teach patient to maintain a weekly record of weight and notify prescriber of weight loss >5 lb
- Caution patient that this drug causes an increase in potassium levels, so foods high in potassium should be avoided; refer to dietician for assistance, planning
- Caution patient not to exercise in hot weather or stand for prolonged periods since orthostatic hypotension will be enhanced
- Teach patient not to use alcohol or any OTC medications without prescriber's approval; serious drug reactions may occur
- Emphasize the need to contact prescriber immediately if muscle cramps, weakness, nausea, dizziness, or numbness occurs
- Teach patient to take own B/P and pulse and record
- Advise patient that dizziness and confusion may occur; avoid driving or other hazardous activities if alertness is decreased
- Teach patient to continue taking medication even if feeling better; this drug controls symptoms but does not cure the condition
- Advise patient with hypertension to continue other medical treatment (exercise, weight loss, relaxation techniques, cessation of smoking)

Evaluation

Positive therapeutic outcome

- Prevention of hypokalemia (diuretic use)
- Decreased edema

A

- Decreased B/P
- Increased diuresis

Treatment of overdose: Lavage if taken orally; monitor electrolytes; administer **IV** fluids; monitor hydration, CV, renal status

amino acid (℞)

(a-mee'noe)

Injection: Aminess, Aminosyn, BranchAmin, NephrAmine, FreAmine HBC, HepatAmine

Solution:

Aminosyn, Aminosyn II, Aminosyn-PF, FreAmine III, Novamine, ProcalAmine, RenAmin, Travasol, Trophamine

Func. class.: Caloric agent

Chem. class.: Nitrogen product

Pregnancy category C

Action: Needed for anabolism to maintain structure; decreases catabolism, promotes healing

➔ **Therapeutic Outcome:** Positive nitrogen balance, decreased catabolism

Uses: Hepatic encephalopathy, cirrhosis, hepatitis, nutritional support in cancer trauma, intestinal obstruction, short bowel syndrome, severe malabsorption

Dosage and routes

Amino acid injection

Adult: **IV** 80-120 g/day; 500 ml of amino acids/500 ml D_{50} given over 24 hr

Amino acid solution

Adult: **IV** 1-1.5 g/kg/day titrated to patient's needs

P ***Child:*** **IV** 2-3 g/kg/day titrated to patient's needs

Available forms: Inj **IV** 2.75%, 3.5%, 4.25%, 5%, 5.5%, 6%, 8.5%, 10%, 11.4%, 15% amino acids

Adverse effects

CNS: *Dizziness, headache,* confusion, **loss of consciousness**

CV: Hypertension, **CHF, pulmonary edema**

ENDO: *Hyperglycemia, rebound hypoglycemia, electrolyte imbalances, hyperosmolar syndrome, hyperosmolar hyperglycemic nonketotic syndrome,* alkalosis, acidosis, hypophosphatemia, hyperammonemia, dehydration, hypocalcemia

GI: Nausea, vomiting, liver fat deposits, abdominal pain

GU: Glycosuria, osmotic diuresis

INTEG: Chills, flushing, warm feeling, rash, urticaria, extravasation necrosis, phlebitis at injection site

Contraindications: Hypersensitivity, severe electrolyte imbalances, anuria, severe liver damage, maple syrup urine disease, PKU

Precautions: Renal disease, P pregnancy **C**, children, diabetes mellitus, CHF

Pharmacokinetics	
Absorption	Complete bioavailability
Distribution	Widely distributed
Metabolism	Anabolism
Excretion	Kidney to urea nitrogen
Half-life	Unknown

Pharmacodynamics

Unknown

Interactions

Drug classifications

Diuretics: ↑ negative nitrogen balance

Glucocorticoids: ↑ negative nitrogen balance

Tetracyclines: ↑ negative nitrogen balance

NURSING CONSIDERATIONS

Assessment

- Monitor electrolytes (potassium, sodium, calcium, chloride, magnesium), blood glucose, ammonia, phosphate, ketones; renal, liver function studies: BUN, creatinine, ALT, AST, bilirubin; urine glucose q6h using Chemstrips, which are not affected by infusion substances; if BUN increases over 15%, therapy may need to be discontinued

- Check injection site for extravasation: redness along vein, edema at site, necrosis, pain; for a hard, tender area
- Monitor respiratory function q4h: auscultate lung fields bilaterally for crackles; monitor respirations for quality, rate, rhythm that indicates fluid overload
- Monitor temperature q4h for increased fever, indicating infection; if infection is suspected, infusion is discontinued and tubing, bottle, catheter tip cultured; blood catheter may be obtained
- ❗ Monitor for impending hepatic coma: asterixis, confusion, fetor, lethargy
- Hyperammonemia: nausea, vomiting, malaise, tremors, anorexia, convulsions; increased ammonia, ketone levels may occur

Nursing diagnoses

- ✓ Nutrition, less than body requirements (uses)
- ✓ Injury, risk for physical (uses, adverse reactions)
- ✓ Infection, risk for (adverse reactions)
- ✓ Knowledge deficit (teaching)

Implementation

- Give up to 40% protein and dextrose (up to 12.5%) via peripheral vein; stronger solutions require central **IV** administration; TPN only mixed with dextrose to promote protein synthesis
- Use immediately after mixing in pharmacy under strict aseptic technique using laminar flowhood; use infusion pump, in-line filter (0.22 μm) unless mixed with fat emulsion and dextrose (3 in 1)
- ❗ Use careful monitoring technique; do not speed up infusion; pulmonary edema, glucose overload will result
- Storage depends on type of solution; consult manufacturer
- Change dressing and **IV** tubing to prevent infection q24-48h or q5-7 days if transparent dressing is used

Y-site compatibilities: Amikacin, aminophylline, amoxicillin, ampicillin, ascorbic acid inj, atracurium, azlocillin, aztreonam, bumetanide, buprenorphine, calcium gluconate, carboplatin, cefamandole, cefazolin, cefonicid, cefoperazone, cefotaxime, cefotetan, cefoxtin, ceftazidime, ceftizoxime, ceftriaxone, cefuroxime, cephalothin, cephapirin, chloramphenicol, chlorpromazine, cimetidine, clindamycin, clonazepam, dexamethasone, diazepam, digoxin, diphenhydramine, dobutamine, dopamine, doxycycline, droperidol, enalaprilat, epinephrine, erythromycin lactobionate, famotidine, fentanyl, flucloxacillin, fluconazole, folic acid, foscarnet, gentamicin, granisetron, haloperidol, heparin, hydrocortisone, hydromorphone, hydroxyzine, idarubicin, ifosfamide, IL-2, imipenem/cilastatin, insulin (regular), isoproterenol, kanamycin, leucovorin, levorphanol, lidocaine, lorazepam, magnesium sulfate, mannitol, meperidine, mesna, methicillin, metronidazole, mezlocillin, miconazole, morphine, moxalactam, multivitamins, nafcillin, netilmicin, nitroglycerin, norepinephrine, octreotide, ofloxacin, ondansetron, oxacillin, paclitaxel, penicillin G, penicillin G potassium, pentobarbital, phenobarbital, piperacillin, potassium chloride, prochlorperazine, ranitidine, salbutamol, sargramostim, tacrolimus, thiotepa, ticarcillin, ticarcillin/clavulanate, tobramycin, trimethoprim/sulfamethoxazole, urokinase, vancomycin, vecuronium, zidovudine

Y-site incompatibilities: Cephradine

Additive compatibilities: Amikacin, aminophylline, aztreonam, calcium gluconate, cefamandole, cefazolin, cefepime, cefotaxime, cefoxitin, cefsulodin, ceftazidime, ceftriaxone, cefuroxime, cimetidine, clindamycin, cyanocobalamin, cyclophosphamide, cyclosporine, cytarabine, dopamine, epoetin, erythromycin, famotidine, folic acid, fosphenytoin, furosemide, heparin, insulin (regular), isoproterenol, lidocaine, meperidine, metaraminol, methicillin, methotrexate, methyldopate, methylprednisolone, metoclopramide, morphine, nafcillin, netilmicin, nizatidine, norepinephrine, ondansetron, oxacillin, penicillin G potassium, penicillin G sodium, phytonadione, polymyxin B, sodium bicarbonate, tacrolimus, tobramycin, vancomycin

Patient/family education

- Teach reason for use of amino acids as part of nutrition (TPN)
- Instruct patient to report at once to prescriber if chills, sweating are experienced

Evaluation

Positive therapeutic outcome

- Weight gain
- Decreased jaundice in liver disorders
- Increased LOC

aminophylline (℞)

(am-in-off'i-lin)

Aminophyllin, Phyllocontin, Truphylline

Func. class.: Bronchodilator, spasmolytic

Chem. class.: Xanthine, ethylenediamine

Pregnancy category C

Action: Relaxes smooth muscle of respiratory system by blocking phosphodiesterase, which increases cyclic AMP; increased cyclic AMP alters intracellular calcium ion movements; produces bronchodilatation, increased pulmonary blood flow, relaxation of respiratory tract

Therapeutic Outcome: Increased ability to breathe

Uses: Bronchial asthma, bronchospasm, Cheyne-Stokes respirations

Investigational uses: Apnea in infancy for respiratory/myocardial stimulation, Cheyne-Stokes respirations as a respiratory stimulant

Dosage and routes

Adult: PO: 6 mg/kg, then 3 mg/kg q6h × 2 doses, then 3 mg/kg q8h maintenance, max 900 mg/day or 13 mg/kg; PO in CHF 6 mg/kg, then 2 mg/kg q8h × 2 doses, then 1-2 mg/kg q12h maintenance; **IV** 4.7 mg/kg, then 0.55 mg/kg/hr × 12 hr, then 0.36 mg/kg/hr maintenance, **IV** in CHF 4.7 mg/kg, then 0.39 mg/kg/hr × 12 hr, then 0.08-0.16 mg/kg/hr maintenance

Elderly and in cor pulmonale: PO 6 mg/kg, then 2 mg/kg q6h × 2 doses, then 2 mg/kg q8h maintenance; **IV** 4.7 mg/kg, then 0.47 mg/kg/hr × 12 hr, then 0.24 mg/kg/hr maintenance

Child 9-16 yr: PO 6 mg/kg, then 3 mg/kg q4h × 3 doses, then 3 mg/kg q6h maintenance, max 18 mg/kg/day 12-16 yr, or 20 mg/kg/day 9-12 yr; **IV** 4.7 mg/kg, then 0.79 mg/kg/hr × 12 hr, then 0.63 mg/kg/hr maintenance

Child 6 mo-9 yr: PO 4 mg/kg q4h × 3 doses, then 4 mg/kg q6h maintenance, max 24 mg/kg/day; **IV** 4.7 mg/kg, then 0.95 mg/kg/hr × 12 hr, then 0.79 mg/kg/hr maintenance

Neonates up to 40 wk premature postconception age: PO/**IV** 1 mg/kg q12hr

Neonates at birth or 40 wk postconception age: PO/**IV** >8 wk postnatal 1-3 mg/kg q6h; 4-8 wk postnatal 1-2 mg/kg q8h; up to 4 wk postnatal 1-2 mg/kg q12h

Hepatic disease

Adult: PO 6 mg/kg, then 2 mg/kg q8h × 2 doses, then 1-2 mg/kg q12h maintenance; **IV** 4.7 mg/kg, then 0.39 mg/kg/hr × 12 hr, then 0.08-0.16 mg/kg/hr maintenance

Available forms: Inj 250 mg/10 ml, 500 mg/21 ml, 100 mg/100 ml in 0.45% NaCl; rec supp 250 mg, 500 mg; oral liq 105 mg/5 ml; tabs 100, 200 mg; cont rel tabs 225 mg

Adverse effects

CNS: Anxiety, restlessness, insomnia, *dizziness,* **seizures,** headache, lightheadedness, muscle twitching

CV: ***Palpitations, sinus tachycardia,*** hypotension, flushing, dysrhythmias, increased respiratory rate

GI: ***Nausea, vomiting,*** anorexia, diarrhea, bitter taste, dyspepsia, anal irritation (suppositories), epigastric pain

GU: Urinary frequency

INTEG: Flushing, urticaria, *rec supp (irritation)*

RESP: Tachypnea

Contraindications: Hypersensitivity to xanthines, tachydysrhythmias

G **Precautions:** Elderly, CHF, cor pulmonale, hepatic disease, active peptic ulcer disease, diabetes mellitus, hyperthyroidism, hypertension, P children, pregnancy **C,** glaucoma, prostatic hypertrophy

Pharmacokinetics

Absorption	Well absorbed (PO), slow (PO–ext rel), erratic (rec)
Distribution	Widely distributed; crosses placenta
Metabolism	Liver to caffeine
Excretion	Kidneys
Half-life	3-12 hr, increased in renal disease, CHF

Pharmacodynamics

	PO	PO–EXT REL	IV
Onset	15-60 min	Unknown	Immediate
Peak	1-2 hr	4-7 hr	Infusion's end
Duration	6-8 hr	8-12 hr	6-8 hr

Interactions

Individual drugs

Adenosine: ↓ aminophylline effect
Allopurinol: ↓ metabolism, ↑ toxicity of aminophylline
Carbamazepine: ↑ or ↓ aminophylline levels
Cimetidine: ↓ metabolism, ↑ toxicity of aminophylline
Clarithromycin: ↑ aminophylline toxicity
Disulfiram: ↓ metabolism, ↑ toxicity of aminophylline
Fluvoxamine: ↑ aminophylline toxicity
Halothane: ↑ risk of dysrhythmias
Interferon: ↓ metabolism, ↑ toxicity of aminophylline
Isoniazid: ↑ or ↓ aminophylline level
Ketoconazole: ↓ effect of aminophylline
Lithium: ↓ effect of lithium
Methotrexate: ↑ effect of aminophylline
Mexiletine: ↓ metabolism, ↑ toxicity
Phenytoin: ↑ metabolism, ↓ effect of aminophylline
Rifampin: ↑ metabolism, ↓ effect of aminophylline
Thiabendazole: ↓ metabolism, ↑ toxicity

Drug classifications

Antibiotics, macrolide: ↑ aminophylline levels
Barbiturates: ↓ effect of aminophylline
β-Adrenergic blockers: ↓ effect of aminophylline
Diuretics, loop: ↑ or ↓ aminophylline levels

Calcium channel blockers: ↑ aminophylline levels
Corticosteroids: ↑ aminophylline toxicity
Fluoroquinolones: ↓ metabolism, ↑ toxicity
Influenza vaccines: ↑ aminophylline toxicity
Oral contraceptives: ↑ aminophylline levels
Sympathomimetics: ↑ CNS, CV adverse reactions

Smoking

↑ Metabolism, ↓ effect

Food/drug

Caffeinated foods (cola, coffee, tea, chocolate): ↑ CNS, CV, adverse reactions
Charcoal-smoked foods: ↓ effect

Herb/drug

Increased effects of ephedra, cola tree

Lab test interferences

↑ Plasma free fatty acids

NURSING CONSIDERATIONS

Assessment

- Monitor theophylline blood levels (therapeutic level is 10-20 μg/ml); toxicity may occur with small increase G above 20 μg/ml, especially elderly; determine whether theophylline was given recently (24 hr); check for toxicity: nausea, vomiting, anxiety, restlessness, insomnia, tachycardia, dysrhythmias, convulsions; notify prescriber immediately
- Monitor I&O; diuresis will occur; G dehydration may result in elderly or P children in whom diuresis is great
- Monitor respiratory rate, rhythm, depth; auscultate lung fields bilaterally; notify prescriber of abnormalities; check ECG for tachycardia, PVCs, PACs in patients with cardiac problems
- Monitor allergic reactions: rash, urticaria; if these occur, drug should be discontinued, prescriber notified

Nursing diagnoses

✓ Airway clearance, ineffective (uses)
✓ Activity intolerance (uses)
✓ Injury, risk for (uses, adverse reactions)
✓ Knowledge deficit (teaching)

Implementation

General

- Give around the clock to maintain blood (theophylline) levels
- If switching from **IV** to PO, give controlled-release dose at time of **IV** infusion discontinuation; if giving tab (immediate release), discontinue **IV** and wait >4 hr

PO route

- Give PO after meals or water to decrease GI symptoms; absorption may be affected with a full glass of water or food
- Do not crush or chew enteric-coated or controlled-release tabs

IV route

- May be diluted for **IV** inf in 100-200 ml in D_5W, $D_{10}W$, $D_{20}W$, 0.9% NaCl, 0.45% NaCl, LR
- Give loading dose over ½ hr, max rate of inf 25 mg/min, use infusion pump; after loading dose, give by cont inf
- Avoid IM injection; pain and tissue damage may occur
- Only clear sol; flush **IV** line before dose; store diluted sol for 24 hr if refrigerated

Syringe compatibilities:

Heparin, metoclopramide, pentobarbital, thiopental

Y-site compatibilities:

Allopurinol, amifostine, amphotericin B sulfate complex, amrinone, aztreonam, ceftazidime, cimetidine, cladribine, doxorubicin liposome, enalaprilat, esmolol, famotidine, filgrastim, fluconazole, fludarabine, foscarnet, gallium, granisetron, heparin sodium with hydrocortisone sodium succinate, labetalol, melphalan, meropenem, morphine, netilmicin, paclitaxel, pancuronium, piperacillin/tazobactam, potassium chloride, propofol, ranitidine, remifentanil, sargramostim, tacrolimus, teniposide, thiotepa, tolazoline, vecuronium, vit B with C

Y-site incompatibilities:
Dobutamine, hydralazine, ondansetron

Additive compatibilities:
Amobarbital, bretylium, calcium gluconate, chloramphenicol, cibenzoline, cimetidine, dexamethasone, diphenhydramine, dopamine, erythromycin lactobionate, esmolol, floxacillin, flumazenil, furosemide, heparin, hydrocortisone, lidocaine, mephentermine, meropenem, methyldopate, metronidazole/sodium bicarbonate, nitroglycerin, pentobarbital, phenobarbital, potassium chloride, ranitidine, secobarbital, sodium bicarbonate, terbutaline

Additive incompatibilities:
Ascorbic acid, bleomycin, cephalothin, cefotaxime, chlorpromazine, cimetidine, clindamycin, codeine, dimenhydrinate, dobutamine, doxorubicin, doxycycline, epinephrine, erythromycin gluceptate, hydralazine, hydroxyzine, insulin, isoproterenol, meperidine, methicillin, morphine, nafcillin, nitroprusside, norepinephrine, oxytetracycline, papaverine, penicillin G, pentazocine, phenobarbital, phenytoin, prochlorperazine, promazine, promethazine, sulfisoxazole, tetracycline, vancomycin

Rectal route
- Rec dose if patient is unable to take PO; retain rec dose for ½ hour

Patient/family education
- Teach patient to take doses as prescribed, not to skip dose; to check OTC medications, current prescription medications for ephedrine, which will increase CNS stimulation; advise patient not to drink alcohol or caffeine products (tea, coffee, chocolate, colas), which will increase action
- Teach patient to avoid hazardous activities; dizziness may occur
- Teach patient if GI upset occurs, to take drug with 8 oz of water or food; absorption may be decreased
- Teach patient to remain in bed 15-20 min after rec supp is inserted to prevent removal
- Instruct patient that smoking increases metabolism; dosage may need to be increased
- Teach patient to obtain blood levels of drug every few months to prevent toxicity; not to change brands, since effect may not be the same
- Teach patient to increase fluids to 2 L/day to decrease viscosity of secretions
- Advise patient to report toxicity: nausea, vomiting, anxiety, insomnia, rapid pulse, seizures, flushing, headache, diarrhea

Evaluation

Positive therapeutic outcome
- Decreased dyspnea
- Respiratory stimulation in infants
- Clear lung fields bilaterally

HIGH ALERT

amiodarone (℞)
(a-mee-oh'da-rone)

Cordarone, Cordarone IV, Pacerone

Func. class.: Antidysrhythmic (Class III)

Chem. class.: Iodinated benzofuran derivative

Pregnancy category D

Action: Prolongs action potential duration and effective refractory period, slows sinus rate with increasing PR and QT intervals, noncompetitive α- and β-adrenergic inhibition; increases PR and QT intervals, decreases sinus rate, decreases peripheral vascular resistance

Therapeutic Outcome: Decreased amount and severity of ventricular dysrhythmias

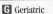

Uses: Severe ventricular tachycardia,

supraventricular tachycardia, ventricular fibrillation or atrial fibrillation not controlled by 1st-line agents

Dosage and routes

Ventricular dysrhythmias

Adult: PO loading dose 800-1600 mg/day for 1-3 wk; then 600-800 mg/day × 1 mo; maintenance 400 mg/day; **IV** loading dose (first rapid) 150 mg over the first 10 min then slow 360 mg over the next 6 hr; maintenance 540 mg given over the remaining 18 hr, decrease rate of the slow infusion to 0.5 mg/min

P **Child:** PO loading dose 10-15 mg/kg/day in 1-2 divided doses for 4-14 days then 5 mg/kg/day (not recommended in children)

Supraventricular tachycardia

Adult: PO 600-800 mg/day × 7 days or until desired response, then 400 mg/day × 21 days, then 200-400 mg/day maintenance

P **Child:** PO 10 mg/kg/day (800 mg/1.72 m^2/day) × 10 days or until desired resposne, then 5 mg/kg/day (400 mg/1.72 m^2/day) × 21-28 days, then 2.5 mg/kg/day (200 mg/1.72 m^2/day) (not recommended in children)

Available forms: Tabs 200, 400 mg; inj 50 mg/ml

Adverse effects

CNS: *Headache, dizziness,* involuntary movement, tremors, peripheral neuropathy, malaise, fatigue, ataxia, paresthesias, insomnia

CV: *Hypotension,* **bradycardia, sinus arrest, CHF, dysrhythmias, SA node dysfunction**

EENT: Blurred vision, halos, photophobia, **corneal microdeposits,** dry eyes

ENDO: Hyperthyroidism or hypothyroidism

GI: Nausea, vomiting, diarrhea, abdominal pain, anorexia, constipation, **hepatotoxicity**

INTEG: Rash, photosensitivity, blue-gray skin discoloration, alopecia, spontaneous ecchymosis, **toxic epidermal necrolysis**

MISC: Flushing, abnormal taste or smell, edema, abnormal salivation, coagulation abnormalities

MS: Weakness, pain in extremities

RESP: **Pulmonary fibrosis,** pulmonary inflammation, **adult respiratory distress syndrome, gasping syndrome in neonates**

Contraindications: Sinus node dysfunction; 2nd- or 3rd- degree AV block; pregnancy **D,** neonates, infants, bradycardia, lactation P

Precautions: Goiter, Hashimoto's thyroiditis, electrolyte imbalances, CHF, severe hepatic, respiratory disease, children P

Do Not Confuse:
Cordarone/Inocor

Pharmacokinetics

Absorption	Slow, variable (PO) up to 65%
Distribution	Body tissues; crosses placenta
Metabolism	Liver
Excretion	Bile, kidney (minimal)
Half-life	15-100 days

Pharmacodynamics

	PO
Onset	1-3 wk
Peak	Unknown
Duration	Up to months

Interactions

Individual drugs

Digoxin: ↑ blood levels, ↑ toxicity
Disopyramide: ↑ levels, ↑ toxicity
Flecainide: ↑ levels, ↑ toxicity

Mexiletine: ↑ levels, ↑ toxicity
Phenytoin: ↑ blood levels
Procainamide: ↑ levels, ↑ toxicity
Quinidine: ↑ levels, ↑ toxicity
Theophylline: ↑ levels
Warfarin: ↑ level, ↑ bleeding

Drug classifications

β-Adrenergic blockers: ↑ dysrhythmias, cardiac arrest
Calcium channel blockers: ↑ dysrhythmias, cardiac arrest

Herb/drug

Aloe: ↑ amiodarone effect
Buckthorn bark/berry: ↑ amiodarone effect
Cascara sagrada bark: ↑ amiodarone effect
Rhubarb root: ↑ amiodarone effect
Senna leaf/fruits: ↑ amiodarone effect

Lab test interference:
↑ T_4

NURSING CONSIDERATIONS

Assessment

- Monitor I&O ratio; monitor electrolytes: potassium, sodium, chloride
- Monitor chest x-ray, thyroid function tests
- Monitor liver function studies: AST, ALT, bilirubin, alkaline phosphatase
- Monitor ECG continuously to determine drug effectiveness; measure PR, QRS, QT intervals; check for PVCs, other dysrhythmias; monitor B/P continuously for hypotension, hypertension; check for rebound hypertension after 1-2 hr
- Monitor for dehydration or hypovolemia
- Assess for CNS symptoms: confusion, psychosis, numbness, depression, involuntary movements; if these occur, drug should be discontinued
- Assess for hypothyroidism: lethargy, dizziness, constipation, enlarged thyroid gland, edema of extremities, cool, pale skin
- Monitor hyperthyroidism: restlessness, tachycardia, eyelid puffiness, weight loss, frequent urination, menstrual irregularities, dyspnea, warm, moist skin
- Assess for pulmonary toxicity including ARDS, pulmonary fibrosis: dyspnea, fatigue, cough, fever, chest pain; drug should be discontinued if these occur
- Monitor cardiac rate, respiration: rate, rhythm, character, chest pain, ventricular tachycardia, supraventricular tachycardia or fibrillation
- Assess sight and vision before treatment and throughout therapy; microdeposits on the cornea may cause blurred vision, halos, and photophobia

Nursing diagnoses

- ✓ Cardiac output, decreased (uses)
- ✓ Gas exchange, impaired (adverse reactions)
- ✓ Knowledge deficit (teaching)

Implementation

Start with patient hospitalized and monitored

PO route

- Give reduced dosage slowly with ECG monitoring only
- Give with meals for GI upset

IV route

Y-site compatibilities: Amikacin, bretylium, clindamycin, dobutamine, dopamine, doxycycline, erythromycin, esmolol, gentamicin, insulin (regular), isoproterenol, labetalol, lidocaine, metaraminol, metronidazole, midazolam, morphine, nitroglycerin, norepinephrine, penicillin G potassium, phentolamine, phenylephrine, potassium chloride, procainamide, tobramycin, vancomycin

Additive compatibilities: Dobutamine, lidocaine, potassium chloride, procainimide, verapamil

Solution compatibilities: D_5W, 0.9% NaCl

Patient/family education

- Instruct patient to report side effects immediately to prescriber

• Instruct patient that skin discoloration is usually reversible but skin may turn bluish on neck, face, arms when used for long periods
• Advise patient that dark glasses may be needed for photophobia
• Instruct patient to use sunscreen and protective clothing to prevent burning associated with photosensitivity
• Instruct patient to take medication as prescribed, not to double doses
• Instruct patient to complete follow-up appointment with health care provider including pulmonary function studies, chest x-ray, ophthalmic examinations

Treatment of overdose: Administer O_2, artificial ventilation, ECG, dopamine for circulatory depression, diazepam or thiopental for convulsions, isoproterenol

amitriptyline (℞)
(a-mee-trip'ti-leen)
amitriptyline HCl, Apo-Amitriptyline ♣, Elavil, Endep, Levate ♣, Novotriptyn ♣
Func. class.: Antidepressant—tricyclic
Chem. class.: Tertiary amine

Pregnancy category C

Action: Blocks reuptake of norepinephrine, serotonin into nerve endings that increase action of norepinephrine, serotonin in nerve cells

Uses: Major depression

Investigational uses: Chronic pain management, prevention of cluster/migraine headaches, fibromyalgia

➡ **Therapeutic Outcome:** Decreased symptoms of depression after 2-3 wk

Dosage and routes

Depression

Adult: PO 75 mg/day in divided doses; may increase to 150 mg qd, not to exceed 300 mg/day; IM 20-30 mg qid, or 80-120 mg hs

P G ***Elderly/Adolescent:*** PO 30mg/day in divided doses; may be increased to 100 mg/day

Cluster/migraine headaches

Adult: PO 50-150 mg/day

Chronic pain

Adult: PO 75-150 mg/day

Fibromyalgia

Adult: PO 10-50 mg qhs

Available forms: Tabs 10, 25, 50, 75, 100, 150 mg; inj IM 10 mg/ml; syrup 10 mg/5 ml

Adverse effects

CNS: Dizziness, drowsiness, confusion, headache, anxiety, tremors, stimulation, weakness, insomnia, G nightmares, EPS (elderly), increased psychiatric symptoms, **hyperthermia**
CV: Orthostatic hypotension, **ECG changes, tachycardia, hypertension,** palpitations, dysrhythmias
EENT: Blurred vision, tinnitus, mydriasis, ophthalmoplegia
GI: Constipation, dry mouth, nausea, vomiting, **paralytic ileus,** increased appetite, cramps, epigastric distress, jaundice, **hepatitis,** stomatitis
GU: Retention
HEMA: **Agranulocytosis, thrombocytopenia, eosinophilia, leukopenia**
INTEG: Rash, urticaria, sweating, pruritus, photosensitivity

Contraindications: Hypersensitivity to tricyclic antidepressants, recovery phase of myocardial infarction, narrow-angle glaucoma, pregnancy **D**

Precautions: Suicidal patients, convulsive disorders, prostatic hypertrophy, schizophrenia, psychosis, severe depression, increased intraocu-

lar pressure, narrow angle glaucoma, urinary retention, cardiac disease, hepatic/renal disease, hyperthyroid-
P ism, electroshock therapy, elective
G surgery, child <12 yr, elderly

Do Not Confuse:
amitriptyline/nortriptyline, Elavil/Mellaril, Elavil/Oruvail

Pharmacokinetics

Absorption	Well absorbed
Distribution	Widely distributed; crosses placenta
Metabolism	Liver, extensively
Excretion	Kidneys, breast milk
Half-life	10-46 hr

Pharmacodynamics

	PO/IM
Onset	45 min
Peak	2-12 hr
Duration	Unknown

Interactions

Individual drugs

Alcohol: ↑ CNS depression
Carbamazepine: ↑ amitriptyline levels
Cimetidine: ↑ levels, ↑ toxicity
Clonidine: ↑ hypertension; avoid use
Fluoxetine: ↑ levels, ↑ toxicity
Guanethidine: ↓ effects

Drug classifications

Antidepressants: ↑ amitriptyline levels
Antidysrhythmics IC: ↑ amitriptyline levels
Antihypertensives: Blocked response to antihypertensives
Antithyroid agents: ↑ risk of agranulocytosis
Barbiturates: ↑ CNS effects
Benzodiazepines: ↑ CNS effects
CNS depressants: ↑ CNS effects
MAOIs: Hypertensive crisis, convulsions
Oral contraceptives: ↑ effects, toxicity
Phenothiazines: ↑ amitriptylline levels, toxicity
Sympathomimetics, indirect acting: ↓ effects

Smoking

↑ Metabolism, ↓ effects

Herb/drug

Belladonna leaf/root: ↑ anticholinergic effect
Henbane leaf: ↑ anticholinergic effect
Kava: ↑ CNS depression
Scopolia root: ↑ amitriptyline action

Lab test interferences

↑ Blood glucose, ↑ alkaline phosphatase

NURSING CONSIDERATIONS

Assessment

- Monitor B/P (with patient lying, standing), pulse q4h; if systolic B/P drops 20 mm Hg, hold drug, notify prescriber; take VS q4h in patients with cardiovascular disease
- Monitor blood studies: CBC, leukocytes, differential, cardiac enzymes if patient is receiving long-term therapy
- Monitor hepatic studies: AST, ALT, bilirubin
- Check weight weekly; appetite may increase with drug
- Assess ECG for flattening of T wave, bundle branch block, AV block, prolongation of QTc interval, dysrhythmias in cardiac patients
- G Assess for EPS primarily in elderly: rigidity, dystonia, akathisia
- Assess mental status: mood, sensorium, affect, suicidal tendencies; increase in psychiatric symptoms: depression, panic
- Monitor urinary retention, P constipation; constipation is more G likely to occur in children or elderly
- Assess for withdrawal symptoms: headache, nausea, vomiting, muscle pain, weakness; do not usually occur unless drug was discontinued abruptly
- Identify alcohol consumption; if alcohol is consumed, hold dose until morning

Nursing diagnoses

- ✓ Coping, ineffective individual (uses)
- ✓ Injury, risk for physical (side effects)
- ✓ Knowledge deficit (teaching)
- ✓ Noncompliance (teaching)

Implementation

PO route

- Give with food or milk for GI symptoms
- Crush if patient is unable to swallow medication whole
- Give dosage hs if oversedation G occurs during day; may take entire dose hs; elderly may not tolerate once/day dosing
- Store at room temp; do not freeze

Patient/family education

- Teach patient that therapeutic effects may take 2-3 wk
- Instruct patient to use caution in driving or other activities requiring alertness because of drowsiness, dizziness, blurred vision; to avoid rising quickly from sitting to standing, G especially elderly
- Advise patient to avoid alcohol ingestion, other CNS depressants; overheating
- Teach patient not to discontinue medication quickly after long-term use; may cause nausea, headache, malaise
- Advise patient to wear sunscreen or large hat, since photosensitivity occurs; hyperthermia can occur
- Teach patient to increase fluids, bulk in diet if constipation, urinary G retention occur, especially elderly
- Teach patient to use gum, hard sugarless candy, or frequent sips of water for dry mouth
- Instruct patient to use contraception during treatment

Evaluation

Positive therapeutic outcome

- Decreased depression
- Absence of suicidal thoughts

Treatment of overdose: ECG monitoring, lavage, administer anticonvulsant, sodium bicarbonate

amlodipine (℞)

(am-loe'di-peen)

Norvasc

Func. class.: Antianginal, calcium channel blocker, antihypertensive

Chem. class.: Dihydropyridine

Pregnancy category C

Action: Inhibits calcium ion influx across cell membrane during cardiac depolarization; produces relaxation of coronary vascular smooth muscle, peripheral vascular smooth muscle; dilates coronary vascular arteries; increases myocardial oxygen delivery in patients with vasospastic angina

➔ **Therapeutic Outcome:** Decreased angina pectoris, dysrhythmias, B/P

Uses: Chronic stable angina pectoris, hypertension, vasospastic angina (Prinzmetal's angina)

Dosage and routes

Adult: PO 5-10 mg qd initially, may increase gradually to max 10 mg qd

G ***Elderly:*** PO 2.5 mg qd

Hepatic dose

Adult: PO 25 mg/day, may ↑ to 10 mg/day (antihypertensive); 5 mg/day, may ↑ to 10 mg/day (antianginal)

Available forms: Tabs 2.5, 5, 10 mg

Adverse effects

CNS: Headache, fatigue, dizziness, anxiety, depression, insomnia, paresthesia, somnolence, asthenia

CV: Dysrhythmia, edema, bradycardia, hypotension, palpitations, syncope, AV block

GI: Nausea, vomiting, diarrhea, gastric upset, constipation, abdominal cramps, flatulence, anorexia, gingival hyperplasia

GU: Nocturia, polyuria
INTEG: Rash, pruritus, urticaria, hair loss
MISC: Flushing, nasal congestion, sweating, shortness of breath, sexual difficulties, muscle cramps, cough, weight gain, tinnitus, epistaxis

Contraindications: Sick sinus syndrome, 2nd- or 3rd-degree heart block, hypotension less than 90 mm Hg systolic, hypersensitivity

Precautions: CHF, hypotension, hepatic injury, pregnancy **C**, lactation, P children, renal disease, G elderly

Do Not Confuse:
Norvasc/Navane

Pharmacokinetics

Absorption	Well absorbed up to 90%
Distribution	Crosses placenta, protein binding 95%
Metabolism	Liver, extensively
Excretion	Kidneys to metabolites (90%)
Half-life	30-50 hr; ↑ in elderly, hepatic disease

Pharmacodynamics

Onset	Unknown
Peak	6-10 hr
Duration	24 hr

Interactions
Individual drugs
Alcohol: ↑ hypotension
Fentanyl: ↑ hypotension
Lithium: ↑ neurotoxicity
Quinidine: ↑ hypotension
Drug classifications
Antihypertensives: ↑ hypotension
Nitrates: ↑ hypotension
NSAIDs: ↓ antihypertensive effect
Food/drug
Grapefruit juice: ↑ hypotension

NURSING CONSIDERATIONS
Assessment
- Assess fluid volume status: I&O ratio and record, weight, distended red veins, crackles in lung, color, quality and sp gr of urine, skin turgor, adequacy of pulses, moist mucous membranes, bilateral lung sounds, peripheral pitting edema; dehydration symptoms of decreasing output, thirst, hypotension, dry mouth and mucous membranes should be reported
- Monitor B/P and pulse; if B/P drops, call prescriber
- Monitor ALT, AST, bilirubin daily; if these are elevated, hepatotoxicity is suspected
- Monitor if platelet count is <150,000/mm^3; drug is usually discontinued and another drug started
- Monitor cardiac status: B/P, pulse, respiration, ECG

Nursing diagnoses
- ✓ Cardiac output, decreased (uses)
- ✓ Knowledge deficit (teaching)

Implementation
- Give once a day, without regard to meals

Patient/family education
- Advise patient to avoid hazardous activities until stabilized on drug, dizziness is no longer a problem
- Instruct patient to avoid alcohol and OTC drugs unless directed by prescriber
- Advise patient to comply in all areas of medical regimen: diet, exercise, stress reduction, smoking cessation, drug therapy; to notify prescriber of irregular heart beat, shortness of breath, swelling of feet and hands, severe dizziness, constipation, nausea, hypotension
- Teach patient to use as directed even if feeling better; may be taken with other cardiovascular drugs (nitrates, β-blockers)

Evaluation
Positive therapeutic outcome
- Decreased anginal pain
- Decreased B/P
- Increased exercise tolerance

Treatment of overdose:
Defibrillation, β-agonists, **IV** calcium

inotropic agents, diuretics, atropine for AV block, vasopressor for hypotension

amoxapine (℞)

(a-mox'a-peen)

amoxapine, Asendin

Func. class.: Antidepressant

Chem. class.: Dibenzoxazepine derivative, secondary amine

Pregnancy category C

Action: Blocks reuptake of norepinephrine, serotonin into nerve endings, thereby increasing action of norepinephrine, serotonin in nerve cells

Therapeutic Outcome: Decreased symptoms of depression after 2-3 wk

Uses: Depression

Dosage and routes

Adult: PO 50 mg tid; may increase to 100 mg tid on 3rd day of therapy; not to exceed 300 mg/day unless lower doses have been given for at least 2 wk; may be given daily dose hs; not to exceed 600 mg/day in hospitalized patients

G ***Elderly:*** PO 25 mg hs, may increase by 25 mg/wk, up to 150 mg/day in divided doses

Available forms: Tabs 25, 50, 100, 150 mg

Adverse effects

CNS: *Dizziness, drowsiness,* confusion, headache, anxiety, tremors, stimulation, weakness, insomnia, G nightmares, EPS (elderly), increased psychiatric symptoms, paresthesia, impairment of sexual functioning, **neuroleptic malignant syndrome**

CV: *Orthostatic hypotension, ECG changes, tachycardia,* hypertension, palpitations

EENT: *Blurred vision,* tinnitus, mydriasis, ophthalmoplegia

GI: *Dry mouth, constipation,* nausea, vomiting, **paralytic ileus,** increased appetite, cramps, epigastric distress, jaundice, **hepatitis,** stomatitis

GU: Retention, **acute renal failure**

HEMA: **Agranulocytosis, thrombocytopenia, eosinophilia, leukopenia**

INTEG: Rash, urticaria, sweating, pruritus, photosensitivity

Contraindications: Hypersensitivity to tricyclic antidepressants, recovery phase of myocardial infarction, convulsive disorders, prostatic hypertrophy, narrow-angle glaucoma

Precautions: Suicidal patients, severe depression, increased intraocular pressure, urinary retention, cardiac disease, hepatic disease, hyperthyroidism, electroshock therapy, G elective surgery, elderly, pregnancy **C**

Do Not Confuse: amoxapine/amoxicillin, amoxapine/Amoxil

Pharmacokinetics

Absorption	Well absorbed
Distribution	Widely distributed; crosses placenta
Metabolism	Liver, extensively
Excretion	Kidneys, breast milk
Half-life	8 hr

Pharmacodynamics

Onset	1-2 wk
Peak	2-6 wk
Duration	6-12 wk

Interactions

Individual drugs

Alcohol: ↑ CNS depression

Cimetidine: ↑ amoxapine levels, ↑ toxicity of amoxapine

Clonidine: Severe hypotension; avoid use

Fluoxetine: ↑ amoxapine levels, ↑ toxicity of amoxapine

Guanethidine: ↓ effects of amoxapine

Paroxetine: ↑ amoxapine level, ↑ toxicity
Sertraline: ↑ amoxapine level, ↑ toxicity

Drug classifications

Barbiturates: ↑ effects of amoxapine
Benzodiazepines: ↑ effects of amoxapine
CNS depressants: ↑ effects of amoxapine
MAOIs: Hypertensive crisis, convulsions
Oral contraceptives: ↑ effects, toxicity of amoxapine
Sympathomimetics, indirect acting: ↓ effects of amoxapine

Smoking

↑ metabolism, ↓ effects

Herb/drug

Belladonna leaf/root: ↑ anticholinergic effect
Henbane leaf: ↑ anticholinergic effect
Kava: ↑ CNS depression
St. John's wort: ↑ CNS depression
Scopolia root: ↑ amoxapine action

Lab test interferences

↑ Blood glucose, ↑ alkaline phosphatase, ↑ prolactin

NURSING CONSIDERATIONS

Assessment

- Monitor B/P (with patient lying, standing), pulse q4h; if systolic B/P drops 20 mm Hg hold drug, notify prescriber; take vital signs q4h in patients with cardiovascular disease
- Monitor blood studies: CBC, leukocytes, differential, cardiac enzymes if patient is receiving long-term therapy
- Monitor blood level: therapeutic 20-100 ng/ml
- Monitor hepatic studies: AST, ALT, bilirubin
- Check weight weekly; appetite may increase with drug
- Assess ECG for flattening of T wave, bundle branch block, AV block, dysrhythmias in cardiac patients
- G Assess for EPS primarily in elderly: rigidity, dystonia, akathisia
- Assess mental status: mood, sensorium, affect, suicidal tendencies; increase in psychiatric symptoms: depression, panic; confusion (elderly) G
- Monitor urinary retention, constipation; constipation is more likely to occur in children and elderly P G
- Assess for withdrawal symptoms: headache, nausea, vomiting, muscle pain, weakness; do not usually occur unless drug was discontinued abruptly
- Identify alcohol consumption; if alcohol is consumed, hold dose until morning

Nursing diagnoses

- ✓ Coping, ineffective individual (uses)
- ✓ Injury, risk for physical (side effects)
- ✓ Knowledge deficit (teaching)
- ✓ Noncompliance (teaching)

Implementation

- Give with food or milk for GI symptoms
- Crush if patient is unable to swallow medication whole
- Store at room temp; do not freeze

Patient/family education

- Teach patient that therapeutic effects may take 2-3 wk
- Instruct patient to use caution in driving or other activities requiring alertness because of drowsiness, dizziness, blurred vision; to avoid rising quickly from sitting to standing, especially elderly G
- Teach patient to avoid alcohol ingestion, other CNS depressants
- Teach patient not to discontinue medication quickly after long-term use: may cause nausea, headache, malaise
- Teach patient to wear sunscreen or large hat, since photosensitivity occurs
- Teach patient to increase fluids, bulk in diet if constipation, urinary retention occur, especially elderly G
- Advise patient to take gum, hard sugarless candy, or frequent sips of water for dry mouth

A

Evaluation

Positive therapeutic outcome
- Decreased depression
- Absence of suicidal thoughts

Treatment of overdose: ECG monitoring, induce emesis, lavage, activated charcoal, administer anticonvulsant

amoxicillin (℞)

(a-mox-i-sill'in)

amoxicillin, Amoxil, Apo-Amoxi ✤, Novamoxin ✤, Nu-Amoxi ✤, Trimox, Wymox

Func. class.: Broad-spectrum antiinfective

Chem. class.: Aminopenicillin

Pregnancy category B

Action: Interferes with cell wall replication of susceptible organisms by binding to the bacterial cell wall; the cell wall, rendered osmotically unstable, swells and bursts from osmotic pressure

➔ **Therapeutic Outcome:** Bactericidal effects for the following organisms: effective for gram-positive cocci *(Streptococcus pyogenes, Streptococcus faecalis, Streptococcus pneumoniae)*, gram-negative cocci *(Neisseria gonorrhoeae, Neisseria meningitidis, Escherichia coli)*, gram-negative bacilli *(Haemophilus influenzae, Proteus mirabilis, Salmonella)*

Uses: Infections of respiratory tract, skin, skin structures, genitourinary tract, otitis media, meningitis, septicemia, sinusitis and bacterial endocarditis prophylaxis

Investigational uses: Lyme disease

Dosage and routes

Renal disease

CrCl 10-50 ml/min dose q12h; CrCl <10 ml/min dose q24h

Systemic infections

Adult: PO 750 mg-1.5 g qd in divided doses q8h

P ***Child:*** PO 20-50 mg/kg/day in divided doses q8h

Gonorrhea/urinary tract infections

Adult: PO 3 g given with 1 g probenecid as a single dose; followed by tetracycline or erythromycin

Chlamydia trachomatis

Adult: PO 500 mg/day × 1 wk

Bacterial endocarditis prophylaxis

P ***Child:*** PO 50 mg/kg/hr before and 25 mg/kg 6 hr after procedure

Helicobacter pylori

Adult: PO 1000 mg bid given with lansoprazole 30 mg bid, clarithromycin 500 mg bid × 2 wk; or 1000 mg bid given with omeprazole 20 mg bid, clarithromycin 500 mg bid × 2 wk; or 1000 mg tid given with lansoprazole 30 mg tid × 2 wk

Available forms: Caps 250, 500 mg; chewable tabs 125, 200, 250, 400, 500, 875; powder for oral susp 50 mg/ml, 125, 250 mg/5 ml; susp pedidrops 50 mg/ml; susp 125, 200, 250, 400 mg/5 ml

Adverse effects

CNS: Headache, fever, **seizures**

GI: *Nausea, vomiting, diarrhea,* increased AST, ALT, abdominal pain, glossitis, colitis, **pseudomembranous colitis**

HEMA: Anemia, increased bleeding time, **bone marrow depression, granulocytopenia**

INTEG: *Urticaria, rash*

SYST: **Anaphylaxis, respiratory distress, serum sickness**

Contraindications: Hypersensitivity to penicillins; P neonates

Precautions: Pregnancy **B**, hypersensitivity to cephalosporins, P neonates, renal disease

Do Not Confuse:
amoxicillin/amoxapine, Amoxil/amoxapine, Amoxil/amoxicillin, Trimox/Diamox, Trimox/Tylox, Wymox/Tylox

Pharmacokinetics

Absorption	Well absorbed (90%)
Distribution	Readily in body tissues, fluids, CSF; crosses placenta
Metabolism	Liver (30%)
Excretion	Breast milk, kidney, unchanged (70%)
Half-life	1-1.3 hr

Pharmacodynamics

Onset	½ hr
Peak	2 hr

Interactions
Individual drugs
Probenecid: ↑ amoxicillin levels, ↓ renal excretion
Warfarin: ↑ anticoagulant effects
Drug classifications
Oral anticoagulants: ↑ anticoagulant effects
Oral contraceptives: ↓ contraceptive effectiveness
Herb/drug
Khat: ↓ absorption, separate by 2 hr
Lab test interferences
False positive: Urine glucose, urine protein, direct Coombs' test

NURSING CONSIDERATIONS
Assessment
- Assess patient for previous sensitivity reaction to penicillins or other cephalosporins; cross-sensitivity between penicillins and cephalosporins is common
- Assess patient for signs and symptoms of infection, including characteristics of wounds, sputum, urine, stool, WBC >10,000/mm^3, earache, fever; obtain baseline information and monitor symptoms during treatment
- Obtain C&S before beginning drug therapy to identify if correct treatment has been initiated
- Assess for allergic reactions during treatment: rash, urticaria, pruritus, chills, fever, joint pain; angioedema may occur a few days after therapy begins; epinephrine and resuscitation equipment should be available for anaphylactic reactions
- Identify urine output; if decreasing, notify prescriber (may indicate nephrotoxicity); also, increased BUN, creatinine, urinalysis, protein, blood
- Monitor blood studies: AST, ALT, CBC, Hct, bilirubin, LDH, alkaline phosphatase, Coombs' test monthly if patient is on long-term therapy
- Monitor electrolytes: potassium, sodium, chloride monthly if patient is on long-term therapy
- Assess bowel pattern qd; diarrhea, cramping, blood in stools; if severe diarrhea occurs, notify prescriber; drug should be discontinued; pseudomembranous colitis may occur
- Monitor for bleeding: ecchymosis, bleeding gums, hematuria, stool guaiac daily if on long-term therapy
- Assess for overgrowth of infection: perineal itching, fever, malaise, redness, pain, swelling, drainage, rash, diarrhea, change in cough, sputum

Nursing diagnoses
- ✓ Infection, risk for (uses)
- ✓ Diarrhea (side effects)
- ✓ Injury, risk for (side effects)
- ✓ Knowledge deficit (teaching)
- ✓ Noncompliance (teaching)

Implementation
- Give in even doses around the clock; if GI upset occurs, give with food; drug must be given for 10-14 days to ensure organism death and prevent superinfection; store in tight container
- The caps may be opened and contents taken with fluids
- Shake susp well before each dose, may be used alone or mixed in drinks,

use immediately; susp may be stored in refrigerator for 14 days

Patient/family education

- Teach patient to report sore throat, bruising, bleeding, joint pain; may indicate blood dyscrasias (rare)
- Advise patient to contact prescriber if vaginal itching, loose, foul-smelling stools, diarrhea, sore throat, fever, fatigue, furry tongue occur; may indicate superinfection or agranulocytopenia
- Instruct patient to take all medication prescribed for the length of time ordered; not to double dose; chew form is available
- Advise patient to notify prescriber of diarrhea with blood or pus, which may indicate pseudomembranous colitis

Evaluation

Positive therapeutic outcome

- Absence of signs/symptoms of infection (WBC <10,000/mm^3, temp WNL, absence of red draining wounds or earache)
- Prevention of endocarditis
- Resolution of ulcer symptoms

Treatment of anaphylaxis: Withdraw drug, maintain airway, administer epinephrine, aminophylline, O_2, **IV** corticosteroids

amoxicillin/clavulanate (℞)

(a-mox-i-sill'in)

Augmentin, Augmentin ES, Clavulin ♣

Func. class.: Broad-spectrum antiinfective (extended spectrum)

Chem. class.: Aminopenicillin-β-lactamase inhibitor

Pregnancy category B

Action: Interferes with cell wall replication of susceptible organisms; the cell wall, rendered osmotically unstable, swells and bursts from osmotic pressure; combination increases spectrum of activity, β-lactamase resistance

Therapeutic Outcome: Bactericidal effects for the following organisms: *Escherichia coli, Proteus mirabilis, Haemophilus influenzae, Streptococcus faecalis, Streptococcus pneumoniae;* and β-lactamase–producing organisms: *Neisseria gonorrhoeae, Neisseria meningitis, Shigella, Salmonella, Enterococcus, Streptococcus*

Uses: Infections of respiratory tract, skin, skin structures, genitourinary tract; otitis media, meningitis, septicemia, sinusitis, and endocarditis prophylaxis

Dosage and routes

Renal dose

CrCl 10-30 ml/min dose q12h; CrCl <10 ml/min dose q24h

Adult: PO 250-500 mg q8h or 500-875 mg q12h depending on severity of infection

P ***Child ≤40 kg:*** PO 20-40 mg/kg/day in divided doses q8h or 25-45 mg/kg/day in divided doses q12h

Available forms: Tabs 250, 500, 875 mg/125 mg clavulanate; chewable tabs 125, 200, 250, 400 mg; powder for oral susp 125, 200, 250, 400 mg/5 ml

Adverse effects

CNS: Headache, fever, **seizures**

GI: Nausea, diarrhea, vomiting, increased AST, ALT, abdominal pain, glossitis, colitis, black tongue, **pseudomembranous colitis**

GU: **Oliguria, proteinuria, hematuria,** *vaginitis, moniliasis,* **glomerulonephritis**

HEMA: Anemia, **bone marrow depression, granulocytopenia, leukopenia, eosinophilia, thrombocytopenic purpura**

INTEG: Rash, urticaria

META: Hyperkalemia, hypokalemia, alkalosis, hypernatremia

SYST: **Anaphylaxis, respiratory distress, serum sickness**

Contraindications: Hypersensitivity to penicillins; neonates P

Precautions: Pregnancy **B**, lactation, hypersensitivity to cephalosporins; neonates P; renal disease

Pharmacokinetics	
Absorption	Well absorbed (90%)
Distribution	Readily in body tissues, fluids, CSF; crosses placenta
Metabolism	Liver (30%)
Excretion	Breast milk; kidney, unchanged (70%), removed by hemodialysis
Half-life	1-1.3 hr

Pharmacodynamics	
Onset	½ hr
Peak	2 hr

Interactions

Individual drugs

Allopurinol: amoxicillin-induced skin rash

Probenecid: ↑ amoxicillin levels, decreased renal excretion

Drug classifications

Oral anticoagulants: ↑ anticoagulant effects

Oral contraceptives: ↓ contraceptive effectiveness

Herb/drug

Khat: ↓ absorption

Lab test interferences

False positive: Urine glucose, urine protein, direct Coombs' test

NURSING CONSIDERATIONS

Assessment

- Assess patient for previous sensitivity reaction to penicillins or other cephalosporins; cross-sensitivity between penicillins and cephalosporins is common
- Assess patient for signs and symptoms of infection, including characteristics of wounds, sputum, urine, stool, WBC >10,000/mm^3, earache, fever; obtain baseline information and during treatment
- Complete C&S before beginning drug therapy to identify if correct treatment has been initiated
- Assess for anaphylaxis: rash, urticaria, pruritus, chills, dyspnea, laryngeal edema, fever, joint pain; angioedema may occur a few days after therapy begins; epinephrine and resuscitation equipment should be available for anaphylactic reaction
- Identify urine output; if decreasing, notify prescriber (may indicate nephrotoxicity)
- Monitor renal studies: urinalysis, protein, blood, BUN, creatinine
- Monitor blood studies: AST, ALT, CBC, Hct, bilirubin, LDH, alkaline phosphatase, Coombs' test monthly if patient is on long-term therapy
- Monitor electrolytes: potassium, sodium, chloride monthly if patient is on long-term therapy
- Assess bowel pattern qd; diarrhea, cramping, blood in stools, report to prescriber; if severe diarrhea occurs, drug should be discontinued; may indicate pseudomembranous colitis
- Monitor for bleeding: ecchymosis, bleeding gums, hematuria, stool guaiac daily if on long-term therapy
- Assess for overgrowth of infection: perineal itching, fever, malaise, redness, pain, swelling, drainage, rash, diarrhea, change in cough, sputum

Nursing diagnoses

- ✓ Infection, risk for (uses)
- ✓ Injury, risk for (side effects)
- ✓ Diarrhea (side effects)
- ✓ Knowledge deficit (teaching)
- ✓ Noncompliance (teaching)

Implementation

- Give in even doses around the clock; if GI upset occurs, give with food; drug must be taken for 10-14 days to ensure organism death and prevent superinfection; store in tight container; cap can be opened and mixed with food or liq; chewable tabs should be chewed

• Administer only as directed; 2 250-mg tabs not equivalent to 1 500-mg tab due to strength of clavulanate

• Shake susp well before each dose; may be used alone or mixed in drinks, use immediately; susp may be stored in refrigerator for 10 days

Patient/family education

• Teach patient to report sore throat, bruising, bleeding, joint pain; may indicate blood dyscrasias (rare)

• Advise patient to contact prescriber if vaginal itching, loose, foul-smelling stools occur; may indicate superinfection

• Instruct patient to take all medication prescribed for the length of time prescribed

• Advise patient to notify prescriber of diarrhea with blood or pus, which may indicate pseudomembranous colitis

• Advise patient to use alternate contraceptive measures if using oral contraceptives

Evaluation

Positive therapeutic outcome

• Absence of signs/symptoms of infection (WBC <10,000/mm^3, temp WNL)

• Reported improvement in symptoms of infection

Treatment of anaphylaxis: Withdraw drug, maintain airway, administer epinephrine, aminophylline, O_2, **IV** corticosteroids

amphetamine (℞)

(am-fet'a-meen)

amphetamine sulfate

Func. class.: Cerebral stimulant

Chem. class.: Amphetamine

Pregnancy category C

Controlled substance schedule II

Action: Increases release of norepinephrine in nerve endings, dopamine in cerebral cortex to reticular activating system; increases CNS, respiratory stimulation, pupillary dilatation, vasoconstriction

Therapeutic Outcome: Increased alertness, decreased fatigue, ability to stay awake (treatment of narcolepsy), increased attention span, decreased hyperactivity (ADHD)

Uses: Narcolepsy, ADHD

Dosage and routes

Narcolepsy

Adult: PO 5-60 mg qd in divided doses

P ***Child >12 yr:*** PO 10 mg qd increasing by 10 mg/day at weekly intervals

P ***Child 6-12 yr:*** PO 5 mg qd increasing by 5 mg/wk, max 60 mg/day

ADHD

P ***Child >6 yr:*** PO 5 mg qd-bid increasing by 5 mg/day at weekly intervals

P ***Child 3-6 yr:*** PO 2.5 mg qd increasing by 2.5 mg/day at weekly intervals

Available forms: Tabs 5, 10 mg

Adverse effects

CNS: *Hyperactivity, insomnia, restlessness, talkativeness,* dizziness, headache, chills, stimulation, dysphoria, irritability, aggressiveness, tremor, dependence, addiction

CV: *Palpitations,* **tachycardia,** hypertension, dysrhythmias, decreased heart rate

GI: Nausea, vomiting, anorexia, dry mouth, diarrhea, constipation, weight loss, metallic taste, cramps
GU: Impotence, change in libido
INTEG: Urticaria

Contraindications: Hypersensitivity to sympathomimetic amines, hyperthyroidism, hypertension, glaucoma, severe arteriosclerosis, drug abuse, cardiovascular disease, anxiety

Precautions: Gilles de la Tourette's P syndrome, lactation, child <6 yr, pregnancy **C**

Pharmacokinetics

Absorption	Well absorbed within 3 hr
Distribution	Widely distributed; crosses placenta; high concentrations in brain
Metabolism	Liver
Excretion	Kidneys: pH dependent, increased pH leads to increased reabsorption; breast milk
Half-life	10-30 hr; increased when urine is alkaline, decreased when urine is acidic

Pharmacodynamics

Onset	½ hr
Peak	1-3 hr
Duration	4-20 hr

Interactions

Individual drugs

Acetazolamide: ↓ excretion, ↑ effect
Ammonium chloride: ↓ effect
Ascorbic acid: ↓ effect
Haloperidol: Altered CNS effect
Meperidine: Hypertensive crisis
Sodium bicarbonate: ↓ excretion, ↑ effect
Thyroid: ↑ effects

Drug classifications

Antidepressants, tricyclic: ↑ dysrhythmias
β-Blockers: ↑ hypertension
Cardiac glycosides: ↑ dysrhythmias
MAOIs: Hypertensive crisis
Phenothiazines: Altered CNS effect
Sympathomimetics: ↑ effect

Food/drug

Cranberries/juice: ↑ amphetamine effect
Caffeine: ↑ amphetamine effect

Herb/drug

Kava: ↓ amphetamine effect

Lab test interferences

↑ Plasma corticosteroids,
Interference: urinary steroids

NURSING CONSIDERATIONS

Assessment

- Monitor VS, B/P, since this drug may reverse antihypertensives; check patients with cardiac disease more often for increased B/P
- Monitor CBC, urinalysis; in diabetes blood glucose, urine glucose; insulin changes may be required, since eating will decrease
- Monitor height and weight q3 mo, P since growth rate in children may be decreased; appetite is suppressed, weight loss is common during the first few months of treatment
- Monitor mental status: mood, sensorium, affect, stimulation, insomnia; aggressiveness may occur; depression with crying spells may occur after drug has worn off
- Assess for physical dependency; should not be used for extended time except in ADHD; should be discontinued gradually to prevent withdrawal symptoms
- Assess for narcoleptic symptoms before medication and after; ability to stay awake should increase significantly
- P In children or adults with ADHD, monitor for improved organizational skills, attention span, attending to tasks, impulse control, socialization, and ability to get along better with others
- Alert: Assess for withdrawal symptoms: headache, nausea, vomiting, muscle pain, weakness; drug tolerance

develops after long-term use; dosage should not be increased if tolerance develops; this medication has a high abuse potential

Nursing diagnoses

- ✓ Thought processes, altered (uses, adverse reactions)
- ✓ Coping, impaired individual (uses)
- ✓ Knowledge deficit (teaching)
- ✓ Family coping, impaired individual (uses)

Implementation

- Give at least 6 hr hs to avoid sleeplessness; titrate to patient's response, lowest dosage should be used to control symptoms
- Use gum, hard candy, frequent sips of water for dry mouth at beginning of treatment; these symptoms tend to lessen with time

Patient/family education

- Advise patient to decrease caffeine consumption (coffee, tea, cola, chocolate), which may increase irritability and stimulation; to avoid OTC preparations unless approved by prescriber; to avoid alcohol ingestion; these may cause serious drug interactions
- Instruct patient to taper off drug over several weeks, or depression, increased sleeping, lethargy may occur
- Advise patient to avoid hazardous activities until stabilized on medication
- Instruct patient not to double doses if medication is missed; prescriber may suggest drug holidays (ADHD) during the school year to assess progress and determine continued drug necessity
- Instruct patient/family to notify health care provider if significant side effects occur: tremors, insomnia, palpitations, restlessness; drug changes may be needed
- Inform patient that if dry mouth occurs to use frequent sips of water, sugarless gum, hard candy during beginning therapy; dry mouth lessens with continued treatment
- Tell patient to get needed rest; patients feel more tired at end of day; to give last dose at least 6 hr hs to avoid insomnia

Evaluation

Positive therapeutic outcome

- Decreased activity in ADHD
- Absence of sleeping during day in narcolepsy

Treatment of overdose:

Administer fluids, hemodialysis, peritoneal dialysis, antihypertensives for increased B/P; ammonium chloride for increased excretion

amphotericin B deoxycholate (℞)

(am-foh-tehr'ih-sin de-ox-ee-kohl'ate)

Fungizone

amphotericin B lipid based (℞)

Abelcet, Amphotec, AmBisome

Func. class.: Antifungal

Chem. class.: Amphoteric polyene

Pregnancy category B

Action: Increases cell membrane permeability in susceptible organisms by binding sterols in fungal cell membrane; decreases potassium, sodium, and nutrients in cell

➔ **Therapeutic Outcome:** Fungistatic against histoplasmosis, blastomycosis, coccidioidomycosis, cryptococcosis, aspergillosis, phycomycosis, candidiasis, sporotrichosis

Uses: Treatment of severe, possibly fatal fungal infections (**IV**); treatment of topical fungal infections (top)

Investigational uses: Candiduria (bladder irrigation)

Dosage and routes

Deoxycholate

Adult: **IV** Give test dose of 1 mg; then 0.5 mg/kg, increase qd slowly to

0.5 mg/kg, may give 1 mg/kg/day or 1.5 mg/kg qid, alternate day dosing may be used

P ***Child:*** **IV** 0.25 mg/kg infused initially, increase by 0.25 mg/kg qod to max of 1 mg/kg/day

P ***Adult and child:*** TOP apply 2-4 × daily

P ***Adult and child:*** 1 ml qid

(Amphotec)

P ***Adult and child:*** **IV** 3-4 mg/kg/day, max 6 mg/kg/day

(Abelcet)

P ***Adult and child:*** **IV** 5 mg/kg/day as a 1 mg/ml inf given 2.5 mg/kg/hr

(AmBisome)

P ***Adult and child:*** **IV** Fungal infections 3-5 mg/kg q24h

Visceral leishmaniasis: 3 mg/kg q24h days 1-5 and 14 and 21; give 4 mg/kg on day 1-5, 10, 17, 24, 31, and 38 to immunocompromised patients

Available forms: ***Amphotericin deoxycholate*** inj 50-mg vial, oral susp 100 mg/ml; cream, ointment, lotion 3%; ***amphotericin B lipid based*** susp for inj 100 mg/20-ml vial

Adverse effects

CNS: *Headache, fever, chills,* peripheral nerve pain, paresthesias, peripheral neuropathy, **convulsions,** dizziness

EENT: Tinnitus, deafness, diplopia, blurred vision

GI: *Nausea, vomiting, anorexia,* diarrhea, cramps, **hemorrhagic gastroenteritis, acute liver failure**

GU: *Hypokalemia,* axotemia, hyposthenuria, **renal tubular acidosis,** nephrocalcinosis, **permanent renal impairment, anuria, oliguria**

HEMA: Normochromic and normocytic anemia, **thrombocytopenia, agranulocytosis, leukopenia, eosinophilia,** hypokalemia, hyponatremia, hypomagnesemia

INTEG: *Burning, irritation,* pain, necrosis at inj site with extravasation, flushing, dermatitis, skin rash (top route)

MS: *Arthralgia, myalgia,* generalized pain, weakness, weight loss

Contraindications: Hypersensitivity, severe bone marrow depression

Precautions: Renal disease, pregnancy **B**

Pharmacokinetics

Absorption	Complete bioavailability (**IV**), rapidly absorbed (top)
Distribution	Body tissues
Metabolism	Liver
Excretion	Kidneys, detectable for several weeks
Half-life	Initial 24-48 hr, terminal 15 days

Pharmacodynamics

	IV	TOP
Onset	Immediate	Unknown
Peak	1-2 hr	Unknown

Interactions

Individual drugs

Mezlocillin: ↑ hypokalemia

Piperacillin: ↑ hypokalemia

Thiazides: ↑ hypokalemia

Ticarcillin: ↑ hypokalemia

Drug classifications

Diuretics: ↑ nephrotoxicity, hypokalemia

Glucocorticoids: ↑ hypokalemia

Nephrotoxic drugs: ↑ nephrotoxicity

Herb/drug

Gossypol: ↑ risk of nephrotoxicity

NURSING CONSIDERATIONS

Assessment

- Monitor VS q15-30 min during first inf; note changes in pulse, B/P
- Monitor blood studies: Hgb, Hct, potassium, sodium, calcium, magnesium q2 wk; BUN, creatinine weekly; decreased Hgb, Hct, and magnesium

are common with increased potassium
- Monitor weight weekly; if weight increases over 2 lb/wk, edema is present; renal damage should be considered
- Monitor for renal toxicity: increasing BUN, serum creatinine; if BUN is >40 mg/dl or if serum creatinine >3 mg/dl, drug may be discontinued or dosage reduced; I&O ratio: watch for decreasing urinary output, change in sp gr; discontinue drug to prevent permanent damage to renal tubules; provide hydration of 2-3 L/day
- Monitor for hepatotoxicity: increasing AST, ALT, alkaline phosphatase, bilirubin
- Monitor for allergic reaction: dermatitis, rash; drug should be discontinued, antihistamines (mild reaction) or epinephrine (severe reaction) administered; check inj site for thrombophlebitis
- Monitor for hypokalemia: anorexia, drowsiness, weakness, decreased reflexes, dizziness, increased urinary output, increased thirst, paresthesias; if these occur, drug should be decreased or discontinued and potassium administered

Topical route
- Monitor for allergic reaction: burning, stinging, swelling, redness

Nursing diagnoses
- ✓ Infection, risk for (uses)
- ✓ Injury, risk for physical (adverse reaction)
- ✓ Knowledge deficit (teaching)

Implementation
Topical route
- Provide enough medication to cover lesions completely; do not cover with occlusive dressing; apply liberally and rub thoroughly into affected area; administer after cleansing with soap, water before each application, dry well (as ordered), wear gloves during application
- Store at room temp in dry place

IV IV route

Deoxycholate
- Give after diluting 50 mg in 10 ml sterile water (no preservatives) (5 mg-1 ml); shake well, further dilute with 500 ml of D_5W to concentration of 0.1 mg/ml; do not use other diluents or sol; use large needle (20 G); change needle for each step; wear gloves
- Use test dosage of 1 mg/20 ml D_5W; give over 10-30 min; if no reaction, drug is administered as ordered
- Administer **IV** using in-line filter (mean pore diameter >1 µm) using distal veins; check for extravasation, necrosis q8h; use an infusion pump; administer over 6 hr; rapid inf may result in circulation collapse; may also be given through central line
- Give acetaminophen and diphenhydramine 30 min before inf to reduce fever, chills, headache
- Give drug only after C&S confirm organism, drug needed to treat condition; make sure drug is used in life-threatening infections
- Store protected from moisture and light; diluted sol is stable for 24 hr at room temp, 1 wk refrigerated

Syringe compatibilities:
Heparin

Y-*site compatibilities:*
Aldesleukin, diltiazem, doxorubicin liposome, famotidine, remifentanil, tacrolimus, teniposide, thiotepa, zidovudine

Y-*site incompatibilities:*
Enalaprilat, fludarabine, foscarnet, ondansetron

Additive compatibilities:
Fluconazole, heparin, hydrocortisone, methylprednisolone, sodium bicarbonate

Solution compatibilities: D_5W

Patient/family education
Topical route
- Teach patient that skin and clothing

may become discolored; to use asepsis (hand washing) before, after each application to prevent further infection
- Instruct patient to apply with glove to prevent further infection; not to cover with occlusive dressing; to continue even if condition improves
- Teach patient to avoid use of OTC creams, ointments, lotions, unless directed by prescriber
- Instruct patient to report increased itching, burning, rash, redness; ointment may irritate most hairy areas; to report if condition worsens

IV route
- Advise patient that long-term therapy may be needed to clear infection (2 wk-3 mo depending on type of infection)
- Teach patient side effects and when to notify prescriber

Evaluation
Positive therapeutic outcome
- Decrease in size, number of lesions (top)
- Decreased fever, malaise, rash
- Negative C&S for infecting organism

ampicillin (℞)
(am-pi-sill'in)
Ampicin ✤, Apo-Ampi ✤, D-Amp ✤, Nu-Ampi ✤, NovoAmpicillin ✤, Penbriten ✤, Polycillin, Principen, Totacillin
Func. class.: Broad-spectrum antiinfective
Chem. class.: Aminopenicillin
Pregnancy category B

Action: Interferes with cell wall replication of susceptible organisms; the cell wall, rendered osmotically unstable, swells, bursts from osmotic pressure

Therapeutic Outcome: Bactericidal effects for the following organisms: effective for gram-positive cocci *(Streptococcus pyogenes, Streptococcus faecalis, Streptococcus pneumoniae)*, gram-negative cocci *(Neisseria gonorrhoeae, Neisseria meningitidis)*, gram-negative bacilli *(Haemophilus influenzae, Proteus mirabilis, Salmonella, Shigella, Listeria monocytogenes)*, gram-positive bacilli

Uses: Infections of respiratory tract, skin, skin structures, genitourinary tract; otitis media, meningitis, septicemia, sinusitis, and endocarditis prophylaxis

Investigational uses: High-risk patients having c-section

Dosage and routes
Renal dose
CrCl 30-50 ml/min dose q6-8hr; CrCl 10-30 ml/min dose q8-12h; <10 ml/min dose q12h

Systemic infections
P ***Adult and child ≥40 kg (88 lb):*** PO 250-500 mg q6h or 1-2 g qd in divided doses q6h; **IV**/IM 250-500 mg q6h, (up to 2 g q4h in severe infections) or 2-8 g qd in divided doses q4-6h

P ***Child <40 kg:*** PO 25-100 mg/kg/day in divided doses q6h; **IV**/IM 25-50 mg/kg/day in divided doses q8h for septicemia or bacterial meningitis

Meningitis
Adult: **IV** 8-14 g/day in divided doses q3-4h × 3 days

P ***Child:*** **IV** 100-200 mg/kg/day in divided doses q3-4h × 3 days

Gonorrhea
P ***Adult and child ≥ 45 kg (99 lb):*** PO 3.5 g given with 1 g probenecid as a single dose or IM/**IV** 500 mg q6h (≥40 kg); IM/**IV** 50 mg/kg/day in divided doses q6-8h (<40 kg)

Available forms: Powder for inj 125, 250, 500 mg, 1, 2, 10 g; **IV** inf 500 mg, 1, 2 g; caps 250, 500 mg; powder for oral susp, 125, 250, 500 mg/5 ml

Adverse effects

CNS: Lethargy, hallucinations, anxiety, depression, twitching, **coma, seizures**
GI: Nausea, vomiting, diarrhea, **pseudomembranous colitis**
GU: Oliguria, proteinuria, hematuria, *vaginitis, moniliasis,* **glomerulonephritis**
HEMA: Anemia, increased bleeding time, **bone marrow depression, granulocytopenia**
INTEG: Rash, urticaria
SYST: **Anaphylaxis, serum sickness**

Contraindications: Hypersensitivity to penicillins

Precautions: Pregnancy **B;** hypersensitivity to cephalosporins; P neonates; renal disease

Do Not Confuse:
Omnipen/imipenem

Pharmacokinetics

Absorption	Moderate, duodenum (35%-50%)
Distribution	Readily in body tissues, fluids, CSF; crosses placenta
Metabolism	Liver (30%)
Excretion	Breast milk; kidney unchanged (70%), removed by dialysis
Half-life	50-110 min

Pharmacodynamics

	PO	IM	IV
Onset	Rapid	Rapid	Rapid
Peak	2 hr	1 hr	Infusion's end

Interactions

Individual drugs

Allopurinol: ↑ ampicillin-induced skin rash
Disulfiram: ↑ ampicillin concentrations
Probenecid: ↑ ampicillin levels, ↓ renal excretion

Drug classifications

Oral contraceptives: ↓ contraceptive effectiveness

Herb/drug

Khat: ↓ absorption, separate by 2 hr

Lab test interferences

False positive: Urine glucose, urine protein

NURSING CONSIDERATIONS

Assessment

- Assess patient for previous sensitivity reaction to penicillins or other cephalosporins; cross-sensitivity between penicillins and cephalosporins is common
- Assess patient for signs and symptoms of infection, including characteristics of wounds, sputum, urine, stool, WBC >10,000/mm^3, earache, fever; obtain baseline information and during treatment
- Obtain C&S before beginning drug therapy to identify if correct treatment has been initiated
- Assess for allergic reactions: rash, urticaria, pruritus, chills, fever, joint pain; angioedema may occur a few days after therapy begins; epinephrine and resuscitation equipment should be on unit for anaphylactic reaction; also, check for ampicillin rash: pruritic, red, raised
- Identify urine output; if decreasing, notify prescriber (may indicate nephrotoxicity)
- Monitor renal studies: urinalysis, protein, blood, BUN, creatinine
- Monitor blood studies: AST, ALT, CBC, Hct, bilirubin, LDH, alkaline phosphatase, Coombs' test monthly if patient is on long-term therapy
- Monitor electrolytes: potassium, sodium, chloride monthly if patient is on long-term therapy
- Assess bowel pattern qd; if severe diarrhea occurs, drug should be discontinued; may indicate pseudomembranous colitis
- Monitor for bleeding: ecchymosis,

bleeding gums, hematuria, stool guaiac daily if on long-term therapy
- Assess for overgrowth of infection: perineal itching, fever, malaise, redness, pain, swelling, drainage, rash, diarrhea, change in cough, sputum

Nursing diagnoses

- ✓ Infection, risk for (uses)
- ✓ Injury, risk for (side effects)
- ✓ Diarrhea (side effects)
- ✓ Knowledge deficit (teaching)
- ✓ Noncompliance (teaching)

Implementation

PO route
- Give in even doses around the clock; drug must be taken for 10-14 days to ensure organism death and prevent superinfection; store caps in tight container
- Tabs may be crushed or caps opened and mixed with water
- Shake susp well before each dose; store in refrigerator for 2 wk or 1 wk at room temp

IM route
- Reconstitute with 125 mg/0.9-1.2 ml; 250 mg/0.9-1.9 ml; 500 mg/1.2-1.8 ml; 1 g/2.4-7.4 ml; 2 g/6.8 ml
- Give deep in large muscle mass

IV **IV route**
- Reconstitute with 125 mg/0.9-1.2 ml; 250 mg/0.9-1.9 ml; 500 mg/1.2-1.8 ml; 1 g/2.4-7.4 ml; 2 g/6.8 ml
- Give by direct **IV** over 3-5 min in lower dosages (125-500 mg) or over 15 min in higher dosages (1-2 g)
- Give by intermittent inf after diluting with 0.9% NaCl, LR, D_5W, D_5/0.45% NaCl; use 50 ml of sol and dilute to concentration of <30 mg/ml

Syringe compatibilities:
Chloramphenicol

Syringe incompatibilities:
Erythromycin, gentamicin, kanamycin, lincomycin, metoclopramide, oxytetracycline, streptomycin, tetracycline

Y-site compatibilities:
Acyclovir, amifostine, allopurinol, aztreonam, cyclophosphamide, doxorubicin liposome, enalaprilat, esmolol, famotidine, filgrastim, fludarabine, foscarnet, granisetron, heparin, regular insulin, labetalol, magnesium sulfate, melphalan, meperidine, morphine, multivitamins, oflaxacin, perphenazine, phytonadione, potassium chloride, propofol, remifentanil, thiotepa, tolazoline, vit B with C

Y-site incompatibilities:
Calcium gluconate, epinephrine, fluconazole, hetastarch, hydromorphone, hydralazine, ondansetron, sargramostim, verapamil, vinorelbine

Additive incompatibilities:
Amikacin, aztreonam, chlorpromazine, dopamine, gentamicin, hydralazine, hydrocortisone, prochlorperazine

Additive compatibilities:
Cefotiam, clindamycin, erythromycin, floxacillin, furosemide, tacrolimus, teniposide, theophylline, verapamil

Patient/family education

- ❗ Teach patient to report sore throat, bruising, bleeding, joint pain; may indicate blood dyscrasias (rare)
- Advise patient to contact prescriber if vaginal itching, loose, foul-smelling stools, furry tongue occur; may indicate superinfection
- Instruct patient to take all medication prescribed for the length of time ordered
- Advise patient to notify prescriber of diarrhea with blood or pus, which may indicate pseudomembranous colitis
- Tab may be crushed; cap may be opened and mixed with water

Evaluation

Positive therapeutic outcome
- Absence of signs/symptoms of infection (WBC <10,000, temp WNL)
- Reported improvement in symptoms of infection

Treatment of anaphylaxis:

Withdraw drug, maintain airway,

administer epinephrine, aminophylline, O_2, **IV** corticosteroids

ampicillin/sulbactam (℞)
(am-pi-sill'in/sul-bak'tam)
Unasyn
Func. class.: Broad-spectrum antiinfective
Chem. class.: Aminopenicillin
Pregnancy category B (ampicillin)

Action: Interferes with cell wall replication of susceptible organisms; the cell wall, rendered osmotically unstable, swells and bursts from osmotic pressure; this combination extends the spectrum of activity and inhibits β-lactamase that may inactivate ampicillin

➔ **Therapeutic Outcome:** Bactericidal against *Pneumococcus, Enterococcus, Streptococcus, Escherichia coli, Proteus mirabilis, Neisseria meningitidis, Neisseria gonorrhoeae, Shigella, Salmonella,* and *Haemophilus influenzae* organisms; use only with β-lactamase–producing strain of infection

Uses: Skin and structure infections, intraabdominal infections, gynecologic infections, soft tissue infections, otitis media, sinusitis, meningitis, septicemia

Dosage and routes
Renal dose
CrCl 15-29 ml/min dose q12h; CrCl 5-14 ml/min dose q24h

Adult and child >40 kg: **IV**/IM 1 g ampicillin and 0.5 g sulbactam or 2 g ampicillin, and 1 g sulbactam q6h, not to exceed 4 g/day sulbactam

P ***Child:*** <40 kg **IV** 300 mg/kg/day (ampicillin component) divided q6h, max 8 g/day

Available forms: Powder for inj 1.5 g (1 g ampicillin, 0.5 g sulbactam), 3 g (2 g ampicillin, 1 g sulbactam)

Adverse effects
CNS: Lethargy, hallucinations, anxiety, depression, twitching, **coma, convulsions**
GI: Nausea, vomiting, diarrhea, increased AST, ALT, abdominal pain, glossitis, colitis, **pseudomembranous colitis**
GU: Oliguria, proteinuria, hematuria, *vaginitis, moniliasis,* **glomerulonephritis**
HEMA: Anemia, increased bleeding time, **bone marrow depression, granulocytopenia**
SYST: **Anaphylaxis**

Contraindications: Hypersensitivity to penicillins, ampicillin, or sulbactam

Precautions: Pregnancy **B,** hypersensitivity to cephalosporins,
P neonates, renal disease

Pharmacokinetics	
Absorption	Well absorbed (IM)
Distribution	Readily in body tissues, fluids, CSF; crosses placenta
Metabolism	Liver (10%-50%)
Excretion	Breast milk; kidney unchanged (75%)
Half-life	50-110 min (ampicillin)

Pharmacodynamics	IM	IV
Onset	Rapid	Immediate
Peak	1 hr	Infusion's end

Interactions
Individual drugs
Allopurinol: ampicillin-induced skin rash
Probenecid: ↑ ampicillin levels, ↓ renal excretion

Drug classifications
Oral contraceptives: ↓ contraceptive effectiveness

Herb/drug
Khat: ↓ absorption, separate by 2 hr

Lab test interferences
False positive: Urine glucose, urine protein

NURSING CONSIDERATIONS
Assessment
- Assess patient for previous sensitivity reaction to penicillins or cephalosporins; cross-sensitivity between penicillins and cephalosporins is common
- Assess patient for signs and symptoms of infection; including characteristics of wounds, sputum, urine, stool, WBC >10,000 mm^3, earache, fever; obtain baseline information and during treatment
- Complete C&S before beginning drug therapy to identify if correct treatment has been initiated
- Assess for allergic reactions: rash, urticaria, pruritus, chills, fever, joint pain; angioedema may occur a few days after therapy begins; epinephrine and resuscitation equipment should be on unit for anaphylactic reaction
- Identify urine output; if decreasing, notify prescriber (may indicate nephrotoxicity)
- Assess renal studies: urinalysis, protein, BUN, creatinine
- Monitor blood studies: AST, ALT, CBC, Hct, bilirubin, LDH, alkaline phosphatase, Coombs' test monthly if patient is on long-term therapy
- Monitor electrolytes: potassium, sodium, chloride monthly if patient is on long-term therapy
- Assess bowel pattern qd; if severe diarrhea occurs, drug should be discontinued; may indicate pseudomembranous colitis
- Monitor for bleeding: ecchymosis, bleeding gums, hematuria, stool guaiac daily if on long-term therapy
- Assess for superinfection: perineal itching, fever, malaise, redness, pain, swelling, drainage, rash, diarrhea, change in cough, sputum

Nursing diagnoses
- ✓ Infection, risk for (uses)
- ✓ Diarrhea (adverse reactions)
- ✓ Injury, risk for (adverse reactions)
- ✓ Knowledge deficit (teaching)
- ✓ Noncompliance (teaching)

Implementation
IM route
- Reconstitute by adding 3.2 ml/1.5 g or 6.4 ml/3 g; use sterile water, 0.5% or 2% lidocaine; give within 1 hr of preparation; give deep in large muscle mass
- Give after C&S completed; on empty stomach

IV route
- Give **IV** after diluting 1.5 g/3.2 ml sterile H_2O for inj; or 3 g/6.4 ml (250 mg ampicillin/125 mg sulbactam); allow to stand until foaming stops; give directly over 15-30 min; dilute further in 50 ml or more of D_5W, D_5/10.45% NaCl, 10% invert sugar in water, LR, 6% sodium lactate, isotonic NaCl; administer within 1 hr after reconstitution; give as an intermittent inf over 15-30 min

Y-*site compatibilities:*
Amifostine, aztreonam, cefepime, enalaprilat, famotidine, filgrastim, fluconazole, fludarabine, granisetron, heparin, regular insulin, meperidine, morphine, paclitaxel, remifentanil, tacrolimus, teniposide, theophylline, thiotepa

Y-*site incompatibilities:*
Idarubicin, ondansetron, sargramostim

Additive compatibilities:
Aztreonam

Additive incompatibilities:
Aminoglycosides

Patient/family education
- Teach patient to report sore throat, bruising, bleeding, joint pain, persis-

A

tent diarrhea; may indicate blood dyscrasias (rare) or superinfection
- Advise patient to contact prescriber if vaginal itching, loose, foul-smelling stools, furry tongue occur; may indicate superinfection
- Instruct patient to use another form of contraception other than oral contraceptives

Evaluation
Positive therapeutic outcome
- Absence of signs/symptoms of infection (WBC <10,000/mm^3, temp WNL, absence of red draining wounds, earache)
- Reported improvement in symptoms of infection

Treatment of overdose:
Withdraw drug, maintain airway, administer epinephrine, aminophylline, O_2, **IV** corticosteroids for anaphylaxis

amprenavir (℞)
(am-pren′-a-ver)
Agenerase
Func. class.: Antiretroviral
Chem. class.: Protease inhibitor
Pregnancy category C

Action: Inhibits HIV protease

➔ **Therapeutic Outcome:** Prevents maturation of the infectious virus

Uses: HIV in combination with other antiretroviral agents

Dosage and routes
Adult: PO (cap) 1200 mg bid

P ***Child 13-16 yr:*** PO (cap) 1200 mg bid

P ***Child 4-12 yr or wt <50 kg:*** PO (cap) 20 mg/kg qd or 15 mg/kg tid, max 2400 mg; PO (oral sol) 22.5 mg/kg bid or 17 mg/kg tid qd, max 2800 mg

Hepatic Dose
Child: PO (Child-Pugh score 5-8) 450 mg bid in combination; (child-Pugh score 9-12) 300 mg bid in combination

Available forms: Cap 50, 150 mg; oral sol 15 mg/ml

Adverse effects
CNS: *Paresthesia*
ENDO: New onset diabetes, hyperglycemia, exacerbation of preexisting diabetes mellitus
GI: *Diarrhea, abdominal pain, nausea,* **hepatotoxicity**
HEMA: **Acute hemolytic anemia**
INTEG: *Rash,* **Stevens-Johnson syndrome**

Contraindications: Hypersensitivity

Precautions: Liver disease, pregnancy **C**, lactation, children, hemophilia, sulfonamide sensitivity, elderly
P G

Pharmacokinetics	
Absorption	Rapidly
Distribution	90% Protein Binding
Metabolism	Unknown
Excretion	Unknown
Half-life	7-10½ hr

Pharmacodynamics
Unknown

Interactions
Individual drugs
Amiodarone: Serious/life threatening reactions
Bepridil: Do not use together
Carbamazepine: ↓ amprenavir levels
Cimetidine: ↑ amprenavir levels
Clarithromycin: ↑ amprenavir levels
Erythromycin: ↑ amprenavir levels
Indinavir: ↑ amprenavir levels
Itraconazole: ↑ amprenavir levels
Lidocaine: Serious/life threatening reactions
Loratadine: Do not use together
Lovastatin: Do not use together
Midazolam: Do not use together
Phenobarbital: ↓ amprenavir levels

Quinidine: Serious/life threatening reactions
Rifampin: Do not use together
Rifamycin: ↓ amprenavir levels
Ritonavir: ↑ amprenavir levels

Drug classifications

Antacids: Decreased amprenavir levels
Ergots: Do not use together
Tricyclics: Serious life-threatening reactions

Herb/drug

St. John's Wort: ↓ amprenavir level

Lab test interferences

Interference: CPK, glucose (low)

NURSING CONSIDERATIONS

Assessment

- Assess for renal/hepatic failure, pregnancy, or those receiving disulfiram, metronidazole; oral sol contains propylene glycol in greater quantities
- Assess signs of infection, anemia
- Monitor liver studies: ALT, AST
- Monitor C&S before drug therapy; drug may be taken as soon as culture is taken; repeat C&S after treatment; determine the presence of other sexually transmitted diseases
- Assess bowel pattern before, during treatment; if severe abdominal pain with bleeding occurs, drug should be discontinued; monitor hydration
- Assess skin eruptions, rash, urticaria, itching
- Assess allergies before treatment, reaction of each medication; place allergies on chart

Nursing diagnoses

✓ Infection, risk for (uses)
✓ Knowledge deficit (teaching)

Implementation

- Caps and oral sol are not interchangeable on a mg/mg basis

Patient/family education

- Advise patient to take as prescribed with or without food, avoid high-fat foods; if dose is missed, take as soon as remembered up to 1 hr before next dose; do not double dose, do not share with others
- Advise patient that drug must be taken in equal intervals around the clock to maintain blood levels for duration of therapy
- Instruct patient that caps and sol are not interchangeable
- Advise patient to use nonhormonal method of contraception during treatment, use condoms
- Advise patient to notify prescriber of diarrhea, nausea, vomiting, rash
- Teach patient that drug does not cure AIDS or prevent transmission to others, only controls symptoms

Evaluation

Positive therapeutic outcome

- Prevention of spread of infection

anagrelide (℞)

(a-na'gre-lide)
Agrylin
Func. class.: Antiplatelet
Chem. class.: Imidazoquinazolinone

Pregnancy cetegory C

Action: Reduces platelet count (mechanism not clear) and prevents early platelet shape changes in response to aggregating agents thus inhibiting platelet aggregation

Therapeutic Outcome: Inhibition of platelet aggregation

Uses: Essential thrombocythemia

Dosage and routes

Adult: PO 0.5 mg qid or 1 mg bid, may be adjusted after 1 wk, max 10 mg/day or 2.5 mg single dose

Available forms: Caps 0.5, 1.0 mg

Adverse effects

CNS: Headache, dizziness, **seizures,** paresthesia, **CVA**
CV: Postural hypotension, tachycardia, palpitations, **CHF, MI,** cardiomyopathy, cardiomegaly, **complete**

heart block, atrial fibrillation, arrhythmia, chest pain
GI: Diarrhea, abdominal pain, nausea, flatulence, vomiting, anorexia, constipation, pancreatitis
GU: Dysuria
HEMA: Anemia, **thrombocytopenia**, ecchymosis, lymphadenoma
INTEG: Rash
MS: Asthenia, back pain
RESP: Dyspnea

Contraindications: Hypersensitivity, hypotension

Precautions: Pregnancy **C**, lactation, child <16 yr, cardiac, renal, hepatic disease

Pharmacokinetics	
Absorption	Unknown
Distribution	Unknown
Metabolism	Liver, extensively
Excretion	Feces/urine
Half-life	1.3 hr

Pharmacodynamics	
Onset	Unknown
Peak	1 hr
Duration	>24 hr

Interactions
Individual drugs
Sucralfate: ↓ absorption
Food/drug
↓ absorption

NURSING CONSIDERATIONS
Assessment
- Monitor B/P, pulse baseline and during treatment until stable; take B/P with patient lying, standing; orthostatic hypotension is common
- Assess cardiac status: chest pain, what aggravates or ameliorates condition
- Monitor platelet counts q2 days × 1 wk, and qwk thereafter, response should begin after 1-2 wk; Hgb, WBC

Nursing diagnoses
☑ Cardiac output, decreased (uses)
☑ Knowledge deficit (teaching)

Implementation
- Give with 8 oz of water; to improve absorption give on an empty stomach
- Store at room temp

Patient/family education
- Teach patient that this medication is not a cure; that drug may have to be taken continuously in evenly spaced doses only as directed; if a dose is missed, take one when remembered up to 4 hr; do not double doses
- Inform patient that it is necessary to quit smoking to prevent excessive vasoconstriction
- Advise patient to rise slowly from sitting or lying down to prevent orthostatic hypotension
- Caution patient not to use alcohol or OTC medication unless approved by prescriber
- Caution patient to avoid hazardous activities until stabilized on medication; dizziness may occur
- Teach patient to report cardiac reactions, ↑ bruising/bleeding
- Advise patient to use contraception (female, child bearing age)

Evaluation
Positive therapeutic outcome
- Absence of thrombocythemia

anakinra
See Appendix A, Selected New Drugs

anastrozole (℞)
(an-ass-stroh'zole)
Arimidex
Func. class.: Antineoplastic
Chem. class.: Aromatase inhibitor

Pregnancy category D

Action: Lowers serum estradiol concentrations; many breast cancers have strong estrogen receptors

➔ Therapeutic Outcome:
Prevention of rapidly growing malignant cells

Uses: Advanced breast carcinoma that has not responded to other therapy in estrogen-receptor-positive patients (usually postmenopausal)

Dosage and routes
Adult: PO 1 mg qd

Available forms: Tab 1 mg

Adverse effects
CNS: Hot flashes, headache, lightheadedness, depression, dizziness, confusion, insomnia, anxiety
CV: Chest pain, hypertension, thrombophlebitis, edema
GI: Nausea, vomiting, altered taste, anorexia, diarrhea, constipation, abdominal pain, dry mouth
GU: Vaginal bleeding, pruritus vulvae, vaginal dryness, pelvic pain
HEMA: **Thrombocytopenia, leukopenia**
INTEG: *Rash,* alopecia
MS: Bone pain, myalgia, asthenia
RESP: Cough, sinusitis, dyspnea

Contraindications: Hypersensitivity, pregnancy **D**

Precautions: Leukopenia, thrombocytopenia, lactation, cataracts, P children, G elderly, liver disease, renal disease

Pharmacokinetics	
Absorption	Adequately absorbed
Distribution	Unknown
Metabolism	Liver
Excretion	Feces, urine
Half-life	50 hr

Pharmacodynamics	
Onset	Unknown
Peak	4-7 hr
Duration	Unknown

Interactions
Lab test interferences
↑ GGT, ↑ AST, ↑ ALT, ↑ alkaline phosphatase, ↑ cholesterol, ↑ LDL

NURSING CONSIDERATIONS
Assessment
- Monitor CBC, differential, platelet count weekly; withhold drug if WBC is <4000/mm^3 or platelet count is <75,000/mm^3; notify prescriber of results; monitor calcium levels (hypercalcemia is common)
- Assess for tumor flare: increase in bone, tumor pain during beginning treatment; give analgesics as ordered to decrease pain
- Assess for bleeding: hematuria, guaiac, bruising or petechiae, mucosa or orifices, q8h; no rec temp

Nursing diagnoses
✓ Injury, risk for (adverse reactions)
✓ Knowledge deficit (teaching)

Implementation
- Give with food or fluids for GI upset; do not break, crush, or chew enteric products; repeat dose may be needed if vomiting occurs
- Store in light-resistant container at room temp

Patient/family education
- Instruct patient to report any complaints, side effects to health care prescriber; if dose is missed, do not double next dose
- Advise patient that vaginal bleeding, pruritus, hot flashes, can occur, and are reversible after discontinuing treatment
- Inform patient about who should be told about tamoxifen therapy
- Advise patient to report vaginal bleeding immediately; that tumor flare—increase in size of tumor, increased bone pain—may occur and will subside rapidly; may take analgesics for pain
- Caution patient to use sunscreen and protective clothing to prevent burns because photosensitivity is common
- Teach patient that hair loss may occur during treatment; a wig or hairpiece may make patient feel better;

new hair may be different in color, texture
- Inform patient that rash or lesions are temporary and may become large during beginning therapy

Evaluation

Positive therapeutic outcome
- Decreased spread of malignant cells in breast cancer

HIGH ALERT

anistreplase (℞)

(an-is-tre-plaze′)

APSAC, Eminase

Func. class.: Thrombolytic enzyme

Chem. class.: Anisoylated plasminogen streptokinase activator complex

Pregnancy category C

Action: Promotes thrombolysis by promoting conversion of plasminogen to plasmin; complex is a combination of plasminogen and streptokinase

➔ Therapeutic Outcome: Thrombolysis in coronary arteries

Uses: Management of acute MI; for lysis of coronary artery thrombi

Dosage and routes

Adult: **IV** inj 30 U over 4-5 min as soon as possible after onset of symptoms

Available forms: Powder, lyophilized 30 U/vial

Adverse effects

CNS: Headache, fever, sweating, agitation, dizziness, paresthesia, tremor, vertigo, **intracranial hemorrhage**

CV: Hypotension, **dysrhythmias,** conduction disorders

GI: Nausea, vomiting

HEMA: Decreased Hct, **GI, GU, intracranial, retroperitoneal,** surface bleeding; **thrombocytopenia**

INTEG: Rash, urticaria, phlebitis at site, itching, flushing

MS: Low back pain, arthralgia

RESP: Altered respirations, dyspnea, **bronchospasm, lung edema**

SYST: **Anaphylaxis (rare)**

Contraindications: Hypersensitivity, active internal bleeding, intraspinal or intracranial surgery, neoplasms of CNS, severe hypertension, cerebral embolism, thrombosis, hemorrhage

Precautions: Arterial emboli from left side of heart, pregnancy **C,** ulcerative colitis/enteritis, renal disease, hepatic disease, hypocoagulation, COPD, subacute bacterial endocarditis, rheumatic valvular disease, intraarterial diagnostic procedure or surgery (10 days), recent major surgery, hypersensitivity to this drug or streptokinase

Pharmacokinetics

Absorption	Complete bioavailability
Distribution	Unknown
Metabolism	Binds to plasmin
Excretion	Kidneys
Half-life	105 min

Pharmacodynamics

Onset	Unknown
Peak	45 min
Duration	Unknown

Interactions

Individual drugs

Abciximab: ↑ bleeding risk
Aspirin: ↑ bleeding risk
Clopidogrel: ↑ bleeding risk
Dipyridamole: ↑ bleeding risk
Eptifibatide: ↑ bleeding risk
Heparin: ↑ bleeding risk
Plicamycin: ↑ bleeding risk
Ticlopidine: ↑ bleeding risk
Tirofiban: ↑ bleeding risk
Valproic acid: ↑ bleeding risk

Drug classifications

Anticoagulants: ↑ bleeding risk
Cephalosporins, some: ↑ bleeding risk
NSAIDs: ↑ bleeding risk

Herb/drug
Bromelain: ↑ bleeding risk
Lab test interferences
↑ PT, ↑ APTT, ↑ TT
↓ Fibrinogen, ↓ plasminogen

NURSING CONSIDERATIONS
Assessment
- Monitor VS, B/P, pulse, respirations, neurologic signs, temp at least q4h, temp >104° F (40° C) or indicators of internal bleeding, cardiac rhythm after intracoronary administration
- Assess for hypersensitivity: fever, rash, itching, chills; mild reaction may be treated with antihistamines; hypersensitivity reactions/dyspnea, wheezing, facial swelling should be treated with epinephrine
- Monitor bleeding during 1st hr of treatment (hematuria, hematemesis, bleeding from mucous membranes, epistaxis, ecchymosis), continue to monitor for 24 hr after treatment; blood studies (Hct, platelets, PTT, PT, TT, APTT) before starting therapy; PT or APTT must be less than 2 × control before starting therapy; TT or PT q3-4h during treatment
- Monitor ECG, treat bradycardia, ventricular changes; assess neurologic status, neurologic change may indicate intracranial bleeding; cardiac enzymes, radionuclide, myocardial scanning/coronary angiography

Nursing diagnoses
- Tissue perfusion, decreased (uses)
- Injury, risk for (uses, adverse reactions)
- Knowledge deficit (teaching)

Implementation
- Give heparin therapy after thrombolytic therapy is discontinued, TT or APTT less than 2 × control (about 3-4 hr)
- Avoid invasive procedures: inj, rec temp; about 10% of patients have high streptococcal antibody titers, requiring increased loading doses
- Treat fever with acetaminophen
- Provide pressure for 30 sec to minor bleeding sites, 30 min to sites of arterial puncture followed by dressing; inform prescriber if hemostasis not attained; apply pressure dressing
- Give after reconstituting single-dose vial/5 ml sterile water for inj (not bacteriostatic water), and roll (not shake) to enhance reconstitution, try to minimize foaming; give over 2-5 min by direct **IV**, give within ½ hr of reconstitution or discard, do not add other meds to vial or syringe; give within 6 hr of thrombi identification for best results; cryoprecipitate or fresh frozen plasma if bleeding occurs; store powder in refrigerator; use within 30 min after reconstitution

Incompatibilities:
Do not mix with other drugs in sol or syringe

Patient/family education
- Teach patient action of drug and expected outcome; alert patient to possible hypersensitivity reactions and symptoms to report
- Advise patient bed rest is needed during entire course of treatment; handle patient as little as possible during therapy

Evaluation
Positive therapeutic outcome
- Absence of thrombolysis in MI
- Improved ventricular function

HIGH ALERT

antihemophilic factor VIII (AHF) (℞)

(an-tee-hee-moe-fill'ik)

Alphanate, antihemophilic factor, Bioclate, Helixate FS, Hemofilm, Humate-P, Hyate:C, Koate-DVI, Kogenate, Kogenate FS, Monoclate-P, Recombinate, ReFacto

Func. class.: Hemostatic, blood factor

Chem. class.: Factor VIII

Pregnancy category C

Action: Necessary for clotting. Activates factor X in conjunction with activated factor IX; transforms prothrombin to thrombin

➔ **Therapeutic Outcome:** Control of hemorrhage or excessive bleeding in factor VIII deficiency

Uses: Hemophilia A, patients with acquired circulating factor VIII inhibitors, factor VIII deficiency

Dosage and routes

Depends on severity of deficiency and level of antihemophilic factor

Massive hemorrhage

P ***Adult and child:*** **IV** 40-50 U/kg, then 20-25 U/kg q8-12h

Bleeding (overt)

P ***Adult and child:*** **IV** 15-25 U/kg, then 8-15 U/kg q8-12h × 4 days

Hemorrhage near vital organs

P ***Adult and child:*** **IV** 15 U/kg, then 8 U/kg q8h × 2 days, then 4 U/kg q8h × 2 days

Minor hemorrhage

P ***Adult and child:*** **IV** 8-10 U/kg/ q24h × 2-3 days or 8 U/kg q12h × 2 days, then q24h × 2 days

Joint bleeding

P ***Adult and child:*** **IV** 5-10 U/kg q8-12h × 1-2 days

Available forms: Inj 250, 500, 1000, 1500 U/vial (number of units noted on label)

Adverse effects

CNS: Headache, *lethargy, chills, fever, flushing*

CV: *Hypotension,* tachycardia

GI: Nausea, vomiting, abdominal cramps, jaundice, **viral hepatitis**

HEMA: **Thrombosis, hemolysis, risk of hepatitis B, HIV**

INTEG: Rash, flushing, *urticaria,* stinging at inj site

RESP: **Bronchospasm**, rhinitis, dyspnea, nosebleeds

Contraindications: Hypersensitivity to mouse, hamster, bovine protein

P **Precautions:** Neonates/ infants, hepatic disease, blood types A, B, AB, pregnancy **C**, factor VIII inhibitor

Pharmacokinetics	
Absorption	Complete availability
Distribution	Plasma
Metabolism	Not metabolized
Excretion	No excretion
Half-life	Biphasic 4 hr, 15 hr

Pharmacodynamics	
Onset	Immediate
Peak	Unknown
Duration	12 hr

Interactions

Drug classifications

NSAIDS: ↑ bleeding

Salicylates: ↑ bleeding

NURSING CONSIDERATIONS

Assessment

- Monitor blood studies (coagulation factors assay by % normal: 5% prevents spontaneous hemorrhage, 30%-50% for surgery, 80%-100% for severe hemorrhage; blood group of patient, donors (if applicable; most factor VIII not from specific blood group donors)
- Monitor I&O, urine color; notify

prescriber if urine becomes orange, red; change in urine color signifying hemolytic reaction; patients other than blood type O are more at risk
- Monitor pulse: discontinue infusion if significant increase
- Obtain test for factor VIII inhibitors before starting treatment, may require concomitant antiinhibitor coagulant complex therapy; Hct, Coombs' test with blood types A, B, AB
- Assess for allergy: fever, rash, itching, jaundice, wheezing, tachycardia, nausea, vomiting; give diphenhydramine (Benadryl); continue therapy if reaction is mild, discontinue if severe; notify prescriber
- Monitor bleeding at ankles, knees, elbows, other joints; check for rebleeding after 15-30 min

Nursing diagnoses

- Tissue perfusion altered (uses)
- Injury, risk for (uses, adverse reactions)
- Knowledge deficit (teaching)

Implementation

- Administer **IV** slowly; use plastic syringe to reconstitute and administer; do not use glass, drug adheres to glass; use another needle as a vent when reconstituting; rotate gently to mix
- Administer after dilution with warm NS, D_5W, LR; give within 3 hr
- Administer by **IV** inf: give at ≤2 ml/min if concentration exceeds 34 U/ml; or over 3 min if concentration is less than 34 U/ml; filter before using
- Store in refrigerator; do not freeze; after reconstitution, do not refrigerate; give within 3 hr

Additive compatibilities:

Do not mix with other drugs in sol or syringe

Patient/family education

- Advise patient to report any signs of bleeding: gums, under skin, urine, stools, emesis; review methods to prevent bleeding; to be checked q2-3 mo for HIV screen
- Instruct patient to avoid salicylates/NSAIDs; increases bleeding tendencies, decreases clotting
- Instruct patient to prepare, administer factor VIII concentrates at first sign of danger
- Instruct patient to advise health professionals of treatment for hemophilia
- Advise patient that immunization for hepatitis B may be given first
- Instruct patient to report hives, urticaria, chest tightness, hypotension; may be monoclonal antibody–derived factor VII; signs of viral hepatitis, AIDS
- Advise patient to carry identification describing disease process, drugs used

Evaluation

Positive therapeutic outcome
- Absence of bleeding
- Prevention of rebleeding

HIGH ALERT

ardeparin (℞)

(are-de-pear′in)

Normiflo

Func. class.: Anticoagulant

Chem. class.: Low molecular weight heparin

Pregnancy category C

Action: Prevents conversion of fibrinogen to fibrin and prothrombin to thrombin by enhancing inhibitory effects of antithrombin III

Therapeutic Outcome:
- Absence of deep vein thrombosis

Uses: Prevention of deep vein thrombosis after knee replacement surgery

Dosage and routes

Adult: SC 50 antifactor XaU/kg q12h beginning the evening of the day of knee replacement surgery or the following AM, continued until patient is fully ambulatory or 2 wk, whichever is first

- To be used SC only

Available forms: Inj 5000, 10,000 anti-XaU/0.5 ml

Adverse effects

CNS: **Intracranial bleeding**, fever, dizziness, headache

CV: Chest pain

GI: Nausea, vomiting, constipation, **hepatotoxicity**

HEMA: **Thrombocytopenia**, anemia

INTEG: Pruritus, superficial wound infection, ecchymosis, rash

RESP: Dyspnea

SYST: Hypersensitivity, **hemorrhage, anaphylaxis** possible

Contraindications: Hypersensitivity to this drug, pork products, heparin, or other anticoagulants; hemophilia, leukemia with bleeding, thrombocytopenic purpura, cerebrovascular hemorrhage, cerebral aneurysm, severe hypertension, other severe cardiac disease

G **Precautions:** Elderly, pregnancy **C**, hepatic disease, severe renal disease, blood dyscrasias, subacute bacterial endocarditis, acute nephritis, lactation, P child, recent childbirth, peptic ulcer disease, pericarditis, pericardial effusion, recent lumbar puncture, vasculitis, other diseases where bleeding is possible

Pharmacokinetics	
Absorption	Well
Distribution	Widely
Metabolism	Unknown
Half-life	Unknown

Pharmacodynamics

Unknown

Interactions

Drug classifications

Anticoagulants, oral: ↑ risk of bleeding

NSAIDs: ↑ risk of bleeding

Platelet inhibitors: ↑ risk of bleeding

Salicylates: ↑ risk of bleeding

NURSING CONSIDERATIONS

Assessment

- Assess for blood studies (Hct, occult blood in stools, CBC, platelets) during treatment since bleeding can occur
- Assess for bleeding gums, petechiae, ecchymosis, black tarry stools, hematuria, epistaxis, decrease in Hct, B/P; may indicate bleeding, possible hemorrhage; notify prescriber immediately, drug should be discontinued; protamine should be equal to dose of drug given; 1 mg protamine = 100 anti-Xa U of drug
- Monitor for hypersensitivity: fever, skin rash, urticaria; notify prescriber immediately

Implementation

- Give by SC only; have patient sit or lie down; SC inj may be around the navel in a U-shape, upper outer side of thigh or upper outer quadrangle of the buttocks; rotate inj sites
- Changing needles is not recommended

Evaluation

- Therapeutic response: absence of deep vein thrombosis

Patient/family education

- Teach patient to avoid OTC preparations that may cause serious drug interactions unless directed by prescriber; may contain aspirin; other anticoagulants, NSAIDs
- Teach patient to use soft-bristle toothbrush to avoid bleeding gums, avoid contact sports, use electric razor, avoid IM injection
- Advise patient to report any signs of bleeding: gums, under skin, urine,

stools; unusual bruising, hematoma at inj site

Treatment of overdose: Protamine sulfate 1% given **IV**

HIGH ALERT

argatroban (℞)

(are-ga-troe'ban)

Acova

Func. class.: Anticoagulant

Chem. class.: Thrombin inhibitor

Pregnancy Category B

Action: Direct inhibitor of thrombin that is derived from L-arginine; it reversibly binds to the thrombin active site

Therapeutic Outcome: Absence or decrease of thrombosis

Uses: Thrombosis, prophylaxis or treatment

Dosage and routes

Adult: **IV** 2 μg/kg/min (1 mg/ml) give at 6 ml/hr for 50 kg of weight, at 8 ml/hr for 70 kg of weight, at 11 ml/hr for 90 kg of weight, at 13 ml/hr for 110 kg of weight, at 16 ml/hr for 130 kg of weight

Available forms: Inj 100 mg/ml

Adverse effects

CNS: Fever

CV: **Atrial fibrillation, ventricular tachycardia**

GI: Nausea, vomiting, abdominal pain, diarrhea, **GI bleeding**

GU: Hematuria, abnormal kidney function, UTI

HEMA: **Hemorrhage, thrombocytopenia**

RESP: Pneumonia, dyspnea

SYST: **Sepsis**

Contraindications: Hypersensitivity, overt major bleeding

Precautions: Intracranial bleeding, renal function impairment, lactation, P children, hepatic disease, pregnancy **B**

Pharmacokinetics

Absorption	Unknown
Distribution	Unknown
Metabolism	Liver
Excretion	Feces
Half-life	39-51 min

Pharmacodynamics

Unknown

Interactions

Drug classifications

Anticoagulants: ↑ risk of bleeding

Thrombolytics: ↑ action of argatroban

NURSING CONSIDERATIONS

Assessment

- Obtain baseline APTT before treatment; do not start treatment if APTT ratio ≥ 2.5, then APTT 4 hr after initiation of treatment and at least qd thereafter; if APTT above target, stop inf for 2 hr, then restart at 50%, take APTT in 4 hr; if below target, increase inf rate by 20%, take APTT in 4 hr, do not exceed inf rate of 0.21 mg/kg/hr without checking for coagulation abnormalities
- Monitor APTT, which should be 1.5-3 × control
- Assess for bleeding gums, petechiae, ecchymosis, black tarry stools, hematuria/epistaxis, B/P, vaginal bleeding and possible hemorrhage
- Fever, skin rash, urticaria

Nursing diagnoses

- ✓ Decreased cardiac output (uses)
- ✓ Diarrhea (adverse reactions)
- ✓ Knowledge deficit (teaching)

Implementation

- Avoid all IM injections that may cause bleeding

IV infusion

- Dilute in 0.9% NaCl, D_5, LR to a final conc 1 mg/ml; dilute each 2.5-ml vial 100-fold by mixing with 250 ml of diluents, mix by repeated inversion of the diluent bag for 1 min; may be slightly hazy

- Dosage adjustment may be made after review of APTT, not to exceed 10 μg/kg/min

Patient/family education

- Advise patient to use soft-bristle toothbrush to avoid bleeding gums, avoid contact sports, use electric razor, avoid IM injection
- Instruct patient to report any signs of bleeding: gums, under skin, urine, stools

Evaluation

Positive therapeutic outcome

- Absence or decrease of thrombosis

HIGH ALERT

arsenic trioxide (℞)

Trisenox

Func. class.: Antineoplastic-miscellaneous

Pregnancy category D

Action: Not understood, causes morphologic changes and DNA fragmentation

➔ **Therapeutic Outcome:** Decrease in malignant cells

Uses: Acute promyelocytic leukemia

Dosage and routes

Induction

Adult: **IV** 0.15 mg/kg/day until bone marrow remission, max 60 doses

Consolidation treatment

Wait 3-6 wk after completion of induction

Adult: **IV** 0.15 mg/kg/day × 25 doses over a period of up to 5 wk

Available forms: Inj 1 mg/ml

Adverse effects

CNS: *Anxiety, confusion, insomnia,* headache, paresthesia, depression, dizziness, tremor, **seizures,** agitation, **coma,** weakness

CV: *Hypotension, hypertension,* prolonged QT interval, other ECG changes, chest pain, *tachycardia,* torsades de pointes

GI: *Abdominal pain, constipation, diarrhea, dyspepsia,* fecal incontinence, **GI hemorrhage,** dry mouth, *nausea, vomiting, anorexia*

GU: Vaginal hemorrhage, **renal failure,** incontinence

HEMA: Leukocytosis, anemia, thrombocytopenia, neutropenia, DIC

META: Increased ALT/AST, hyperkalemia, hypokalemia, hypomagnesemia, hyperglycemia

MISC: Weight gain or decrease, fatigue, severe edema, rigors, herpes simplex/zoster

RESP: **Pleural effusion,** dyspnea, cough, epistaxis, hypoxia, sinusitis, wheezing, rales, tachypnea

Contraindications: Hypersensitivity, pregnancy **D**

G P **Precautions:** Elderly, lactation, children

Pharmacokinetics	
Absorption	Unknown
Distribution	Stored in liver, kidney, heart, lung, hair, nails
Metabolism	Liver
Excretion	Kidneys
Half-life	Unknown

Pharmacodynamics

Unknown

Interactions

None known

NURSING CONSIDERATIONS

Assessment

! Monitor for APL differentiation syndrome: fever, dyspnea, pulmonary infiltrates, pleural or pericardial effusions, weight gain; this condition can be fatal; give high-dose steroids

- Assess for ECG changes: QT interval prolongation, complete AV block; obtain baseline ECG prior to drug therapy

- Monitor electrolytes: potassium, calcium, magnesium, creatine

Nursing diagnoses
✓ Risk for infection (adverse reactions)
✓ Altered nutrition: less than body requirements (adverse reactions)
✓ Knowledge deficit (teaching)

Implementation
IV **IV route**
- Dilute with 100-250 ml D_5 or 0.9% NaCl immediately after withdrawing from ampule, give over 1-2 hr; may give over 4 hr if reactions occur

Patient/family education
- Teach patient to report planned or suspected pregnancy
- Inform patient that fertility impairment has not been studied

Evaluation
Positive therapeutic outcome
- Decrease in malignant cells

Treatment of overdose:
- Dimercaprol 3 mg/kg IM q4h, then 250 mg penicillamine PO, max 4 ×/day (≤1 g/day)

ascorbic acid (vitamin C) (OTC, ℞)
(as-kor'bic)

Apo-C ✦, ascorbic acid, Ascorbicap, C-Span, Cebid, Cecon, Cecore 500, Cemill, Cenolate, Cetane, Cevalin, Cevi-Bid, Ce-Vi-Sol, C-Crystals, Flavorcee, Kamu-Jay ✦, Mega-C/A Plus, Ortho/CS, Sunkist

Func. class.: Vitamin C, water-soluble vitamin

Pregnancy category C

Action: Needed for wound healing, collagen synthesis, antioxidant, carbohydrate metabolism, protein, lipid synthesis, prevention of infection

➔ **Therapeutic Outcome:** Replacement and supplementation of vit C

Uses: Vit C deficiency, scurvy, delayed wound and bone healing, chronic disease, urine acidification, before gastrectomy; increased need: lactation, pregnancy, hyperthyroidism, emotional stress, trauma, burns

Investigational uses: Acidification of urine, common cold prevention

Dosage and routes
RDA

P ***Neonates and up to 6 mo:*** 30 mg

P ***Infants 6 mo-1 yr:*** 35 mg

P ***Child 1-3 yr:*** 40 mg

P ***Child 4-10 yr:*** 45 mg

P ***Child 11-14 yr:*** 50 mg

P ***Adult and child ≥15 yr:*** 60 mg

Pregnancy: 70 mg

Lactation: 90 mg

Scurvy

Adult: PO/SC/IM/**IV** 100 mg-500 mg qd × 2 wk, then 50 mg or more qd

P ***Child:*** PO/SC/IM/**IV** 100-300 mg qd × 2 wk, then 35 mg or more qd

Wound healing/chronic disease/fracture

Adult: SC/IM/**IV**/PO 200-500 mg qd

P ***Child:*** SC/IM/**IV**/PO 100-200 mg added doses

Urine acidification

Adult: 4-12 g qd in divided doses

P ***Child:*** 500 mg q6-8h

Available forms: Tabs 25, 50, 100, 250, 500, 1000, 1500 mg; effervescent tabs 1000 mg; chewable tabs 100, 250, 500 mg; timed release tabs 500, 750, 1000, 1500 mg; timed release caps 500 mg; crystals 4 g/tsp; powder 4 g/tsp; liq 35 mg/0.6 ml; sol 100 mg/ml; syr 20 mg/ml, 500 mg/5 ml; inj SC, IM, **IV** 100, 250, 500 mg/ml

Adverse effects
CNS: Headache, insomnia, dizziness, fatigue, flushing

GI: Nausea, vomiting, diarrhea, anorexia, heartburn, cramps
GU: Polyuria, urine acidification, oxalate or urate renal stones, dysuria
***HEMA:* Hemolytic anemia in patients with G6PD**
INTEG: Inflammation at inj site

Contraindications: None significant

Precautions: Gout, pregnancy **C**, diabetes, renal calculi (large doses)

Pharmacokinetics

Absorption	Readily absorbed (PO)
Distribution	Widely distributed; crosses placenta
Metabolism	Oxidation
Excretion	Kidneys, inactive; breast milk
Half-life	Unknown

Pharmacodynamics

Unknown

Interaction

Individual drugs

Deferoxamine: ↑ iron toxicity
Iron, oral: ↑ effect of oral iron
Mexiletine: ↑ excretion in acidic urine
Primadone: ↑ requirements for vit C

Drug classifications

Anticoagulants, oral: ↓ action of anticoagulants (large doses)
Antidepressants, tricyclic: ↑ excretion in acidic urine
Estrogens: ↑ effect of estrogen
Salicylates: ↑ requirements of vit C

Smoking

Smoking decreases vitamin C levels

Lab test interferences

↓ Bilirubin, ↓ urine oxalate, ↓ cysteine
False positive: negatives in glucose tests (Clinitest, Tes-Tape)
False negative: occult blood (large dose)

NURSING CONSIDERATIONS

A

Assessment

- Assess nutritional status for inclusion of foods high in vit C: citrus fruits, cantaloupe, tomatoes
- Assess for vit C deficiency before, during, and after treatment; scurvy (gingivitis, bleeding gums, loose teeth); poor bone development
- Monitor I&O ratio, polyuria; in patients receiving large doses renal stones may occur
- Monitor ascorbic acid levels throughout treatment if continued deficiency is suspected
- Assess inj sites for inflammation, pain, redness

Nursing diagnoses

✓ Nutrition, less than body requirements (uses)
✓ Knowledge deficit (teaching)

Implementation

IV IV route

- Give undiluted by *direct* **IV** 100 mg over at least 1 min, rapid inf may cause fainting
- Give by intermittent inf after diluting with D_5W, $D_{10}W$, 0.9% NaCl, 0.45% NaCl, LR, Ringer's sol, dextrose/saline, dextrose/Ringer's combinations; temperature will increase pressure in ampules; wrap with gauze before breaking

Syringe compatibilities:
Metoclopramide

Syringe incompatibilities:
Cefazolin, doxapram

Additive compatibilities:
Amikacin, calcium chloride, calcium gluceptate, calcium gluconate, cephalothin, chloramphenicol, chlorpromazine, colistimethate, cyanocobalamin, diphenhydramine, heparin, kanamycin, methicillin, methyldopate, penicillin G potassium, polymyxin B, prednisolone, procaine, prochlorperazine, promethazine, verapamil

Additive incompatibilities: Bleomycin, cephapirin, nafcillin, sodium bicarbonate, warfarin

Y-site compatibilities: Warfarin

PO route
- Mix oral sol with foods or fluids; ext rel caps should be swallowed whole
- Do not crush, break, or chew ext rel tab/cap

IM route
- Not to be diluted; give deep in large muscle mass

Patient/family education
- Teach patient necessary foods to be included in diet that are rich in vit C: citrus fruits, cantaloupe, tomatoes, chili peppers (red)
- Teach patient that smoking decreases vit C levels; not to exceed prescribed dose; increases will be excreted in urine, except time release
- Teach patient not to exceed RDA recommended dose, urinary stones may occur
- Teach patient using ascorbic acid for acidification of urine to test urine pH periodically

Evaluation
Positive therapeutic outcome
- Absence of anorexia, irritability, pallor, joint pain, hyperkeratosis, petechiae, poor wound healing
- Reversal of scurvy: bleeding gums, gingivitis, loose teeth

HIGH ALERT

asparaginase (℞)
(a-spar'a-gin-ase)
Elspar, Kidrolase
Func. class.: Antineoplastic
Chem. class.: Escherichia coli enzyme
Pregnancy category C

Action: Indirectly inhibits protein synthesis in tumor cells; without amino acids, DNA, RNA synthesis is halted; asparagine, protein synthesis is halted; G_1 phase of cell cycle specific; a nonvesicant

Therapeutic Outcome: Prevention of rapidly growing malignant cells in leukemia

Uses: Acute lymphocytic leukemia in combination with other antineoplastics unresponsive to other agents

Dosage and routes
In combination
Adult/child: **IV** 1000 IU/kg/day × 10 days given over 30 min; IM 6000 IU/m²/day

Sole induction
Adult/child: **IV** 200 IU/kg/day × 28 days

Desensitization
Adult/child: **IV**/ID test dose of 2 IU ID, then 1 IU, then double dose q10 min, until total dose is administered or reaction occurs

Available forms: Inj 10,000 IU with mannitol

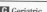

Adverse effects
CNS: Neuritis, dizziness, headache, **coma,** depression, fatigue, confusion, hallucinations, lethargy, drowsiness, agitation, Parkinson-like syndrome, **seizures**
CV: Chest pain
ENDO: Hyperglycemia
GI: *Nausea, vomiting, anorexia, cramps, stomatitis,* diarrhea, weight loss, **hepatotoxicity, pancreatitis**
GU: Urinary retention, **renal failure,** glycosuria, polyuria, azotemia, proteinuria, uric acid neuropathy
HEMA: **Thrombocytopenia, leukopenia, myelosuppression, anemia, decreased clotting factors** (V, VII, VIII, IX), decreased fibrinogen
INTEG: *Rash,* urticaria, chills, fever, perspiration
RESP: **Fibrosis, pulmonary infiltrate**
SYST: **Anaphylaxis**

A

Contraindications: Hypersensitivity, infants, lactation, pancreatitis

Precautions: Renal disease, hepatic disease, pregnancy **C**

Pharmacokinetics

Absorption	Complete bioavailability (**IV**)
Distribution	Intravascular spaces
Metabolism	Unknown
Excretion	Reticuloendothelial system
Half-life	8-30 hr (**IV**), 39-49 hr (IM)

Pharmacodynamics

	IV	IM
Onset	Immediate	Immediate
Peak	14-24 hr	Unknown
Duration	3-5 wk	3-5 wk

Interactions

Individual drugs

Methotrexate: Blocked action of methotrexate

Vincristine: ↑ neurotoxicity

Drug classifications

Glucocorticosteroids: ↑ hyperglycemia

Hepatotoxic agents: ↑ hepatotoxicity

Live virus vaccines: ↓ response of vaccines

Lab test interferences

↓ Thyroid function tests

NURSING CONSIDERATIONS

Assessment

- Assess for signs and symptoms of pancreatitis (nausea, vomiting, severe abdominal pain), anaphylaxis (bronchospasm, dyspnea), cyanosis; monitor amylase, glucose; more toxic in adults than children
- Assess symptoms indicating severe allergic reaction: rash, pruritus, urticaria, purpuric skin lesions, itching, flushing; joint pain, bronchospasm, hypotension; epinephrine and emergency equipment should be nearby
- Monitor for frequency of stools, characteristics: cramping, acidosis; signs of dehydration: rapid respirations, poor skin turgor, decreased urine output, dry skin, restlessness, weakness
- Monitor CBC, differential, platelet count weekly; withhold drug if WBC is <4000/mm^3 or platelet count is <100,000/mm^3, notify prescriber of results; also monitor PT, PTT, and TT, which may be increased
- Monitor pulmonary function tests, chest x-ray studies before, during therapy; chest x-ray film should be obtained q2 wk during treatment
- Monitor renal function studies: BUN, serum uric acid, ammonia urine CrCl, electrolytes before, during therapy
- Check I&O ratio; report fall in urine output of 30/ml/hr
- Monitor temperature q4h; may indicate beginning infection
- Obtain liver function tests before, during therapy (bilirubin, AST, ALT, LDH) as needed or monthly
- Monitor RBC, Hct, Hgb, since these may be decreased; serum, urine glucose levels
- Assess for bleeding: hematuria, guaiac, bruising or petechiae, mucosa, or orifices q8h
- Assess for dyspnea, rales, nonproductive cough, chest pain, tachypnea, fatigue, increased pulse, pallor, lethargy, or swelling around eyes or lips; anaphylaxis may occur
- Assess for yellowing of skin and sclera, dark urine, clay-colored stools, itchy skin, abdominal pain, fever, diarrhea

Nursing diagnoses

✓ Injury, risk for (uses, adverse reactions)

✓ Body image disturbance (adverse reactions)

Implementation

- Give after intradermal skin testing and desensitization, give 0.1 ml (2 IU) intradermally after reconstituting with 5 ml sterile H_2O or 0.9% NaCl for inj; then add 0.1 ml of reconstituted drug to 9.9 ml diluent (20 IU/ml); observe for 1 hr, check for wheal

- Use allopurinol or sodium bicarbonate to reduce uric acid levels, alkalinization of urine

IM route

- Reconstitute with 2 ml 0.9% NaCl/10,000 IU/vial, refrigerate, use within 8 hr, discard sooner if sol becomes cloudy

IV **IV route**

- Give by **IV** inf using 21-, 23-, 25-gauge needle; administer by slow **IV** inf via Y-tube or 3-way stopcock of flowing D_5W or 0.9% NaCl inf over 30 min after diluting 10,000 IU/5 ml of sterile H_2O or 0.9% NaCl (no preservatives) (2000 IU/ml); use of filter may be necessary if fibers are present

Y-site compatibilities: Methotrexate, sodium bicarbonate

Patient/family education

- Teach patient to report any complaints or side effects to nurse or physician
- Teach patient to report any changes in breathing or coughing

Evaluation

Positive therapeutic response

- Decreased replication of leukemia cells

Treatment of anaphylaxis: Administer epinephrine, diphenhydramine, **IV** corticosteroids, O_2

aspirin (OTC)

(as'pir-in)

Acuprin, Artria S.R., A.S.A., Aspergum, Aspirin ♣, Aspir-Low, Aspirtab, Astrin ♣, Bayer Aspirin, Coryphen ♣, Easprin, Ecotrin, 8-Hour Bayer Timed Release, Empirin, Entrophen ♣, Halfprin, Norwich Extra-Strength, Novasen ♣, PMS-ASA ♣, Sloprin, St. Joseph Children's Supasa ♣, Therapy Bayer, ZORprin

Func. class.: Nonnarcotic analgesic

Chem. class.: Salicylate

Pregnancy category D (3rd trimester)

Action: Blocks pain impulses in CNS, inhibition of prostaglandin synthesis; antipyretic action results from vasodilatation of peripheral vessels; decreases platelet aggregation

Therapeutic Outcome: Decreased pain, inflammation, fever; absence of MI, transient ischemic attacks, thrombosis

Uses: Mild to moderate pain or fever including rheumatoid arthritis, osteoarthritis, thromboembolic disorders, transient ischemic attacks in men, rheumatic fever, post-MI, prophylaxis of MI

Investigational uses: Prevention of cataracts (long-term use), prevention of pregnancy loss in women with clotting disorders

Dosage and routes

Arthritis

Adult: PO 2.6-5.2 g/day in divided doses q4-6h

P ***Child:*** PO 90-130 mg/kg/day in divided doses q4-6h

Kawasaki disease

P ***Child:*** PO 80-120 mg/kg/day in 4 divided doses, maintenance 3-8 mg/kg/day as a single dose × 8 wk

MI, stroke prophylaxis
Adult: PO 81-650 mg/day
Pain/fever
Adult: PO/REC 325-650 mg q4h prn, not to exceed 4 g/day
P ***Child:*** PO/REC 40-100 mg/kg/day in divided doses q4-6h prn
Thromboembolic disorders
Adult: PO 325-650 mg/day or bid
Transient ischemic attacks
Adult: PO 650 mg qid or 325 mg qid

Available forms: Tabs 81, 162.5, 325, 500, 650, 975 mg; chewable tabs 80, 81 mg; supp 60, 120, 125, 130, 150, 160, 195, 200, 300, 320, 325, 600, 640, 650 mg, 1.2 g; cream; gum 227.5 mg; dispersible tabs 325, 500 mg; tabs delayed release, enteric coated 80, 165, 300, 325, 500, 600, 650, 975 mg; ext rel 325, 650, 800 mg; del rel caps 325, 500 mg

Adverse effects

CNS: Stimulation, drowsiness, dizziness, confusion, **convulsion,** headache, flushing, hallucinations, **coma**
CV: Rapid pulse, pulmonary edema
EENT: Tinnitus, hearing loss
ENDO: Hypoglycemia, hyponatremia, hypokalemia
GI: *Nausea, vomiting,* **GI bleeding,** diarrhea, heartburn, anorexia, **hepatitis**
HEMA: **Thrombocytopenia, agranulocytosis, leukopenia, neutropenia, hemolytic anemia,** increased pro-time, PTT, bleeding time
INTEG: *Rash,* urticaria, bruising
RESP: Wheezing, hyperpnea
P ***SYST:*** **Reye's syndrome (children)**

Contraindications: Hypersensitivity to salicylates, tartrazine (FDC yellow dye #5), GI bleeding, bleeding P disorders, children <12 yr, children with flulike symptoms, pregnancy **D** (3rd trimester), lactation, vitamin K deficiency, peptic ulcer

Precautions: Anemia, hepatic disease, renal disease, Hodgkin's disease, pre/postoperatively, gastritis, asthmatic patients with nasal polyps or aspirin sensitivity

Pharmacokinetics

Absorption	Well absorbed, small intestine (PO); erratic (enteric); slow (rec)
Distribution	Rapidly, widely distributed; crosses placenta
Metabolism	Liver, extensively
Excretion	Inactive metabolites, kidney; breast milk
Half-life	2-3 hr (low doses); 30 hr (high doses)

Pharmacodynamics

	PO	REC
Onset	15-30 min	Slow
Peak	1-2 hr	4-5 hr
Duration	4-6 hr	6-7 hr

Interactions

Individual drugs
Alcohol: ↑ bleeding
Ammonium chloride: ↑ salicylate level
Cefamandole: ↑ bleeding
Furosemide: ↑ toxic effects
Heparin: ↑ bleeding
Insulin: ↑ effects of insulin
Methotrexate: ↑ effects of methotrexate
Nizatidine: ↑ salicylate level
PABA: ↑ toxic effects
Phenytoin: ↑ effects of phenytoin
Plicamycin: ↑ bleeding
Probenecid: ↓ effects of probenecid
Spironolactone: ↓ effects
Sulfinpyrazone: ↓ effects
Drug classifications
Antacids: ↓ effects of aspirin
Anticoagulants: ↑ bleeding
Carbonic anhydrase inhibitors: ↑ toxic effects
Corticosteroids: ↓ effects of aspirin
NSAIDs: ↑ gastric ulcers

Penicillins: ↑ effects of penicillins
Salicylates: ↓ blood sugar levels
Steroids: ↓ effects of aspirin, ↑ gastric ulcers
Sulfonylamides: ↓ effects of sulfonylamides
Urinary acidifiers: ↑ salicylate levels
Urinary alkalizers: ↓ effects of aspirin

Herb/drug
Horse chestnut: ↑ risk of bleeding
Kelpware: ↑ risk of bleeding

Lab test interferences
↑ Coagulation studies, ↑ liver function studies, ↑ serum uric acid, ↑ amylase, ↑ CO_2, ↑ urinary protein
↓ Serum potassium, ↓ PBI, ↓ cholesterol
Interference: Urine catecholamines, pregnancy test, urine glucose tests (Clinistix, Tes-Tape)

NURSING CONSIDERATIONS
Assessment
- Monitor liver function studies: AST, ALT, bilirubin, creatinine if patient is on long-term therapy
- Monitor renal function studies: BUN, urine creatinine if patient is on long-term therapy
- Monitor blood studies: CBC, Hct, Hgb, pro-time if patient is on long-term therapy
- Check I&O ratio; decreasing output may indicate renal failure (long-term therapy)
- (Alert) Assess hepatotoxicity: dark urine, clay-colored stools, yellowing of the skin and sclera, itching, abdominal pain, fever, diarrhea if patient is on long-term therapy
- Assess for allergic reactions: rash, urticaria; if these occur, drug may have to be discontinued
- Assess for ototoxicity: tinnitus, ringing, roaring in ears; audiometric testing needed before, after long-term therapy
- Assess for visual changes: blurring, halos; corneal, retinal damage
- Check edema in feet, ankles, legs
- Identify prior drug history; there are many drug interactions
- Monitor pain: location, duration, type, intensity, before dose and 1 hr after
- Monitor musculoskeletal status: ROM before dose
- Identify fever: length of time and related symptoms

Nursing diagnoses
- ✓ Pain (uses)
- ✓ Mobility, impaired physical (uses)
- ✓ Injury, risk for (side effects)
- ✓ Knowledge deficit (teaching)

Implementation
PO route
- Administer to patient crushed or whole; chewable tab may be chewed
- (Do Not Crush) Do not crush enteric product
- Give with food or milk to decrease gastric symptoms; give 30 min before or 2 hr pc; absorption may be slowed
- Give antacids 1-2 hr after enteric products

Patient/family education
- Teach patient to report any symptoms of hepatotoxicity, renal toxicity, visual changes, ototoxicity, allergic reactions, bleeding (long-term therapy)
- Instruct patient to take with 8 oz of water and sit upright for 30 min after dose; to discard tabs if vinegar-like smell is present
- Instruct patient not to exceed recommended dosage; acute poisoning may result
- Advise patient to read label on other OTC drugs; many contain aspirin
- Inform patient that the therapeutic response takes 2 wk (arthritis); give ½ hr before planned exercise
- Teach patient to report tinnitus, confusion, diarrhea, sweating, hyperventilation
- Advise patient to avoid alcohol ingestion; GI bleeding may occur
- Advise patient with allergies that allergic reactions may develop

- Instruct patient to avoid buffered or effervescent products

P • Teach patient not to give to children or teens with flu-like symptoms or chicken pox; Reye's syndrome may develop

Evaluation

Positive therapeutic outcome

- Decreased pain
- Decreased inflammation
- Decreased fever
- Absence of MI
- Absence of transient ischemic attacks, thrombosis

Treatment of overdose: Lavage, activated charcoal, monitor electrolytes, VS

atenolol (℞)

(a-ten'oh-lole)

Apo-Atenolol ♣, atenolol, Novo-Atenol ♣, Tenormin

Func. class.: Antihypertensive

Chem. class.: β-Blocker; β_1-; β_2-blocker (high doses)

Pregnancy category D

Action: Competitively blocks stimulation of β-adrenergic receptor within vascular smooth muscle; produces negative chronotropic activity, positive inotropic activity (decreases rate of SA node discharge, increases recovery time), slows conduction of AV node, decreases heart rate, decreases O_2 consumption in myocardium; also decreases renin-aldosterone-angiotensin system at high doses, inhibits β_2-receptors in bronchial system at higher doses

➔ **Therapeutic Outcome:** Decreased B/P, heart rate, prevention of angina pectoris, MI

Uses: Mild to moderate hypertension; prophylaxis of angina pectoris; suspected or known MI (**IV** use)

Investigational uses: Dysrhythmia, mitral valve prolapse, pheochromocytoma, hypertrophic cardiomyopathy, vascular headaches, thyrotoxicosis, tremors, alcohol withdrawal

Dosage and routes

Adult: **IV** 5 mg; repeat in 10 min if initial dose is well tolerated, then start PO dose 10 min after last **IV** dose

Adult: PO 50 mg qd, increasing q1-2 wk to 100 mg qd; may increase to 200 mg qd for angina

G ***Elderly:*** PO 25 mg/day initially

Renal dose

CrCl 15-35 ml/min, max 50 mg/day; CrCl <15 ml/min max 50 mg qod; hemodialysis 25-50 mg after dialysis

Available forms: Tabs 25, 50, 100 mg; **IV** 5 mg/10 ml

Adverse effects

CNS: *Insomnia, fatigue, dizziness, mental changes,* memory loss, hallucinations, depression, lethargy, drowsiness, strange dreams, catatonia

CV: **Profound hypotension, bradycardia, CHF, cold extremities, postural hypotension, 2nd- or 3rd-degree heart block**

EENT: Sore throat, dry burning eyes

ENDO: Increased hypoglycemic response to insulin

GI: *Nausea, diarrhea,* vomiting, **mesenteric arterial thrombosis, ischemic colitis**

GU: Impotence

HEMA: **Agranulocytosis, thrombocytopenia, purpura**

INTEG: Rash, fever, alopecia

RESP: **Bronchospasm,** dyspnea, wheezing

Contraindications: Hypersensitivity to β-blockers, cardiogenic shock, 2nd- or 3rd-degree heart block, sinus bradycardia, CHF, cardiac failure, pregnancy **D**

Precautions: Major surgery, lactation, diabetes mellitus, renal disease, thyroid disease, COPD, asthma, well-compensated heart failure

Do Not Confuse:
atenolol/albuterol, Tenormin/thiamine

Pharmacokinetics	
Absorption	50%-60% (PO)
Distribution	Crosses placenta; protein binding (5%-15%)
Metabolism	Not metabolized
Excretion	Breast milk, kidneys (50%), feces (50%—unabsorbed drug)
Half-life	6-7 hr

Pharmacodynamics	
	PO
Onset	1 hr
Peak	2-4 hr
Duration	24 hr

Interactions

Individual drugs

Alcohol: ↑ hypotension (large amounts)
Diltiazem: ↑ hypotension, bradycardia
Epinephrine: α-Adrenergic stimulation
Hydralazine: ↑ hypotension, bradycardia
Indomethacin: ↓ antihypertensive effect
Insulin: ↑ hypoglycemia
Methyldopa: ↑ hypotension, bradycardia
Prazosin: ↑ hypotension, bradycardia
Reserpine: ↑ hypotension, bradycardia
Thyroid: ↓ effectiveness of atenolol
Verapamil: ↑ myocardial depression

Drug classifications

Antidiabetics, oral: ↑ hypoglycemia
Antihypertensives: ↑ hypertension
β_2-Agonist: ↓ bronchodilatation
Cardiac glycosides: ↑ bradycardia
Nitrates: ↑ hypotension
Theophyllines: ↓ bronchodilatation

Lab test interferences

↑ Uric acid, ↑ potassium, ↑ triglyceride, ↑ lipoproteins
Interference: Glucose, insulin tolerance tests

NURSING CONSIDERATIONS

Assessment

- Monitor B/P during beginning treatment, periodically thereafter; pulse q4h; note rate, rhythm, quality: apical/radial pulse before administration; notify prescriber of any significant changes (pulse <50 bpm)
- Check for baselines in renal, liver function tests before therapy begins
- Assess for edema in feet, legs daily; monitor I&O, daily weight; check for jugular vein distention, rales bilaterally, dyspnea (CHF)
- Monitor skin turgor, dryness of mucous membranes for hydration status, especially elderly [G]

Nursing diagnoses

- ✓ Cardiac output, decreased (uses)
- ✓ Injury, risk for physical (side effects)
- ✓ Knowledge deficit (teaching)
- ✓ Noncompliance (teaching)

Implementation

PO route

- Given ac, hs, tablet may be crushed or swallowed whole; give with food to prevent GI upset; reduced dosage in renal dysfunction
- Store protected from light, moisture; place in cool environment

[IV] **IV route**

- Give **IV** direct over 5 min or diluted in 10-50 ml D_5W, 0.9% NaCl, and give at prescribed rate

Y-site compatibilities:
Meperidine, meropenem, morphine

Patient/family education

- [Alert] Teach patient not to discontinue drug abruptly; taper over 2 wk; may cause precipitate angina if stopped abruptly
- Teach patient not to use OTC products containing α-adrenergic

stimulants (such as nasal decongestants, OTC cold preparations); to limit alcohol, smoking; to limit sodium intake as prescribed
- Teach patient how to take pulse and B/P at home; advise when to notify prescriber
- Instruct patient to comply with weight control, dietary adjustments, modified exercise program
- Advise patient to carry/wear Medic Alert ID for drugs and allergies; tell patient drug controls symptoms but does not cure
- Caution patient to avoid hazardous activities if dizziness, drowsiness is present
- Teach patient to report symptoms of CHF: difficult breathing, especially on exertion or when lying down, night cough, swelling of extremities or bradycardia, dizziness, confusion, depression, fever
- Teach patient to take drug as prescribed, not to double doses, skip doses; take any missed doses as remembered if at least 6 hr until next dose
- Advise patient that drug may mask symptoms of hypoglycemia in diabetic patients
- Advise patient to use contraception while taking this drug

Evaluation

Positive therapeutic outcome
- Decreased B/P in hypertension (after 1-2 wk)
- Absence of dysrhythmias
- Absence of MI
- Decreased angina

Treatment of overdose:
Lavage, **IV** atropine for bradycardia, **IV** theophylline for bronchospasm, digitalis, O_2, diuretic for cardiac failure, hemodialysis, **IV** glucose for hyperglycemia, **IV** diazepam (or phenytoin) for seizures

atorvastatin (℞)
(at-or′va-sta-tin)
Lipitor
Func. class.: Antilipidemic
Chem. class.: HMG-CoA reductase inhibitor

Pregnancy category X

Action: Inhibits HMG-CoA reductase enzyme, which reduces cholesterol synthesis

➔ Therapeutic Outcome: Decreased cholesterol levels and LDLs, increased HDLs

Uses: As an adjunct in primary hypercholesterolemia (types Ia, Ib), dysbetalipoproteinemia, elevated triglyceride levels

Dosage and routes
Adult: PO 10 mg qd, usual range 10-80, dosage adjustments may be made in 2-4 wk intervals

Available forms: Tabs 10, 20, 40 mg

Adverse effects
CNS: Headache
EENT: Lens opacities
GI: Dyspepsia, flatus, *liver dysfunction,* pancreatitis
INTEG: Rash, pruritus, alopecia
MS: Myalgia

Contraindications: Hypersensitivity, pregnancy **X**, lactation, active liver disease

Precautions: Past liver disease, alcoholism, severe acute infections, trauma, hypotension, uncontrolled seizure disorders, severe metabolic disorders, electrolyte imbalance

Pharmacokinetics	
Absorption	Unknown
Distribution	Unknown
Metabolism	Liver
Excretion	Bile, feces, kidneys
Half-life	14 hr

Pharmacodynamics
Unknown

Interactions
Individual drugs
Cholestyramine: ↓ action of atorvastatin
Clofibrate: ↑ risk of rhabdomyolysis
Colestipol: ↓ action of atorvastatin
Cyclosporine: ↑ risk of rhabdomyolysis
Digoxin: ↑ action of digoxin
Erythromycin: ↑ risk of rhabdomyolysis
Gemfibrozil: ↑ risk of rhabdomyolysis
Niacin: ↑ risk of rhabdomyolysis
Warfarin: ↑ action of warfarin
Drug classifications
Azole antifungals: Possible rhabdomyolysis
Oral contraceptives: ↑ action

NURSING CONSIDERATIONS
Assessment
- Assess nutrition: fat, protein, carbohydrates; nutritional analysis should be completed by dietician before treatment
- Assess for muscle pain, tenderness, obtain CPK if these occur, drug may need to be discontinued
- Monitor bowel pattern daily; diarrhea may be a problem
- Monitor triglycerides, cholesterol at baseline and throughout treatment; LDL and VLDL should be watched closely; if increased, drug should be discontinued
- Monitor liver function studies q1-2 mo during the first 1½ yr of treatment; AST, ALT, liver function tests may be increased
- Monitor renal studies in patients with compromised renal system: BUN, I&O ratio, creatinine
- Assess eyes via ophthalmic exam 1 mo after treatment begins, annually

Nursing diagnoses
✓ Diarrhea (adverse reactions)
✓ Knowledge deficit (teaching)
✓ Noncompliance (teaching)

Implementation
- Administer total daily dose at any time of day
- Store in cool environment in airtight, light-resistant container

Patient/family education
- Inform patient that compliance is needed for positive results to occur, not to double doses
- Teach patient that risk factors should be decreased: high-fat diet, smoking, alcohol consumption, absence of exercise
- Advise patient to notify prescriber if the GI symptoms of diarrhea, abdominal or epigastric pain, nausea, vomiting; chills, fever, sore throat; muscle pain, weakness occur
- Advise patient that treatment will take several years
- Advise patient that blood work and eye exam will be necessary during treatment
- Advise not to take if pregnant
- Advise patient to stay out of the sun or use sunscreen to prevent photosensitivity (rare)

Evaluation
Positive therapeutic outcome
- Decreased cholesterol levels, serum triglyceride
- Improved ratio of HDLs

atovaquone (℞)
(a-toe'va-kwon)
Mepron
Func. class.: Antiprotozoal
Chem. class.: Aromatic diamide derivative; analog of ubiquinone

Pregnancy category C

Action: Interferes with DNA/RNA synthesis in protozoa, specifically ATP and nucleic acid synthesis

➔ Therapeutic Outcome: Antiprotozoal for *Pneumocystis carinii* only

Uses: *Pneumocystis carinii* infections in patients intolerant of trimethoprim/sulfamethoxazole (co-trimoxazole)

Dosage and routes

Adult and adolescents 13-16 yr: PO 750 mg bid with food tid for 21 days

Available forms: 750 mg/5 ml

Adverse effects

CNS: *Dizziness, headache, anxiety,* insomnia

CV: Hypotension

GI: *Nausea, vomiting, diarrhea,* anorexia, increased AST and ALT, acute pancreatitis, constipation, abdominal pain

HEMA: Anemia, **leukopenia, neutropenia**

INTEG: Pruritus, urticaria, *rash,* oral monilia

META: Hyperkalemia, hypoglycemia, hyponatremia

Contraindications: Hypersensitivity or history of developing life-threatening allergic reactions to any component of the formulation

Precautions: Blood dyscrasias, hepatic disease, diabetes mellitus, P pregnancy **C,** lactation, children, G elderly

Do Not Confuse:
Mepron (U.S.)/Mepron (meprobamate in Australia)

Pharmacokinetics

Absorption	Poor; increased when taken with fatty foods
Distribution	Unknown
Metabolism	Hepatic recycling
Excretion	Feces, unchanged (94%)
Half-life	2-3 days

Pharmacodynamics

Onset	Unknown
Peak	1-8 hr

Interactions

Individual drugs

Rifampin: ↓ effectiveness of atovaquone

Rifabutin: ↓ effectiveness of atovaquone

Drug classifications

Use cautiously with highly protein-bound drugs

Food/drug

↑ absorption of drug, especially fatty foods

NURSING CONSIDERATIONS

Assessment

- Assess for *Pneumocystis carinii:* monitor WBC, bilateral lung sounds, sputum for C&S; these should be checked before, periodically during, and after treatment; after collection of 1st sputum, therapy may begin
- Monitor for symptoms of hyponatremia: *CV:* increased B/P, cold, clammy skin, hypovolemia or hypervolemia; *GI:* anorexia, nausea, vomiting, diarrhea, abdominal cramps; *neuro:* lethargy, increased ICP, confusion, headache, seizures, coma, fatigue, tremors, hyperreflexia
- Monitor for symptoms of hypoglycemia/hyperglycemia in diabetic patients
- Monitor blood studies: blood glucose, CBC, platelets; I&O ratio; ECG for cardiac dysrhythmias, check B/P; liver studies: AST, ALT
- Monitor for signs of infection; anemia; monitor bowel pattern before, during treatment
- Monitor respiratory status: rate, character, wheezing, dyspnea
- Assess for dizziness, confusion, hallucination
- Assess for allergies before treatment, reaction of each medication; place allergies on chart; notify all people giving drugs

Nursing diagnoses
- ✓ Infection, risk for (uses)
- ✓ Diarrhea (adverse reactions)
- ✓ Knowledge deficit (teaching)

Implementation
- Give with food (preferably fatty); increased absorption of the drug and higher plasma concentrations will occur; give tid × 3 wk

Patient/family education
- Instruct patient to take with food, preferably fatty foods, to increase plasma concentrations
- Advise patient to take drug exactly as prescribed

Evaluation
Positive therapeutic outcome
- Decreased temperature
- Ability to breathe
- Three negative sputum cultures

HIGH ALERT

atropine ◊ (℞)
(a'troe-peen)

Atro-Pen

Methotrexate: ↑ blood levels, ↑ toxicity

Func. class.: Antidysrhythmic, anticholinergic parasympatholytic, mydriatic

Chem. class.: Belladonna alkaloid

Pregnancy category C

Action: Blocks acetylcholine at parasympathetic neuroeffector sites; increases cardiac output, heart rate by blocking vagal stimulation in heart; dries secretions, decreases sweating, salivation in low doses; mydriasis, increased heart rate and cycloplegia occur at moderate doses; motility of GI, GU systems at high dose

➔ **Therapeutic Outcome:** Drying of secretions, increased heart rate, cycloplegia, mydriasis

Uses: Bradycardia, bradydysrhythmia, reversal of anticholinesterase agents, insecticide poisoning, blocking cardiac vagal reflexes, decreasing secretions before surgery, antispasmodic with GU and biliary surgery, bronchodilator; opthalmically for cycloplegia, mydriasis

Dosage and routes
Bradycardia/ bradydysrhythmias
Adult: **IV** bol 0.5-1 mg given q3-5 min, not to exceed 2 mg

P ***Child:*** **IV** bol 0.01-0.03 mg/kg up to 0.4 mg or 0.3 mg/m^2; may repeat q4-6h, min dose 0.1 mg to avoid paradoxical reaction

Organophosphate poisoning
P ***Adult and child:*** IM/**IV** 2 mg qh until muscarinic symptoms disappear; may need 6 mg qh

Before surgery
Adult: SC/IM/**IV** 0.4-0.6 mg before anesthesia

P ***Child:*** SC 0.1-0.4 mg 30 min before surgery

Cycloplegic refraction
Adult: OPHTH i-ii gtt of 1% sol 1 hr before exam

P ***Child:*** OPHTH i-ii gtt of 0.5% sol bid-tid for up to 3 days before and 1 hr after exam

GI disorders
Adult: PO 0.3-1.2 mg q4-6h

Available forms: Inj 0.05, 0.1, 0.3, 0.4, 0.5, 0.8, 1 mg/ml; 2 mg/0.7 ml autoinjector; tabs 0.4 mg

Adverse effects
CNS: Headache, dizziness, involuntary movement, confusion, psychosis, anxiety, coma, flushing, drowsiness, G insomnia, weakness, delirium (elderly)

CV: Hypotension, paradoxic bradycardia, angina, PVCs, hypertension, tachycardia, ectopic ventricular beats

EENT: Blurred vision, photophobia, glaucoma, eye pain, pupil dilatation, nasal congestion

A

GI: Dry mouth, nausea, vomiting, abdominal pain, anorexia, constipation, paralytic ileus, abdominal distention, altered taste
GU: Retention, hesitancy, impotence, dysuria
INTEG: Rash, urticaria, contact dermatitis, dry skin, flushing
MISC: Suppression of lactation, decreased sweating

Contraindications: Hypersensitivity to belladonna alkaloids, angle closure glaucoma, GI obstructions, myasthenia gravis, thyrotoxicosis, ulcerative colitis, prostatic hypertrophy, tachycardia/tachydysrhythmias, asthma, acute hemorrhage, hepatic disease, myocardial ischemia

Precautions: Pregnancy **C**, renal disease, lactation, CHF, tachydysrhythmias, hyperthyroidism, COPD, hepatic disease, **P** child <6 yr, hypertension, **G** elderly, intraabdominal infections, Down syndrome, spastic paralysis, gastric ulcer

Pharmacokinetics

Absorption	Well absorbed(PO, SC, IM)
Distribution	Crosses blood-brain barrier, placenta
Metabolism	Liver
Excretion	Kidneys, unchanged (70%-90%); breast milk
Half-life	13-40 hr

Pharmacodynamics

	PO	IM/SC	IV	OPHTH
Onset	½ hr	15 min	2-4 min	½ hr
Peak	½-1 hr	30 min	2-4 min	30-60 min
Duration	4-6 hr	4-6 hr	4-6 hr	1-2 wk

Interactions
Individual drugs
Disopyramide: ↑ anticholinergic effect
Ketoconazole: ↓ absorption
Levodopa: ↓ absorption
Potassium chloride, oral: ↑ GI lesions

Drug classifications
Antacids: ↓ absorption of atropine
Anticholinergics: ↑ anticholinergic effect
Antidepressants, tricyclic: ↑ anticholinergic effect
Antihistamines: ↑ anticholinergic effect
Antiparkinson agents: ↑ anticholinergic effects

Herb/drug
Aloe: ↑ atropine action
Buckthorn bark/berry: ↑ atropine action
Cascara sagrada bark: ↑ atopine action
Rhubarb root: ↑ atropine action
Senna leaf/fruits: ↑ atropine action

NURSING CONSIDERATIONS
Assessment
- Monitor I&O ratio; check for urinary retention and daily output in **G** elderly or postoperative patients
- Monitor ECG for ectopic ventricular beats, PVC, tachycardia in cardiac patients
- Monitor for bowel sounds; check for constipation; abdominal distention and constipation may occur
- Monitor respiratory status: rate, rhythm, cyanosis, wheezing, dyspnea, engorged neck veins
- Monitor for increased intraocular pressure: eye pain, nausea, vomiting, blurred vision, increased tearing; discontinue use if pain occurs (optic)
- Monitor cardiac rate: rhythm, character, B/P continuously
- Monitor allergic reaction: rash, urticaria

Nursing diagnoses
✓ Cardiac output, decreased (uses)
✓ Sensory-perceptual alteration: visual (adverse reactions)
✓ Constipation (adverse reactions)
✓ Knowledge deficit (teaching)

Implementation
IV **IV route**
- Give **IV** undiluted or diluted with

10 ml sterile H_2O; give at a rate of 0.6 mg/min; give through Y-tube or 3-way stopcock; do not add to **IV** sol; may cause paradoxic bradycardia lasting 2 min

Syringe compatibilities:
Benzquinamide, butorphanol, chlorpromazine, cimetidine, dimenhydrinate, diphenhydramine, droperidol, fentanyl, glycopyrrolate, heparin, hydromorphone, hydroxyzine, meperidine, metoclopramide, midazolam, milrinone, morphine, nalbuphine, pentazocine, perphenazine, prochlorperazine, promazine, promethazine, propiomazine, ranitidine, scopolamine, sufentanil, vit B with C

Y-site compatibilities:
Amrinone, etomidate, famotidine, heparin, hydrocortisone sodium succinate, meropenem, nafcillin, potassium chloride, sufentanil, vit B/C

Additive compatibilities:
Dobutamine, furosemide, meropenem, netilmicin, sodium bicarbonate, verapamil

PO route
- PO 30 min ac
- Give increased bulk, water in diet if constipation occurs (anticholinergic effect)

IM route
- Expect atropine flush 15-20 min after inj; it may occur in children and is not harmful

Patient/family education
- Advise patient not to perform strenuous activity in high temperatures; heat stroke may result
- Instruct patient to take as prescribed; not to skip doses
- Instruct patient to report change in vision; blurring or loss of sight; trouble breathing; sweating; flushing, chest pain, allergic reactions, constipation, urinary retention
- Caution patient not to operate machinery if drowsiness occurs
- Advise patient not to take OTC products without approval of physician

Ophthalmic route
- Teach patient method of instillation: pressure on lacrimal sac for 1 min; do not touch dropper to eye
- Instruct patient that blurred vision will decrease with repeated use of drug; to omit next instillation if side effects are present
- Instruct patient not to perform hazardous tasks until able to see
- Advise patient to wait 5 min to use other drops; not to blink more than usual; use sunglasses to protect eyes

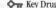

Evaluation
Positive therapeutic outcome
- Decreased dysrhythmias
- Increased heart rate
- Decreased secretions, GI, GU spasms
- Bronchodilatation
- Decrease in inflammation (iritis) or cycloplegic refraction (ophthalmic)

Treatment of overdose: O_2, artificial ventilation, ECG; administer dopamine for circulatory depression; administer diazepam or thiopental for convulsion; assess need for antidysrhythmics

attapulgite (OTC)
(at-a-pull'gite)

Diar Aid, Diasorb, Fowler's Diarrhea Tablets ✤, Hydrated Magnesium Silicate, Kaopectate, Kaopectate Advanced Formula, Kaopectate Maximum Strength, Parepectolin, Rheaban, St. Joseph Antidiarrheal

Func. class.: Antidiarrheal
Chem. class.: Hydrous magnesium aluminum silicate

Pregnancy class C

Action: Decreases gastric motility, water content of stool; adsorbent, demulcent

Therapeutic Outcome: Decreased diarrhea

Uses: Diarrhea (cause undetermined), mild to moderate

Dosage and routes

Adult: PO 60-120 ml (45-90 ml conc) after each loose bowel movement

P ***Child >12 yr:*** PO 60 ml after each loose bowel movement

P ***Child 6-12 yr:*** PO 30-60 ml (30 ml conc) after each loose bowel movement

P ***Child 3-6 yr:*** PO 15-30 ml (15 ml conc) after each loose bowel movement

Available forms: Susp kaolin 0.87 g/5 ml, pectin 43 mg/5 ml; kaolin 0.98 g/5 ml, pectin 21.7 mg/5 ml

Adverse effects

GI: Constipation (chronic use)

Precautions: Pregnancy **C**

Pharmacokinetics	
Absorption	Not absorbed
Distribution	Unknown
Metabolism	Unknown
Excretion	Unknown
Half-life	Unknown

Pharmacodynamics

Unknown

Interactions

All drugs: ↓ action of all other drugs

Nursing diagnoses

- ✓ Diarrhea (uses)
- ✓ Constipation (adverse reactions)
- ✓ Knowledge deficit (teaching)

NURSING CONSIDERATIONS

Assessment

- Assess bowel pattern before, during, and after treatment; check for rebound constipation
- P Monitor for dehydration in children

Implementation

- For 48 hr only after each diarrhea stool

Patient/family education

- Advise patient not to exceed recommended dosage; notify prescriber if symptoms continue
- Instruct patient to shake well before administration

Evaluation

Positive therapeutic outcome

- Decreased diarrhea

azathioprine (℞)

(ay-za-thye'oh-preen)

Imuran

Func. class.: Immunosuppressant

Chem. class.: Purine analog

Pregnancy category D

Action: Produces immunosuppression by inhibiting purine synthesis, DNA, RNA in cells

Therapeutic Outcome: Absence of graft rejection, slowing of rheumatoid arthritis

Uses: Renal transplants to prevent graft rejection, often used with corticosteroids, cytotoxics; refractory rheumatoid arthritis, refractory ITP, glomerulonephritis, nephrotic syndrome, bone marrow transplant

Investigational uses: Myasthenia gravis, chronic ulcerative colitis, Crohn's disease, Behçet's syndrome

Dosage and routes

Renal dose

CrCl 10-50 ml/min 75% of dose; CrCl <10 ml/min 50% of dose

Preventlon of rejection

P ***Adult and child:*** PO, **IV** 3-5 mg/kg/day, then maintenance (PO) of at least 1-2 mg/kg/day

Refractory rheumatoid arthritis

Adult: PO 1/mg/kg/day; may increase dosage after 2 mo by 0.5 mg/kg/day; not to exceed 2.5 mg/kg/day

Available forms: Tabs 50 mg; inj **IV** 100 mg

Adverse effects

GI: Nausea, vomiting, stomatitis, esophagitis, **pancreatitis, hepatotoxicity, jaundice**

HEMA: **Leukopenia, thrombocytopenia, anemia, pancytopenia**

INTEG: Rash, alopeia

MS: Arthralgia, muscle wasting

Contraindications: Hypersensitivity, pregnancy **D**

Precautions: Severe renal disease, G severe hepatic disease, elderly

Do Not Confuse:
Imuran/Imferon

Pharmacokinetics

Absorption	Readily (PO)
Distribution	Crosses placenta
Metabolism	Liver to mercaptopurine
Excretion	Kidney, minimal
Half-life	3 hr

Pharmacodynamics

	PO	IV
Onset	Unknown	Unknown
Peak	4 hr	Unknown
Duration	Unknown	Unknown

Interactions

Individual drugs

Allopurinol: ↑ toxicity
Cyclosporine: ↑ myelosuppression
Warfarin: ↓ action of warfarin

Drug classifications

ACE inhibitors: ↑ leukopenia
Antineoplastics: ↑ myelosuppression
Vaccines: ↓ immune response

Lab test interferences

↓ Uric acid, ↑ LFTs
Interference: CBC, diff count

NURSING CONSIDERATIONS

Assessment

- Assess symptoms of rheumatoid arthritis: pain in joints, stiffness, poor range of motion, inflammation
- Monitor blood studies: Hgb, WBC, platelets during treatment monthly; if leukocytes are <3000/mm^3 or platelets <100,000/mm^3, drug should be discontinued or reduced; decreased Hgb level may indicate bone marrow suppression
- Monitor liver function studies: alkaline phosphatase, AST, ALT, amylase, bilirubin; and for hepatotoxicity: dark urine, jaundice, itching, light-colored stools; drug should be discontinued
- Monitor I&O, weight qd, report decreasing urine output, toxicity may occur
- Asses for infection: increased temp, WBC; sputum, urine

Nursing diagnoses

✓ Mobility, impaired (uses)
✓ Infection, risk for (uses)
✓ Knowledge deficit (teaching)

Implementation

PO route

- Give all medications PO if possible, avoiding IM injections, since bleeding may occur
- Give with meals to reduce GI upset; nausea is common
- For several days before transplant surgery, patients should be placed in protective isolation

IV **IV route**

- Prepare in biologic cabinet using gown, gloves, mask; give after diluting 100 mg/10 ml of sterile water for inj; rotate to dissolve; may further dilute with 50 ml or more saline or glucose in saline given over >30 min (intermittent inf)

Solution compatibilities: D_5W, NaCl 0.9%, NaCl 0.45%

Patient/family education

- Teach patient to take as prescribed,

do not miss doses, if dose is missed on qd regimen, skip dose, if on multiple dosing/day, take as soon as remembered

- Teach patient that therapeutic response may take 3-4 mo in rheumatoid arthritis, to continue with prescribed exercise, rest, other medications; that drug is needed for life in renal transplant
- Instruct patient to report fever, rash, severe diarrhea, chills, sore throat, fatigue, since serious infections may occur; or clay-colored stools and cramping (hepatotoxicity)
- Advise patient to use contraceptive measures during treatment for 12 wk after ending therapy; drug is teratogenic
- Advise patient to avoid vaccinations
- Tell patient to avoid crowds and persons with known infections to reduce risk of infection
- Instruct patient not to use OTC medications without approval of prescriber
- Advise patient to use soft-bristled toothbrush to prevent bleeding

Evaluation

Positive therapeutic outcome

- Absence of graft rejection
- Immunosuppression in autoimmune disorders
- Increased joint mobility without pain in rheumatoid arthritis

azelastine (℞)

(ay'ze-lass-teen)

Astelin

Func. class.: Leukotriene synthesis inhibitor

Chem. class.: Phthalazinone derivative

Pregnancy category C

Action: Inhibits the synthesis and release of leukotrienes; antagonizes action of acetylcholine, histamine, serotonin

→ Therapeutic Outcome: Decreased nasal stuffiness, itching, swollen eyes

Uses: Seasonal allergic rhinitis

Dosage and routes

P ***Adult and child ≥12 yr:*** Nasal 2 sprays/nostril bid

Available forms: Spray 137 μg/actuation

Adverse effects

CNS: Sedation (more common with increased dosages), drowsiness

MISC: Weight increase, myalgia

Contraindications: Hypersensitivity

Precautions: Pregnancy **C**

Pharmacokinetics	
Absorption	Unknown
Distribution	Unknown
Metabolism	Liver, extensively
Excretion	Feces
Half-life	25-42 hr

Pharmacodynamics	
Onset	Unknown
Peak	4-5 hr
Duration	Unknown

Interactions

Individual drugs

Alcohol: ↑ CNS depression

Drug classifications

CNS depressants: ↑ CNS depression

Narcotics: ↑ CNS depression

Sedative/hypnotics: ↑ CNS depression

NURSING CONSIDERATIONS

Assessment

- Assess respiratory status: rate, rhythm, increase in bronchial secretions, wheezing, chest tightness; provide fluids to 2 L/day to decrease secretion thickness

Nursing diagnoses

✓ Airway clearance, ineffective (uses)

✓ Knowledge deficit (teaching)
✓ Noncompliance (teaching, overuse)

Implementation

- Remove cap/safety clip from spray pump
- Prime pump if using for first time, push 4 times quickly, away from face, blow your nose, then place tip of pump into one nostril, while holding other nostril closed, tilt head forward, and spray into nostril
- Put cover/safety clip back on

Patient/family education

- Teach patient all aspects of drug uses; to notify prescriber if confusion, sedation occur; to avoid driving and other hazardous activity if drowsiness occurs; to avoid alcohol and other CNS depressants that may potentiate effect
- Caution patient not to exceed recommended dosage; dysrhythmias may occur

Evaluation

Positive therapeutic outcome

- Absence of running or congested nose

azithromycin (℞)

(ay-zi-thro-my′sin)

Zithromax

Func. class.: Antiinfective

Chem. class.: Macrolide (azalide)

Pregnancy category B

Action: Binds to 50S ribosomal subunits of susceptible bacteria and suppresses protein synthesis; much greater spectrum of activity than erythromycin

➔ **Therapeutic Outcome:** Bacteriostatic against the following susceptible organisms: *Moraxella catarrhalis, Streptococcus pneumoniae, Streptococcus pyogenes, Staphylococcus aureus, Haemophilus influenzae, Clostridium, Legionella pneumophila, Chlamydia trachomatis, Mycoplasma;* no effect on methicillin-resistant *S. aureus;* P in children: acute otitis media *(H. influenzae, M. catarrhalis, S. pneumoniae)* PO, acute pharyngitis/tonsillitis (group A streptococcal) PO; acute skin/soft tissue infections (PO); community-acquired pneumonia *(C. pneumoniae, H. influenzae, M. pneumoniae, S. pneumoniae)* PO; pharyngitis/tonsillitis *(S. pyogenes)*

Uses: Mild to moderate infections of the upper respiratory tract, lower respiratory tract; uncomplicated skin and skin structure infections, nongonococcal urethritis, or cervicitis; prophylaxis of disseminated *Mycobacterium avium* complex (MAC)

Investigational uses: Bacterial endocarditis prevention

Dosage and routes

Adult: PO 500 mg on day 1, then 250 mg qd on days 2-5 for a total dose of 1.5 g; may give a one-time dose of 1 g for chlamydial infections; 1200 mg qwk for MAC prophylaxis; **IV** 500 mg qd ≥2 days, then 500 mg qd to complete 7-10 day therapy (community-acquired pneumonia); 500 mg qd × 3 days (upper/lower respiratory infections) **IV** 500 mg qd × 2 days, then 250 mg qd to complete 7-day therapy (pelvic inflammatory disease [PID])

P ***Child ≥2 yr:*** PO 12 mg/kg qd for 5 days

P ***Child <6 mo:*** PO 10 mg/kg on day 1, then 5 mg/kg qd

Lower respiratory tract infections, acute skin/soft tissue infections, acute pharyngitis/tonsillitis, acute otitis media

P ***Child:*** PO 3-day regimen, 10 mg/kg qd × 3 days

Prevention of acute otitis media

P ***Child:*** PO 10 mg/kg qwk × 6 mo

Available forms: Tabs 250, 600 mg; powder for inj 500 mg; powder for oral susp 1 g/packet; susp 100, 200 mg/5 ml

Adverse effects

CNS: Dizziness, headache, vertigo, somnolence
CV: Palpitations, chest pain
GI: Nausea, vomiting, diarrhea, **hepatotoxicity,** abdominal pain, stomatitis, heartburn, dyspepsia, flatulence, melena, **cholestatic jaundice**
GU: Vaginitis, moniliasis, nephritis
INTEG: Rash, urticaria, pruritus, photosensitivity

Contraindications: Hypersensitivity to azithromycin, erythromycin, or any macrolide

Precautions: Pregnancy **B,** lactation, hepatic/renal/cardiac disease, G elderly, child <6 mo for otitis media, P child <2 yr for pharyngitis, tonsillitis

Do Not Confuse:
Zithromax/Zinacef

Pharmacokinetics

Absorption	Rapid, (PO) up to 50%
Distribution	Widely distributed
Metabolism	Unknown, minimal metabolism
Excretion	Unchanged (bile); kidneys, minimal
Half-life	11-70 hr

Pharmacodynamics

Onset	Unknown
Peak	2-4 hr
Duration	24 hr

Interactions

Individual drugs

Astemizole: ↑ toxicity, fatal reaction
Carbamazepine: ↑ toxicity
Ergotamine: ↑ toxicity
Phenytoin: ↑ effects of oral anticoagulants
Pimozide: ↑ toxicity, fatal reaction
Tacrolimus: ↑ effects of tocrolimus
Theophylline: ↑ toxicity
Triazolam: ↓ clearance of triazolam

Drug classifications

Aluminum antacids: ↓ peak serum
Anticoagulants, orals: ↑ effect of oral anticoagulants
Magnesium antacids: ↓ levels of azithromycin

Lab test interferences

↑ Bilirubin, ↑ LDH, ↑ alkaline phosphatase, ↑ CPK, ↑ K, ↑ pro-time, ↑ BUN, ↑ creatinine, ↑ blood glucose, ↑ AST, ↑ ALT

NURSING CONSIDERATIONS

Assessment

- Assess for signs and symptoms of infection: drainage, fever, increased WBC >10,000/mm^3, urine culture positive, sore throat, sputum culture positive
- Monitor respiratory status: rate, character, wheezing, tightness in chest; discontinue drug if these occur
- Monitor allergies before treatment, reaction of each medication; place allergies on chart, notify all people giving drugs; skin eruptions, itching
- Monitor I&O ratio, renal studies; report hematuria, oliguria in renal disease; check urinalysis, protein, blood
- Monitor liver studies: AST, ALT, bilirubin, LDH, alkaline phosphatase; CBC with differential
- Monitor C&S before drug therapy; drug may be taken as soon as culture is taken; C&S may be repeated after treatment
- Monitor bowel pattern before, during treatment
- Assess for superinfection: sore throat, mouth, tongue; fever, fatigue, diarrhea, anogenital pruritus

Nursing diagnoses

- ✓ Infection, risk for (uses)
- ✓ Diarrhea (adverse reactions)
- ✓ Knowledge deficit (teaching)

Implementation

PO route

- Provide adequate intake of fluids (2 L) during diarrhea episodes
- Give with a full glass of water; give susp 1 hr before or 2 hr pc; tabs may be taken without regard to food; do not give with fruit juices
- Store at room temperature
- Reconstitute 1 g packet for susp with 60 ml water, mix, rinse glass with more water and have patient drink to consume all medication

IV **IV route**

- Reconstitute 500 mg drug/4.8 ml sterile water for inj (100 mg/ml), shake, dilute with ≥250 ml 0.9% NaCl, 0.45% NaCl, or LR to 1-2 mg/ml
- Give 500 mg/1 hr or more, never give IM or as a bol

Patient/family education

- Instruct patient to report sore throat, black furry tongue, fever, loose foul-smelling stool, vaginal itching, discharge, fatigue; may indicate superinfection
- Caution patient not to take aluminum/magnesium-containing antacids or food simultaneously with this drug; blood levels of azithromycin will be decreased
- Instruct patient to notify prescriber of diarrhea stools, dark urine, pale stools, yellow discoloration of eyes or skin, severe abdominal pain; cholestatic jaundice is a severe adverse reaction
- Teach patient complete dosage regimen; to notify prescriber if symptoms continue
- Teach patient that if pregnancy is suspected to notify prescriber
- Inform patient that sunburns may occur; wear protective clothing and sunscreen

Evaluation

Positive therapeutic outcome

- C&S negative for infection
- WBC within 5,000-10,000/mm^3

aztreonam (℞)

(az-tree'oh-nam)

azactam

Func. class.: Misc. antiinfective

Chem. class.: Monobactam

Pregnancy category B

Action: Inhibits organisms by inhibiting bacterial cell wall synthesis, which causes death of organism (bactericidal)

➔ **Therapeutic Outcome:** Bactericidal action against susceptible organisms, specifically gram-negative aerobic organisms: *Escherichia coli, Serratia, Klebsiella, Enterobacter, Haemophilus influenzae, Shigella, Providencia, Salmonella, Neisseria gonorrhoeae, Pseudomonas aeruginosa,* including strains resistant to other drugs

Uses: Urinary tract infection; septicemia; skin, muscle, bone, lower respiratory tract, intraabdominal infections, and other infections caused by gram-negative organisms

Investigational uses: May be used for acute uncomplicated gonorrhea in patients with penicillin-resistant gonococci, instead of spectinomycin

Dosage and routes

Urinary tract infections

Adult: **IV**/IM 500 mg-1 g q8-12h

Systemic infections

Adult: **IV**/IM 1-2 g q8-12h

P ***Child:*** **IV**/IM 90-120 mg/kg/day divided q6-8h

Severe systemic infections

Adult: **IV**/IM 2 g q6-8h; do not exceed 8 g/day

Continue treatment for 48 hr after negative culture or until patient is asymptomatic

Available forms: Powder for inj 500 mg, 1, 2 g

A

Adverse effects

CNS: Lethargy, hallucinations, fever (pediatric), anxiety, depression, twitching, **coma, convulsions,** malaise
EENT: Tinnitus, diplopia, nasal congestion
GI: *Nausea, vomiting, diarrhea,* increased AST, ALT, abdominal pain, glossitis, colitis, pseudomembranous colitis
GU: Vaginal candidiasis, vaginitis, breast tenderness, increased BUN, creatinine
HEMA: Anemia, increased bleeding time, **bone marrow depression, granulocytopenia**
INTEG: Rash (pediatric)

Contraindications: Hypersensitivity

Precautions: Pregnancy **B,** lactation, children, impaired renal/hepatic function, elderly

Pharmacokinetics

Absorption	Well absorbed (IM)
Distribution	Widely distributed; crosses placenta
Metabolism	Liver, minimal
Excretion	Kidneys, unchanged (60%-70%); breast milk
Half-life	1.7 hr; increased in renal disease

Pharmacodynamics

	IM	IV
Onset	Rapid	Rapid
Peak	1 hr	Infusion's end

Interactions

Individual drugs

Cefoxitin: ↑ antagonist effect
Clindamycin: ↓ action of clindamycin
Furosemide: ↑ levels
Imipenem: ↑ antagonist effect
Probenecid: ↑ levels

Drug classifications

Aminoglycosides: ↑ nephrotoxicity
Antiinfectives: ↑ antagonist effect
Penicillins: ↑ or ↓ action of penicillins

Lab test interferences

↑ ALT, AST, alkaline phosphatase, PT, PTT
Interference: Urine glucose using Clinitest/Benedict's reagent
False positive: Coombs' test

NURSING CONSIDERATIONS

Assessment

- Assess patient for previous sensitivity reaction to penicillins or cephalosporins; cross-sensitivity between penicillins, cephalosporins and this drug is common
- Assess patient for signs and symptoms of infection including characteristics of wounds, sputum, urine, stool, WBC >10,000/mm^3, fever; obtain baseline information before and during treatment
- Complete C&S before beginning drug therapy to identify if correct treatment has been initiated
- Identify urine output; if decreasing, notify prescriber (may indicate nephrotoxicity); note color, character, pH of urine if drug is administered for urinary tract infection; output should be 800 ml less than intake; if urine is highly acidic, alkalinization may be needed
- Assess renal studies: urinalysis, protein, blood, serum creatinine, BUN
- Monitor blood studies: AST, ALT, CBC, Hct, bilirubin, LDH, alkaline phosphatase, Coombs' test monthly if patient is on long-term therapy
- Monitor electrolytes: potassium, sodium, chloride monthly if patient is on long-term therapy
- Assess bowel pattern daily; if severe diarrhea occurs, drug should be discontinued; may indicate pseudomembranous colitis
- Monitor for bleeding: ecchymosis, bleeding gums, hematuria, stool guaiac daily if on long-term therapy
- Assess for overgrowth of infection: perineal itching, fever, malaise, red-

ness, pain, swelling, drainage, rash, diarrhea, change in cough, sputum

Nursing diagnoses

- ✓ Infection, risk for (uses)
- ✓ Diarrhea (side effects)
- ✓ Injury, risk for (side effects)
- ✓ Knowledge deficit (teaching)
- ✓ Noncompliance (teaching)

Implementation

IM route

- Reconstitute 1 g/3 ml or more of sterile water for inj 0.9% NaCl; may be diluted with 0.5% or 1% lidocaine to prevent pain; give deep in large muscle mass, massage; sol stable 1 wk refrigerated, room temp 8 hr; discard if precipitate forms

IV **IV route**

- Check for irritation, extravasation, phlebitis daily; change **IV** site q72h
- For direct **IV**, dilute 1 g/10 ml or 2 g/20 ml sterile water for injection, shake, let stand until clear; give over 3-5 min into running **IV**
- For intermittent inf, further dilute with 50-100 ml D_5W, $D_{10}W$, D_5/0.25% NaCl, D_5/0.45% NaCl, D_5/0.9% NaCl, 0.9% NaCl, D_5/LR, D_5/0.02%, sodium bicarbonate, Ringer's or LR; give over 15-60 min into running **IV**

Syringe compatibilities:

Clindamycin

Y-*site compatibilities:*

Allopurinol, amifostine, amikacin, aminophylline, ampicillin, ampicillin/sulbactam, bleomycin, bumetanide, buprenorphine, butorphanol, calcium gluconate, carboplatin, carmustine, cefazolin, cefepime, cefonicid, cefoperazone, cefotaxime, cefotetan, cefoxitin, ceftazidime, ceftizoxime, ceftriaxone, cefuroxime, cimetidine, ciprofloxacin, cisatracurium, cisplatin, clindamycin, cyclophosphamide, cytarabine, dacarbazine, dactinomycin, dexamethasone, diltiazem, diphenhydramine, dobutamine, dopamine, doxorubicin, doxorubicin liposome, doxycycline, droperidol, enalaprilat, etoposide, famotidine, filgrastim, floxuridine, fluconazole, fludarabine, fluorouracil, foscarnet, furosemide, gallium, gentamicin, granisetron, haloperidol, heparin, hydrocortisone, hydromorphone, hydroxyzine, idarubicin, ifosfamide, imipenem-cilastatin, insulin (regular), leucovorin, magnesium sulfate, mannitol, mechlorethamine, melphalan, meperidine, mesna, methotrexate, methylprednisolone, metoclopramide, mezlocillin, minocycline, morphine, nalbuphine, netilmicin, ondansetron, piperacillin, piperacillin/tazobactam, plicamycin, potassium chloride, promethazine, propofol, ranitidine, remifentanil, sargramostim, sodium bicarbonate, teniposide, theophylline, thiotepa, ticarcillin, ticarcillin/clavulanate, tobramycin, trimethoprim-sulfamethoxazole, vinblastine, vincristine, vinorelbine, zidovudine

Y-*site incompatibilities:*

Vancomycin

Additive compatibilities:

Ampicillin/sulbactam, cefazolin, ciprofloxacin, clindamycin, gentamicin, tobramycin

Additive incompatibilities:

Nafcillin, cephradine, metronidazole

Patient/family education

- Teach patient to report sore throat, bruising, bleeding, joint pain; may indicate blood dyscrasias (rare)
- Advise patient to contact prescriber if vaginal itching, loose, foul-smelling stools, furry tongue occur; may indicate superinfection; report itching, rash, pruritus, urticaria
- Instruct patient to take all medication prescribed for the length of time ordered; drug must be taken around the clock to maintain blood levels; do not give medication to others
- Advise patient to notify prescriber of diarrhea with blood or pus

B

Evaluation

Positive therapeutic outcome

- Absence of signs/symptoms of infection (WBC <10,000/mm^3, temp WNL, absence of red draining wounds), inflammation, temp
- Reported improvement in symptoms of infection

balsalazide (℞)

(ball-sal'a-zide)

Colazal

Func. class.: Antiinflammatory

Chem. class.: Salicylate derivative

Pregnancy category B

Action: Delivered intact to the colon, bioconverted to 4-aminobenzoyl-β-alanine

Therapeutic Outcome: Decreased inflammation in colon

Uses: Active, mild to moderate ulcerative colitis

Dosage and routes

Adult: PO 750 mg tid × 8 wk, may take up to 12 wk

Available forms: Tabs 750 mg

Adverse effects

CNS: Headache, insomnia, fatigue, fever, dizziness

EENT: Dry mouth, dry eyes, rhinitis, sinusitis, watery eyes, blurred vision

GI: Nausea, vomiting, abdominal pain, diarrhea, rectal bleeding, flatulence, dyspepsia, dry mouth, constipation

MS: Arthralgia, back pain, myalgia

SYST: **Anaphylaxis**

Contraindications: Hypersensitivity to salicylates

P Precautions: Pregnancy **B,** child <14 yr, lactation, pyloric stenosis

Pharmacokinetics

Absorption	Low, variable
Distribution	Plasma protein binding 99%
Metabolism	Unknown
Excretion	Kidneys, as metabolites
Half-life	Unknown

Pharmacodynamics

Unknown

Interactions

None known

Lab test interferences

False positive: Urinary glucose test

NURSING CONSIDERATIONS

Assessment

- Monitor kidney function studies: BUN, creatinine, urinalysis (long-term therapy)
- Assess for allergic reaction: rash, dermatitis, urticaria, pruritus, dyspnea, bronchospasm

Nursing diagnoses

☑ Injury, risk for (uses)
☑ Knowledge deficit (teaching)

Implementation

- Give with food in evenly divided doses
- Use with resuscitative equipment available; severe allergic reactions may occur
- Give total daily dose evenly spaced to minimize GI intolerance
- Store in tight, light-resistant container at room temp

Evaluation

Positive therapeutic outcome

- Absence of fever, mucus in stools, resolution of symptoms of ulcerative colitis

HIGH ALERT

basiliximab (℞)
(bas-ih-liks'ih-mab)
Simulect
Func. class.: Immunosuppressive
Chem. class.: Murine/human monoclonal antibody (interleukin-2) receptor antagonist

Pregnancy category B

Action: Binds to and blocks the IL-2 receptor, which is selectively expressed on the surface of activated T-lymphocytes; impairs the immune system to antigenic challenges

Therapeutic Outcome: Prevention of graft rejection

Uses: Acute allograft rejection in renal transplant patients when used with cyclosporine and corticosteroids

Dosage and routes
***Adult:* IV** 20 mg × 2 doses; 1st dose within 2 hr before transplant surgery; 2nd dose given 4 days after transplantation

P ***Child 2-15 yr:* IV** 12 mg/m^2 × 2 doses; 1st dose within 2 hr before transplant surgery; 2nd dose given 4 days after transplantation

Available forms: Powder for inj 20 mg

Adverse effects
CNS: *Pyrexia, chills, tremors, headache, insomnia, weakness*
CV: *Chest pain,* angina, **cardiac failure,** hypotension, hypertension, edema
GI: *Vomiting, nausea, diarrhea,* constipation, abdominal pain, GI bleeding, gingival hyperplasia, stomatitis
INTEG: *Acne*
META: Acidosis, hypercholesterolemia, hyperuricemia, hyperkalemia, hypocalcemia, hypokalemia, hypophosphatemia
MISC: Infection, moniliasis
MS: Arthralgia, myalgia
RESP: *Dyspnea, wheezing, cough,* **pulmonary edema**

Contraindications: Hypersensitivity

P G **Precautions:** Pregnancy **B,** infections, elderly, lactation, children

Pharmacokinetics	
Absorption	Unknown
Distribution	Unknown
Metabolism	Unknown
Excretion	Unknown
Half-life	7 days (adult)
	P 9½ days (child)

Pharmacodynamics	
Onset	Unknown
Peak	½ hr (adults)
Duration	Unknown

Interactions
None known

NURSING CONSIDERATIONS
Assessment
- Assess for infection, increased temp, WBC, sputum, urine
- Monitor blood studies: Hgb, WBC, platelets during treatment qmo; if leukocytes are <3000/mm^3, drug should be discontinued
- Monitor liver function studies: alkaline phosphatase, AST, ALT, bilirubin
- Assess hepatotoxicity: dark urine, jaundice, itching, light-colored stools; drug should be discontinued

Nursing diagnoses
✓ Infection, risk for (adverse reactions)
✓ Knowledge deficit (teaching)

Implementation
- Administer all medications PO if possible; avoid IM injection, since infection may occur

IV route
- After adding 5 ml sterile water for inj, shake gently to dissolve, reconsti-

tute to a vol of 50 ml with 0.9% NaCl or D_5, gently invert bag, do not shake, do not admix

Patient/family education

- Instruct patient to report fever, chills, sore throat, fatigue, since serious infection may occur; avoid crowds, persons with known upper respiratory infections; use contraception during treatment

Evaluation

Positive therapeutic outcome

- Absence of graft rejection

beclomethasone (℞)

(be-kloe-meth'a-sone)

Beclodisk ♣, Becloforte Inhaler ♣, Beclovent, Qvar, Vanceril

Func. class.: Synthetic glucocorticoid (long acting)

Chem. class.: Beclomethasone diester

Pregnancy category C

Action: Antiinflammatory; vasoconstrictive properties; also immunosuppressive

➔ **Therapeutic Outcome:** Decreased inflammation and normal immunity

Uses: Seasonal, perennial allergic rhinitis, nasal polyps, chronic steroid-dependent asthma

Dosage and routes

P ***Adult and child >12 yr:*** INSTILL 1-2 sprays in each nostril bid-qid; INH 2-4 puffs tid-qid (42 µg/actuations), max 20 inh/day; inh 2 puffs bid, max 10 inh/day (84 µg/actuation)

P ***Child 6-12 yrs:*** INSTILL 1 spray in each nostril tid; INH 1-2 puffs tid-qid (42 µg/actuation); 2 puffs bid, max 5 inh/day (84 µg/actuation)

Available forms: Aero 42 µg/spray (nasal); aero for inh 42, 50, 84, 250 µg/activation; aerosol for nasal inh 0.042%; inh cap 100, 200 µg

Adverse effects

CNS: *Headache,* paresthesia

EENT: *Dryness, nasal irritation, burning, sneezing,* secretions with blood, nasal ulcerations, **perforation of nasal septum,** candidal infection, earache, *hoarseness*

ENDO: **Adrenal suppression**

GI: Dry mouth, dyspepsia

INTEG: Rash, urticaria, pruritus

MISC: **Angioedema adrenal insufficiency,** facial edema

RESP: **Acute status asthmaticus,** wheezing, cough

Contraindications: Hypersensitivity, systemic corticosteroid therapy

P **Precautions:** Pregnancy **C,** children <12, nasal ulcers, recurrent epistaxis

Pharmacokinetics

Absorption	Locally only
Distribution	Not distributed
Metabolism	Lungs, liver, GI system (by CYP3A)
Excretion	Feces, urine
Half-life	2.8 hr

Pharmacodynamics

	INH	NASAL
Onset	10 min	10 min
Peak	Unknown	Unknown
Duration	Unknown	Unknown

NURSING CONSIDERATIONS

Assessment

- Assess adrenal suppression: 17-KS, plasma cortisol for decreased levels, adrenal function periodically for HPA axis suppression during prolonged therapy; monitor growth and development
- Assess blood studies, neutrophils, decreased platelets; WBC with diff baseline and q3 mo, if neutrophils <1000/mm³, discontinue treatment
- Check nasal passages during

zlong-term treatment for changes in mucus; check for burning, stinging; assess for glucocorticoid withdrawal: dizziness, hypotension, fatigue, muscle/joint pain; notify prescriber immediately
- Assess respiratory status: rest, rhythm, characteristics; auscultate lung bilaterally before and throughout treatment
- Assess for fungal infections in mucous membranes

Nursing diagnoses

- ✓ Airway clearance, ineffective (uses)
- ✓ Oral mucous membranes, altered (adverse reactions)
- ✓ Knowledge deficit (teaching)
- ✓ Noncompliance (teaching)

Implementation

- Give PO, using a spacer device for proper dose
- Use after cleaning aerosol top daily with warm water; dry thoroughly
- Store in cool environment; do not puncture or incinerate container

Patient/family education

- Teach patient to gargle/rinse mouth after each use to prevent oral fungal infections
- Teach patient that in times of stress, systemic corticosteroids may be needed to prevent adrenal insufficiency; do not discontinue oral drug abruptly, taper slowly
- Teach patient to continue using product even if mild nasal bleeding occurs; is usually transient
- Teach patient method of instillation after providing written instructions from manufacturer
- Teach patient to clear nasal passages before administration; use decongestant if needed; shake inhaler, invert, tilt head backward, insert nozzle into nostril, away from septum; hold other nostril closed and depress activator, inhale through nose, exhale through mouth

Evaluate

Positive therapeutic outcome

- Decrease in runny nose, improved symptoms of bronchial asthma

benazepril (℞)

(ben-a'za-pril)

Lotensin

Func. class.: Antihypertensive

Chem. class.: ACE inhibitor

Pregnancy category

C (1st trimester)

D (2nd/3rd trimesters)

Action: Selectively suppresses renin-angiotensin-aldosterone system; inhibits ACE, preventing conversion of angiotensin I to angiotensin II

➔ **Therapeutic Outcome:** Decreased B/P in hypertension

Uses: Hypertension, alone or in combination with thiazide diuretics

Dosage and routes

Adult: PO 10 mg qd initially, then 20-40 mg/day divided bid or qd (without a diuretic); 5 mg PO qd (with a diuretic)

Renal dose

5 mg qd with CrCl <30 ml/min/1.73 m^2; increase as needed to maximum of 40 mg/day

G ***Elderly:*** PO 5-10 mg/day initially

Available forms: Tabs 5, 10, 20, 40 mg

Adverse effects

CNS: Anxiety, hypertonia, insomnia, paresthesia, headache, dizziness, fatigue

CV: Hypotension, postural hypotension, syncope, palpitations, angina

GI: Nausea, constipation, vomiting, gastritis, melena

GU: Increased BUN, creatinine, decreased libido, impotence, urinary tract infection

HEMA: **Neutropenia, agranulocytosis**

B

INTEG: Rash, flushing, sweating
MISC: **Angioedema**
META: Hyperkalemia, hyponatremia
MS: Arthralgia, arthritis, myalgia
RESP: Cough, asthma, bronchitis, dyspnea, sinusitis

Contraindications: Hypersensitivity to ACE inhibitors, pregnancy **D** (2nd/3rd trimesters), lactation, P children

Precautions: Impaired renal/liver function, dialysis patients, hypovolemia, blood dyscrasias, CHF, COPD, G asthma, elderly, bilateral renal artery stenosis; pregnancy **C** (1st trimester)

Do Not Confuse:
Lotensin/Lioresal, Lotensin/Loniten

Pharmacokinetics

Absorption	<40%
Distribution	Unknown; crosses placenta
Metabolism	Liver metabolites; serum protein binding 97%
Excretion	Kidney, breast milk (minimal)
Half-life	10-11 hr (metabolite); increased in renal disease

Pharmacodynamics

Onset	Unknown
Peak	½-1 hr
Duration	Unknown

Interactions

Individual drugs

Alcohol: ↑ hypotension (large amounts)
Lithium: ↑ serum levels

Drug classifications

Antihypertensives: ↑ hypotension
Diuretics: ↑ hypotension
Diuretics, potassium-sparing: ↑ hyperkalemia
Potassium supplements: ↑ toxicity
Sympathomimetics: ↑ toxicity

Lab test interferences

↑ BUN, ↑ creatinine, ↑ LFTs, ↑ bilirubin, ↑ uric acid, ↑ blood glucose

NURSING CONSIDERATIONS

Assessment

- Monitor blood studies: neutrophils, decreased platelets
- Monitor B/P at peak/trough level of drug, check for orthostatic hypotension, syncope; if changes occur, dosage change may be required
- Monitor renal studies: protein, BUN, creatinine; watch for increased levels that may indicate nephrotic syndrome and renal failure; monitor urine for protein; monitor renal symptoms: polyuria, oliguria, frequency, dysuria
- Establish baselines in renal, liver function tests before therapy begins
- Check potassium levels throughout treatment, although hyperkalemia rarely occurs
- Assess for allergic reactions: rash, fever, pruritus, urticaria; drug should be discontinued if antihistamines fail to help

Nursing diagnoses

✓ Cardiac output, decreased (uses)
✓ Injury, potential for (side effects)
✓ Knowledge deficit (teaching)
✓ Noncompliance (teaching)

Implementation

PO route

- Store in air-tight container at 86° F (30° C) or less
- Severe hypotension may occur after 1st dose of this medication; decreased hypotension may be prevented by reducing or discontinuing diuretic therapy 3 days before beginning benazepril therapy

Patient/family education

- Instruct patient not to discontinue drug abruptly; advise patient to tell all persons associated with care
- Teach patient not to use OTC products (cough, cold, allergy) unless directed by prescriber; serious side effects can occur; xanthines such as coffee, tea, chocolate, cola can prevent action of drug
- Emphasize the importance of complying with dosage schedule, even

if feeling better; to continue with medical regimen to decrease B/P: exercise, cessation of smoking, decreasing stress, diet modifications

- Emphasize the need to rise slowly to sitting or standing position to minimize orthostatic hypotension; not to exercise in hot weather because increased hypotension can occur
- Teach patient to notify prescriber of mouth sores, sore throat, fever, swelling of hands or feet, irregular heartbeat, chest pain, coughing, shortness of breath
- Caution patient to report excessive perspiration, dehydration, vomiting, diarrhea; may lead to fall in B/P
- Caution patient that drug may cause dizziness, fainting, light-headedness; may occur during 1st few days of therapy; to avoid activities that may be hazardous
- Teach patient how to take B/P; teach normal readings for age group; ensure patient takes own B/P
- Advise patient to notify prescriber of pregnancy, drug will need to be discontinued

Evaluation

Positive therapeutic outcome

- Decreased B/P in hypertension

Treatment of overdose: 0.9% NaCl **IV** inf, hemodialysis

benztropine 🔑 (℞)

(benz'troe-peen)

Apo-Benztropin 🍁, benztropine mesylate, Cogentin

Func. class.: Cholinergic blocker, antiparkinson agent

Chem. class.: Tertiary amine

Pregnancy category C

Action: Blockade of central acetylcholine receptors in the CNS, neurotransmitters are balanced

➡ **Therapeutic Outcome:** Decreased involuntary movements

Uses: Parkinsonian symptoms, extrapyramidal symptoms associated with neuroleptic drugs, acute dystonia

Dosage and routes

Drug-induced extrapyramidal symptoms

Adult: IM/**IV** 1-4 mg qd/bid; give PO dose as soon as possible; PO 1-2 mg bid/tid; increase by 0.5 mg q5-6 days

P ***Child:*** IM/**IV** 0.02-0.05 mg/kg/dose 1-2 × 1 day

G ***Elderly:*** PO 0.5 mg qd/bid, increase by 0.5 mg q5-6 days

Parkinsonian symptoms

Adult: PO 1-2 mg qd, in divided doses; increased 0.5 mg q5-6 days titrated to patient response

Acute dystonic reactions

Adult: IM/**IV** 1-2 mg, may increase to 1-2 mg bid (PO)

Available forms: Tabs 0.5, 1, 2 mg; inj IM, **IV** 1 mg/ml

Adverse effects

CNS: Confusion, anxiety, restlessness, irritability, delusions, hallucinations, headache, sedation, depression, incoherence, dizziness, memory loss; G delirium (elderly)

CV: Palpitations, tachycardia, hypotension, bradycardia

EENT: Blurred vision, photophobia, dilated pupils, difficulty swallowing, dry eyes, mydriasis, increased intraocular tension, angle closure glaucoma

GI: *Dryness of mouth, constipation,* nausea, vomiting, abdominal distress, **paralytic ileus**, epigastric distress

GU: Hesitancy, retention, dysuria

INTEG: Rash, urticaria, dermatoses

MISC: Increased temperature, flushing, decreased sweating, **hyperthermia, heat stroke,** numbness of fingers

MS: Muscular weakness, cramping

Contraindications: Hypersensitivity, narrow angle glaucoma, myasthenia gravis, GI/GU obstruction, P child

<3 yr, peptic ulcer, megacolon, prostate hypertrophy

G **Precautions:** Pregnancy **C**, elderly, lactation, tachycardia, liver, kidney disease, drug abuse history, dysrhythmias, hypotension, hypertension, P psychiatric patients, children

Pharmacokinetics

Absorption	Well (PO, IM), completely (**IV**) absorbed
Distribution	Unknown
Metabolism	Unknown
Excretion	Unknown
Half-life	Unknown

Pharmacodynamics

	IM/IV	PO
Onset	15 min	1 hr
Peak	Unknown	Unknown
Duration	6-10 hr	6-10 hr

Interactions

Individual drugs

Disopyramide: ↑ anticholinergic effects
Quinidine: ↑ anticholinergic effects

Drug classifications

Antacids: ↓ absorption of benzotropine
Antidepressants, tricyclic: ↑ anticholinergic effects
Antidiarrheals: ↓ absorption
Antihistamines: ↑ anticholinergic effects
Phenothiazines: ↑ anticholinergic effects

NURSING CONSIDERATIONS

Assessment

- Monitor I&O ratio; retention commonly causes decreased urinary output, distention, frequency, incontinence
- Assess for parkinsonism, extrapyramidal symptoms: shuffling gait, muscle rigidity, involuntary movements, loss of balance, pill rolling, muscle spasms, drooling before and during treatment
- Monitor for urinary hesitancy, retention; palpate bladder if retention occurs
- Monitor for constipation, cramping, pain in abdomen, abdominal distention; increase fluids, bulk, exercise if this occurs
- Assess for tolerance over long-term therapy; dosage may have to be increased or changed
- Assess for mental status: affect, mood, CNS depression, worsening of mental symptoms during early therapy
- Assess for benztropine "buzz" or "high," patients may imitate EPS

Nursing diagnoses

✓ Mobility, impaired (uses)
✓ Knowledge deficit (teaching)
✓ Noncompliance (teaching)

Implementation

PO route

- Give with or after meals to prevent GI upset; may give with fluids other than water; hard candy, frequent drinks, gum to relieve dry mouth
- Give hs to avoid daytime drowsiness in patient with parkinsonism
- May be crushed and mixed with food
- Store at room temperature

IM route

- Give in large muscle mass for dystonic symptoms

IV **IV route**

- Give parenteral dose with patient recumbent to prevent postural hypotension; give undiluted 1 mg/1 min

Syringe compatibilities: Chlorpromazine, fluphenazine, metoclopramide, perphenazine, thiothixene

Y-*site compatibilities:* Fluconazole, tacrolimus

Patient/family education

- Teach patient to use caution in hot weather; drug may increase susceptibility to stroke since perspiration is decreased; patient should remain indoors

- Advise patient not to discontinue this drug abruptly; to taper off over 1 wk to prevent withdrawal symptoms (insomnia, involuntary movements, anxiety, tachycardias)
- Caution patient to avoid driving or other hazardous activities; drowsiness, dizziness may occur
- Teach patient to avoid OTC medication: cough, cold preparations with alcohol, antihistamines unless directed by prescriber; increased CNS depression may occur
- Advise patient to rise from sitting or recumbent position slowly to minimize orthostatic hypotension
- Teach patient to use gum, hard candy, frequent sips of water to decrease dry mouth; if dry mouth continues, saliva substitutes may be prescribed
- Instruct patient that doses should not be doubled, but missed dose may be taken up to 2 hr before next dose
- Advise patient to use good oral hygiene, use frequent sips of water, sugarless gum for dry mouth

Evaluation

Positive therapeutic outcome

- Absence of involuntary movements (pill rolling, tremors, muscle spasms)

bepridil (℞)

(be′pri-dil)

Bepadin, Vascor

Func. class.: Calcium channel blocker, antianginal, antihypertensive

Pregnancy category C

Action: Inhibits calcium ion influx across cell membrane during cardiac depolarization; produces relaxation of coronary vascular smooth muscle, peripheral vascular smooth muscle; dilates coronary vascular arteries; increases myocardial oxygen delivery in patients with vasospastic angina

Therapeutic Outcome: Decreased angina pectoris

Uses: Chronic stable angina, used alone or in combination with propranolol

Dosage and routes

Adult: PO 200 mg qd, after 10 days may increase dose if needed; max dose 400 mg/day

Available forms: Tabs, film-coated, 200, 300, 400 mg

Adverse effects

CNS: Headache, fatigue, drowsiness, dizziness, anxiety, depression, weakness, insomnia, confusion, lightheadedness, nervousness

CV: **Dysrhythmias,** edema, **CHF,** bradycardia, hypotension, palpitations, **AV block, torsades de pointes**

GI: Nausea, vomiting, diarrhea, gastric upset, constipation, increased levels in liver function studies, gingival hyperplasia

GU: Nocturia, polyuria

HEMA: **Agranulocytosis**

Contraindications: Sick sinus syndrome, 2nd- or 3rd-degree heart block, Wolff-Parkinson-White syndrome, hypotension less than 90 mm Hg systolic, cardiogenic shock, history of serious ventricular arrhythmias

Precautions: CHF, hypotension, hepatic injury, pregnancy **C,** lactation, P children, renal disease, IHSS, concomitant β-blocker therapy

Do Not Confuse:
bepridil/Prepidil

Pharmacokinetics	
Absorption	Well absorbed
Distribution	Plasma protein bound (99%), crosses placenta
Metabolism	Liver
Excretion	Urine, feces
Half-life	42 hr

Pharmacodynamics	
Onset	1 hr
Peak	2-3 hr
Duration	24 hr

Interactions
Individual drugs
Fentanyl: ↑ hypotension
Drug classifications
Antidysrhythmics: ↑ prolongation of QT interval, depression of AV node
β-Adrenergic blockers: ↑ adverse reactions
Cardiac glycosides: ↑ prolongation of QT, depression of AV node
Food/drug
Grapefruit: ↑ hypotension
Lab test interferences
↑ Liver function tests, ↑ aminotransferase, ↑ CPK, ↑ LDH

NURSING CONSIDERATIONS
Assessment
- Assess fluid volume status: I&O ratio and record, weight, distended red veins, crackles in lung, color, quality, and sp gr of urine, skin turgor, adequacy of pulses, moist mucous membranes, bilateral lung sounds, peripheral pitting edema
- Assess cardiac status: B/P, pulse, respiration, ECG intervals (PR, QRS, QT), dysrhythmias; may prolong QT interval, alter T wave
- Obtain digoxin levels if cardiac glycosides are given with bepridil

Nursing diagnoses
✓ Cardiac output, decreased (uses)
✓ Knowledge deficit (teaching)

Implementation
- Give once a day, with food for GI symptoms; adjust dose no more frequently than q10 days
- ⊘ Do not break, chew, crush tabs

Patient/family education
- Instruct patient to avoid hazardous activities until stabilized on drug and dizziness is no longer a problem
- Instruct patient to limit caffeine consumption; to avoid alcohol and OTC drugs unless directed by prescriber
- Advise patient to comply in all areas of medical regimen: diet, exercise, stress reduction, drug therapy; to notify prescriber of irregular heart beat, shortness of breath, swelling of feet and hands, pronounced dizziness, constipation, nausea, hypotension
- Teach patient to use as directed even if feeling better; may be taken with other cardiovascular drugs (nitrates, β-blockers)
- Teach patient to notify prescriber of swelling, weight gain, dyspnea, irregular heart beat
- Advise patient to maintain good oral hygiene to prevent gingival hyperplasia

Evaluation
Positive therapeutic outcome
- Decreased anginal pain
- Increased activity tolerance

Treatment of overdose:
Defibrillation, atropine for AV block, vasopressor for hypotension

betamethasone (℞)
(bay-tah-meth'ah-sone)
Betnelan ♣, Betnesol ♣, Celestone, Selestoject ♣
Func. class.: Corticosteroid, synthetic; glucocorticoid, long acting

Pregnancy category C

Action: Decreases inflammation by suppression of migration of polymorphonuclear leukocytes, fibroblasts, reversal of increased capillary permeability and lysosomal stabilization

➔ **Therapeutic Outcome:** Decreased inflammation and normal immunity

Uses: Immunosuppression, severe P inflammation, prevention of neonatal respiratory distress syndrome (by administration to mother), chronic asthma, rhinitis (inh); psoriasis, eczema, contact dermatitis, pruritus (top)

Dosage and routes

Adult: PO 0.6-7.2 mg qd; IM/**IV** 0.6-7.2 mg qd in joint or soft tissue (sodium phosphate)

P ***Child:*** PO 17.5 μg/kg/day in 3 divided doses; IM 17.5 μg/kg/day in 3 divided doses every 3rd day or 5.8-8.75 μg/kg/day as a single dose (adrenal insufficiency)

P ***Child:*** PO 62.5-250 μg/kg/day in 3 divided doses; IM 20.8-125 μg/kg/day of the base q12-24h (other uses)

P ***Adult and child:*** TOP apply to affected area qid

Adult: INH 2-4 puffs tid-qid; not to exceed 20 inh/day

P ***Child: 6-12 yr:*** INH 1-2 puffs tid-qid; not to exceed 10 inh/day

P ***Adult and child >12 yr:*** INSTILL 1-2 sprays in each nostril bid-qid

Available forms: Tabs 500, 600 μg; tabs, effervescent 500 μg (Canada); syrup 600 μg/5 ml; ext rel tab 1 mg; sol for inj (phosphate) 3 mg/ml; susp for inj (phosphate/acetate) 6 mg/ml

Adverse effects

CNS: *Depression, flushing, sweating,* headache, ecchymosis, bruising, mood changes

CV: *Hypertension,* **circulatory collapse, thrombophlebitis, embolism,** tachycardia, **necrotizing angiitis, CHF**

EENT: Fungal infections, increased intraocular pressure, blurred vision

GI: *Diarrhea, nausea, abdominal distention,* **GI hemorrhage,** increased appetite, **pancreatitis**

HEMA: **Thrombocytopenia**

INTEG: *Acne, poor wound healing, ecchymosis, bruising,* petechiae

MS: Fractures, osteoporosis, weakness

Contraindications: Psychosis, hypersensitivity, idiopathic thrombocytopenia, acute glomerulonephritis, amebiasis, fungal infections, nonasthmatic bronchial disease, P child <2 yr, AIDS, TB

Precautions: Pregnancy **C**, diabetes mellitus, glaucoma, osteoporosis, seizure disorders, ulcerative colitis, CHF, myasthenia gravis, renal disease, esophagitis, peptic ulcer

Pharmacokinetics

Absorption	Well absorbed (PO); systemic (top)
Distribution	Crosses placenta
Metabolism	Liver, extensively
Excretion	Kidney, breast milk
Half-life	3-5 hr, adrenal suppression 3-4 days

Pharmacodynamics

	PO	IM	IV	TOP
Onset	1-2 hr	Unknown	Rapid	Unknown
Peak	2 hr	4-8 hr	4-8 hr	Unknown
Duration	3 days	1-1½ days	1-1½ days	Unknown

Interactions

Individual drugs

Alcohol: ↑ GI bleeding
Amphotericin B: ↑ hypokalemia
Insulin: ↑ need for insulin
Mezlocillin: ↑ hypokalemia
Phenytoin: ↓ action, ↑ metabolism
Rifampin: ↓ action, ↑ metabolism
Ticarcillin: ↑ hypokalemia

Drug classifications

Barbiturates: ↓ action, ↑ metabolism
Diuretics: ↑ hypokalemia
Hypoglycemic agents: ↑ need for hypoglycemic agents
NSAIDs: ↑ GI bleeding
Salicylates: ↑ GI bleeding
Toxoids/vaccines: ↓ immune response

Herb/drug

Aloe: ↑ hypokalemia

Buckthorn bark/berry: ↑ hypokalemia
Cascara sagrada (bark): ↑ hypokalemia, chronic use/abuse
Lily of the valley: ↑ side effects
Pheasant's eye: ↑ side effects
Rhubarb root: ↑ hypokalemia
Senna leaf/fruits: ↑ hypokalemia
Squill: ↑ side effects

Lab test interferences
↑ Cholesterol, ↑ sodium, ↑ blood glucose, ↑ uric acid, ↑ calcium, ↑ urine glucose
↓ calcium, ↓ potassium, ↓ T_4, ↓ T_3, ↓ thyroid ^{131}I uptake test, ↓ urine 17-OHCS, ↓ 17-KS, ↓ PBI
False negative: Skin allergy tests

NURSING CONSIDERATIONS
Assessment
Systemic route
- Monitor potassium, blood glucose, urine glucose while on long-term therapy; hypokalemia and hyperglycemia; check weight daily; notify prescriber of weekly gain >5 lb
- Monitor B/P q4h, pulse; notify prescriber if chest pain occurs
- Monitor I&O ratio; be alert for decreasing urinary output and increasing edema
- Check plasma cortisol levels during long-term therapy (normal level: 138-635 nmol/L [SI units] when drawn at 8 AM); adrenal function periodically for HPA axis suppression
- Assess for symptoms of infection: increase temperature, WBC even after withdrawal of medication; drug masks infection symptoms
- Assess for symptoms of potassium depletion: paresthesias, fatigue, nausea, vomiting, depression, polyuria, dysrhythmias, weakness
- Monitor for edema, hypertension, cardiac symptoms
- Assess for mental status: affect, mood, behavioral changes, aggression

Topical route
- Check temperature; if fever develops, drug should be discontinued
- Assess for systemic absorption: increased temperature, inflammation, irritation

Nursing diagnoses
✓ Infection, risk for (adverse reactions)
✓ Knowledge deficit (teaching)
✓ Noncompliance (teaching)

Implementation
IV IV route
- Give **IV** (only sodium phosphate product); give over >1 min; may be given by **IV** inf in compatible sol after shaking susp (parenteral)
- Give titrated dose; use lowest effective dose

Y-site compatibilities:
Heparin, hydrocortisone, potassium chloride, vit B/C

IM route
- Give IM injection deep in large mass, rotate sites, avoid deltoid, use 21-G needle; in one dose in AM to prevent adrenal suppression; avoid SC administration; may damage tissue

PO route
- Give with food or milk to decrease GI symptoms

Inhalation route
- Give inh with water to decrease possibility of fungal infections; titrated dose; use lowest effective dose
- Use after cleaning aerosol top daily with warm water; dry thoroughly
- Store in cool environment; do not puncture or incinerate container

Topical route
- Apply only to affected areas; do not get in eyes; apply medication, then cover with occlusive dressing (only if prescribed), seal to normal skin, change q12h; systemic absorption may occur
- Apply only to dermatoses; do not use on weeping, denuded, or infected area
- Cleanse before applying drug; use treatment for a few days after area has cleared
- Store at room temperature

Patient/family education

Systemic route

- Advise patient that long-term therapy may be needed to clear infection (1-2 mo depending on type of infection); that ID as steroid user should be carried; dosage adjustment may be needed
- Instruct patient to notify prescriber if therapeutic response decreases; caution patient not to discontinue abruptly; adrenal crisis can result
- Instruct patient to avoid OTC products: salicylates, alcohol in cough products, cold preparations unless directed by prescriber
- Teach patient all aspects of drug usage including cushingoid symptoms
- Teach patient symptoms of adrenal insufficiency: nausea, anorexia, fatigue, dizziness, dyspnea, weakness, joint pain

Topical route

- Caution patient to avoid sunlight on affected area; burns may occur

Evaluation

Positive therapeutic outcome

- Ease of respirations, decreased inflammation (systemic)
- Absence of severe itching, patches on skin, flaking (top)

bethanechol (℞)

(be-than′e-kol)

bethanechol chloride, Duvoid, Urebeth, Urecholine

Func. class.: Cholinergic agonist

Chem. class.: Synthetic choline ester

Pregnancy category C

Action: Stimulates muscarinic acetylcholine receptors directly; mimics effects of parasympathetic nervous system stimulation; stimulates gastric motility, micturition; increases lower esophageal sphincter pressure

Therapeutic Outcome: Absence of continued urinary retention

Uses: Urinary retention (postoperative, postpartum), neurogenic atony of bladder with retention

Dosage and routes

Adult: PO 25-50 mg bid-qid; SC 5-10 mg tid-qid prn

Child: PO 0.6 mg/kg/day divided in 3-4 doses/day; SC 0.06 mg/kg tid or 0.15 mg/kg qid

Test dose

Adult: SC 2.5 mg repeated 15-30 min intervals × 4 doses to determine effective dose

Available forms: Tabs 5, 10, 25, 50 mg; inj SC 5 mg/ml

Adverse effects

CNS: Dizziness

CV: Hypotension, bradycardia, orthostatic hypotension, reflex tachycardia, **cardiac arrest, circulatory collapse**

EENT: Miosis, increased salivation, lacrimation, blurred vision

GI: *Nausea, bloody diarrhea, belching, vomiting, cramps, fecal incontinence*

GU: Urgency

INTEG: Rash, urticaria, flushing, increased sweating

RESP: **Acute asthma, dyspnea, bronchoconstriction**

Contraindications: Hypersensitivity, severe bradycardia, asthma, severe hypotension, hyperthyroidism, peptic ulcer, parkinsonism, seizure disorders, CAD, COPD, coronary occlusion, mechanical obstruction, peritonitis, recent urinary or GI surgery

Precautions: Hypertension, pregnancy **C**, lactation, child <8 yr, urinary retention

B

Pharmacokinetics

Absorption	Poorly absorbed (PO); well absorbed (SC)
Distribution	Does not cross blood-brain barrier
Metabolism	Unknown
Excretion	Kidneys
Half-life	Unknown

Pharmacodynamics

	PO	SC
Onset	30-90 min	5-15 min
Peak	1 hr	15-30 min
Duration	1-6 hr	2 hr

Interactions

Individual drugs

Donepezil: ↑ action of bethanechol
Procainamide: ↓ action of bethanechol
Quinidine: ↓ action of bethanechol

Drug classifications

Cholinergic agonists: ↑ action, ↑ toxicity
Ganglionic blockers: ↑ severe hypotension

Lab test interferences

↑ AST, ↑ lipase/amylase, ↑ bilirubin

NURSING CONSIDERATIONS

Assessment

- Monitor B/P, pulse, respirations; observe after parenteral dose for 1 hr
- Check I&O ratio; check for urinary retention or incontinence; if bladder emptying does not occur, notify prescriber; catheterization may be needed
- Assess for bradycardia, hypotension, bronchospasm, headache, dizziness, convulsions, sweating, cramping, respiratory depression; drug should be discontinued if toxicity occurs; atropine administration

Nursing diagnoses

✓ Urinary elimination, altered patterns (uses)
✓ Injury, risk for (adverse reactions)
✓ Knowledge deficit (teaching)

Implementation

SC route

- ⚠ Give parenteral dose by SC route; use of IM, **IV** may result in cardiac arrest or cholinergic crisis (diarrhea with blood, cramping, hypotension, circulatory collapse)
- ⚠ Administer only with atropine sulfate available for cholinergic crisis; give only after all other cholinergics have been discontinued
- Do not use sol with a precipitate, or if discolored

PO route

- Give increased doses if tolerance occurs as prescribed
- To avoid nausea and vomiting, take on an empty stomach; 1 hr ac or 2 hr pc
- Store at room temperature

Patient/family education

- Instruct patient to take drug exactly as prescribed; 1 hr ac or 2 hr pc; do not double doses; if dose is missed take within 1 hr of scheduled dose
- Caution patient to make position changes slowly; orthostatic hypotension may occur
- Instruct patient to report cramping, diarrhea with blood, flushing to prescriber

Evaluation

Positive therapeutic outcome

- Absence of urinary retention
- Absence of abdominal distention

Treatment of overdose:

Administer atropine 0.6-1.2 mg **IV** or IM (adult)

bexarotene (℞)

(bex-air'-oo-teen)

Targretin

Func. class.: Retinoid, 2nd generation

Pregnancy category X

Action: Selectively binds and activates retinoid X receptors (RXRs) that are partially responsible for cellular proliferation and differentiation; inhibits some tumor cells

Therapeutic Outcome: Decreased size and number of lesions

Uses: Cutaneous T-cell lymphoma

Investigational uses: Breast cancer

Dosage and routes

Adult: PO 300 mg/day/mm^2, may increase to 400 mg/day with proper monitoring

Available forms: Cap 75 mg

Adverse effects

CNS: *Headache,* fatigue, lethargy

GI: *Nausea, abdominal pain, diarrhea,* **acute pancreatitis**

HEMA: **Leukopenia, neutropenia, anemia**

INTEG: Rash, asthenia, dry skin

SYST: Infection, hypothyroidism

Contraindications: Hypersensitivity to retinoids, pregnancy **X**

Precautions: Lactation, sunburn, hepatic, renal disease, children

Pharmacokinetics

Absorption	Unknown
Distribution	Unknown
Metabolism	Unknown
Excretion	Kidneys
Half-life	Unknown

Pharmacodynamics

Unknown

Interactions

Individual drugs

Phenytoin: ↓ bexarotene levels

Tamoxifen: ↓ action of tamoxifen

Vitamin A: limit intake to ≤15,000 IU/day

Drug classifications

Antidiabetics: ↑ action of antidiabetics

Azole antiinfectives: ↑ bexarotene levels

Barbiturates: ↓ bexarotene levels

Oral contraceptives: ↓ action of oral contraceptives

Rifampins: ↓ bexarotene levels

Food/drug

Grapefruit juice: ↑ bexarotene levels

NURSING CONSIDERATIONS

Assessment

- Assess part of body involved, including time involved, what helps or aggravates condition, cysts, dryness, itching
- Assess cholesterol, HDL, triglycerides; these may be elevated
- Monitor CBC for leukopenia, neutropenia, anemia

Nursing diagnoses

- ✓ Skin integrity, impaired (uses)
- ✓ Body image disturbances (uses)
- ✓ Knowledge deficit (teaching)

Implementation

- Administer with food

Patient/family education

- Advise patient to avoid sunlight, sunlamps or to use protective clothing or sunscreen to prevent burns
- Instruct patient to avoid pregnancy while taking this drug and ≥1 mo after discontinuing therapy
- Teach patient to limit vit A to ≤15,000 IU/day to prevent toxicity
- Advise diabetic patients on insulin to watch for hypoglycemia

Evaluation

Positive therapeutic outcome

- Decrease in size and number of lesions

B

bicalutamide (℞)

(bi-kal-yut'ah-mide)

Casodex

Func. class.: Antineoplastic hormone

Chem. class.: Non-steroidal antiandrogen

Pregnancy category X

Action: Competitively inhibits the action to androgens by binding to cytosol androgen receptors in target tissue

➔ **Therapeutic Outcome:** Prevention of growth of malignant cells

Uses: Prostate cancer in combination with luteinizing hormone-releasing hormone (LHRH) analog

Dosage and routes

Adult: PO 50 mg qd with LHRH

Available forms: Tab 50 mg

Adverse effects

CV: Hot flashes, hypertension, chest pain, **CHF**, edema

CNS: Dizziness, paresthesia, insomnia, anxiety, neuropathy, headache

GI: *Diarrhea, constipation, nausea,* vomiting, increased liver enzyme test, anorexia, dry mouth, abdominal pain

GU: Nocturia, **hematuria,** UTI, impotence, gynecomastia, urinary incontinence, frequency, dysuria, retention, urgency, breast tenderness, decreased libido, hot flashes

INTEG: Rash, sweating, dry skin, pruritus, alopecia

MISC: Infection, anemia, dyspnea, bone pain, headache, asthenia, *back pain,* flu syndrome

Contraindications: Hypersensitivity, pregnancy **X**

Precautions: Renal, hepatic G disease, elderly, lactation

Pharmacokinetics

Absorption	Well absorbed
Distribution	Unknown
Metabolism	Liver
Excretion	Urine, feces
Half-life	5.2 days

Pharmacodynamics

Unknown

Interactions

Drug classifications

Anticoagulants: May be displaced from their binding sites

Lab test interferences

↑ AST, ↑ ALT, ↑ bilirubin, ↑ BUN, ↑ creatinine

↓ Hgb, ↓ WBC

NURSING CONSIDERATIONS

Assessment

- Assess for diarrhea, constipation, nausea, vomiting
- Assess for hot flashes, gynecomastia; assure patient that these are common side effects
- Monitor PSA (prostate specific antigen), liver function studies

Nursing diagnoses

✓ Injury, risk for (uses, adverse reactions)

✓ Knowledge deficit (teaching)

Implementation

- Give at same time each day (for both drugs) either AM or PM with or without food
- Give only with LHRH treatment

Patient/family education

- Teach patient to recognize and report signs of anemia, hepatotoxicity, renal toxicity
- Advise patient that hair may be lost, but is reversible after therapy is discontinued
- Advise patient not to use other products unless approved by prescriber
- Advise patient to use contraception

Evaluation

Positive therapeutic outcome

- Decreased tumor size, spread of malignancy

biperiden (℞)

(bye-per'i-den)

Akineton

Func. class.: Cholinergic blocker, antiparkinsonian agent

Pregnancy category C

Action: Centrally acting competitive anticholinergic; blocks cholinergic responses in the CNS

Therapeutic Outcome: Decreased involuntary movements

Uses: Parkinsonian symptoms, extrapyramidal symptoms secondary to neuroleptic drug therapy

Dosage and routes

Extrapyramidal symptoms

Adult: PO 2 mg qd-tid; IM/**IV** 2 mg q30 min, if needed, not to exceed 8 mg/24 hr

P ***Child:*** IM 40 μg/kg or 1.2 mg/m^2, may repeat q½h

Parkinsonian symptoms

Adult: PO 2 mg tid-qid; max 16 mg/24 hr

Available forms: Tabs 2 mg; inj IM/**IV** 5 mg/ml (lactate)

Adverse effects

CNS: Confusion, anxiety, restlessness, irritability, delusions, hallucinations, headache, sedation, depression, incoherence, dizziness, euphoria, tremors, memory loss

CV: Palpitations, tachycardia, postural hypotension, bradycardia

EENT: *Blurred vision,* photophobia, dilated pupils, difficulty swallowing, mydriasis, increased intraocular tension, angle closure glaucoma

GI: *Dryness of mouth, constipation,* nausea, vomiting, abdominal distress, **paralytic ileus**

GU: Hesitancy, retention, dysuria

INTEG: Rash, urticaria, dermatoses

MISC: Increased temperature, flushing, decreased sweating, **hyperthermia, heat stroke,** numbness of fingers

MS: Weakness, cramping

Contraindications: Hypersensitivity, narrow-angle glaucoma, myasthenia gravis, GI/GU obstruction, megacolon, stenosing peptic ulcers, prostatic hypertrophy

G **Precautions:** Pregnancy **C,** elderly, lactation, tachycardia, dysrhythmias, liver, kidney disease, drug abuse, hypotension, hypertension, psychiatric P patients, children

Pharmacokinetics

Absorption	Well absorbed (PO, IM)
Distribution	Unknown
Metabolism	Unknown
Excretion	Unknown
Half-life	18-24 hr

Pharmacodynamics

	IM/IV	PO
Onset	15 min	1 hr
Peak	Unknown	Unknown
Duration	6-10 hr	6-10 hr

Interactions

Individual drugs

Alcohol: ↑ sedation

Amantadine: ↑ anticholinergic effects

Haloperidol: ↑ schizophrenic symptoms

Quinidine: ↑ anticholinergic action

Drug classifications

Antacids: ↓ biperiden absorption

Antidepressants, tricyclic: ↑ anticholinergic effects

Antidiarrheals: ↓ biperiden absorption

Antihistamines: ↑ anticholinergic effects

Phenothiazines: ↑ anticholinergic effects

NURSING CONSIDERATIONS

Assessment

- Monitor I&O ratio; retention commonly causes decreased urinary output, distention, frequency, incontinence
- Assess for parkinsonism, extrapyramidal symptoms: shuffling gait, muscle rigidity, involuntary movements, pill rolling, muscle spasms, drooling before and during treatment
- Assess patient response if anticholinergics are given
- Monitor for urinary hesitancy, retention; palpate bladder if retention occurs
- Monitor for constipation, cramping, pain in abdomen, abdominal distention; increase fluids, bulk, exercise if this occurs
- Assess for tolerance over long-term therapy; dosage may have to be increased or changed
- Assess for mental status: affect, mood, CNS depression, worsening of mental symptoms during early therapy

Nursing diagnoses

✓ Mobility, impaired (uses)
✓ Knowledge deficit (teaching)

Implementation

PO route

- Give with food or pc to prevent GI upset; may give with fluids other than water; hard candy, frequent drinks, gum to relieve dry mouth
- Give hs to avoid daytime drowsiness in patients with parkinsonism
- Store at room temp

IV route

- Give parenteral dose with patient recumbent to prevent postural hypotension; give undiluted 2 mg or less over 1 min or more

Patient/family education

- Teach patient to use caution in hot weather; drug may increase susceptibility to heat stroke since perspiration is decreased; patient should remain indoors
- Teach patient not to discontinue this drug abruptly; to taper off over 1 wk to prevent withdrawal symptoms (insomnia, involuntary movements, anxiety, tachycardias)
- Teach patient to avoid driving or other hazardous activities; drowsiness, dizziness may occur
- Teach patient to avoid OTC medication: cough, cold preparations with alcohol, antihistamines unless directed by prescriber; increased CNS depression may occur
- Caution patient to rise from sitting or recumbent position slowly to minimize orthostatic hypotension
- Teach patient to use gum, hard candy, frequent sips of water to decrease dry mouth; if dry mouth continues, saliva substitutes may be prescribed
- Instruct patient that doses should not be doubled, but missed dose may be taken up to 2 hr before next dose

Evaluation

Positive therapeutic outcome

- Absence of involuntary movements (pill rolling, tremors, muscle spasms)

bisacodyl (OTC)

(bis-a-koe'dill)

Bisc-Evac ✱, Bisacolax ✱, Bisco-Lax ✱, Carter's Little Pills, Dacodyl, Deficol, Dulcagen, Dulcolax, Fleet Bisacodyl, Fleet Laxative, Therelax

Func. class.: Laxative, stimulant
Chem. class.: Diphenylmethane

Pregnancy category C

Action: Acts directly on intestine by increasing motor activity; thought to irritate colonic intramural plexus; increases water in the colon

Therapeutic Outcome: Decreased constipation

Uses: Short-term treatment of constipation, bowel or rectal preparation for surgery, examination

Dosage and routes

P ***Adult* ≥*12 yr:*** PO 5-15 mg in PM or AM; may use up to 30 mg for bowel or rec preparation; REC 10 mg (single dose)

P ***Child* >*3 yr:*** PO 5-10 mg as a single dose; REC 10 mg as a single dose

P ***Child* <*2 yr:*** REC 5 mg as a single dose

Available forms: Enteric coated tabs 5 mg; supp 5, 10 mg; rec sol 10 mg/37 ml; enema 0.33 mg/ml, 10 mg/5 ml; powder for rec sol 1.5 mg bisacodyl/2.5 g tannic acid

Adverse effects

CNS: Muscle weakness

GI: *Nausea, vomiting, anorexia, cramps,* diarrhea, rectal burning (supp)

META: Protein-losing enteropathy, alkalosis, hypokalemia, ***tetany,*** electrolyte and fluid imbalances

Contraindications: Hypersensitivity, rectal fissures, abdominal pain, nausea, vomiting, appendicitis, acute surgical abdomen, ulcerated hemorrhoids, acute hepatitis, fecal impaction, intestinal/biliary tract obstruction

Precautions: Pregnancy **C**

Pharmacokinetics

Absorption	Poor
Distribution	Unknown
Metabolism	Liver, minimally
Excretion	Kidneys
Half-life	Unknown

Pharmacodynamics

	PO	RECT
Onset	6-10 hr	15-60 min
Peak	Unknown	Unknown
Duration	Unknown	Unknown

Interactions

Drug classifications

Antacids: ↓ of enteric coating of drugs

H_2-blockers: ↑ gastric irritation

Herb/drug

Lily of the valley: ↑ action/side effects

Pheasant's eye: ↑ action/side effects

Squill: ↑ action/side effects

NURSING CONSIDERATIONS

Assessment

- Monitor blood, urine electrolytes if used often by patient; check I&O ratio to identify fluid loss
- Assess cramping, rectal bleeding, nausea, vomiting; if these symptoms occur, drug should be discontinued; identify cause of constipation; identify whether fluids, bulk, or exercise missing from lifestyle

Nursing diagnoses

✓ Constipation (uses)
✓ Diarrhea (side effects)
✓ Knowledge deficit (teaching)
✓ Noncompliance (teaching)

Implementation

PO route

- Give alone with water only for better absorption; do not take within 1 hr of antacids, milk
- Administer in AM or PM (oral dose)
- Do not chew; swallow tabs whole

Rectal route

- Lubricate before insertion, patient should retain for ½ hr

Patient/family education

- Discuss with the patient that adequate fluid and bulk consumption is necessary
- Advise patient that normal bowel movements do not always occur daily
- Teach patient not to use in presence of abdominal pain, nausea, vomiting; tell patient to notify prescriber if constipation unrelieved or if symptoms of electrolyte imbalance occur: muscle cramps, pain, weakness, dizziness, excessive thirst

Evaluation

Positive therapeutic outcome

- Decreased constipation within 3 days

bismuth subsalicylate (OTC)
(bis'meth sub-sa-li'si-late)

Bismatrol, Bismatrol Extra Strength, Bismed, Pepto-Bismol, Pepto-Bismol Maximum Strength, Pink Bismuth, PMS-Bismuth Subsalicylate

Func. class.: Antidiarrheal
Chem. class.: Salicylate

Pregnancy category C

Action: Inhibits prostaglandin synthesis responsible for GI hypermotility; stimulates absorption of fluid and electrolytes; antimicrobial, antisecretory effects

Therapeutic Outcome: Absence of loose, watery stools

Uses: Diarrhea (cause undetermined); prevention of diarrhea when traveling; may be included to treat *Helicobacter pylori*

Dosage and routes
Antidiarrheal

Adult: PO 524 mg q½h or 1048 mg q1h, max 4.2 g/24 hr

Child 9-12 yr: PO 15 ml; 262 mg q½-1h, max 2.1 g/24 hr

Child 6-9 yr: PO 174.6 mg q½-1h, max 1.4 g/24 hr

Child 3-6 yr: PO 88 mg q½-1h, max 704 mg/24 hr

Available forms: Chewable tabs 262 mg; susp 262, 300, 524 mg/15 ml

Adverse effects
CNS: Confusion, twitching
EENT: Hearing loss, tinnitus, metallic taste, blue gums
GI: Increased fecal impaction (high doses), dark stools, constipation
HEMA: Increased bleeding time

P Contraindications: Child <3 yr; impaction, children, teens with flulike symptoms, hypersensitivity (aspirin), history of GI bleeding, renal disease

Precautions: Anticoagulant therapy, pregnancy **C**, elderly, lactation, gout, diabetes mellitus, immobility

Pharmacokinetics

Absorption	Salicylate >90%
Distribution	None
Metabolism	None
Excretion	Feces (unchanged)
Half-life	Unknown

Pharmacodynamics

Onset	1 hr
Peak	2 hr
Duration	4 hr

Interactions
Individual drugs
Aminosalicylic acid: ↑ side effects, ↑ toxicity
Tetracycline: ↓ absorption
Drug classifications
Anticoagulants, oral: ↑ effect of anticoagulants
Antidiabetics, oral: ↑ effect of antidiabetics
Salicylates: ↑ risk of salicylate toxicity
Lab test interferences
Interference: Radiographic studies of GI system

NURSING CONSIDERATIONS
Assessment
- Monitor skin turgor; dehydration may occur in severe diarrhea; monitor electrolytes (potassium, sodium, chloride) if diarrhea is severe or continues long term
- Assess bowel pattern (frequency, consistency, shape, volume, color) before drug therapy, after treatment; check weight, bowel sounds; identify factors contributing to diarrhea (bacteria, diet, medications, tube feedings)

Nursing diagnoses
- ✓ Diarrhea (uses)
- ✓ Constipation (adverse reactions)
- ✓ Knowledge deficit (teaching)

Implementation
- Shake susp before use; chewable tabs should not be swallowed whole

Patient/family education
- Teach patient to stop use if symptoms do not improve within 2 days or become worse, or if diarrhea is accompanied by high fever
- Teach patient to increase fluids for rehydration
- Tell patient to chew or dissolve chewable tabs in mouth; do not swallow whole; shake susp before using
- Tell patient to avoid other salicylates unless directed by prescriber; not to P give to children because of possibility of Reye's syndrome
- Tell patient that stools may turn gray; tongue may darken; impaction may occur in debilitated patients

Evaluation
Positive therapeutic outcome
- Decreased diarrhea

bisoprolol (℞)
(bis-oh'pro-lole)
Zebeta
Func. class.: Antihypertensive
Chem. class.: β_1-Blocker (selective)
Pregnancy category C

Action: Preferentially and competitively blocks stimulation of β_1-adrenergic receptor within cardiac muscle (decreases rate of SA node discharge, increases recovery time), slows conduction of AV node, decreases heart rate, which decreases O_2 consumption in myocardium; decreases renin-aldosterone-angiotensin system; inhibits β_2-receptors in bronchial and vascular smooth muscle at high doses

Therapeutic Outcome: Decreased B/P, heart rate

Uses: Mild to moderate hypertension

Investigational uses: Angina pectoris, supraventricular tachycardia

Dosage and routes
Renal/hepatic dose
2.5 mg PO, titrate upward

Hypertension
Adult: PO 5 mg qd; may increase if necessary to 20 mg once daily; may need to reduce dose in presence of renal or hepatic impairment

Available forms: Tabs 5, 10 mg

Adverse effects
CNS: Vertigo, headache, insomnia, fatigue, dizziness, mental changes, memory loss, hallucinations, depression, lethargy, drowsiness, strange dreams, catatonia, peripheral neuropathy
CV: **Ventricular dysrhythmias, profound hypotension, bradycardia, CHF,** cold extremities, postural hypotension, 2nd- or 3rd-degree heart block
EENT: Sore throat, dry burning eyes
ENDO: Increased hypoglycemic response to insulin
GI: Nausea, diarrhea, vomiting, **mesenteric arterial thrombosis,** ischemic colitis, flatulence, gastritis, gastric pain
GU: Impotence, decreased libido
HEMA: **Agranulocytosis, thrombocytopenia,** purpura, **eosinophilia**
INTEG: Rash, fever, alopecia, pruritus, sweating
MISC: Facial swelling, weight gain, decreased exercise tolerance
MS: Joint pain, arthralgia
RESP: **Bronchospasm,** dyspnea, wheezing, cough, nasal stuffiness

Contraindications: Hypersensitivity to β-blockers, cardiogenic shock, heart block (2nd or 3rd degree), sinus bradycardia, CHF, cardiac failure

Precautions: Major surgery, P pregnancy **C,** lactation, children, diabetes mellitus, renal or hepatic disease, thyroid disease, COPD, asthma, well-compensated heart failure, aortic or mitral valve disease, peripheral vascular disease, myasthenia gravis

Do Not Confuse:

Zebeta/Diabeta

Pharmacokinetics

Absorption	Well absorbed
Distribution	Unknown; protein binding (30%)
Metabolism	Liver, inactive metabolites
Excretion	Urine, unchanged (50%)
Half-life	9-12 hr

Pharmacodynamics

Onset	Unknown
Peak	2-4 hr
Duration	24 hr

Interactions

Individual drugs

Alcohol: (large amounts) ↑ hypotension
Clonidine: Fatal reactions after discontinuing clonidine
Epinephrine: ↑ hypertension, then bradycardia
Flecainide: ↑ effects of both drugs
Guanethidine: ↑ hypotension
Haloperidol: ↑ effects of both drugs
Hydralazine: ↑ hypotension, bradycardia
Lidocaine: ↑ lidocaine toxicity
Quinidine: ↑ hypotension, bradycardia
Prazosin: ↑ hypotension, bradycardia
Reserpine: ↑ hypotension
Theophylline: ↓ bronchodilatation

Drug classifications

Barbiturates: ↓ antihypertensive effects
Calcium channel blockers: ↑ hypotension, myocardial depression
Diuretics, loop: ↑ CV effects
MAOIs: ↑ bradycardia
NSAIDs: ↓ antihypertensive effect
Oral contraceptives: ↑ hypotension
Penicillins: ↓ antihypertensive effects
Salicylates: ↓ antihypertensive effects
Sulfonylureas: ↓ hypoglycemic effect

Lab test interferences

↑ AST, ↑ ALT
Interference: Glucose/insulin tolerance tests

NURSING CONSIDERATIONS

Assessment

- Monitor B/P during beginning treatment, periodically thereafter; pulse q4h: note rate, rhythm, quality; apical/radial pulse before administration; notify prescriber of any significant changes (pulse <50 bpm)
- Check for baselines in renal, liver function tests before therapy begins
- Assess for edema in feet, legs daily, monitor I&O, daily weight; check for jugular vein distention, rales bilaterally, dyspnea (CHF)
- Monitor skin turgor, dryness of mucous membranes for hydration G status, especially elderly

Nursing diagnoses

- ✓ Cardiac output, decreased (uses)
- ✓ Injury, risk for (side effects)
- ✓ Knowledge deficit (teaching)
- ✓ Noncompliance (teaching)

Implementation

- Give qd; give with food to prevent GI upset; may be crushed
- Store protected from light, moisture; place in cool environment

Patient/family education

- Teach patient not to discontinue drug abruptly; may cause precipitate angina if stopped abruptly, evaluate noncompliance
- Teach patient not to use OTC products containing α-adrenergic stimulants (such as nasal decongestants, cold preparations); to avoid alcohol, smoking and to limit sodium intake as prescribed
- Teach patient how to take pulse and

B/P at home; advise when to notify prescriber
- Instruct patient to comply with weight control, dietary adjustments, modified exercise program
- Tell patient to carry/wear Medic Alert ID to identify drug being taken, allergies; tell patient drug controls symptoms but does not cure
- Caution patient to avoid hazardous activities if dizziness, drowsiness present
- Teach patient to take drug as prescribed, not to double doses, skip doses; take any missed doses as soon as remembered if at least 8 hr until next dose
- Advise patient to report bradycardia, dizziness, confusion, depression, fever, cold extremities

Evaluation
Positive therapeutic outcome
- Decreased B/P in hypertension (after 1-2 wk)

Treatment of overdose:
Lavage, **IV** atropine for bradycardia, **IV** theophylline for bronchospasm, digitalis, O_2, diuretic for cardiac failure, hemodialysis, **IV** glucose for hypoglycemia, **IV** diazepam (or phenytoin) for seizures

HIGH ALERT

bivalirudin (℞)
(bye-val-i-rue′din)
Angiomax
Func. class.: Anticoagulant
Chem. class.: Thrombin inhibitor
Pregnancy category B

Action: Direct inhibitor of thrombin that is highly specific

➡ **Therapeutic Outcome:** Anticoagulation in percutaneous transluminal coronary angioplasty (PTCA)

Uses: Unstable angina in patients undergoing PTCA

Dosage and routes
Adult: **IV** bol 1 mg/kg, then **IV** inf 2.5 mg/kg/hr for 4 hr; another **IV** inf may be used at 0.2 mg/kg/hr for ≤20 hr; this drug is intended to be used with aspirin (325 mg qd) adjusted to body weight

Available forms: Inj, lyophilized 250 mg

Adverse effects
CV: *Hypo/hypertension, bradycardia*
CNS: *Headache, insomnia, anxiety, nervousness, fever*
GI: *Nausea, vomiting, abdominal pain, dyspepsia*
HEMA: **Hemorrhage**
MS: *Back pain*
MISC: Pain at inj site, pelvic pain, urinary retention

Contraindications: Hypersensitivity, active bleeding

Precautions: Renal function **P** impairment, lactation, children, hepatic disease, pregnancy **B**

Pharmacokinetics
Absorption	Unknown
Distribution	Unknown
Metabolism	Unknown
Excretion	Kidneys
Half-life	25 min

Pharmacodynamics
Unknown

Interactions
Drug classifications
Anticoagulants: ↑ risk of bleeding
Thrombolytics: ↑ risk of bleeding

NURSING CONSIDERATIONS
Assessment
❗ Assess for fall in B/P or Hct that may indicate hemorrhage
- Assess for fever, skin rash, urticaria

Nursing diagnoses
✓ Decreased cardiac output (uses)
✓ Knowledge deficit (teaching)

Implementation

- To each 250-mg vial add 5 ml of sterile water for inj, swirl until dissolved, further dilute reconstituted vial with 50 ml of D_5W or 0.9% NaCl (5 mg/ml); the dose is adjusted to body weight
- Give reduced dose in renal impairment

Patient/family education

- Explain reason for drug and expected results

Evaluation

Positive therapeutic outcome

- Anticoagulation in PTCA

HIGH ALERT

bleomycin (℞)

(blee-oh-mye'sin)

Blenoxane

Func. class.: Antineoplastic, antibiotic

Chem. class.: Glycopeptide

Pregnancy category D

Action: Inhibits synthesis of DNA, RNA, protein; derived from *Streptomyces verticillus;* replication is decreased by binding to DNA, which causes strand splitting; phase specific in the G_2 and M phases; a nonvesicant

Therapeutic Outcome: Prevention of rapidly growing malignant cells

Uses: Cancer of head, neck, penis, cervix, vulva of squamous cell origin, Hodgkin's disease, lymphosarcoma, reticulum cell sarcoma, testicular carcinoma, malignant pleural effusion

Dosage and routes

P ***Adult and child:*** SC/**IV**/IM 0.25-0.5 U/kg q1-2 wk or 10-20 U/m^2; then 1 U/day or 5 U/wk; may also be given intraarterially; do not exceed total dose, 400 U in lifetime

Available forms: Powder for inj 15 U/vial

Adverse effects

CNS: Fever, chills, pain at tumor site, headache, confusion

CV: Hypotension, peripheral vasoconstriction

GI: *Nausea, vomiting, anorexia, stomatitis, weight loss,* ulceration of mouth, lips

HEMA: Hypotension, peripheral vasoconstriction

IDIOSYNCRATIC REACTION: Hypotension, confusion, fever, chills, wheezing

INTEG: *Rash, hyperkeratosis, nail changes, alopecia,* fever and chills, pruritus, acne, striae, peeling

RESP: **Fibrosis,** pneumonitis, wheezing, **pulmonary toxicity**

SYST: **Anaphylaxis,** radiation recall, Raynaud's phenomenon

Contraindications: Hypersensitivity, pregnancy **D**

Precautions: Renal, hepatic, respiratory disease

Pharmacokinetics	
Absorption	Well absorbed (IM, SC, intrapleural, intraperitoneal)
Distribution	Widely distributed
Metabolism	Liver, 30%
Excretion	Kidneys, unchanged (50%)
Half-life	2 hr; ↑ in renal disease

Pharmacodynamics

Unknown

Interactions

Individual drugs

Phenytoin: ↓ phenytoin levels

Radiation: ↑ toxicity, bone marrow suppression

Drug classifications

Anesthetics, general: ↑ toxicity

Antineoplastics: ↑ toxicity, bone marrow suppression

NURSING CONSIDERATIONS

Assessment

- Assess buccal cavity q8h for dryness, sores or ulceration, white patches, oral pain, bleeding, dysphagia; obtain prescription for viscous lidocaine (Xylocaine)
- Assess symptoms indicating anaphylaxis: rash, pruritus, urticaria, purpuric skin lesions, itching, flushing, wheezing, hypotension; have emergency equipment available
- Monitor CBC, differential, platelet count weekly; withhold drug if WBC <4000/mm^3 or platelet count <100,000/mm^3; notify prescriber of results if WBC <20,000/mm^3, platelets <150,000/mm^3
- Monitor temp q4h (may indicate beginning of infection)
- Monitor liver function tests before and during therapy (bilirubin, AST, ALT, LDH) as needed or monthly
- Assess for bleeding: hematuria, stool guaiac, bruising or petechiae, mucosa or orifices q8h; inflammation of mucosa, breaks in skin
- Identify dyspnea, rales, unproductive cough, chest pain, tachypnea
- Identify effects of alopecia on body image; discuss feelings about body changes; if edema in feet, joint pain, stomach pain, shaking present, prescriber should be notified; identify inflammation of mucosa, breaks in skin

Nursing diagnoses

- Injury, risk for (adverse reactions)
- Body image disturbance (adverse reactions)
- Infection, risk for (adverse reactions)
- Knowledge deficit (teaching)

Implementation

- Avoid contact with skin, very irritating; wash completely to remove
- Give fluids **IV** or PO before chemotherapy to hydrate patient
- Give antacid before oral agent; give antiemetic 30-60 min before giving drug to prevent vomiting and prn and antibiotics for prophylaxis of infection
- Provide liq diet: carbonated beverages, gelatin may be added if patient is not nauseated or vomiting
- Rinsing of mouth tid-qid with water, club soda; brushing of teeth bid-qid with soft brush or cotton-tipped applicators for stomatitis; use unwaxed dental floss

SC/IM route

- IM test dose in lymphoma
- Reconstitute with 1-5 ml sterile water for inj; D_5W, 0.9% NaCl, rotate inj sites

IV route

- Drug should be prepared by experienced personnel using proper precautions
- Two test doses 2-5 U before initial dose in lymphoma; monitor for anaphylaxis
- Give by direct **IV** after reconstituting 15 U or less/5 ml or more of D_5W or 0.9% NaCl; give 15 U or less/10 min through Y-tube or 3-way stopcock initial dose; monitor for anaphylaxis

Intermittent infusion

- Administer after diluting 50-100 ml 0.9% NaCl, D_5W and giving at prescribed rate

Intrapleural route

- Give 60 U/50-100 ml of 0.9% NaCl, administered by physician through thoracotomy tube

Syringe compatibilities:

Cisplatin, cyclophosphamide, doxorubicin, droperidol, fluorouracil, furosemide, heparin, leucovorin, methotrexate, metoclopramide, mitomycin, vinblastine, vincristine

Y-site compatibilities:

Allopurinol, amisostine, aztreonam, cisplatin, cyclophosphamide, doxorubicin, doxorubicin liposome, droperidol, filgrastim, fludarabine, fluorouracil, granisetron, heparin, leucovorin, melphalan, methotrexate, metoclopramide, mitomycin, ondansetron, paclitaxel, piperacillin/

tazobactam, sargramostim, teniposide, thiotepa, vinblastine, vincristine, vinorelbine

Additive compatibilities: Amikacin, cephapirin, dexamethasone, diphenhydramine, fluorouracil, gentamicin, heparin, hydrocortisone, phenytoin, streptomycin, tobramycin, vinblastine, vincristine

Additive incompatibilities: Aminophylline, ascorbic acid inj, carbenicillin, cefazolin, cephalothin, diazepam, hydrocortisone, methotrexate, mitomycin, nafcillin, penicillin G sodium, terbutaline

Solution compatibilities: 0.9% NaCl

Patient/family education

- Teach patient to avoid use of products containing aspirin or ibuprofen, razors, commercial mouthwash; bleeding may occur; to report symptoms of bleeding (hematuria, tarry stools)
- Instruct patient to report signs of anemia (fatigue, headache, irritability, faintness, shortness of breath)
- Instruct patient to report any changes in breathing or coughing even several months after treatment; to avoid crowds and persons with respiratory tract or other infections
- Inform patient that hair may be lost during treatment; a wig or hairpiece may make patient feel better; new hair may be different in color, texture
- Caution patient not to have any vaccinations without the advice of the prescriber; serious reactions can occur
- Advise patient contraception is needed during treatment and for several months after completion of therapy

Evaluation

Positive therapeutic outcome

- Prevention of rapid division of malignant cells

bosentan

See Appendix A, Selected New Drugs

HIGH ALERT

bretylium (℞)

(bre-til'ee-um)

Bretylate ♣, bretylium tosylate, Bretylol

Func. class.: Antidysrhythmic (Class III)

Chem. class.: Quaternary ammonium compound

Pregnancy category C

Action: After a transient release of norepinephrine, inhibits further release by postganglionic nerve endings; prolongs action potential, duration, and effective refractory period

➔ **Therapeutic Outcome:** Absence of dysrhythmias

Uses: Life-threatening ventricular tachycardia, cardioversion, ventricular fibrillation; for short-term use only

Dosage and routes

Renal dose

CrCl 10-50 ml/min 25%-50% dose; CrCl <10 ml/min avoid use

Severe ventricular fibrillation

Adult: **IV** bol 5 mg/kg; increase to 10 mg/kg repeated q15 min, up to 30 mg/kg; **IV** inf 1-2 mg/min or give 5-10 mg/kg over 10 min q6h (maintenance)

Ventricular tachycardia

Adult: **IV** inf 500 mg diluted in 50 ml D_5W or NS; infuse over 10-30 min; may repeat in 1 hr; maintain with 1-2 mg/min or 5-10 mg/kg over 10-30 min q6h; IM 5-10 mg/kg undiluted; repeat in 1-2 hr if needed; maintain with same dose q6-8h

P ***Child:*** 2-5 mg/kg/dose

Available forms: Inj 50 mg/ml; 1, 2, 4 mg/ml prefilled syringes

Adverse effects

CNS: *Syncope, dizziness,* confusion, psychosis, anxiety

CV: *Hypotension, postural hypotension, bradycardia,* angina, PVCs, substernal pressure, transient hypertension, precipitation of angina

GI: *Nausea, vomiting*

RESP: **Respiratory depression**

Contraindications: Hypersensitivity, digitalis toxicity, aortic stenosis, P pulmonary hypertension, children

Precautions: Renal disease, P pregnancy **C**, lactation, children

Pharmacokinetics	
Absorption	Complete bioavailability (**IV**)
Distribution	Unknown
Metabolism	Not metabolized
Excretion	Kidneys, unchanged
Half-life	4-17 hr

Pharmacodynamics	IV	IM
Onset	5 min	½-2 hr
Peak	Infusion's end	Unknown
Duration	6-24 hr	6-24 hr

Interactions

Individual drugs

Caffeine: ↓ effects of adenosine

Carbamazepine: ↑ heart block

Dopamine: ↑ pressor effects

Norepinephrine: ↑ pressor effects

Drug classifications

Cardiac glycosides: ↑ toxicity

Sympathomimetics: ↑ sympathomimetic effect

Herb/drug

Aloe: ↑ bretylium effect

Buckthorn bark/berry: ↑ bretylium effect

Cascara sagrada: ↑ bretylium effect

Rhubarb root: ↑ bretylium effect

Senna leaf/roots: ↑ bretylium effect

NURSING CONSIDERATIONS

Assessment

- Monitor ECG continuously to determine drug effectiveness; measure PR, QRS, QT intervals; check for PVCs, other dysrhythmias; monitor B/P continuously for hypotension, hypertension; check for rebound hypertension after 1-2 hr

Nursing diagnoses

- ✓ Cardiac output, decreased (uses)
- ✓ Gas exchange, impaired (adverse reactions)
- ✓ Knowledge deficit (teaching)

Implementation

IM route

- Give in large muscle mass, rotate sites to prevent necrosis

IV **IV route**

Direct

- Give **IV** bol undiluted; give 6 mg or less over 1 min; if using an **IV** line, use port near insertion site, flush with normal saline (50 ml)

Intermittent infusion

- Give by intermittent inf after diluting 500 mg/50 ml or more with 0.9% NaCl, D_5W, D_5/0.45% NaCl, D_5/0.9% NaCl, LR, ⅙ mol/L sodium lactate; run over >8 min

Continuous infusion

- Give by cont inf diluted in sol; give 1-2 mg/min; use inf site
- Store at room temp; sol should be clear

Additive compatibilities:
Aminophylline, atracurium, calcium chloride, calcium gluconate, digoxin, dopamine, esmolol, regular insulin, lidocaine, potassium chloride, quinadine verapamil

Y-site compatibilities:
Amiodarone, amrinone, cisatracurium, diltiazem, dobutamine, famotidine, isoproterenol, ranitidine, remifentanil

Additive incompatibilities: Phenytoin

Evaluation

Positive therapeutic outcome

- Decreased B/P, dysrhythmias, heart rate; normal sinus rhythm

bromocriptine (℞)

(broe-moe-krip'teen)

Alti-Bromocriptine ♣, Apo-Bromocriptine ♣, Parlodel

Func. class.: Antiparkinsonian agent; dopamine receptor agonist

Chem. class.: Ergot alkaloid derivative

Pregnancy category B

Action: Inhibits prolactin release by activating postsynaptic dopamine receptors; activation of striatal dopamine receptors may be reason for improvement in Parkinson's disease

Therapeutic Outcome: Decreased involuntary movements in Parkinson's disease; decreased lactation; decreased hormone levels in acromegaly; absence of amenorrhea in hyperprolactinemia

Uses: Adjunct with levodopa in Parkinson's disease, amenorrhea/galactorrhea caused by hyperprolactinemia, acromegaly

Investigational uses: Pituitary adenomas, neuroleptic malignant syndrome

Dosage and routes

Hyperprolactinemia

Adult: PO 1.25-2.5 mg with meals; may increase by 2.5 mg q3-7 days; usual dosage 5-7.5 mg

Acromegaly

Adult: PO 1.25-2.5 mg/day × 3 days hs; may increase by 1.25-2.5 mg q3-7 days; usual range 20-30 mg/day; max 100 mg/day

Parkinson's disease

Adult: PO 1.25 mg bid with meals; may increase q2-4 wk by 2.5 mg/day; not to exceed 100 mg/day

Pituitary adenoma

Adult: PO 1.25 mg bid-tid, may increase over several weeks

Neuroleptic malignant syndrome

Adult: PO 5 mg qd, max 20 mg/day

Available forms: Caps 5 mg; tabs 2.5 mg

Adverse effects

CNS: *Headache,* depression, restlessness, anxiety, nervousness, confusion, **convulsions,** hallucinations, *dizziness,* fatigue, drowsiness, abnormal involuntary movements, psychosis

CV: *Orthostatic hypotension,* decreased B/P, palpitations, extrasystole, **shock,** dysrhythmias, bradycardia, **MI**

EENT: Blurred vision, diplopia, burning eyes, nasal congestion

GI: *Nausea, vomiting, anorexia,* cramps, constipation, diarrhea, dry mouth, GI hemorrhage

GU: Frequency, retention, incontinence, diuresis

INTEG: *Rash on face, arms,* alopecia, coolness, pallor of fingers, toes

Contraindications: Hypersensitivity to ergot, severe ischemic disease, severe peripheral vascular disease

Precautions: Lactation, hepatic disease, renal disease, children, pituitary tumors, pregnancy **B**

Do Not Confuse:
Parlodel/pindolol

Pharmacokinetics

Absorption	Poorly absorbed
Distribution	Unknown
Metabolism	Liver, completely
Excretion	85%-98% feces
Half-life	4 hr (initial); 50 hr (terminal)

Pharmacodynamics

Onset	½-1½ hr
Peak	1-3 hr
Duration	8-12 hr

Interactions

Individual drugs

Alcohol: ↑ disulfiram-like reaction
Haloperidol: ↓ levels of bromocriptine
Levodopa: ↑ neurologic effects
Loxapine: ↓ bromocriptine
Methyldopa: ↓ levels of bromocriptine
Metoclopramide: ↓ bromocriptine
Reserpine: ↓ effects of bromocriptine

Drug classifications

Analgesics, opioid: ↑ CNS depression
Antidepressants, tricyclic: ↓ levels of bromocriptine
Antihistamines: ↑ CNS depression
Antihypertensives: ↑ hypotension
Estrogens: ↓ bromocriptine effect
MAOIs: ↓ bromocriptine
Oral contraceptives: ↓ bromocriptine
Phenothiazines: ↓ levels of bromocriptine
Progestins: ↓ bromocriptine
Sedative/hypnotics: ↑ CNS depression

☒ *Herb/drug*

Chaste tree fruit: ↓ bromocriptine effect

Lab test interferences

↑ Growth hormone, ↑ AST, ↑ ALT, ↑ BUN, ↑ uric acid, ↑ alkaline phosphatase

NURSING CONSIDERATIONS

Assessment

- Assess symptoms of Parkinson's disease (extrapyramidal symptoms): shuffling gait, muscle rigidity, involuntary movements, pill rolling, muscle spasms, drooling before and during treatment
- Assess for resolution of symptoms of neuroleptic malignant syndrome: decreased temp, seizures, sweating, pulse
- Monitor for change in size of soft tissue volume in acromegaly
- Monitor B/P; establish baseline, compare with other readings; this drug decreases B/P; patient should remain recumbent for 2-4 hr after first dose; supervise ambulation

Nursing diagnoses

✓ Mobility, impaired (uses)
✓ Knowledge deficit (teaching)

Implementation

- Give with meals or milk to prevent GI symptoms; crush tab if patient has swallowing difficulty
- Give hs so dizziness, orthostatic hypotension do not occur
- Store at room temp in air-tight container

Patient/family education

- Advise patient to change position slowly to prevent orthostatic hypotension
- Tabs may be crushed and mixed with food
- Caution patient to use contraceptives during treatment with this drug; pregnancy may occur; to use methods other than oral contraceptives
- Teach patient that therapeutic effect for Parkinson's disease may take 2 mo: galactorrhea, amenorrhea
- Caution patient to avoid hazardous activity if dizziness, drowsiness occurs during treatment start-up
- Advise patient to avoid alcohol and OTC medication unless approved by prescriber
- Teach patients with acromegaly to notify prescriber immediately if severe headache, nausea, vomiting, blurred vision occur; indicates change in enlargement of tumor
- Advise patient to report symptoms of MI immediately

B

Evaluation

Positive therapeutic outcome

- Parkinson's disease: decreased dyskinesia, decreased slow movements, decreased drooling
- Decreased breast engorgement with accompanied pain, tenderness
- Acromegly: decreased growth hormone levels

brompheniramine (OTC, ℞)

(brome-fen-eer'a-meen)

Bromfenac, brompheniramine, Chlorphed, Dehist, Diamine T.D., Dimetane, Dimetane Extentabs, Dimetapp Allergy Liqui-Gels, Nasahist-B

Func. class.: Antihistamine

Chem. class.: Alkylamine, H_1-receptor antagonist

Pregnancy category B

Action: Acts on blood vessels, GI, respiratory system by competing with histamine for H_1-receptor site; decreases allergic response by blocking histamine

➡ **Therapeutic Outcome:** Absence of allergy symptoms and rhinitis

Uses: Allergy symptoms, rhinitis, allergic dermatoses, nasal allergies, hypersensitivity reactions including blood transfusion reactions, anaphylaxis

Dosage and routes

Adult and child >12 yr: PO 4-8 mg tid-qid, not to exceed 36 mg/day; TIME REL 8-12 mg bid-tid, not to exceed 36 mg/day; IM/**IV**/SC 5-20 mg q6-12h, not to exceed 40 mg/day

P ***Child 6-12 yr:*** PO 2 mg tid-qid, not to exceed 12 mg/day; IM/**IV**/SC 0.5 mg/kg/day divided tid or qid

P ***Child 2-6 yr:*** 1 mg q4-6h (not to exceed 6 mg/day)

Available forms: Tabs 4 mg; elix 2 mg/5 ml; inj 10 mg/ml; caps 4 mg

Adverse effects

CNS: *Dizziness, drowsiness,* poor coordination, fatigue, anxiety, euphoria, confusion, paresthesia, neuritis

CV: Hypotension, palpitations, tachycardia

EENT: Blurred vision, dilated pupils, tinnitus, nasal stuffiness, dry nose, throat, mouth

GI: Nausea, vomiting, anorexia, constipation, diarrhea

GU: Retention, dysuria, frequency, impotence

HEMA: **Thrombocytopenia, agranulocytosis, hemolytic anemia**

INTEG: Photosensitivity

RESP: Increased thick secretions, wheezing, chest tightness

Contraindications: Hypersensitivity to H_1-receptor antagonists, acute asthma attack, lower respiratory tract P disease, child <2 yr

Precautions: Increased intraocular pressure, renal disease, cardiac disease, hypertension, bronchial asthma, seizure disorder, stenosed peptic ulcers, hyperthyroidism, prostatic hypertrophy, bladder neck obstruction, pregnancy **B**

Pharmacokinetics

Absorption	Well absorbed (PO, IM)
Distribution	Widely distributed; crosses blood-brain barrier
Metabolism	Liver, extensively
Excretion	Kidneys, metabolite; breast milk (minimal)
Half-life	12-34 hr

Pharmacodynamics

	PO	SC/IM	IV
Onset	15-30 min	30 min	Immediate
Peak	2-5 hr	Unknown	Unknown
Duration	6-12 hr	8-12 hr	8-12 hr

Interactions

Individual drugs

Alcohol: ↑ CNS depression

Drug classifications

CNS depressants: ↑ CNS depression
MAOIs: ↑ anticholinergic effect
Opiates: ↑ CNS depression
Sedative/hypnotics: ↑ CNS depression

Herb/drug

Henbane leaf: ↑ anticholinergic effect
Kava: ↑ CNS depression

Lab test interferences

False negative: Skin allergy tests (discontinue antihistamines before testing)

NURSING CONSIDERATIONS

Assessment

- Assess respiratory status: rate, rhythm, increase in bronchial secretions, wheezing, chest tightness; provide fluids to 2 L/day to decrease secretion thickness
- Monitor I&O ratio: be alert for urinary retention, frequency, dysuria, especially elderly; drug should be discontinued if these occur
- Monitor CBC during long-term therapy; blood dyscrasias may occur but are rare
- **IV** administration may result in rapid drop in B/P, sweating, dizziness, especially in elderly

Nursing diagnoses

✓ Airway clearance, ineffective (uses)
✓ Injury, risk for (side effects)
✓ Knowledge deficit (teaching)
✓ Noncompliance (teaching, overuse)

Implementation

PO route

- May give with food to prevent GI upset; absorption is not altered by food
- Store in tight, light-resistant container

IV route

- Give undiluted or dilute 10 mg/ml using 0.9% NaCl at a rate of 1 min or more
- May be further diluted in 0.9% NaCl, D_5W; give as intermittent inf at prescribed rate

Patient/family education

- Teach patient all aspects of drug use; to notify prescriber if confusion, sedation, hypotension occur; to avoid driving or other hazardous activity if drowsiness occurs; to avoid alcohol or other CNS depressants that may potentiate effect
- Instruct patient not to exceed recommended dosage; dysrhythmias may occur
- Teach patient hard candy, gum, frequent rinsing of mouth may be used for dryness

Evaluation

Positive therapeutic outcome

- Absence of running or congested nose, rashes

Treatment of overdose:

Administer ipecac syrup or lavage, diazepam, vasopressors, barbiturates (short acting)

bumetanide (Rx)

(byoo-met'a-nide)

Bumex

Func. class: Loop diuretic, antihypertensive

Chem. class.: Sulfonamide derivative

Pregnancy category C

Action: Acts on the ascending loop of Henle in the kidney to inhibit the reabsorption of the electrolytes sodium and chloride, causing excretion of sodium, calcium, magnesium, chloride, water, and some potassium; also decreases reabsorption of sodium and chloride and increases the excretion of potassium in the distal tubule of the kidney; responsible for antihypertensive effect and peripheral vasodilatation

B

Therapeutic Outcome: Decreased edema in lung tissue and peripherally; decreased B/P

Uses: Edema in congestive heart failure, nephrotic syndrome, ascites caused by hepatic disease, hepatic cirrhosis

Investigational uses: May be used alone or as adjunct with antihypertensives such as spironolactone, triamterene

Dosage and routes

Adult: PO 0.5-2 mg qd; may give 2nd or 3rd dose at 4-5 hr intervals; not to exceed 10 mg/day; may be given on alternate days or intermittently; **IV**/IM 0.5-1 mg/day; may give 2nd or 3rd dose at 2-3 hr intervals; not to exceed 10 mg/day

P ***Child:*** PO/IM/**IV** 0.02-0.1 mg/kg q12h, max 10 mg/day

Available forms: Tabs 0.5, 1, 2 mg; inj 0.25 mg/ml

Adverse effects

CNS: Headache, fatigue, weakness, vertigo, paresthesias

CV: *Orthostatic hypotension,* chest pain, ECG changes, circulatory collapse

EENT: Ear pain, tinnitus, blurred vision

ELECT: *Hypokalemia, hypochloremic alkalosis, hypomagnesia, hyperuricemia, hypocalcemia, hyponatremia, metabolic alkalosis*

ENDO: *Hyperglycemia*

GI: *Nausea,* diarrhea, dry mouth, vomiting, anorexia, cramps, oral and gastric irritations, pancreatitis

GU: *Polyuria,* **renal failure,** *glycosuria*

HEMA: **Thrombocytopenia, leukopenia, anemia**

INTEG: *Rash, pruritus, purpura, urticaria*

MS: Cramps, stiffness

Contraindications: Hypersensitivity to sulfonamides, anuria, electrolyte depletion

Precautions: Diabetes mellitus, dehydration, severe renal disease, pregnancy **C**, lactation

Do Not Confuse:
Bumex/Buprenex

Pharmacokinetics	
	PO/IM
Absorption	Rapidly, completely absorbed
	PO/IM/IV
Distribution	Crosses placenta
Metabolism	Liver (30%-40%)
Excretion	Breast milk, urine, feces
Half-life	1-1½ hr

Pharmacodynamics			
	PO	IM	IV
Onset	½-1 hr	40 min	5 min
Peak	1-2 hr	Unknown	½ hr
Duration	4 hr	4 hr	2-3 hr

Interactions

Individual drugs

Alcohol: ↑ orthostatic hypotension
Ethacrynic acid: Combination may cause ↑ chance of arrhythmias (do not use together)
Indomethacin: ↓ diuretic and antihypertensive effects of bumetanide
Lithium: ↓ renal clearance causing ↑ toxicity
Metolazone: ↑ diuresis, electrolyte loss
Mezlocillin: ↑ hypokalemia
Probenecid: ↓ effect of bumetanide
Piperacillin: ↑ hypokalemia
Ticarcillin: ↑ hypokalemia

Drug classifications

Aminoglycosides: ↑ ototoxicity
Digitalis glycosides: ↑ potassium loss with relating arrhythmias
Glucocorticoids: ↑ hypokalemia
NSAIDs: ↓ diuretic effect
Potassium-wasting drugs: ↑ hypokalemia

NURSING CONSIDERATIONS
Assessment

- Assess patient for tinnitus, hearing loss, ear pain; periodic testing of hearing is needed when high doses of this drug are given by **IV** route
- Monitor for manifestations of hypokalemia: *RENAL:* acidic urine, reduced urine osmolality, nocturia, polyuria, polydipsia; *CV:* hypotension, broad T wave, U wave, ectopy, tachycardia, weak pulse; *NEURO:* muscle weakness, altered LOC, drowsiness, apathy, lethargy, confusion, depression; *GI:* anorexia, nausea, cramps, constipation, distention, paralytic ileus; *RESP:* hypoventilation, respiratory muscle weakness
- Monitor for manifestations of hypocalcemia: *CNS:* personality changes, anxiety, disturbances, depression, psychosis; *GI:* nausea, vomiting, constipation, abdominal pain from muscle spasm; *CV:* decreased contractility, decreased cardiac output, hypotension, lengthened ST segment, prolonged QT interval; *INTEG:* scaling eczema, alopecia, hyperpigmentation; *NEURO:* tetany, muscle twitching, cramping, grimacing, seizure, altered deep tendon reflexes, spasm
- Monitor for manifestations of hypomagnesemia: *CNS:* agitation; *NEURO:* muscle twitching, paresthesias, hyperactive reflexes, positive Babinski's reflex, dysphagia, nystagmus, seizures, tetany; *GI:* nausea, vomiting, diarrhea, anorexia, abdominal distention; *CV:* ectopy, tachycardia, broad, flat, or inverted T waves, depressed ST segment, prolonged QT, decreased cardiac output, hypotension
- Monitor for manifestations of hyponatremia: *CV:* increased B/P, cold, clammy skin, hypovolemia or hypervolemia; *GI:* anorexia, nausea, vomiting, diarrhea, abdominal cramps; *NEURO:* lethargy, increased ICP, confusion, headache, seizures, coma, fatigue, tremors, hyperreflexia
- Monitor for manifestations of hyperchloremia: *NEURO:* weakness, lethargy, coma; *RESP:* deep rapid breathing
- Assess fluid volume status: I&O ratio and record, distended red veins, crackles in lung, color, quality and sp gr of urine, skin turgor, adequacy of pulses, moist mucous membranes, bilateral lung sounds, peripheral pitting edema; dehydration symptoms of decreasing output, thirst, hypotension, dry mouth and mucous membranes should be reported; if urinary output decreases or azotemia occurs, drug should be discontinued
- Monitor electrolytes: potassium, sodium, calcium, magnesium; also include BUN, blood pH, ABGs, uric acid, CBC, blood sugar
- Assess B/P before and during therapy with patient lying, standing, and sitting as appropriate; orthostatic hypotension can occur rapidly
- Monitor for digoxin toxicity in patients taking digoxin; lithium toxicity in those taking lithium

Nursing diagnoses

- ✓ Altered urinary elimination (side effects)
- ✓ Fluid volume deficit (side effects)
- ✓ Fluid volume excess (uses)
- ✓ Knowledge deficit (teaching)

Implementation

- Give in AM to avoid interference with sleep
- Potassium replacement if potassium level is <3.0 mg/dl whole, or use oral solutions; drug may be crushed if patient is unable to swallow

PO route

- With food, if nausea occurs; absorption may be reduced; the safest dosage schedule is on alternate days

IV **IV route**

- Do not use solution that is yellow or has a precipitate or crystals

IV **Direct IV**

- Give undiluted through Y-tube or 3-way stopcock; give 20 mg or less/min

Intermittent infusion

- May be added to 0.9% NaCl, D_5W, $D_{10}W$, $D_{20}W$, invert sugar 10% in electrolyte #1, LR, sodium lactate ⅙ mol/L; use within 24 hr to ensure compatibility; give through Y-tube or 3-way stopcock; give at 4 mg/min or less; use infusion pump

Syringe compatibility:
Doxapram

Y-site compatibilities:
Allopurinol, amifostine, aztreonam, cefepime, cisatracurium, cladribine, diltiazem, filgrastim, granisetron, lorazepam, morphine, piperacillin/tazobactam, propofol, remifantanil, teniposide, thiotepa, vinorelbine

Additive compatibilities:
Floxacillin, furosemide

Patient/family education

- Teach patient to take the medication early in the day to prevent nocturia
- Instruct the patient to take with food or milk if GI symptoms of nausea and anorexia occur
- Teach patient to maintain weekly record of weight and notify prescriber of weight loss of >5 lb
- Caution the patient that this drug causes a loss of potassium so food rich in potassium should be added to the diet; refer to a dietician for assistance in planning
- Caution the patient not to exercise in hot weather or stand for prolonged periods since orthostatic hypotension will be enhanced
- Teach patient not to use alcohol or any OTC medications without prescriber's approval; serious drug reactions may occur
- Emphasize the need to contact prescriber immediately if muscle cramps, weakness, nausea, dizziness, or numbness occurs
- Teach patient to take own B/P and pulse and record
- Caution the patient that orthostatic hypotension may occur; patient should rise slowly from sitting or reclining positions and lie down if dizziness occurs
- Teach patient to continue taking medication even if feeling better; this drug controls symptoms but does not cure the condition
- Advise the patient with hypertension to continue other medical treatment (exercise, weight loss, relaxation techniques, cessation of smoking)

Evaluation

Positive therapeutic outcome

- Decreased edema
- Decreased B/P
- Increased diuresis

buprenorphine (℞)

(byoo-pre-nor'feen)

Buprenex

Func. class.: Opioid analgesic
Chem. class.: Thebaine derivative

Pregnancy category C

Controlled substance schedule V

Action: Inhibits ascending pain pathways in limbic system, thalamus, midbrain, hypothalamus by binding to opiate receptor sites; this alters pain perception and response; generalized CNS depression

➡ **Therapeutic Outcome:** Relief of pain

Uses: Moderate to severe pain

Dosage and routes

Adult: IM/**IV** 0.3 mg q6h prn; may repeat dose after ½ hr; reduce dosage G in elderly, may repeat after ½ hr; epidural 60-180 µg over 48 hr

G ***Elderly:*** PO 0.15 mg q6h prn

Available forms: Inj 0.3 mg/ml (1-ml vials)

Adverse effects

CNS: Drowsiness, dizziness, confusion, headache, sedation, euphoria,

increased intracranial pressure, amnesia
CV: Palpitations, bradycardia, change in B/P, tachycardia
EENT: Tinnitus, blurred vision, *miosis,* diplopia
GI: Nausea, vomiting, anorexia, constipation, cramps, dry mouth
GU: Increased urinary output, dysuria, urinary retention
INTEG: Rash, urticaria, bruising, flushing, diaphoresis, pruritus
***RESP:* Respiratory depression,** dyspnea, hypo-/hyperventilation

Contraindications: Hypersensitivity, addiction (narcotic)

Precautions: Addictive personality, pregnancy **C**, lactation, increased intracranial pressure, MI (acute), severe heart disease, respiratory depression, hepatic disease, renal disease

Do Not Confuse:
Buprenex/Bumex

Pharmacokinetics

Absorption	Well absorbed (IM)
Distribution	Crosses placenta
Metabolism	Liver, extensively
Excretion	Kidneys, feces, breast milk
Half-life	2½-3½ hr

Pharmacodynamics

	IM	IV
Onset	10-15 min	Immediate
Peak	1 hr	5 min
Duration	4 hr	2-5 hr

Interactions
Individual drugs
Alcohol: ↑ respiratory depression, hypotension, sedation
Drug classifications
Antihistamines: ↑ respiratory depression, hypotension
CNS depressants: ↑ respiratory depression, hypotension
MAOIs: Do not use within 2 wk
Opioids: ↑ CNS depression
Sedative/hypnotics: ↑ respiratory depression, hypotension
Herb/drug
Kava: ↑ CNS depression

NURSING CONSIDERATIONS
Assessment
- Assess pain characteristics: location, intensity, type, severity before medication administration and after treatment
- Monitor VS after parenteral route; note muscle rigidity, drug history, liver, kidney function tests, respiratory dysfunction: respiratory depression, character, rate, rhythm; notify prescriber if respirations are <10/min
- Monitor CNS changes: dizziness, drowsiness, hallucinations, euphoria, LOC, pupil reaction; withdrawal in opioid-dependent persons; if dependence occurs within 2 wk of discontinuing drug, withdrawal symptoms will occur
- Monitor allergic reactions: rash, urticaria

Nursing diagnoses
✓ Pain (uses)
✓ Sensory-perceptual alteration: visual, auditory (adverse reactions)
✓ Breathing pattern, ineffective (adverse reactions)
✓ Knowledge deficit (teaching)

Implementation
- Give by inj (IM, **IV**), only with resuscitative equipment available; give slowly to prevent rigidity

IM route
- Give deep in large muscle mass; rotate sites of inj

IV route
- Give **IV** direct undiluted over 3-5 min (0.3 mg/2 min); give slowly

Syringe compatibility:
Midazolam

Y-site compatibilities:
Allopurinol, amifostine, aztreonam, cefepime, cisatracurium, cladribine, filgrastim, granisetron, melphalan,

piperacillin/tazobactam, propofol, remifentanil, teniposide, thiotepa, vinorelbine

Additive compatibilities: Atropine, bupivacaine, diphenhydramine, droperidol, glycopyrrolate, haloperidol, hydroxyzine, promethazine, scopolamine

Additive incompatibilities: Diazepam, floxacillin, furosemide, lorezepam

Patient/family education

• Instruct patient to report any symptoms of CNS changes, allergic reactions

• Caution patients to avoid CNS depressants: alcohol, sedative/hypnotics for at least 24 hr after taking this drug

• Discuss with patient that dizziness, drowsiness, and confusion are common; to avoid getting up without assistance, to avoid hazardous activities

• Discuss in detail all aspects of the drug

• Instruct patient to change position slowly to prevent orthostatic hypotension

• Teach patient to turn, cough, deep breathe after surgery to prevent atelectasis

Evaluation

Positive therapeutic outcome

• Relief of pain

bupropion (℞)

(byoo-proe'pee-on)

Wellbutrin, Wellbutrin SR, Zyban

Func. class.: Misc. antidepressant, smoking deterrent

Chem. class.: Aminoketone

Pregnancy category B

Action: Inhibits reuptake of dopamine, serotonin, norepinephrine

Therapeutic Outcome: Decreased symptoms of depression after 2-3 wk

Uses: Depression (Wellbutrin), smoking cessation (Zyban)

Dosage and routes

Depression

Adult: PO 100 mg bid initially, then increase after 3 days to 100 mg tid if needed; may increase after 1 mo to 150 mg tid

G ***Elderly:*** PO 50-100 mg/day, may increase by 50-100 mg q3-4 days

Smoking cessation

Adult: PO 150 mg bid, begin with 150 mg qd x 3 days then 300 mg/day continue for 7-12 wk

Available forms: Tabs 75, 100 mg; tabs, sus rel 50, 100, (Zyban) 150 mg

Adverse effects

CNS: *Headache, agitation, confusion,* **seizures**, delusions, *insomnia,* sedation, tremors

CV: **Dysrhythmias,** hypertension, palpitations, tachycardia, hypotension

EENT: Blurred vision, auditory disturbance

GI: *Nausea, vomiting, dry mouth,* increased appetite, constipation

GU: Impotence, frequency, retention

INTEG: Rash, pruritus, sweating

Contraindications: Hypersensitivity, eating disorders

Precautions: Renal and hepatic disease, recent MI, cranial trauma, P pregnancy **B,** lactation, children <18 G yr, seizure disorders, elderly

Pharmacokinetics

Absorption	Well absorbed; bioavailability poor
Distribution	Unknown
Metabolism	Liver extensively
Excretion	Kidneys
Half-life	14 hr, steady state 1½-5 wk

Pharmacodynamics	
Onset	Up to 4 wk
Peak	Unknown
Duration	Unknown

Interactions
Individual drugs
Alcohol: ↑ risk of seizures
Carbamazepine: ↓ bupropion effect
Cimetidine: ↑ levels, ↑ toxicity
Levodopa: ↑ risk of seizures
Phenytoin: ↑ toxicity
Ritonavir: ↑ bupropion toxicity
Theophylline: ↑ risk of seizures
Drug classifications
Antidepressants: ↑ risk of seizures
Antihistamines: ↑ CNS depression
Barbiturates: ↓ bupropion effects
Benzodiazepines: ↑ risk of seizures
CNS depressants: ↑ effects
MAOIs: Acute toxicity, risk of seizures
Phenothiazines: ↑ toxicity, risk of seizures
Steroids, systemic: ↑ risk of seizures
Herb/drug
Kava: ↑ CNS depression
Belladonna leaf/root: ↑ anticholinergic effect
Lab test interferences
↑ Serum bilirubin, ↑ blood glucose, ↑ alkaline phosphatase
↓ VMA, ↓ 5-HIAA
False positive: Urinary catecholamines

NURSING CONSIDERATIONS
Assessment
- Monitor B/P (with patient lying, standing), pulse q4h; if systolic B/P drops 20 mm Hg hold drug, notify prescriber; take vital signs q4h in patients with cardiovascular disease
- Assess smoking cessation progress after 7-12 wk, if progress has not been made, drug should be discontinued
- Assess for increased risk of seizures; if patient has used CNS depressant or CNS stimulants, dosage of bupropion should not be exceeded
- Monitor blood studies: CBC, leukocytes, differential, cardiac enzymes if patient is receiving long-term therapy
- Monitor hepatic studies: AST, ALT, bilirubin if on long-term treatment
- Check weight weekly; appetite may increase with drug
- Assess ECG for flattening of T wave, bundle branch block, AV block, dysrhythmias in cardiac patients
- G Assess for EPS primarily in elderly: rigidity, dystonia, akathisia
- Assess mental status: mood, sensorium, affect, suicidal tendencies; increase in psychiatric symptoms: depression, panic
- P G Monitor urinary retention, constipation; constipation is more likely to occur in children or elderly
- Identify alcohol consumption; if alcohol was consumed, hold dose

Nursing diagnoses
- ✓ Coping, ineffective individual (uses)
- ✓ Injury, risk for (side effects)
- ✓ Knowledge deficit (teaching)
- ✓ Noncompliance (teaching)

Implementation
- Give with food or milk for GI symptoms
- Store at room temp; do not freeze

Patient/family education
- Teach patient that therapeutic effects may take 2-3 wk; not to increase dose without prescriber's approval; that treatment for smoking cessation lasts 7-12 wk
- G Teach patient to use caution in driving or other activities requiring alertness because of drowsiness, dizziness, blurred vision; to avoid rising quickly from sitting to standing, especially elderly
- Teach patient to avoid alcohol ingestion, obtain approval for other drugs
- G Teach patient to increase fluids, bulk in diet if constipation, urinary retention occur, especially elderly
- Teach patient to take gum, hard

sugarless candy, or frequent sips of water for dry mouth
- Advise patient not to use with nicotine patches unless directed by prescriber, may increase B/P
- Teach patient that risk of seizures increases when dose is exceeded, or if patient has seizure disorder
- Teach patient to notify prescriber if pregnancy is suspected or planned

Evaluation
Positive therapeutic outcome
- Decrease in depression
- Absence of suicidal thoughts
- Smoking cessation

Treatment of overdose: ECG monitoring, induce emesis, lavage, activated charcoal, administer anticonvulsant

buspirone (℞)
(byoo-spye'rone)
BuSpar
Func. class.: Antianxiety, sedative
Chem. class.: Azaspirodecanedione
Pregnancy category B

Action: Acts by inhibiting the action of serotonin (5-HT) by binding to serotonin and dopamine receptors; also increases norepinephrine metabolism; has shown little potential for abuse

➔ **Therapeutic Outcome:** Decreased anxiety

Uses: Management and short-term relief of anxiety disorders

Dosage and routes
Adult: PO 5 mg tid; may increase by 5 mg/day q2-3 days; not to exceed 60 mg/day

Available forms: Tabs 5, 10, 15 mg

Adverse effects
CNS: *Dizziness, headache, depression, stimulation, insomnia, nervousness, light-headedness, numbness, paresthesia, incoordination, tremors,* excitement, involuntary movements, confusion, akathisia
CV: *Tachycardia, palpitations,* hypotension, hypertension, **CVA, CHF, MI**
EENT: *Sore throat, tinnitus, blurred vision, nasal congestion,* red, itching eyes, change in taste, smell
GI: *Nausea, dry mouth, diarrhea, constipation,* flatulence, increased appetite, rectal bleeding
GU: Frequency, hesitancy, menstrual irregularity, change in libido
INTEG: *Rash,* edema, pruritus, alopecia, dry skin
MISC: *Sweating,* fatigue, weight gain, fever
MS: *Pain, weakness,* muscle cramps, spasms
RESP: Hyperventilation, chest congestion, shortness of breath

Contraindications: Hypersensitivity, P child <18 yr

Precautions: Pregnancy **B,** lactation, G elderly, impaired hepatic/renal function

Pharmacokinetics

Absorption	Rapidly absorbed
Distribution	Unknown
Metabolism	Liver, extensively
Excretion	Feces
Half-life	2-3 hr

Pharmacodynamics
Unknown

Interactions
Individual drugs
Alcohol: ↑ CNS depression
Rifampin: ↓ buspirone effect
Drug classifications
MAOIs: ↑ B/P, do not use together
Psychotropics: ↑ CNS depression
Food/drug
Grapefruit juice: ↑ buspirone effect
Herb/drug
Kava: ↑ CNS depression

NURSING CONSIDERATIONS

Assessment

- Assess anxiety reaction: inability to sleep, apprehension, dread, foreboding, or uneasiness related to unidentified source of danger
- Assess for previous drug dependence or tolerance; if patient is drug dependent or tolerant, amount of medication should be restricted
- Monitor B/P (lying, standing), pulse; if systolic B/P drops 20 mm Hg, hold drug, notify prescriber; check I&O; may indicate renal dysfunction
- Monitor mental status: mood, sensorium, affect, sleeping patterns, drowsiness, dizziness, suicidal tendencies
- Assess for CNS reaction, some reactions may be unpredictable

Nursing diagnoses

✓ Anxiety (uses)
✓ Knowledge deficit (teaching)
✓ Noncompliance (teaching)

Implementation

- Give with food or milk for GI symptoms; sugarless gum, hard candy, frequent sips of water for dry mouth
- May be crushed

Patient/family education

- Teach patient that drug may be taken with food; if dose is missed take as soon as remembered; do not double doses
- Caution patient to avoid OTC preparations unless approved by the prescriber; to avoid alcohol ingestion and other psychotropic medications unless prescribed; that 1-2 wk of therapy may be required before therapeutic effects occur
- Caution patient to avoid driving and activities requiring alertness since drowsiness may occur; until medication response is known, tell patient that drowsiness may worsen at beginning of treatment
- Instruct patient not to discontinue medication abruptly after long-term use
- Advise patient to rise slowly or fainting may occur, especially in G elderly

Evaluation

Positive therapeutic outcome

- Increased well-being
- Decreased anxiety, restlessness, sleeplessness, dread

Treatment of overdose:

Gastric lavage, VS, supportive care

HIGH ALERT

busulfan (℞)

(byoo-sul'fan)

Myleran

Func. class.: Antineoplastic alkylating agent

Chem. class.: Nitrosourea

Pregnancy category D

Action: Changes essential cellular ions to covalent bonding with resultant alkylation; this interferes with normal biologic function of DNA; activity is not phase specific; action is due to myelosuppression

➔ **Therapeutic Outcome:** Prevention of rapid growth of malignant cells in chronic myelocytic leukemia

Uses: Chronic myelocytic leukemia

Dosage and routes

Adult: PO 4-8 mg/day initially until WBC levels fall to 10,000/mm^3; then drug is stopped until WBC levels rise over 50,000/mm^3; then 1-3 mg/day; **IV** 0.8 mg/kg q6h × 4 days, given with cyclophosphamide

P ***Child:*** PO 0.06-0.12 mg/kg or 1.8-4.6 mg/m^2/day; dosage is titrated to maintain WBC levels at 20,000/mm^3

Available forms: Tabs 2 mg; sol for inj 6 mg/ml

Adverse effects

PO route

GI: Nausea, vomiting, *diarrhea, weight loss*

GU: Impotence, sterility, amenorrhea, gynecomastia, **renal toxicity,** hyperuremia, adrenal insufficiency–like syndrome
HEMA: **Thrombocytopenia, leukopenia, pancytopenia, severe bone marrow depression**
INTEG: Dermatitis, hyperpigmentation, alopecia
MISC: **Chromosomal aberrations**
RESP: **Irreversible pulmonary fibrosis,** pneumonitis

IV **IV route**
CNS: **Cerebral hemorrhage, coma, seizures,** *anxiety, depression, dizziness, headache,* encephalopathy, weakness, mental changes
CV: Hypotension, **thrombosis,** *chest pain,* tachycardia, **atrial fibrillation, heart block**
EENT: Pharyngitis, epistaxis
GI: Anorexia, constipation, diarrhea, dry mouth, nausea, vomiting
RESP: **Alveolar hemorrhage, atelectasis,** cough, hemoptysis, hypoxia, pleural effusion, pneumonia, sinusitis

Contraindications: Radiation, chemotherapy, lactation, pregnancy **D** (3rd trimester), blastic phase of chronic myelocytic leukemia, hypersensitivity

Precautions: Childbearing age men and women, leukopenia, thrombocytopenia, anemia, hepatotoxicity, renal toxicity

Pharmacokinetics

Absorption	Rapidly absorbed
Distribution	Unknown; crosses placenta
Metabolism	Liver, extensively
Excretion	Kidneys, breast milk
Half-life	2.5 hr

Pharmacodynamics

Unknown

Interactions

Individual drugs

Radiation: ↑ toxicity, bone marrow suppression

Drug classifications

Anticoagulants: ↑ risk of bleeding
Antineoplastics: ↑ toxicity, bone marrow suppression
Salicylates: ↑ risk of bleeding

Lab test interferences

False positive: Breast, bladder, cervix, lung cytology tests

NURSING CONSIDERATIONS

Assessment

- Monitor CBC, differential, platelet count weekly; withhold drug if WBC <4000/mm^3 or platelets <75,000/mm^3; notify prescriber of results if WBC <15,000/mm^3, platelets <150,000/mm^3; institute thrombocytopenia precautions
- Monitor pulmonary function tests, chest x-ray films before, during therapy; chest film should be obtained q2 wk during treatment; check for dyspnea, rales, nonproductive cough, chest pain, tachypnea; pulmonary fibrosis may occur up to 10 yr after treatment with busulfan
- Assess for increased uric acid levels, swelling, joint pain primarily in extremities; patient should be well hydrated to prevent urate deposits
- Monitor renal function studies: BUN, serum uric acid, urine CrCl before, during therapy; I&O ratio; report fall in urine output of 30 ml/hr; check for decreased hyperuricemia
- Monitor for cold, fever, sore throat (may indicate beginning infection); identify edema in feet, joint or stomach pain, shaking; prescriber should be notified
- Assess for bleeding: hematuria, guaiac, bruising or petechiae, mucosa or orifices q8h; no rectal temps

Nursing diagnoses

- ✓ Injury, risk for (adverse reactions)
- ✓ Body image disturbance (adverse reactions)

✓ Infection, risk for (adverse reactions)
✓ Knowledge deficit (teaching)

Implementation

• Give 1 hr before or 2 hr pc to lessen nausea and vomiting; give at same time qd
• Increase fluid intake to 2-3 L/day to prevent urate deposits, calculus formation
• Administer antibiotics for prophylaxis of infection; may be prescribed since infection potential is high
• Store in tight container

IV route

• Prepare in biologic cabinet using gloves, gown, mask; dilute with 10 times volume of drug using D_5W or 0.9% NaCl (0.5 mg/ml); when withdrawing drug, use needle with 5-µ filter provided, remove amount needed, remove filter, and inject drug into diluent; always add drug to diluent, not vice versa; stable for 8 hr at room temp using D_5W or 0.9% NaCl; give by central venous catheter over 2 hr q6h × 4 days, use infusion pump, do not admix
• Give antiemetic before **IV** route
• Give phenytoin before **IV** to prevent seizures

Patient/family education

• Teach patient to avoid use of products containing aspirin or ibuprofen, razors, commercial mouthwash since bleeding may occur; to report symptoms of bleeding (hematuria, tarry stools)
• Instruct patient to report signs of anemia (fatigue, headache, irritability, faintness, shortness of breath)
• Instruct patient to report any changes in breathing or coughing even several months after treatment; to avoid crowds and persons with respiratory tract or other infections
• Teach patient that hair loss may occur; discuss the use of wigs or hair pieces
• Caution patient not to have any vaccinations without the advice of the prescriber; serious reactions can occur
• Advise patient that contraception is needed during treatment and for several months after the completion of therapy

Evaluation

Positive therapeutic outcome

• Decreased leukocytes to normal limits
• Absence of sweating at night
• Increased appetite, increased weight

butorphanol (℞)

(byoo-tor'fa-nole)
Stadol, Stadol NS
Func. class.: Opiate analgesic

Pregnancy category C

Controlled substance schedule IV

Action: Inhibits ascending pain pathways in limbic system, thalamus, midbrain, hypothalamus by binding to opiate receptor sites; this alters pain perception and response

➔ **Therapeutic Outcome:** Relief of pain

Uses: Moderate to severe pain, analgesia during labor, sedation preoperatively

Investigational uses: Migraine headache, pain

Dosage and routes

Adult: IM 1-4 mg q3-4h prn; **IV** 0.5-2 mg q3-4h prn; nasal spray in 1 nostril; may give another dose 1-1½ hr later; may repeat q3-4h

G ***Elderly:*** ½ adult dose at 2× the interval

Renal dose

CrCl 10-50 ml/min 75% dose; CrCl <10 ml/min 50% dose

Available forms: Inj 1, 2 mg/ml; intranasal 10 mg/ml

B

Adverse effects

CNS: Drowsiness, dizziness, confusion, headache, sedation, euphoria, weakness, hallucinations
CV: Palpitations, bradycardia, change in B/P
EENT: Tinnitus, blurred vision, miosis, diplopia
GI: Nausea, vomiting, anorexia, constipation, cramps
GU: Increased urinary output, dysuria, urinary retention
INTEG: Rash, urticaria, bruising, flushing, diaphoresis, pruritus
RESP: **Respiratory depression,** pulmonary hypertension

Contraindications: Hypersensitivity, addiction (narcotic), CHF, MI

Precautions: Addictive personality, pregnancy **C,** lactation, increased intracranial pressure, respiratory depression, hepatic disease, renal disease, P child <18 yr

Do Not Confuse:
Stadol/Haldol

Pharmacokinetics

Absorption	Well absorbed (IM, nasal); complete (**IV**)
Distribution	Crosses placenta
Metabolism	Liver, extensively
Excretion	Feces (10%-15%); kidneys, unchanged (small amounts)
Half-life	3-4 hr

Pharmacodynamics

	IM	IV	NASAL
Onset	10-30 min	1 min	15 min
Peak	½ hr	5 min	1-2 hr
Duration	3-4 hr	2-4 hr	4-5 hr

Interactions

Individual drugs

Alcohol: ↑ respiratory depression, hypotension, sedation

Drug classifications

Antihistamines: ↑ respiratory depression, hypotension
CNS depressants: ↑ respiratory depression, hypotension
MAOIs: Do not use 2 wk before butorphanol, fatal reaction
Sedative/hypnotics: ↑ respiratory depression, hypotension

Herb/drug

Kava: ↑ CNS depression

NURSING CONSIDERATIONS

Assessment

- Monitor VS after parenteral route; note muscle rigidity, drug history, liver, kidney function tests, respiratory dysfunction: respiratory depression, character, rate, rhythm; notify prescriber if respirations are <10/min
- Monitor CNS changes: dizziness, drowsiness, hallucinations, euphoria, LOC, pupil reaction
- Monitor allergic reactions: rash, urticaria

Nursing diagnoses

- ✓ Pain (uses)
- ✓ Sensory-perceptual alteration: visual, auditory (adverse reactions)
- ✓ Injury, risk for (adverse reactions)
- ✓ Knowledge deficit (teaching)

Implementation

- Store in light resistant container at room temp

IM route

- Give deeply in large muscle mass; rotate injection sites

Intranasal

- Give 1 spray in nostril

IV route

- Give **IV** undiluted at a rate of ≤2 mg/>3-5 min; titrate to patient response

Syringe compatibilities:

Atropine, chlorpromazine, cimetidine, diphenhydramine, droperidol, fentanyl, hydroxyzine, meperidine, methotrimeprazine, metoclopramide, midazolam, morphine, pentazocine, perphenazine, prochlorperazine, promethazine, scopolamine, thiethylperazine

Syringe incompatibilities: Dimenhydrinate, pentobarbital

Y-site compatibilities: Allopurinol, amifostine, azetreonam, cefepime, cisatracurium, cladribine, doxorubicin liposome, enalaprilat, esmolol, filgrastim, fludarabine, granisetron, labetalol, melphalan, paclitaxel, piperacillin/tazobactam, propofol, remifentanil, sargramostim, teniposide, thiotepa, vinorelbine

Patient/family education

- Instruct patient to report any symptoms of CNS changes, allergic reactions; to avoid CNS depressants: alcohol, sedative/hypnotics for at least 24 hr after taking this drug
- Discuss with patient that dizziness, drowsiness, and confusion are common; to avoid getting up without assistance
- Discuss in detail all aspects of the drug

Nasal route

- Teach patient to blow nose to clear both nostrils before using; remove clip and cover, prime before using until spray appears; pump must be re-primed q48h; close nostril with finger and spray once quickly; have patient sniff
- Patient should replace clip and cover after use; caution patient not to shake medication

Evaluation

Positive therapeutic outcome

- Pain relief

Treatment of overdose:

Narcan 0.2-0.8 **IV**, O_2, **IV** fluids, vasopressors

calcitonin (human) (℞)

(kal-sih-toh'nin)

Cibacalcin

calcitonin (salmon) (℞)

Calcimir, Miacalcin, Miacalin Nasal Spray, Osteocalcin, Salmonine

Func. class.: Parathyroid agents (calcium regulator)

Chem. class.: Polypeptide hormone

Pregnancy category C

Action: Decreases bone resorption, blood calcium levels by direct action on bone, GI system, and kidney; increases deposits of calcium in bones; renal excretion of calcium occurs; opposes parathyroid hormone

➔ **Therapeutic Outcome:** Lowered calcium level, decreasing symptoms of Paget's disease

Uses: Paget's disease, postmenopausal osteoporosis, hypercalcemia

Dosage and routes

Human

Paget's disease

Adult: SC 0.5 mg/day initially; may require 0.5 mg bid × 6 mo, then decrease until symptoms reappear

Salmon

Postmenopausal osteoporosis

Adult: SC/IM 100 IU/day; nasal 200 IU (1 spray) alternating nostrils qd, activate pump before 1st dose

Paget's disease

Adult: SC/IM 100 IU qd, maintenance 50-100 IU qd or qod

Hypercalcemia

Adult: SC/IM 4 IU/kg q6h, increase to 8 IU/kg q6h if response is unsatisfactory

Available forms: **Human:** Inj (SC) 0.5 mg/vial; **Salmon:** Inj 100 IU, 200 IU/ml, nasal spray 200 IU/actuation

Adverse effects

CNS: Headache, **tetany,** chills, weakness, dizziness, fever

CV: Chest pressure

EENT: Nasal congestion, eye pain
GI: Nausea, diarrhea, vomiting, anorexia, abdominal pain, salty taste, epigastric pain
GU: Diuresis, nocturia, urine sediment, frequency
INTEG: Rash, flushing, pruritus of earlobes, edema of feet, inj site reaction
MS: Swelling, tingling of hands
RESP: Dyspnea
SYST: **Anaphylaxis**

Contraindications: Hypersensitivity

Precautions: Renal disease, P children, lactation, osteogenic sarcoma, pregnancy **C**, pernicious anemia

Pharmacokinetics

Absorption	Completely absorbed
Distribution	Unknown
Metabolism	Rapid; kidneys, tissue, blood
Excretion	Kidneys, inactive metabolite
Half-life	1 hr

Pharmacodynamics

	SC
Onset	15 min
Peak	4 hr
Duration	8-24 hr

Interactions: None

NURSING CONSIDERATIONS
Assessment

• Assess for GI symptoms, polyuria, flushing, head swelling, tingling, headache; may indicate hypercalcemia; nervousness, irritability, twitching, seizures, spasm, paresthesia indicate hypocalcemia during beginning of treatment
• Identify nutritional status; check diet for sources of vit D (milk, some seafood), calcium (dairy products, dark green vegetables), phosphates
• Monitor BUN, creatinine, uric acid, chloride, electrolytes, urine pH, urinary calcium, magnesium, phosphate, urinalysis (calcium should be kept at 9-10 mg/dl; vit D 50-135 IU/dl), alkaline phosphatase baseline and q3-6 mo; check urine sediment for casts throughout treatment
• Assess for increased drug level, since toxic reactions occur rapidly; have calcium chloride or gluconate on hand if calcium level drops too low; check for tetany

Nursing diagnoses

✓ Injury, risk for (adverse reactions)
✓ Pain, chronic (uses)
✓ Knowledge deficit (teaching)

Implementation

• Store at <77° F (25° C); protect from light

SC route (human)
• Give by SC route only; rotate inj sites; use within 6 hr of reconstitution; give hs to minimize nausea, vomiting

IM route (salmon)
• After test dose of 10 IU/ml, 0.1 ml intradermally; watch 15 min; give only with epinephrine and emergency meds available
• IM injection in deep muscle mass slowly; rotate sites

Nasal route
• Use alternating nostrils for nasal spray

Patient/family education

• Teach method of inj if patient will be responsible for self-medication
• Instruct patient to notify prescriber for hypercalcemic relapse: renal calculi, nausea, vomiting, thirst, lethargy, deep bone or flank pain
• Teach patient that warmth and flushing occur and last 1 hr
• Provide a low-calcium diet as prescribed (Paget's disease, hypercalcemia)
• Advise patients with osteoporosis to increase calcium and vit D in diet and to continue with moderate exercise to prevent continued bone loss
• Advise patients to report difficulty

swallowing or change in side effects to prescriber immediately

Evaluation

Positive therapeutic outcome

- Calcium levels 9-10 mg/dl
- Decreasing symptoms of Paget's disease, including pain
- Decreased bone loss in osteoporosis

calcitriol (℞)

(kal-si-tree'ole)

Calcijex, Rocaltrol, Vitamin D_3

Func. class.: Parathyroid agent (calcium regulator)

Chem. class.: Vitamin D hormone

Pregnancy category C

Action: Increases intestinal absorption of calcium, provides calcium for bones, increases renal tubular resorption of phosphate

Therapeutic Outcome: Calcium at normal level

Uses: Hypocalcemia in chronic renal disease, hypoparathyroidism, pseudohypoparathyroidism

Dosage and routes

Hypocalcemia

Adult: **IV** 0.5 µg tid, initially; may increase by 0.25-0.5 µg/dose q2-4 wk; 0.5-3 µg tid maintenance

Predialysis

Adult: PO 0.25 µg/day, max 0.5 µg/day

P ***Child:*** PO 0.25 µg/day, max 0.5 µg/day

P ***Child <3 yr: PO 1015 µg/kg/day***

Hypocalcemia during chronic dialysis

Adult: PO 0.5-3 µg/day

P ***Child:*** PO 0.25-2 µg/day

Renal osteodystrophy

Adult: PO 0.25 µg qod-3 µg/day

P ***Child:*** PO 0.014-0.041 µg/kg/day

Hypoparathyroidism

Adult: PO 0.25-2.7 µg/day

P ***Child:*** PO 0.04-0.08 µg/kg/day

Available forms: Caps 0.25, 0.5 µg

Adverse effects

CNS: Drowsiness, headache, vertigo, fever, lethargy, weakness

CV: Palpitations

EENT: Blurred vision, photophobia

GI: Nausea, diarrhea, vomiting, jaundice, anorexia, dry mouth, constipation, cramps, metallic taste

GU: Polyuria, hypercalciuria, hyperphosphatemia, hematuria, thirst

MS: Myalgia, arthralgia, decreased bone development

Contraindications: Hypersensitivity, hyperphosphatemia, hypercalcemia, vit D toxicity

Precautions: Pregnancy **C**, renal calculi, lactation, CV disease

Do Not Confuse:
calcitriol/Calciferol

Pharmacokinetics	
Absorption	Well absorbed
Distribution	To liver, crosses placenta
Metabolism	Liver
Excretion	Bile
Half-life	3-6 hr

Pharmacodynamics	
Onset	2-6 hr
Peak	10-12 hr
Duration	Up to 5 days

Interactions

Individual Drugs

Cholestyramine: ↓ absorption of calcitriol

Phenytoin: ↑ vit D metabolism

Verapamil: ↑ dysrhythmias

Drug classifications

Antacids: ↑ hypermagnesemia

Diuretics, thiazide: ↑ hypercalcemia

Calcium supplements: ↑ hypercalcemia
Cardiac glycosides: ↑ dysrhythmias
Vitamin D products: ↑ toxicity
Vitamins, fat-soluble: ↓ calcitriol absorption
Food/drug:
Large amounts of high-calcium foods may cause hypercalcemia
Lab test interferences
False: ↑ Cholesterol
Interference: Alkaline phosphatase, electrolytes

NURSING CONSIDERATIONS
Assessment
- Assess GI symptoms, polyuria, flushing, head swelling, tingling, headache; may indicate hypercalcemia
- Identify nutritional status; check diet for sources of vit D (milk, some seafood), calcium (dairy products, dark green vegetables), phosphates
- Monitor BUN, creatinine, uric acid, chloride, electrolytes, urine pH, urinary calcium, magnesium, phosphate, urinalysis (calcium should be kept at 9-10 mg/dl; vit D 50-135 IU/dl), alkaline phosphatase baseline and q3-6 mo
- ❗ Assess for increased drug level, since toxic reactions occur rapidly; have calcium chloride on hand if calcium level drops too low; check for tetany

Nursing diagnoses
- ✓ Injury, risk for (adverse reactions)
- ✓ Pain, chronic (uses)
- ✓ Knowledge deficit (teaching)

Implementation
PO route
- Give with meals for GI symptoms
- ⊘ Do not crush or chew caps

IV route
- Give by direct **IV** over 1 min

Patient/family education
- Teach patient the symptoms of hypercalcemia and about foods rich in calcium
- Advise patient to avoid products with sodium: cured meats, dairy products, cold cuts, olives, beets, pickles, soups, meat tenderizers in chronic renal failure
- Advise patient to avoid products with potassium: oranges, bananas, dried fruit, peas, dark green leafy vegetables, milk, melons, beans in chronic renal failure
- Advise patient to avoid OTC products containing calcium, potassium, or sodium in chronic renal failure
- Instruct patient to avoid all preparations containing vit D
- Instruct patient to monitor weight weekly

Evaluation
Positive therapeutic outcome
- Calcium levels 9-10 mg/dl

calcium carbonate
(PO-OTC, IV-℞)

Alka-Mints, Amitone, Apo-Cal ✤, BioCal, Calcarb, Calci-Chew, Calcilac, Calci-Mix, Calcite ✤, Calglycine ✤, Cal-Plus, Calsan ✤, Caltrate 600, Caltrate Jr., Chooz, Dicarbosil, Equilet, Gencalc, LIquid-Cal, Liquid-Cal-600, Maalox Antacid Caplets, Mallamint, Mylanta Lozenges ✤, Nephro-Calci, Nu-Cal ✤, Os-Cal 500, Oysco 500, Oystercal 500, Oyst-Cal 500, Rolaids Calcium Rich, Titralac, Tums, Tums E-X Extra Strength

Func. class.: Antacid, calcium supplement
Chem. class.: Calcium product

Pregnancy category C

Action: Neutralizes gastric acidity

➔ **Therapeutic Outcome:** Neutralized gastric acidity; calcium at normal levels

Uses: Antacid, calcium supplement; not suitable for chronic therapy

Dosage and routes

Antacid

Adult: PO 350 mg-1.5 g or 2 pieces of gum 1 hr pc and hs

Osteoporosis

Adult: PO 1-2 g bid-tid

Available forms: Chewable tabs 350, 420, 500, 750, 850, 1000, 1250 mg; tabs 500, 600, 650, 1000, 1250 mg; gum 500 mg; susp 1250 mg/5 ml; lozenges 600 mg

Adverse effects

GI: *Constipation,* anorexia, nausea, vomiting, flatulence, diarrhea, rebound hyperacidity, eructation

Contraindications: Hypersensitivity, hypercalcemia, hyperparathyroidism, bone tumors

G **Precautions:** Elderly, fluid restriction, decreased GI motility, GI obstruction, dehydration, renal disease, pregnancy **C**, lactation

Pharmacokinetics	
Absorption	⅓ absorbed by small intestine
Distribution	Unknown
Metabolism	Unknown
Excretion	Feces, urine, crosses placenta
Half-life	Unknown

Pharmacodynamics	
Onset	20 min
Peak	Unknown
Duration	20-180 min

Interactions

Drug Classifications

Azole antiinfectives: ↓ levels of azole antiinfectives

Calcium channel blockers: ↓ levels of calcium channel blockers

Iron products: ↓ levels of iron products

Salicylates: ↓ levels of salicylates

NURSING CONSIDERATIONS

Assessment

- Monitor Ca^+ (serum, urine), Ca^+ should be 8.5-10.5 mg/dl, urine Ca^+ should be 150 mg/day, monitor weekly
- (Alert) Assess for milk-alkali syndrome: nausea, vomiting, disorientation, headache
- Assess for constipation; increase bulk in the diet if needed
- Assess for hypercalcemia: headache, nausea, vomiting, confusion

Implementation

PO route

- Administer as antacid 1 hr pc and hs
- Administer as supplement 1½ hr pc and hs
- Administer only with regular tablets or capsules; do not give with enteric-coated tablets
- Administer laxatives or stool softeners if constipation occurs

Evaluation

- Therapeutic response: absence of pain, decreased acidity

Patient/family education

- Advise patient to increase fluids to 2 L unless contraindicated, to add bulk to diet for constipation; notify prescriber of constipation
- Advise patient not to switch antacids unless directed by prescriber, not to use as antacid for >2 wk without approval by prescriber
- Teach patient that therapeutic dose recommendations are figured as elemental calcium

calcium chloride
calcium gluceptate
calcium gluconate
calcium lactate
(PO, OTC; IV, ℞)

Func. class.: Electrolyte replacement—calcium product

Pregnancy category C

Action: Cation needed for maintenance of nervous, muscular, skeletal systems, enzyme reactions, normal cardiac contractility, coagulation of blood; affects secretory activity of endocrine, exocrine glands

➔ **Therapeutic Outcome:** Calcium at normal level, absence of increased magnesium, potassium

Uses: Prevention and treatment of hypocalcemia, hypermagnesemia, P hypoparathyroidism, neonatal tetany, cardiac toxicity caused by hyperkalemia, lead colic, hyperphosphatemia, vit D deficiency

Dosage and routes

Calcium chloride

Adult: **IV** 500 mg-1 g q1-3 days as indicated by serum calcium levels; give at <1 ml/min; IAV 200-800 mg injected in ventricle of heart

P ***Child:*** **IV** 25 mg/kg over several min

Calcium gluceptate

Adult: **IV** 5-20 ml; IM 2-5 ml

P ***Newborn:*** 0.5 ml/100 ml of blood transfused

Calcium gluconate

Adult: PO 0.5-2 g bid-qid; **IV** 0.5-2 g at 0.5 ml/min (10% sol)

P ***Child:*** PO/**IV** 500 mg/kg/day in divided doses

Calcium lactate

Adult: PO 325 mg-1.3 g tid with meals

P ***Child:*** PO 500 mg/kg/day in divided doses

Available forms: Many; check product listings

Adverse effects

CV: Shortened QT interval, heart block, hypotension, bradycardia, dysrhythmias; **cardiac arrest (IV)**

GI: Vomiting, nausea, constipation

HYPERCALCEMIA: Drowsiness, lethargy, muscle weakness, headache, constipation, **coma,** anorexia, nausea, vomiting, polyuria, thirst

INTEG: Pain, burning at **IV** site, severe venous thrombosis, necrosis, extravasation

Contraindications: Hypercalcemia, digitalis toxicity, ventricular fibrillation, renal calculi

Precautions: Pregnancy **C**, lactation, P children, renal disease, respiratory disease, cor pulmonale, digitalized patient, respiratory failure

Pharmacokinetics

Absorption	Complete bioavailability (**IV**)
Distribution	Readily extracellular; crosses placenta
Metabolism	Liver
Excretion	Feces (80%), kidney (20%), breast milk
Half-life	Unknown

Pharmacodynamics

	PO	IV
Onset	Unknown	Immediate
Peak	Unknown	Rapid
Duration	Unknown	½-1½ hr

Interactions

Individual drugs

Atenolol: ↓ effects of atenolol

Tetracycline: ↓ absorption of tetracycline (PO)

Verapamil: ↓ effects of verapamil

Drug classifications

Antacids: Milk-alkali syndrome (renal disease)

Cardiac glycosides: ↑ toxicity

Diuretics, thiazide: ↑ hypercalcemia

Fluoroquinolones: ↓ absorption of fluoroquinolones
Iron salts: ↓ absorption of iron

Food/drug

Calcium (dairy products): ↑ hypercalcemia

Lab test interferences

False: ↓ Magnesium, ↓ 17-OHCS

NURSING CONSIDERATIONS

Assessment

- Monitor ECG for decreased QT interval and T-wave inversion: in hypercalcemia, drug should be reduced or discontinued
- Monitor calcium levels during treatment (9-10 mg/dl is normal level)
- Assess cardiac status: rate, rhythm, CVP (PWP, PAWP if being monitored directly)

Nursing diagnoses

✓ Injury, risk for (uses, adverse reactions)
✓ Knowledge deficit (teaching)

Implementation

IV IV route

- Administer **IV** undiluted or diluted with equal amounts of 0.9% NaCl for inj to a 5% sol; give 0.5-1 ml/min
- Give through small-bore needle into large vein; if extravasation occurs, necrosis will result (**IV**); IM injection may cause severe burning, necrosis, and tissue sloughing; warm sol to body temp before administering (only gluconate/gluceptate)
- Provide seizure precautions: padded side rails, decreased stimuli (noise, light); place airway suction equipment, padded mouth gag if calcium levels are low

Calcium chloride

Syringe compatibilities:

Milrinone

Y-site compatibilities:

Amrinone, dobutamine, epinephrine, esmolol, morphine, paclitaxel

Additive compatibilities:

Amikacin, ascorbic acid, bretylium, cephapirin, chloramphenicol, dopamine, hydrocortisone, isoproterenol, lidocaine, methicillin, norepinephrine, penicillin G potassium, penicillin G sodium, pentobarbital, phenobarbital, sodium bicarbonate, verapamil, vit B/C

Calcium gluceptate

Additive compatibilities:

Ascorbic acid inj, isoproterenol, lidocaine, norepinephrine, phytonadione, sodium bicarbonate

Calcium gluconate

Syringe compatibilities:

Aldesleukin, allopurinol, amifostine, aztreonam, cefazolin, cefepime, ciprofloxacin, cladribine, dobutamine, enalaprilat, epinephrine, famotidine, filgrastim, granisetron, heparin/hydrocortisone, labetalol, melphalan, midazolam, netilmicin, piperacillin/tazobactam, potassium chloride, prochlorperazine, propofol, sargramostim, tacrolimus, teniposide, thiotepa, tolazoline, vinorelbine, vit B/C

Additive compatibilities:

Amikacin, aminophylline, ascorbic acid inj, bretylium, cephapirin, chloramphenicol, corticotropin, dimenhydrinate, erythromycin, furosemide, heparin, hydrocortisone, lidocaine, magnesium sulfate, methicillin, norepinephrine, penicillin G potassium, penicillin G sodium, phenobarbital, potassium chloride, tobramycin, vancomycin, verapamil, vit B/C

PO route

- Give PO with or following meals to enhance absorption
- Store at room temp

Patient/family education

- Advise patient to remain recumbent 30 min after **IV** dose
- Caution patient to add food high in vit D content; to add calcium-rich foods to diet: dairy products, shellfish, dark green leafy vegetables; decrease oxalate-rich and zinc-rich foods: nuts, legumes, chocolate, spinach, soy

- Advise patient to prevent injuries, avoid immobilization

Evaluation

Positive therapeutic outcome

- Decreased twitching, paresthesias, muscle spasms
- Absence of tremors, convulsions, dysrhythmias, dyspnea, laryngospasm, negative Chvostek's sign, negative Trousseau's sign

calcium polycarbophil (OTC)

(pol-i-kar'boe-fil)

Equalactin, Fiberall, FiberCon, Fiber-Lax, Mitrolan

Func. class.: Laxative, bulk-forming

Pregnancy category C

Action: Attracts water, expands in intestine to increase peristalsis; also absorbs excess water in stool; decreases diarrhea

Therapeutic Outcome: Absence of constipation or diarrhea in irritable bowel syndrome

Uses: Constipation, irritable bowel syndrome (diarrhea), acute, nonspecific diarrhea

Dosage and routes

Adult: PO 1 g qd-qid prn, not to exceed 6 g/24 hr

P ***Child 6-12 yr:*** PO 500 mg bid prn, not to exceed 3 g/24 hr

P ***Child 3-6 yr:*** PO 500 mg bid prn, not to exceed 1.5 g/24 hr

Available forms: Chewable tabs 500, 1000 mg; tabs 500 mg

Adverse effects

GI: **Obstruction,** abdominal distention, flatus, laxative dependence

Contraindications: Hypersensitivity, GI obstruction

Precautions: Pregnancy **C**

Pharmacokinetics

Absorption	None
Distribution	None
Metabolism	Unknown
Excretion	Feces
Half-life	Not known

Pharmacodynamics

Onset	12-24 hr
Peak	1-3 days
Duration	Unknown

Interactions

Individual drugs

Tetracycline: ↓ absorption of tetracycline

NURSING CONSIDERATIONS

Assessment

- Monitor blood, urine electrolytes if used often by patient; check I&O ratio to identify fluid loss
- Assess cramping, rectal bleeding, nausea, vomiting; if these symptoms occur, drug should be discontinued; identify cause of constipation; identify whether fluids, bulk, or exercise is missing from lifestyle

Nursing diagnoses

- ✓ Constipation (uses)
- ✓ Diarrhea (side effects)
- ✓ Knowledge deficit (teaching)
- ✓ Noncompliance (teaching)

Implementation

- Give alone for better absorption; give after mixing with water immediately before use; administer with 6-8 oz of water or juice followed by another 8 oz of fluid
- Administer in AM or PM

Patient/family education

- Discuss with the patient that adequate fluid consumption is necessary; not to use laxatives long-term, laxative dependence will result
- Teach patient that normal bowel movements do not always occur daily
- Teach patient not to use in presence of abdominal pain, nausea, vomiting;

tell patient to notify prescriber if constipation is unrelieved or if symptoms of electrolyte imbalance occur: muscle cramps, pain, weakness, dizziness, excessive thirst

Evaluation

Positive therapeutic outcome

- Decreased constipation within 3 days
- Decreased diarrhea in colitis within 1 wk

candesartan (℞)

(can-deh-sar'tan)

Atacand

Func. class.: Antihypertensive

Chem. class.: Angiotensin II receptor (Type AT_1)

Pregnancy category C, 1st trimester; D, 2nd/3rd trimesters

Action: Blocks the vasoconstrictor and aldosterone-secreting effects of angiotensin II; selectively blocks the binding of angiotensin II to the AT_1 receptor found in tissues

Therapeutic Outcome: Decreased B/P

Uses: Hypertension, alone or in combination

Dosage and routes

Adult: PO (single agent) 16 mg qd initially in patients who are not volume depleted, range 8-32 mg/day; with diuretic or volume depletion 2-32 mg/day as a single dose or divided bid

Available forms: Tabs 4, 8, 16, 32 mg

Adverse effects

CNS: *Dizziness,* fatigue, headache

CV: Chest pain, peripheral edema

EENT: Sinusitis, rhinitis, pharyngitis

GI: *Diarrhea,* nausea

MS: Arthralgia, pain

RESP: *Cough, upper respiratory infection*

SYST: **Angioedema**

Contraindications:

Hypersensitivity; pregnancy **D** (2nd and 3rd trimesters)

Precautions: Hypersensitivity to ACE inhibitors; pregnancy **C** 1st trimester; lactation; [P] children; [G] elderly

Pharmacokinetics

Absorption	Well
Distribution	Bound to plasma proteins
Metabolism	Extensive
Excretion	Feces, urine, breast milk
Half-life	9 hr

Pharmacodynamics

Onset	Unknown
Peak	2 hr
Duration	24 hr

Interactions

None significant

NURSING CONSIDERATIONS

Assessment

- Assess B/P, pulse q4h; note rate, rhythm, quality
- Monitor electrolytes: potassium, sodium, chloride; total CO_2
- Obtain baselines in renal, liver function tests before therapy begins
- Assess blood studies: BUN, creatinine, LFTs before treatment
- Monitor for edema in feet, legs daily
- Assess for skin turgor, dryness of mucous membranes for hydration status, for angioedema; facial swelling, dyspnea
- Assess for pregnancy, this drug can cause fetal death when given in pregnancy
- Assess for adverse reactions, especially in renal disease
- Monitor for severe hypotension, place supine, give 0.9% NaCl **IV**

Nursing diagnoses

✓ Fluid volume deficit (side effects)

✓ Noncompliance (teaching)
✓ Knowledge deficit (teaching)

Implementation

PO route

- Administer without regard to meals

Patient/family education

- Teach patient not to take the drug if breastfeeding or pregnant, or have had an allergic reaction to this drug
- If a dose is missed, instruct patient to take as soon as possible, unless it is within an hour before next dose
- Advise patient to comply with dosage schedule, even if feeling better
- Teach patient to notify prescriber of fever, swelling of hands or feet, irregular heartbeat, chest pain
- Advise patient excessive perspiration, dehydration, diarrhea may lead to fall in blood pressure—consult prescriber if these occur
- Inform patient that drug may cause dizziness, fainting; lightheadedness may occur
- Caution patient to rise slowly to sitting or standing position to minimize orthostatic hypotension
- Advise patient to avoid all OTC medications unless approved by prescriber; to inform all health care providers of medication use
- Teach proper technique for obtaining B/P and acceptable parameters

Evaluation

Positive therapeutic outcome

- Decreased B/P

capecitabine (℞)

(cap-eh-sit'ah-bean)

Xeloda

Func. class.: Antineoplastic, antimetabolite

Chem. class.: Fluoropyrimidine carbamate

Pregnancy category D

Action: Competes with physiologic substrate of DNA synthesis, thus interfering with cell replication in the S phase of cell cycle (before mitosis); drug is converted to 5-fluorouracil (5-FU)

Therapeutic Outcome: Decreasing symptoms of breast cancer

Uses: Metastatic breast, colorectal cancer

Dosage and routes:
Adult: PO 2500 mg/m^2/day in 2 divided doses q12h at end of meal × 2 wk, then 1 wk rest period; given in 3 wk cycles

Available forms: Tabs 150, 500 mg

Adverse effects

CNS: Dizziness, headache, *paresthesia, fatigue,* insomnia

GI: *Nausea, vomiting, anorexia, diarrhea, stomatitis, abdominal pain, constipation, anorexia, dyspepsia,* **intestinal obstruction**

HEMA: **Neutropenia, lymphopenia, thrombocytopenia, myelosuppression,** anemia

INTEG: *Hand and foot syndrome,* dermatitis, nail disorder

MISC: Hyperbilirubinemia, eye irritation, pyrexia, edema, myalgia, limb pain, *pyrexia,* dehydration

Contraindications: Hypersensitivity to 5-FU, infants [P], pregnancy **D,** severe renal impairment (CrCl <30 ml/min)

Precautions: Renal disease, hepatic disease, lactation, children [P], elderly [G]

Pharmacokinetics	
Absorption	Readily, food ↓
Distribution	Unknown
Metabolism	Liver, extensively
Excretion	Kidneys
Half-life	45 min

Pharmacodynamics	
Onset	Unknown
Peak	1½ hr
Duration	Unknown

Interactions
Individual drugs
Leucovorin: ↑ toxicity
Warfarin: ↑ risk of bleeding
Drug classifications
Antacids: ↑ capecitabine

NURSING CONSIDERATIONS
Assessment
- Assess buccal cavity q8h for dryness, sores or ulceration, white patches, pain, bleeding, dysphagia; obtain prescription for viscous lidocaine (Xylocaine)
- Assess symptoms indicating severe allergic reation: rash, pruritus, urticaria, purpuric skin lesions, itching, flushing; drug should be discontinued
- Monitor CBC, differential, platelet count weekly; withhold drug if WBC <4000/mm^3 or platelet count is <100,000/mm^3; notify prescriber of results if WBC <20,000/mm^3, platelet count <150,000/mm^3
- Monitor temp q4h (may indicate beginning of infection)
- Assess for hand/foot syndrome: paresthesia, tingling, painful/painless swelling, blistering, erythema with severe pain of hands/feet
- Assess for toxicity: severe diarrhea, nausea, vomiting, stomatitis
- Assess GI symptoms: frequency of stools, cramping; if severe diarrhea occurs, fluids/electrolytes may need to be given
- Monitor liver function tests before and during therapy (bilirubin, AST, ALT, LDH) as needed or monthly; note jaundice of skin or sclera, dark urine, clay-colored stools, itchy skin, abdominal pain, fever, diarrhea
- Assess for bleeding: hematuria, stool guaiac, bruising or petechiae, mucosa or orifices q8h; inflammation of mucosa, breaks in skin

Nursing diagnoses
- ✓ Injury, risk for (adverse reactions)
- ✓ Body image disturbance (adverse reactions)
- ✓ Infection, risk for (adverse reactions)
- ✓ Knowledge deficit (teaching)

Implementation
PO route
- Give antiemetic 30-60 min before giving drug to prevent vomiting and prn; give antibiotics for prophylaxis of infection
- Provide liq diet: carbonated beverages; gelatin may be added if patient is not nauseated or vomiting
- Help patient to rinse mouth tid-qid with water or club soda, brush teeth bid-qid with soft brush or cotton-tipped applicators for stomatitis, use unwaxed dental floss

Patient/family education
- Contraceptive measures are recommended during therapy; drug is teratogenic to fetus
- Advise patient to avoid use of products containing aspirin or ibuprofen, razors, commercial mouthwash, since bleeding may occur; to report symptoms of bleeding (hematuria, tarry stools)
- Instruct patient to report signs of anemia (fatigue, headache, irritability, faintness, shortness of breath)
- Advise patient not to become pregnant while taking this drug; to avoid using while lactating
- Advise patient not to double dose, if dose is missed
- Advise patient to report immediately severe diarrhea, vomiting, stomatitis, fever ≥100° F, hand/foot syndrome, anorexia

Evaluation
Positive therapeutic outcome
- Prevention of rapid division of malignant cells

C

captopril (℞)

(kap'toe-pril)

Capoten, Novo-Captopril ✦

Func. class.: Antihypertensive

Chem. class.: Angiotensin-converting enzyme (ACE) inhibitor

Pregnancy category C (1st trimester); D (2nd/3rd trimester)

Action: Selectively suppresses renin-angiotensin-aldosterone system; inhibits ACE; prevents conversion of angiotensin I to angiotensin II

Therapeutic Outcome: Decreased B/P in hypertension; decreased preload, afterload in CHF

Uses: Hypertension, CHF, left ventricular dysfunction (LVD) after MI, diabetic nephropathy

Dosage and routes

Malignant hypertension

Adult: PO 25 mg increasing q2h until desired response; not to exceed 450 mg/day

Hypertension

Adult: Initial dose: PO 12.5 mg bid-tid; may increase to 50 mg bid-tid at 1-2 wk intervals; usual range 25-150 mg bid-tid; max 450 mg

P ***Child:*** PO 0.3-0.5 mg/kg/dose, titrate up to 6 mg/kg/day in 2-4 divided doses

P ***Neonate:*** PO 10 μg (0.01 mg)/kg bid-tid, may increase as needed

CHF

Adult: PO 12.5 mg bid-tid given with a diuretic; may increase to 50 mg bid-tid; after 14 days may increase to 150 mg tid if needed

LVD after MI

Adult: PO 50 mg tid, may begin treatment 3 days after MI; give 6.25 mg as a single dose, then 12.5 mg tid, increase to 25 mg tid for several days, then 50 mg tid

Diabetic nephropathy

Adult: PO 25 mg tid

Renal dose

Adult: PO 6.25-12.5 mg bid-tid

P ***Child:*** PO 150 μg (0.15)/kg tid

Available forms: Tabs 12.5, 25, 50, 100 mg

Adverse effects

CNS: Fever, chills

CV: *Hypotension,* postural hypotension, *tachycardia,* angina

GI: Loss of taste

GU: Impotence, dysuria, nocturia, **proteinuria, nephrotic syndrome, acute reversible renal failure,** polyuria, oliguria, frequency

HEMA: **Neutropenia, agranulocytosis, pancytopenia, thrombocytopenia,** anemia

INTEG: Rash, **angioedema**

MISC: **Angioedema,** hyperkalemia

RESP: **Bronchospasm,** *dyspnea, cough*

Contraindications: Hypersensitivity, lactation, heart block, children, P potassium-sparing diuretics, bilateral renal artery stenosis, pregnancy **D** (2nd/3rd trimester)

Precautions: Dialysis patients, hypovolemia, leukemia, scleroderma, LE, blood dyscrasias, CHF, diabetes mellitus, pregnancy **C** (1st trimester), renal disease, thyroid disease, COPD, asthma

Pharmacokinetics	
Absorption	Well absorbed
Distribution	Widely distributed; crosses placenta
Metabolism	Liver (50%)
Excretion	Kidneys, unchanged (50%)
Half-life	1½-2 hr

Pharmacodynamics	
Onset	¼-1 hr
Peak	1 hr
Duration	6-12 hr

Interactions

Individual drugs

Alcohol, acute ingestion: ↑ hypotension (large amounts)
Allopurinol: ↑ hypersensitivity
Digoxin: ↑ serum levels
Indomethacin: ↓ antihypertensive effect
Insulin: ↑ hypoglycemia
Lithium: ↑ serum levels, toxicity
Tetracycline: ↓ absorption of tetracycline

Drug classifications

Antacids: ↓ absorption
Antidiabetics, oral: ↑ hypoglycemia
Antihypertensives: ↑ hypotension
Diuretics: ↑ hypotension
Diuretics, potassium-sparing: ↑ toxicity
Nitrates: ↑ hypotension
NSAIDs: ↓ captopril effect
Phenothiazines: ↑ hypotension
Potassium supplements: ↑ toxicity

Food/drug

- Decreased perindopril to perindoprilat conversion

Lab test interferences

False positive: Urine acetone, ANA titer

NURSING CONSIDERATIONS

Assessment

- May be crushed and mixed with food
- Monitor blood studies: decreased platelets; WBC with diff baseline and periodically q3 mo, if neutrophils <1000/mm^3, discontinue treatment
- Monitor B/P, check for orthostatic hypotension, syncope; if changes occur, dosage change may be required
- Monitor renal studies: protein, BUN, creatinine; watch for increased levels that may indicate nephrotic syndrome and renal failure; monitor renal symptoms: polyuria, oliguria, frequency, dysuria
- Establish baselines in renal, liver function tests before therapy begins and check periodically; monitor for increased liver function studies; watch for increased uric acid, glucose
- Check potassium levels throughout treatment, although hyperkalemia rarely occurs
- Check for edema in feet, legs daily; monitor weight daily in CHF
- Assess for allergic reactions: rash, fever, pruritus, urticaria; drug should be discontinued if antihistamines fail to help

Nursing diagnoses

- ✓ Cardiac output, decreased (uses)
- ✓ Injury, risk for (side effects)
- ✓ Knowledge deficit (teaching)
- ✓ Noncompliance (teaching)

Implementation

- Store in air-tight container at 86° F (30° C) or less
- Severe hypotension may occur after 1st dose of this medication; decreasing hypotension may be prevented by reducing or discontinuing diuretic therapy 3 days before beginning captopril therapy
- Administer 1 hr ac or 1½ hr pc

Patient/family education

- Caution patient not to discontinue drug abruptly; advise patient to tell all persons associated with care
- Teach patient not to use OTC products (cough, cold, allergy) unless directed by prescriber; serious side effects can occur; xanthines such as coffee, tea, chocolate, cola can prevent action of drug
- Teach patient importance of complying with dosage schedule, even if feeling better; to continue with medical regimen to decrease B/P: exercise, cessation of smoking, decreasing stress, diet modifications
- Emphasize the need to rise slowly to sitting or standing position to minimize orthostatic hypotension; not to exercise in hot weather or increased hypotension can occur
- Teach patient to notify prescriber of mouth sores, sore throat, fever, swelling of hands or feet, irregular

heartbeat, chest pain, coughing, shortness of breath

- Caution patient to report excessive perspiration, dehydration, vomiting, diarrhea; may lead to fall in B/P
- Caution patient that drug may cause dizziness, fainting, lightheadedness; may occur during 1st few days of therapy; to avoid activities that may be hazardous
- Teach patient how to take B/P, and teach normal readings for age group; ensure patient takes regularly
- Advise patient to tell prescriber if pregnancy is suspected or planned

Evaluation

Positive therapeutic outcome

- Decreased B/P in hypertension

Treatment of overdose: 0.9% NaCl **IV** infusion, hemodialysis

carbamazepine (℞)

(kar-ba-maz'e-peen)

Apo-Carbamazepine ♣, Atretol, Carbatrol, Epitol, Mazepine ♣, PMS-Carbamazepine ♣, Tegretol, Tegretol CR ♣, Tegretol-XR

Func. class.: Anticonvulsant

Chem. class.: Iminostilbene derivative

Pregnancy category C

Action: Inhibits nerve impulses by limiting influx of sodium ions across cell membrane in motor cortex

➔ **Therapeutic Outcome:** Absence of seizures; decreased trigeminal neuralgia pain

Uses: Tonic-clonic, complex-partial, mixed seizures; trigeminal neuralgia, diabetic neuropathy

Investigational uses: Diabetes insipidus, bipolar disorder, neurogenic pain, schizophrenia, psychotic behavior with dementia, rectal administration

Dosage and routes

Seizures

P ***Adult and child >12 yr:*** PO 200 mg bid; may be increased by 200 mg/day in divided doses q6-8h; maintenance 800-1200 mg/day; maximum 1200 mg/day; adjustment is needed to minimum dose to control seizures; ext rel give bid; rec administration of oral susp 200 mg/10 ml or 6 mg/kg as a single dose

P ***Child 6-12 yr:*** PO tabs 100 mg bid or susp 50 mg qid; may increase by 100 mg qwk; ext rel tabs qd-bid

P ***Child <6 yr:*** PO 10-20 mg/kg/day in 2-3 divided doses, may increase by 100 mg/day qwk

Trigeminal neuralgia

Adult: PO 100 mg/bid; may increase 100 mg q12h until pain subsides; not to exceed 1.2 g/day; maintenance is 200-400 mg bid

Available forms: Chewable tabs 100, 200 mg; tabs 200 mg; oral susp 100 mg/5 ml; ext rel 100, 200, 400 ♣ mg

Adverse effects

CNS: *Drowsiness,* dizziness, confusion, fatigue, **paralysis,** headache, hallucinations, **worsening of seizures**

CV: **Hypertension, CHF,** hypotension, aggravation of CAD, dysrhythmias

EENT: Tinnitus, dry mouth, blurred vision, diplopia, nystagmus, conjunctivitis

ENDO: Syndrome of inappropriate antidiuretic hormone (SIADH) G (elderly)

GI: *Nausea, constipation, diarrhea,* anorexia, vomiting, abdominal pain, stomatitis, glossitis, increased liver enzymes, **hepatitis**

GU: Frequency, retention, albuminuria, glycosuria, impotence

HEMA: **Thrombocytopenia, agranulocytosis, leukocytosis, neutropenia, aplastic anemia, eosinophilia,** increased pro-time

INTEG: *Rash,* **Stevens-Johnson syndrome,** urticaria
RESP: Pulmonary hypersensitivity (fever, dyspnea, pneumonitis)

Contraindications: Hypersensitivity to carbamazepine or tricyclic antidepressants, bone marrow depression, concomitant use of MAOIs

Precautions: Glaucoma, hepatic disease, renal disease, cardiac disease, psychosis, pregnancy **C,** lactation, P child <6 yr

Do Not Confuse:
Tegretol/Toradol

Pharmacokinetics

Absorption	Slow; completely absorbed
Distribution	Widely distributed
Metabolism	Extensively, liver
Excretion	Urine, feces, breast milk
Half-life	14-16 hr or more

Pharmacodynamics

Onset	2-4 day
Peak	4-8 hr
Duration	Unknown

Interactions

Individual drugs

Acetaminophen: ↑ metabolism, ↓ action
Benzodiazepines: ↓ effect of benzodiazepine
Clarithromycin: ↑ toxicity
Danazol: ↑ carbamazepine effect
Diltiazem: ↑ toxicity
Doxycycline: ↓ half-life
Felbamate: ↑ carbamazepine effect
Fluoxetine: ↑ carbamazepine effect
Fluvoxamine: ↑ carbamazepine effect
Haloperidol: ↓ serum levels, ↓ therapeutic efficacy
Lithium: ↑ CNS toxicity
Oral contraceptives: ↓ effect of oral contraceptives
Phenobarbital: ↑ effect
Phenytoin: ↑ and ↓ plasma levels, ↓ carbamazepine plasma levels
Quinine: ↑ carbamazepine levels
Theophylline: ↓ effect of theophylline, carbamazepine
Thyroid hormones: ↓ effect of thyroid hormones
Valproic acid: ↓ plasma levels, ↑ half-life of carbamazepine
Verapamil: ↑ toxicity
Warfarin: ↓ effect of warfarin

Drug classifications

Barbiturates: ↓ serum levels of carbamazepine
MAOIs: Fatal reaction; do not use together
Nondepolarizing muscle relaxants: Resistance to or reversal of effects of these agents
Posterior pituitary hormones: Potentiates antidiuretic effects
Succinimides: ↓ plasma levels

Food/drug

Grapefruit juice: ↓ carbamazepine level

Lab test interferences

↓ Thyroid function tests

NURSING CONSIDERATIONS

Assessment

- Monitor liver function tests (AST, ALT) and urine function tests, BUN, urine protein periodically during treatments
- Check blood levels during treatment or when changing dose; therapeutic level 4-12 μg/ml
- Assess for blood dyscrasias: fever, sore throat, bruising, rash, jaundice, epistaxis (long-term treatment only)
- Assess seizure activity including type, aura, location, duration, and character; provide seizure precaution

Nursing diagnoses

- ✓ Injury, risk for (side effects)
- ✓ Knowledge deficit (teaching)

Implementation

- Give with food for GI symptoms
- Chew tab: tell patient to chew, not swallow whole
- Shake oral susp before use
- Mix an equal amount of water, D_5W,

0.9% NaCl when giving by NG tube, flush tube with 100 ml of above sol

Patient/family education

- Teach patient to carry Medic Alert ID stating patient's name, drugs taken, condition, prescriber's name, phone number
- Caution patient to avoid driving, other activities that require alertness until stabilized on medication
- Teach patient not to discontinue medication quickly after long-term use
- Teach patient to use a nonhormonal type of contraception to prevent harm to the fetus
- Advise patient to use sunscreen to prevent burns
- Teach patient to take exactly as prescribed, do not double or omit doses, not to crush, break, or chew extended release products

Evaluation

Positive therapeutic outcome

- Decreased seizure activity

Treatment of overdose:
Lavage, VS

carbidopa-levodopa (℞)

(kar-bi-doe'pa lee-voe-doe'pa)

carbidopa/levodopa, Sinemet, Sinemet CR

Func. class.: Antiparkinsonism agent
Chem. class.: Catecholamine

Pregnancy category C

Action: Decarboxylation of levodopa to periphery is inhibited by carbidopa; more levodopa is made available for transport to brain and conversion to dopamine in the brain

Therapeutic Outcome: Absence of involuntary movements

Uses: Parkinsonism, restless leg syndrome, chronic manganese intoxication, cerebral arteriosclerosis

Dosage and routes

Beginning therapy for those not taking levodopa

Adult: PO 10 mg carbidopa/100 mg levodopa tid-qid or 25 mg carbidopa/100 mg levodopa tid, may increase qd to desired response

For those not taking levodopa ER

Adult: PO 50 mg carbidopa/200 mg levodopa bid

For those taking levodopa ER

Adult: Begin treatment with 10% more levodopa/day given PO q8h, may increase or decrease dose q3 days

For those taking levodopa <1.5 g/day

Adult: PO 25 mg carbidopa/100 mg levodopa tid-qid, may increase qd to desired response

For those taking levodopa >1.5 g/day

Adult: PO 25 mg carbidopa/250 mg levodopa tid-qid, may increase qd to desired response

Available forms: Tabs 10/100, 25/100, 25 mg carbidopa/250 mg levodopa; ext rel tab: 25 mg/100 mg, 50 mg/200 mg carbidopa/levodopa (Sinemet CR)

Adverse effects

CNS: *Involuntary choreiform movements, hand tremors, fatigue, headache, anxiety, twitching, numbness, weakness, confusion, agitation, insomnia, nightmares,* psychosis, hallucination, hypomania, severe depression, dizziness
CV: *Orthostatic hypotension,* tachycardia, hypertension, palpitation
EENT: Blurred vision, diplopia, dilated pupils
GI: *Nausea, vomiting, anorexia, abdominal distress, dry mouth, flatulence, dysphagia, bitter taste, diarrhea, constipation*
HEMA: **Hemolytic anemia, leukopenia, agranulocytosis**

INTEG: Rash, sweating, alopecia
MISC: Urinary retention, incontinence, weight change, dark urine

Contraindications: Hypersensitivity, narrow-angle glaucoma, malignant melanoma, history of malignant melanoma, or undiagnosed skin lesions resembling melanoma

Precautions: Renal disease, cardiac disease, hepatic disease, respiratory disease, MI with dysrhythmias, wide angle glaucoma, convulsions, peptic ulcer, pregnancy **C**

Pharmacokinetics

Absorption	Well absorbed (PO); ER dose slow
Distribution	Widely distributed
Metabolism	Liver, extensively
Excretion	Kidneys, metabolites
Half-life	Levodopa (1 hr); carbidopa (1-2 hr)

Pharmacodynamics

	PO	PO-ER
Onset	Unknown	Unknown
Peak	1 hr	2½ hr
Duration	6-24 hr	Unknown

Interactions

Individual drugs

Metoclopramide: ↑ effects of levodopa
Papaverine: ↓ effects of levodopa
Pyridoxine: ↓ effects of levodopa

Drug classifications

Antacids: ↑ effects of levodopa
Anticholinergics: ↓ effects of levodopa
Antidepressants, tricyclic: ↑ hypotension
Benzodiazepines: ↓ effects of levodopa
Hydantoins: ↓ effects of levodopa
MAOIs: Hypertensive crisis

Lab test interferences

↑ Uric acid, ↑ urine protein
↓ VMA, ↓ BUN, ↓ creatinine
False positive: Urine ketones
False negative: Urine glucose

Food/drug

Protein: ↓ absorption of levodopa

Herb/drug

Kava: ↑ Parkinson's symptoms

NURSING CONSIDERATIONS

Assessment

- Assess B/P, respiration, orthostatic B/P
- Monitor I&O ratio; retention commonly causes decreased urinary output, distention, frequency, incontinence; palpate bladder if retention occurs
- Assess for muscle twitching, blepharospasm that may indicate toxicity
- Monitor renal, liver, hematopoietic studies, also for diabetes, acromegaly during long-term therapy
- Assess for parkinsonism, shuffling gait, muscle rigidity, involuntary movements, pill rolling, muscle spasms, drooling before and during treatment
- Monitor for constipation, cramping, pain in abdomen, abdominal distention; increase fluids, bulk, exercise if this occurs
- Assess for tolerance over long-term therapy; dose may have to be increased or changed
- Assess for mental status: affect, mood, CNS depression, worsening of mental symptoms during early therapy

Nursing diagnoses

✓ Physical mobility, impaired (uses)
✓ Knowledge deficit (teaching)

Implementation

PO route

- Give drug until NPO before surgery; check with prescriber for continuing drug
- Adjust dosage depending on patient response
- Give with meals or pc to prevent GI symptoms; limit protein taken with drug
- Give only after MAOIs have been discontinued for 2 wk; if previously on

levodopa, discontinue for at least 8 hr before change to levodopa-carbidopa
- Controlled-release tabs should be swallowed whole, not crushed or chewed

Patient/family education

- Teach patient to change positions slowly to prevent orthostatic hypotension
- Teach patient to report side effects: twitching, eye spasms, grimacing, protrusion of tongue, personality changes that indicate overdose
- Instruct patient to use drug exactly as prescribed; if drug is discontinued abruptly, parkinsonian crisis may occur; do not double doses; take missed dose as soon as remembered up to 2 hr before next dose
- Teach patient that urine, sweat may darken and is harmless
- Advise patient to use physical activities to maintain mobility and lessen spasms
- Instruct patient that OTC medications should not be used unless approved by prescriber
- Advise patient that drowsiness, dizziness are common; to avoid hazardous activities until response is known
- Explain that sips of water, hard candy, or gum may lessen dry mouth
- Teach patient to take with meals to prevent GI symptoms; to limit protein intake, which impairs drug's absorption

Evaluation

Positive therapeutic outcome

- Decrease in akathisia
- Improved mood
- Decreased involuntary movements

HIGH ALERT

carboplatin (℞)

(kar'boe'pla-tin)

Paraplatin, Paraplatin-AQ ✤

Func. class.: Antineoplastic alkylating agent

Chem. class.: Platinum coordination compound

Pregnancy category D

Action: Produces interstrand DNA cross-links and to a lesser extent DNA-protein cross-links; activity is not cell cycle phase specific

Therapeutic Outcome: Prevention of rapidly growing malignant cells

Uses: Initial treatment of ovarian cancer in combination with other agents; palliative treatment of recurrent ovarian carcinoma after treatment with other antineoplastic agents, including cisplatin

Dosage and routes

(single agent)

Adult: **IV** inf initially 300 mg/m^2 given with cyclophosphamide, q4-6 wk; refractory tumors 360 mg/m^2 single dose, may repeat q4 wk, as needed

Renal dose

CrCl 41-59 ml/min 250 mg/m^2, CrCl 16-40 ml/min 200 mg/m^2

Available forms: Inj 50, 150, 450 mg/vial

Adverse effects

CNS: **Convulsions, central neurotoxicity,** peripheral neuropathy, dizziness, confusion

CV: Cardiac abnormalities

EENT: Tinnitus, hearing loss, ***vestibular toxicity,*** visual changes

GI: Severe nausea, vomiting, diarrhea, weight loss, mucositis, anorexia, constipation, taste change

GU: **Renal tubular damage,** renal

insufficiency, impotence, sterility, amenorrhea, gynecomastia
***HEMA:* Thrombocytopenia, leukopenia, pancytopenia, neutropenia,** anemia, bleeding
INTEG: Alopecia, dermatitis, rash, erythema, pruritus, urticaria
META: Hypomagnesemia, hypocalcemia, hypokalemia, hyponatremia, hyperuremia
***SYST:* Anaphylaxis**

Contraindications: Hypersensitivity to this drug, platinum products, mannitol; severe bone marrow depression, significant bleeding, pregnancy **D**

Precautions: Radiation therapy within 1 mo, chemotherapy within 1 mo, lactation, liver disease

Do Not Confuse:
carboplatin/cisplatin

Pharmacokinetics

Absorption	Complete
Distribution	Unknown
Metabolism	Liver
Excretion	Kidneys
Half-life	Initial 1-2 hr; postdistribution 2½-6 hr; increased in renal disease

Pharmacodynamics

Onset	½ hr
Peak	Unknown
Duration	4-6 hr

Interactions
Individual drugs
Aspirin: ↑ risk of bleeding
Phenytoin: ↓ phenytoin level
Radiation: ↑ toxicity, bone marrow suppression
Drug classifications
Aminoglycosides: ↑ nephrotoxicity
Antineoplastics: ↑ toxicity, bone marrow suppression
Bone marrow–suppressing drugs: ↑ bone marrow suppression
Diuretics, loop: ↑ ototoxicity
Myelosuppressives: ↑ myelosuppression
Lab test interferences
↑ AST, ↑ BUN, ↑ alkaline phosphatase, ↑ bilirubin, ↑ creatinine

NURSING CONSIDERATIONS
Assessment
- Monitor CBC, differential, platelet count weekly; withhold drug if neutrophil count is <2000/mm^3 or platelet count is <100,000/mm^3; notify prescriber of results if WBC <20,000/mm^3, platelets <150,000/mm^3
- Assess for anaphylaxis: pruritus, wheezing, tachycardia; notify physician after discontinuing drugs; resuscitation equipment should be available
- Monitor renal function studies: BUN, creatinine, serum uric acid, urine CrCl before and during therapy; I&O ratio; report fall in urine output to <30 ml/hr
- Monitor temp q4h (may indicate beginning of infection)
- Monitor liver function tests before and during therapy (bilirubin, AST, ALT, LDH) as needed or monthly; note jaundice of skin or sclera, dark urine, clay-colored stools, itchy skin, abdominal pain, fever, diarrhea
- Assess for bleeding: hematuria, stool guaiac, bruising or petechiae, mucosa or orifices q8h; inflammation of mucosa, breaks in skin
- Identify dyspnea, rales, unproductive cough, chest pain, tachypnea
- Identify effects of alopecia on body image; discuss feelings about body changes

Nursing diagnoses
✓ Injury, risk for (adverse reactions)
✓ Body image disturbance (adverse reactions)
✓ Infection, risk for (adverse reactions)
✓ Knowledge deficit (teaching)

Implementation
- Antiemetic 30-60 min before giving drug to prevent vomiting, and prn

IV IV route

• Give **IV** after diluting 10 mg/ml of sterile water for inj, D_5W, 0.9% NaCl (10 mg/ml); then further dilute with the same sol 1-4 mg/ml; give over 15 min or more (intermittent inf)

• Give **IV** inf over 5-6 hr; do not use needles or **IV** administration sets containing aluminum; may cause precipitate or loss of potency; diuretic (furosemide 40 mg **IV**) after inf

• Store protected from light at room temp; reconstituted sol is stable for 8 hr at room temp

Y-site compatibilities: Allopurinol, amifostine, aztreonam, cefepime, cladribine, doxorubicin liposome, filgrastim, fludarabine, granisetron, melphalan, ondansetron, paclitaxel, piperacillin/tazobactam, propofol, sargramostim, teniposide, thiotepa, vinorelbine

Additive compatibilities: Cisplatin, etoposide, floxuridine, ifosfamide, ifosfamide/etoposide, paclitaxel

Additive incompatibilities: Fluorouracil, mesna

Solution compatibilities: D_5/0.2% NaCl, D_5/0.45% NaCl, D_5/0.9% NaCl, 0.9% NaCl, D_5W, sterile water for inj

Solution incompatibilities: Sodium bicarbonate

Patient/family education

• Teach patient to avoid use of products containing aspirin or ibuprofen, razors, commercial mouthwash, since bleeding may occur; to report symptoms of bleeding (hematuria, tarry stools)

• Instruct patient to report signs of anemia (fatigue, headache, irritability, faintness, shortness of breath); sore throat, bleeding, bruising

• Instruct patient to report any changes in breathing or coughing even several months after treatment; to avoid crowds and persons with respiratory tract or other infections

• Advise patient that hair may be lost during treatment; a wig or hairpiece may make patient feel better; new hair may be different in color, texture

• Caution patient not to have any vaccinations without the advice of the prescriber; serious reactions can occur

• Teach patient that contraception is needed during treatment and for several months after the completion of therapy; not to breast feed during treatment

Evaluation

Positive therapeutic outcome

• Prevention of rapid division of malignant cells

carboprost (℞)

(kar'boe-prost)

Hemabate, Prostin/15M ✱

Func. class.: Oxytocic, abortifacient

Chem. class.: Prostaglandin

Pregnancy category C

Action: Stimulates uterine contractions, causing complete abortion in approximately 16 hr

➲ **Therapeutic Outcome:** Loss of fetus; decreased postpartum bleeding

Uses: Abortion between 13-20 wk gestation; postpartum hemorrhage caused by uterine atony not controlled by other methods

Dosage and routes

To induce abortion

Adult: IM 250 μg, then 250 μg q1½-3½h, may increase to 500 μg if no response, not to exceed 12 mg total dose

Postpartum hemorrhage

Adult: IM 250 μg, repeat at 15-90 min intervals, max total dosage 2 mg

Available forms: Inj 250 μg/ml

Adverse effects
CNS: Fever, chills, headache
GI: Nausea, vomiting, diarrhea

Contraindications: Hypersensitivity, severe hepatic disease, severe renal disease, PID, respiratory disease, cardiac disease

Precautions: Asthma, anemia, jaundice, diabetes mellitus, convulsive disorders, past uterine surgery, pregnancy **C**

Pharmacokinetics	
Absorption	Well absorbed (nasal)
Distribution	Widely distributed (extracellular fluid)
Metabolism	Liver—rapidly
Excretion	Kidneys
Half-life	3-9 min

Pharmacodynamics	
Onset	Unknown
Peak	16 hr
Duration	Unknown

Interactions
Drug classifications
Oxytocics: ↑ effects
Herb/drug
Ephedra: ↑ B/P, hypertension

NURSING CONSIDERATIONS
Assessment
- Monitor B/P, pulse; watch for change that may indicate hemorrhage
- Monitor respiratory rate, rhythm, depth; notify physician of abnormalities
- For length, duration of contraction; notify physician of contractions lasting over 1 min or absence of contractions
- Assess for incomplete abortion, pregnancy must be terminated by another method; drug is teratogenic

Nursing diagnoses
✓ Knowledge deficit (teaching)

Implementation
- Give IM in deep muscle mass; rotate injection sites if additional doses are given
- Have crash cart available on unit

Patient/family education
- Advise patient to report increased blood loss, abdominal cramps, increased temperature or foul-smelling lochia

Evaluation
Positive therapeutic outcome
- Loss of fetus
- Control of bleeding

carisoprodol (℞)
(kar-i-soe-proe′dole)
carisoprodol, Sodol, Soma, Vanadom
Func. class.: Skeletal muscle relaxant, central acting
Chem. class.: Meprobamate congener

Pregnancy category C

Action: Depresses CNS by blocking interneuronal activity in descending reticular formation of spinal cord, producing sedation

Therapeutic Outcome: Relaxation of skeletal muscles

Uses: Relieving pain, stiffness in musculoskeletal disorders

Dosage and routes
P ***Adult and child >12 yr:*** PO 350 mg tid-qid
P ***Child 6-12 yr:*** PO 6.25 mg/kg qid

Available forms: Tabs 350 mg

Adverse effects
CNS: Dizziness, weakness, drowsiness, headache, tremor, depression, insomnia, ataxia, irritability
CV: Postural hypotension, tachycardia
EENT: Diplopia, temporary loss of vision
GI: Nausea, vomiting, hiccups, epigastric discomfort
HEMA: Eosinophilia

INTEG: Rash, pruritus, fever, facial flushing, **erythema multiforme**
RESP: Asthmatic attack
SYST: **Angioedema, anaphylaxis**

Contraindications: Hypersensitivity, child <12 yr, intermittent porphyria

Precautions: Renal disease, hepatic disease, addictive personality, pregnancy **C**, elderly

Pharmacokinetics	
Absorption	Well absorbed
Distribution	Crosses placenta
Metabolism	Liver, partially
Excretion	Kidney, unchanged; breast milk
Half-life	8 hr

Pharmacodynamics	
Onset	½ hr
Peak	4 hr
Duration	4-6 hr

Interactions
Individual drugs
Alcohol: ↑ CNS depression
Drug classifications
Antidepressants, tricyclic: ↑ CNS depression
Barbiturates: ↑ CNS depression
Opioids: ↑ CNS depression
Sedative/hypnotics: ↑ CNS depression
Herb/drug
Kava: ↑ CNS depression
Lab test interferences
↑ AST, ↑ alkaline phosphatase, ↑ blood glucose

NURSING CONSIDERATIONS
Assessment
- Monitor ROM, atrophy, stiffness, and pain in muscles; assess throughout treatment
- Assess for idiosyncratic reaction within a few min or hr of administration (disorientation, restlessness, weakness, blurred vision); patient should be reassured that reaction is temporary
- Check for allergic reactions: rash, fever

Nursing diagnoses
✓ Mobility, impaired (uses)
✓ Injury, risk for (adverse reactions)
✓ Knowledge deficit (teaching)

Implementation
PO route
- Give with meals for GI symptoms
- Have patient use gum, frequent sips of water for dry mouth
- Store in tight container at room temp

Patient/family education
- Caution patient not to take with alcohol, other CNS depressants
- Advise patient to avoid altering activities while taking this drug
- Caution patient to avoid hazardous activities if drowsiness or dizziness occurs
- Caution patient to avoid using OTC medication such as cough preparations, antihistamines, unless directed by prescriber

Evaluation
Positive therapeutic outcome
- Decreased pain, spasticity

Treatment of overdose:
Induce emesis of conscious patient, lavage, dialysis

HIGH ALERT

carmustine (℞)
(kar-mus'teen)
BiCNU, BCNU, Gliadel
Func. class.: Antineoplastic alkylating agent
Chem. class.: Nitrosourea
Pregnancy category D

Action: Alkylates DNA, RNA; inhibits enzymes that allow synthesis of amino acids in proteins; also responsible for cross-linking DNA strands; activity is not cell cycle phase specific

Therapeutic Outcome: Prevention of rapidly growing malignant cells

Uses: Brain tumors such as glioblastoma, medulloblastoma, astrocytoma; multiple myeloma, Hodgkin's disease, other lymphomas; GI, breast, bronchogenic, and renal carcinomas, other lymphomas

Dosage and routes

Adult: **IV** 75-100 mg/m² over 1-2 hr × 2 days or 150-200 mg/m² × 1 dose q6-8 wk or 40 mg/m²/day × 5 days q6 wk; if WBC 3000-3999/mm³ give 50% of dose; if WBC is 2000-2999/mm³ and platelet count is 25,000-75,000/mm³ give 25% of dose; withhold dose if WBC <2000/mm³ and platelets <25,000/mm³

Adult: Intracavitary 8 wafers inserted into resection cavity

Available forms: Powder for inj 100 mg; wafer 7.7 mg

Adverse effects

GI: Nausea, vomiting, anorexia, stomatitis, **hepatotoxicity**
GU: Azotemia, **renal failure**
HEMA: **Thrombocytopenia, leukopenia, myelosuppression, anemia**
INTEG: Burning, hyperpigmentation at inj site, alopecia
RESP: **Fibrosis, pulmonary infiltrate**

Contraindications: Hypersensitivity, leukopenia, thrombocytopenia, pregnancy **D**

Pharmacokinetics

Absorption	Completely absorbed
Distribution	Readily penetrates CSF
Metabolism	Liver, rapid
Excretion	Kidneys, breast milk
Half-life	Unknown

Pharmacodynamics

Unknown

Interactions

Individual drugs

Aspirin: ↑ risk of bleeding
Cimetidine: ↑ toxicity
Phenytoin: ↑ metabolism, ↓ effect
Radiation: ↑ toxicity, bone marrow suppression

Drug classifications

Anticoagulants: ↑ risk of bleeding
Antineoplastics: ↑ toxicity, bone marrow suppression
Bone marrow–suppressing drugs: ↑ bone marrow suppression
Live vaccines: ↑ adverse reactions, ↓ antibody reaction

NURSING CONSIDERATIONS

Assessment

- Assess buccal cavity q8h for dryness, sores or ulceration, white patches, pain, bleeding, dysphagia; obtain prescription for viscous lidocaine (Xylocaine)
- Assess symptoms indicating severe allergic reaction: rash, pruritus, urticaria, purpuric skin lesions, itching, flushing; drug should be discontinued
- Monitor CBC, differential, platelet count weekly; withhold drug if WBC <4000/mm³ or platelet count is <100,000/mm³; notify prescriber of results if WBC <20,000/mm³, platelets <150,000/mm³
- Monitor renal function studies: BUN, creatinine, urine CrCl before and during therapy; I&O ratio; report fall in urine output to <30 ml/hr
- Monitor temp q4h (may indicate beginning of infection)
- Monitor liver function tests before and during therapy (bilirubin, AST, ALT, LDH) as needed or monthly; note yellowing of skin or sclera, dark urine, clay-colored stools, itchy skin, abdominal pain, fever, diarrhea; hepatotoxicity can be serious and fatal
- Assess for bleeding: hematuria, stool guaiac, bruising or petechiae, mucosa or orifices q8h; inflammation of mucosa, breaks in skin

• Identify effects of alopecia on body image; discuss feelings about body changes

Nursing diagnoses

✓ Injury, risk for (adverse reactions)
✓ Body image disturbance (adverse reactions)
✓ Infection, risk for (adverse reactions)
✓ Knowledge deficit (teaching)

Implementation

• Blood transfusion or RBC colony-stimulating factors to counter anemia may be required
• Give fluids **IV** or PO before chemotherapy to hydrate patient
• Provide antiemetic 30-60 min before giving drug to prevent vomiting, and prn; antibiotics for prophylaxis of infection
• Provide liq diet (carbonated beverages); gelatin may be added if patient is not nauseated or vomiting
• Give all medications PO, if possible, avoid IM inj if platelets <100,000/mm^3

Wafer

• Foil pouches may be kept at room temp for 6 hr, if unopened
• If wafers are broken in several pieces, do not use

IV **IV route**

• Administer after diluting 100 mg/3 ml ethyl alcohol (provided); then further dilute 27 ml sterile water for inj; then dilute with 100-500 ml 0.9% NaCl or D_5W; give over 1 hr or more; use only glass containers; reduce rate if discomfort is felt
• Store reconstituted sol in refrigerator for 24 hr or room temp for 8 hr

Y-site compatibilities:
Amifostine, aztreonam, cefepime, filgrastim, fludarabine, granisetron, melphalan, ondansetron, piperacillin/tazobactam, sargramostim, teniposide, thiotepa, vinorelbine

Additive incompatibilities:
Sodium bicarbonate

Patient/family education

• Teach patient to avoid use of products containing aspirin or ibuprofen, razors, commercial mouthwash, since bleeding may occur; to report symptoms of bleeding (hematuria, tarry stools)
• Advise patient to avoid foods with citric acid, hot or rough texture if stomatitis is present
• Instruct patient to report signs of anemia (fatigue, headache, irritability, faintness, shortness of breath)
• Advise patient that hair may be lost during treatment; a wig or hairpiece may make patient feel better; new hair may be different in color, texture
• Caution patient not to have any vaccinations without the advice of the prescriber; serious reactions can occur
• Advise patient that contraception is needed during treatment and for several months after completion of therapy; drug has teratogenic properties

Evaluation

Positive therapeutic outcome

• Prevention of rapid division of malignant cells

carteolol (℞)

(kar-tee'oe-lole)
Cartrol
Func.class.: Antihypertensive
Chem. class.: Nonselective β-blocker

Pregnancy category C

Action: Produces fall in B/P without reflex tachycardia or significant reduction in heart rate through mixture of α-blocking, β-blocking effects and intrinsic sympathomimetic activity; elevated plasma renins are reduced; decreased intraocular pressure in glaucoma and intraocular hypertension

Therapeutic Outcome: Decreased B/P, heart rate; decreased intraocular pressure

Uses: Mild to moderate hypertension; oph intraocular hypertension, open-angle glaucoma (see Appendix C)

Dosage and routes

Adult: PO 2.5 mg qd initially; may gradually increase to de- sired response, max 10 mg/day; ophth i gtt bid

Renal dose

CrCl >60 ml/min give dose q24h, CrCl 20-60 ml/min give dose q48h, CrCl <20 ml/min give dose q72h

Available forms: Tabs 2.5, 5 mg

Adverse effects

CNS: Dizziness, mental changes, drowsiness, fatigue, headache, catatonia, depression, anxiety, nightmares, paresthesia, lethargy, insomnia, decreased concentration

CV: Orthostatic hypotension, **bradycardia, CHF, chest pain, ventricular dysrhythmias, AV block, peripheral vascular insufficency,** palpitations

EENT: Tinnitus, visual changes, sore throat, double vision, dry, burning eyes

GI: Nausea, vomiting, diarrhea, dry mouth, flatulence, constipation, anorexia

GU: Impotence, dysuria, ejaculatory failure, urinary retention

HEMA: **Agranulocytosis, thrombocytopenic purpura (rare)**

INTEG: Rash, alopecia, urticaria, pruritus, fever

MISC: Facial swelling, decreased exercise tolerance, weight change, Raynaud's disease, lupus-like syndrome

MS: Joint pain, arthralgia, muscle cramps, pain

RESP: **Bronchospasm,** dyspnea, wheezing, nasal stuffiness, pharyngitis

Contraindications: Hypersensitivity to β-blockers, cardiogenic shock, heart block (2nd or 3rd degree), sinus bradycardia, bronchial asthma

Precautions: Major surgery, pregnancy **C,** lactation, CHF, diabetes mellitus, renal disease, thyroid disease, COPD, well-compensated heart failure, nonallergic bronchospasm

Do Not Confuse:
Ocupress/Ocufen

Pharmacokinetics	
Absorption	80%-90%
Distribution	Unknown; protein binding 23%-30%
Metabolism	Liver to active metabolite
Excretion	Kidneys, unchanged (50%-75%)
Half-life	Carteolol (6-8 hr); metabolite (8-12 hr); ↑ renal disease

Pharmacodynamics	PO	OPHTH
Onset	Unknown	Unknown
Peak	1-3 hr	Unknown
Duration	Unknown	Unknown

Interactions

Individual drugs

Alcohol: ↑ hypotension (large amounts)
Clonidine: ↑ hypotension, bradycardia
Dopamine: ↓ CV effect
Dobutamine: ↓ CV effect
Epinephrine: α-Adrenergic stimulation
Insulin: ↑ hypoglycemia
Phenytoin (IV): ↑ myocardial depression
Reserpine: ↑ hypotension, bradycardia
Thyroid agents: ↓ effectiveness of carteolol
Verapamil: ↑ myocardial depression

Drug classifications

Amphetamines: ↑ hypertension, bradycardia
Anesthetics, general: ↑ hypotension

Antidiabetics, oral: ↑ hypoglycemia
Antihypertensives: ↑ hypertension
β_2-Agonists: ↓ bronchodilatation
Cardiac glycosides: ↑ bradycardia
MAOIs: ↑ hypertension
Nitrates: ↑ hypotension
NSAIDs: ↓ antihypertensive action
Theophyllines: ↓ bronchodilatation

NURSING CONSIDERATIONS

Assessment

- Monitor B/P during beginning treatment, periodically thereafter; pulse q4h; note rate, rhythm, quality: apical/radial pulse before administration; notify prescriber of any significant changes (pulse <50 bpm)
- Monitor blood glucose in those taking insulin, oral antidiabetics, dosage adjustment may be needed
- Check for baselines in renal, liver function tests before therapy begins
- Assess for edema in feet, legs daily; monitor I&O, daily weight; check for jugular vein distention and rales bilaterally, dyspnea (CHF)
- Monitor skin turgor, dryness of mucous membranes for hydration G status, especially elderly

Nursing diagnoses

- ✓ Cardiac output, decreased (uses)
- ✓ Injury, risk for (side effects)
- ✓ Knowledge deficit (teaching)
- ✓ Noncompliance (teaching)

Implementation

PO route

- Give ac, hs; tab may be crushed or swallowed whole; give with food to prevent GI upset
- Store protected from light, moisture; placed in cool environment

Patient/family education

- Teach patient not to discontinue drug abruptly; taper over 2 wk; may cause precipitate dysrhythmias, hypertension if stopped abruptly
- Teach patient not to use OTC products containing α-adrenergic stimulants (such as nasal decongestants, cold preparations); to avoid alcohol, smoking and to limit sodium intake as prescribed
- Teach patient how to take pulse and B/P at home; advise when to notify prescriber
- Instruct patient to comply with weight control, dietary adjustments, modified exercise program
- Advise patient to carry/wear Medic Alert ID to identify drug being taken, allergies; tell patient drug controls symptoms but does not cure
- Caution patient to avoid hazardous activities if dizziness, drowsiness present
- Teach patient to report symptoms of CHF; difficult breathing, especially on exertion or when lying down, night cough, swelling of extremities or bradycardia, dizziness, confusion, depression, fever
- Teach patient to take drug as prescribed, not to double doses, skip doses; take any missed doses as soon as remembered if at least 4 hr until next dose

Evaluation

Positive therapeutic outcome

- Decreased B/P in hypertension (after 1-2 wk)

Treatment of overdose:

Lavage, **IV** atropine for bradycardia; **IV** theophylline for bronchospasm, digitalis, O_2, diuretic for cardiac failure; **IV** glucose for hypoglycemia; **IV** diazepam (or phenytoin) for seizures

carvedilol (℞)

(kar-veh′dee-lol)

Coreg

Func. class.: Antihypertensive α/β blocker

Pregnancy category C

Action: A mixture of nonselective β-blocking and α-blocking activity;

decreases cardiac output, exercise-induced tachycardia, reflex orthostatic tachycardia; causes reduction in peripheral vascular resistance and vasodilation

➔ **Therapeutic Outcome:** Decreased B/P in hypertension

Uses: Essential hypertension alone or in combination with other antihypertensives, CHF

Investigational uses: Angina pectoris, idiopathic cardiomyopathy

Dosage and routes

Essential hypertension

Adult: PO 6.25 mg bid × 7-14 days if tolerated well, then increase to 12.5 mg bid × 7-14 days if tolerated well, may be increased if needed to 25 mg bid, max 50 mg qd

Congestive heart failure

Adult: PO 3.125 mg bid × 2 wk; if well tolerated, give 6.25 mg bid × 2 wk, then double qwk to max dose 25 mg bid <85 kg or 80 mg bid >85 kg

Angina pectoris

Adult: PO 25-50 mg bid

Idiopathic cardiomyopathy

Adult: PO 6.25-25 mg bid

Available forms: Tabs 3.125, 6.25, 12.5, 25 mg

Adverse effects

CNS: *Dizziness,* somnolence, insomnia, ataxia, hypesthesia, paresthesia, vertigo, depression, fatigue, weakness

CV: *Bradycardia, postural hypotension,* dependent edema, peripheral edema, **AV block, extrasystoles,** hypertension, hypotension, palpitations, peripheral ischemia, **CHF,** pulmonary edema

GI: *Diarrhea,* abdominal pain, ↑ alkaline phosphatase, ↑ ALT/AST

GU: Decreased libido, *impotence*

MISC: Fatigue, injury, back pain, UTI, viral infection, hypertriglyceridemia, **thrombocytopenia,** *hyperglycemia*

RESP: Rhinitis, pharyngitis, dyspnea

Contraindications: Hypersensitivity, bronchial asthma, class IV decompensated cardiac failure, 2nd or 3rd degree heart block, cardiogenic shock, severe bradycardia

Precautions: Cardiac failure, hepatic injury, peripheral vascular disease, anesthesia, major surgery, diabetes mellitus, thyrotoxicosis, G elderly, pregnancy **C,** lactation, P children, emphysema, chronic bronchitis, renal disease

Pharmacokinetics

Absorption	Readily and extensively absorbed
Distribution	>98% protein binding
Metabolism	Extensively liver
Excretion	Via bile into feces
G **Half-life**	Terminal half-life 7-10 hr, increased in the elderly, hepatic disease

Pharmacodynamics

Unknown

Interactions

Individual drugs

Alcohol, acute ingestion: ↑ toxicity
Cimetidine: ↑ toxicity
Clonidine: ↓ heart rate, B/P
Digoxin: ↑ concentrations of digoxin
Reserpine: ↑ hypotension, bradycardia
Rifampin: ↓ levels of carvedilol

Drug classifications

Antidiabetic agents: ↑ hypoglycemia
Calcium channel blockers: ↑ conduction disturbance
MAOIs: ↑ bradycardia, hypotension
Nitrates: ↑ toxicity
NSAIDS: ↓ levels of carvedilol

NURSING CONSIDERATIONS

Assessment

- Monitor renal studies including protein, BUN, creatinine; watch for increased levels that may indicate nephrotic syndrome; obtain baselines in renal and liver function studies before beginning treatment; if liver

function studies are elevated, drug should be discontinued
- Monitor I&O, weight daily
- Monitor B/P during beginning treatment and periodically thereafter, pulse q4h, note rate, rhythm, quality
- Monitor apical/radial pulse before administration; notify prescriber of significant changes
- Assess for edema in feet and legs daily, fluid overload: dyspnea, weight gain, jugular vein distention, fatigue, rales, crackles

Nursing diagnoses

✓ Cardiac output, decreased (uses)
✓ Injury, risk for (adverse reactions)
✓ Knowledge deficit (teaching)
✓ Noncompliance (teaching)

Implementation

- Give PO ac, hs; tablets may be crushed or swallowed whole, give with food to decrease orthostatic hypotension
- Administer reduced dosage in renal dysfunction

Patient/family education

- Tell patient to comply with dosage schedule even if feeling better, that improvement may take several weeks
- Teach patient to rise slowly to sitting or standing position to minimize orthostatic hypotension
- Encourage patient to report bradycardia, dizziness, confusion, depression, fever, weight gain, shortness of breath, cold extremities, rash, sore throat, bleeding, bruising
- Teach patient to take pulse at home; advise when to notify prescriber
- Encourage patient not to discontinue drug abruptly, taper over 1-2 wk
- Advise patient to avoid hazardous activities until stabilized on medication; dizziness may occur
- Advise patient to avoid all OTC medications unless approved by prescriber
- Advise patient to carry Medic Alert ID with drug name, prescriber at all times
- Advise patient to inform all health care providers of drugs taken

Evaluation

Positive therapeutic outcome
- Decreased B/P
- Decreased symptoms of CHF or angina

cascara sagrada/ cascara sagrada aromatic fluid extract/ cascara sagrada fluid extract (OTC)

(kas-kar'a)

Func. class.: Laxative
Chem. class.: Anthraquinone

Pregnancy category C

Action: Direct chemical irritation in colon; increases propulsion of stool; increases fluid in colon

➔ **Therapeutic Outcome:** Decreased constipation; removal of bowel contents before surgery or diagnostic tests

Uses: Constipation; bowel or rectal preparation for surgery or examination

Dosage and routes

Adult: PO 325 mg hs; fluid 1 ml qd; aromatic fluid 5 ml qd

P ***Child 2-12 yr:*** PO/fluid/aromatic fluid ½ adult dose

P ***Child < 2 yr:*** PO/fluid/aromatic fluid ¼ adult dose

Available forms: Tabs 325 mg; fluid extract 1 g/ml; aromatic fluid extract 1 g/ml

Adverse effects

GI: *Nausea, vomiting, anorexia, cramps, diarrhea*
META: Hypocalcemia, enteropathy, alkalosis, hypokalemia, **tetany**

Contraindications: Hypersensitivity, GI bleeding, obstruction, CHF, lactation, abdominal pain, nausea/vomiting, appendicitis, acute surgical abdomen, alcoholics (aromatic fluid extract)

Precautions: Pregnancy **C**

Pharmacokinetics

Absorption	Minimal
Distribution	Unknown
Metabolism	Liver, minimally
Excretion	Kidneys, feces, breast milk
Half-life	Not known

Pharmacodynamics

Onset	Unknown
Peak	6-12 hr
Duration	Unknown

Interactions

Individual drugs

Digitalis: ↓ absorption
Nitrofurantoin: ↓ absorption

Drug classifications

Antibiotics: ↓ absorption
Oral anticoagulants: ↓ absorption
Salicylates: ↓ absorption
Tetracyclines: ↓ absorption

Herb/drug

Lily of the valley: ↑ action, side effects
Pheasant's eye: ↑ action, side effects
Squill: ↑ action, side effects

NURSING CONSIDERATIONS

Assessment

- Monitor blood, urine electrolytes if drug used often by patient; check I&O ratio to identify fluid loss
- Assess cramping, rectal bleeding, nausea, vomiting; if these symptoms occur, drug should be discontinued; identify cause of constipation; identify whether fluids, bulk, or exercise is missing from lifestyle

Nursing diagnoses

- ✓ Bowel elimination, altered: constipation (uses)
- ✓ Bowel elimination, altered: diarrhea (side effects)
- ✓ Knowledge deficit (teaching)
- ✓ Noncompliance (teaching)

Implementation

- Give alone with water only for better absorption; do not administer with food; do not take within 1 hr of antacids, milk, or cimetidine
- Do not crush; swallow tabs whole
- Give in AM or PM (oral dose); evacuation will occur 6-12 hr later

Patient/family education

- Discuss with the patient that adequate fluid consumption is necessary
- Teach patient that normal bowel movements do not always occur daily
- Teach patient not to use in presence of abdominal pain, nausea, vomiting; tell patient to notify prescriber if constipation unrelieved or if symptoms of electrolyte imbalance occur: muscle cramps, pain, weakness, dizziness, excessive thirst

Evaluation

Positive therapeutic outcome

- Decreased constipation in 6-12 hr
- Removal of bowel contents

cefaclor
See cephalosporins—2nd generation
cefadroxil
See cephalosporins—1st generation
cefamandole
See cephalosporins—2nd generation
cefazolin
See cephalosporins—1st generation
cefdinir
See cephalosporins—3rd generation
cefepime
cefixime
See cephalosporins—3rd generation
cefmetazole
cefonicid
See cephalosporins—2nd generation
cefoperazone
cefotaxime
See cephalosporins—3rd generation
cefotetan
cefoxitin
See cephalosporins—2nd generation
cefpodoxime
See cephalosporins—3rd generation
cefprozil
See cephalosporins—2nd generation
ceftazidime
ceftibuten
ceftizoxime
ceftriaxone
See cephalosporins—3rd generation
cefuroxime
See cephalosporins—2nd generation
cephalexin
See cephalosporins—1st generation

cefditoren pivoxil
See Appendix A, Selected New Drugs

celecoxib (℞)

(cel-eh-cox'ib)
Celebrex
Func. class.: Nonsteroidal antiinflammatory
Chem. class.: COX-2 inhibitor
Pregnancy category C

Action: Inhibits prostaglandin synthesis by decreasing enzyme needed for biosynthesis; analgesic, antiinflammatory, antipyretic properties

➔ **Therapeutic Outcome:** Decreased pain, inflammation

Uses: Acute, chronic rheumatoid arthritis, osteoarthritis, familial adenomatous polyposis (FAP)

Investigational uses: Colorectal polyps

Dosage and routes

Osteoarthritis
Adult: PO 200 mg/day as a single dose or 100 mg bid

Rheumatoid arthritis
Adult: PO 100-200 mg bid

FAP
Adult: PO 400 mg bid

Colorectal polyps
Adult: PO 400 mg bid × 6 mo

Available forms: Caps 100, 200 mg

Adverse effects
CNS: *Fatigue, anxiety, depression, nervousness, paresthesia,* dizziness, insomnia
CV: **Tachycardia,** angina, **MI,** palpitations, dysrhythmias, hypertension, fluid retention
EENT: Tinnitus, hearing loss, blurred vision, glaucoma, cataract, conjunctivitis, eye pain
GI: *Nausea, anorexia, vomiting, constipation, dry mouth,* diverticulitis, gastritis, gastroenteritis, hemorrhoids, hiatal hernia, stomatitis, **GI bleeding**

GU: **Nephrotoxicity: dysuria, hematuria, oliguria, azotemia, cystitis, UTI**
HEMA: *Blood dyscrasias,* epistaxis, bruising, anemia
INTEG: Purpura, rash, pruritus, sweating, erythema, petechiae, photosensitivity, alopecia
RESP: Pharyngitis, shortness of breath, pneumonia, coughing

Contraindications: Hypersensitivity to aspirin, iodides, other NSAIDs, sulfonamides, 3rd trimester of pregnancy asthma

Precautions: Pregnancy **C**, renal, hepatic, hypertension, severe dehydration, P children <18 yr, lactation, bleeding, GI, cardiac disorders, hypersensitivity to other antiinflammatories, glucocorticoids, anticoagulants, elderly

Do Not Confuse:
Celebrex/Celexa

Pharmacokinetics	
Absorption	Well absorbed (PO)
Distribution	Crosses placenta, bound to plasma proteins
Metabolism	Liver
Excretion	Kidneys
Half-life	Unknown

Pharmacodynamics	
Onset	Unknown
Peak	3 hr
Duration	Unknown

Interactions
Individual drugs
Aspirin: ↓ effectiveness, ↑ adverse reactions
Fluconazole: ↑ celecoxib level
Furosemide: ↓ effect of furosemide
Lithium: ↑ toxicity
Warfarin: ↑ anticoagulant effects
Drug classifications
ACE inhibitors: may ↓ effects of ACE inhibitors
Anticoagulants: ↑ risk of bleeding
Antineoplastics: ↑ risk of hematologic toxicity
Glucocorticoids: ↑ adverse reactions
NSAIDs: ↑ adverse reactions
Thiazide diuretics: ↓ effectiveness of diuretics

NURSING CONSIDERATIONS
Assessment
- Assess for pain of rheumatoid arthritis, osteoarthritis; check ROM, inflammation of joints, characteristics of pain
- Monitor blood counts during therapy; watch for decreasing platelets; if low, therapy may need to be discontinued, restarted after hematologic recovery; and for blood dyscrasias (thrombocytopenia): bruising, fatigue, bleeding, poor healing
- Assess FAP patient for decreasing number of polyps

Nursing diagnoses
✓ Pain (uses)
✓ Mobility, impaired physical (uses)
✓ Injury, risk for (side effects)
✓ Knowledge deficit (teaching)

Implementation
PO route
- Administer with food or milk to decrease gastric symptoms
- Do not crush, dissolve, or chew caps; do not ↑ dose

Patient/family education
- Teach patient that drug must be continued for prescribed time to be effective; to avoid other NSAIDs, sulfonamides
- Caution patient to report bleeding, bruising, fatigue, malaise, since blood dyscrasias do occur; to report GI symptoms: black tarry stools, cramping
- Teach patient to take with a full glass of water to enhance absorption; do not crush, break, or chew
- Teach patient to check with prescriber to determine when drug should be discontinued before

surgery; advise patient to notify prescriber if pregnancy is planned or suspected

Evaluation

Positive therapeutic outcome

- Decreased pain in arthritic conditions
- Decreased inflammation in arthritic conditions
- Decreased number of polyps (FAP)

CEPHALOSPORINS—1ST GENERATION

cefadroxil (℞)
(sef-a-drox'ill)
cefadroxil, Duricef, Ultracef

cefazolin (℞)
(sef-a'zoe-lin)
Ancef, cefazolin, Kefzol

cephalexin (℞)
(sef-a-lex'in)
Apo-Cephalex*, Cefanex, C-Lexin, cephalexin, Keflex, Keftab, Novo-Lexin*, Nu-Cephalex*

cephalothin (℞)
(sef-a-loe'thin)
cephalothin, Keflin

cephapirin (℞)
(sef-a-pye'rin)
Cefadyl, cephapirin

cephradine (℞)
(sef'ra-deen)
cephradine, Velosef

Func. class.: Antiinfective
Chem. class.: Cephalosporin (1st generation)

Action: Inhibits bacterial cell wall synthesis, rendering cell wall osmotically unstable, leading to cell death by binding to cell wall membrane

cefadroxil

Therapeutic Outcome: Bactericidal effects for the following: gram-negative bacilli *Escherichia coli, Proteus mirabilis, Klebsiella* (UTI only); gram-positive organisms *Streptococcus pneumoniae, Streptococcus pyogenes, Staphylococcus aureus*

Uses: Upper, lower respiratory tract, urinary tract, skin infections; otitis media; tonsillitis, pharyngitis; particularly for UTI

cefazolin

Therapeutic Outcome Bactericidal effects for the following: gram-negative organisms *Enterobacter* sp., *Haemophilus influenzae, Escherichia coli, Proteus mirabilis, Klebsiella;* gram-positive organisms *Streptococcus pneumoniae, Streptococcis pyogenes, Staphylococcus aureus*

Uses: Upper, lower respiratory tract, urinary tract, skin infections; bone, joint, biliary, genital infections; endocarditis, surgical prophylaxis, septicemia

cephalexin

Therapeutic Outcome: Bactericidal effects for the following: gram-negative organisms *Haemophilus influenzae, Escherichia coli, Proteus mirabilis, Klebsiella;* gram-positive organisms *Streptococcus pneumoniae, Streptococcus pyogenes, Staphylococcus aureus*

Uses: Upper, lower respiratory tract, urinary tract, skin, bone infections; otitis media

cephalothin

Therapeutic Outcome: Bactericidal effects for the following: gram-negative bacilli *Haemophilus influenzae, Escherichia coli, Proteus mirabilis, Klebsiella, Salmonella, Shigella;* gram-positive organisms *Streptococcus pneumoniae, Streptococcus pyogenes, Staphylococcus aureus*

Uses: Lower respiratory tract, urinary tract, skin and bone infections;

septicemia, endocarditis; bacterial peritonitis

cephapirin

Therapeutic Outcome: Bactericidal effects for the following: gram-negative bacilli *Haemophilus influenzae, Escherichia coli, Proteus mirabilis, Klebsiella;* gram-positive organisms *Streptococcus pneumoniae, Streptococcus viridans, Staphylococcus aureus*

Uses: Lower respiratory tract, urinary tract, skin infections; septicemia, endocarditis, bacterial peritonitis

cephradine

Therapeutic Outcome: Bactericidal effects for the following: gram-negative bacilli *Haemophilus influenzae, Escherichia coli, Proteus mirabilis, Klebsiella;* gram-positive organisms *Streptococcus pneumoniae, Streptococcus pyogenes, Staphylococcus aureus*

Uses: Serious respiratory tract, urinary tract, skin infections; otitis media

Dosage and routes

cefadroxil

Adult: PO 1-2 g qd or q12h in divided doses, give a loading dose of 1 g initially

P ***Child:*** PO 30 mg/kg/day in divided doses bid

Renal dose: CrCl 25-50 ml/min 1 g, then 500 mg q1/2h; CrCl 10-24 ml/min 500 mg q24h, CrCl <10 ml/min 500 mg q36h

Endocarditis prophylaxis: 2 g 1 hr before procedure

Available forms: Caps 500 mg; tabs 1 g; oral susp 125, 250, 500 mg/5 ml

cefazolin

Life-threatening infections

Adult: IM/**IV** 1-2 g q6h

P ***Child >1 mo:*** IM/**IV** 100 mg/kg in 3-4 divided doses

Mild/moderate infections

Adult: IM/**IV** 250 mg-1 g q8h

P ***Child >1 mo:*** IM/**IV** 25-50 mg/kg in 3-4 equal doses

Renal dose: CrCl 35-54 ml/min 250-1000 mg q12h; CrCl 10-34 ml/min 125-500 mg q12h; CrCl <10 ml/min 125-500 mg q24h

Available forms: Inj 500 mg, 1, 5, 10, 20 g

cephalexin

Renal dose: CrCl <40 ml/min q8-12h; CrCl 5-10 ml/min q12h; CrCl <5 ml/min q24h

Moderate infections

Adult: PO 250-500 mg q6h

P ***Child:*** PO 25-50 mg/kg/day in 4 equal doses

Moderate skin infections

Adult: PO 500 mg q12h

Severe infections

Adult: PO 500 mg-1 g q6h

P ***Child:*** PO 50-100 mg/kg/day in 4 equal doses

Available forms: Caps 250, 500 mg; tabs 250, 500 mg, 1 g; oral susp 125, 250 mg/5 ml

cephalothin

Renal dose: CrCl 26-50 ml/min 1.5 g q6h; CrCl 10-25 ml/min 1 g q6h; CrCl <10 ml/min 500 mg q6h

Moderate infections

Adult: IM/**IV** 500 mg-1 g q4-6h

P ***Child:*** IM/**IV** 14-27 mg/kg q4h or 20-40 mg/kg q6h

Uncomplicated gonorrhea

Adult: IM 2 g as a single dose

Severe infections

Adult: IM/**IV** 1-2 g q4h

P ***Child:*** IM/**IV** 80-160 mg/kg/day in divided doses q4h

Available forms: Powder for inj 1, 2, 20 g

C

cephapirin

Adult: IM/**IV** 500 mg-1 g q4-6h

P ***Child:*** IM/**IV** 40-80 mg/kg/day in divided doses q6h or 10-20 mg/kg q6h

Renal dose: CrCl <10 ml/min give q12h

Available forms: Powder for inj 500 mg, 1, 2, 20 g; **IV** only 1, 2, 4 g

cephradine

Adult: PO 250 mg-1 g q6-12h

P ***Child >1 yr:*** PO 6-12 mg/kg q6h

Renal dose: CrCl >20 ml/min 500 mg q6h; CrCl 5-20 ml/min 250 mg q6h

Available forms: Caps 250, 500 mg; oral susp 125, 250 mg/5 ml

Side effects/adverse reactions

CNS: Headache, dizziness, weakness, paresthesia, fever, chills

GI: Nausea, vomiting, *diarrhea, anorexia,* pain, glossitis, bleeding; increased AST, ALT, bilirubin, LDH, alkaline phosphatase; abdominal pain, **pseudomembranous colitis**

GU: Proteinuria, vaginitis, pruritus, candidiasis, increased BUN, **nephrotoxicity, renal failure**

HEMA: **Leukopenia, thrombocytopenia, agranulocytosis,** anemia, **neutropenia, lymphocytosis, eosinophilia, pancytopenia, hemolytic anemia**

INTEG: Rash, urticaria, dermatitis, **anaphylaxis**

RESP: Dyspnea

Contraindications: Hypersensitivity to cephalosporins, P infants <1 mo

Precautions: Hypersensitivity to penicillins, pregnancy **B,** lactation, renal disease

Do Not Confuse: cephalexin/cefaclor, cephapirin/cephradine, Kefzol/Cefzil

cefadroxil

Pharmacokinetics

Absorption	Well absorbed
Distribution	Widely distributed; crosses placenta
Metabolism	Not metabolized
Excretion	Unchanged by kidneys; enters breast milk
Half-life	1½-2 hr

Pharmacodynamics

	PO
Onset	Rapid
Peak	1½-2 hr
Duration	12-24 hr

cefazolin

Pharmacokinetics

Absorption	Well absorbed
Distribution	Widely distributed; crosses placenta
Metabolism	Not metabolized
Excretion	Unchanged by kidneys; enters breast milk
Half-life	1½-2½ hr

Pharmacodynamics

	IM	IV
Onset	Rapid	10 min
Peak	1-2 hr	Infusion's end
Duration	6-12 hr	

cephalexin

Pharmacokinetics

Absorption	Well absorbed
Distribution	Widely distributed; crosses placenta
Metabolism	Not metabolized
Excretion	Kidneys, unchanged; enters breast milk
Half-life	½-1 hr; increased in renal disease

Pharmacodynamics

Onset	15-30 min
Peak	1 hr
Duration	6-12 hr

cephalothin

Pharmacokinetics

Absorption	Well absorbed
Distribution	Widely distributed; crosses placenta
Metabolism	Not metabolized
Excretion	Kidneys, unchanged; enters breast milk
Half-life	½-1 hr

Pharmacodynamics

	IM	IV
Onset	Rapid	Immediate
Peak	½ hr	Infusion's end
Duration	Unknown	

cephapirin

Pharmacokinetics

Absorption	Well absorbed
Distribution	Widely distributed; crosses placenta
Metabolism	Not metabolized
Excretion	Kidneys, unchanged; enters breast milk
Half-life	½-1 hr

Pharmacodynamics

	IM	IV
Onset	Rapid	Immediate
Peak	½ hr	Infusion's end
Duration	4-6 hr	

cephradine

Pharmacokinetics

Absorption	Well absorbed
Distribution	Widely distributed; crosses placenta
Metabolism	Not metabolized
Excretion	Kidneys, unchanged; enters breast milk
Half-life	1-2 hr

Pharmacodynamics

	PO/IM	IV
Onset	Rapid	Immediate
Peak	1 hr	Infusion's end
Duration	6-12 hr	

Interactions

Individual drugs

Probenecid: ↓ excretion of drug and ↑ blood levels
Vancomycin: ↑ toxicity

Drug classifications

Aminoglycosides: ↑ toxicity
Diuretics, loop: ↑ toxicity
Oral contraceptives: ↑ toxicity

Lab test interferences

False: ↑ Creatinine (serum urine), ↑ urinary 17-KS
False positive: Urinary protein, direct Coombs' test, urine glucose
Interference: Cross-matching

NURSING CONSIDERATIONS

Assessment

- Assess patient for previous sensitivity reaction to penicillins or other cephalosporins; cross-sensitivity between penicillins and cephalosporins is common
- Assess patient for signs and symptoms of infection including characteristics of wounds, sputum, urine, stool, WBC >10,000/mm^3, earache, fever; obtain baseline information and during treatment
- Obtain C&S before beginning drug therapy to identify if correct treatment has been initiated
- Assess for anaphylaxis: rash, urticaria, pruritus, chills, fever, joint pain; angioedema may occur a few days after therapy begins; epinephrine and resuscitation equipment should be available for anaphylactic reaction
- Identify urine output; if decreasing, notify prescriber (may indicate nephrotoxicity); also check for increased BUN, creatinine
- Monitor blood studies: AST, ALT, CBC, Hct, bilirubin, LDH, alkaline phosphatase, Coombs' test monthly if patient is on long-term therapy
- Monitor electrolytes: potassium, sodium, chloride monthly if patient is on long-term therapy
- Assess bowel pattern qd; if severe diarrhea occurs, drug should be

discontinued; may indicate pseudomembranous colitis
- Monitor for bleeding: ecchymosis, bleeding gums, hematuria, stool guaiac daily if on long-term therapy
- Assess for superinfection: perineal itching, fever, malaise, redness, pain, swelling, drainage, rash, diarrhea, change in cough, sputum

Nursing diagnoses

- ✓ Infection, risk for (uses)
- ✓ Diarrhea (side effects)
- ✓ Fluid volume deficit, risk for (side effects)
- ✓ Injury, risk for (side effects)
- ✓ Knowledge deficit (teaching)
- ✓ Noncompliance (teaching)

cefadroxil

Implementation

- Give in even doses around the clock; if GI upset occurs, give with food; drug must be given for 10-14 days to ensure organism death and prevent superinfection
- Shake susp, refrigerate, discard after 2 wk

cefazolin

Implementation

IM route

- Reconstitute 250-500 mg of drug with 2 ml sterile or bacteriostatic water for inj, or 0.9% NaCl; reconstitute 1 g of drug with 2.5 ml; give deep in large muscle mass, massage

IV route

- Check for irritation, extravasation, phlebitis daily, change site q72h
- For direct **IV** dilute in 10 ml of sterile water for inj; give over 5 min
- For intermittent inf dilute reconstituted sol (500 mg or 1 mg) in 50-100 ml D_5W, $D_{10}W$, D_5/0.25% NaCl, D_5/0.45% NaCl, D_5/0.9% NaCl, D_5/LR, or LR, 0.9% NaCl; give over 30-60 min; may be refrigerated up to 96 hr or stored 24 hr at room temp

Syringe compatibilities:
Heparin, vit B complex

Syringe incompatibilities:
Ascorbic acid injection, cimetidine, lidocaine, vit B/C

Y-site compatibilities:
Acyclovir, allopurinol, amifostine, atracurium, aztreonam, calcium gluconate, cyclophosphamide, diltiazem, enalaprilat, esmolol, famotidine, filgrastim, fluconazole, fludarabine, foscarnet, heparin, labetalol, lidocaine, magnesium sulfate, melphalan, meperidine, midazolam, morphine, multivitamins, ondansetron, perphenazine, pancuronium, regular insulin, sargramostim, tacrolimus, teniposide, theophylline, thiotepa, vecuronium, vit B/C

Y-site incompatibilities:
Amiodarone, hetastarch, hydromorphone, idarubicin, vinorelbine tartrate

Additive compatibilities:
Aztreonam, clindamycin, famotidine, fluconazole, metronidazole, verapamil

Additive incompatibilities:
Amikacin, amobarbital, bleomycin, calcium gluceptate, calcium gluconate, colistimethate, erythromycin, kanamycin, oxytetracycline, pentobarbital, polymyxin B, tetracycline

cephalexin

Implementation

- Advise not to crush or chew caps
- Give in even doses around the clock; if GI upset occurs, give with food; drug must be taken for 10-14 days to ensure organism death and prevent superinfection
- Shake susp, refrigerate, discard after 2 wk

cephalothin

Implementation

IM route

- Reconstitute 1 g/4 ml sterile water for inj; give deep in large muscle mass and massage
- IM route not preferred; causes intense pain and induration

IV route

- Check for irritation, extravasation,

phlebitis daily; change site q72h

- For direct **IV** dilute in 1 g/10 ml or more sterile water for inj, D_5W, 0.9% NaCl; give over 3-5 min
- For intermittent inf, reconstitute 1-2 mg/50 ml sterile water for inj, D_5W, $D_{10}W$, D_5/LR, D_5/0.9% NaCl; 0.9% NaCl; may be further diluted in 50-100 ml D_5W, $D_{10}W$, 0.9% NaCl, or LR; give over 15-30 min
- For cont inf may be diluted in 500-1000 ml and run at prescribed rate; may use hydrocortisone 10-25 mg added to inf containing 4-6 g or more of cephalothin to decrease the incidence of thrombophlebitis
- Store refrigerated 96 hr, room temp 24 hr

Syringe compatibilities:
Cimetidine

Syringe incompatibilities:
Metoclopramide

Y-site compatibilities:
Cyclophosphamide, famotidine, heparin, hydromorphone, magnesium sulfate, meperidine, morphine, multivitamins, perphenazine, potassium chloride, vit B/C

Y-site incompatibilities:
Hetastarch

Additive compatibilities:
Ascorbic acid, chloramphenicol, clindamycin, fluorouracil, hydrocortisone, isoproterenol, magnesium sulfate, metaraminol, methicillin, methotrexate, potassium chloride, prednisolone, procaine, sodium bicarbonate, vit B/C

Additive incompatibilities:
Aminoglycosides, amikacin, aminophylline, amobarbital, bleomycin, calcium chloride, calcium gluceptate, calcium gluconate, colistimethate, diphenhydramine, doxorubicin, erythromycin, gentamicin, kanamycin, oxytetracycline, pentobarbital, penicillin G sodium, phenobarbital, polymyxin B, prochlorperazine, tetracycline

cephapirin
Implementation

IM route

- Reconstitute 1-2 g/1-2 ml of sterile water for inj; give deep in large muscle mass and massage

IV **IV route**

- Check for irritation, extravasation, phlebitis daily; change site q72h
- For intermittent inf, reconstitute 250 mg/2.4 ml, 500 mg/4.8 ml, 1 g/9.6 ml, 2 gm/19.2 ml sterile water for inj, D_5W, 0.9% NaCl; do not use sol P with benzyl alcohol for neonates; may be further diluted in 50-100 ml D_5W, $D_{10}W$, 0.9% NaCl, or LR; give over 30-60 min
- Store refrigerated 96 hr, room temp 24 hr

Y-site compatibilities:
Acyclovir, cyclophosphamide, famotidine, heparin, hydrocortisone, hydromorphone, magnesium sulfate, meperidine, morphine, multivitamins, perphenazine, potassium chloride, vit B/C

Additive compatibilities:
Bleomycin, calcium chloride, calcium gluconate, chloramphenicol, diphenhydramine, ergonovine maleate, heparin, hydrocortisone, metaraminol, oxacillin, penicillin G potassium, pentobarbital, phenobarbital, phytonadione, potassium chloride, sodium bicarbonate, succinylcholine, verapamil, warfarin, vit B complex

Additive incompatibilities:
Aminoglycosides, amikacin, ascorbic acid, epinephrine, gentamicin, kanamycin, mannitol, norepinephrine, oxytetracycline, phenytoin, tetracycline, thiopental

cephradine
Implementation

PO route

- May be given with food for GI symptoms
- When giving susp, shake well; refrigerate unused portion

IM route

- Reconstitute 250 mg/1.2 ml, 500 mg/ml, 1 g/4 ml sterile or bacteriostatic water for inj; give deep in large muscle mass, massage

IV **IV route**

- Check for irritation, extravasation, phlebitis daily; change site q72h
- For direct **IV** route, reconstitute 250-500 mg/5 ml sterile water, 0.9% NaCl, D_5W, or 1 g/10 ml, 2 g/20 ml; give over 3-5 min
- For intermittent inf, dilute 1 g/10 ml or more sterile water for inj, D_5W, $D_{10}W$, or D_5/0.9% NaCl; give over 30-60 min
- Store refrigerated 96 hr, room temp 24 hr

Additive incompatibilities:
Other antibiotics, calcium salts, D_5W, epinephrine, lidocaine, Ringer's or LR sol, NormosolR, 0.9% NaCl, TPN #61, tetracycline

Patient/family education

- Teach patient to report sore throat, bruising, bleeding, joint pain; may indicate blood dyscrasias (rare)
- Advise patient to contact prescriber if vaginal itching, loose, foul-smelling stools, furry tongue occur; may indicate superinfection
- Instruct patient to take all medication prescribed for the length of time ordered
- Advise patient to notify prescriber of diarrhea with blood or pus, which may indicate pseudomembranous colitis

Evaluation

Positive therapeutic outcome

- Absence of signs/symptoms of infection (WBC <10,000/mm^3, temp WNL, absence of red draining wounds, earache)
- Reported improvement in symptoms of infection
- Negative C&S

Treatment of anaphylaxis:
Epinephrine, antihistamines, resuscitate if needed

CEPHALOSPORINS—2ND GENERATION

cefaclor (℞)
(sef'a-klor)
Ceclor

cefamandole (℞)
(sef-a-man'dole)
Mandol

cefmetazole (℞)
(sef-met'a-zole)
Zefazone

cefonicid (℞)
(se-fon'i-sid)
Monocid

cefotetan (℞)
(sef'oh-tee-tan)
Cefotan

cefoxitin (℞)
(se-fox'i-tin)
Mefoxin

cefprozil (℞)
(sef-proe'zill)
Cefzil

loracarbef (℞)
(lor-a-kar'beff)
Lorabid

Func. class.: Antiinfective
Chem. class.: Cephalosporin (2nd generation)

Action: Inhibits bacterial cell wall synthesis, rendering cell wall osmotically unstable, leading to cell death by binding to cell wall membrane

cefaclor

Therapeutic Outcome: Bactericidal effects for the following: gram-negative bacilli *Haemophilus influenzae, Escherichia coli, Proteus mirabilis, Klebsiella;* gram-positive organisms *Streptococcus pneumoniae, Staphylococcus* β-hemolytic; streptococci, anaerobes, bacteroides sp.

Uses: Upper and lower respiratory tract, urinary tract, skin infections;

C

otitis media; increased bone, joint, gynecologic infections; septicemia

cefamandole

Therapeutic Outcome: Bactericidal effects for the following: anaerobes *Bacteroides* sp., *Clostridium* sp., *Fusobacterium* sp., *Peptococcus* sp., *Peptostreptococcus* sp.; gram negative organisms *Haemophilus influenzae, Escherichia coli, Proteus mirabilis, Klebsiella;* gram-positive organisms *Streptococcus pneumoniae, Streptococcus pyogenes, Staphylococcus aureus; Enterobacter* sp., *Morganella morganii, Proteus vulgaris, Providencia rettgeri*

Uses: Upper, lower respiratory tract, urinary tract, skin infections; peritonitis, septicemia, surgical prophylaxis

cefmetazole

Therapeutic Outcome: Bactericidal effects for the following: anaerobes, *Clostridium, Bacteroides* sp., *Fusobacterium* sp.; gram-negative organisms *Morganella morganii, Haemophilus influenzae, Escherichia coli, Proteus, Klebsiella, Bacteroides fragilis;* gram-positive organisms *Streptococcus pneumoniae, Streptococcus pyogenes, Staphylococcus aureus*

Uses: Infections of lower respiratory tract, urinary tract, skin, bone; intraabdominal infections

cefonicid

Therapeutic Outcome: Bactericidal effects for the following: gram-negative organisms *Morganella morganii, Proteus vulgaris, Providencia rettgeri, Haemophilus influenzae, Escherichia coli, Proteus mirabilis, Klebsiella;* gram-positive organisms *Streptococcus pneumoniae, Streptococcus pyogenes, Staphylococcus aureus*

Uses: Lower respiratory tract, urinary tract, skin, bone, joint infections; otitis media, peritonitis, septicemia, preoperative prophylaxis

cefotetan

Therapeutic Outcome: Bactericidal effects for the following: gram-negative organisms *Haemophilus influenzae, Escherichia coli, Enterobacter aerogenes, Proteus mirabilis, Klebsiella, Morganella morganii, Proteus vulgaris, Providencia, Enterobacter, Salmonella, Shigella, Acinetobacter, Bacteroides fragilis, Neisseria, Serratia;* gram-positive organisms *Streptococcus pneumoniae, Streptococcus pyogenes, Staphylococcus aureus;* anaerobes *Bacteroides, Clostridium, Fusobacterium, Peptococcus, Peptostreptococcus*

Uses: Serious upper or lower respiratory tract, urinary tract, gynecologic, skin, bone, joint, gonococcal, intraabdominal infections

cefoxitin

Therapeutic Outcome: Bactericidal effects for the following: gram-negative bacilli *Haemophilus influenzae, Escherichia coli, Proteus, Klebsiella, Providencia, Neisseria gonorrhoeae;* gram-positive organisms *Streptococcus pneumoniae, Streptococcus pyogenes, Staphylococcus aureus;* anaerobes including *Clostridium, Bacteroides, Peptococcus, Peptostreptococcus*

Uses: Lower respiratory tract, urinary tract, skin, bone, gynecologic, gonococcal infections; septicemia, peritonitis

cefprozil

Therapeutic Outcome: Bactericidal effects for the following: gram-negative bacilli *Haemophilus influenzae, Escherichia coli;* gram-positive organisms *Streptococcus pneumoniae, Streptococcus pyogenes, Staphylococcus aureus*

Uses: Upper and lower respiratory

tract, urinary tract, skin infections; otitis media

loracarbef

Therapeutic Outcome: Bactericidal effects for the following: gram-negative organisms *Haemophilus influenzae, Escherichia coli, Proteus mirabilis, Klebsiella;* gram-positive organisms *Streptococcus pneumoniae, Streptococcus pyogenes, Staphyloccus aureus*

Uses: Upper and lower respiratory tract, urinary tract, skin infections; otitis media, pharyngitis, tonsillitis

Dosage and routes

cefaclor

Adult: PO 250-500 mg q8h, not to exceed 4 g/day or 375-500 mg (ext rel) q12h × 7-10 days

P ***Child <1 mo:*** PO 20-40 mg/kg qd in divided doses q8h, or total daily dose may be divided and given q12h, not to exceed 1 g/day

Acute bacterial exacerbations of chronic bronchitis or acute bronchitis

Adult: 500 mg/12 hr × 1 wk (ext rel)

Pharyngitis/tonsillitis

Adult: 375 mg/12 hr × 10 days (ext rel)

Available forms: Caps 250, 500 mg; oral susp 125, 187, 250, 375 mg/5 ml; tabs, ext rel 375, 500 mg

cefamandole

Adult: IM/**IV** 500 mg-1 g q4-8h; may give up to 2 g q4h for severe infections

P ***Child >1 mo:*** IM/**IV** 8.3-16.7 mg/kg q4h, not to exceed adult dose

Renal dose: Dosage reduction indicated in renal impairment (CrCl <50 ml/min)

Available forms: Inj 1, 2, 10 g

cefmetazole

Adult: **IV** 2 g divided q6-12h × 5-14 days

Renal dose: CrCl <50 ml/min 1-2 g q12h; CrCl 10-29 ml/min 1-2 g q48h

Available forms: Powder for inj 1, 2 g/vial

cefonicid

Life-threatening infections

Adult: IM/**IV** bol or inf 0.5-2 g/24 hr; divide in two doses if giving 2 g

• Dosage reduction indicated in renal impairment

Available forms: Inj 500 mg, 1, 10 g

cefotetan

Adult: **IV**/IM 1-2 g q12h × 5-10 days

Renal dose: CrCl 10-30 ml/min q24h; CrCl <10 ml/min q48h

Perioperative proplylaxis

Adult: **IV** 1-2 g ½-1 hr before surgery

Available forms: Inj 1, 2, 10 g

cefoxitin

Adult: IM/**IV** 1-2 g q6-8h

Renal dose: CrCl <50 ml/min q8-12h; CrCl 10-29 ml/min q24h; CrCl <10 ml/min q24-48h

• Dosage reduction indicated in renal impairment (CrCl <50 ml/min)

• Uncomplicated gonorrhea 2 g IM as single dose with 1 g PO probenecid at same time

Severe infections

Adult: IM/**IV** 2 g q4h

P ***Child ≥3 mo:*** IM/**IV** 80-160 mg/kg/day divided q4-6h; max 12 g/day

Available forms: Powder for inj 1, 2, 10 g

cefprozil

Renal dose: CrCl <30 ml/min 50% of dose

Upper respiratory infections
Adult: PO 250-500 mg q24h × 10 days

Otitis media
P ***Child 6 mo-12 yr:*** PO 15 mg/kg q12h × 10 days

Lower respiratory infections
Adult: PO 500 mg q12h × 10 days

Skin/skin structure infections
Adult: PO 250-500 mg q12h × 10 days

Available forms: Tabs 250, 500 mg; susp 125, 250 mg/5 ml

loracarbef
P ***Adult and child >13 yr:*** PO 200-400 mg q12h

P ***Child to 12 yr:*** PO 15-30 mg/kg/day in 2 divided doses q12h

Renal dose: CrCl 10-49 ml/min 50% of dose; CrCl <10 ml/min q3-5 days

Available forms: Tabs 125, 500 mg; inj 150, 750 mg, 1.5, 7.5 g; inj 750 mg; 1.5 g powder; susp 125, 250 mg/5 ml

Side effects/adverse reactions:
CNS: Dizziness, headache, fatigue, paresthesia, fever, chills, confusion
GI: *Diarrhea,* nausea, vomiting, anorexia, dysgeusia, glossitis, bleeding; increased AST, ALT, bilirubin, LDH, alkaline phosphatase; abdominal pain, loose stools, flatulence, heartburn, stomach cramps, colitis, jaundice
GU: Vaginitis, pruritus, candidiasis, increased BUN, **nephrotoxicity, renal failure,** pyuria, dysuria, reversible interstitial nephritis
HEMA: **Leukopenia, thrombocytopenia, agranulocytosis,** anemia, **neutropenia, lymphocytosis, eosinophilia, pancytopenia, hemolytic anemia, leukocytosis, granulocytopenia**
INTEG: Rash, urticaria, dermatitis, **Stevens-Johnson syndrome**
RESP: Dyspnea
SYST: **Anaphylaxis, serum sickness**

Contraindications Hypersensitivity to cephalosporins or related antibiotics, seizures

Precautions: Pregnancy **B,** lactation, P children, renal disease

Do Not Confuse:
cefaclor/cephalexin, Cefotan/Ceftin, cefprozil/Cafazolin, cefprozil/cefuroxime, Cefzil/Ceftin, Cefzil/Kefzol

cefaclor

Pharmacokinetics	
Absorption	Well absorbed
Distribution	Widely distributed; crosses placenta
Metabolism	Not metabolized
Excretion	Unchanged by kidneys (60%-80%); enters breast milk
Half-life	36-54 min; increased in renal disease

Pharmacodynamics	
Onset	15 min
Peak	½-1 hr

cefamandole

Pharmacokinetics	
Absorption	Well absorbed
Distribution	Widely distributed; crosses placenta
Metabolism	Not metabolized
Excretion	Unchanged by kidneys (60%-80%); enters breast milk
Half-life	½ to 1½ hr

Pharmacodynamics	IM	IV
Onset	Rapid	Immediate
Peak	½-2 hr	Infusion's end

C

cefmetazole

Pharmacokinetics

Absorption	Complete
Distribution	Widely distributed; crosses placenta
Metabolism	Not metabolized
Excretion	Kidneys, unchanged (85%); enters breast milk
Half-life	½-2 hr; increased in renal disease

Pharmacodynamics

Onset	Rapid
Peak	Infusion's end

cefonicid

Pharmacokinetics

Absorption	Well absorbed (IM)
Distribution	Widely distributed; crosses placenta
Metabolism	Not metabolized
Excretion	Kidneys, unchanged; enters breast milk
Half-life	4½ hr; increased in renal disease

Pharmacodynamics

	IM	IV
Onset	Rapid	5 min
Peak	1 hr	Infusion's end

cefotetan

Pharmacokinetics

Absorption	Well absorbed (IM)
Distribution	Widely distributed; crosses placenta
Metabolism	Not metabolized
Excretion	Kidneys, unchanged; enters breast milk
Half-life	5 hr; increased in renal disease

Pharmacodynamics

	IM	IV
Onset	Rapid	Immediate
Peak	1-3 hr	Infusion's end

cefoxitin

Pharmacokinetics

Absorption	Well absorbed (IM)
Distribution	Widely distributed; crosses placenta
Metabolism	Not metabolized
Excretion	Kidneys, unchanged; enters breast milk
Half-life	½-1 hr; increased in renal disease

Pharmacodynamics

	IM	IV
Onset	Rapid	Immediate
Peak	½ hr	Infusion's end

cefprozil

Pharmacokinetics

Absorption	Well absorbed (PO)
Distribution	Widely distributed; crosses placenta
Metabolism	Not metabolized
Excretion	Kidneys, unchanged; enters breast milk
Half-life	1-1½ hr; increased in renal disease

Pharmacodynamics

	PO
Onset	Unknown
Peak	Unknown

loracarbef

Pharmacokinetics

Absorption	Well absorbed
Distribution	Widely distributed; crosses placenta
Metabolism	Not metabolized
Excretion	Kidneys, unchanged; enters breast milk
Half-life	1 hr; increased in renal disease

Pharmacodynamics

Onset	Rapid
Peak	1 hr

Interactions

Individual drugs

Alcohol: Disulfiram reaction if ingested within 48-72 hr of cephalosporin
Plicamycin: ↑ bleeding
Probenecid: ↓ excretion of drug and ↑ blood levels
Sulfinpyrazone: ↑ toxicity
Valproic acid: ↑ bleeding
Vancomycin: ↑ toxicity

Drug classifications

Aminoglycosides: ↑ toxicity
Anticoagulants: ↑ bleeding
Thrombolytics: ↑ bleeding

Lab test interferences

False ↑ Creatinine (serum urine), false ↑ urinary 17-KS
False positive: Urinary protein, direct Coombs' test, urine glucose
Interference: Cross-matching

NURSING CONSIDERATIONS

Assessment

- Assess patient for previous sensitivity reaction to penicillins or other cephalosporins; cross-sensitivity between penicillins and cephalosporins is common
- Assess patient for signs and symptoms of infection including characteristics of wounds, sputum, urine, stool, WBC >10,000/mm^3, earache, fever; obtain baseline information and during treatment
- Obtain C&S before beginning drug therapy to identify if correct treatment has been initiated
- Assess for anaphylaxis: rash, urticaria, pruritus, dyspnea, chills, fever, joint pain; angioedema may occur a few days after therapy begins; epinephrine and resuscitation equipment should be available for anaphylactic reaction
- Identify urine output; if decreasing, notify prescriber (may indicate nephrotoxicity); also check for increased BUN, creatinine
- Monitor blood studies: AST, ALT, CBC, Hct, bilirubin, LDH, alkaline phosphatase, Coombs' test monthly if patient is on long-term therapy
- Monitor electrolytes: potassium, sodium, chloride monthly if patient is on long-term therapy
- Assess bowel pattern qd; if severe diarrhea occurs, drug should be discontinued; may indicate pseudomembranous colitis
- Monitor for bleeding: ecchymosis, bleeding gums, hematuria, stool guaiac daily if on long-term therapy
- Assess for overgrowth of infection: perineal itching, fever, malaise, redness, pain, swelling, drainage, rash, diarrhea, change in cough, sputum

Nursing diagnoses

✓ Infection, risk for (uses)
✓ Diarrhea (side effects)
✓ Fluid volume deficit, risk for (side effects)
✓ Injury, risk for (side effects)
✓ Knowledge deficit (teaching)
✓ Noncompliance (teaching)

Implementation

cefaclor

- Give in even doses around the clock; if GI upset occurs, give with food; drug must be given for 10-14 days to ensure organism death and prevent superinfection
- Shake susp, refrigerate, discard after 2 wk
- ⊘ Do not crush, cut, or chew ext rel tabs

cefamandole

IM route

- Reconstitute with 3 ml of sterile or bacteriostatic water for inj, 0.9% NaCl, or 0.5%-2.0% lidocaine HCl; give deep in large muscle mass, massage; check for redness, abscess at inj site

IV **IV route**

- Check for irritation, extravasation, phlebitis daily; change site q72h
- Direct **IV**: Dilute each g of drug with 10 ml of D_5W, 0.9% NaCl, or sterile water for inj; give over 5 min
- For intermittent inf further dilute with 100 ml of D_5W, $D_{10}W$, $D_5/0.25\%$

NaCl, D_5/0.45% NaCl, D^5/0.9% NaCl, D_5 LR, 0.9% NaCl; give over 15-30 min; may be refrigerated up to 96 hr or 24 hr at room temp

- For cont inf dilute with 500-1000 ml of above solutions; give over prescribed rate

Syringe compatibilities:
Heparin

Syringe incompatibilities:
Cimetidine, gentamicin, tobramycin

Y-site compatibilities:
Acyclovir, cyclophosphamide, hydromorphone, magnesium sulfate, meperidine, morphine, perphenazine

Y-site incompatibilities:
Amiodarone, hetastarch

Additive compatibilities:
Clindamycin, floxacillin, furosemide, metronidazole, or verapamil

Additive incompatibilities:
Aminoglycosides, calcium gluceptate, calcium gluconate, cimetidine, gentamicin

cefmetazole

- Check for irritation, extravasation, phlebitis daily; change site q72h
- For intermittent inf, reconstitute with sterile, bacteriostatic water for inj or 0.9% NaCl; may be further diluted with 0.9% NaCl, LR, D_5W (1-20 mg/ml); give over 30-60 min; may be refrigerated for 1 wk or stored 24 hr at room temp

Additive compatibilities:
Famotidine, clindamycin, KCl

cefonicid

IM route

- Reconstitute 500 mg/2 ml of sterile water for inj (220 mg/ml) or 1000 mg/2.5 ml (325 mg/ml)
- Give deep in large muscle mass, massage

IV **IV route**

- Check for irritation, extravasation, phlebitis daily; change site q72h
- For direct **IV** give over 5 min
- For intermittent inf reconstituted sol should be further diluted in 50-100 ml of D_5W, $D_{10}W$, D_5/LR, D_5/0.25% NaCl, D_5/0.45% NaCl, D_5/0.9% NaCl, 0.9% NaCl; or Ringer's, LR; give over 30 min; may be refrigerated up to 96 hr or stored 24 hr at room temp

C

Y-site compatibilities:
Acyclovir, amifostine, aztreonam, teniposide, thiotepa

Y-site incompatibilities:
Hetastarch, sargramostim

Additive compatibilities:
Clindamycin

Additive incompatibilities:
Aminoglycosides

cefotetan

IM route

- Reconstitute 1 g/2 ml or 2 g/3 ml of sterile or bacteriostatic water for inj; may be diluted with 0.5% of 1% lidocaine to prevent pain; give deep in large muscle mass, massage

IV **IV route**

- May be stored 96 hr refrigerated or 24 hr room temp
- Check for irritation, extravasation, phlebitis daily; change site q72h
- For direct **IV** dilute in 1 g/10 ml or more and give over 5 min
- For intermittent inf further dilute in 50-100 ml of 0.9% NaCl or D_5W; give over 3-5 min; discontinue primary line while running intermittent inf

Syringe incompatibilities:
Doxapram

Y-site compatibilities:
Allopurinol, amifostine, aztreonam, diltiazem, famotidine, filgrastim, fluconazole, fludarabine, heparin, regular insulin, melphalan, meperidine, morphine, paclitaxel, sargramostim, tacrolimus, teniposide, theophylline, thiotepa

Additive incompatibilities:
Aminoglycosides, tetracyclines, heparin

cefoxitin

IM route

- Reconstitute 1 g/2 ml of sterile water for inj; may be diluted with 0.5% or 1% lidocaine to prevent pain; give deep in large muscle mass, massage

IV **IV route**

- Check for irritation, extravasation, phlebitis daily; change site q72h
- For direct **IV**, dilute 1 g/10 ml or 2 g/20 ml of sterile water for inj; shake, let stand until clear; give over 3-5 min
- For intermittent inf further dilute with 50-100 ml of D_5W, $D_{10}W$, D_5/0.25% NaCl, D_5/0.45% NaCl, D_5/0.9% NaCl, 0.9% NaCl D_5/LR, D_5/0.02%, sodium bicarbonate, Ringer's, or LR; give over 15-30 min; may store 96 hr refrigerated or 24 hr room temp
- For cont inf dilute in 500-1000 ml; give over prescribed rate

Syringe compatibilities:
Heparin, insulin

Y-site compatibilities:
Acyclovir, amifostine, aztreonam, cyclophosphamide, diltiazem, famotidine, fluconazole, foscarnet, hydromorphone, magnesium sulfate, meperidine, morphine, ondansetron, perphenazine, temiposide, thiotepa

Y-site incompatibilities:
Hetastarch

Additive compatibilities:
Amikacin, cimetidine, clindamycin, gentamicin, kanamycin, multivitamins, sodium bicarbonate, tobramycin, verapamil, vit B/C

Additive incompatibilities:
Aztreonam

cefprozil

IM route

- Reconstitute with 1 g/2 ml or 2 g/3 ml of sterile or bacteriostatic water for inj; may be diluted with 0.5% or 1% lidocaine to prevent pain; give deep in large muscle mass, massage

IV **IV route**

- Check for irritation, extravasation, phlebitis daily; change site q72h
- For direct **IV**, dilute 1 g/10 ml or more and give over 5 min
- For intermittent inf further dilute with 50-100 ml of 0.9% NaCl or D_5W; give over 3-5 min; discontinue primary line while running intermittent infusion

Syringe incompatibilities:
Doxapram

Y-site compatibilities:
Famotidine, fluconazole, fludarabine, regular insulin, meperidine, morphine, sargramostim

Additive incompatibilities:
Aminoglycosides, tetracyclines, heparin

loracarbef

- Give on an empty stomach, 1 hr ac or 2 hr pc
- Do not crush, chew caps
- Oral susp should be shaken before administration; store for 2 wk at room temp, discard after 2 wk

Patient/family education

- Teach patient to report sore throat, bruising, bleeding, joint pain; may indicate blood dyscrasias (rare)
- Advise patient to contact prescriber if vaginal itching, loose, foul-smelling stools, furry tongue occur; may indicate superinfection
- Instruct patient to take all medication prescribed for the length of time ordered
- Advise patient to notify prescriber of diarrhea with blood or pus, which may indicate pseudomembranous colitis

Evaluation

Positive therapeutic outcome

- Absence of signs/symptoms of infection (WBC <10,000/mm^3, temp WNL, absence of red draining wounds, earache)
- Reported improvement in symptoms of infection
- Negative C&S

Treatment of anaphylaxis:
Epinephrine, antihistamines, resuscitate if needed

C

CEPHALOSPORINS—3RD GENERATION

cefdinir (℞)
(sef'dih-ner)
Omnicef
cefepime (℞)
(sef'e-peem)
Maxipime
cefixime (℞)
(sef-icks'ime)
Suprax
cefoperazone (℞)
(sef-oh-per'a-zone)
Cefobid
cefotaxime (℞)
(sef-oh-taks'eem)
Claforan
cefpodoxime (℞)
(sef-poe-docks'eem)
Vantin
ceftazidime (℞)
(sef'tay-zi-deem)
Ceptaz, Fortaz, Magnacef ✦, Pentacef, Tazicef, Tazidime
ceftibuten (℞)
(sef-ti-byoo'tin)
Cedax
ceftizoxime (℞)
(sef-ti-zox'eem)
Cefizox
ceftriaxone (℞)
(sef-try-ax'one)
Rocephin
moxalactam (℞)
(mox'a-lak-tam)
Moxam
Func. class.: Broad-spectrum antibiotic
Chem. class.: Cephalosporin (3rd generation)

Action: Inhibits bacterial cell wall synthesis, rendering cell wall osmotically unstable, leading to cell death

cefdinir

Therapeutic Outcome: Bactericidal effects for the following: gram-negative organisms *Haemophilus influenzae,* gram-positive organisms *Streptococcus pneumoniae, Streptococcus pyogenes, Staphylococcus aureus*

Uses: Uncomplicated skin and skin structure infections, community-acquired pneumonia, acute exacerbations of chronic bronchitis, acute maxillary sinusitis, pharyngitis, tonsillitis

cefepime

Therapeutic Outcome: Bactericidal effects for the following: gram-negative bacilli, *Escherichia coli, Proteus, Klebsiella;* gram-positive organisms *Streptococcus pneumoniae, Streptococcus pyogenes, Staphylococcus aureus*

Uses: Lower respiratory tract, urinary tract, skin, bone, gonococcal infections; septicemia, peritonitis

cefixime

Therapeutic Outcome: Bactericidal effects for the following: *Escherichia coli, Proteus mirabilis, Streptococcus pyogenes, Streptococcus pneumoniae, Haemophilus influenzae, Moraxella catarrhalis*

Uses: Uncomplicated UTI, pharyngitis and tonsillitis, otitis media, acute bronchitis, and acute/exacerbations of chronic bronchitis

cefoperazone

Therapeutic Outcome: Bactericidal effects for the following: gram-negative organisms *Acinetobacter, Morganella morganii, Neisseria gonorrhea, Proteus vulgaris;* gram-positive organisms *Staphylococci,* Streptococci, Streptococci (β-hemolytic), *Streptococcus pneumoniae, Haemophilus influenzae, Escherichia coli, Proteus mirabilis, Klebsiella, Enterobacter, Serratia, Citrobacter, Providencia, Pseudomo-*

nas aeruginosa; anaerobes *Bacteroides, Clostridium, Eubacterium, Fusobacterium, Peptococcus, Peptostreptococcus*

Uses: Lower respiratory tract, urinary tract, skin, bone infections; bacterial septicemia, peritonitis, PID, endometritis

cefotaxime

Therapeutic Outcome: Bactericidal effects for the following: gram-negative organisms *Haemophilus influenzae, Escherichia coli, Neisseria meningitidis, Proteus mirabilis, Klebsiella, Citrobacter, Serratia, Salmonella, Shigella;* gram-positive organisms *Streptococcus pneumoniae, Streptococcus pyogenes, Staphylococcus aureus*

Uses: Lower serious respiratory tract, urinary tract, skin, bone, gonococcal infections; bacteremia, septicemia, meningitis

cefpodoxime

Therapeutic Outcome: Bactericidal effects for the following: gram-negative organisms *Neisseria gonorrhoeae, Haemophilus influenzae, Escherichia coli, Proteus mirabilis, Klebsiella;* gram-positive organisms *Streptococcus pneumoniae, Streptococcus pyogenes, Staphylococcus aureus*

Uses: Upper and lower respiratory tract, urinary tract, skin infections; otitis media, sexually transmitted diseases

ceftazidime

Therapeutic Outcome: Bactericidal effects for the following: gram-negative organisms *Haemophilus influenzae, Escherichia coli, Enterobacter aerogenes, Proteus mirabilis, Klebsiella, Citrobacter, Enterobacter, Pseudomonas aeruginosa, Shigella, Acinetobacter, Bacteroides fragilis, Neisseria;* gram-positive organisms *Streptococcus pneumoniae, Streptococcus pyogenes, Staphylococcus aureus*

Uses: Serious upper or lower respiratory tract, urinary tract, skin, gynecologic, bone, joint, intraabdominal infections; septicemia, meningitis

ceftibuten

Therapeutic Outcome: Bactericidal effects for the following: gram-negative bacilli *Haemophilus influenzae, Escherichia coli;* gram-positive organisms *Streptococcus pneumoniae, Streptococcus pyogenes, Staphylococcus aureus*

Uses: Upper and lower respiratory tract infections; otitis media

ceftizoxime

Therapeutic Outcome: Bactericidal effects for the following: gram-negative organisms *Haemophilus influenzae, Escherichia coli, Enterobacter aerogenes, Proteus mirabilis, Klebsiella, Acinetobacter, Neisseria gonorrhea, Providencia rettgeri, Pseudomonas aeruginosa, Serratia, Enterobacter;* gram-positive organisms *Streptococcus pneumoniae, Streptococcus pyogenes, Staphylococcus aureus;* anaerobes *Bacteroides, Peptococcus, Peptostreptococcus*

Uses: Serious lower respiratory tract, urinary tract, skin, intraabdominal infections; septicemia, meningitis; bone, joint infections; PID caused by *Neisseria gonorrhoeae*

ceftriaxone

Therapeutic Outcome: Bactericidal effects on the following: gram-negative organisms *Haemophilus influenzae, Escherichia coli, Enterobacter aerogenes, Proteus mirabilis, Klebsiella, Citrobacter, Enterobacter, Pseudomonas aeruginosa, Neisseria, Serratia;* gram-positive organisms *Streptococcus pneumoniae, Streptococcus pyogenes, Staphylococcus aureus;* anaerobes *Bacteroides*

Uses: Serious lower respiratory tract, urinary tract, skin, gonococcal, intraabdominal infections; septicemia, meningitis; bone, joint infections

moxalactam

➔ **Therapeutic Outcome:** Bactericidal effects for the following gram-negative organisms: *Haemophilus influenzae, Escherichia coli, Proteus mirabilis, Klebsiella, Citrobacter, Salmonella, Shigella, Serratia;* gram-positive organisms: *Streptococcus pneumoniae, Streptococcus pyogenes, Staphylococcus aureus*

Uses: Serious lower respiratory tract, urinary tract, skin, bone infections; septicemia, meningitis, intraabdominal infections

Dosage and routes

cefdinir

Uncomplicated skin and skin structure infections/ community-acquired pneumonia

P ***Adult and child ≥13 yr:*** PO 300 mg q12h × 10 days

Acute exacerbations of chronic bronchitis/acute maxillary sinusitis

P ***Adult and child ≥13 yr:*** PO 300 mg q12h or 600 mg q24h × 10 days or 300 mg bid × 5 days in some infections

Pharyngitis/tonsillitis

P ***Adult and child ≥13 yr:*** PO 300 mg q12h or 600 mg q24h × 10 days or 300 mg bid × 5 days in some infections

Available forms: Caps 300 mg, oral susp 125 mg/ml

cefepime

Urinary tract infections (mild to moderate)

Adult: **IV**/IM 0.5-1 g q12h × 7-10 days

Urinary tract infections (severe)

Adult: **IV** 2 g q12h × 10 days

Pneumonia (moderate to severe)

Adult: **IV** 1-2 g q12h × 10 days

Dosage reduction indicated in renal impairment (CrCl <50 ml/min)

Uncomplicated gonorrhea

- IM 2 g as a single dose with 1 g PO probenecid at the same time

Available forms: Powder for inj 500 mg, 1, 2 g

cefixime

Adult: PO 400 mg qd as a single dose or 200 mg q12h

P ***Child >50 kg or >12 yr:*** PO use adult dosage

P ***Child <50 kg or <12 yr:*** PO 8 mg/kg/day as a single dose or 4 mg/kg q12h

Renal dose: CrCl 21-60 ml/min 75% of dose; CrCl <20 ml/min 50% of dose

Available forms: Tabs 200, 400 mg; powder for oral susp 100 mg/5 ml

cefoperazone

Adult: IM/**IV** 1-2 g q12h

Severe infections

Adult: IM/**IV** 6-12 g/day divided in 2-4 equal doses

Hepatic dose: Give 50% of dose

Mild/moderate infections

Available forms: Inj 1, 2 g

cefotaxime

Adult: IM/**IV** 1-2 g q12h as a single dose

P ***Child 1 mo-12 yr:*** IM/**IV** 50-180 mg/kg/day divided q6h

Severe infections

Adult: IM/**IV** 2 g q4h, not to exceed 12 g/day

P ***Child 1 mo-12 yr:*** IM/**IV** 50 mg/kg q6h

Uncomplicated gonorrhea
Adult: IM 1 g; dosage reduction indicated for severe renal impairment (CrCl <30 ml/min)

Available forms: Powder for inj 1, 2, 10 g; frozen inj 20, 40 mg/ml

cefpodoxime

P ***Adult >13 yr:*** *Pneumonia:* 200 mg q12h for 14 days; *uncomplicated gonorrhea:* 200 mg single dose; *skin and skin structure:* 400 mg q12h for 7-14 days; *pharyngitis and tonsillitis:* 100 mg q12h for 10 days; *uncomplicated UTI:* 100 mg q12h for 7 days; dosing interval increased in presence of severe renal impairment

P ***Child 5 mo-12 yr: Acute otitis media:*** 5 mg/kg q12h for 10 days; *pharyngitis/tonsillitis:* 5 mg/kg q12h (max 100 mg/dose or 200 mg/day) × 5-10 days

Renal dose: Reduce dose in renal disease

Available forms: Tabs 100, 200 mg/granules for susp 50, 100 mg/5 ml

ceftazidime
Adult: **IV**/IM 1-2 g q8-12h × 5-10 days

P ***Child:*** **IV** 30-50 mg/kg q8h not to exceed 6 g/day

P ***Neonate:*** **IV** 30-50 mg/kg q12h

Renal dose: CrCl <50 ml/min q12h; CrCl 10-30 ml/min q24h; CrCl <10 ml/min q48h

Available forms: Inj 500 mg, 1, 2, 6 g

ceftibuten
Adult: PO 400 mg qd × 10 days

P ***Child 6 mo-12 yr:*** PO 9 mg/kg qd × 10 days

Renal dose: CrCl <50 ml/min 200 mg q24h; CrCl 5-20 ml/min 100 mg q24h

Available forms: Caps 400 mg; 90, 180 mg/5 ml

ceftizoxime
Adult: IM/**IV** 1-2 g q8-12h, may give up to 4 g q8h in life-threatening infections

P ***Child <6 mo:*** IM/**IV** 50 mg/kg q6-8h

Renal dose: CrCl <80 ml/min 500-1500 mg q8h; CrCl 10-49 ml/min 250-1000 mg q12h

PID
Adult: **IV** 2 g q8h, may increase to 4 g q8h in severe infections

Available forms: Powder for inj 500 mg, 1, 2, 10 g; premixed 1 g, 2 g/50 ml

ceftriaxone
Reduce dosage in severe renal impairment (CrCl <10 ml/min)

Adult: IM/**IV** 1-2 g qd, max 2 g q12h

P ***Child:*** IM/**IV** 50-75 mg/kg/day in equal doses q12h

Uncomplicated gonorrhea
Adult: 250 mg IM as single dose

Meningitis
P ***Adult and child:*** IM/**IV** 100 mg/kg/day in equal doses q12h, max 4 g/day

Surgical prophylaxis
Adult: **IV** 1 g ½-2 hr preop

Available forms: Inj 500 mg, 1, 2, 10 g

moxalactam
Adult: IM/**IV** 2-4 g q8-12h

Mild infections
Adult: IM/**IV** 250-500 mg q8-12h

Severe infections
Dosage reduction indicated even for mild renal impairment (CrCl <80 ml/min)

Adult: IM/**IV** 2-6 g q8h

P ***Child:*** IM/**IV** 50 mg/kg q6-8h

Available forms: Powder for inj 1, 2, 10 g

C

Adverse effects

CNS: Headache, dizziness, weakness, paresthesia, fever, chills, seizures
GI: *Nausea, vomiting, diarrhea, anorexia,* pain, glossitis, **bleeding;** increased AST, ALT, bilirubin, LDH, alkaline phosphatase; abdominal pain, **pseudomembranous**
GU: **Proteinuria,** vaginitis, pruritus, candidiasis, increased BUN, **nephrotoxicity, renal failure**
HEMA: **Leukopenia, thrombocytopenia, agranulocytosis,** anemia, **neutropenia, lymphocytosis, eosinophilia, pancytopenia, hemolytic anemia**
INTEG: Rash, urticaria, dermatitis
RESP: Dyspnea
SYST: **Anaphylaxis,** serum sickness

Contraindications: Hypersensitivity to cephalosporins, P infants <1 mo

Precautions: Hypersensitivity to penicillins, pregnancy **B,** lactation, P renal disease, children

Do Not Confuse: ceftazidime/ceftizoxime, Vantin/Ventolin

cefdinir

Pharmacokinetics

Absorption	Well absorbed
Distribution	Widely distributed; crosses placenta
Metabolism	Not metabolized
Excretion	Kidneys, unchanged; enters breast milk
Half-life	Unknown

Pharmacodynamics

	PO
Onset	Unknown
Peak	Unknown

cefepime

Pharmacokinetics

Absorption	Well absorbed (IM)
Distribution	Widely distributed; crosses placenta
Metabolism	Not metabolized
Excretion	Kidneys, unchanged; enters breast milk
Half-life	2 hr; increased in renal disease

Pharmacodynamics

	IM	IV
Onset	Rapid	Immediate
Peak	79 min	Infusion's end

cefixime

Pharmacokinetics

Absorption	40%-50% (PO: tab)
Distribution	Widely distributed
Metabolism	Not metabolized
Excretion	Kidneys, unchanged (50%); bile (10%); enters breast milk
Half-life	3-4 hr, increased in renal disease

Pharmacodynamics

Onset	15-30 min
Peak	1-2 hr

cefoperazone

Pharmacokinetics

Absorption	Well absorbed (IM)
Distribution	Widely distributed; crosses placenta
Metabolism	Not metabolized
Excretion	Bile; enters breast milk
Half-life	2 hr

Pharmacodynamics

	IM	IV
Onset	Rapid	5 min
Peak	1-2 hr	Infusion's end

cefotaxime

Pharmacokinetics

Absorption	Widely distributed
Distribution	Breast milk, small amounts
Metabolism	Liver, active metabolites
Excretion	40%-65% unchanged, kidney
Half-life	1 hr

Pharmacodynamics

	IV	IM
Onset	5 min	30 min
Peak	Unknown	Unknown
Duration	Unknown	Unknown

cefpodoxime

Pharmacokinetics

Absorption	Well absorbed (PO)
Distribution	Widely distributed; crosses placenta
Metabolism	Not metabolized
Excretion	Kidneys, unchanged; enters breast milk
Half-life	2-3 hr, increased in renal disease

Pharmacodynamics

	PO
Onset	Unknown
Peak	Unknown

ceftazidime

Pharmacokinetics

Absorption	Well absorbed (IM)
Distribution	Widely distributed; crosses placenta
Metabolism	Not metabolized
Excretion	Kidneys, unchanged; enters breast milk
Half-life	½-1 hr; increased in renal disease

Pharmacodynamics

	IM	IV
Onset	Rapid	Immediate
Peak	1 hr	Infusion's end

ceftibuten

Pharmacokinetics

Absorption	Well absorbed
Distribution	Widely distributed; crosses placenta
Metabolism	Not metabolized
Excretion	Kidneys, unchanged; enters breast milk
Half-life	1-1½ hr; increased in renal disease

Pharmacodynamics

Onset	Unknown
Peak	Unknown

ceftizoxime

Pharmacokinetics

Absorption	Well absorbed (IM)
Distribution	Widely distributed; crosses placenta
Metabolism	Not metabolized
Excretion	Kidneys, unchanged; enters breast milk
Half-life	1½-2 hr; increased in renal disease

Pharmacodynamics

	IM	IV
Onset	Rapid	Immediate
Peak	1 hr	Infusion's end

ceftriaxone

Pharmacokinetics

Absorption	Well absorbed
Distribution	Widely distributed; crosses placenta; enters CSF
Metabolism	Liver
Excretion	Kidneys, partly
Half-life	5-8 hr

Pharmacodynamics

	IM	IV
Onset	Rapid	Immediate
Peak	1 hr	Infusion's end

moxalactam

Pharmacokinetics

Absorption	Widely distributed
Distribution	Placenta, breast milk
Metabolism	Not metabolized
Excretion	60%-97% unchanged, urine
Half-life	1½-2½ hr

Pharmacodynamics

	IV	IM
Onset	5 min	½-2 hr
Peak	Unknown	Unknown
Duration	Unknown	Unknown

Interactions
Individual drugs
Probenecid: ↓ excretion of drug and ↑ blood levels
Vancomycin: ↑ toxicity
Drug classifications
Aminoglycosides: ↑ toxicity
Lab test interferences
False: ↑ Creatinine (serum urine), ↑ urinary 17-KS
False positive: Urinary protein, direct Coombs' test, urine glucose
Interference: Cross-matching

NURSING CONSIDERATIONS
Assessment
- Assess patient for previous sensitivity reaction to penicillins or other cephalosporins; cross-sensitivity between penicillins and cephalosporins is common
- Assess patient for signs and symptoms of infection including characteristics of wounds, sputum, urine, stool, WBC >10,000/mm^3, fever; obtain baseline information and during treatment
- Obtain C&S before beginning drug therapy to identify if correct treatment has been initiated
- Assess for anaphylaxis: rash, urticaria, pruritus, chills, fever, joint pain; angioedema may occur a few days after therapy begins; epinephrine and resuscitation equipment should be available for anaphylactic reaction
- Identify urine output; if decreasing, notify prescriber (may indicate nephrotoxicity); also check for increased BUN, creatinine
- Monitor blood studies: AST, ALT, CBC, Hct, bilirubin, LDH, alkaline phosphatase, Coombs' test monthly if patient is on long-term therapy
- Monitor electrolytes: potassium, sodium, chloride monthly if patient is on long term therapy
- Assess bowel pattern qd; if severe diarrhea occurs, drug should be discontinued; may indicate pseudomembranous colitis
- Monitor for bleeding: ecchymosis, bleeding gums, hematuria, stool guaiac daily if on long-term therapy
- Assess for overgrowth of infection: perineal itching, fever, malaise, redness, pain, swelling, drainage, rash, diarrhea, change in cough, sputum

Nursing diagnoses
✓ Infection, risk for (uses)
✓ Injury, risk for (side effects)
✓ Diarrhea (side effects)
✓ Knowledge deficit (teaching)

Implementation
cefdinir
PO route
- Give oral suspension after adding 39 ml water to the 60 ml bottle; 65 ml water to the 12.0 ml bottle; discard unused portion after 10 days

cefepime
IM route
- Reconstitute 1 g/2 ml of sterile water for inj; may be diluted with 0.5% or 1% lidocaine to prevent pain; give deep in large muscle mass, massage

IV **IV route**
- Check for irritation, extravasation, phlebitis daily; change site q72h
- For intermittent inf dilute with 50-100 ml of D_5W, give over 30 min

Solution compatibilities: 0.9% NaCl, D_5, 0.5, 1.0% lidocaine, bacte-

C

riostatic water for inj with parabens/ benzyl alcohol

cefixime

- Give in even doses around the clock; if GI upset occurs, give with food; drug must be given for 10-14 days to ensure organism death and prevent superinfection
- Shake suspension

cefoperazone

IM route

- Reconstitute 1 g/2.8 ml of sterile or bacteriostatic water for inj, or 2 g/5.4 ml; may be diluted further with 1 ml or 1.8 ml of 2% lidocaine to prevent pain; give deep in large muscle mass, massage

IV **IV route**

- Check for irritation, extravasation, phlebitis daily; change site q72h
- For intermittent inf, reconstituted sol should be further diluted 1 g/20-40 ml of 0.9% NaCl, D_5W, D_5/ 0.9% NaCl, D_5/LR, or LR; give over 15-30 min; may be refrigerated up to 96 hr or stored 24 hr at room temp
- For cont inf, final concentration is 2-25 mg/ml, give at prescribed rate

Syringe compatibilities: Heparin

Syringe incompatibilities: Doxapram

Y-site compatibilities: Acyclovir, allopurinol, aztreonam, cyclophosphamide, enalaprilat, esmolol, famotidine, foscarnet, fludarabine, hydromorphone, magnesium sulfate, melphalan, morphine, teniposide, thiotepa

Y-site incompatibilities: Gentamicin, hetastarch, labetalol, meperidine, ondansetron, perphenazine, sargramostim, tobramycin, vinorelbine tartrate

Additive compatibilities: Cimetidine, clindamycin, furosemide

Additive incompatibilities: Aminoglycosides

cefotaxime

IV **IV route**

- Dilute 1 g/10 ml D_5W, NS, sterile H_2O for inj and give over 3-5 min by Y-tube or 3-way stopcock; may be diluted further with 50-100 ml of 0.9% NaCl or D_5W; run over ½-1 hr; discontinue primary inf during administration; or may be diluted in larger volume of sol and given as a cont inf over 6-24 hr
- Give for 10-14 days to ensure organism death, prevent superinfection

Syringe compatibilities: Heparin, oflaxacin

Y-site compatibilities: Acyclovir, amifostine, aztreonam, cyclophosphamide, diltiazem, famotidine, fludarabine, hydromorphone, lorazepam, magnesium sulfate, melphalan, meperidine, midazolam, morphine, ondansetron, perphenazine, sargramostim, teniposide, thiotepa, tolazoline, vinorelbine

Additive compatibilities: Clindamycin, metronidazole, verapamil

cefpodoxime

IM route

- Reconstitute 1 g/2 ml or 2 g/3 ml of sterile or bacteriostatic water for inj; may be diluted with 0.5% of 1% lidocaine to prevent pain; give deep in large muscle mass, massage

IV **IV route**

- Check for irritation, extravasation, phlebitis daily; change site q72h
- For direct **IV** dilute in 1 g/10 ml or more and give over 5 min
- For intermittent inf further dilute in 50-100 ml of 0.9% NaCl or D_5W; give over 3-5 min; discontinue primary line while running intermittent inf

Syringe incompatibilities: Doxapram

Y-site compatibilities: Famotidine, fluconazole, fludarabine, regular insulin, meperidine, morphine, sargramostim

Additive incompatibilities: Aminoglycosides, heparin, tetracyclines

ceftazidime

IM route

- Reconstitute 500 mg/1.5 ml or 1 g/3 ml of sterile or bacteriostatic water for inj; may be diluted with 0.5% or 1% lidocaine to prevent pain; give deep in large muscle mass, massage

IV **IV route**

- Check for irritation, extravasation, phlebitis daily; change site q72h
- For direct **IV** dilute 500 mg/5 ml or 1 g/10 ml sterile water for inj; give over 3-5 min; do not use sol with P benzyl alcohol for neonates
- For intermittent inf further dilute 1 g/10 ml or more 0.9% NaCl, D_5W, $D_{10}W$, D_5/0.25% NaCl, D_5/0.45% NaCl, D_5/0.9% NaCl, or LR; give over 30-60 min
- Store for 96 hr refrigerated, 24 hr room temp

Y-site compatibilities: Acyclovir, allopurinol, amifostine, aztreonam, ciprofloxacin, diltiazem, enalaprilat, esmolol, famotidine, filgrastim, fludarabine, foscarnet, granisetron, heparin, hydromorphone, labetalol, meperidine, melphalan, morphine, ondansetron, paclitaxel, rantidine, tacrolimus, teniposide, theophylline, thiotepa, vinorelbine tartrate, zidovudine

Y-site incompatibilities: Amsacrine, fluconazole, idarubicin, sargramostim

Additive compatibilities: Ciprofloxacin, clindamycin, fluconazole, metronidazole, ofloxacin

Additive incompatibilities: Aminoglycosides, sodium bicarbonate

ceftibuten

- Administer for 10 days to ensure organism death, prevent superimposed infection
- Administer after C&S

ceftizoxime

IM route

- Reconstitute 250 mg/0.9 ml, 500 mg/1.8 ml, 1 g/3.6 ml, 2 g/7.2 ml; may be diluted with 0.5% or 1% lidocaine to prevent pain; give deep in large muscle mass, massage

IV **IV route**

- Check for irritation, extravasation, phlebitis daily; change site q72h
- For intermittent inf reconstitute 250 mg/2.4 ml, 500 mg/4.8 ml, 1 g/9.6 mg/2 g/19.2 ml sterile water for inj, D_5W, or 0.9% NaCl; do not use sol P with benzyl alcohol for neonates; may be further diluted in 50-100 ml of D_5W, $D_{10}W$, 0.9% NaCl, or LR; give over 30-60 min
- May store 96h refrigerated, 24h room temp

Y-site compatibilities: Acyclovir, allopurinol, amifostine, aztreonam, enalaprilat, esmolol, famotidine, fludarabine, foscarnet, hydromorphone, labetalol, melphalan, meperidine, morphine, ondansetron, sargramostim, teniposide, thiotepa, vinorelbine

Additive compatibilities: Clindamycin, metronidazole

Additive incompatibilities: Aminoglycosides

ceftriaxone

- Give for 10-14 days to ensure organism death, prevent superinfection

IV **IV route**

- Give **IV** after diluting 250 mg/2.4 ml of D_5W, H_2O for inj, 0.9% NaCl; may be further diluted with 50-100 ml of 0.9% NaCl, D_5W, $D_{10}W$, shake; run over ½-1 hr

Y-site compatibilities: Acyclovir, allopurinol, aztreonam, cisatracurium, diltiazem, doxorubicin liposome, fludarabine, foscarnet, heparin, melphalan, meperidine, methotrexate, morphine, paclitaxel, remifentanil, sargramostim, tacroli-

C

mus, teniposide, theophylline, vinorelbine, warfarin, zidovudine

Additive compatibilities: Amino acids or sodium bicarbonate, metronidazole

moxalactam

• Give for 10-14 days to ensure organism death, prevent superinfection

IV **IV route**

• Dilute 1 g/10 ml sterile H_2O, D_5, 0.9% NaCl; give through Y-tube over 3-5 min; may be further diluted 1 g/20 ml in D_5, 0.9% NaCl, give over ½ hr; may be added to 500-1000 ml, give over 6-24 hr

• Give vit K for bleeding (10 mg/wk)

Additive compatibilities: Metronidazole, ranitidine, verapamil

Syringe compatibilities: Heparin

Y-site compatibilities: Cyclophosphamide, hydromorphone, magnesium sulfate, meperidine, morphine, perphenazine

Patient/family education

• Teach patient to report sore throat, bruising, bleeding, joint pain; may indicate blood dyscrasias (rare)

• Advise patient to contact prescriber if vaginal itching, loose foul-smelling stools, furry tongue occur; may indicate superinfection

• Advise patient to notify prescriber of diarrhea with blood or pus, may indicate pseudomembranous colitis

Evaluation

Positive therapeutic outcome

• Absence of signs/symptoms of infection (WBC <10,000/mm^3, temp WNL, absence of red draining wounds, earache)

• Reported improvement in symptoms of infection

• Negative C&S

Treatment of anaphylaxis: Epinephrine, antihistamines, resuscitate if needed

cephalothin
cephapirin
cephradine

See cephalosporins—1st generation

cetirizine (℞)

(se-tear′i-zeen)

Zyrtec

Func. class: Antihistamine, peripherally selective (2nd generation)

Chem. class.: Piperazine, H_1 histamine antagonist

Pregnancy category B

Action: Acts on blood vessels, GI, respiratory system by competing with histamine for H_1-receptor site; decreases allergic response by blocking pharmacologic effects of histamine; less sedation rate than with other antihistamines; causes increased heart rate, vasodilatation, increased secretions

Therapeutic Outcome: Absence of allergy symptoms and rhinitis

Uses: Rhinitis, allergy symptoms

Dosage and routes

P *Adult and child >12 yr:* PO 5-10 mg qd

P *Child 6-12 yr:* PO 5-10 mg qd

P *Child 2-6 yr:* PO 2.5 mg qd, may increase to 5 mg qd or 2.5 mg bid

G *Elderly:* PO 5 mg qd, may increase to 10 mg/day

Renal/hepatic dose

CrCl 11-31 ml/min 5 mg qd

Available forms: Tabs 5, 10 mg; syrup 5 mg/5 ml

C

Adverse effects
CNS: *Headache,* stimulation, *drowsiness,* sedation, *fatigue,* confusion, blurred vision, tinnitus, restlessness, P tremors, parodoxical excitation in G children or elderly
CV: Hypotension, palpitations, bradycardia, tachycardia, dysrhythmias (rare)
GI: *Nausea, diarrhea,* abdominal pain, *vomiting, constipation,* appetite increase, dry mouth
GU: Frequency, dysuria, urinary retention, impotence
***HEMA:* Hemolytic anemia, thrombocytopenia, leukopenia, agranulocytosis, pancytopenia**
INTEG: Rash, eczema, photosensitivity, urticaria
RESP: *Thickening of bronchial secretions;* dry nose, throat

Contraindications: Hypersensitivity to this drug or hydroxyzine, P newborn or premature infants, lactation, severe hepatic disease

G **Precautions:** Pregnancy **B**, elderly, P children, respiratory disease, narrow-angle glaucoma, prostatic hypertrophy, bladder neck obstruction, asthma

Pharmacokinetics	
Absorption	Well absorbed
Distribution	Protein binding 93%
Metabolism	Liver
Excretion	Kidneys
Half-life	8.3 hr, ↓ in children, ↑ in hepatic/renal disease

Pharmacodynamics	
Onset	½ hr
Peak	1-2 hr
Duration	24 hr

Interactions
Individual drugs
Alcohol: ↑ CNS depression
Drug classifications
Anticoagulants, oral: ↓ action
CNS depressants: ↑ CNS depression
MAOIs: ↑ anticholinergic effect
Opioids: ↑ CNS depression
Sedative/hyponotics: ↑ CNS depression
Herb/drug
Kava: ↑ CNS depression
Food/drug
↓ absorption by 1.7 hr
Lab test interferences
False negative: Skin allergy tests (discontinue antihistamine 3 days before testing)

NURSING CONSIDERATIONS
Assessment
- Assess respiratory status: rate, rhythm; increase in bronchial secretions, wheezing, chest tightness; provide fluids to 2 L/day to decrease secretion thickness
- Assess for allergy symptoms: pruritus, urticaria, watering eyes, baseline and during treatment

Nursing diagnoses
- ✓ Airway clearance, ineffective (uses)
- ✓ Injury, risk for (side effects)
- ✓ Knowledge deficit (teaching)
- ✓ Noncompliance (teaching overuse)

Implementation
- Give without regard to meals
- Store in tight, light-resistant container

Patient/family education
- Teach all aspects of drug uses; to notify prescriber if confusion, sedation, hypotension occur; to avoid driving or other hazardous activity if drowsiness occurs; to avoid alcohol or other CNS depressants that may potentiate effect
- Instruct patient to take 1 hr before or 2 hr pc to facilitate absorption
- Instruct patient not to exceed recommended dose; dysrhythmias may occur
- Teach patient hard candy, gum, frequent rinsing of mouth may be used for dryness
- Advise patient to avoid using if breast feeding

• Advise patient to avoid exposure to sunlight; burns may occur

Evaluation

Positive therapeutic outcome

• Absence of running or congested nose, rashes

Treatment of overdose: Administer ipecac syrup or lavage diazepam, vasopressors, barbiturates (short acting)

cetrorelix (℞)

(set-roe-ree′lix)

Cetrotide

Func. class.: Gonadotropin-releasing hormone antagonist

Chem. class.: Synthetic decapeptide

Pregnancy category X

Action: Inhibitor of pituitary gonadotropin secretion; initially increases LH and FSH, induces a rapid suppression of gonadotropin secretion

Therapeutic Outcome: Pregnancy

Uses: For inhibition of premature LH surges in women undergoing controlled ovarian hyperstimulation

Dosage and routes

Single-dose regimen

Adult: SC 3 mg when serum estradiol level is at appropriate stimulation response, usually on stimulation day 7; if hCG has not been given within 4 days after inj of 3 mg cetrorelix, give 0.25 mg qd until day of hCG administration

Multiple-dose regimen

Adult: SC 0.25 mg is given on stimulation day 5 (either morning or evening) or 6 (morning) and continued qd until day hCG is given

Available forms: Inj 0.25, 3 mg

Adverse effects

CNS: Headache

ENDO: Ovarian hyperstimulation syndrome, abdominal pain (gyn)

GI: Nausea

INTEG: Pain on injection; local site reactions

SYST: Fetal death

Contraindications: Hypersensitivity, pregnancy **X**, latex allergy, lactation

Pharmacokinetics

Absorption	Unknown
Distribution	Protein binding 86%
Metabolism	Liver to metabolites
Excretion	Feces/urine
Half-life	Depends on dosage

Pharmacodynamics

Unknown

Interactions

None known

NURSING CONSIDERATIONS

Assessment

• Assess for suspected pregnancy; drug should not be used

• Assess for latex allergy; drug should not be used

• Monitor ALT, AST, GGT, alkaline phosphatase

Nursing diagnoses

✓ Knowledge deficit (teaching)

Implementation

• Give SC using abdomen, around navel or upper thigh, swab inj area with disinfectant, clean a 2 in circle and allow to dry, pinch up area between thumb and finger, insert needle at 45-90° to surface; if blood is drawn into the syringe, reposition needle without removing it

• Do not administer if patient is pregnant

• Protect from light

Patient/family education

• Instruct to report abdominal pain, vaginal bleeding

• Teach self-administration technique if needed

Evaluation

Positive therapeutic outcome

- Pregnancy

chloral hydrate (℞)

(klor'al hye'drate)

Aquachloral, chloral hydrate, Novo-Chlorhydrate ✽, PMS-Chloral Hydrate

Func. class.: Sedative/hypnotic
Chem. class.: Chloral derivative

Pregnancy category C

Controlled substance schedule IV (USA), **schedule** F (Canada)

Action: Reduced to product trichloroethanol, which produces mild cerebral depression, causing sleep; generalized CNS depression

➔ **Therapeutic Outcome:** Ability to sleep, sedation

Uses: Sedation, short-term treatment of insomnia, preoperative reduction of anxiety

Dosage and routes

Sedation

Adult: PO/rec 250 mg tid pc

P ***Child:*** PO 25-50 mg/kg tid, not to exceed 500 mg tid

Procedure sedation

P ***Child:*** PO/REC 25-50 mg/kg, not to exceed 100 mg/kg or 2 g

Insomnia

Adult: PO/REC 500 mg-1g 30 min before hs

P ***Child:*** PO/REC 50-75 mg/kg (one dose)

Renal dose

CrCl <50 ml/min avoid use

Available forms: Caps 250, 500, 650 mg; syr 250, 500 mg/5 ml; supp 325, 500 mg

Adverse effects

CNS: *Drowsiness,* dizziness, stimulation, nightmares, ataxia, hangover (rare), lightheadedness, headache, paranoia

CV: Hypotension, **dysrhythmias**

GI: *Nausea, vomiting, flatulence, diarrhea,* unpleasant taste, **gastric necrosis**

HEMA: **Eosinophilia, leukopenia**

INTEG: Rash, urticaria, **angioedema,** fever, purpura, eczema

RESP: **Depression**

Contraindications: Hypersensitivity to this drug or triclofos, severe renal disease, severe hepatic disease, GI disorders (oral forms), gastritis

Precautions: Severe cardiac disease, depression, suicidal individuals, asthma, intermittent porphyria, pregnancy **C,** lactation, G elderly

Pharmacokinetics

Absorption	Well absorbed (PO, rec)
Distribution	Widely distributed; crosses placenta
Metabolism	Liver to trichloroethanol
Excretion	Kidneys (inactive metabolite), feces, breast milk
Half-life	8-10 hr; active metabolite

Pharmacodynamics

	PO	REC
Onset	½-1 hr	Slow
Peak	Unknown	Unknown
Duration	4-8 hr	4-8 hr

Interactions

Individual drugs

Alcohol: ↑ CNS depression
Fluoxetine: ↑ action
Furosemide: ↑ diaphoresis, flushing
Propoxyphene: ↑ action

Drug classifications

Analgesics, opioid: ↑ CNS depression
Anticoagulants, oral: ↑ action of anticoagulants
Antidepressants: ↑ CNS depression
Antihistamines: ↑ CNS depression
Sedative/hypnotics: ↑ CNS depression

Herb/drug

Kava: ↑ CNS depression

Lab test interferences

Interferences: Urine catecholamines, urinary 17-OHCS

NURSING CONSIDERATIONS

Assessment

- Assess patient's sleep pattern and note physical (sleep apnea, obstructed airway, pain/discomfort, urinary frequency) and psychologic (fear, anxiety) circumstances that interrupt sleep
- Assess patient's bedtime routine, presleep cues/props
- Assess potential for abuse; this drug may lead to physical and psychologic dependency; amount of drug should be limited
- Monitor blood studies: Hct, Hgb, RBCs, serum folate (if on long-term therapy), pro-time in patients receiving anticoagulants since action of anticoagulant may be increased
- Monitor mental status: mood, sensorium, affect, memory (long, short)
- Monitor physical dependency: more frequent requests for medication, shakes, anxiety, pinpoint pupils
- Monitor respiratory dysfunction: respiratory depression, character, rate, rhythm; hold drug if respirations are <10/min or if pupils are dilated (rare)
- Assess for blood dyscrasias: fever, sore throat, bruising, rash, jaundice, epistaxis (rare)
- Assess previous history of substance abuse, cardiac disease, or gastritis

Nursing diagnoses

✓ Sleep pattern disturbance (uses)
✓ Anxiety (uses)
✓ Knowledge deficit (teaching)
✓ Noncompliance (teaching)

Implementation

General

- Regulate environmental stimuli (light, noise, temperature), remove foods and fluids that interfere with sleep
- Place side rails up after giving medication for hypnotic; remove cigarettes/matches from patient's environment to prevent fires

PO route

- Give ½-1 hr before hs for sleeplessness; give on empty stomach with full glass of water or juice for best absorption and to decrease corrosion (do not chew); after meals to decrease GI symptoms if used for sedation; dilute syr in 4 oz water or juice
- Do not crush, chew caps
- Check dose of syrup carefully, fatal overdoses have occurred

Rectal route

- Store supp in dark container, in refrigerator; remove outer wrapper before insertion

Patient/family education

- Caution patient to avoid driving and other activities requiring alertness; to avoid alcohol ingestion or CNS depressants; serious CNS depression may result plus tachycardia, flushing, headache, hypotension
- Instruct patient not to discontinue medication quickly after long-term use; drug should be tapered over 1-2 wk; that benefits may take 2 nights to be noticed; withdrawal symptoms include tremors, anxiety, hallucinations, delirium
- Teach patient alternate measures to improve sleep (reading, exercise several hours before hs, warm bath, warm milk, TV, self-hypnosis, deep breathing)
- Instruct the patient about factors that contribute to sleep pattern disturbances (lifestyle, shift work, long work hours, environmental factors, frequent napping)
- Teach patient to take drug as prescribed, not to double doses

Evaluation

Positive therapeutic outcome

- Ability to sleep at night

- Decreased amount of early morning awakening if taking drug for insomnia
- Sedation

Treatment of overdose: Lavage, activated charcoal; monitor electrolytes, VS

chlorambucil (℞)

(klor-am'byoo-sil)

Leukeran

Func. class.: Antineoplastic alkylating agent

Chem. class.: Nitrogen mustard

Pregnancy category D

Action: Alkylates DNA, RNA; inhibits enzymes that allow synthesis of amino acids in proteins; activity is not cell cycle phase specific

Therapeutic Outcome: Prevention of rapidly growing malignant cells

Uses: Chronic lymphocytic leukemia, Hodgkin's disease, other lymphomas, macroglobulinemia, nephrotic syndrome, breast carcinoma, choreocarcinoma, ovarian carcinoma

Dosage and routes

Adult: PO 0.1-0.2 mg/kg/day × 3-6 wk initially, then 2-6 mg/day; maintenance 0.2 mg/kg × 2-4 wk; course may be repeated at 2-4 wk intervals or 0.4 mg/kg (12 mg/m^2) 2 ×/wk, may increase by 0.1 mg/kg (3 mg/m^2) q2 wk, adjust as needed

G ***Elderly:*** PO initially ≤2-4 mg/day

P ***Child:*** PO 0.1-0.2 mg/kg/day (4.5 mg/m^2/day) in divided doses or 4.5 mg/m^2/day as 1 dose or in divided doses

Available forms: Tabs 2 mg

Adverse effects

P *CNS:* **Convulsions**

GI: Nausea, vomiting, diarrhea, weight loss, **hepatotoxicity,** *jaundice*

GU: Hyperuremia

HEMA: **Thrombocytopenia, leukopenia, pancytopenia** (prolonged use), **permanent bone marrow suppression**

INTEG: Alopecia (rare), dermatitis, rash, **Stevens-Johnson syndrome**

RESP: **Fibrosis, pneumonitis**

Contraindications: Radiation therapy within 1 mo, chemotherapy within 1 mo, thrombocytopenia, smallpox vaccination, pregnancy **D**

Precautions: *Pneumococcus* vaccination

Do Not Confuse:

Leukeran/leucovorin, Leukeran/Leukine

Pharmacokinetics

Absorption	Rapidly, completely absorbed
Distribution	Crosses placenta
Metabolism	Liver, extensively
Excretion	Kidneys
Half-life	2 hr

Pharmacodynamics

Unknown

Interactions

Individual drugs

Radiation: ↑ toxicity, bone marrow suppression

Drug classifications

Anticoagulants: ↑ risk of bleeding

Antineoplastics: ↑ toxicity, bone marrow suppression

Bone marrow–suppressing drugs: ↑ bone marrow suppression

Live vaccines: ↑ adverse reactions, ↓ antibody reaction

Salicylates: ↑ risk of bleeding

Lab test interferences

↑ Uric acid

NURSING CONSIDERATIONS

Assessment

- Monitor CBC, differential, platelet count weekly; withhold drug if WBC is <2000/mm^3 or granulocyte count <1000/mm^3 notify prescriber of results if WBC <20,000/mm^3, platelets <50,000/mm^3

- Monitor pulmonary function tests, chest x-ray films before, during therapy; chest film should be obtained q2 wk during treatment; check for dyspnea, rales, unproductive cough, chest pain, tachypnea
- Assess for increased uric acid levels, swelling, joint pain primarily in extremities; patient should be well hydrated to prevent urate deposits
- Monitor renal function studies: BUN, serum uric acid, urine CrCl before, during therapy; I&O ratio; report fall in urine output of 30 ml/hr; monitor for decreased hyperuricemia
- Assess for jaundice of skin, sclera, dark urine, clay-colored stools, itchy skin, abdominal pain, fever, diarrhea
- Monitor for cold, fever, sore throat (may indicate beginning infection); identify edema in feet, joint, stomach pain, shaking; prescriber should be notified
- Assess for bleeding: hematuria, guaiac, bruising or petechiae, mucosa or orifices q8h, no rect temp

Nursing diagnoses

✓ Injury, risk for (adverse reactions)
✓ Body image disturbance (adverse reactions)
✓ Infection, risk for (adverse reactions)
✓ Knowledge deficit (teaching)

Implementation

- Give 1 hr ac or 2 hr pc to lessen nausea and vomiting or antacid before oral agent, give drug after evening meal, before hs or 1 hr before breakfast; antiemetic 30-60 min before giving drug to prevent vomiting
- Give allopurinol to maintain uric acid levels, alkalinization of urine; increase fluid intake to 2-3 L/day to prevent urate deposits, calculus formation
- Antibiotics for prophylaxis of infection may be prescribed, since infection potential is high
- Give all drugs PO if possible, avoid IM inj when platelets <150,000/mm^3
- Store in tight container

Patient/family education

- Teach patient to avoid use of products containing aspirin or ibuprofen, razors, commercial mouthwash, since bleeding may occur; to report symptoms of bleeding (hematuria, tarry stools)
- Instruct patient to report signs of anemia (fatigue, headache, irritability, faintness, shortness of breath)
- Instruct patient to report any changes in breathing or coughing even several mo after treatment; to avoid crowds and persons with respiratory tract or other infections
- Advise patient hair loss is common; discuss the use of wigs or hairpieces
- Instruct patient to drink 2-3 L of fluid qd unless contraindicated
- Caution patient not to have any vaccinations without the advice of the prescriber; serious reactions can occur
- Advise patient contraception is needed during treatment and for several months after the completion of therapy, may cause irreversible gonadal suppression

Evaluation

Positive therapeutic outcome

- Decreased size of tumor
- Decreased spread of malignancy
- Improved blood values
- Absence of sweating at night
- Increased appetite, increased weight

C

chloramphenicol (℞)
(klor-am-fen'i-kole)

Ak-Chlor, Chloracol, Chlorofair, chloramphenicol, Chloromycetin, Chloroptic, EconoChlor, Fenicol ♣, I-Chlor, Novochlorocap ♣, Pentamycetin ♣

Func. class.: Antiinfective, misc.
Chem. class.: Dichloroacetic acid derivative

Pregnancy category C

Action: Binds to 50S ribosomal subunit, which interferes with or inhibits protein synthesis

➔ **Therapeutic Outcome:** Bactericidal for *Haemophilus influenzae, Salmonella typhi, Rickettsia, Neisseria, Mycoplasma*

Uses: Meningitis, bacteremia, abdominal, skin, soft tissue infections; local infections of skin, ear, eye; not to be used if less-toxic drugs can be used

Dosage and routes

Adult: PO/**IV** 12.5 mg/kg q6h, not to exceed 4 g/day

P ***Children and infants >2 wk:*** **IV**/PO 12 mg/kg q6h or 2.5 mg/kg q2hr

P ***Infants <2 wk and premature:*** **IV**/PO 6.25 mg/kg q6h

P ***Adult and child:*** OPHTH 1-2 gtt of sol or ointment q3-6 mo; otic 2-3 gtt bid or tid; top 1% cream tid or qid

P ***Premature infants and neonates:*** **IV**/PO 25 mg/kg/day in divided doses q6h

Available forms: Inj **IV** 100 mg/ml in 1-g vial; caps 250 mg; ophth ointment 10 mg/g; ophth sol 25 mg/15 ml, 5 mg/ml; top cream 1%; otic sol 0.5%

Adverse effects

CNS: Headache, **depression**, confusion, peripheral neuritis

CV: **Gray syndrome in newborns: failure to feed, pallor, cyanosis, abdominal distention, irregular respiration, vasomotor collapse**

EENT: Optic neuritis, blindness

GI: Nausea, vomiting, diarrhea, abdominal pain, xerostomia, glossitis, colitis, pruritus ani

HEMA: **Anemia, bone marrow depression, thrombocytopenia, aplastic anemia, granulocytopenia, leukopenia** (rare)

INTEG: Itching, urticaria, contact dermatitis, rash

Contraindications: Hypersensitivity, severe renal disease, severe hepatic disease, minor infections

Precautions: Hepatic disease, P renal disease, infants, children, bone marrow depression (drug-induced), pregnancy **C**, lactation

Pharmacokinetics

Absorption	Well (PO) Completely (**IV**)
Distribution	Wide
Metabolism	Liver
Excretion	Kidneys, unchanged
Half-life	1½-4 hr

Pharmacodynamics

	PO	IV	TOP	OPHTH	OTIC
Onset	15 min	Rapid	Unkn	Unkn	Unkn
Peak	1-2 hr	Inf end	Unkn	Unkn	Unkn

Interactions

Individual drugs

Folic acid: ↓ action of folic acid
Iron: ↑ action of iron
Phenytoin: ↑ action of phenytoin
Rifampin: ↓ action of rifampin
Vitamin B_{12}: ↓ action of vitamin B_{12}

Drug classifications

Anticoagulants: ↑ prothrombin time
Antidiabetics: ↑ action of antidiabetics
Barbiturates: ↑ levels of barbiturates
Penicillins: ↑ synergism

NURSING CONSIDERATIONS

Assessment

- Assess patient for previous sensitivity reaction to other antiinfectives; cross-sensitivity between penicillins and cephalosporins is common
- Assess patient for signs and symptoms of infection including characteristics of wounds, sputum, urine, stool, WBC >10,000/mm^3, fever; obtain baseline information and during treatment
- Perform C&S testing before starting drug therapy to identify if correct treatment has been initiated
- Monitor drug level in impaired hepatic, renal systems; peak 15-20 mg/ml 3 hr after dose, trough 5-10 mg/ml before next dose
- Monitor blood studies: platelets q2 days, CBC
- Assess bowel pattern qd; if severe diarrhea occurs, drug should be discontinued
- Monitor for bleeding: ecchymosis, bleeding gums, hematuria, stool guaiac daily if on long-term therapy
- Assess for overgrowth of infection: perineal itching, fever, malaise, redness, pain, swelling, drainage, rash, diarrhea, change in cough, sputum

Nursing diagnoses

✓ Infection, risk for (uses)
✓ Diarrhea (adverse reaction)
✓ Injury, risk for (side effects)
✓ Knowledge deficit (teaching)
✓ Noncompliance (teaching)

Implementation

Topical route

- Wash hands, clean area to be treated with soap and water before application

Ophthalmic route

- Apply a small amount of ointment in lower lid
- Have patient tilt head back before application

IV **IV route**

- Give after diluting 1 g/10 ml of sterile H_2O for inj or D_5W (10% sol); give >1 min
- May be further diluted in 50-100 ml of D_5W; give through Y-tube, 3-way stopcock, or additive infusion set; run over ½-1 hr; store reconstituted sol at room temp for up to 30 days

Syringe compatibilities:
Ampicillin, cloxacillin, heparin, methicillin, penicillin G sodium

Y-site compatibilities:
Acyclovir, cyclophosphamide, enalaprilat, esmolol, foscarnet, hydromorphone, labetalol, magnesium sulfate, meperidine, morphine, perphenazine, tacrolimus

Y-site incompatibilities:
Fluconazole

Additive compatibilities:
Amikacin, aminophylline, ascorbic acid, calcium chloride/gluconate, cephalothin, cephapirin, colistimethate, corticotropin, cyanocobalamin, dimenhydrinate, dopamine, ephedrine, heparin, hydrocortisone, kanamycin, lidocaine, magnesium sulfate, metaraminol, methicillin, methyldopate, methylprednisolone, metronidazole, nafcillin, oxacillin, oxytocin, penicillin G potassium, penicillin G sodium, pentobarbital, phenylephrine, phytonadione, plasma protein fraction, potassium chloride, promazine, ranitidine, sodium bicarbonate, thiopental, verapamil, vit B

PO route

- Give oral form on empty stomach with full glass of water
- ⊘ Do not crush or chew caps
- Store cap in airtight container at room temp

Patient/family education

- Teach patient all aspects of drug therapy; need to complete entire course of medication to ensure organism death (10-14 days); culture may be taken after complete course of medication
- Advise patient to report sore throat,

fever, fatigue, unusual bleeding, or bruising; could indicate bone marrow depression (may occur weeks or months after termination of drug)
- Tell patient that drug must be taken at regular intervals around the clock to maintain blood levels

Evaluation
Positive therapeutic outcome
- Decreased symptoms of infection

chlordiazepoxide (℞)
(klor-dye-az-e-pox′ide)
Apo-Chlordiazepoxide ✤, chlordiazepoxide HCl, Libritabs, Librium, Novopoxide ✤
Func. class.: Antianxiety
Chem. class.: Benzodiazepine

Pregnancy category D

Controlled substance schedule IV

Action: Potentiates the actions of GABA, an inhibitory neurotransmitter, especially in the limbic system reticular formation, which depresses the CNS

Therapeutic Outcome: Decreased anxiety, successful alcohol withdrawal, relaxation

Uses: Short-term management of anxiety, acute alcohol withdrawal, preoperative relaxation

Dosage and routes
Mild anxiety
Adult: PO 5-10 mg tid-qid
P ***Child >6 yr:*** PO 5 mg bid-qid, not to exceed 10 mg bid-tid

Severe anxiety
Adult: PO 20-25 mg tid-qid

Preoperatively
Adult: PO 5-10 mg tid-qid on day before surgery; IM 50-100 mg 1 hr before surgery

Alcohol withdrawal
Adult: PO/IM/**IV** 50-100 mg, not to exceed 300 mg/day

Available forms: Caps 5, 10, 25 mg; tabs 5, 10, 25 mg; IM inj 100 mg

Adverse effects
CNS: *Dizziness, drowsiness,* confusion, headache, anxiety, tremors, stimulation, fatigue, depression, insomnia, hallucinations
CV: *Orthostatic hypotension,* **ECG changes, tachycardia,** hypotension
EENT: *Blurred vision,* tinnitus, mydriasis
GI: Constipation, dry mouth, nausea, vomiting, anorexia, diarrhea
INTEG: Rash, dermatitis, itching

Contraindications: Hypersensitivity to benzodiazepines, narrow-angle glaucoma, psychosis, pregnancy **D**, P child <6 yr

G **Precautions:** Elderly, debilitated, hepatic disease, renal disease

Do Not Confuse:
Librium/Librax

Pharmacokinetics

Absorption	Well absorbed (PO); slow, erratic (IM)
Distribution	Widely distributed; crosses placenta, blood-brain barrier
Metabolism	Liver extensively
Excretion	Kidneys, breast milk
G **Half-life**	5-30 hr (increased in elderly)

Pharmacodynamics

	PO	IM	IV
Onset	30 min	15-30 min	1-5 min
Peak	½ hr	Unknown	Unknown
Duration	4-6 hr	Unknown	Up to 1 hr

Interactions
Individual drugs
Alcohol: ↑ CNS depression
Cimetidine: ↑ action of cimetidine
Disulfiram: ↑ action of disulfiram
Fluoxetine: ↑ action of fluoxetine

Isoniazid: ↑ action of isoniazid
Ketoconazole: ↑ action of ketoconazole
Levodopa: ↓ action of levodopa
Metoprolol: ↑ action of metoprolol
Propoxyphene: ↑ action of propoxyphene
Propranolol: ↑ action of propranolol
Rifampin: ↓ action of chlordiazepoxide
Theophylline: ↓ sedative effects
Valproic acid: ↑ action of valproic acid

Drug classifications
Analgesics, opioid: ↑ CNS depression
Antidepressants: ↑ CNS depression
Antihistamines: ↑ CNS depression
Barbiturates: ↓ effect of chlordiazepoxide
Contraceptives, oral: ↑ effect of contraceptive

Herb/drug
Kava: ↑ CNS depression

Lab test interferences
↑ AST/ALT, serum bilirubin, ↑ 17-OHCS
↓ Radioactive iodine uptake
False positive: Pregnancy test (some methods)

NURSING CONSIDERATIONS
Assessment
- Assess anxiety reaction: inability to sleep, apprehension, dread, foreboding, or uneasiness related to unidentified source of danger
- Assess for previous drug dependence or tolerance; if drug dependent or tolerant, amount of medication should be restricted
- Monitor B/P (with patient lying, standing), pulse; if systolic B/P drops 20 mm Hg, hold drug, notify prescriber
- Monitor blood studies: CBC during long-term therapy; blood dyscrasias have occurred rarely
- Monitor hepatic studies: AST, ALT, bilirubin, creatinine, LDH, alkaline phosphatase during long-term therapy
- Monitor mental status: mood, sensorium, affect, sleeping patterns, drowsiness, dizziness, suicidal tendencies

Nursing diagnoses
- ✓ Anxiety (uses)
- ✓ Knowledge deficit (teaching)
- ✓ Noncompliance (teaching)

Implementation
PO route
- Give with food or milk for GI symptoms, crushed if patient unable to swallow medication whole; do not open capsules; provide sugarless gum, hard candy, frequent sips of water for dry mouth

IM route
- Reconstitute with diluent provided (2 ml); agitate slowly, do not shake; give deep in large muscle mass to prevent severe pain; do not use IM diluent for **IV** route

IV route
- Reconstitute 100 mg/5 ml sterile water for inj or 0.9% NaCl; give over at least 1 min to prevent cardiac arrest, apnea, bradycardia
- Keep powder from light; refrigerate, mix when ready to use

Y-site compatibilities:
Heparin, hydrocortisone, potassium chloride, vit B with C

Solution compatibilities:
D_5W, 0.9% NaCl

Patient/family education
- Instruct patient that drug may be taken with food; if dose is missed take as soon as remembered; do not double doses
- Tell patient to avoid OTC preparations unless approved by prescriber; to avoid alcohol ingestion or other psychotropic medications unless directed by a prescriber
- Caution patient to avoid driving and activities requiring alertness, since drowsiness may occur; until medica-

tion response is known, tell patient that drowsiness may worsen at beginning of treatment
- Instruct patient not to discontinue medication abruptly after long-term use, drug should be tapered over 1 wk
- Caution patient to rise slowly or fainting may occur, especially in G elderly
- Advise patient that drug should be avoided during pregnancy

Evaluation

Positive therapeutic outcome
- Increased well being
- Decreased anxiety, restlessness, sleeplessness, dread
- Successful alcohol withdrawal

Treatment of overdose: Lavage, VS, supportive care

chloroquine (℞)

(klor'oh-kwin)

Aralen HCl, Aralen Phosphate, chloroquine phosphate

Func. class.: Antimalarial

Chem. class.: Synthetic 4-aminoquinoline derivative

Pregnancy category C

Action: Inhibits parasite replications, transcription of DNA to RNA by forming complexes with DNA of parasite

Therapeutic Outcome: Decreased symptoms of malaria, amebiasis

Uses: Malaria caused by *Plasmodium vivax, Plasmodium malariae, Plasmodium ovale, Plasmodium falciparum* (some strains), amebiasis

Dosage and routes

Malaria suppression

P ***Adult and child:*** PO 5 mg base/kg/wk on same day of week, not to exceed 300 mg base; treatment should begin 1-2 wk before exposure and for 8 wk after; if treatment begins after exposure, 600 mg base for adult and P 10 mg base/kg for children in 2 divided doses 6 hr apart

Extraintestinal amebiasis

Adult: IM 160-200 mg base qd × 10-12 days or PO (HCl) 600 mg base qd × 2 days, then 300 mg base qd × 2-3 wk (phosphate)

P ***Child:*** IM/PO 10 mg/kg qd (HCl) × 2-3 wk, not to exceed 300 mg/day

Available forms: Tabs 250 mg (150 mg base), 500 mg (300 mg base) phosphate; inj 50 mg (40 mg base)/ml HCl

Adverse effects

CNS: Headache, stimulation, fatigue, **convulsion**, psychosis

CV: Hypotension, **heart block, asystole with syncope,** ECG changes

EENT: Blurred vision, corneal changes, retinal changes, difficulty focusing, tinnitus, vertigo, deafness, photophobia, corneal edema

GI: Nausea, vomiting, anorexia, diarrhea, cramps

HEMA: **Thrombocytopenia, agranulocytosis, hemolytic anemia, leukopenia**

INTEG: Pruritus, pigmentary changes, skin eruptions, lichen planus–like eruptions, eczema, **exfoliative dermatitis**

Contraindications: Hypersensitivity, retinal field changes, porphyria

Precautions: Pregnancy **C**, children, blood dyscrasias, severe GI disease, neurologic disease, alcoholism, hepatic disease, G6PD deficiency, psoriasis, eczema, lactation, porphyria

Pharmacokinetics	
Absorption	Well absorbed
Distribution	Widely
Metabolism	Liver
Excretion	Kidneys, feces
Half-life	3-5 days

Pharmacodynamics

	PO	IM
Onset	Rapid	Rapid
Peak	1-3 hr	30 min
Duration	6-8 hr	Unknown

Interactions

Individual drugs

Cimetidine: ↓ absorption
Kaolin: ↓ absorption

Drug classifications

Antacids, aluminum: ↓ absorption

NURSING CONSIDERATIONS

Assessment

- Monitor liver studies weekly: ALT, AST, bilirubin; renal status: before exposure, monthly thereafter: BUN, creatinine, output, sp gr, urinalysis
- Assess mental status often: affect, mood, behavioral changes; psychosis may occur
- Assess hepatic status: decreased appetite, jaundice, dark urine, fatigue
- Assess for toxicity: blurring vision, difficulty focusing, headache, dizziness, decreased knee, ankle reflexes, drug should be discontinued immediately

Nursing diagnoses

✓ Infection, risk for (uses)
✓ Diarrhea (side effects)
✓ Knowledge deficit (teaching)
✓ Noncompliance (teaching)
✓ Injury, risk for (side effects)

Implementation

PO route

- Give with meals to decrease GI symptoms; better to take on empty stomach 1 hr ac or 2 hr pc
- Give antiemetic if vomiting occurs
- Give after C&S is completed; monthly to detect resistance

IM route

- Give IM after aspirating to prevent inj into bloodstream

Additive compatibility: Promethazine

Patient/family education

- Advise patient that compliance with dosage schedule, duration is necessary
- Instruct patient that scheduled appointments must be kept or relapse may occur
- Caution patient to avoid alcohol while taking drug
- Instruct diabetic to use blood glucose monitor to obtain correct result
- Teach patient to report weakness, fatigue, loss of appetite, nausea, vomiting, yellowing of skin or eyes, tingling/numbness of hands/feet
- Advise patient that urine may turn rust brown color
- Instruct patient to use sunglasses in bright sunlight to prevent photophobia

Evaluation

Positive therapeutic outcome

- Decreased symptoms of malaria

Treatment of overdose:

Induce vomiting, gastric lavage, administer barbiturate (ultrashort-acting), vasopressor; tracheostomy may be necessary

chlorothiazide (℞)

(klor-oh-thye'a-zide)

Diurigen, Diuril, Diuril Sodium, Diurigen

Func. class.: Diuretic, antihypertensive

Chem. class.: Thiazide; sulfonamide derivative

Pregnancy category B

Action: Acts on the distal tubule and thick ascending limb of the loop of Henle in the kidney, increasing excretion of sodium, water, chloride, magnesium, potassium, and bicarbonate

➔ **Therapeutic Outcome:** Decreased BP, decreased edema in tissues peripherally, diuresis

Uses: Edema in CHF, nephrotic

syndrome; may be used alone or as adjunct with antihypertensives; also for edema in corticosteroids, estrogen therapy

Dosage and routes
Edema, hypertension
Adult: PO/**IV** 500 mg-2 g qd; may divide bid
Diuresis
P ***Child >6 mo:*** PO 10-20 mg/kg/day may divide bid
P ***Child <6 mo:*** PO up to 40 mg/kg/day; may divide bid

Available forms: Tabs 250, 500 mg; oral susp 250 mg/5 ml; inj 500 mg

Adverse effects
CNS: Drowsiness, paresthesia, anxiety, depression, headache, *dizziness, fatigue, weakness, fever, insomnia*
CV: Irregular pulse, orthostatic hypotension, palpitations, volume depletion
EENT: Blurred vision
ELECT: Hypokalemia, hypercalcemia, hyponatremia, hypochloremia, hypophosphatemia, hypomagnesemia, hyperlipidemia
GI: Nausea, vomiting, anorexia, constipation, diarrhea, cramps, pancreatitis, GI irritation, ***hepatitis***
GU: Frequency, polyuria, ***uremia,*** glucosuria, hematuria
HEMA: Aplastic anemia, hemolytic anemia, leukopenia, agranulocytosis, thrombocytopenia, neutropenia
INTEG: Rash, urticaria, purpura, photosensitivity, alopecia
META: Hyperglycemia, *hyperuricemia,* hypomagnesemia, increased creatinine, BUN

Contraindications: Hypersensitivity to thiazides or sulfonamides, anuria, renal decompensation, lactation, hepatic coma

Precautions: Hypokalemia, renal disease, hepatic disease, gout, COPD, LE, diabetes mellitus, pregnancy **B,**
G elderly, hyperlipidemia

Do Not Confuse:
chlorothiazide/chlorpromazine, chlorothiazide/chlorpropamide, chlorothiazide/chlorthalidone

Pharmacokinetics

	PO
Absorption	GI tract (10%-20%)
Distribution	Extracellular spaces; crosses placenta
Metabolism	Liver
Excretion	Urine, unchanged; breast milk
Half-life	1-2 hr

Pharmacodynamics

	PO	IV
Onset	2 hr	15 min
Peak	4 hr	½ hr
Duration	6-12 hr	2 hr

Interactions
Individual drugs
Allopurinol: ↑ toxicity
Cholestyramine: ↓ absorption of chlorothiazide
Colestipol: ↓ absorption of chlorothiazide
Digitalis: ↑ toxicity
Lithium: ↑ toxicity
Mezlocillin: ↑ hypokalemia
Piperacillin: ↑ hypokalemia
Ticarcillin: ↑ hypokalemia
Drug classifications
Anticoagulants: ↓ effects
Antihypertensives: ↑ antihypertensive effect
Glucocorticoids: ↑ hypokalemia
Nitrates: ↑ hypotension
NSAIDs: ↓ diuretic action, ↑ risk of NSAID-induced renal failure
Nondepolarizing skeletal muscle relaxants: ↑ toxicity
Food/drug
↑ Absorption
Herb/drug
Aloe: ↑ hypokalemia
Buckthorn bark/berry: ↑ hypokalemia

Cascara sagrada bark: ↑ hypokalemia
Licorice root: ↑ hypokalemia
Senna pod/leaf: ↑ hypokalemia

Lab test interferences
↑ BSP retention, calcium, amylase, parathyroid test
↓ PBI, ↓ PSP
False negative: Phentolamine and tyramine tests
Interference: Urine steroid tests

NURSING CONSIDERATIONS
Assessment

- Assess glucose in urine if patient is diabetic
- Monitor improvement in CVP q8h
- Check for rashes, temp elevation qd
- Assess for confusion, especially in G elderly; take safety precautions if needed
- Monitor manifestations of hypokalemia; *RENAL:* acidic urine, reduced urine osmolality, nocturia; *CV:* hypotension, broad T wave, U wave, ectopy, tachycardia, weak pulse; *NEURO:* muscle weakness, altered LOC, drowsiness, apathy, lethargy, confusion, depression; *GI:* anorexia, nausea, cramps, constipation, distention, paralytic ileus; *RESP:* hypoventilation, respiratory muscle weakness
- Monitor for manifestations of hypomagnesemia; *CNS:* agitation, muscle twitching, paresthesias, hyperactive reflexes, positive Babinski's reflex, dysphagia, nystagmus, seizures, tetany; *GI:* nausea, vomiting, diarrhea, anorexia, abdominal distention; *CV:* ectopy, tachycardia, broad, flat, or inverted T waves, depressed ST segment, prolonged QT interval, decreased cardiac output, hypotension
- Monitor for manifestations of hyponatremia: *CV:* increased B/P, cold, clammy skin, hypovolemia or hypervolemia; *GI:* anorexia, nausea, vomiting, diarrhea, abdominal cramps; *NEURO:* lethargy, increased ICP, confusion, headache, seizures, coma, fatigue, tremors, hyperreflexia
- Monitor for manifestations of hyperchloremia: *NEURO:* weakness, lethargy, coma; *RESP:* coma, deep rapid breathing
- Assess fluid volume status: I&O ratios and record, count or weigh diapers as appropriate, weight, distended red veins, crackles in lung, color, quality and sp gr of urine, skin turgor, adequacy of pulses, moist mucous membranes, bilateral lung sounds, peripheral pitting edema; dehydration symptoms of decreasing output, thirst, hypotension, dry mouth and mucous membranes should be reported
- Monitor electrolytes: potassium, sodium, calcium, magnesium; also include BUN, blood pH, ABGs, uric acid, CBC, blood sugar
- Assess B/P before and during therapy with patient lying, standing, and sitting as appropriate; orthostatic hypotension can occur rapidly

Nursing diagnoses

- ✓ Altered urinary elimination (adverse reactions)
- ✓ Fluid volume deficit
- ✓ Fluid volume excess (uses)
- ✓ Knowledge deficit (teaching)

Implementation

- Give in AM to avoid interference with sleep
- Potassium replacement if potassium level is 3.0 mg/dl
- Give whole, or use oral sol; drug may be crushed if patient is unable to swallow

PO route

- Give with food; if nausea occurs, absorption may be increased

IV **IV route**

- Do not use sol that is yellow, has a precipitate, or crystals
- Administer **IV** after diluting 0.5 g/18 ml or more of sterile water for inj; may be diluted further with dextrose or NaCl: give over 5 min; sol is stable at room temp for 24 hr

Additive compatibilities: Cimetidine, lidocaine, nafcillin, sodium bicarbonate

Additive incompatibilities: Amikacin, blood, blood products, chlorpromazine, codeine, hydralazine, insulin, levorphanol, methadone, morphine, multivitamins, norepinephrine, polymyxin B, procaine, prochlorperazine, promazine, promethazine, streptomycin, tetracycline, triflupromazine, vancomycin

Patient/family education

- Teach patient to take medication early in the day to prevent nocturia
- Instruct patient to take with food or milk if GI symptoms of nausea and anorexia occur
- Teach patient to maintain a weekly record of weight and notify prescriber of weight loss >5 lb
- Caution patient that this drug causes a loss of potassium, so food rich in potassium should be added to the diet; refer to a dietician for assistance in planning
- Caution patient not to exercise in hot weather or stand for prolonged periods, since orthostatic hypotension will be enhanced; to use sunscreen to prevent burning
- Teach patient not to use alcohol or any OTC medications without prescriber's approval; serious drug reactions may occur
- Emphasize the need to contact prescriber immediately if muscle cramps, weakness, nausea, dizziness, or numbness occurs
- Teach patient to take own B/P and pulse and record
- Caution patient that orthostatic hypotension may occur; patient should rise slowly from sitting or reclining positions and lie down if dizziness occurs
- Teach patient to continue taking medication even if feeling better; this drug controls symptoms but does not cure the condition
- Advise the patient with hypertension to continue other medical treatment (exercise, weight loss, relaxation techniques, cessation of smoking)

Evaluation

Positive therapeutic outcome

- Decreased edema
- Decreased B/P
- Increased diuresis

Treatment of overdose: Lavage if taken orally, monitor electrolytes; administer dextrose in saline; monitor hydration, CV, renal status

chlorpheniramine (OTC, Ph)

(klor-fen-ir'a-meen)

Aller-Chlor, Allergy, Chlo-Amine, Chlorate, chlorpheniramine maleate, Chlor-Trimeton, Chlor-Tripolon ✤, Gon-Allerate, Novo-Pheniram ✤, PediaCare Allergy Formula, Phenetron, Teldrin

Func. class.: Antihistamine (1st generation, nonselective)

Chem. class.: Alkylamine, H_1-receptor antagonist

Pregnancy category B

Action: Acts on blood vessels, GI, respiratory system by competing with histamine for H_1-receptor site; decreases allergic response by blocking histamine

➔ **Therapeutic Outcome:** Absence of allergy symptoms and rhinitis

Uses: Allergy symptoms, rhinitis, allergic dermatoses, nasal allergies, hypersensitive reactions including blood transfusion reactions, anaphylaxis

Dosage and routes

Adult/child ≥12 yr: PO 2-4 mg tid-qid, not to exceed 24 mg/day; time rel 8-12 mg bid-tid, not to exceed 36

mg/day; IM/**IV**/SC 5-40 mg/day, max 40 mg/day

P ***Child 6-12 yr:*** PO 2 mg q4-6h, not to exceed 12 mg/day; sus rel 8 mg hs or qd; sus rel not recommended for child <6 yr; SC 87.5 μg/kg or 2.5 mg/m^2 q6h

P ***Child 2-5 yr:*** PO 1 mg q4-6h, not to exceed 4 mg/day

Available forms: Chewable tabs 2 mg; tabs 4 mg; time rel tabs 8, 12 mg; time rel caps 8, 12 mg; syr 1, 2, 2.5 mg/5 ml; inj 10, 100 mg/ml

Adverse effects

CNS: *Dizziness, drowsiness,* poor coordination, fatigue, anxiety, euphoria, confusion, paresthesia, neuritis
EENT: Blurred vision, dilated pupils, tinnitus, nasal stuffiness, dry nose, throat, mouth
GI: Nausea, anorexia, diarrhea
GU: *Retention,* dysuria, frequency
HEMA: **Thrombocytopenia, agranulocytosis, hemolytic anemia**
INTEG: Photosensitivity
RESP: Increased thick secretions, wheezing, chest tightness

Contraindications: Hypersensitivity to H_1-receptor antagonists, acute asthma attack, lower respiratory tract disease, stenosed peptic ulcers, bladder neck obstruction

Precautions: Increased intraocular pressure, renal disease, cardiac disease, hypertension, bronchial asthma, seizure disorder, hyperthyroidism, prostatic hypertrophy, pregnancy **B**, G elderly

Do Not Confuse:

Teldrin/Tedral

Pharmacokinetics

Absorption	Well absorbed (PO, SC, IM, **IV**)
Distribution	Widely distributed; crosses blood-brain barrier
Metabolism	Liver, mostly
Excretion	Kidneys, metabolite; breast milk (minimal)
Half-life	12-15 hr

Pharmacodynamics

	PO	PO-ER	SC	IM	IV
Onset	15-30 min	Unknown	Unknown	Unknown	Immediate
Peak	1-2 hr	Unknown	Unknown	Unknown	Unknown
Duration	4-12 hr	8-24 hr	4-12 hr	4-12 hr	4-12 hr

Interactions

Individual drugs

Alcohol: ↑ CNS depression
Atropine: ↑ anticholinergic reactions
Disopyramide: ↑ anticholinergic reactions
Haloperidol: ↑ anticholinergic reactions
Quinidine: ↑ anticholinergic reactions

Drug classifications

Antidepressants: ↑ anticholinergic reactions
Antihistamines: ↑ anticholinergic reactions
CNS depressants: ↑ CNS depression
MAOIs: ↑ anticholinergic effect
Opiates: ↑ CNS depression
Phenothiazines: ↑ anticholinergic reactions
Sedative/hypnotics: ↑ CNS depression

Herb/drug

Henbane leaf: ↑ anticholinergic effect
Kava: ↑ CNS depression

Lab test interferences

False negative: Skin allergy tests (discontinue antihistamines 3 days before testing)

C

NURSING CONSIDERATIONS
Assessment
- Assess respiratory status: rate, rhythm, increase in bronchial secretions, wheezing, chest tightness; provide fluids to 2 L/day to decrease secretion thickness
- Monitor I&O ratio: be alert for urinary retention, frequency, dysuria, G especially elderly; drug should be discontinued if these occur
- **IV** administration may result in rapid drop in B/P, sweating, dizziness, G especially in elderly

Nursing diagnoses
✓ Airway clearance, ineffective (uses)
✓ Injury, risk for (side effects)
✓ Knowledge deficit (teaching)
✓ Noncompliance (teaching, overuse)

Implementation
PO route
- May give with food to decrease GI upset; chewable tabs should be chewed and not swallowed whole; caps, time rel tabs should be swallowed whole
- ⊘ Do not open or chew time rel tabs
- Store in tight, light-resistant container

SC/IM route
- Use only 20 and 100 mg/ml strengths; does not need to be reconstituted or diluted

IV **IV route**
Give undiluted by direct **IV** (10 mg/ml strength only); administer 10 mg over 1 min or more

Additive incompatibilities:
Calcium chloride, kanamycin, norepinephrine, pentobarbital

Patient/family education
- Teach all aspects of drug use; to notify prescriber if confusion, sedation, hypotension, or difficulty voiding occurs; to avoid driving and other hazardous activity if drowsiness occurs; to avoid alcohol and other CNS depressants that may potentiate effect
- Teach patient not to exceed recommended dosage; dysrhythmias may occur
- Advise patient hard candy, gum, frequent rinsing of mouth may be used for dryness

Evaluation
Positive therapeutic outcome
- Absence of running or congested nose, rashes

Treatment of overdose:
Administer ipecac syrup or lavage, diazepam, vasopressors, barbiturates (short acting)

chlorpromazine
🗝 (℞)
(klor-proe'ma-zeen)
chlorpromazine HCl, Chlorpromanyl ✤, Thorazine, Thor-Prom
Func. class.: Antipsychotic/neuroleptic/antiemetic
Chem. class.: Phenothiazine, aliphatic

Pregnancy category C

Action: Depresses cerebral cortex, hypothalamus, limbic system, which control activity aggression; blocks neurotransmission produced by dopamine at synapse; exhibits a strong α-adrenergic, anticholinergic blocking action; mechanism for antipsychotic effects is unclear

⇒ **Therapeutic Outcome:** Decreased signs and symptoms of psychosis; control of nausea, vomiting, intractable hiccups, decreased anxiety preoperatively

Uses: Psychotic disorders, Tourette's syndrome, mania, schizophrenia, anxiety, intractable hiccups (adults), nausea, vomiting, preoperative relaxation, acute intermittent porphyria, P behavioral problems in children, nonpsychotic patients with dementia

Investigational uses: Vascular headache

Dosage and routes

Psychosis

Adult: PO 10-50 mg q1-4h initially, then increase up to 2 g/day if necessary; IM 10-50 mg q1-4h

G ***Elderly:*** Use lowest effective dose

P ***Child:*** PO 0.5 mg/kg q4-6h; IM 0.5 mg/kg q6-8h; REC 1 mg/kg q6-8h

Nausea and vomiting

Adult: PO 10-25 mg q4-6h prn; IM 25-50 mg q3h prn; rec 50-100 mg q6-8h prn, not to exceed 400 mg/day; **IV** 25-50 mg qd-qid

P ***Child ≥6 mo:*** PO 0.55 mg/kg q4-6h; IM q6-8h; REC 1.1 mg/kg q6-8h, max IM ≤5 yr or ≤22.7 kg 40 mg; max IM 5-10 yr or 22.7-45.5 kg 75 mg; **IV** 0.55 mg/kg q6-8h

Intractable hiccups

Adult: PO 25-50 mg tid-qid; IM 25-50 mg (used only if PO dose does not work); **IV** 25-50 mg in 500-1000 ml saline (only for severe hiccups)

Available forms: Tabs 10, 25, 50, 100, 200 mg; sus rel caps 30, 75, 150, 200, 300 mg; syr 10, 25, 100 mg/5 ml; conc 30, 40, 100 mg/ml; supp 25, 100 mg; inj 25 mg/ml

Adverse effects

CNS: **Neuroleptic malignant syndrome,** *extrapyramidal symptoms: pseudoparkinsonism, akathisia, dystonia, tardive dyskinesia,* seizures, *headache*

CV: *Orthostatic hypotension,* hypertension, **cardiac arrest,** ECG changes, **tachycardia**

EENT: Blurred vision, glaucoma, dry eyes

GI: *Dry mouth, nausea, vomiting, anorexia, constipation,* diarrhea, jaundice, weight gain

GU: Urinary retention, enuresis, impotence, amenorrhea, gynecomastia, breast engorgement

HEMA: Anemia, **leukopenia, leukocytosis, agranulocytosis**

INTEG: *Rash,* photosensitivity, dermatitis

RESP: **Laryngospasm,** dyspnea, **respiratory depression**

Contraindications: Hypersensitivity, circulatory collapse, liver damage, cerebral arteriosclerosis, coronary disease, severe hypertension/hypotension, blood dyscrasias, coma, P child <6 mo, brain damage, bone marrow depression, alcohol and barbiturate withdrawal, narrow-angle glaucoma

Precautions: Pregnancy **C,** lactation, seizure disorders, hypertension, hepatic disease, cardiac disease, G elderly, prostate enlargement

Do Not Confuse:
chlorpromazine/chlorothiazide, chlorpromazine/chlorpropamide, chlorpromazine/chlrothalidone, chlorpromazine/prochlorperazine

Pharmacokinetics

Absorption	Variable (PO); well absorbed (IM)
Distribution	Widely distributed; crosses placenta
Metabolism	Liver, GI mucosa extensively
Excretion	Kidneys
Half-life	30 hr

Pharmacodynamics

	PO	REC	IM	IV
Onset	½-1 hr	12 hr	Unkn	Rapid
Peak	Unkn	Unkn	Unkn	Unkn
Duration	4-6 hr*	3-4 hr	4-8 hr	Unkn

*Duration PO ext rel is 10-12 hr.

Interactions

Individual drugs

Alcohol: ↑ effects of both drugs, oversedation

Aluminum hydroxide: ↓ absorption

Bromocriptine: ↓ antiparkinsonian activity

Disopyramide: ↑ anticholinergic effects
Epinephrine: ↑ toxicity
Guanethidine: ↓ antihypertensive response
Levodopa: ↓ antiparkinsonian activity
Lithium: ↓ chlorpromazine levels, ↑ extrapyramidal symptoms, masking of lithium toxicity
Magnesium hydroxide: ↓ absorption
Norepinephrine: ↓ vasoresponse, ↑ toxicity
Phenobarbital: ↓ effectiveness, ↑ metabolism
Valproic acid: ↑ valproic acid level
Warfarin: ↓ anticoagulant effect

Drug classifications
Antacids: ↓ absorption
Anticholinergics: ↑ anticholinergic effects
Anticonvulsants: ↓ seizure threshold
Antidepressants: ↑ CNS depression
Antidiarrheals, adsorbent: ↓ absorption
Antihistamines: ↑ CNS depression
Antihypertensives: ↑ hypotension
Antithyroid agents: ↑ agranulocytosis
Barbiturate anesthetics: ↑ CNS depression
β-Adrenergic blockers: ↑ effects of both drugs
General anesthetics: ↑ CNS depression
MAOIs: ↑ CNS depression
Opioids: ↑ CNS depression
Sedative/hypnotics: ↑ CNS depression

Herb/drug
Kava: ↑ CNS depression
Henbane leaf: ↑ anticholinergic effect

Lab test interferences
↑ Liver function tests, ↑ cardiac enzymes, ↑ cholesterol, ↑ blood glucose, ↑ prolactin, ↑ bilirubin, ↑ PBI, ↑ cholinesterase I, ↑ alkaline phosphatase, ↑ leukocytes, ↑ granulocytes, ↑ platelets
↓ Hormones (blood and urine)
False positive: Pregnancy tests, PKU, urine bilirubin
False negative: Urinary steroids, 17-OHCS

NURSING CONSIDERATIONS

Assessment

- Assess mental status: orientation, mood, behavior, presence of hallucinations, and type before initial administration and monthly; this drug should significantly reduce psychotic behavior
- Assess any potentially reversible cause of behavior problems in the elderly before and during therapy
- Check for swallowing of PO medication; check for hoarding or giving of medication to other patients
- Monitor I&O ratio; palpate bladder if low urinary output occurs, especially in elderly; urinalysis recommended before, during prolonged therapy
- Monitor bilirubin, CBC, liver function studies monthly
- Assess affect, orientation, LOC, reflexes, gait, coordination, sleep pattern disturbances
- Monitor B/P with patient sitting, standing, and lying; take pulse and respirations q4h during initial treatment; establish baseline before starting treatment; report drops of 30 mm Hg; obtain baseline ECG, Q wave, and T wave changes
- Check for dizziness, faintness, palpitations, tachycardia on rising; severe orthostatic hypotension is common
- Identify for neuroleptic malignant syndrome: hyperpyrexia, muscle rigidity, increased CPK, altered mental status; drug should be discontinued
- Assess for extrapyramidal symptoms including akathisia (inability to sit still, no pattern to movements), tardive dyskinesia (bizarre movements of the jaw, mouth, tongue, extremities), pseudoparkinsonism (rigidity, tremors, pill rolling, shuffling gate); an antiparkinsonian drug should be prescribed

• Assess for constipation, urinary retention daily; if these occur, increase bulk, water in diet

Nursing diagnoses

✓ Thought processes, altered (uses)
✓ Coping, ineffective individual (uses)
✓ Knowledge deficit (teaching)
✓ Noncompliance (teaching)

Implementation

PO route

• Give drug in liquid form mixed in glass of juice or cola if hoarding is suspected

• Periodically attempt dosage reduction in patients with behavioral problems

• Give with full glass of water, milk; or give with food to decrease GI upset

• Do not crush, break, or chew time rel caps

• Store in tight, light-resistant container, oral sol in amber bottle

Rectal route

• Give after placing in refrigerator for 30 min if too soft to insert; this route is used for nausea, vomiting, hiccups

IM route

• Inject in deep muscle mass; do not give SC; may be diluted with 0.9% NaCl, 2% procaine as prescribed; do not administer sol with a precipitate

IV route

• Give by direct **IV** by diluting with 0.9% NaCl to a concentration of 1 mg/1 ml; administer at a rate of 1 mg/2 min

• Give by cont inf after diluting 50 mg/500-1000 ml of D_5W, $D_{10}W$, 0.9% NaCl, 0.45% NaCl, LR, Ringer's or combinations (used for intractable hiccups)

Syringe compatibilities: Atropine, benztropine, butorphanol, diphenhydramine, doxapram, droperidol, fentanyl, glycopyrrolate, hydromorphone, hydroxyzine, meperidine, metoclopramide, midazolam, morphine, pentazocine, perphenazine, prochlorperazine, promazine, promethazine, scopolamine

Syringe incompatibilities: Cimetidine, dimenhydrinate, heparin, pentobarbital, thiopental

Y-site compatibilities: Amsacrine, cisatracurium, cisplatin, cladribine, cyclophosphamide, cytarabine, doxorubicin, doxorubicin liposome, famotidine, filgrastim, fluconazole, granisetron, heparin, hydrocortisone, ondansetron, potassium chloride, propofol, teniposide, thiotepa, vinorelbine

Additive compatibilities: Ascorbic acid, ethacrynate, netilmicin, theophylline, vit B/C

Additive incompatibilities: Aminophylline, amphotericin B, ampicillin, chloramphenicol, chlorothiazide, methicillin, methohexital, penicillin G, phenobarbital

Patient/family education

• Teach patient to use good oral hygiene; frequent rinsing of mouth, sugarless gum for dry mouth

• Caution patient to avoid hazardous activities until drug response is determined; dizziness, blurred vision may occur

• Inform patient that orthostatic hypotension occurs often and to rise from sitting or lying position gradually, to remain lying down after IM injection for at least 30 min; tell patient to avoid hot tubs, hot showers, tub baths, since hypotension may occur; tell patient that in hot weather heat stroke may occur; take extra precautions to stay cool

• Advise patient to avoid abrupt withdrawal of this drug, or extrapyramidal symptoms may result; drug should be withdrawn slowly

• Teach patient to avoid OTC preparations (cough, hay fever, cold) unless approved by prescriber, since serious drug interactions may occur; avoid use with alcohol, CNS depressants, since increased drowsiness may occur

C

34• Caution patient to use sunscreen and sunglasses to prevent burns
• Teach patient about extrapyramidal symptoms and necessity of meticulous oral hygiene, since oral candidiasis may occur
• Instruct patient to take antacids 2 hr before or after taking this drug
• Instruct patient to report sore throat, malaise, fever, bleeding, mouth sores; if these occur, CBC should be drawn and drug discontinued
• Teach that urine may turn pink or red
• Teach patient to use contraceptive measures

Evaluation

Positive therapeutic outcome
• Decrease in emotional excitement, hallucinations, delusions, paranoia
• Reorganization of patterns of thought, speech
• Increase in target behaviors

Treatment of overdose: Lavage if orally ingested; provide airway, *do not induce vomiting or use epinephrine*

chlorthalidone (℞)

(klor-tha'li-doan)

Apo-Chlorthalidone ✤, Hygroton, Thalitone, Uridon ✤

Func. class.: Diuretic, antihypertensive

Chem. class.: Thiazide-like phthalimindine derivative

Pregnancy category B

Action: Acts on the distal tubule and thick ascending limb of the loop of Henle in the kidney, increasing excretion of sodium, water, chloride, magnesium, potassium, and bicarbonate, possible arteriolar dilation

➔ **Therapeutic Outcome:** Decreased B/P, decreased edema in lung tissues and peripherally, diuresis

Uses: Edema in congestive heart failure, nephrotic syndrome; may be used alone or as adjunct with antihypertensives; also for edema in corticosteroid, estrogen therapy

Dosage and routes

Adult: PO 25-200 mg/day or 200 mg every other day

G ***Elderly:*** PO 12.5 mg qd, initially

P ***Child:*** PO 2 mg/kg or 60 mg/m^2 3 ×/wk

Available forms: Tabs 25, 50, 100 mg

Adverse effects

CNS: Paresthesia, headache, *dizziness, fatigue, weakness,* fever

EENT: Blurred vision

ELECT: *Hypokalemia,* hypercalcemia, hyponatremia, hypochloremia, hypomagnesemia

GI: *Nausea, vomiting, anorexia,* constipation, diarrhea, cramps, pancreatitis, GI irritation, **hepatitis**

GU: *Frequency,* polyuria, **uremia,** glucosuria

HEMA: **Aplastic anemia, leukopenia, agranulocytosis, thrombocytopenia, neutropenia**

INTEG: Rash, urticaria, purpura, photosensitivity

META: *Hyperglycemia, hyperuricemia,* increased creatinine, BUN

Contraindications: Hypersensitivity to thiazides or sulfonamides, anuria, renal decompensation, lactation

Precautions: Hypokalemia, hepatic disease, gout, COPD, LE, diabetes G mellitus, elderly, pregnancy **B,** hyperlipidemia

Do Not Confuse:
chlorthalidone/chlorothiazide,
chlorthalidone/chlorpromazine,
chlorthalidone/chlorpropamide,
Hygroton/Regroton, Uridon ✤/Vicodin

Pharmacokinetics

Absorption	Well absorbed
Distribution	Extracellular spaces; crosses placenta
Metabolism	Liver
Excretion	Urine, unchanged (30%-60%)
Half-life	40 hr

Pharmacodynamics

Onset	2 hr
Peak	6 hr
Duration	24-72 hr

Interactions
Individual drugs
Alcohol: ↑ hypotensive effect
Allopurnol: ↑ toxicity
Amphotericin B: ↑ hypokalemia
Cholestyramine: ↓ absorption of chlorothalidone
Colestipol: ↓ absorption of chlorothalidone
Diazoxide: ↑ hyperglycemia, hyperuricemia, hypotension
Digitalis: ↑ toxicity
Lithium: ↑ toxicity
Mezlocillin: ↑ hypokalemia
Piperacillin: ↑ hypokalemia
Ticarcillin: ↑ hypokalemia
Drug classifications
Antihypertensives: ↑ antihypertensive effect
Nitrates: ↑ hypotension
Nondepolarizing skeletal muscle relaxants: ↑ toxicity
Glucocorticoids: ↑ hypokalemia
Sulfonylureas: ↓ effect of sulfonylurea
Food/drug
↑ Absorption
Herb/drug
Aloe: Potassium deficiency
Buckthorn bark/berry: Potassium deficiency
Cascara sagrada bark: Potassium deficiency
Licorice root: Potassium deficiency
Senna pod/leaf: Potassium deficiency

Lab test interferences
↑ BSP retention, ↑ triglycerides, ↑ calcium, ↑ amylase
↓ PBI, ↓ PSP

NURSING CONSIDERATIONS
Assessment
- Monitor manifestations of hypokalemia; *CV:* hypotension, broad T wave, U wave, ectopy, tachycardia, weak pulse; *GI:* anorexia, nausea, cramps, constipation, distention, paralytic ileus; *NEURO:* muscle weakness, altered LOC, drowsiness, apathy, lethargy, confusion, depression; *RENAL:* acidic urine, reduced urine, osmolality, nocturia; *RESP:* hypoventilation, respiratory muscle weakness
- Monitor for manifestations of hypomagnesemia; *CNS:* agitation, muscle twitching, paresthesias, hyperactive reflexes, positive Babinski's reflex, dysphagia, nystagmus seizures, tetany; *CV:* ectopy, tachycardia, broad, flat or inverted T waves, depressed ST segment, prolonged QT, decreased cardiac output, hypotension; *GI:* nausea, vomiting, diarrhea, anorexia, abdominal distention
- Monitor for manifestations of hyponatremia; *CV:* increased B/P, cold, clammy skin, hypovolemia or hypervolemia; *GI:* anorexia, nausea, vomiting, diarrhea, abdominal cramps; *NEURO:* lethargy, increased ICP, confusion, headache, seizures, coma, fatigue, tremors, hyperreflexia
- Monitor for manifestations of hyperchloremia; *NEURO:* weakness, lethargy, coma; *RESP:* coma, deep rapid breathing
- Assess fluid volume status: I&O ratios and record, count or weigh diapers as appropriate, weight, distended red veins, crackles in lung, color, quality and sp gr of urine, skin turgor, adequacy of pulses, moist mucous membranes, bilateral lung sounds, peripheral pitting edema; dehydration symptoms of decreasing output, thirst, hypotension, dry mouth,

and mucous membranes should be reported
- Monitor electrolytes: potassium, sodium, calcium, magnesium; also include BUN, blood pH, ABGs, uric acid, CBC, blood sugar
- Assess B/P before and during therapy with patient lying, standing, and sitting as appropriate; orthostatic hypotension can occur rapidly

Nursing diagnoses

✓ Altered urinary elimination (side effect)
✓ Fluid volume deficit (adverse reactions)
✓ Fluid volume excess (uses)
✓ Knowledge deficit (teaching)

Implementation

- Brand names Thalitone/Hygroton should not be used interchangeably
- Give in AM to avoid interference with sleep
- Provide potassium replacement if potassium level is 3.0 mg/dl; give whole, or use oral solutions lightly; drug may be crushed if patient is unable to swallow
- Give with food; if nausea occurs, may crush tab and mix with fluids or applesauce for swallowing

Patient/family education

General

- Teach patient to take the medication early in the day to prevent nocturia
- Instruct patient to take with food or milk if GI symptoms of nausea and anorexia occur
- Teach patient to maintain weekly record of weight and notify prescriber of weight loss >5 lb
- Caution patient that this drug causes a loss of potassium, so foods rich in potassium should be added to the diet; refer to a dietician for assistance in planning
- Caution the patient not to exercise in hot weather or stand for prolonged periods, since orthostatic hypotension will be enhanced; to use sunscreen to prevent burns
- Teach patient not to use alcohol, or any OTC medications without prescriber's approval; serious drug reactions may occur
- Emphasize the need to contact prescriber immediately if muscle cramps, weakness, nausea, dizziness, or numbness occurs
- Teach patient to take own B/P and pulse and record
- Caution patient that orthostatic hypotension may occur; patient should rise slowly from sitting or reclining positions and lie down if dizziness occurs
- Teach patient to continue taking medication even if feeling better; this drug controls symptoms but does not cure the condition
- Advise patient with hypertension to continue other medical treatment (exercise, weight loss, relaxation techniques, cessation of smoking)

Evaluation

Positive therapeutic outcome

- Decreased edema
- Decreased B/P
- Increased diuresis

Treatment of overdose:

Lavage if taken orally, monitor electrolytes; administer dextrose in saline; monitor hydration, CV, renal status

cholecalciferol

See vitamin D

C

cholestyramine

Key Drug (℞)

(koe-less-tear′a-meen)

LoCholest Light, Prevalite, Questran, Questran Light

Func. class.: Antilipemic

Chem. class.: Bile acid sequestrant

Pregnancy category C

Action: Absorbs, combines with bile acids to form an insoluble complex that is excreted through feces; loss of bile acids lowers cholesterol levels

Therapeutic Outcome: Decreasing cholesterol levels and low-density lipoproteins, decreased pruritus

Uses: Primary hypercholesterolemia, pruritus associated with biliary obstruction, diarrhea caused by excess bile acid, xanthomas

Dosage and routes

Adult: PO 4 g ac and hs, not to exceed 32 g/day

P ***Child:*** PO 240 mg/kg/day in 3 divided doses; administer with food or drink, max 8 g/day

Available forms: Powder 4 g/ cholestyramine of 9 g

Adverse effects

CNS: Headache, dizziness, drowsiness, vertigo, tinnitus

GI: *Constipation, abdominal pain, nausea,* fecal impaction, hemorrhoids, flatulence, vomiting, steatorrhea, peptic ulcer

HEMA: **Bleeding,** decreased pro-time

INTEG: Rash, irritation of perianal area, tongue, skin

META: Decreased vit A, D, K, red cell folate content, **hyperchloremic acidosis**

MS: Muscle, joint pain

Contraindications: Hypersensitivity, biliary obstruction

Precautions: Pregnancy **C,** lactation, children P

Pharmacokinetics

Absorption	Not absorbed
Distribution	Not distributed
Metabolism	Not metabolized
Excretion	Binds with bile acids, feces
Half-life	Unknown

Pharmacodynamics

Onset	24-48 hr
Peak	1-3 wk
Duration	2-4 wk

Interactions

Individual drugs

Acetaminophen: ↓ absorption

Iron: ↓ absorption

Thyroid hormones: ↓ absorption

Drug classifications

Anticoagulants, oral: ↓ absorption

β-Adrenergic blockers: ↓ absorption

Cardiac glycosides: ↓ absorption

Vitamins A, D, E, K: ↓ absorption

Lab test interferences

Interference: Cholecystography

NURSING CONSIDERATIONS

Assessment

- Assess nutrition: fat, protein, carbohydrates, nutritional analysis should be completed by dietician
- Assess skin integrity after patient has been receiving drug; itching, pruritus often occur from bile deposits on skin
- Monitor cardiac glycoside level if both drugs are being administered; cardiac glycoside levels will be decreased
- Monitor for signs of vit A, D, E, K deficiency; fasting LDL, HDL, total cholesterol, triglyceride levels, electrolytes if on extended therapy
- Monitor bowel pattern daily; increase bulk, water in diet if constipation develops

Nursing diagnoses

- ✓ Constipation (adverse reactions)
- ✓ Knowledge deficit (teaching)
- ✓ Noncompliance (teaching)

Implementation

- Give drug ac, hs; give all other medications 1 hr before cholestyramine or 4 hr after cholestyramine to avoid poor absorption; do not take dry; mix drug with applesauce or stir into beverage (2-6 oz); let stand for 2 min; avoid inhaling powder
- Provide supplemental doses of vit A, D, E, K, if levels are low

Patient/family education

- Teach patient symptoms of hypoprothrombinemia: bleeding mucous membranes, dark tarry stools, hematuria, petechiae; report immediately
- Teach patient importance of compliance
- Teach patient that risk factors should be decreased: high-fat diet, smoking, alcohol consumption, absence of exercise
- Have patient mix drug with 6 oz of milk, water, fruit juice; do not mix with carbonated beverages; rinse glass to make sure all medication is taken or may mix drug in applesauce; allow to stand for 2 min before mixing

Evaluation

Positive therapeutic outcome

- Decreased cholesterol level (hyperlipidemia)
- Decreased diarrhea, pruritus (excess bile acids)

choline salicylate (℞)

(koe'leen sa-lis'ih-late)

Arthropan, Teejel ✱

choline/magnesium salicylates (℞)

CMT, Tricosal, Trilisate

Func. class.: Nonnarcotic analgesic

Chem. class.: Salicylate

Pregnancy category C

Action: Blocks pain impulses in CNS that occur in response to inhibition of prostaglandin synthesis; antipyretic action results from inhibition of hypothalamic heat-regulating center to produce vasodilatation to allow heat dissipation

Therapeutic Outcome: Decreased pain, inflammation, fever

Uses: Mild to moderate pain or fever including arthritis, juvenile rheumatoid arthritis

Dosage and routes

Choline salicylate

Adult and child >12 yr: PO 870-1740 mg qid; max 6×/day

Pain/fever

Adult: PO 435-870 mg q3-4h prn

Choline/magnesium salicylates

Adult: PO 2-3 g salicylate/day divided bid-tid

Child >37 kg: PO 2.2 g of salicylate/day divided bid

Child <37 kg: PO 50 mg of salicylate/kg/day divided bid

Available forms: Choline salicylate liq 870 mg/5 ml; choline/magnesium salicylate tabs 500, 750, 1000 mg; liq 500 mg/5 ml

Adverse effects

CNS: Stimulation, drowsiness, dizziness, confusion, **convulsion,** headache, flushing, hallucinations, **coma**

CV: Rapid pulse, pulmonary edema

EENT: Tinnitus, hearing loss

ENDO: Hypoglycemia, hyponatremia, hypokalemia

GI: *Nausea, vomiting, GI bleeding, diarrhea, heartburn,* anorexia, **hepatitis, hepatotoxicity**

HEMA: **Thrombocytopenia, agranulocytosis, leukopenia, neutropenia, hemolytic anemia,** increased pro-time

INTEG: *Rash,* urticaria, bruising, sweating

RESP: Wheezing, hyperpnea, hyperventilation

Contraindications: Hypersensitivity to salicylates, GI bleeding, **P** bleeding disorders, children <3 yr, vit **P** K deficiency, children with flulike symptoms

Precautions: Anemia, hepatic disease, renal disease, Hodgkin's disease, pregnancy **C**, lactation

Pharmacokinetics

Absorption	Well absorbed
Distribution	Widely distributed; crosses placenta
Metabolism	Liver, extensively
Excretion	Kidney, active metabolites; breast milk
Half-life	2-3 hr (low doses); 15-30 hr (high doses)

Pharmacodynamics

Onset	15-30 min
Peak	1-3 hr
Duration	3-6 hr

Interactions

Individual drugs

Alcohol: ↑ bleeding
Cefamandole: ↑ bleeding
Furosemide: ↑ toxic effects
Heparin: ↑ bleeding
Insulin: ↑ effects
Methotrexate: ↑ effects
PABA: ↑ toxic effects
Penicillins: ↑ effects
Phenytoin: ↑ effects
Plicamycin: ↑ bleeding
Probenecid: ↓ effects
Spironolactone: ↓ effects
Sulfinpyrazone: ↓ effects
Valproic acid: ↑ effects, ↑ bleeding
Vancomycin: ↑ ototoxicity

Drug classifications

Antacids: ↓ effects of choline salicylate
Anticoagulants: ↑ effects
Carbonic anhydrase inhibitors: ↑ toxic effects
NSAIDs: ↑ gastric ulcers
Penicillins: ↑ effects
Salicylates: ↓ blood sugar levels
Steroids: ↓ effects of choline salicylate, ↑ gastric ulcers
Sulfonylamides: ↓ effects
Urinary acidifiers: ↑ salicylate levels
Urinary alkalizers: ↓ effects of choline salicylate

Food/drug

Foods that acidify the urine ↑ salicylate level

Lab test interferences

↑ Coagulation studies, ↑ liver function studies, ↑ serum uric acid, ↑ amylase, ↑ CO_2, ↑ urinary protein, ↓ Serum potassium, ↓ PBI, ↓ cholesterol
Interference: Urine catecholamines, pregnancy test, urine glucose tests (Clinistix, Tes-Tape)

NURSING CONSIDERATIONS

Assessment

- Monitor pain: location, duration, type, intensity, before dose and 1 hr after
- Monitor musculoskeletal status: ROM before dose
- Identify fever, length of time and related symptoms
- Monitor liver function studies: AST, ALT, bilirubin, creatinine if patient is on long-term therapy
- Monitor renal function studies: BUN, urine creatinine if patient is on long-term therapy
- Monitor blood studies: CBC, Hct, Hgb, pro-time if patient is on long-term therapy
- Check I&O ratio; decreasing output may indicate renal failure (long-term therapy)
- (Alert) Assess hepatotoxicity: dark urine, clay-colored stools, yellowing of the skin and sclera, itching, abdominal pain, fever, diarrhea if patient is on long-term therapy
- Assess for allergic reactions: rash, urticaria; if these occur, drug may have to be discontinued
- Assess for ototoxicity: tinnitus, ringing, roaring in ears; audiometric testing needed before, after long-term therapy

- Assess for visual changes: blurring, halos; corneal, retinal damage
- Check edema in feet, ankles, legs
- Identify prior drug history; there are many drug interactions

Nursing diagnoses

✓ Pain (uses)
✓ Mobility, impaired physical (uses)
✓ Knowledge deficit (teaching)
✓ Injury, risk for (side effects)

Implementation

- Administer to patient crushed or whole
- Give with food or milk to decrease gastric symptoms; give 30 min ac or 2 hr pc; absorption may be slowed
- Give antacids 1-2 hr after enteric products

Patient/family education

- Teach patient to report any symptoms of hepatotoxicity, renal toxicity, visual changes, ototoxicity, allergic reactions, bleeding (long-term therapy)
- Advise patient to take with 8 oz of water and sit upright for 30 min after dose
- Caution patient not to exceed recommended dosage; acute poisoning may result
- Caution patient to read label on other OTC drugs; many contain aspirin products
- Inform patient that the therapeutic response takes 2 wk (arthritis)
- Teach patient to report tinnitus, confusion, diarrhea, sweating, hyperventilation
- Caution patient to avoid alcohol ingestion; GI bleeding may occur
- Teach patient that patients who have allergies may develop allergic reactions
- Caution patient to avoid buffered or effervescent products
- Teach patient not to give to P children; Reye's syndrome may develop

Evaluation

Positive therapeutic outcome

- Decreased pain
- Decreased inflammation
- Decreased fever
- Increased mobility

Treatment of overdose:

Lavage, activated charcoal, monitor electrolytes, VS

choriogonadotropin

(℞)

(chore-i-oh-gon′a-doe-troe-pin)

Ovidrel

Func. class.: Ovulation stimulant

Pregnancy category X

Action: hCG is an analog of LH and binds to LH/hCG receptor

➔ **Therapeutic Outcome:** Fertility

Uses: Final follicular maturation ovulation induction

Dosage and routes

Infertile women undergoing ovulation induction

Adult: SC 250 μg single dose after last dose of FS agent

Infertile women undergoing assisted reproduction therapy

Adult: SC 250 μg/day after last dose of FS agent

Available forms: Powder for inj, lyophilized 285 μg r-hCG

Adverse effects

CV: Vasomotor flushing, phlebitis, ***deep-vein thrombosis***

CNS: Headache, depression, restlessness, anxiety, nervousness, fatigue, insomnia, dizziness, flushing, lability

GI: *Nausea, vomiting, abdominal pain, bloating,* diarrhea

GU: Polyuria, urinary frequency, birth defects, spontaneous abortions,

multiple ovulation, breast pain, oliguria, abnormal uterine bleeding
INTEG: Rash

Contraindications: Hypersensitivity, pregnancy **X,** hepatic disease, undiagnosed uterine bleeding, uncontrolled thyroid or adrenal dysfunction, intracranial lesion, ovarian cysts

Precautions: Hypertension, depression, convulsions, diabetes mellitus

Pharmacokinetics

Absorption	Unknown
Distribution	Unknown
Metabolism	Unknown
Excretion	Unknown
Half-life	29 hr

Pharmacodynamics

Unknown

Interactions

None known

Lab test interferences:

↑ FSH/LH, ↑ ALT

NURSING CONSIDERATIONS

Nursing diagnoses

✓ Knowledge deficit (teaching)

Implementation

- After reconstituting with 1 ml sterile water for inj, discard unused portion, store vial at room temp, protect from light

Patient/family education

- Advise that multiple births are common
- Advise to notify prescriber immediately if low abdominal pain occurs; may indicate ovarian cyst, cyst rupture
- Teach the method for taking, recording basal body temp to determine whether ovulation has occurred
- Teach if ovulation can be determined (there is a slight decrease in temp, then a sharp increase for ovulation), to attempt coitus 3 days before and qod until after ovulation
- Teach if pregnancy is suspected, to notify prescriber immediately

Evaluation

Positive therapeutic outcome

- Fertility

cidofovir (℞)

(si-doh-foh′veer)

Vistide

Func. class.: Antiviral

Chem. class.: Nucleotide analog

Pregnancy category C

Action: Suppresses cytomegalovirus (CMV) replication by selective inhibition of viral DNA synthesis

➔ **Therapeutic Outcome:** Decreased symptoms of CMV

Uses: CMV retinitis in patients with HIV, used with probenecid

Dosage and routes

Dilute in 100 ml 0.9% NaCl sol before administration; probenecid must be given PO 2 g 3 hr before the cidofovir inf and 1 g at 2 and 8 hr after ending the cidofovir inf; give 1 L of 0.9% NaCl before sol **IV** with each inf of cidovovir, give saline inf over 1-2 hr period immediately before cidofovir; patient should be given a second L if the patient can tolerate the fluid load; second L given at time of cidofovir or immediately afterward and should be given over a 1-3 hr period

Renal dose

CrCl <50 ml/min reduce dose

Induction

Adult: IV inf initially 5 mg/kg given over 1 hr at a constant rate qwk × 2 consecutive wk

Maintenance

Adult: IV inf 5 mg/kg given over 1 hr q2 wk

Available forms: Inj

Adverse effects

CNS: Fever, chills, **coma,** confusion,

abnormal thought, *dizziness,* bizarre dreams, *headache,* psychosis, tremors, somnolence, paresthesia, *amnesia, anxiety, insomnia,* **seizures**
CV: **Dysrhythmias,** hypertension/hypotension
EENT: Retinal detachment in CMV retinitis
GI: Abnormal LFTs, nausea, vomiting, anorexia, diarrhea, abdominal pain, **hemorrhage**
GU: **Hematuria,** increased creatinine, BUN, **nephrotoxicity**
HEMA: **Granulocytopenia, thrombocytopenia, irreversible neutropenia, anemia, eosinophilia**
INTEG: Rash, alopecia, pruritus, acne, urticaria, pain at inj site, phlebitis
RESP: Dyspnea

Contraindications: Hypersensitivity to this drug or probenecid, sulfa drugs

Precautions: Preexisting cytopenias, renal function impairment, P pregnancy **C**, lactation, children G <6 mo, elderly, platelet count <25,000/mm^3

Pharmacokinetics

Unknown

Pharmacodynamics

Unknown

Interactions

Individual drugs

Amphotericin B: ↑ nephrotoxicity
Foscarnet: ↑ nephrotoxicity
Pentamidine IV: ↑ nephrotoxicity

Drug classifications

Aminoglycosides: ↑ nephrotoxicity
NSAIDS: ↑ nephrotoxicity

NURSING CONSIDERATIONS

Assessment

- Obtain culture before treatment is initiated; cultures of blood, urine, and throat may all be taken; CMV is not confirmed by this method; the diagnosis is made by an ophthalmic exam
- Monitor kidney, liver function, increased hemopoietic studies and BUN; serum creatinine, AST, ALT, creatinine, creatinine clearance, A-G ratio, baseline and drip treatment, blood counts should be done q2wk; watch for decreasing granulocytes, Hgb; if low, therapy may have to be discontinued and restarted after hematologic recovery; blood transfusions may be required
- Assess for GI symptoms: severe nausea, vomiting, diarrhea; severe symptoms may necessitate discontinuing drug
- Assess electrolytes and minerals: calcium, phosphorous, magnesium, sodium, potassium; watch closely for tetany during first administration
- Assess for symptoms of blood dyscrasias (anemia, granulocytopenia); bruising, fatigue, bleeding, poor healing
- Assess allergic reactions: flushing, rash, urticaria, pruritus
- Assess for leukopenia, neutropenia, thrombocytopenia: WBCs, platelets q2 days during 2 ×/day dosing and qwk thereafter; check for leukopenias, with qd WBC count in patients with prior leukopenia, with other nucleoside analogs, or for whom leukopenia counts are <1000 cells/mm^3 at start of treatment
- Monitor serum creatinine or creatinine clearance at least q2 wk; give only to those with creatinine levels ≤1.5 mg/dl, CrCl >55 ml/min, urine protein <100 mg/dl

Nursing diagnoses

✓ Infection, risk for (uses)

Implementation

- Mix under strict aseptic conditions using gloves, gown and mask, and using precautions for antineoplastics
- Administer after diluting in 100 ml of 0.9% NaCl

• Give slowly; do not give by bolus **IV**, **IV**, SC inj
• Use diluted sol within 12 hr, do not refrigerate or freeze; do not use sol with particulate matter or discoloration

Patient/family education
• Advise to notify prescriber if sore throat, swollen lymph nodes, malaise, fever occur, may indicate other infections
• Advise to report perioral tingling, numbness in extremities, and paresthesias
• Teach that serious drug interactions may occur if OTC products are ingested; check first with prescriber
• Teach that drug is not a cure, but will control symptoms
• Advise that regular ophthalmic exams must be continued
• Advise that major toxicities may necessitate discontinuing drug
• Advise to use contraception during treatment and that infertility may occur; men should use barrier contraception for 90 days after treatment

Evaluation
Positive therapeutic outcome
• Decreased symptoms of CMV

Treatment of overdose: Discontinue drug; use hemodialysis, and increase hydration

cilastatin
See imipenem/cilastatin

cilostazol
(sil-oo-stay'zole)
Pletal
Func. class.: Platelet aggregation inhibitor
Chem. class.: Quinolinone derivative
Pregnancy category C

Action: Inhibits cellular phosphodiesterase; reversibly inhibits platelet aggregation induced by thrombin, ADP, collagen, arachidonic acid, epinephrine, and shear stress

➔ **Therapeutic Outcome:** Increased walking distance

Uses: Intermittent claudication

Dosage and routes
Adult: PO 100 mg bid taken ≥30 min ac or 2 hr pc breakfast and dinner or 50 mg bid, if using drugs that inhibit CYP3A4; 12 wk of treatment may be needed

Available forms: Tab 50, 100 mg

Adverse effects
CNS: *Dizziness,* headache
CV: *Palpitations, tachycardia,* **nodal arrhythmia,** postural hypotension
EENT: Blindness, diplopia, ear pain, tinnitus, retinal hemorrhage
GI: *Nausea, vomiting, diarrhea, GI disorder,* colitis, cholelithiasis, ulcer, esophagitis, gastritis, anorexia, flatulence, dyspepsia
GU: Cystitis, frequency, vaginitis, **vaginal hemorrhage**
HEMA: **Bleeding (epistaxis, hematuria, retinal hemorrhage, GI bleeding), thrombocytopenia,** anemia, polycythemia
INTEG: *Rash,* urticaria, dry skin
MISC: *Back pain, infection, myalgia, peripheral edema,* chills, fever, malaise, diabetes mellitus
RESP: *Cough, pharyngitis, rhinitis,* asthma, pneumonia

Contraindications: Hypersensitivity, CHF

Precautions: Past liver disease, renal disease, [G] elderly, pregnancy **C**, lactation, [P] children, increased bleeding risk, low platelet count, platelet dysfunction, active bleeding

Pharmacokinetics

Absorption	Unknown
Distribution	95%-98% protein binding
Metabolism	Hepatic extensively by cytochrome P450 enzymes
Excretion	Urine (74%), feces (20%)
Half-life	11-13 hrs

Pharmacodynamics

Unknown

Interactions

Individual drugs

Diltiazem: ↑ cilostazol levels
Erythromycin: ↑ cilostazol levels
Fluconazole: May ↑ cilostazol levels; reduce dose to 50 mg bid
Fluoxetine: May ↑ cilostazol levels; reduce dose to 50 mg bid
Fluvoxamine: May ↑ cilostazol levels; reduce dose to 50 mg bid
Itraconazole: May ↑ cilostazol levels; reduce dose to 50 mg bid
Ketoconazole: May ↑ cilostazol levels; reduce dose to 50 mg bid
Nefazodone: May ↑ cilostazol levels; reduce dose to 50 mg bid
Omeprazole: May ↑ cilostazol levels; reduce dose to 50 mg bid

Drug classifications

Anticoagulants: May ↑ bleeding tendencies

Food/drug

- Do not use with grapefruit juice

NURSING CONSIDERATIONS

Assessment

- Assess for underlying CV disease since cardiovascular risk is great
- Assess for CV lesions with repeated oral administration
- Assess for CHF
- Monitor blood studies: CBC, Hct, Hgb, pro-time if patient is on long-term therapy; thrombocytopenia, neutropenia may occur

Nursing diagnoses

✓ Injury, risk for (uses)
✓ Knowledge deficit (teaching)

Implementation

- Give bid ≥1 hr ac or 2 hr pc; do not give with grapefruit juice

Patient/family education

- Advise patient to report any unusual bleeding to prescriber
- Caution patient to report side effects such as diarrhea, skin rashes, subcutaneous bleeding
- Teach patient that effects may take 2-4 wk, treatment of up to 12 wk may be required for necessary effect
- Teach patients with CHF about potential risks
- Advise patient to take ≥30 min ac or 2 hr pc
- Advise patient that reading patient package insert is necessary

Evaluation

Positive therapeutic outcome

- Increased walking distance and duration
- Decreased pain

cimetidine (℞, OTC)

(sye-met'i-deen)

Apo-Cimetidine ♣, cimetidine, Novocimetine ♣, Peptol ♣ Tagamet, Tagamet HBL

Func. class.: H_2-receptor antagonist
Chem. class.: Imidazole derivative

Pregnancy category B

Action: Inhibits histamine at H_2-receptor site in the gastric parietal cells, which inhibits gastric acid secretion

➔ Therapeutic Outcome: Healing of duodenal or gastric ulcers; prevention of duodenal ulcers; decreases symptoms of gastroesophageal reflux disease (GERD) and Zollinger-Ellison syndrome

Uses: Short-term treatment of duodenal and gastric ulcers and maintenance; management of GERD and Zollinger-Ellison syndrome

Investigational uses: Prevention of aspiration pneumonitis, stress ulcers, upper GI bleeding, herpes infection, hirsutism, urticaria, cutaneous/nongenital warts, weight loss

Dosage and routes

Treatment of active ulcers

P ***Adult and child:*** PO 300 mg qid with meals, hs × 8 wk or 400 mg bid, 800 mg hs; after 8 wk give hs dose only; **IV** bol 300 mg/20 ml 0.9% NaCl over 1-2 min q6h; **IV** inf 300 mg/50 ml D_5W over 15-20 min; IM 300 mg q6h, not to exceed 2400 mg

P ***Child:*** PO 20-40 mg/kg/day; IM/**IV** 5-10 mg/kg q6-8h

Prophylaxis of duodenal ulcer

P ***Adult and child >16 yr:*** 400 mg hs

GERD

Adult: PO 800-1600 mg/day in divided doses

Hypersecretory conditions (Zollinger-Ellison syndrome)

Adult: PO/IM/**IV** 300-600 mg q6h; may increase to 12 g/day if needed

Upper GI bleeding prophylaxis

Adult: **IV** 50 mg/hr; lowered in renal disease

Aspiration pneumonitis prophylaxis

Adult: **IV** 300 mg 1 hr before anesthesia, then 300 mg **IV** q4h until patient is alert, max 2400 mg/day

Weight loss

Adult: PO 200-400 mg tid × 8-12 wk

Warts

Adult: PO 400-800 mg tid × 12 wk or 30-40 mg/kg/day given tid × 3 mo

Hirsutism

Adult: PO 300 mg × 5 times/day or 1600 mg qd up to 6 mo

Renal dose

CrCl 20-40 ml/min 300 mg q8h; CrCl <20 ml/min 300 mg q12h

Available forms: Tabs 100, 200, 300, 400, 800 mg; liq 200, 300 mg/5 ml; inj 300 mg/2 ml, 300 mg/50 ml 0.9% NaCl

Adverse effects

CNS: *Confusion, headache,* depression, dizziness, anxiety, weakness, psychosis, tremors, **convulsions**
CV: Bradycardia, tachycardia, **dysrhythmias**
GI: *Diarrhea,* abdominal cramps, **paralytic ileus,** *jaundice*
GU: Gynecomastia, galactorrhea, impotence, increase in BUN, creatinine
HEMA: **Agranulocytosis, thrombocytopenia, neutropenia, aplastic anemia, increase in pro-time**
INTEG: Urticaria, rash, alopecia, sweating, flushing, **exfoliative dermatitis**

Contraindications: Hypersensitivity

Precautions: Pregnancy **B,** lactation, P child <16 yr, organic brain syndrome, hepatic disease, renal disease, G elderly

Pharmacokinetics

Absorption	Well absorbed (PO, IM); completely absorbed (**IV**)
Distribution	Widely distributed; crosses placenta
Metabolism	Liver (30%)
Excretion	Kidneys, unchanged (70%); breast milk
Half-life	1½-2 hr; increased in renal disease

Pharmacodynamics

	PO	IV/IM
Onset	½ hr	10 min
Peak	45-90 min	½ hr
Duration	4-5 hr	4-5 hr

Interactions

Individual drugs

Carbamazepine: ↑ toxicity (cytochrome P450 pathway)
Chloroquine: ↑ toxicity (cytochrome P450 pathway)
Ketoconazole: ↓ absorption of cimetidine
Lidocaine: ↑ toxicity
Metronidazole: ↑ toxicity (cytochrome P450 pathway)
Moricizine: ↑ toxicity (cytochrome P450 pathway)
Procainamide: ↑ toxicity
Quinidine: ↑ toxicity
Quinine: ↑ toxicity (cytochrome P450 pathway)
Warfarin: ↑ toxicity
Valproic acid: ↑ toxicity (cytochrome P450 pathway)

Drug classifications

Antacids: ↓ absorption of cimetidine
Antidepressants, tricyclic: ↑ toxicity
Benzodiazepines: ↑ toxicity
β-Adrenergic blockers: ↑ toxicity
Calcium channel blockers: ↑ toxicity (cytochrome P450 pathway)
Iron salts: ↓ absorption of iron salts
Phenytoins: ↑ toxicity
Sulfonylureas: ↑ toxicity (cytochrome P450 pathway)
Theophyllines: ↑ toxicity

Lab test interferences

↑ Alkaline phosphatase, ↑ AST, ↑ creatinine, prolactin
False positive: Gastroccult **False negative:** Skin allergy tests

NURSING CONSIDERATIONS

Assessment

- Assess patient with ulcers or suspected ulcers: epigastric or abdominal pain, hematemesis, occult blood in stools, blood in gastric aspirate before and/or throughout treatment; monitor gastric pH (5 or > should be maintained)
- Monitor I&O ratio, BUN, creatinine, CBC with differential periodically

Nursing diagnoses

☑ Pain (uses)
☑ Knowledge deficit (teaching)

Implementation

PO route

- Give with meals for lengthened drug effect; antacids 1 hr before or 1 hr after cimetidine

IV **IV route**

- Give by direct **IV** after diluting 300 mg/20 ml of 0.9% NaCl for inj; give over 5 min or more
- Give intermittent **IV** by diluting 300 mg/50 ml of D_5W; run over 15-20 min
- Give by cont inf after using total daily dose (900 mg) diluted in 100-1000 ml D_5W given over 24 hr
- Store diluted sol at room temp up to 48 hr

Syringe compatibilities:
Atropine, butorphanol, cephalothin, diazepam, diphenhydramine, doxapram, droperidol, fentanyl, glycopyrrolate, heparin, hydromorphone, hydroxyzine, lorazepam, meperidine, midazolam, morphine, nafcillin, nalbuphine, penicillin G sodium, pentazocine, perphenazine, prochlorperazine, promazine, promethazine, scopolamine

Syringe incompatibilities:
Cefamandole, cefazolin, chlorpromazine, pentobarbital, secobarbital

Y-site compatibilities:
Acyclovir, amifostine, aminophylline, amrinone, atracurium, aztreonam, cisatracurium, cisplatin, cladribine, cyclosphosphamide, cytarabine, diltiazem, doxorubicin, doxorubicin liposome, enalaprilat, esmolol, filgrastim, fluconazole, fludarabine, foscarnet, gallium, granisetron,

haloperidol, heparin, hetastarch, idarubicin, labetalol, melphalan, meropenem, methotrexate, midazolam, ondansetron, paclitaxel, pancuronium, piperacillin/tazobactam, propofol, sargramostim, tacrolimus, teniposide, theophylline, thiotepa, tolazoline, vecuronium, vinorelbine, zidovudine

Y-site incompatibilities: Amsacrine

Additive compatibilities: Acetazolamide, amikacin, aminophylline, atracurium, cefoperazone, cefoxitin, chlorothiazide, clindamycin, colistimethate, dexamethasone, digoxin, epinephrine, erythromycin, ethacrynate, floxacillin, flumazenil, furosemide, gentamicin, insulin, isoproterenol, lidocaine, lincomycin, meropenem, metaraminol, methylprednisolone, norepinephrine, penicillin G potassium, phytonadione, polymyxin B, potassium chloride, protamine, quinidine, tacrolimus, tetracycline, vancomycin, verapamil, vit B complex, vit B/C

Additive incompatibilities: Amphotericin B

Patient/family education

- Advise patient that any gynecomastia or impotence that develops is reversible after treatment is discontinued
- Caution patient to avoid driving, other hazardous activities until stabilized on this medication; drowsiness or dizziness may occur
- Advise patient to avoid black pepper, caffeine, alcohol, harsh spices, extremes in temp of food; tell patient to avoid OTC preparations: aspirin, cough, cold preparations; condition may worsen
- Advise patient that smoking decreases the effectiveness of the drug; smoking cessation should be considered
- Teach patient that drug must be continued for prescribed time to be effective and taken exactly as prescribed; doses are not to be doubled; to take missed dose when remembered up to 1 hr before next dose
- Instruct patient to report bruising, fatigue, malaise; blood dyscrasias may occur
- Have patient report to prescriber immediately any diarrhea, black tarry stools, sore throat, dizziness, confusion, or delirium

Evaluation

Positive therapeutic outcome

- Decreased pain in abdomen
- Healing of ulcers
- Absence of gastroesophageal reflux
- Gastric pH of ≥5

ciprofloxacin (Key Drug) (℞)

(sip-ro-floks'a-sin)

Cipro, Cipro IV

Func. class.: Urinary antiinfectives

Chem. class.: Fluoroquinolone

Pregnancy category C

Action: Interferes with conversion of intermediate DNA fragments into high-molecular-weight DNA in bacteria; DNA gyrase inhibitor

Therapeutic Outcome: Bactericidal action against the following: gram-positive organisms *Staphylococcus epidermidis,* methicillin-resistant strains of *Staphylococcus aureus, Streptococcus pyogenes, Streptococcus pneumoniae;* gram-negative organisms *Escherichia coli, Klebsiella* species, *Enterobacter, Salmonella, Shigella, Proteus vulgaris, Providencia stuartii, Providencia rettgeri, Morganella morganii, Pseudomonas aeruginosa, Serratia, Haemophilus, Acinetobacter, Neisseria gonorrhoeae, Neisseria meningitidis, Branhamella catarrhalis, Yersinia, Vibrio, Brucella, Campylobacter, Aeromonas*

Uses: Adult urinary tract infections (including complicated); chronic bacterial prostatitis; acute sinusitis; lower respiratory, skin, bone, joint infections; infectious diarrhea, exposure to inhalation anthrax; conjunctivitis, corneal ulcers (ophthalmic)

Dosage and routes

Uncomplicated urinary tract infections

Adult: PO 250 mg q12h; **IV** 200 mg q12h

Complicated/severe urinary tract infections

Adult: PO 500 mg q12h; **IV** 400 mg q12h

Respiratory, bone, skin, joint infections

Adult: PO 500 mg q12h

Corneal ulcers, conjunctivitis

Adult: Ophth 1-2 gtt q15-30 min until infection is controlled, then 1-2 gtt 4-6 times daily

Renal dose

CrCl <50 ml/min PO 250-500 mg q12h; CrCl 5-29 ml/min PO 250-500 mg q18h; **IV** 200-400 mg q18-24h

Available forms: Tabs 250, 500, 750 mg; inj 200 mg/20 ml, 400 mg/40 ml, 200 mg/100 ml D_5, 400 mg/200 ml D_5; oral susp 250, 500 mg/5 ml

Adverse effects

CNS: Headache, dizziness, fatigue, insomnia, depression, *restlessness*

GI: Nausea, constipation, increased ALT, AST, flatulence, insomnia, heartburn, *vomiting, diarrhea,* oral candidiasis, dysphagia, **pseudomembranous colitis**

INTEG: Rash, pruritus, urticaria, photosensitivity, flushing, fever, chills

MISC: **Anaphylaxis, Stevens-Johnson syndrome**

MS: Tremor, arthralgia, tendon rupture

Contraindications: Hypersensitivity to quinolones

Precautions: Pregnancy **C**, lactation, children, renal disease

C

Pharmacokinetics

Absorption	Well absorbed (75%) (PO)
Distribution	Widely distributed
Metabolism	Liver (15%)
Excretion	Kidneys (40%-50%)
Half-life	3-4 hr; increased in renal disease

Pharmacodynamics

	PO	IV
Onset	Rapid	Immediate
Peak	1 hr	Infusion's end

Interactions

Individual drugs

Caffeine: ↑ caffeine levels
Cyclosporine: ↑ nephrotoxicity
Didanosine: ↓ absorption of ciprofloxacin
Enteral feeding: ↓ absorption of ciprofloxacin
Glyburide: ↑ hypoglycemia
Probenecid: ↑ blood levels of ciprofloxacin
Sucralfate: ↓ absorption of ciprofloxacin
Theophylline: ↑ theophylline levels
Warfarin: ↑ warfarin effect
Zinc sulfate: ↓ absorption of ciprofloxacin

Drug classifications

Antacids: ↓ absorption of ciprofloxacin
Anticoagulants, oral: ↑ effect of anticoagulants
Antineoplastics: ↓ ciprofloxacin levels
Iron salts: ↓ absorption of ciprofloxacin

Herb/drug

Yerba mate: ↑ toxicity

Food/drug

Dairy products: ↓ absorption
Food: ↓ absorption

Lab test interferences

↑ AST, ↑ ALT, ↑ BUN, ↑ creatinine, ↑ alkaline phosphatase

NURSING CONSIDERATIONS

Assessment

- Assess patient for previous sensitivity reaction
- Assess patient for signs and symptoms of infection including characteristics of wounds, sputum, urine, stool, WBC >10,000/mm^3, fever; obtain baseline information before and during treatment
- Obtain C&S before beginning drug therapy to identify if correct treatment has been initiated
- Assess for anaphylaxis: rash, urticaria, pruritus, chills, fever, joint pain; may occur a few days after therapy begins; epinephrine and resuscitation equipment should be available for anaphylactic reaction
- Identify urine output; if decreasing, notify prescriber (may indicate nephrotoxicity); also check for increased BUN, creatinine
- Monitor blood studies: AST, ALT, CBC, Hct, bilirubin, LDH, alkaline phosphatase, Coombs' test monthly if patient is on long-term therapy
- Monitor electrolytes: potassium, sodium, chloride monthly if patient is on long-term therapy
- Assess bowel pattern qd; if severe diarrhea occurs, drug should be discontinued
- Monitor for bleeding: ecchymosis, bleeding gums, hematuria, stool guaiac daily if on long-term therapy
- Assess for overgrowth of infection: perineal itching, fever, malaise, redness, pain, swelling, drainage, rash, diarrhea, change in cough, sputum

Nursing diagnoses

✓ Infection, risk for (uses)
✓ Diarrhea (side effects)
✓ Injury, risk for (side effects)
✓ Knowledge deficit (teaching)
✓ Noncompliance (teaching)

Implementation

PO route

- Give around the clock to maintain proper blood levels
- Administer 2 hr before or 2 hr after antacids, zinc, iron, calcium

IV **IV route**

- Check for irritation, extravasation, phlebitis daily
- For intermittent inf, dilute to 1-2 mg/ml of D_5W, 0.9% NaCl; give over 60 min; it will remain stable under refrigeration for 2 wk

Y-site compatibilities:
Amifostine, amino acids, aztreonam, calcium gluconate, ceftazidime, cisatracurium, digoxin, diltiazem, diphenhydramine, dobutamine, dopamine, doxorubicin liposome, gallium, gentamicin, granisetron, hydroxyzine, lidocaine, lorazepam, metoclopramide, midazolam, midodrine, piperacillin, potassium acetate, potassium chloride, potassium phosphates, prednisolone, promethazine, propofol, ranitidine, remifentanil, Ringer's, sodium chloride, tacrolimus, teniposide, thiotepa, tobramycin, verapamil

Y-site incompatibilities:
Heparin, mezlocillin

Additive compatibilities:
Amikacin, aztreonam, ceftazidime, cyclosporine, gentamicin, metronidazole, netilmicin, piperacillin, potassium acetate, potassium chloride, potassium phosphates, prednisolone, promethazine, propofol, ranitidine, Ringer's, sodium chloride, tobramycin, vit B/C

Additive incompatibilities:
Aminophylline, amoxicillin, clindamycin, floxacillin, mezlocillin

Patient/family education

- Teach patient to report sore throat, bruising, bleeding, joint pain; may indicate blood dyscrasias (rare)
- Teach patient to contact prescriber if adverse reaction occurs or if inflammation or pain in tendon occurs

- Advise patient to contact prescriber if vaginal itching, loose, foul-smelling stools, furry tongue occur; may indicate superinfection; report itching, rash, pruritus, urticaria
- Instruct patient to take all medication prescribed for the length of time ordered; drug must be taken around the clock to maintain blood levels; do not give medication to others
- Advise patient to notify prescriber of diarrhea with blood or pus
- Advise patient to rinse mouth frequently, use sugarless candy or gum for dry mouth

Evaluation

Positive therapeutic outcome

- Absence of signs/symptoms of infection (WBC <10,000/mm^3, temp WNL, absence of red draining wounds)
- Reported improvement in symptoms of infection

cisatracurium (℞)

(sis-a-tra-cyoor'ee-um)

Nimbex

Func. class.: Neuromuscular blocker (nondepolarizing)

Pregnancy category B

Action: Inhibits transmission of nerve impulses by binding with cholinergic receptor sites, antagonizing action of acetylcholine

➔ **Therapeutic Outcome:** Paralysis of body for administration of anesthesia

Uses: Facilitation of endotracheal intubation, skeletal muscle relaxation during mechanical ventilation surgery, or general anesthesia

Dosage and routes

Adult: **IV** 0.15 and 0.2 mg/kg depending on desired time to intubate and length of surgery: use peripheral nerve stimulation to evaluate dosage

P ***Child 2-12 yr:*** **IV** 0.1 mg/kg over 5-10 sec with halothane or opioid anesthesia

Available forms: Inj 2, 10 mg/ml

Adverse effects

CV: Bradycardia, tachycardia; increased, decreased B/P

EENT: Increased secretions

RESP: **Prolonged apnea, bronchospasm, cyanosis, respiratory depression**

INTEG: Rash, flushing, pruritus, urticaria

Contraindications: Hypersensitivity

Precautions: Pregnancy **B**, cardiac disase, lactation, P children <2 yr electrolyte imbalances, dehydration, neuromuscular disease, respiratory disease

Pharmacokinetics

Unknown

Pharmacodynamics

Onset	1-3 min
Peak	2-5 min
Duration	30-40 min

Interactions

Individual drugs

Carbamazepine: ↓ duration of neuromuscular blockade

Lithium: ↑ neuromuscular blockade

Isoflurane: ↑ neuromuscular blockade

Phenytoin: ↓ duration of neuromuscular blockade

Succinylcholine: ↓ neuromuscular blockade

Drug classifications

Aminoglycosides: ↑ neuromuscular blockade

Antibiotics, polymix: ↑ neuromuscular blockade

β-Adrenergic blockers: ↑ neuromuscular blockade

Opioids: ↑ neuromuscular blockade

C

NURSING CONSIDERATIONS

Assessment

- Assess for electrolyte imbalances (K, Mg), may lead to increased action of this drug
- Assess vital signs (B/P, pulse, respirations, airway) until fully recovered; rate, depth, pattern of respirations; strength of handgrip
- Assess I&O ratio: check for urinary retention, frequency, hesitancy
- Assess recovery: decreased paralysis of face, diaphragm, legs, arms, rest of body
- Assess allergic reactions: rash, fever, respiratory distress, pruritus; drug should be discontinued

Nursing diagnoses

✓ Breathing pattern, ineffective (uses)
✓ Communication, impaired (adverse reactions)
✓ Knowledge deficit (teaching)

Implementation

IV route

- Use nerve stimulator by anesthesiologist to determine neuromuscular blockade
- Give anticholinesterase to reverse neuromuscular blockade
- Give by slow **IV** only by qualified person, do not administer IM
- Store in light-resistant area
- Reassure if communication is difficult during recovery from neuromuscular blockage

Evaluation

Positive therapeutic outcome

- Paralysis of jaw, eyelid, head, neck, rest of body

Treatment of overdose:

Edrophonium or neostigmine, atropine, monitor VS; mechanical ventilation

HIGH ALERT

cisplatin (℞)

(sis'pla-tin)

Platinol, Platinol-AQ

Func. class.: Antineoplastic alkylating agent

Chem. class.: Inorganic heavy metal

Pregnancy category D

Action: Alkylates DNA, RNA; inhibits enzymes that allow synthesis of amino acids in proteins; activity is not cell cycle phase specific

Therapeutic Outcome: Prevention of rapidly growing malignant cells

Uses: Advanced bladder cancer; adjunctive in metastatic testicular cancer and metastatic ovarian cancer; head, neck, esophageal, prostatic, lung, and cervical cancer; lymphoma

Dosage and routes

Dosage protocols may vary

Testicular cancer

Adult: **IV** 20 mg/m^2 qd × 5 days, repeat q3 wk for 3 cycles or more, depending on response

Bladder cancer

Adult: **IV** 50-70 mg/m^2 q3-4 wk

Metastatic ovarian cancer

Adult: **IV** 100 mg/m^2 q4 wk or 50 mg/m^2 q3 wk with cyclophosphamide therapy; mix with 2 L of NaCl and 37.5 g mannitol over 6 hr

Available forms: Inj 0.5 mg/ml 🍁; powder for inj 10, 50 mg vials

Adverse effects

CNS: **Seizures,** peripheral neuropathy

CV: Cardiac abnormalities

EENT: *Tinnitus, hearing loss, vestibular toxicity*

GI: *Severe nausea, vomiting, diarrhea, weight loss*

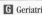

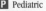

GU: **Renal tubular damage,** renal insufficiency, impotence, sterility,

amenorrhea, gynecomastia, hyperuremia
HEMA: **Thrombocytopenia, leukopenia, pancytopenia**
INTEG: *Alopecia,* dermatitis
META: Hypomagnesemia, hypocalcemia, hypokalemia, hypophosphatemia
RESP: **Fibrosis**
SYST: **Anaphylaxis**

Contraindications: Radiation therapy within 1 mo, chemotherapy within 1 mo, thrombocytopenia, smallpox vaccination, pregnancy **D**

Precautions: Pneumococcal vaccination

Do Not Confuse:
cisplatin/carboplatin

Pharmacokinetics

Absorption	Complete
Distribution	Widely distributed, accumulates in body tissues for several months
Metabolism	Liver
Excretion	Kidneys
Half-life	30-100 hr

Pharmacodynamics

Unknown

Interactions

Individual drugs

Aspirin: ↑ risk of bleeding
Radiation: ↑ toxicity, bone marrow suppression

Drug classifications

Aminoglycosides: ↑ nephrotoxicity
Antineoplastics: ↑ toxicity, bone marrow suppression
Bone marrow–suppressing drugs: ↑ bone marrow suppression
Diuretics, loop: ↑ ototoxicity
NSAIDs: ↑ risk of bleeding
Vaccines, live virus: ↓ antibody response

Lab test interferences

↑ Uric acid, ↑ BUN, ↑ creatinine, ↓ creatinine clearance, ↓ calcium, ↓ phosphate, ↓ potassium, ↓ magnesium
Positive: Coombs' test

NURSING CONSIDERATIONS

Assessment

- Monitor for bone marrow depression: CBC, differential, platelet count weekly; withhold drug if WBC count is <4000/mm^3 or platelet count is <100,000/mm^3; notify prescriber of results if WBC <20,000/mm^3, platelets <150,000/mm^3
- Monitor renal function studies: BUN, creatinine, serum uric acid, urine CrCl before and during therapy; I&O ratio; report fall in urine output to <30 ml/hr; dose should not be given if BUN <25 mg/dl; creatinine <1.5 mg/dl
- Assess for anaphylaxis: wheezing, tachycardia, facial swelling, fainting; discontinue drug and report to prescriber, resuscitation equipment should be nearby
- Monitor temp q4h (may indicate beginning of infection)
- Monitor liver function tests before and during therapy (bilirubin, AST, ALT, LDH) as needed or monthly; note yellowing of skin or sclera, dark urine, clay-colored stools, itchy skin, abdominal pain, fever, diarrhea
- Assess for increased uric acid levels, swelling, joint pain primarily in extremities; patient should be well hydrated to prevent urate deposits
- Assess for bleeding: hematuria, stool guaiac, bruising or petechiae, mucosa or orifices q8h; note inflammation of mucosa, breaks in skin
- Identify dyspnea, rales, nonproductive cough, chest pain, tachypnea
- Identify effects of alopecia on body image; discuss feelings about body changes
- Identify edema in feet, joint pain, stomach pain, shaking; prescriber should be notified

Nursing diagnoses

- ✓ Injury, risk for (adverse reactions)
- ✓ Body image disturbance (adverse reactions)
- ✓ Infection, risk for (adverse reactions)
- ✓ Knowledge deficit (teaching)

Implementation

- Hydrate patient with 0.9% NaCl over 8-12 hr before treatment
- Give all medications PO, if possible; avoid IM inj when platelets <100,000/mm^3
- Give epinephrine, antihistamines, corticosteroids for hypersensitivity reaction; antiemetic 30-60 min before giving drug to prevent vomiting, and prn; allopurinol or sodium bicarbonate to maintain uric acid level, alkalinization of urine; antibiotics for prophylaxis of infection; diuretic (furosemide 40 mg **IV**) or mannitol after infusion
- After diluting 10 mg/10 ml or 50 mg/50 ml sterile water for inj; withdraw prescribed dose, dilute ½ dose with 1000 ml D_5 0.2 NaCl or D_5 0.45 NaCl with 37.5 g mannitol; **IV** inf is given over 3-4 hr; use a 0.45 μm filter; total dose 2000 ml over 6-8 hr; check site for irritation, phlebitis; do not use equipment containing aluminum
- Prepare in biologic cabinet using gown, gloves, mask; do not allow drug to come in contact with skin, use soap and water if contact occurs

Syringe compatibilities:

Bleomycin, cyclophosphamide, doxapram, doxorubicin, droperidol, fluorouracil, furosemide, heparin, leucovorin, methotrexate, metoclopramide, mitomycin, vinblastine, vincristine

Y-*site compatibilities:*

Allopurinol, aztrenonam, bleomycin, chlorpromazine, cimetidine, cladribine, cyclophosphamide, dexamethasone, diphenhydramine, doxapram, doxorubicin, doxorubicin liposome, droperidol, famotidine, filgrastim, fludarabine, fluorouracil, furosemide, ganciclovir, granisetron, heparin, hydromorphone, leucovorin, lorazepam, melphalan, methotrexate, methylprednisolone, metoclopramide, mitomycin, morphine, ondansetron, paclitaxel, prochlorperazine, promethazine, propofol, ranitidine, sargramostim, teniposide, vinblastine, vincristine, vinorelbine

Additive compatibilities:

Carboplatin, cyclophosphamide with etoposide, etoposide, etoposide with floxuridine, floxuridine, floxuridine with leucovorin, hydroxyzine, ifosfamide, ifosfamide with etoposide, leucovorin, magnesium sulfate, mannitol, ondansetron

Additive incompatibilities:

Fluorouracil, mesna, thiotepa

Solution compatibilities:

D_5/0.225% NaCl, D_5/0.45% NaCl, D_5/0.9% NaCl, D_5/0.45% NaCl with mannitol 1.875%, D_5/0.33% NaCl with mannitol 1.875%, D_5/0.33% NaCl with KCl 20 mEq and mannitol 1.875%, 0.9% NaCl, 0.45% NaCl, 0.3% NaCl, 0.225% NaCl, water

Solution incompatibilities:

Sodium bicarbonate 5%, 0.1% NaCl, water

Patient/family education

- Teach patient to avoid use of products containing aspirin or ibuprofen, NSAIDs, alcohol (may cause GI bleeding), razors, commercial mouthwash; to report symptoms of bleeding (hematuria, tarry stools)
- Advise patient to report numbness, tingling in face or extremities, poor hearing or joint pain, swelling
- Instruct patient to report signs of anemia (fatigue, headache, irritability, faintness, shortness of breath)
- Instruct patient to report any changes in breathing or coughing even several months after treatment; to avoid crowds and persons with respiratory tract or other infections
- Advise patient that hair may be lost during treatment; a wig or hair piece

may make patient feel better; new hair may be different in color, texture

- Tell patient not to have any vaccinations without the advice of the prescriber; serious reactions can occur
- Caution patient contraception is needed during treatment and for several months after the completion of therapy

Evaluation

Positive therapeutic outcome

- Prevention of rapid division of malignant cells

citalopram (℞)

(sigh-tal'oh-pram)

Celexa

Func. class.: Antidepressant

Chem class.: Selective serotonin reuptake inhibitor (SSRI)

Pregnancy category B

Action: Inhibits CNS neuron uptake of serotonin but not of norepinephrine

Therapeutic Outcome: Decreased symptoms of depression after 2-3 wk

Uses: Major depressive disorder

Investigational uses: Fibromyalgia, premenstrual disorders

Dosage and routes

Adult: PO 20 mg qd AM or PM, may increase if needed to 40 mg/day after 1 wk; maintenance: after 6-8 wk of initial treatment, continue for 24 wk (32 wk total), reevaluate long-term usefulness (max 60 mg/day)

G ***Elderly:*** PO 20 mg qd initially, max 40 mg/day

Fibromyalgia

Adult: PO 20 mg qd × 4 wk, increase dose to 40 mg qd × 4 wk

Hepatic dose

Adult: PO 20 mg/day, may increase to 40 mg/day if no response

Available forms: Tabs 20, 40 mg

Adverse effects

CNS: *Headache, nervousness, insomnia, drowsiness, anxiety, tremor, dizziness, fatigue, sedation, poor concentration, abnormal dreams, agitation,* **seizures**

CV: *Hot flashes, palpitations,* angina pectoris, **hemorrhage,** hypertension, first-degree tachycardia

EENT: Visual changes, ear/eye pain, photophobia, tinnitus

GI: *Nausea, diarrhea, dry mouth, anorexia, dyspepsia, constipation, cramps, vomiting, taste changes, flatulence, decreased appetite*

GU: *Dysmenorrhea, decreased libido, urinary frequency, urinary tract infection,* amenorrhea, cystitis, impotence

INTEG: *Sweating, rash, pruritus,* acne, alopecia, urticaria

MS: *Pain,* arthritis, twitching

RESP: *Infection, pharyngitis, nasal congestion, sinus headache, sinusitis, cough, dyspnea, bronchitis,* asthma, hyperventilation, pneumonia

SYST: *Asthenia, viral infection, fever, allergy, chills*

Contraindications: Hypersensitivity

P G **Precautions:** Pregnancy **B,** lactation, children, elderly

Pharmacokinetics	
Absorption	Well absorbed
Distribution	Unknown
Metabolism	Liver
Excretion	Kidneys, steady state 28-35 days
Half-life	Unknown

Pharmacodynamics	
Onset	Unknown
Peak	Unknown
Duration	Unknown

Interactions
Individual drugs
Alcohol: ↑ CNS depression
Carbamazepine: ↑ toxicity
Lithium: ↑ toxicity
Drug classifications
Antifungals, azole: ↑ citalopram levels
Barbiturates: ↑ CNS depression
Benzodiazepines: ↑ CNS depression
β-Adrenergic blockers: ↑ plasma levels of β-blockers
CNS depressants: ↑ CNS depression
Macrolides: ↑ citalopram levels
MAOIs: Hypertensive crisis, seizures, fatal reactions
Sedative/hypnotics: ↑ CNS depression
Herb/drug
St. John's wort: do not use with citalopram

Lab test interferences:
↑ Serum bilirubin, ↑ blood glucose, ↑ alkaline phosphatase,
↓ VMA, ↓ 5-HIAA, ↓ blood glucose
False: ↑ Urinary catecholamines

NURSING CONSIDERATIONS
Assessment
- Monitor B/P (lying, standing), pulse q4h; if systolic B/P drops 20 mm Hg, hold drug and notify prescriber; take vital signs q4h in patients with cardiovascular disease
- Monitor blood studies: CBC, leukocytes, differential, cardiac enzymes if patient is receiving long-term therapy; check platelets, bleeding can occur
- Monitor hepatic studies: AST, ALT, bilirubin
- Check weight qwk; appetite may increase with drug
- Assess ECG for flattening of T wave, bundle branch block, AV block, dysrhythmias in cardiac patients
- G Assess EPS primarily in elderly: rigidity, dystonia, akathisia
- Assess mental status: mood, sensorium, affect, suicidal tendencies; increase in psychiatric symptoms: depression, panic
- Monitor urinary retention, P G constipation; constipation is more likely to occur in children or elderly
- Alert: Assess for withdawal symptoms: headache, nausea, vomiting, muscle pain, weakness; usually do not occur unless drug is discontinued abruptly
- Identify patient's alcohol consumption; if alcohol is consumed, hold dose until AM

Nursing diagnoses
- ✓ Coping, ineffective individual (uses)
- ✓ Injury, risk for (side effects)
- ✓ Knowledge deficit (teaching)
- ✓ Noncompliance (teaching)

Implementation
- Give with food or milk for GI symptoms
- Give dosage hs if oversedation occurs during day
- Store at room temp; do not freeze

Patient/family education
- Teach patient that therapeutic effects may take 2-3 wk
- Instruct patient to use caution in driving or other activities requiring alertness because of drowsiness, dizziness, blurred vision; to avoid rising quickly from sitting to standing, G especially elderly
- Caution patient to avoid alcohol ingestion, other CNS depressants
- Advise patient not to discontinue medication quickly after long-term use: may cause nausea, headache, malaise
- Instruct patient to increase fluids, bulk in diet if constipation, urinary G retention occur, especially elderly
- Advise patient to take gum, hard sugarless candy, or frequent sips of water for dry mouth

Evaluation
Positive therapeutic outcome
- Decrease in depression
- Absence of suicidal thoughts

C

clarithromycin (℞)

(clare-i-thro-mye'sin)

Biaxin, Biaxin XL

Func. class.: Antiinfective

Chem. class.: Macrolide

Pregnancy category C

Action: Binds to 50S ribosomal subunits of susceptible bacteria and suppresses protein synthesis

➔ **Therapeutic Outcome:** Bactericidal action against the following: *Streptococcus pneumoniae, Streptococcus pyogenes, Mycoplasma pneumoniae, Corynebacterium diphtheriae, Bordetella pertussis, Listeria monocytogenes, Haemophilus influnzae, Staphylococcus aureus, Mycobacterium avium (MAC), Mycobacterium intracellulare,* complex infections in AIDS patients, *Helicobacter pylori* in combination with omeprazole

Uses: Mild to moderate infections of the upper respiratory tract, lower respiratory tract; uncomplicated skin and skin structure infections

Dosage and routes

Adult: PO 250-500 mg q12h × 7-14 days; 500 mg q12h continues for MAC

P ***Child:*** PO 15 mg/kg/day (max 1000 mg) divided q12h × 10 days

H. pylori infection

Adult: PO 500 mg qd plus omeprazole 2 × 20 mg q AM (day 1-14) then omeprazole 20 mg q AM (days 15-28)

Acute maxillary sinusitis/ acute bacterial bronchitis

Adult: PO 500 mg q12h × 10 days

Available forms: Tabs 250, 500 mg; granules for oral susp 125, 250 mg/5 ml; ext rel tab 500 mg

Adverse effects

CV: Ventricular dysrhythmias

GI: Nausea, vomiting, diarrhea, **hepatotoxicity,** abdominal pain, stomatitis, heartburn, anorexia, abnormal taste, **pseudomembranous colitis**

GU: Vaginitis, moniliasis

HEMA: Leukopenia, thrombocytopenia, increased INR

INTEG: Rash, urticaria, pruritus, **Stevens-Johnson syndrome**

MISC: Headache

Contraindications: Hypersensitivity

Precautions: Pregnancy **C,** lactation, hepatic/renal disease

Pharmacokinetics

Absorption	50%
Distribution	Widely distributed
Metabolism	Liver
Excretion	Kidneys, unchanged (20%-30%)
Half-life	4-6 hr

Pharmacodynamics

Onset	Unknown
Peak	2 hr

Interactions

Individual drugs

Carbamazepine: ↑ toxicity, from ↑ levels of carbamazepine

Delavirdine: ↑ clarithromycin levels

Digoxin: ↑ blood levels of digoxin, ↑ digoxin effects

Fluconazole: ↑ clarithromycin levels

Pimozide: ↑ effect, ↑ dysrhythmias

Tacrolimus: ↑ effects of tacrolimus

Theophylline: ↑ toxicity from ↑ levels of theophylline

Triazolam: ↑ effects of triazolam

Zidovudine: ↑ or ↓ action

Drug classifications

Oral anticoagulants: ↑ effects of oral anticoagulants

Lab test interferences

↑ 17-OHCS/17-KS, ↑ AST, false ↑ ALT, BUN, creatinine, LDH, total bilirubin

↓ Folate assay

NURSING CONSIDERATIONS
Assessment
- Assess patient for signs and symptoms of infection including characteristics of wounds, sputum, urine, stool, WBC >10,000/mm^3, earache, fever; obtain baseline information before and during treatment
- Obtain C&S before beginning drug therapy to identify if correct treatment has been initiated
- Monitor blood studies: AST, ALT, CBC, Hct, bilirubin, LDH, alkaline phosphatase, Coombs' test monthly if patient is on long-term therapy
- Assess bowel pattern qd; if severe diarrhea occurs, drug should be discontinued
- Assess for overgrowth of infection: perineal itching, fever, malaise, redness, pain, swelling, drainage, rash, diarrhea, change in cough, sputum

Nursing diagnoses
✓ Infection, risk for (uses)
✓ Diarrhea (side effects)
✓ Knowledge deficit (teaching)
✓ Noncompliance (teaching)

Implementation
- Ensure adequate fluid intake (2 L) during diarrhea episodes
- Give q12h to maintain serum level

Patient/family education
- Advise patient to contact physician if vaginal itching, loose, foul-smelling stools, furry tongue occur; may indicate superinfection
- Instruct patient to take all medication prescribed for the length of time ordered, do not crush
- Advise prescriber if pregnancy is planned or suspected

Evaluation
Positive therapeutic outcome
- Absence of signs/symptoms of infection (WBC <10,000/mm^3, temp WNL, absence of red draining wounds)
- Reported improvement in symptoms of infection

clavulanate
See amoxicillin/clavulanate, ticarcillin/clavulanate

clemastine (℞)
(klem'as-teen)
Antihist-1, Contac Allergy 12 Hour, Tavist
Func. class.: Antihistamine
Chem. class.: Ethanolamine derivative, H_1-receptor antagonist
Pregnancy category B

Action: Acts on blood vessels, GI, respiratory system by competing with histamine for H_1-receptor site; decreases allergic response by blocking histamine

→ Therapeutic Outcome: Absence of allergy symptoms and rhinitis

Uses: Allergy symptoms, rhinitis, allergic dermatoses, nasal allergies, hypersensitive reactions including blood transfusion reactions, anaphylaxis

Dosage and routes
P ***Adult and child >12 yr:*** PO 1.34-2.68 mg bid-tid, not to exceed 8.04 mg/day

Available forms: Tabs 1.34, 2.68 mg; syr 0.67 mg/ml

Adverse effects
CNS: *Dizziness, drowsiness,* poor coordination, fatigue, anxiety, euphoria, confusion, paresthesia, neuritis, paradoxic excitement (child)
CV: Hypotension, palpitations, tachycardia
EENT: *Blurred vision,* dilated pupils, tinnitus, nasal stuffiness, dry nose, throat, *mouth*
GI: *Constipation,* dry mouth, nausea, vomiting, anorexia, diarrhea
GU: *Retention,* dysuria, frequency
HEMA: **Thrombocytopenia, agranulocytosis, hemolytic anemia**

INTEG: Rash, urticaria, photosensitivity, sweating
RESP: Increased thick secretions, wheezing, chest tightness

Contraindications: Hypersensitivity to H_1-receptor antagonists, acute asthma attack, lower respiratory tract disease

Precautions: Increased intraocular pressure, renal disease, cardiac disease, hypertension, bronchial asthma, seizure disorder, stenosed peptic ulcers, hyperthyroidism, prostatic hypertrophy, bladder neck obstruction, pregnancy **B**, G elderly

Pharmacokinetics

Absorption	Well absorbed
Distribution	Widely distributed
Metabolism	Liver, extensively
Excretion	Kidneys, breast milk (high)
Half-life	Unknown

Pharmacodynamics

Onset	15-60 min
Peak	1-2 hr
Duration	12 hr

Interactions

Individual drugs

Alcohol: ↑ CNS depression

Drug classifications

CNS depressants: ↑ CNS depression
MAOIs: ↑ anticholinergic effect
Opioids: ↑ CNS depression
Sedative/hypnotics: ↑ CNS depression

Herb/drug

Henbane leaf: ↑ anticholinergic effect
Kava: ↑ CNS depression

Lab test interferences

False negative: Skin allergy tests (discontinue antihistamines 3 days before testing)

NURSING CONSIDERATIONS

Assessment

- Assess respiratory status: rate, rhythm, increase in bronchial secretions, wheezing, chest tightness; provide fluids to 2 L/day to decrease secretion thickness
- Monitor I&O ratio: be alert for urinary retention, frequency, dysuria, G especially elderly; drug should be discontinued if these occur

Nursing diagnoses

✓ Airway clearance, ineffective (uses)
✓ Injury, risk for (side effects)
✓ Knowledge deficit (teaching)
✓ Noncompliance (teaching, overuse)

Implementation

- May give with food to decrease GI upset
- Do not crush or chew caps
- Store in tight, light-resistant container

Patient/family education

- Teach all aspects of drug uses; to notify prescriber if confusion, sedation, hypotension occur; to avoid driving and other hazardous activity if drowsiness occurs; to avoid alcohol and other CNS depressants that may potentiate effect
- Instruct patient to take 1 hr ac or 2 hr pc to facilitate absorption
- Caution patient not to exceed recommended dosage; dysrhythmias may occur
- Teach patient hard candy, gum, frequent rinsing of mouth may be used for dryness
- Tell patient if EENT or CNS symptoms occur (blurred vision, severe dry mouth, dry throat, confusion, dizziness, poor coordination, euphoria), prescriber should be notified

Evaluation

Positive therapeutic outcome

- Absence of running or congested nose, rashes

Treatment of overdose:

Administer ipecac syrup or lavage, diazepam, vasopressors, barbiturates (short acting)

clindamycin HCl (℞)
(klin-dah-my'sin)
Cleocin HCl

clindamycin palmitate (℞)
Cleocin Pediatric, Dalacin C Palmitate

clindamycin phosphate (℞)
Cleocin Phosphate, Dalacin C, Dalacin C Phosphate

Func. class.: Antiinfective, misc.
Chem. class.: Lincomycin derivative

Pregnancy category B

Action: Binds to 50S subunit of bacterial ribosomes; suppresses protein synthesis

➡ **Therapeutic Outcome:** Absence of infection

Uses: Infections caused by staphylococci, streptococci, *Rickettsia, Fusobacterium, Actinomyces, Peptococcus, Clostridium*

Dosage and routes

Adults: PO 150-450 mg q6h, max 1.8 g/day; IM/**IV** 1.2-1.8 g/day in 2-4 divided doses q6-12h, not to exceed 4800 mg/day

P ***Child <1 mo:*** 15-20 mg/kg/day divided q6-8h

P ***Child >1 mo:*** PO 8-20 mg/kg/day in divided doses q6-8h; IM/**IV** 20-40 mg/kg/day in divided doses q6-8h in 3-4 equal doses

Vaginal route

Adult: 5 g applicatorful at bedtime × 1 wk

Topical route

Adult: Sol 1% apply bid

PID

Adult: **IV** 600 mg q6h plus gentamicin or 900 mg q8h

Bacterial endocarditis prophylaxis

Adult: 600 mg 1 hr before procedure

Available forms: Phosphate: inj 150, 300, 600 mg base/4 ml; 900 mg base/ml; 900 mg base/60 ml; inj inf in D_5 300, 600, 900 mg; HCl: caps 75, 150, 300 mg; palmitate: oral sol 75 mg/ml

Adverse effects

EENT: Rash, urticaria, pruritus, erythema, pain, abscess at injection site

GI: *Nausea, vomiting, abdominal pain, diarrhea,* **pseudomembranous colitis,** *anorexia, weight loss*

GU: Increased AST, ALT, bilirubin, alkaline phosphatase, jaundice, *vaginitis,* urinary frequency

HEMA: **Leukopenia, eosinophilia, agranulocytosis, thrombocytopenia, polyarthritis**

Contraindications: Hypersensitivity to this drug or lincomycin, tartrazine dye, ulcerative colitis/enteritis

Precautions: Renal disease, liver G disease, GI disease, elderly, pregnancy **B,** lactation, tartrazine sensitivity, pseudomembranous colitis

Pharmacokinetics

Absorption	Well absorbed (PO, IM), minimal (top)
Distribution	Widely distributed; crosses placenta
Metabolism	Liver, extensively
Excretion	Kidneys, breast milk
Half-life	2½ hr

Pharmacodynamics

	PO	IM	IV	TOP	VAG
Onset	Rapid	Rapid	Rapid	Rapid	Rapid
Peak	½-1 hr	1½ hr	Infusion's end	Unknown	Unknown

Interactions

Individual drugs

Chloramphenicol: ↓ action of chloramphenicol

Erythromycin: ↓ action of clindamycin

Kaolin: ↓ absorption

Drug classifications

Neuromuscular blockers: ↑ neuromuscular blockade

Lab test interferences

↑ Alkaline phosphatase, ↑ bilirubin, ↑ CPK, ↑ AST, ↑ ALT

NURSING CONSIDERATIONS

Assessment

- Assess any patient with compromised renal system; drug is excreted slowly in poor renal system function; toxicity may occur rapidly
- Assess patient for signs and symptoms of infection including characteristics of wounds, sputum, urine, stool, WBC >10,000/mm^3, fever; obtain baseline information before and during treatment
- Complete C&S testing before beginning drug therapy; this will identify if correct treatment has been initiated
- Assess for allergic reactions: rash, urticaria, pruritus, chills, fever, joint pain; may occur a few days after therapy begins; epinephrine and resuscitation equipment should be available in case of an anaphylactic reaction
- Identify urine output; if decreasing, notify prescriber (may indicate nephrotoxicity); also look for increased BUN and creatinine levels
- Monitor blood studies: AST, ALT, CBC, Hct, bilirubin, LDH, alkaline phosphatase, Coombs' test monthly if patient is on long-term therapy
- Monitor electrolytes: potassium, sodium, chloride monthly if patient is on long-term therapy
- Assess bowel pattern qd; if severe diarrhea occurs, drug should be discontinued; may indicate pseudomembranous colitis
- Monitor for bleeding: ecchymosis, bleeding gums, hematuria, stool guaiac daily if on long-term therapy
- Assess for overgrowth of infection: perineal itching, fever, malaise, redness, pain, swelling, drainage, rash, diarrhea, change in cough, sputum

Nursing diagnoses

- ✓ Infection, risk for (uses)
- ✓ Diarrhea (adverse reactions)
- ✓ Injury, risk for (adverse reaction)
- ✓ Knowledge deficit (teaching)
- ✓ Noncompliance (teaching)

Implementation

PO route

- Give with 8 oz of water; give with meals for GI symptoms
- Shake liquids well
- Do not refrigerate oral preparations; stable at room temperature for 2 wk
- ⊘ Do not crush, chew caps

IM route

- If more than 600 mg must be given, divide into 2 injections
- Give deeply in large muscle mass; rotate sites

IV IV route

- Give by inf only; do not administer bolus dose; dilute 300 mg or more/50 ml or more of D_5W, 0.9% NaCl
- May be further diluted in greater amounts of D_5W, 0.9% NaCl and given as a cont inf in acute PID; give first dose 10 mg/min over ½ hr, then 0.75 mg/min; increased rates may be used to keep serum blood levels higher; run over >10 min; no more than 120 mg in a 1 hr inf

Syringe compatibilities:

Amikacin, aztreonam, gentamicin, heparin

Syringe incompatibilities:

Tobramycin

Y-site compatibilities:

Amifostine, amiodarone, amphotericin B cholesteryl, amsacrine, aztreonam, cisatracurium, cyclophosphamide, diltiazem, doxorubicin liposome, enalaprilat, esmolol, fludarabine, foscarnet, granisetron, heparin, hydromorphone, labetolol, magnesium sulfate, melphalan, meperidine, midazolam, morphine, multivitamins, odansetron, perphenazine, piperacillin/tazobactam, propofol,

C

remifentanil, sargramostim, tacrolimus, teniposide, theophylline, thiotepa, vinorelbine, vit B/C, zidovudine

Y-site incompatibilities: Idarubicin

Additive compatibilities Amikacin, ampicillin, aztreonam, cefamandole, cefazolin, cefepine, cefonicid, cefoperazone, cefotaxime, cefoxitin, ceftazidime, ceftizoxime, cefuroxime, cephalothin, cimetidine, fluconazole, heparin, hydrocortisone, kanamycin, methylprednisolone, metoclopramide, metronidazole, netilmicin, ofloxacin, penicillin G, pipercillin, potassium chloride, sodium bicarbonate, tobramycin, verapamil, vit B/C

Additive incompatibilities: Ciprofloxacin

Topical route

- Avoid contact with eyes, mucous membranes, and open cuts during topical application; if accidental contact occurs, rinse with cool water
- Wash affected areas with warm water and soap, rinse, pat dry before application

Patient/family education

- Tell patient to take oral drug with full glass of water; may take with food if GI symptoms occur; antiperistaltic drugs may worsen diarrhea
- Teach patient aspects of drug therapy: need to complete entire course of medication to ensure organism death (10-14 days); culture may be taken after medication course has been completed
- Advise patient to report sore throat, fever, fatigue; may indicate superimposed infection
- Advise patient that drug must be taken at equal intervals around clock to maintain blood levels

Evaluation

Positive therapeutic outcome

- Decreased temperature, negative C&S

Treatment of hypersensitivity: Withdraw drug; maintain airway; administer epinephrine, aminophylline, O_2, **IV** corticosteroids

clomiphene (℞)

(kloe'mi-feen)

Clomid, clomiphene citrate, Milophene, Serophene

Func. class.: Ovulation stimulant

Chem. class.: Nonsteroidal antiestrogenic

Pregnancy category X

Action: Increases LH, FSH release from the pituitary, which increase maturation of ovarian follicle, ovulation, development of corpus luteum

Therapeutic Outcome: Pregnancy

Uses: Female infertility (ovulatory failure)

Dosage and routes

Adult: PO 50-100 mg qd × 5 days or 50-100 mg qd beginning on day 5 of cycle; may be repeated until conception occurs or 3 cycles of therapy have been completed

Available forms: Tabs 50 mg

Adverse effects

CNS: *Headache, depression,* restlessness, anxiety, nervousness, fatigue, insomnia, dizziness, flushing

CV: Vasomotor flushing, phlebitis, **deep vein thrombosis**

EENT: Blurred vision, diplopia, photophobia

GI: *Nausea, vomiting, constipation,* abdominal pain, bloating

GU: Polyuria, frequency of urination, **birth defects, spontaneous abortions,** multiple ovulation, breast pain, oliguria, abnormal uterine bleeding

INTEG: *Rash, dermatitis,* urticaria, alopecia

Contraindications: Hypersensitivity, pregnancy **X**, hepatic disease, undiagnosed uterine bleeding, uncontrolled thyroid or adrenal dysfunction, intracranial lesion, ovarian cysts

Precautions: Hypertension, depression, convulsions, diabetes mellitus

Do Not Confuse:
clomiphene/clomipramine

Pharmacokinetics

Absorption	Well distributed
Distribution	Unknown
Metabolism	Liver, extensively
Excretion	Feces
Half-life	5 days

Pharmacodynamics

Unknown

Interactions: None

Lab test interferences

↑ FSH/LH, ↑ BSP, ↑ thyroxine, ↑ TBG

NURSING CONSIDERATIONS

Assessment

- Determine liver function tests before therapy: AST, ALT, alkaline phosphatase
- Monitor serum progesterone, urinary excretion of pregnanediol to identify occurrence of ovulation
- Pelvic examination should be done to determine ovarian size, cervical condition
- Endometrial biopsy may be done in women over 35 to rule out endometrial carcinoma

Nursing diagnoses

✓ Sexual dysfunction (uses)
✓ Knowledge deficit (teaching)

Implementation

- Give after discontinuing estrogen therapy
- Give at same time qd to maintain drug level; begin on 5th day of menstrual cycle

Patient/family education

- Advise patient that multiple births are common after drug is taken
- Instruct patient to notify prescriber immediately if low abdominal pain occurs; may indicate ovarian cyst, cyst rupture
- Advise patient to notify prescriber of photophobia, blurred vision, diplopia
- Teach patient if dose is missed, double at next time; if more than one dose is missed, call prescriber
- Instruct patient that response usually occurs 4-10 days after last day of treatment
- Teach patient method for taking, recording basal body temp to determine whether ovulation has occurred; if ovulation can be determined (there is a slight decrease in temp, then a sharp increase for ovulation), to attempt coitus 3 days before and qod until after ovulation
- Teach patient if pregnancy is suspected, to notify prescriber immediately

Evaluation

Positive therapeutic outcome

- Fertility

clomipramine (℞)

(klom-ip′ra-meen)

Anafranil

Func. class.: Tricyclic antidepressant

Chem. class.: Tertiary amine

Pregnancy category C

Action: Potent inhibitor of serotonin and norepinephrine uptake; also increases dopamine metabolism

Therapeutic Outcome: Decreased signs and symptoms of obsessive-compulsive disorder, decreased depression

Uses: Obsessive-compulsive disorder, depression, dysphoria, anxiety, agoraphobia and other phobias

Dosage and routes

Obsessive-compulsive disorder

Adult: PO 25 mg hs; increase gradually over 4 wk to a dosage of 75-300 mg/day in divided doses

P ***Child 10-18 yr:*** PO 25-50 mg/day gradually increased or 3 mg/kg/day whichever is smaller; not to exceed 200 mg/day

Depression

Adult: PO 50-150 mg/day in a single or divided dose

Anxiety/agoraphobia

Adult: PO 25-75 mg/day

Available forms: Caps 10, 25, 50, 75 mg

Adverse effects

CNS: *Dizziness, tremors, mania,* **seizures,** aggressiveness

CV: Hypotension, tachycardia, **cardiac arrest**

ENDO: Galactorrhea, hyperprolactinemia

GI: *Constipation, dry mouth, nausea, dyspepsia*

GU: *Delayed ejaculation, anorgasmia,* retention

HEMA: **Agranulocytosis, neutropenia, pancytopenia**

INTEG: Diaphoresis

META: Hyponatremia

Contraindications: Hypersensitivity, immediately after MI

Precautions: Seizures, suicidal G patients, elderly, cardiac disease, pregnancy **C**

Do Not Confuse: clomipramine/clomiphene, clomipramine/desipramine

Pharmacokinetics

Absorption	Well absorbed
Distribution	Widely distributed
Metabolism	Liver, extensively
Excretion	Kidneys, breast milk
Half-life	19-37 hr; steady state 1-2 wk

Pharmacodynamics

Onset	≥2 wk
Peak	2-6 hr

Interactions

Individual drugs

Alcohol: ↑ CNS depression

Carbamazepine: ↓ clomipramine action

Cimetidine: ↑ clomipramine level; do not use together

Clonidine: Severe hypertension; avoid use

Epinephrine: Severe hypertension, avoid use

Fluoxetine: ↑ clomipramine level; do not use together

Fluvoxamine: ↑ clomipramine level; do not use together

Guanethidine: ↓ effects

Norepinephrine: Severe hypertension, avoid use

Phenytoin: ↓ clomipramine action

Sertraline: ↑ clomipramine level; do not use together

Drug classifications

Barbiturates: ↓ clomipramine levels

Benzodiazepines: ↑ effects; do not use together

CNS depressants: ↑ effects; do not use together

MAOIs: Hypertensive crisis, convulsions; do not use together

Sympathomimetics, indirect-acting: ↓ effects

Oral contraceptives: ↑ effects, toxicity

Herb/drug

Belladonna leaf/root: ↑ anticholinergic effect

Henbane leaf: ↑ anticholinergic effect

Kava: ↑ CNS depression

Scopolia root: ↑ clomipramine effect

Lab test interferences

↑ Serum bilirubin, ↑ blood glucose, ↑ alkaline phosphatase

↓ VMA, ↓ 5-HIAA

False positive: Urinary catecholamines

NURSING CONSIDERATIONS

Assessment

- Monitor B/P (with patient lying, standing), pulse q4h; if systolic B/P drops 20 mm Hg hold drug, notify prescriber; take VS q4h in patients with cardiovascular disease
- Monitor blood studies: CBC, leukocytes, differential, cardiac enzymes if patient is receiving long-term therapy
- Monitor hepatic studies: AST, ALT, bilirubin
- Check weight weekly; appetite may increase with drug
- Assess ECG for flattening of T wave, QTc prolongation bundle branch block, AV block, dysrhythmias in cardiac patients
- G Assess for EPS primarily in elderly: rigidity, dystonia, akathisia
- Assess mental status: mood, sensorium, affect, suicidal tendencies; increase in psychiatric symptoms: depression, panic, frequency of obsessive-compulsive behaviors
- Monitor urinary retention, P constipation; constipation is more G likely to occur in children or elderly
- Assess for withdrawal symptoms: headache, nausea, vomiting, muscle pain, weakness; do not usually occur unless drug was discontinued abruptly
- Identify alcohol consumption; if alcohol is consumed, hold dose until morning

Nursing diagnoses

✓ Coping, ineffective individual (uses)
✓ Injury, risk for physical (side effects)
✓ Knowledge deficit (teaching)
✓ Noncompliance (teaching)

Implementation

- Give with food or milk for GI symptoms
- ⊘ Do not crush, chew caps
- Store at room temp; do not freeze

Patient/family education

- Teach patient that therapeutic effects may take 2-3 wk
- Teach patient to use caution in driving or other activities requiring alertness because of drowsiness, dizziness, blurred vision; to avoid rising quickly from sitting to standing, G especially elderly
- Teach patient to avoid alcohol ingestion, other CNS depressants
- Teach patient not to discontinue medication quickly after long-term use: may cause nausea, headache, malaise
- Teach patient to wear sunscreen or large hat, since photosensitivity occurs
- Teach patient to increase fluids, bulk in diet if constipation, urinary G retention occur, especially elderly
- Teach patient to take gum, hard sugarless candy, or frequent sips of water for dry mouth

Evaluation

Positive therapeutic outcome

- Decrease in depression
- Absence of suicidal thoughts

Treatment of overdose: ECG monitoring, induce emesis, lavage, activated charcoal, administer anticonvulsant

clonazepam (℞)

(kloe-na'zi-pam)

Klonopin, Rivotril, Syn-Clonazepam ✤

Func. class.: Anticonvulsant

Chem. class.: Benzodiazepine derivative

Pregnancy category C

Controlled substance schedule IV

Action: Inhibits spike, wave formation in absence seizures (petit mal), decreases amplitude, frequency, duration, spread of discharge in minor motor seizures

➔ **Therapeutic Outcome:** Decreased frequency, severity of seizures

Uses: Absence, atypical absence,

akinetic, myoclonic seizures, Lennox-Gastaut syndrome

Investigational uses: Parkinsonian dysarthrias, acute mania, adjunct in schizophrenia, neuralgias, multifocal tic disorders, restless leg syndrome, rectal administration

Dosage and routes

Adult: PO not to exceed 1.5 mg/day in 3 divided doses; may be increased 0.5-1 mg q3 days until desired response; not to exceed 20 mg/day; rec 0.02 mg/kg

P ***Child <10 yr or 30 kg:*** PO 0.01-0.03 mg/kg/day in divided doses q8h, not to exceed 0.05 mg/kg/day; may be increased 0.25-0.5 mg q3 days until desired response; not to exceed 0.1-0.2 mg/kg/day; rec 0.05-0.1 mg/kg

Available forms: Tabs 0.5, 1, 2 mg; oral susp; **IV** sol

Adverse effects

CNS: *Drowsiness,* dizziness, confusion, behavioral changes, tremors, insomnia, headache, suicidal tendencies, slurred speech

CV: Palpitations, bradycardia

EENT: *Increased salivation, nystagmus, diplopia,* abnormal eye movements

GI: *Nausea, constipation,* polyphagia, anorexia, xerostomia, diarrhea, gastritis, sore gums

GU: Dysuria, enuresis, nocturia, retention

HEMA: **Thrombocytopenia, leukocytosis, eosinophilia**

INTEG: Rash, alopecia, hirsutism

RESP: **Respiratory depression,** dyspnea, congestion

Contraindications: Hypersensitivity to benzodiazepines, acute narrow-angle glaucoma

Precautions: Open-angle glaucoma, chronic respiratory disease, G renal/hepatic disease, elderly, pregnancy **C**

Do Not Confuse:
Klonopin/clonidine

Pharmacokinetics

Absorption	Well absorbed
Distribution	Crosses blood-brain barrier, placenta
Metabolism	Liver
Excretion	Kidneys
Half life	18-50 hr

Pharmacodynamics

Onset	½-1 hr
Peak	1-2 hr
Duration	6-12 hr

Interactions

Individual drugs

Alcohol: ↑ CNS depression
Carbamazepine: ↓ effectiveness
Cimetidine: ↓ metabolism, ↑ action
Disulfiram: ↓ metabolism, ↑ action
Fluoxetine: ↓ metabolism, ↑ action
Isoniazid: ↓ metabolism, ↑ action
Ketoconazole: ↓ metabolism, ↑ action
Metoprolol: ↓ metabolism, ↑ action
Phenytoin: ↓ clonazepam levels
Propoxyphene: ↓ metabolism, ↑ action
Propranolol: ↓ metabolism, ↑ action
Valproic acid: ↑ seizures

Drug classifications

Antidepressants: ↑ CNS depression
Anticonvulsants: ↑ CNS depression
Antihistamines: ↑ CNS depression
Barbiturates: ↑ CNS depression, ↓ effect of clonazepam
General anesthetics: ↑ CNS depression **Opiates:** ↑ CNS depression
Oral contraceptives: ↓ metabolism, ↑ action
Sedatives/hypnotics: ↑ CNS depression

Herb/drug

Kava: ↑ CNS depression

Lab test interferences

↑ AST, ↑ alkaline phosphatase

NURSING CONSIDERATIONS
Assessment
- Assess mental status: mood, sensorium, affect, memory (long, short), especially elderly
- Assess for blood dyscrasias: fever, sore throat, bruising, rash, jaundice, epistaxis (long-term treatment only)
- Monitor blood level: therapeutic level 20-80 ng/ml
- Assess seizure activity including type, location, duration, and character; provide seizure precaution
- Assess renal studies: urinalysis, BUN, urine creatinine
- Monitor blood studies: RBCs, Hct, Hgb, reticulocyte counts weekly for 4 wk then monthly
- Monitor hepatic studies: ALT, AST, bilirubin, creatinine
- Monitor drug levels during initial treatment
- Assess for signs of physical withdrawal if medication suddenly discontinued
- Assess eye problems: need for ophthalmic examinations before, during, after treatment (slit lamp, fundoscopy, tonometry)
- Assess allergic reaction: red raised rash; if this occurs, drug should be discontinued
- Monitor for toxicity: bone marrow depression, nausea, vomiting, ataxia, diplopia, cardiovascular collapse

Nursing diagnoses
✓ Injury, risk for (side effects)
✓ Knowledge deficit (teaching)

Implementation
PO route
- Give on empty stomach for best absorption

Rectal route
- **IV** sol may be used rectally, 1 ml syringe inserted 3 cm into rectum
- Oral susp may be used rectally (1 mg/ml of drug with 1 ml of water), use plastic tube (volume 2.2-3.3 ml)

Patient/family education
- Teach patient to carry ID card or Medic Alert bracelet stating patient's name, drugs taken, condition, physician's name, phone number
- Caution patient to avoid driving, other activities that require alertness
- Caution patient to avoid alcohol ingestion or CNS depressants; increased sedation may occur
- Teach patient not to discontinue medication quickly after long-term use; taper off over several weeks

Evaluation
Positive therapeutic outcome
- Decreased seizure activity

Treatment of overdose:
Lavage, activated charcoal, VS, monitor electrolytes

clonidine (℞)
(klon'i-deen)

Catapres, Catapres-TTS, clonidine HCl, Dixarit ✦, Duraclon

Func. class.: Antihypertensive, analgesic (centrally acting)

Chem. class.: Central α-adrenergic agonist

Pregnancy category C

Action: Inhibits sympathetic vasomotor center in CNS, which reduces impulses in sympathetic nervous system; B/P, pulse rate, cardiac output decreased; prevents pain signal transmission in CNS by α-adrenergic receptor stimulation of the spinal cord

Therapeutic Outcome: Decreased B/P in hypertension

Uses: Mild to moderate hypertension; used alone or in combination

Investigational uses: Narcotic withdrawal, prevention of vascular headaches, treatment of menopausal symptoms, dysmenorrhea, attention deficit hyperactivity disorder (ADHD)

Dosage and routes

Hypertension

Adult: PO/trans 0.1 mg bid, then increase by 0.1-0.2 mg/day until desired response; range 0.2-0.8 mg/day in divided doses

G ***Elderly:*** PO 0.1 mg hs, may increase gradually

P ***Child:*** PO 5-10 μg/kg/day in divided doses q8-12h, max 0.9 mg/day

Opioid withdrawal

Adult: PO 0.3-1.2 mg/day; may decrease by 50% × 3 days then decrease by 0.1-0.2 mg/day or discontinue

Severe pain

Adult: Cont epidural inf 30 μg/hr

Menopausal symptoms

Adult: TD 0.1 mg patch q1 wk; PO 0.05-0.4 mg bid

ADHD

P ***Child:*** PO 0.05 mg/day; titrate up to max 0.4 mg/day

Available forms: Tabs 0.025 ✦, 0.1, 0.2, 0.3 mg; trans sys 2.5, 5, 7.5 mg delivering 0.1, 0.2, 0.3 mg/24 hr, respectively; inj 100, 500 μg/ml

Adverse effects

CNS: *Drowsiness, sedation, headache, fatigue,* nightmares, insomnia, mental changes, anxiety, depression, hallucinations, delirium

CV: *Orthostatic hypotension, palpitations,* **CHF**, ECG abnormalities

EENT: Taste change, parotid pain

ENDO: Hyperglycemia

GI: *Nausea, vomiting, malaise,* constipation, *dry mouth*

GU: Impotence, dysuria, *nocturia,* gynecomastia

INTEG: *Rash,* alopecia, facial pallor, pruritus, hives, edema, burning papules, excoriation (trans patches)

MISC: *Withdrawal symptoms*

MS: Muscle, joint pain, leg cramps

Contraindications: Hypersensitivity; (epidural) bleeding disorders, anticoagulants

Precautions: MI (recent), diabetes mellitus, chronic renal failure, Raynaud's disease, thyroid disease, P depression, COPD, child <12 yr (transdermal), asthma, pregnancy **C**, G lactation, elderly, noncompliant patients

Do Not Confuse: Catapres/Cataflam, clonidine/Klonopin

Pharmacokinetics

Absorption	Well absorbed (PO, trans)
Distribution	Widely distributed; crosses blood-brain barrier
Metabolism	Liver, extensively
Excretion	Kidneys, unchanged (30%)
Half-life	12-21 hr

Pharmacodynamics

	PO	TD
Onset	½-1 hr	3 days
Peak	2-4 hr	Unknown
Duration	8-12 hr	8 hr (after removal)

Interactions

Individual drugs

Alcohol: ↑ CNS depression

Levodopa: ↓ levodopa effect

Verapamil: AV block

Drug classifications

Amphetamines: ↓ hypotensive effects

Anesthetics: ↑ CNS depression

Antidepressants, tricyclic: ↓ hypotensive effects

β-Adrenergic blockers: ↑ bradycardia

Cardiac glycosides: ↑ bradycardia

Diuretics: ↑ hypotensive effects

Nitrates: ↑ hypotensive effects

Opiates: ↑ CNS depression

Sedatives/hypnotics: ↑ CNS depression

Lab test interferences

↑ Blood glucose

↓ VMA, ↓ urinary catecholamines, ↓ aldosterone

NURSING CONSIDERATIONS

Assessment

- Assess pain: location, intensity,

character, alleviating, aggravation factors, baseline and frequency
- Perform blood studies: neutrophils, decreased platelets
- Perform renal studies: protein, BUN, creatinine; watch for increased levels that may indicate nephrotic syndrome: polyuria, oliguria, frequency
- Monitor baselines for renal, liver function tests before therapy begins; check potassium levels, although hyperkalemia rarely occurs
- Monitor B/P, pulse if the drug is being used for hypertension; notify prescriber of changes
- Assess for opiate withdrawal in patients receiving the drug for opioid withdrawal, including fever, diarrhea, nausea, vomiting, cramps, insomnia, shivering, dilated pupils, weakness
- Check for edema in feet, legs daily; monitor I&O; check for decreasing output
- Note allergic reaction: rash, fever, pruritus, urticaria; drug should be discontinued if antihistamines fail to help
- Note allergic reaction from patches: rash, urticaria, angioedema; should not continue to use
- Assess for symptoms of CHF: edema, dyspnea, wet rales, B/P, weight gain, report significant changes

Nursing diagnoses

✓ Injury, potential for physical (side effects)
✓ Knowledge deficit (teaching)
✓ Noncompliance (teaching)

Implementation

PO route
- PO: give last dose at hs

Transdermal route
- Apply patch weekly; remove old patch and wash off residue; apply to site without hair; best absorption over chest or upper arm; rotate sites with each application; clean site before application; apply firmly, especially around edges
- Store patches in cool environment, tabs in tight container

Patient/family education

- Instruct patient not to discontinue drug abruptly, or withdrawal symptoms may occur: anxiety, increased B/P, headache, insomnia, increased pulse, tremors, nausea, sweating
- Caution patient not to use OTC (cough, cold, or allergy) products unless directed by prescriber
- Teach patient to comply with dosage schedule even if feeling better; drug controls symptoms, does not cure
- Caution patient to change position slowly, to rise slowly to sitting or standing position to minimize ortho- G static hypotension, especially elderly
- Instruct patient to notify physician of mouth sores, sore throat, fever, swelling of hands or feet, irregular heartbeat, chest pain, signs of angioedema, increased weight
- Teach patient about excessive perspiration, dehydration, vomiting; diarrhea may lead to fall in B/P; consult prescriber if these occur
- Tell patient that drug may cause dizziness, fainting; light-headedness may occur during 1st few days of therapy; use hard candy, saliva product, or frequent rinsing of mouth for dry mouth
- Advise patient that compliance is necessary; not to skip or stop drug unless directed by prescriber
- Teach patient that drug may cause skin rash or impaired perspiration
- Teach patient that response may take 2-3 days if drug is given TD; instruct on administration of patch; return demonstration
- Teach patient to avoid hazardous activities, since drug may cause drowsiness, dizziness
- Teach patient to administer 1 hr ac

Evaluation

Positive therapeutic outcome
- Decrease in B/P in hypertension
- Decrease in withdrawal symptoms

- Decrease in pain
- Decrease in vascular headaches
- Decrease in dysmenorrhea
- Decrease in menopausal symptoms

Treatment of overdose: Supportive treatment; administer tolazoline, atropine, dopamine prn

clopidogrel (℞)

(klo-pid'oh-grel)

Plavix

Func. class.: Platelet aggregation inhibitor

Chem. class.: Thienopyridine derivative

Pregnancy category B

Action: Inhibits first and second phases of ADP-induced effects in platelet aggregation

➔ **Therapeutic Outcome:** Decreased possibility of stroke, MI by decreasing platelet aggregation

Uses: Reducing the risk of stroke in high-risk patients

Investigational uses: Loading dose

Dosage and routes

Adult: PO 75 mg qd with or without food

Loading dose

Adult: PO 150-600 mg then 75-150 mg qd

Available forms: Tabs 75 mg

Adverse effects

CNS: Headache, dizziness

CV: Edema, hypertension

GI: Nausea, vomiting, diarrhea, GI discomfort, **GI bleeding**

HEMA: *Epistaxis*, purpura, **bleeding, neutropenia**

INTEG: Rash, pruritus

MISC: UTI, depression, hypercholesterolemia, chest pain, fatigue, **intracranial hemorrhage**

MS: Arthralgia, back pain

RESP: Upper respiratory tract infection, dyspnea, rhinitis, bronchitis, cough

Contraindications: Hypersensitivity, active bleeding

Precautions: Past liver disease, P pregnancy **B**, lactation, children, increased bleeding risk, neutropenia, agranulocytosis

Pharmacokinetics

Absorption	Rapidly absorbed
Distribution	Unknown
Metabolism	Liver, extensively
Excretion	Kidneys, unchanged drug
Half-life	Platelets 11 days

Pharmacodynamics

Onset	Unknown
Peak	1-3 hr
Duration	Unknown

Interactions

Individual drugs

Abciximab: ↑ bleeding tendencies
Aspirin: ↑ bleeding tendencies
Eptifibatide: ↑ bleeding tendencies
Fluvastatin: ↑ action of fluvastatin
Phenytoin: ↑ action of phenytoin
Tamoxifen: ↑ action of tamoxifen
Ticlopidine: ↑ bleeding tendencies
Tirofiban: ↑ bleeding tendencies
Tolbutamide: ↑ action of tolbutamide
Torsemide: ↑ action of torsemide
Warfarin: ↑ action of warfarin

Drug classifications

Anticoagulants: ↑ bleeding tendencies
NSAIDs: ↑ bleeding tendencies
Thrombolytics: ↑ bleeding tendencies

NURSING CONSIDERATIONS

Assessment

- Assess for symptoms of stroke, MI during treatment
- Monitor liver function studies: AST, ALT, bilirubin, creatinine if patient is on long-term therapy (4 mo or more)

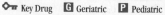

• Monitor blood studies: CBC, Hct, Hgb, pro-time, cholesterol if patient is on long-term therapy; thrombocytopenia, neutropenia may occur

Nursing diagnoses

✓ Injury, risk for (uses)
✓ Knowledge deficit (teaching)

Implementation

• Give with food to decrease gastric symptoms

Patient/family education

• Advise patient that blood work will be necessary during treatment
• Advise patient to report any unusual bleeding to prescriber
• Instruct patient to take with food or just after eating to minimize GI discomfort
• Caution patient to report side effects such as diarrhea, skin rashes, subcutaneous bleeding

Evaluation

Positive therapeutic outcome

• Absence of stroke

clorazepate (℞)

(klor-az′e-pate)

APO-Clorazepate ✤, clorazepate, Gen-XENE, Novo-Clopate, Tranxene, Tranxene-SD

Func. class.: Antianxiety, anticonvulsant, sedative/hypnotic

Chem. class.: Benzodiazepine

Pregnancy category D

Controlled substance schedule IV

Action: Potentiates the actions of GABA; especially in limbic system, reticular formation has anticonvulsant effects

➡ **Therapeutic Outcome:** Decreased anxiety, restlessness, insomnia

Uses: Anxiety, acute alcohol withdrawal, adjunct in seizure disorders

Dosage and routes

Anxiety

Adult: PO 15-60 mg/day

G ***Elderly:*** PO 7.5 mg qd bid

Alcohol withdrawal

Adult: PO 30 mg then day 1, 30-60 mg in divided doses; day 2, 45-90 mg in divided doses; day 3, 22.5-45 mg in divided doses; day 4, 15-30 mg in divided doses; then reduce daily dose to 7.5-15 mg

Seizure disorders

P ***Adult and child >12 yr:*** PO 7.5 mg tid; may increase by 7.5 mg/wk or less, not to exceed 90 mg/day

P ***Child 9-12 yr:*** PO 7.5 mg bid; may increase by 7.5 mg/wk or less, not to exceed 60 mg/day

Available forms: Caps 3.75, 7.5, 15 mg; tabs 3.75, 7.5, 15 mg

Adverse effects

CNS: Dizziness, drowsiness, confusion, headache, anxiety, tremors, stimulation, fatigue, depression, insomnia, hallucinations, lethargy

CV: Orthostatic hypotension, **ECG changes, tachycardia,** hypotension

EENT: Blurred vision, tinnitus, mydriasis

GI: Constipation, dry mouth, nausea, vomiting, anorexia, diarrhea

INTEG: Rash, dermatitis, itching

Contraindications: Hypersensitivity to benzodiazepines, narrow-angle glaucoma, psychosis, pregnancy **D,**
P child <9 yr

G **Precautions:** Elderly, debilitated, hepatic disease, renal disease

Pharmacokinetics	
Absorption	Well absorbed
Distribution	Widely distributed; crosses placenta
Metabolism	Liver
Excretion	Kidneys, breast milk
Half-life	30-100 hr

Pharmacodynamics	
Onset	1 hr
Peak	1-2 hr
Duration	Up to 24 hr

Interactions

Individual drugs

Alcohol: ↑ CNS depression
Cimetidine: ↑ effects of clorazepate
Disulfiram: ↑ effects of clorazepate
Fluoxetine: ↑ clorazepate effects
Isoniazid: ↑ clorazepate action
Ketoconazole: ↑ clorazepate effects
Propoxyphene: ↑ clorazepate action
Rifampin: ↓ action of clorazepate
Valproic acid: ↑ effects of clorazepate

Drug classifications

β-Blockers, some: ↓ clorazepate action
CNS depressants: ↑ CNS depression
MAOIs: ↑ effects of clorazepate
Oral contraceptives: ↑ effects of clorazepate

Herb/drug

Kava: ↑ CNS depression

Lab test interferences

↑ AST/ALT

NURSING CONSIDERATIONS

Assessment

- Assess seizures: duration, location, intensity, aura
- Monitor B/P (with patient lying, standing), pulse; if systolic B/P drops 20 mm Hg, hold drug, notify prescriber
- Monitor blood studies: CBC during long-term therapy; blood dyscrasias have occurred rarely
- Monitor hepatic studies: AST, ALT, bilirubin, creatinine, LDH, alkaline phosphatase
- Monitor I&O; may indicate renal dysfunction
- Monitor mental status: mood, sensorium, affect, sleeping pattern, drowsiness, dizziness, physical dependency; withdrawal symptoms: headache, nausea, vomiting, muscle pain, weakness after long-term use; suicidal tendencies

Nursing diagnoses

✓ Coping, ineffective individual (uses)
✓ Knowledge deficit (teaching)
✓ Noncompliance (teaching)

Implementation

- Give with food or milk for GI symptoms
- Do not chew, crush caps
- Use sugarless gum, hard candy, frequent sips of water for dry mouth
- Check to see PO medication has been swallowed

Patient/family education

- Teach patient that drug may be taken with food
- Teach patient not to use for everyday stress or longer than 4 mo, unless directed by a prescriber; not to take more than prescribed amount; may be habit forming
- Caution patient to avoid OTC preparations unless approved by a prescriber
- Caution patient to avoid driving, activities that require alertness; drowsiness may occur, especially in elderly
- Advise patient to avoid alcohol ingestion or other psychotropic medications, unless prescribed
- Advise patient not to discontinue medication abruptly after long-term use
- Advise patient to rise slowly or fainting may occur
- Teach patient that drowsiness may worsen at beginning of treatment

Evaluation

Positive therapeutic outcome

- Decreased anxiety, restlessness
- Decreased seizure activity

Treatment of overdose:

Lavage, VS, supportive care, flumazenil

cloxacillin (℞)

(klox-a-sill'in)

Apo-Cloxi ✤, Bactopen ✤, cloxacillin, Cloxapen, Novo-cloxin ✤, Orbenin ✤

Func. class.: Broad-spectrum antiinfective

Chem. class.: Penicillinase-resistant penicillin

Pregnancy category B

Action: Interferes with cell wall replication of susceptible organisms; the cell wall, rendered osmotically unstable, swells, bursts from osmotic pressure; resists the penicillinase action that inactivates penicillins

➔ **Therapeutic Outcome:** Bactericidal effects for the following: gram-positive cocci *Staphylococcus aureus, Staphylococcus epidermidis,* penicillinase-producing staphylococci

Uses: Penicillinase-producing staphylococci, streptococci; respiratory tract, skin, skin structure infections; sinusitis

Dosage and routes

Adult: PO 1-4 g/day in divided doses q6h or 250 mg-1 g q6h

P ***Child:*** PO 50-100 mg/kg in divided doses q6h, max 4 g/day

Available forms: Caps 250, 500 mg; oral sol 125 mg/5 ml

Adverse effects

CNS: Lethargy, hallucinations, anxiety, depression, muscle twitching, **coma, seizures**

GI: Nausea, vomiting, diarrhea, increased AST, ALT, abdominal pain, glossitis, **pseudomembranous colitis**

GU: **Oliguria, proteinuria,** hematuria, *vaginitis, moniliasis,* **glomerulonephritis**

HEMA: Anemia, **increased bleeding time, bone marrow depression, granulocytopenia**

SYST: **Anaphylaxis, serum sickness**

Contraindications: Hypersensitivity to penicillins; neonates, severe renal, hepatic disease P

Precautions: Pregnancy **B,** hypersensitivity to cephalosporins

Pharmacokinetics	
Absorption	Moderate (35%-60%)
Distribution	Widely distributed; crosses placenta
Metabolism	Liver (up to 22%)
Excretion	Breast milk; kidneys, unchanged (30%-45%)
Half-life	0.5-1.1 hr, increased in hepatic/renal disease

Pharmacodynamics	
Onset	½ hr
Peak	½-2 hr

Interactions

Individual drugs

Probenecid: ↑ cloxacillin concentrations, ↓ renal excretion

Drug classifications

Oral anticoagulants: ↑ anticoagulant effects

Food/drug

Food, carbonated drinks, citrus fruit juices: ↓ absorption

Herb/drug

Khat: ↓ absorption, separate by ≥2 hr

Lab test interferences

False positive: Urine glucose, urine protein

NURSING CONSIDERATIONS

Assessment

- Assess patient for previous sensitivity reaction to penicillins or other cephalosporins; cross-sensitivity between penicillins and cephalosporins is common
- Assess patient for signs and symptoms of infection including characteristics of wounds, sputum, urine, stool, WBC >10,000/mm^3, fever; obtain

baseline information and during treatment
- Obtain C&S before beginning drug therapy to identify if correct treatment has been initiated
- Assess for anaphylaxis: rash, urticaria, pruritus, chills, fever, joint pain may occur a few days after therapy begins; epinephrine and resuscitation equipment should be available for anaphylactic reaction
- Identify urine output; if decreasing, notify prescriber (may indicate nephrotoxicity); also check for increased BUN, creatinine
- Monitor blood studies: AST, ALT, CBC, Hct, bilirubin, LDH, alkaline phosphatase, Coombs' test monthly if patient is on long-term therapy
- Monitor electrolytes: potassium, sodium, chloride monthly if patient is on long-term therapy
- Assess bowel pattern qd; if severe diarrhea occurs, drug should be discontinued; may indicate pseudomembranous colitis
- Monitor for bleeding: ecchymosis, bleeding gums, hematuria, stool guaiac daily if on long-term therapy
- Assess for overgrowth of infection: perineal itching, fever, malaise, redness, pain, swelling, drainage, rash, diarrhea, change in cough, sputum

Nursing diagnoses
- ✓ Infection, risk for (uses)
- ✓ Diarrhea (side effects)
- ✓ Injury, risk for (side effects)
- ✓ Knowledge deficit (teaching)
- ✓ Noncompliance (teaching)

Implementation
- Give in even doses around the clock; if GI upset occurs, give with food; drug must be given for 10-14 days to ensure organism death and prevent superinfection; store in airtight container
- Do not crush, chew caps
- Shake susp well before each dose; store in refrigerator for 2 wk, 3 days at room temp

Patient/family education
- Teach patient to report sore throat, bruising, bleeding, joint pain; may indicate blood dyscrasias (rare)
- Advise patient to contact prescriber if vaginal itching, loose, foul-smelling stools, furry tongue occur; may indicate superinfection
- Instruct patient to take all medications prescribed for the length of time ordered
- Advise patient to notify prescriber of diarrhea with blood or pus, which may indicate pseudomembranous colitis

Evaluation
Positive therapeutic outcome
- Absence of signs/symptoms of infection (WBC $<10,000/mm^3$, temp WNL, absence of red, draining wounds)
- Reported improvement in symptoms of infection

Treatment of anaphylaxis:
Withdraw drug, maintain airway, administer epinephrine, aminophylline, O_2, **IV** corticosteroids

clozapine (℞)
(kloz′a-peen)
clozapine, Clozaril
Func. class.: Antipsychotic
Chem. class.: Tricyclic dibenzodiazepine derivative
Pregnancy category B

Action: Interferes with dopamine receptor binding with lack of extrapyramidal symptoms and tardive dyskinesia; also acts as an adrenergic, cholinergic, histaminergic, serotonergic antagonist

Therapeutic Outcome: Decreased psychotic behavior

Uses: Management of psychotic symptoms in schizophrenic patients for whom other antipsychotics have failed

C

Dosage and routes

Adult: PO 25 mg qd or bid; may increase by 25-50 mg/day; normal range 300-450 mg/day after 2 wk; do not increase dosage more than 2 times/wk; do not exceed 900 mg/day; use lowest dosage to control symptoms

Available forms: Tabs 25, 100 mg

Adverse effects

CNS: *Sedation, salivation, dizziness, headache, tremors, sleep problems, akinesia, fever,* **seizures,** *sweating, akathisia, confusion, fatigue, insomnia, depression, slurred speech, anxiety,* **neuroleptic malignant syndrome**

CV: *Tachycardia, hypotension, hypertension,* chest pain, ECG changes

GI: *Drooling or excessive salivation, constipation, nausea, abdominal discomfort, vomiting, diarrhea,* anorexia

GU: *Urinary abnormalities,* incontinence, ejaculation dysfunction, frequency, urgency, retention, dysuria

HEMA: **Leukopenia, neutropenia, agranulocytosis, eosinophilia, thrombocytopenia**

MS: Weakness; pain in back, neck, legs; spasm

RESP: Dyspnea, nasal congestion, throat discomfort

Contraindications: Hypersensitivity, myeloproliferative disorders, severe granulocytopenia, CNS depression, coma

Precautions: Pregnancy **B,** lactation, children <16 yr, hepatic, renal, cardiac disease, seizures, prostatic enlargement, elderly, narrow-angle glaucoma

Do Not Confuse:
Clozaril/Clinoril

Pharmacokinetics

Absorption	Well absorbed
Distribution	Widely distributed; crosses blood-brain barrier, placenta; 95% bound to plasma proteins
Metabolism	Liver
Excretion	Kidneys, feces (metabolites)
Half-life	8-12 hr

Pharmacodynamics

Onset	Unknown
Peak	Steady state 2½ hr
Duration	4-12 hr

Interactions

Individual drugs

Alcohol: ↑ effects of both drugs, oversedation
Digoxin: ↑ plasma concentration of digoxin
Phenytoin: ↓ phenytoin action
Warfarin: ↑ plasma concentrations

Drug classifications

Antacids: ↓ absorption
Anticholinergics: ↑ anticholinergic effects
Antidepressants: ↑ CNS depression
Antihistamines: ↑ CNS depression
Antihypertensives: ↑ hypotension
Antineoplastics: ↑ bone marrow suppression
Nitrates: ↑ hypotension

Food/drug

Caffeine: ↓ clozapine levels

Herb/drug

Kava: ↑ CNS depression
St. John's wort: ↑ CNS depression

Lab test interferences

↑ Liver function tests, ↑ cardiac enzymes, ↑ cholesterol, ↑ blood glucose, ↑ prolactin, ↑ bilirubin, ↑ PBI, ↑ cholinesterase, ↑ ^{131}I
False positive: Pregnancy tests, PKU
False negative: Urinary steroids, 17-OHCS

NURSING CONSIDERATIONS

Assessment

- Assess mental status: orientation, mood, behavior, presence of hallucinations, and type before initial administration and monthly; this drug should significantly reduce psychotic behavior

- Check for swallowing of PO medication; check for hoarding or giving of medication to other patients
- Monitor I&O ratio, palpate bladder if low urinary output occurs, especially G in elderly; urinalysis recommended before, during prolonged therapy
- Monitor bilirubin, CBC, liver function studies monthly; discontinue treatment if WBC <3000/mm^3 or if ANC <1500/mm^3; test qwk; may resume when normal; if WBS <2000/mm^3 or ANC <1000/mm^3, discontinue
- Assess affect, orientation, LOC, reflexes, gait, coordination, sleep pattern disturbances
- Monitor B/P with patient sitting, standing, and lying; take pulse and respirations q4h during initial treatment; establish baseline before starting treatment; report drops of 30 mm Hg
- Check for dizziness, faintness, palpitations, tachycardia on rising
- Assess for neuroleptic malignant syndrome: hyperpyrexia, muscle rigidity, increased CPK, altered mental status; drug should be discontinued
- Assess for extrapyramidal symptoms including akathisia (inability to sit still, no pattern to movements), tardive dyskinesia (bizarre movements of the jaw, mouth, tongue, extremities), pseudoparkinsonism (rigidity, tremors, pill rolling, shuffling gate)
- Assess for constipation, urinary retention daily; if these occur, increase bulk, water in diet

Nursing diagnoses

✓ Thought processes, altered (uses)
✓ Coping, ineffective individual (uses)
✓ Knowledge deficit (teaching)
✓ Noncompliance (teaching)

Implementation

- G Decrease dosage in elderly since metabolism is slowed
- Give with full glass of water, milk; or give with food to decrease GI upset
- Store in tight, light-resistant container; oral sol in amber bottle

Patient/family education

- Teach patient to use good oral hygiene; frequent rinsing of mouth, sugarless gum for dry mouth
- Caution patient to avoid hazardous activities until drug response is determined
- Inform patient that orthostatic hypotension occurs often and to rise from sitting or lying position gradually
- Caution patient to avoid hot tubs, hot showers, tub baths, since hypotension may occur
- Teach patient to avoid OTC preparations (cough, hay fever, cold) unless approved by prescriber, since serious drug interactions may occur; avoid use with alcohol, CNS depressants; increased drowsiness may occur
- Teach patient about extrapyramidal symptoms and necessity of meticulous oral hygiene, since oral candidiasis may occur
- Teach patient to report sore throat, malaise, fever, bleeding, mouth sores; if these occur, CBC should be performed and drug discontinued
- Advise patient that in hot weather, heat stroke may occur; take extra precautions to stay cool
- Teach patient symptoms of agranulocytosis and need for blood test qwk for 6 mo, then q2wk; report flu-like symptoms

Evaluation

Positive therapeutic outcome

- Decrease in emotional excitement, hallucinations, delusions, paranoia
- Reorganization of patterns of thought, speech

Treatment of anaphylaxis:

Withdraw drug, maintain airway

HIGH ALERT

coagulation factor VIIa, recombinant (℞)

NovoSeven

Func. class.: Antihemophilic

Pregnancy category C

Action: Promotes hemostasis by activating the intrinsic pathway of coagulation

Uses: Bleeding in hemophilia A or B, with inhibitors to factor VIII or IX

Dosage and routes

Adult: **IV** bol 90 μg/kg q2h until hemostasis occurs, or until therapy is deemed to be inadequate; posthemostatic doses q3-6h may be required

Available forms: Lyophilized powder 1.2 mg/vial (1200 μg/vial) recombinant human coagulation factor VIIa (rFVIIa); 4.8 mg/vial (4800 μg/vial) recombinant human coagulation factor VIIa (rFVIIa)

Adverse effects

CNS: Fever, headache

INTEG: Pain, redness at inj site, pruritus, purpura, rash

SYST: **Hemorrhage not otherwise specified, hemarthrosis, fibrinogen plasma decreased,** hypertension, bradycardia, **DIC, coagulation disorder, thrombosis**

Contraindications: Hypersensitivity to this product or mouse, hamster, or bovine products

Precautions: Pregnancy **C**, lactation, children

P

Pharmacokinetics

Half-life	2-3 hr

Pharmacodynamics

Unknown

Interactions

Individual drugs

Activated prothrombin complex concentrate: Do not use together

Prothrombin complex concentrate: Do not use together

NURSING CONSIDERATIONS

Assessment

- Assess VS, B/P, pulse, respirations, neurologic signs, temperature at least q4h, temperature 104° F (40° C) or indicators of internal bleeding, cardiac rhythm
- Monitor pro time, APTT, plasma FVII clotting
- Monitor for thrombosis, dose should be reduced or stopped

Implementation

IV route

- Bring to room temp; for 1.2 mg vial/2.2 ml sterile water for inj; 4.8 mg vial/8.5 ml sterile water for injection; remove caps from stopper, cleanse stopper with alcohol, allow to dry, draw back plunger of sterile syringe and allow air into syringe, insert needle of syringe into sterile water for inj, inject the air and withdraw amount required, insert syringe needle with diluent into drug vial, aim to side so liquid runs down vial wall, gently swirl until dissolved, use within 3 hr, give by bol over 3-5 min
- Do not admix, keep refrigerated until ready to use, avoid sunlight

Evaluation

Positive therapeutic outcome

- Therapeutic response: hemostasis

codeine ⊶ (℞)
(koe'deen)
Paveral ♣, Codeine
Narcotic analgesics
Func. class.: Opiate, phenanthrene derivative

Pregnancy category C

Controlled substance schedule II, III, IV, V
(depends on route)

Action: Depresses pain impulse transmission at the spinal cord level by interacting with opioid receptors; decreases cough reflex, GI motility

Therapeutic Outcome: Pain relief, decreased cough, decreased diarrhea depending on route

Uses: Moderate to severe pain, nonproductive cough

Investigational uses: Diarrhea

Dosage and routes

Pain

Adult: PO 15-60 mg q4h prn; IM/SC 15-60 mg q4h prn

P ***Child:*** PO 3 mg/kg/day in divided doses q4h prn

Cough

Adult: PO 10-20 mg q4-6h, not to exceed 120 mg/day

P ***Child:*** PO 1-1.5 mg/kg/day in 4 divided doses, not to exceed 60 mg/day

Diarrhea

Adult: PO 30 mg; may repeat qid prn

Renal dose

CrCl 10-50 ml/min 75% of dose; CrCl <10 ml/min 50% of dose

Available forms: Inj 30, 60 mg/ml; tabs 15, 30, 60 mg; oral sol 10 mg/5 ml, 15 mg/5 ml

Adverse effects

CNS: *Drowsiness, sedation,* dizziness, agitation, dependency, lethargy, restlessness, euphoria, **seizures**

CV: Bradycardia, palpitations, orthostatic hypotension, tachycardia, **circulatory collapse**

GI: *Nausea, vomiting, anorexia, constipation*

GU: Urinary retention

INTEG: Flushing, rash, urticaria, pruritus

RESP: **Respiratory depression, respiratory paralysis**

SYST: **Anaphylaxis**

Contraindications: Hypersensitivity to opiates, respiratory depression, increased intracranial pressure, seizure disorders, severe respiratory disorders

G **Precautions:** Elderly, cardiac dysrhythmias, pregnancy **C**

Do Not Confuse:
codeine/Lodine

Pharmacokinetics

Absorption	Complete (IM)
Distribution	Widely distributed; crosses placenta
Metabolism	Liver, extensively
Excretion	Kidneys (up to 15%), breast milk
Half-life	3-4 hr

Pharmacodynamics

	PO	IM	SC
Onset	30-45 min	15-30 min	15-30 min
Peak	1-2 hr	30-60 min	Unknown
Duration	4 hr	4 hr	4 hr

Interactions

Individual drugs

Alcohol: ↑ respiratory depression, hypotension, ↑ sedation

Drug classifications

Antihistamines: ↑ respiratory depression, hypotension

CNS depressants: ↑ respiratory depression, hypotension

MAOIs: ↑ toxicity

Phenothiazines: ↑ respiratory depression, hypotension

Sedative/hypnotics: ↑ respiratory depression, hypotension

Herb/drug

Kava: ↑ CNS depression

Lab test interferences

↑ Amylase, ↑ lipase

NURSING CONSIDERATIONS

Assessment

- Assess pain: intensity, type, alleviating factors
- Assess GI function: nausea, vomiting, constipation
- Monitor VS after parenteral route; note muscle rigidity, drug history, liver, kidney function tests, respiratory dysfunction: respiratory depression, character, rate, rhythm; notify prescriber if respirations are <10/min
- Monitor CNS changes: dizziness, drowsiness, hallucinations, euphoria, LOC, pupil reaction
- Monitor allergic reactions: rash, urticaria

Nursing diagnoses

- ✓ Pain (uses)
- ✓ Sensory perceptual alteration: visual, auditory (adverse reactions)
- ✓ Breathing pattern, ineffective (adverse reactions)
- ✓ Knowledge deficit (teaching)

Implementation

- Give with antiemetic if nausea, vomiting occur
- Administer when pain is beginning to return, determine dosage interval by patient response; continuous dosing of medication is more effective given prn; explain analgesic effect
- Medication should be slowly withdrawn after long-term use to prevent withdrawal symptoms
- Store in light-resistant container at room temp

PO route

- May be given with food or milk to lessen GI upset

IM/SC route

- Do not give if cloudy, or a precipitate has formed

IV route

- Give slowly by direct inj

Syringe compatibilities:
Glycopyrrolate, hydroxyzine

Y-site compatibilities:
Cefmetazole

Additive incompatibilities:
Aminophylline, amobarbital, chlorothiazide, heparin, methicillin, pentobarbital, phenobarbital, phenytoin, secobarbital, thiopental

Patient/family education

- Teach patient to report any symptoms of CNS changes, allergic reactions; to avoid CNS depressants: alcohol, sedative/hypnotics for at least 24 hr after taking this drug
- Discuss with patient that dizziness, drowsiness, and confusion are common
- Advise patient to avoid getting up without assistance
- Discuss in detail all aspects of the drug

Evaluation

Positive therapeutic outcome

- Decreased pain
- Decreased cough
- Decreased diarrhea

Treatment of overdose:

Naloxone 0.2-0.8 **IV**, O_2, **IV** fluids, vasopressors

colchicine (℞)

(kol'chi-seen)

Func. class.: Antigout agent

Chem. class.: Colchicum autumnale alkaloid

Pregnancy category
C (PO), D (IV)

Action: Inhibits microtubule formation of lactic acid in leukocytes, which decreases phagocytosis and inflammation in joints

Therapeutic Outcome: Decreased pain, inflammation of joints

Uses: Gout, gouty arthritis (prevention, treatment); to arrest progression of neurologic disability in multiple sclerosis

Investigational uses: Hepatic cirrhosis, familial Mediterranean fever, pericarditis

Dosage and routes

Prevention

Adult: PO 0.5-1.8 mg qd depending on severity; **IV** 0.5-1 mg qd-bid

Treatment

Adult: PO 0.5-1.2 mg, then 0.5-1.2 mg q1h, until pain decreases or side effects occur; **IV** 2 mg, then 0.5 mg q6h, not to exceed 4 mg/24 hr

Pericarditis

Adult: PO 0.5-3 mg qd × 3 days, then 1 mg qd up to 1 yr

Available forms: Tabs 0.5, 0.6 mg; inj **IV** 1 mg/2 ml

Adverse effects

GI: *Nausea, vomiting, anorexia, malaise,* metallic taste, cramps, peptic ulcer, diarrhea
GU: Hematuria, **oliguria, renal damage**
HEMA: **Agranulocytosis, thrombocytopenia, aplastic anemia, pancytopenia**
INTEG: Chills, dermatitis, pruritus, purpura, erythema
MISC: Myopathy, alopecia, reversible azoospermia, peripheral neuritis

Contraindications: Hypersensitivity; serious GI, renal, hepatic, cardiac disorders; blood dyscrasias, pregnancy **D (IV)**

Precautions: Severe renal disease, blood dyscrasias, pregnancy **C** (PO), hepatic disease, elderly [G], lactation, children [P]

Pharmacokinetics

Absorption	Well absorbed
Distribution	WBCs
Metabolism	Deacetylates in liver
Excretion	Feces (metabolites/active drug)
Half-life	20 min

Pharmacodynamics

	PO
Onset	Unknown
Peak	½-2 hr
Duration	Unknown

Interactions

Individual drugs

Cyclosporine: ↑ bone marrow depression
Erythromycin: ↑ colchicine effect
Phenylbutazone: ↑ blood dyscrasias
Radiation: ↑ bone marrow depression
Vitamin B_{12}: ↓ action of vit B_{12}, may cause reversible malabsorption

Drug classifications

Acidifiers: ↓ action of colchicine
Alkalinizers: ↑ action of colchicine
Bone marrow depressants: ↑ bone marrow depression
CNS depressants: ↑ action of CNS depressants
Diuretics, loop: ↓ colchicine effect
NSAIDs: ↑ GI effects
Sympathomimetics: ↑ action of sympathomimetics

Lab test interferences

↑ Alkaline phosphatase, ↑ AST/ALT
False positive: RBC, Hgb

NURSING CONSIDERATIONS

Assessment

- Assess pain and mobility of joints
- Monitor I&O ratio; observe for decrease in urinary output; CBC, platelets, reticulocytes before, during therapy (q3 mo): Coombs' test to determine Coombs' negative hemolytic anemia
- Assess for toxicity: weakness, abdominal pain, nausea, vomiting, diarrhea

Nursing diagnoses
- ✓ Pain, chronic (uses)
- ✓ Immobility, impaired (uses)
- ✓ Knowledge deficit (teaching)

Implementation
PO route
- Give on empty stomach (1 hr ac or 2 hr pc) for better absorption

IV **IV route**
- Give **IV** undiluted or diluted 1 mg/10-20 ml normal saline or sterile water for inj; give over 2-5 min
- Do not give IM or SC
- Wait ≥1 wk after giving a full course of **IV** colchicine, before giving more doses

Patient/family education
- Teach patient to increase fluids to 3-4 L/day
- Caution patient to avoid alcohol, OTC preparations that contain alcohol; skin rashes have occurred
- Instruct patient to report any pain, redness, or hard area, usually in legs
- Teach patient importance of complying with medical regimen; bone marrow depression may occur

Evaluation
Positive therapeutic outcome
- Decreased stone formation on x-ray
- Decreased pain in kidney region
- Absence of hematuria
- Decreased pain in joints

Treatment of overdose:
D/C medication, may need opioids to treat diarrhea

colesevelam (℞)
(coal-see-vel'am)
Welchol
Func. class.: Antilipemic
Chem. class.: Bile acid sequestrant
Pregnancy category C

Action: Absorbs, combines with bile acids to form insoluble complex that is excreted through feces; loss of bile acids lowers cholesterol levels

➔ **Therapeutic Outcome:** Decreasing LDL cholesterol

Uses: Elevated LDL cholesterol, alone or in combination with HMG-CoA reductase inhibitor

Dosage and routes
Adult: PO monotherapy: 3 625 mg tabs bid with meals or 6 tabs qd with a meal; may increase to 7 tabs if needed

Combination therapy
3 tabs bid with meals or 6 tabs qd with a meal given with an HMG-CoA reductase inhibitor

Available forms: Tabs 625 mg

Adverse effects
CNS: Headache, dizziness, drowsiness, vertigo, tinnitus
GI: Constipation, abdominal pain, nausea, fecal impaction, hemorrhoids, flatulence, vomiting, steatorrhea, peptic ulcer
INTEG: Rash, irritation of perianal area, tongue, skin
HEMA: Decreased vit A, D, K, red cell folate content; ***hyperchloremic acidosis, bleeding,*** decreased pro-time
MS: Muscle, joint pain

Contraindications: Hypersensitivity, biliary obstruction

Precautions: Pregnancy **C,** lactation, children (P)

Pharmacokinetics

Absorption	Unknown
Distribution	Unknown
Metabolism	Unknown
Excretion	Feces
Half-life	Unknown

Pharmacodynamics
Unknown

Interactions
Individual drugs
Cephalexin: ↓ absorption of cephalexin

Chenodiol: ↓ absorption of chenodiol
Clindamycin: ↓ absorption of clindamycin
Digitalis: ↓ absorption of digitalis
Folic acid: ↓ absorption of folic acid
Iron: ↓ absorption of iron
Penicillin G: ↓ absorption of penicillin G
Phenobarbital: ↓ absorption of phenobarbital
Phenylbutazone: ↓ absorption of phenylbutazone
Thyroid hormones: ↓ absorption of thyroid
Trimethoprim: ↓ absorption of trimethoprim
Warfarin: ↓ absorption of warfarin

Drug classifications

Fat-soluble vitamins: ↓ absorption of fat-soluble vitamins
Tetracyclines: ↓ absorption of tetracyclines
Thiazides: ↓ absorption of thiazides

Lab test interferences

↑ Liver function studies, ↑ Cl, ↑ PO_4

NURSING CONSIDERATIONS

Assessment

- Assess cardiac glycoside level if both drugs are being administered
- Assess for signs of vit A, D, K deficiency
- Monitor fasting LDL, HDL, total cholesterol, triglyceride levels, electrolytes if on extended therapy
- Monitor bowel pattern daily; increase bulk, H_2O in diet for constipation

Nursing diagnoses

✓ Constipation (adverse reactions)
✓ Knowledge deficit (teaching)
✓ Noncompliance (teaching)

Implementation

- Give drug ac, hs; give all other medications 1 hr before colesevalam or 4 hr after colesevalam to avoid poor absorption
- Give supplemental doses of vit A, D, K, if levels are low

Patient/family education

(Alert) Teach the symptoms of hypoprothrombinemia: bleeding mucous membranes, dark tarry stools, hematuria, petechiae; report immediately
- Teach the importance of compliance; toxicity may result if doses missed
- Teach that risk factors should be decreased: high-fat diet, smoking, alcohol consumption, absence of exercise
- Advise not to discontinue suddenly

Evaluation

Positive therapeutic outcome

- Decreased cholesterol level (hyperlipidemia); diarrhea, pruritus (excess bile acids)

colestipol (℞)

(koe-les′ti-pole)

Colestid

Func. class.: Antilipemic

Chem. class.: Bile acid sequestrant

Pregnancy category B

Action: Absorbs, combines with bile acids to form an insoluble complex that is excreted through feces; loss of bile acids lowers cholesterol levels

Therapeutic Outcome: Decreasing cholesterol levels and low-density lipoproteins, decreased pruritus

Uses: Primary hypercholesterolemia, xanthomas, digitalis toxicity, pruritus due to biliary obstruction, diarrhea due to bile acids

Dosage and routes

Adult: PO tabs 2 g qd-bid, may increase by 1 g/mo, max 16 g/day; granules 5 g qd-bid, may increase qmo, max 30 g/day

Available forms: Granules 300 g, 500 g bottles, 5 g packets, tabs 1 g

C

Adverse effects

GI: Constipation, abdominal pain, nausea, fecal impaction, hemorrhoids, flatulence, vomiting, steatorrhea, peptic ulcer
HEMA: **Bleeding, decreased protime**
INTEG: Rash, irritation of perianal area, tongue, skin
META: Decreased vit A, D, E, K, red folate content; **hyperchloremic acidosis**

Contraindications: Hypersensitivity, biliary obstruction

Precautions: Pregnancy **B,**
P lactation, children, bleeding disorders

Pharmacokinetics

Absorption	Not absorbed
Distribution	Not distributed
Metabolism	Not metabolized
Excretion	Binds with bile acids, feces
Half-life	Unknown

Pharmacodynamics

Onset	24-48 hr
Peak	30 days
Duration	30 days

Interactions

Individual drugs

Acetaminophen: ↓ absorption of acetominophen
Amiodarone: ↓ absorption of amiodarone
Methotrexate: ↓ absorption of methotrexate
Naproxen: ↓ absorption of naproxen
Phenylbutazone: ↓ absorption of phenylbutazone
Piroxicam: ↓ absorption of piroxicam
Propranolol: ↓ absorption of propanolol
Thyroid hormone: ↓ absorption of thyroid
Ursodiol: ↓ absorption of ursodiol

Drug classifications

Anticoagulants, oral: ↓ absorption
Antidiabetics, oral: antagonize colestipol
Cardiac glycosides: ↓ absorption
Diuretics, thiazide: ↓ absorption
NSAIDs: ↓ absorption
Vitamins A, D, E, K: ↓ absorption

Lab test interferences

↑ Liver function studies, ↑ Cl, ↑ PO_4

NURSING CONSIDERATIONS

Assessment

- Assess nutrition: fat, protein, carbohydrates; nutritional analysis should be completed by dietician
- Assess skin integrity after patient has been receiving drug; itching, pruritus often occur from bile deposits on skin
- Monitor cardiac glycoside level, if both drugs are being administered; cardiac glycoside levels will be decreased
- Monitor for signs of vit A, D, E, K deficiency; check serum cholesterol, triglyceride levels, electrolytes if on extended therapy
- Monitor bowel pattern daily; increase bulk, water in diet if constipation develops

Nursing diagnoses

✓ Constipation (adverse reactions)
✓ Knowledge deficit (teaching)
✓ Noncompliance (teaching)

Implementation

- Give drug ac, hs; give all other medications 1 hr before or 4 hr after colestipol to avoid poor absorption; give drug mixed with applesauce or stirred into beverage (2-6 oz), let stand for 2 min; do not take dry
- Provide supplemental doses of vit A, D, E, K, if levels are low
- ⊘ Tabs should be swallowed whole; do not crush, chew

Patient/family education

- Teach patient symptoms of hypoprothrombinemia: bleeding mucous membranes, dark, tarry stools, hematuria, petechiae; report immediately
- Teach patient importance of compliance, not to miss or double doses

- Teach patient that risk factors should be decreased: high-fat diet, smoking, alcohol consumption, absence of exercise
- Tell patient to mix drug with 6 oz of milk, water, fruit juice; may be mixed with carbonated beverages; rinse glass to make sure all medication is taken or may mix drug in applesauce; allow to stand for 2 min before mixing

Evaluation

Positive therapeutic outcome

- Decreased cholesterol level (hyperlipidemia)
- Decreased diarrhea, pruritus (excess bile acids)

cortisone (Key Drug) (℞)

(kor'ti-sone)

Cortone (Canada), cortone acetate

Func. class.: Corticosteroid, synthetic

Chem. class.: Short-acting glucocorticoid

Pregnancy category D

Action: Decreases inflammation by suppression of migration of polymorphonuclear leukocytes, fibroblasts, reversal of increased capillary permeability, and lysosomal stabilization; suppresses adrenal function with long-term use

Therapeutic Outcome: Replacement of cortisol in adrenal insufficiency

Uses: Inflammation, severe allergy, adrenal insufficiency, collagen disorders, respiratory and dermatologic disorders

Dosage and routes

Adult: PO/IM 25-300 mg qd or q2 days, titrated to patient response

P ***Child:*** PO 2.5-10 mg/kg/day; IM 1-5 mg/kg/day

Available forms: Tabs 5, 10, 25 mg; inj 50 mg/ml

Adverse effects

CNS: *Depression, flushing, sweating,* headache, mood changes

CV: *Hypertension,* **circulatory collapse, thrombophlebitis, embolism,** tachycardia, **necrotizing angiitis, CHF,** edema

EENT: Fungal infections, increased intraocular pressure, blurred vision

GI: *Diarrhea, nausea, abdominal distention,* **GI hemorrhage,** increased appetite, **pancreatitis**

HEMA: **Thrombocytopenia**

INTEG: Acne, poor wound healing, ecchymosis, bruising, petechiae

MS: Fractures, osteoporosis, weakness

Contraindications: Psychosis, hypersensitivity, idiopathic thrombocytopenia, acute glomerulonephritis, amebiasis, fungal infections, nonasthmatic bronchial disease, P child <2 yr, AIDS, TB, pregnancy **D**

Precautions: Diabetes mellitus, glaucoma, osteoporosis, seizure disorders, ulcerative colitis, CHF, myasthenia gravis, renal disease, esophagitis, peptic ulcer

Pharmacokinetics

Absorption	Slowly IM
Distribution	Widely, crosses placenta
Metabolism	Liver
Excretion	Unknown
Half-life	½ hr

Pharmacodynamics

	PO	IM
Onset	Unknown	Unknown
Peak	2 hr	20-48 hr
Duration	1½ days	1½ days

Interactions

Individual drugs

Amphotericin B: ↑ hypokalemia

Insulin: ↑ need for insulin

Mezlocillin: ↑ hypokalemia

Phenobarbital: ↓ effectiveness of cortisone

Phenytoin: ↓ effectiveness of cortisone

Drug classifications
Contraceptives, oral: blocked metabolism of cortisone
Diuretics, potassium-wasting: ↑ side effects
NSAIDs: ↑ GI symptoms
Salicylates: ↑ GI symptoms

Herb/drug
Aloe: ↑ potassium deficiency
Buckthorn bark/berry: ↑ potassium deficiency
Cascara sagrada bark: ↑ potassium deficiency, chronic use
Rhubarb root: ↑ potassium deficiency
Senna leaf/fruits: ↑ potassium deficiency

Lab test interferences
↑ Cholesterol, ↑ sodium, ↑ blood glucose, ↑ uric acid, ↑ calcium, ↑ urine glucose
↓ Calcium, ↓ potassium, ↓ T_4, ↓ T_3, ↓ thyroid ^{131}I uptake test, ↓ urine 17-OHCS, ↓ 17-KS, ↓ PBI
False negative: Skin allergy tests

NURSING CONSIDERATIONS
Assessment
- Assess for adrenal insufficiency symptoms: weakness, nausea, vomiting, confusion, anxiety, restlessness, decreased B/P, weight loss; check before and during treatment
- Monitor potassium, blood glucose, urine glucose for patient on long-term therapy; hypokalemia and hyperglycemia can occur
- Check B/P, pulse q4h; notify prescriber if chest pain occurs
- Monitor I&O ratio and weight daily; be alert for decreasing urinary output and increasing edema with bilateral rales, dyspnea, weight gain
- Monitor plasma cortisol levels during long-term therapy (normal level: 138-635 nmol/L if checked at 8 AM)
- Assess for symptoms of infection: increased temp, WBC even after withdrawal of medication; drug masks symptoms of infection
- Monitor for potassium depletion: paresthesias, fatigue, nausea, vomiting, depression, polyuria, dysrhythmias, weakness, edema, hypertension, cardiac symptoms, weight daily; notify prescriber of weekly gain >5 lb
- Assess for mental changes: affect, mood, behavioral changes, aggression; depression, psychoses may occur

Nursing diagnoses
- ✓ Infection, risk for (adverse reactions)
- ✓ Injury, risk for (adverse reactions)
- ✓ Knowledge deficit (teaching)

Implementation
IM route
- Give after shaking susp (parenteral); titrate dose; use lowest effective dosage
- Give IM inj deep in large muscle mass; rotate sites; avoid deltoid; use a 21 G needle
- Administer in 1 dose in AM to prevent adrenal suppression; avoid SC administration; damage may be done to tissue; do not give **IV**

PO route
- Administer with food or milk to decrease GI symptoms

Patient/family education
- Advise patient that ID as steroid user should be carried at all times
- Instruct patient to notify prescriber if therapeutic response decreases; dosage adjustment may be needed; teach not to discontinue this medication abruptly or adrenal crisis can result; teach all aspects of drug usage, including cushingoid symptoms
- Caution patient to avoid OTC products: salicylates, potassium, alcohol in cough products, cold preparations unless directed by prescriber
- Teach patient symptoms of adrenal insufficiency: nausea, anorexia, fatigue, dizziness, dyspnea, weakness, joint pain, tarry stools, bruising, blurred vision
- Advise patient to avoid persons with known infections; report probable infection rapidly; drug masks infection

• Caution patient that diet modification is necessary if on long-term treatment: increased calcium, potassium, and protein; also low sodium and carbohydrates

Evaluation

Positive therapeutic outcome

• Ease of respirations, decreased inflammation

cotrimoxazole

See trimethoprim/sulfamethoxazole

cyclobenzaprine (℞)

(sye-kloe-ben′za-preen)

cyclobenzaprine HCl, Cycloflex, Flexeril

Func. class.: Skeletal muscle relaxant, central acting

Chem. class.: Tricyclic amine salt

Pregnancy category B

Action: Unknown; may be related to antidepressant effects

Therapeutic Outcome: Relaxation of skeletal muscle

Uses: Adjunct for relief of muscle spasm and pain in musculoskeletal conditions

Dosage and routes

Musculoskeletal disorders

Adult: PO 10 mg tid × 1 wk, not to exceed 60 mg/day × 3 wk

P ***Child:*** PO 20-40 mg/kg/day in 2-4 divided doses

Fibromyalgia

Adult: PO 10-40 mg hs

Available forms: Tabs 10 mg

Adverse effects

CNS: *Dizziness, weakness, drowsiness,* headache, tremor, depression, insomnia, confusion, paresthesia

CV: Postural hypotension, tachycardia, **dysrhythmias**

EENT: Diplopia, temporary loss of vision

GI: *Nausea,* vomiting, hiccups, dry mouth, constipation

GU: Urinary retention, frequency, change in libido

INTEG: Rash, pruritus, fever, facial flushing, sweating

Contraindications: Acute recovery phase of MI, dysrhythmias, heart P block, CHF, hypersensitivity, child <12 yr, intermittent porphyria, thyroid disease

Precautions: Renal disease, hepatic disease, addictive personality, G pregnancy **B**, elderly

Do Not Confuse:
cyclobenzaprine/cyproheptadine

Pharmacokinetics	
Distribution	Well
Metabolism	Liver, partially
Excretion	Kidney (unchanged)
Half-life	1-3 days

Pharmacodynamics	
Onset	1 hr
Peak	3-8 hr
Duration	12-24 hr

Interactions

Individual drugs

Alcohol: ↑ CNS depression

Drug classifications

Antidepressants, tricyclic: ↑ CNS depression

Antihistamines: ↑ CNS depression

Barbiturates: ↑ CNS depression

MAOIs: Do not use within 14 days

Opiates: ↑ CNS depression

Sedative/hypnotics: ↑ CNS depression

Herb/drug

Kava: ↑ CNS depression

NURSING CONSIDERATIONS

Assessment

• Assess pain periodically: location, duration, mobility, stiffness, baseline

- Monitor ECG in epileptic patients; poor seizure control has occurred in patients taking this drug
- Check for allergic reactions: rash, fever, respiratory distress
- Check for severe weakness, numbness, in extremities
- Assess for CNS depression: dizziness, drowsiness, psychiatric symptoms

Nursing diagnoses

✓ Physical mobility, impaired uses
✓ Injury, risk for (adverse reactions)
✓ Knowledge deficit (teaching)

Implementation

- Give with meals for GI symptoms
- Store in airtight container at room temp

Patient/family education

- Teach patient not to discontinue medication quickly; insomnia, nausea, headache, spasticity, tachycardia will occur; drug should be tapered off over 1-2 wk
- Caution patient not to take with alcohol, other CNS depressants
- Advise to avoid altering activities while taking this drug
- Caution patient to avoid hazardous activities if drowsiness/dizziness occurs
- Caution patient to avoid using OTC medication: cough preparations, antihistamines, unless directed by prescriber
- Teach patient to use gum, frequent sips of water for dry mouth

Evaluation

Positive therapeutic outcome

- Decreased pain, spasticity; muscle spasms of acute, painful musculoskeletal conditions are generally short term; long-term therapy is seldom warranted

Treatment of overdose: Empty stomach with emesis, gastric lavage, then administer activated charcoal; use anticonvulsants if indicated; monitor cardiac function

HIGH ALERT

cyclophosphamide

(℞)

(sye-kloe-foss'fa-mide)

Cytoxan, Neosar, Procytox ✤

Func. class.: Antineoplastic alkylating agent

Chem. class.: Nitrogen mustard

Pregnancy category D

Action: Alkylates DNA, RNA; inhibits enzymes that allow synthesis of amino acids in proteins; is also responsible for cross-linking DNA strands; activity is not cell cycle phase specific

Therapeutic Outcome: Prevention of rapidly growing malignant cells

Uses: Hodgkin's disease, lymphomas, leukemia, multiple myeloma, neuroblastoma, retinoblastoma, Ewing's sarcoma, cancer of female reproductive tract, breast, lung, prostate

Dosage and routes

Adult: PO initially 1-5 mg/ kg over 2-5 days; maintenance 1-5 mg/kg; **IV** initially 40-50 mg/kg in divided doses over 2-5 days; maintenance 10-15 mg/kg q7-10 days, or 3-5 mg/kg q3 days

P ***Child:*** PO/**IV** 2-8 mg/kg or 60-250 mg/m^2 in divided doses × 6 or more days; maintenance **IV** 10-15 mg/kg q7-10 days or 30 mg/kg q3-4 wk; or PO 2-5 mg/kg 2×/wk dose should be reduced by half when bone marrow suppression occurs

Renal dose

CrCl 25-50 ml/min 50% of dose; CrCl <25 ml/min avoid use

Available forms: Powder for inj **IV** 100, 200, 500, 750 mg, 1, 2 g; tabs 25, 50 mg

Adverse effects

CNS: Headache, dizziness

CV: **Cardiotoxicity** (high doses)

ENDO: Syndrome of inappropriate antidiuretic hormone (SIADH), gonadal suppression
GI: *Nausea, vomiting, diarrhea, weight loss,* colitis, **hepatotoxicity**
GU: **Hemorrhagic cystitis, hematuria, neoplasms, amenorrhea, azoospermia, sterility, ovarian fibrosis**
HEMA: **Thrombocytopenia, leukopenia, pancytopenia, myelosuppression**
INTEG: *Alopecia,* dermatitis
META: Hyperuricemia
MISC: Secondary neoplasms
RESP: **Fibrosis**

Contraindications: Lactation, pregnancy **D**

Precautions: Radiation therapy

Do Not Confuse:
cyclophosphamide/cyclosporine, Cytoxan/Cytosar, Cytoxan/Cytotec

Pharmacokinetics

Absorption	Well absorbed (PO)
Distribution	Widely distributed; crosses placenta, blood-brain barrier (50%)
Metabolism	Liver to active drug
Excretion	Kidneys, unchanged (30%)
Half-life	4-6½ hr

Pharmacodynamics

Unknown

Interactions

Individual drugs

Allopurinol: ↑ bone marrow suppression
Chloramphenicol: ↓ cyclophosphamide
Doxorubicin: ↑ cardiotoxicity
Insulin: ↑ hypoglycemia
Phenobarbital: ↑ toxicity
Radiation: ↑ toxicity, bone marrow suppression
Rifampin: ↑ toxicity, bone marrow suppression
Succinylcholine: ↑ neuromuscular blockade

Drug classifications

Aminoglycosides: ↑ nephrotoxicity
Anticoagulants, oral: ↑ bleeding
Antineoplastics: ↑ toxicity, bone marrow suppression
Barbiturates: ↑ toxicity of cyclophosphamide
Bone marrow–suppressing drugs: ↑ bone marrow suppression
Corticosteroids: ↓ cyclophosphamide effect
Diuretics, loop: ↑ ototoxicity
Live virus vaccines: ↓ antibody reaction

Lab test interferences

↑ Uric acid
↓ Pseudocholinesterase
False positive: Pap smear
False negative: PPD, mumps trichophytin, *Candida*

NURSING CONSIDERATIONS

Assessment

- Assess symptoms indicating severe allergic reaction: rash, pruritus, urticaria, purpuric skin lesions, itching, flushing
- Assess for tachypnea, ECG changes, dyspnea, edema, fatigue
- Monitor CBC, differential, platelet count weekly; withhold drug if WBC count is <2500/mm^3 or platelet count is <75,000/mm^3; notify prescriber of results
- Assess for hemorrhagic cystitis: renal function studies including BUN, creatinine, serum uric acid, urine CrCl before and during therapy; I&O ratio; report fall in urine output to <30 ml/hr
- Monitor temp q4h (may indicate beginning of infection)
- Monitor liver function tests before and during therapy (bilirubin, AST, ALT, LDH) as needed or monthly; note jaundice of skin or sclera, dark urine, clay-colored stools, itchy skin, abdominal pain, fever, diarrhea
- Assess for bleeding: hematuria,

stool guaiac, bruising or petechiae, mucosa or orifices q8h
- Identify dyspnea, rales, unproductive cough, chest pain, tachypnea
- Identify effects of alopecia on body image; discuss feelings about body changes

Nursing diagnoses

✓ Injury, risk for (adverse reactions)
✓ Body image disturbance (adverse reactions)
✓ Infection, risk for (adverse reactions)
✓ Knowledge deficit (teaching)

Implementation

- Give fluids **IV** or PO before chemotherapy to hydrate patient
- Give antacid before oral agent, pc PM, before hs; antiemetic 30-60 min before giving drug to prevent vomiting, and prn; antibiotics for prophylaxis of infection
- Give top or syst analgesics for pain; give in AM so drug can be eliminated before hs

IV route

- Give **IV** after diluting 100 mg/5 ml of sterile or bacteriostatic water; shake; let stand until clear; may be further diluted in up to 250 ml D_5 0.9% NaCl, 0.45% NaCl, LR, Ringer's; give 100 mg or less/min through 3-way stopcock of glucose or saline inf
- Use 21, 23, 25 G needle; check site for irritation, phlebitis

Syringe compatibilities:

Bleomycin, cisplatin, doxapram, doxorubicin, droperidol, fluorouracil, furosemide, heparin, leucovorin, methotrexate, metoclopramide, mitomycin, mitoxantrone, vinblastine, vincristine

Y-*site compatibilities:*

Amifostine, amikacin, ampicillin, azlocillin, aztreonam, bleomycin, cefamandole, cefazolin, cefepime, cefoperazone, cefotaxime, cefoxitin, cefuroxime, cephalothin, cephapirin, chloramphenicol, chlorpromazine, cimetidine, cisplatin, cladribine, clindamycin, dexamethasone, diphenhydramine, doxorubicin, doxycycline, droperidol, erythromycin, famotidine, filgrastim, fludarabine, fluorouracil, furosemide, gallium, ganciclovir, gentamicin, granisetron, heparin, hydromorphone, idarubicin, kanamycin, leucovorin, lorazepam, melphalan, methotrexate, methylprednisolone, metoclopramide, metronidazole, mezlocillin, minocycline, mitomycin, moxalactam, nafcillin, ondansetron, oxacillin, paclitaxel, penicillin G potassium, piperacillin, piperacillin/tazobactam, prochlorperazine, promethazine, propofol, ranitidine, sargramostim, sodium bicarbonate, teniposide, tetracycline, thiotepa, ticarcillin, ticarcillin-clavulanate, tobramycin, trimethoprim-sulfamethoxazole, vancomycin, vinblastine, vincristine, vinorelbine

Additive compatibilities:

Cisplatin with etoposide, hydroxyzine, methotrexate, methotrexate with fluorouracil, mitoxantrone, ondansetron

Solution compatibilities:

Amino acids 4.25%/D_{25}, D_5/0.9% NaCl, D_5W, 0.9% NaCl

Patient/family education

- Teach patient to avoid use of products containing aspirin or ibuprofen, razors, commercial mouthwash, since bleeding may occur; to report symptoms of bleeding (hematuria, tarry stools)
- Instruct patient to report signs of anemia (fatigue, headache, irritability, faintness, shortness of breath)
- Teach patient to report any changes in breathing or coughing even several months after treatment
- Advise patient that hair may be lost during treatment; a wig or hairpiece may make patient feel better; new hair may be different in color, texture
- Teach patient not to have any vaccinations without the advice of the

prescriber; serious reactions can occur
- Advise patient contraception is needed during treatment and for several months after the completion of therapy

Evaluation

Positive therapeutic outcome
- Prevention of rapid division of malignant cells
- Increased appetite, increased weight

cyclosporine (℞)
(sye-kloe-spor'een)
Neoral, Sandimmune, SangCya
Func. class.: Immunosuppressant
Chem. class.: Fungus-derived peptide
Pregnancy category C

Action: Produces immunosuppression by inhibiting T lymphocytes

Therapeutic Outcome: Absence of transplant rejection

Uses: Organ transplants (liver, kidney, heart) to prevent rejection, rheumatoid arthritis, psoriasis

Investigational uses: Recalcitrant ulcerative colitis

Dosage and routes

Prevention of transplant rejection

P ***Adult and child:*** PO 15 mg/kg several hr before surgery, daily for 2 wk, reduce dosage by 2.5 mg/kg/wk to 5-10 mg/kg/day; **IV** 5-6 mg/kg several hr before surgery, daily, switch to PO form as soon as possible

Rheumatoid arthritis

Adult: PO 2.5 mg/kg/day divided bid, may increase 0.5-0.75 mg/kg/day after 8-12 wk, max 4 mg/kg/day

Psoriasis

Adult: PO 2.5 mg/kg/day divided bid × 4 wk, then increase by 0.5 mg/kg/day q2 wk, max 4 mg/kg/day

Available forms: Microemulsion oral sol (Neoral) 100 mg/ml; microemulsion soft get cap (Neoral) 25, 100 mg; soft gel caps 25, 100 mg; oral sol 100 mg/ml; inj 50 mg/ml

Adverse effects

CNS: Tremors, headache, **seizures**
GI: Nausea, vomiting, diarrhea, *oral Candida, gum hyperplasia,* **hepatotoxicity,** pancreatitis
GU: **Albuminuria, hematuria, proteinuria, renal failure**
INTEG: Rash, acne, ***hirsutism***
META: Hyperkalemia, hypomagnesemia, hyperlipidemia, hyperuricemia
MISC: Gingival hyperplasia, infection

Contraindications: Hypersensitivity

Precautions: Severe renal disease, severe hepatic disease, pregnancy **C**

Do Not Confuse:
cyclosporine/Cycloserine, cyclosporine/cyclophosphamide

Pharmacokinetics

Absorption	Poorly absorbed (PO)
Distribution	Crosses placenta
Metabolism	Liver to mercaptopurine
Excretion	Kidney, minimal
Half-life	Biphasic 1.2 hr, 25 hr

Pharmacodynamics

	PO
Onset	Unknown
Peak	4 hr
Duration	Unknown

Interactions

Individual drugs

Amphotericin B: ↑ cyclosporine toxicity
Carvedilol: ↑ cyclosporine toxicity
Cimetidine: ↑ cyclosporine toxicity
Digoxin: ↑ digoxin level
Etoposide: ↑ etoposide level
Fluconazole: ↑ cyclosporine toxicity
Ketoconazole: ↑ cyclosporine toxicity

Melphalan: ↑ cyclosporine toxicity
Phenytoin: ↓ cyclosporine action
Rifampin: ↓ cyclosporine action
Tacrolimus: Do not use with cyclosporine

Drug classifications:

Androgens: ↑ cyclosporine levels
Antifungals, azole: ↑ cyclosporine level
Calcium channel blockers: ↑ cyclosporine levels
Corticosteroids: ↑ cyclosporine level
Live virus vaccines: ↓ antibody reaction
Macrolides: ↑ cyclosporine toxicity
Neoral products: ↓ absorption
NSAIDs: ↑ cyclosporine toxicity
Oral contraceptives: ↑ cyclosporine toxicity
Rifamycins: ↓ cyclosporine levels

Food/drug

Grapefruit juice: ↑ CNS side effects

NURSING CONSIDERATIONS

Assessment

- Monitor renal studies: BUN, creatinine at least monthly during treatment, 3 mo after treatment
- Monitor liver function studies: alkaline phosphatase, AST, ALT, bilirubin
- Monitor drug blood levels during treatment
- Assess for hepatotoxicity: dark urine, jaundice, itching, light-colored stools; drug should be discontinued
- Assess for nephrotoxicity: 6 wk postop, CyA trough level >200 ng/ml, intracapsular pressure <40 mm Hg, rise in creatinine 0.15 mg/dl/day

Nursing diagnoses

✓ Mobility, impaired (uses)
✓ Infection, risk for (uses)
✓ Knowledge deficit (teaching)

Implementation

PO route

- Use pipette provided to draw up oral sol; may mix with milk or juice, wipe pipette, do not wash
- Give for several days before transplant surgery with corticosteroids
- Microemulsion products (Neoral) and other products are not interchangeable
- Give with meals for GI upset or drug placed in chocolate milk
- Do not crush, chew caps
- Give with oral antifungal for *Candida* infections

IV route

- Give **IV** after diluting each 50 mg/20-100 ml of 0.9% NaCl or D_5W; run over 2-6 hr; use an infusion pump, glass inf bottles only; may give as cont inf over 24 hr

Additive compatibilities:

Ciprofloxacin

Y-site compatibility:

Cefmetazole, propofol, sargramostim

Solution compatibilities:

D_5W, NaCl 0.9%

- Give for several days before transplant surgery
- Give with corticosteroids

Patient/family education

- Advise patient to report fever, rash, severe diarrhea, chills, sore throat, fatigue, since serious infections may occur; also to report clay-colored stools, cramping (may indicate hepatotoxicity); tremors, bleeding gums, increased B/P
- Caution patient to use contraceptive measures during treatment and for 12 wk after ending therapy; drug is teratogenic
- Caution patient to avoid crowds and persons with known infections to reduce risk of infection

Evaluation

Positive therapeutic outcome

- Absence of graft rejection

cyproheptadine (℞)

(si-proe-hep′ta-deen)
cyproheptadine HCl, Periactin, PMS-Cyproheptadine

Func. class.: Antihistamine, H_1-receptor antagonist
Chem. class.: Piperidine

Pregnancy category B

Action: Acts on blood vessels, GI, respiratory system by competing with histamine for H_1-receptor site; decreases allergic response by blocking histamine; blocks serotonin to increase appetite and relieve vascular headaches

Therapeutic Outcome: Absence of allergy symptoms and rhinitis

Uses: Allergy symptoms, rhinitis, pruritus, cold urticaria

Investigational uses: Appetite stimulant, management of vascular headache, nightmares, post-traumatic stress disorder

Dosage and routes

Adult: PO 4 mg tid-qid, not to exceed 0.5 mg/kg/day

P ***Child 7-14 yr:*** PO 4 mg bid-tid, not to exceed 16 mg/day

P ***Child 2-6 yr:*** PO 2 mg bid-tid, not to exceed 12 mg/day

Nightmares, post-traumatic stress disorder

Adult: PO 4-12 mg qhs, max 32 mg

Available forms: Tabs 4 mg; syr 2 mg/5 ml

Adverse effects

CNS: *Dizziness, drowsiness,* poor coordination, fatigue, anxiety, euphoria, confusion, paresthesia, neuritis
CV: Hypotension, palpitations, tachycardia
EENT: *Blurred vision,* dilated pupils; tinnitus; nasal stuffiness; dry nose, throat, mouth
GI: *Constipation, dry mouth,* nausea, vomiting, anorexia, diarrhea, weight gain
GU: *Retention,* dysuria, frequency, increased appetite
HEMA: **Hemolytic anemia, leukopenia, thrombocytosis, agranulocytosis**
INTEG: Rash, urticaria, photosensitivity
MISC: **Anaphylaxis**
RESP: Increased thick secretions, wheezing, chest tightness

Contraindications: Hypersensitivity to H_1-receptor antagonist, acute asthma attack, lower respiratory tract disease

Precautions: Increased intraocular pressure, renal disease, cardiac disease, hypertension, bronchial asthma, seizure disorder, stenosed peptic ulcers, hyperthyroidism, prostatic hypertrophy, bladder neck obstruction, pregnancy **B,** G elderly

Do Not Confuse:
cyproheptadine/cyclobenzaprine

Pharmacokinetics	
Absorption	Well absorbed
Distribution	Unknown
Metabolism	Liver, complete
Excretion	Kidneys
Half-life	Unknown

Pharmacodynamics	
Onset	15-60 min
Peak	1-2 hr
Duration	8 hr

Interactions

Individual drugs

Alcohol: ↑ CNS depression

Drug classifications

CNS depressants: ↑ CNS depression
MAOIs: ↑ anticholinergic effect
Opiates: ↑ CNS depression
Sedative/hypnotics: ↑ CNS depression

C

Herb/drug

Henbane leaf: ↑ anticholinergic effect
Kava: ↑ CNS depression

Lab test interferences

False negative: Skin allergy tests (discontinue antihistamine 3 days before testing)

NURSING CONSIDERATIONS

Assessment

- Assess respiratory status: rate, rhythm, increase in bronchial secretions, wheezing, chest tightness; provide fluids to 2 L/day to decrease secretion thickness
- Monitor I&O ratio: be alert for urinary retention, frequency, dysuria, G especially elderly; drug should be discontinued if these occur; monitor food intake, weight if using as an appetite stimulant

Nursing diagnoses

✓ Airway clearance, ineffective (uses)
✓ Injury, risk for (side effects)
✓ Knowledge deficit (teaching)
✓ Noncompliance (teaching, overuse)

Implementation

- May give with food to decrease GI upset
- Syrup may be used for patients with P difficulty swallowing or children
- Store in tight, light-resistant container

Patient/family education

- Teach all aspects of drug uses; tell patient to notify prescriber if confusion, sedation, hypotension occur; to avoid driving and other hazardous activity if drowsiness occurs; to avoid alcohol and other CNS depressants that may potentiate effect
- Caution patient not to exceed recommended dosage; dysrhythmias may occur
- Teach patient hard candy, gum, frequent rinsing of mouth may be used for dryness

Evaluation

Positive therapeutic outcome

- Absence of running or congested nose, rashes

Treatment of overdose:

Administer ipecac syrup or lavage, diazepam, vasopressors, barbiturates (short acting)

HIGH ALERT

cytarabine (℞)

(sye-tare'a-been)

Ara-C, Cytosar ✤, Cytosar-U, cytosine arabinoside, Depo Cyt, Tarabine PFS

Func. class.: Antineoplastic, antimetabolite

Chem. class.: Pyrimidine nucleoside

Pregnancy category D

Action: Competes with physiologic substrate of DNA synthesis, thus interfering with cell replication in the S phase of the cell cycle (before mitosis)

➔ **Therapeutic Outcome:** Prevention of rapidly growing malignant cells

Uses: Acute myelocytic leukemia, acute lymphocytic leukemia, chronic myelocytic leukemia, lymphomatous meningitis (IT), and in combination for non-Hodgkin's lymphomas in P children

Dosage and routes

Acute myelocytic leukemia

Adult: **IV** inf 200 mg/m^2/day × 5 days q2 wk as single agent or 2-6 mg/kg/day (100-200 mg/m^2/day) as single dose or 2-3 divided doses for 5-10 days until remission, used in combination; maintenance 70-200 mg/m^2/day for 2-5 days qmo; SC maintenance 1 mg/kg 1-2×/wk

Lymphomatous meningitis Liposomal (DepoCyt)

Adult: IT 50 mg q14 days × 2 doses (wk 1, 3) then 50 mg q14 days × 3

doses (wk 5, 7, 9) followed by 1 dose wk 13; then 50 mg q28 days × 4 doses (wk 17, 21, 25, 29); if neurotoxicity occurs, reduce dose to 25 mg, if it persists, discontinue use

In combination

P ***Child:*** **IV** inf 100 mg/m²/day × 5-10 days

Available forms: Powder for inj 100, 500 mg, 1, 2 g; liposomal for IT use 10 mg/ml

Adverse effects

CNS: Neuritis, dizziness, headache, personality changes, ataxia, mechanical dysphasia, **coma; chemical arachnoiditis** (IT)

CV: Chest pain, **cardiopathy**

CYTARABINE SYNDROME: Fever, myalgia, bone pain, chest pain, rash, conjunctivitis, malaise (6-12 hr after administration)

EENT: Sore throat, conjunctivitis

GI: *Nausea, vomiting, anorexia, diarrhea, stomatitis,* **hepatotoxicity,** abdominal pain, hematemesis, **GI hemorrhage**

GU: Urinary retention, **renal failure, hyperuricemia**

HEMA: **Thrombophlebitis, bleeding, thrombocytopenia, leukopenia, myelosuppression, anemia**

INTEG: *Rash, fever,* freckling, cellulitis

META: Hyperuricemia

RESP: **Pneumonia,** dyspnea, **pulmonary edema** (high doses)

SYST: **Anaphylaxis**

Contraindications: Hypersensitivity, infants, pregnancy **D** (P)

Precautions: Renal disease, hepatic disease

Do Not Confuse:

Cytosar/Cytovene, Cytosar/Cytoxan

Pharmacokinetics

Absorption	Complete
Distribution	Widely distributed; crosses blood-brain barrier, placenta
Metabolism	Liver, extensively
Excretion	Kidneys
Half-life	1-3 hr; IT 100-236 hr

Pharmacodynamics

Unknown

Interactions

Individual drugs

Cyclophosphamide: ↑ cardiotoxicity, CHF

Radiation: ↑ toxicity, bone marrow suppression

Drug classifications

Antineoplastics: ↑ toxicity, bone marrow suppression

NURSING CONSIDERATIONS

Assessment

- Assess buccal cavity q8h for dryness, sores or ulceration, white patches, pain, bleeding, dysphagia; obtain prescription for viscous lidocaine (Xylocaine)
- Assess symptoms indicating anaphylaxis: rash, pruritus, urticaria, purpuric skin lesions, itching, flushing, resuscitation equipment should be nearby
- (Alert) Assess for chemical arachnoiditis (IT): headache, nausea, vomiting, fever; neck rigidity/pain, meningism, CSF pleocytosis; may be decreased by dexamethasone
- Assess tachypnea, dyspnea, edema, fatigue; identify dyspnea, rales, unproductive cough, chest pain, tachypnea; pulmonary edema may be fatal (rare)
- (Alert) Assess for cytarabine syndrome 6-12 hr after inf: fever, myalgia, bone pain, chest pain, rash, conjunctivitis, malaise; corticosteroid may be ordered
- Monitor CBC, differential, platelet count weekly; withhold drug if WBC

count is <1000/mm³ or platelet count is <50,000/mm³
- Assess for increased uric acid levels, swelling, joint pain primarily in extremities; patient should be well hydrated to prevent urate deposits
- Monitor renal function studies: BUN, creatinine, serum uric acid, urine CrCl before and during therapy; I&O ratio; report fall in urine output to <30 ml/hr
- Monitor temp q4h (may indicate beginning of infection)
- Monitor liver function tests before and during therapy (bilirubin, AST, ALT, LDH) as needed or monthly; note yellowing of skin or sclera, dark urine, clay-colored stools, pruritus, abdominal pain, fever, diarrhea; an antispasmodic may be used for GI symptoms
- Assess for bleeding: hematuria, stool guaiac, bruising or petechiae, mucosa or orifices q8h; identify inflammation of mucosa, breaks in skin

Nursing diagnoses

- ✓ Injury, risk for (adverse reactions)
- ✓ Body image disturbance (adverse reactions)
- ✓ Infection, risk for (adverse reactions)
- ✓ Knowledge deficit (teaching)

Implementation

- Avoid contact with skin; very irritating; wash completely to remove
- Give fluids **IV** or PO before chemotherapy to hydrate patient
- Give antiemetic 30-60 min before giving drug to prevent vomiting, and prn; antibiotics for prophylaxis of infection
- Give top or syst analgesics for pain
- Give in AM so drug can be eliminated before hs
- Provide liquid diet: carbonated beverages; gelatin may be added if patient is not nauseated or vomiting
- Provide rinsing of mouth tid-qid with water, club soda; brushing of teeth bid-qid with soft brush or cotton-tipped applicators for stomatitis; use unwaxed dental floss
- Give **IV** direct after diluting 100 mg/5 ml of sterile water for inj; give by direct **IV** over 1-3 min through free-flowing tubing

IV **IV infusion**

- May be further diluted in 50-100 ml 0.9% NaCl or D_5W and given over 30 min to 24 hr depending on dosage; may be given by cont inf also

Syringe compatibilities:

Metoclopramide

Y-site compatibilities:

Amifostine, amsacrine, aztreonam, cefepime, chlorpromazine, cimetidine, cladribine, dexamethasone, diphenhydramine, droperidol, famotidine, filgrastim, fludarabine, gentamicin, granisetron, heparin, hydrocortisone, hydromorphone, idarubicin, lorazepam, melphalan, methotrexate, methylprednisolone, metoclopramide, morphine, ondansetron, paclitaxel, piperacillin/tazobactam, prochlorperazine, promethazine, propofol, ranitidine, sargramostim, sodium bicarbonate, teniposide, thiotepa, vinorelbine

Additive compatibilities:

Corticotropin, daunorubicin with etoposide, etoposide, hydroxyzine, lincomycin, mitoxantrone, potassium chloride, prednisolone, ondansetron, sodium bicarbonate, vincristine

Additive incompatibilities:

Carbenicillin, fluorouracil, heparin, regular insulin, nafcillin, oxacillin, penicillin G sodium

Solution compatibilities:

Amino acids, 4.25%/D_{25}, D_5/LR, D_5/0.2% NaCl, D_5/0.9% NaCl, D_{10}/0.9% NaCl, D_5W, invert sugar 10% in electrolyte #1, Ringer's LR, 0.9% NaCl, sodium lactate 1/6 mol/L, TPN #57

Intrathecal route

- Liposomal: withdraw drug immediately before use; use within 4 hr, do not save unused portions, or use

in-line filter; give directly into CSF by intraventricular reservoir or by direct inj into lumbar site
- Give slowly over 1-5 min, follow with lumbar puncture, instruct patient to lie flat, give dexamethasone 4 mg bid PO or **IV** × 5 days beginning on day of liposomal inj

SC/IM route
- Reconstitute 100 mg/5 ml or 500 mg/10 ml with bacteriostatic water for inj with benzyl alcohol 0.9%; do not use sol with precipitate; stable for 48 hr

Patient/family education
- Advise patient that contraceptive measures are recommended during and 4 mo after therapy
- Teach patient to avoid use of products containing aspirin or ibuprofen, NSAIDs, razors, commercial mouthwash, since bleeding may occur; to report symptoms of bleeding (hematuria, tarry stools)
- Advise patient to continue using dexamethasone with IT administration, that fever, headache, nausea, vomiting are likely to occur
- Advise patient to report signs of anemia (fatigue, headache, irritability, faintness, shortness of breath)
- Advise patient to avoid foods with citric acid, hot or rough texture if stomatitis is present, use sponge brush and rinse with water after each meal; to report stomatitis: any bleeding, white spots, ulcerations in mouth; tell patient to examine mouth qd, report any symptoms
- Instruct patient to report any changes in breathing or coughing even several months after treatment; to avoid crowds and persons with respiratory tract or other infections; neurotoxicity
- Caution patient not to have any vaccinations without the advice of the prescriber; serious reactions can occur
- Advise patient to take fluids 3 L/day to prevent renal damage

Evaluation
Positive therapeutic outcome
- Prevention of rapid division of malignant cells

HIGH ALERT

dacarbazine (℞)
(da-kar'ba-zeen)

dacarbazine, DTIC ♣, DTIC-Dome

Func. class.: Antineoplastic misc agent

Chem. class.: Imidazole

Pregnancy category C

Action: Alkylates DNA, RNA; inhibits enzymes that allow synthesis of amino acids in proteins; also responsible for cross-linking DNA strands; activity is not cell cycle phase specific

Therapeutic Outcome: Prevention of rapidly growing malignant cells

Uses: Hodgkin's disease, sarcomas, neuroblastoma, malignant melanoma

Investigational uses: Metastatic sarcoma

Dosage and routes
Malignant melanoma

Adult: **IV** 2-4.5 mg/kg or 70-160 mg/m^2 qd × 10 days; repeat q4 wk depending on response or 250 mg/m^2 qd × 5 days; repeat q3 wk

Hodgkin's disease

Adult: **IV** 150 mg/m^2 qd × 5 days with other agents, repeat q4 wk or 375 mg/m^2 on day 1 when given in combination, repeat q15 days

Available forms: Inj 100, 200 mg

Adverse effects
CNS: Facial paresthesia, flushing, fever, malaise

GI: *Nausea, anorexia, vomiting,* **hepatotoxicity** (rare)

HEMA: **Thrombocytopenia, leukopenia,** anemia
INTEG: *Alopecia,* dermatitis, pain at inj site
SYST: **Anaphylaxis**

Contraindications: Lactation

Precautions: Radiation therapy, pregnancy (1st trimester) **C**

Pharmacokinetics

Absorption	Complete bioavailability (**IV**)
Distribution	Widely distributed; concentrates in liver
Metabolism	Liver (50%, 5% protein bound)
Excretion	Kidneys, unchanged (50%)
Half-life	Initial 35 min, terminal 5 hr

Pharmacodynamics

Unknown

Interactions

Individual drugs

Phenobarbital: ↑ toxicity
Phenytoin: ↑ metabolism, ↓ effect
Radiation: ↑ toxicity, bone marrow suppression

Drug classifications

Aminoglycosides: ↑ nephrotoxicity
Anticoagulants: ↑ risk of bleeding
Antineoplastics: ↑ toxicity, bone marrow suppression
Bone marrow–suppressing drugs: ↑ bone marrow suppression, toxicity
Diuretics, loop: ↑ ototoxicity
Live virus vaccines: ↑ adverse reactions, ↓ antibody reaction
Salicylates: ↑ risk of bleeding

NURSING CONSIDERATIONS

Assessment

- Assess symptoms indicating severe allergic reaction: rash, pruritus, urticaria, purpuric skin lesions, itching, flushing; drug should be discontinued
- Monitor CBC, differential, platelet count weekly; withhold drug if WBC is <4000/mm^3 or platelet count is <100,000/mm^3
- Monitor renal function studies: BUN, creatinine, urine CrCl before and during therapy; I&O ratio; report fall in urine output to <30 ml/hr
- Monitor temp q4h (may indicate beginning of infection)
- Monitor liver function tests before and during therapy (bilirubin, AST, ALT, LDH) as needed or monthly; note jaundice of skin or sclera, dark urine, clay-colored stools, itchy skin, abdominal pain, fever, diarrhea; hepatoxicity can be serious and fatal
- Assess for bleeding: hematuria, stool guaiac, bruising or petechiae, mucosa or orifices q8h; check for inflammation of mucosa, breaks in skin
- Identify effects of alopecia on body image; discuss feelings about body changes

Nursing diagnoses

- ✓ Injury, risk for (adverse reactions)
- ✓ Body image disturbance (adverse reactions)
- ✓ Infection, risk for (adverse reactions)
- ✓ Knowledge deficit (teaching)

Implementation

- Give fluids **IV** or PO before chemotherapy to hydrate patient
- Give antiemetic 30-60 min before giving drug to prevent vomiting, and prn; antibiotics for prophylaxis of infection
- Provide liquid diet: carbonated beverages; gelatin may be added if patient is not nauseated or vomiting
- After diluting 100 mg/9.9 ml of sterile water for inj (10 mg/ml), give by direct **IV** over 1 min through Y-tube or 3-way stopcock
- May be further diluted in 50-250 ml of D_5W or normal saline for inj and given over 30 min
- Watch for extravasation; give 3-5 ml of mixture of 4 ml sodium thiosulfate 10% plus 5 ml of sterile water SC as prescribed

D

Y-site compatibilities:
Amifostine, aztreonam, filgrastim, fludarabine, granisetron, melphalan, ondansetron, paclitaxel, sargramostim, teniposide, thiotepa, vinorelbine

Additive compatibilities:
Bleomycin, carmustine, cyclophosphamide, cytarabine, dactinomycin, doxorubicin, fluorouracil, mercaptopurine, methotrexate, ondansetron, vinblastine

Additive incompatibilities:
Hydrocortisone sodium succinate, cysteine

Patient/family education

- Teach patient to avoid use of products containing aspirin or ibuprofen, razors, commercial mouthwash, since bleeding may occur; to report symptoms of bleeding (hematuria, tarry stools)
- Instruct patient to report signs of anemia (fatigue, headache, irritability, faintness, shortness of breath)
- Advise patient that hair may be lost during treatment; a wig or hairpiece may make patient feel better; new hair may be different in color, texture
- Caution patient not to have any vaccinations without the advice of prescriber; serious reactions can occur
- Advise patient contraception is needed during treatment and for several months after the completion of therapy; drug has teratogenic properties

Evaluation

Positive therapeutic outcome

- Prevention of rapid division of malignant cells

HIGH ALERT

daclizumab (℞)
(dah-kliz'uh-mab)
Zenapax
Func. class.: Immunosuppressive
Chem class.: Humanized IgGl monoclonal antibody

Pregnancy category C

Action: Binds to the IL-2 receptor antagonist

Therapeutic Outcome: Prevention of graft rejection

Uses: Acute allograft rejection in renal transplant patients

Dosage and routes

Adult: **IV** 1 mg/kg as part of a regimen that includes cyclosporine and corticosteroids, mix calculated vol with 50 ml of 0.9% NaCl and give via peripheral/central vein over 15 min

Available forms: Inj 25 mg/ml

Adverse effects

CNS: *Chills, tremors,* headache, prickly sensation
CV: Hypertension, **tachycardia, thrombosis, bleeding**
GI: Vomiting, nausea, diarrhea, constipation, abdominal pain, pyrosis
GU: Oliguria, dysuria, **renal tubular necrosis, renal damage, hydronephrosis**
INTEG: Impaired wound healing
RESP: *Dyspnea, wheezing,* **pulmonary edema,** coughing, atelectasis, congestion, hypoxia

Contraindications: Hypersensitivity

Precautions: Pregnancy **C,** child <2 yr, lactation, elderly

Pharmacokinetics

Unknown

Pharmacodynamics

Unknown

Interactions
Unknown

NURSING CONSIDERATIONS
Assessment
- Monitor blood studies: Hgb, WBC, platelets during treatment qmo; if leukocytes are <3000/mm^3, drug should be discontinued
- Monitor liver function studies: alkaline phosphatase, AST, ALT, bilirubin
- Assess for hepatotoxicity: dark urine, jaundice, itching, light-colored stools; drug should be discontinued
- Assess for anaphylaxis: have corticosteroids, epinephrine available

Nursing diagnoses
✓ Injury, risk for (uses)
✓ Knowledge deficit (teaching)

Implementation
- Give all other medications PO if possible; avoid IM inj, since infection may occur

IV **IV route**
- Solution compatibilities 0.9% NaCl
- Protect undiluted sol from direct light; should be used with drugs for immunosuppression

Patient/family education
- Teach patient to report fever, chills, sore throat, fatigue, since serious infection may occur
- Instruct patient to use contraception (women), before, during, and for 4 mo after treatment
- Advise patient to avoid vaccinations during treatment
- Advise patient to drink fluids during treatment

Evaluation
Positive therapeutic outcome
- Absence of graft rejection

HIGH ALERT

dactinomycin (℞)
(dak-ti-noe-mye'sin)
actinomycin D, Cosmegen
Func. class.: Antineoplastic, antibiotic

Pregnancy category C

Action: Inhibits DNA, RNA, protein synthesis; derived from *Streptomyces parvulus;* replication is decreased by binding to DNA, which causes strand splitting; cell cycle nonspecific; a vesicant

➔ **Therapeutic Outcome:** Prevention of rapidly growing malignant cells, immunosuppression

Uses: Sarcomas, melanomas, trophoblastic tumors in women, testicular cancer, Wilms' tumor, rhabdomyosarcoma

Dosage and routes
Adult: **IV** 500 μg/m^2/day × 5 days; stop drug for 2-4 wk; then repeat cycle

P ***Child:*** **IV** 15 μg/kg/day × 5 days, not to exceed 500 μg/day; stop drug until bone marrow recovery, then repeat cycle

Available forms: Inj 0.5 mg/vial

Adverse effects
CNS: Malaise, fatigue, lethargy, fever
EENT: Cheilitis, dysphagia, esophagitis
GI: *Nausea, vomiting, anorexia, stomatitis,* **hepatotoxicity,** abdominal pain, diarrhea
HEMA: **Thrombocytopenia, leukopenia, aplastic anemia**
INTEG: *Rash,* alopecia, pain at inj site, folliculitis, acne, desquamation, *extravasation*
MS: Myalgia

Contraindications: Hypersensitivity, herpes infections, P child <6 mo

Precautions: Renal, hepatic disease, pregnancy **C,** lactation, bone marrow suppression

Pharmacokinetics

Absorption	Complete bioavailability
Distribution	Widely distributed; crosses placenta
Metabolism	Unknown
Excretion	Bile; feces, unchanged (50%); kidneys (10%)
Half-life	36 hr

Pharmacodynamics

Unknown

Interactions

Individual drugs

Radiation: ↑ toxicity, bone marrow suppression

Drug classifications

Antineoplastics: ↑ toxicity, bone marrow suppression

Bone marrow–suppressing drugs: ↑ bone marrow suppression

Live virus vaccines: ↓ antibody reaction

Lab test interferences

↑ Uric acid

NURSING CONSIDERATIONS

Assessment

- Assess buccal cavity q8h for dryness, sores or ulceration, white patches, pain, bleeding, dysphagia; obtain prescription for viscous lidocaine (Xylocaine)
- (Alert) Assess symptoms indicating severe allergic reaction: rash, pruritus, urticaria, purpuric skin lesions, itching, flushing; drug should be discontinued
- Monitor CBC, differential, platelet count weekly; withhold drug if WBC is <4000/mm^3 or platelet count is <100,000/mm^3; notify prescriber of results if WBC <20,000/mm^3, platelets <150,000/mm^3
- Monitor renal function studies: BUN, creatinine, serum uric acid, urine CrCl before and during therapy; I&O ratio; report fall in urine output to <30 ml/hr
- Monitor temp q4h (may indicate beginning of infection)
- Monitor liver function tests before and during therapy (bilirubin, AST, ALT, LDH) as needed or monthly; note jaundice of skin or sclera, dark urine, clay-colored stools, itchy skin, abdominal pain, fever, diarrhea
- Assess for bleeding: hematuria, stool guaiac, bruising or petechiae, mucosa or orifices q8h; check for inflammation of mucosa, breaks in skin
- Identify effects of alopecia on body image; discuss feelings about body changes

Nursing diagnoses

- ✓ Injury, risk for (adverse reactions)
- ✓ Body image disturbance (adverse reactions)
- ✓ Oral mucous membranes, altered (adverse reactions)
- ✓ Infection, risk for (adverse reactions)
- ✓ Knowledge deficit (teaching)

Implementation

- Provide antacid before oral agent; give drug pc PM, before hs; antiemetic 30-60 min before giving drug to prevent vomiting, and prn; antibiotics for prophylaxis of infection
- Provide liquid diet: carbonated beverages; gelatin may be added if patient is not nauseated or vomiting
- Help patient rinse mouth tid-qid with water, club soda, brush teeth bid-qid with soft brush or cotton-tipped applicators for stomatitis, use unwaxed dental floss
- Drug should be prepared by experienced personnel using proper precautions
- Give after diluting 0.5 mg/1.1 ml of sterile water for inj without preservative; use 2.2 ml (0.25 mg/ml), give by direct **IV** at 0.5 mg or less/min through Y-tube or 3-way stopcock of inf in progress

Intermittent infusion

- May be further diluted in 50 ml of D_5W or 0.9% NaCl for inf; run over 10-15 min
- Give hydrocortisone, sodium

thiosulfate to infiltration area, and ice compress after stopping inf

- Store in darkness in cool environment

Y-site compatibilities:
Allopurinol, amifostine, aztreonam, cefepime, fludarabine, granisetron, melphalan, ondansetron, sargramostim, teniposide, thiotepa, vinorelbine

Patient/family education

- Teach patient to avoid use of products containing aspirin or ibuprofen, razors, commercial mouthwash, since bleeding may occur; to report symptoms of bleeding (hematuria, tarry stools)
- Instruct patient to report signs of anemia (fatigue, headache, irritability, faintness, shortness of breath)
- Advise patient that hair may be lost during treatment; a wig or hairpiece may make patient feel better; new hair may be different in color, texture
- Caution patient not to have any vaccinations without the advice of the prescriber, serious reactions can occur
- Advise patient that contraception is needed during treatment and for several months after the completion of therapy
- Advise patient to increase fluids to 3 L/day

Evaluation

Positive therapeutic outcome

- Prevention of rapid division of malignant cells

HIGH ALERT

dalteparin (℞)

(dahl'ta-pear-in)
Fragmin
Func. class.: Anticoagulant
Chem. class.: Low molecular weight heparin

Pregnancy category B

Action: Prevents conversion of fibrinogen to fibrin and prothrombin to thrombin by enhancing inhibitory effects of antithrombin III

➔ **Therapeutic Outcome:** Absence of deep vein thrombosis

Uses: Unstable angina/non-Q-wave MI; prevention of deep vein thrombosis in abdominal surgery patients

Investigational uses: Systemic anticoagulation in venous/arterial thromboembolic complications

Dosage and routes

Hip replacement surgery
Adult: SC 2500 IU 2 hr before surgery and 2nd dose in the evening the day of surgery, then 5000 IU SC 1st postop day and qd 5-10 days

Unstable angina/ non-Q-wave MI
Adult: SC 120 IU/kg, do not exceed 10,000 IU q12h with concurrent aspirin, continue until stable

Systemic anticoagulation
Adult: SC 200 IU/kg qd or 100 IU/kg bid

Deep vein thrombosis, prophylaxis
Adult: SC 2500 IU qd, 1-2 hr before abdominal surgery and repeat qd × 5-10 days; in high-risk patients 5000 IU may be used

Available forms: Prefilled syringes, 2500, 5000 IU/0.2 ml; 10,000 IU multidose vials

Adverse effects

CNS: **Intracranial bleeding**
HEMA: **Thrombocytopenia**
INTEG: Pruritus, superficial wound infection
SYST: Hypersensitivity, **hemorrhage, anaphylaxis** possible

Contraindications: Hypersensitivity to this drug, heparin, or other anticoagulants; hemophilia, leukemia with bleeding, thrombocytopenic purpura, cerebrovascular hemorrhage, cerebral aneurysm, severe hypertension, other severe cardiac disease

G **Precautions:** Elderly, pregnancy **B,** hepatic disease, severe renal disease, blood dyscrasias, subacute bacterial endocarditis, acute nephritis,
P lactation, child, recent childbirth, peptic ulcer disease, pericarditis, pericardial effusion, recent lumbar puncture, vasculitis, other diseases where bleeding is possible

Pharmacokinetics	
Absorption	87%
Distribution	Unknown
Metabolism	Liver
Excretion	Kidney
Half-life	2 hr

Pharmacodynamics	
Onset	Unknown
Peak	4 hr
Duration	Unknown

Interactions

Drug classifications

Anticoagulants: ↑ risk of bleeding
Platelet inhibitors: ↑ risk of bleeding
Salicylates: ↑ risk of bleeding

Herb/drug

Bromelain, cinchona: ↑ risk of bleeding

NURSING CONSIDERATIONS

Assessment

- Assess for bleeding (Hct, occult blood in stools) during treatment since bleeding can occur
- (Alert) Assess for bleeding gums, petechiae, ecchymosis, black tarry stools, hematuria, epistaxis, decrease in Hct, B/P; may indicate bleeding, possible hemorrhage; notify prescriber immediately, drug should be discontinued
- Assess for hypersensitivity: fever, skin rash, urticaria; notify prescriber immediately
- Assess for needed dosage change q1-2 wk; dose may need to be decreased if bleeding occurs

Nursing diagnoses

- ✓ Injury, risk for (uses, adverse reactions)
- ✓ Tissue perfusion (uses) altered
- ✓ Knowledge deficit (teaching)

Implementation

SC route

- Do not give IM or **IV** drug route; approved is SC only; do not mix with other inj or sol
- Give by SC only; have patient sit or lie down; SC inj may be 2 in from umbilicus in a U-shape, upper outer side or high or upper outer quadrangle of the buttocks; rotate inj sites
- Changing needles is not recommended

Patient/family education

- Advise patient to avoid OTC preparations that contain aspirin, other anticoagulants; serious drug interaction may occur; if dose is missed, take as soon as possible, but not if almost time for next dose
- Advise patient to use soft-bristle toothbrush to avoid bleeding gums, avoid contact sports, use electric razor, avoid IM injection
- Instruct patient to report any signs of bleeding: gums, under skin, urine, stools; unusual bruising

Evaluation

Positive therapeutic outcome

- Absence of deep vein thrombosis

Treatment of overdose:
Protamine sulfate 1% given **IV**; 1 mg protamine/100 anti-Xa IU of dalteparin given

HIGH ALERT

danaparoid (℞)
(dan-a-pair'oid)
orgaran
Func. class.: Anticoagulant
Chem. class.: Low molecular weight heparin
Pregnancy category B

Action: Prevents conversion of fibrinogen to fibrin and prothrombin to thrombin by enhancing inhibitory effects of antithrombin III

➔ **Therapeutic Outcome:** Absence of deep vein thrombosis

Uses: Prevention of vein thrombosis in hemodialysis, stroke, elective surgery for malignancy or total hip replacement, hip fracture surgery

Dosage and routes
Prevention of venous thrombosis
Adult: SC 750 anti-Xa units bid × 7-10 days, begin 1-4 hr presurgery and restart 2 hr after surgery
Hemodialysis
Adult: **IV** 2400-4800 anti-Xa units given predialysis

Available forms: Inj 750 anti-Xa units in 0.6 ml H_2O for injection

Adverse effects
CNS: Insomnia, headache
GI: Nausea, vomiting, constipation
HEMA: **Thrombocytopenia**
INTEG: Rash, pruritis, inj site pain
MS: Asthenia
SYST: Hypersensitivity, **hemorrhage**

Contraindications: Hypersensitivity to this drug, sulfites, pork; hemophilia, leukemia with bleeding; thrombocytopenia purpura; cerebrovascular hemorrhage, cerebral aneurysm, severe hypertension, other severe cardiac disease

Precautions: Hypersensitivity
G to heparin, elderly, pregnancy **B**, hepatic disease, severe renal disease, blood dyscrasias, subacute bacterial endocarditis, acute nephritis, lacta-
P tion, child, recent childbirth, peptic ulcer disease, pericarditis, pericardial effusion, recent lumbar puncture, vasculitis, other diseases where bleeding is possible

Pharmacokinetics	
Absorption	100%
Distribution	Unknown
Metabolism	Unknown
Excretion	Kidneys
Half-life	24 hr

Pharmacodynamics	
Onset	Unknown
Peak	4 hr
Duration	Unknown

Interactions
Individual drugs
Aspirin: ↑ risk of bleeding
Dextran: ↑ risk of bleeding
Penicillin: ↑ risk of bleeding
Drug classifications
Anticoagulants, oral: ↑ risk of bleeding
NSAIDs: ↑ risk of bleeding
Platelet inhibitors: ↑ risk of bleeding
Salicylates: ↑ risk of bleeding
Herb/drug
Bromelain: ↑ risk of bleeding
Cinchona bark: ↑ risk of bleeding

NURSING CONSIDERATIONS
Assessment
- Monitor blood studies (Hct, CBC, occult blood in stools) during treatment since bleeding can occur; APTT, ACT, antifactor Xa test, platelets
- Assess for bleeding gums, petechiae, ecchymosis, black tarry stools,

hematuria, epistaxis, decrease in Hct, B/P; may indicate bleeding, possible hemorrhage; notify prescriber immediately, drug should be discontinued
- Assess for hypersensitivity: fever, skin rash, urticaria; notify prescriber immediately
- Assess for needed dosage change q1-2 wk; dose may need to be decreased if bleeding occurs

Nursing diagnoses
✓ Tissue perfusion, altered (uses)
✓ Injury, risk for (adverse reactions)
✓ Knowledge deficit (teaching)

Implementation
SC route
- Have patient sit or lie down; SC inj may be around the navel in a U-shape, upper outer side of thigh or upper outer quadrangle of the buttocks; rotate inj sites
- Changing needles is not recommended

Patient/family education
- Advise patient to avoid OTC preparations that may cause serious drug interactions unless directed by prescriber; may contain aspirin, other anticoagulants
- Advise patient to use soft-bristle toothbrush to avoid bleeding gums, avoid contact sports, use electric razor, avoid IM inj
- Advise patient to report any signs of bleeding: gums, under skin, urine, stools; unusual bruising

Evaluation
Positive therapeutic outcome
- Absence of deep vein thrombosis

Treatment of overdose:
Protamine sulfate 1% given **IV**; 1 mg protamine/100 anti-Xa IU of dalteparin sodium given

danazol (℞)
(da′na-zole)
Cyclomen ✦, danazol, Danocrine
Func. class.: Androgen, anabolic steroid
Chem. class.: α-Ethinyl testosterone derivative
Pregnancy category X

Action: Atrophy of endometrial tissue; decreases FSH, LH, which are controlled by pituitary; this leads to amenorrhea/anovulation; has weak androgen, anabolic activity

➔ **Therapeutic Outcome:** Decreased pain and nodules/fibrocystic breast disease; correction in hereditary angioedema; atrophy of endometrial tissue (ectopic)

Uses: Endometriosis, prevention of hereditary angioedema, fibrocystic breast disease

Dosage and routes
Endometriosis
Adult: PO 100-500 mg bid, uninterrupted for 3-9 mo

Fibrocystic breast disease
Adult: PO 100-400 mg qd in 2 divided doses × 2-6 mo

Hereditary angioedema prevention
Adult: PO 200 mg bid-tid until desired response, then decrease dose to 100 mg at 1-3 mo intervals

Available forms: Caps 50, 100, 200 mg

Adverse effects
CNS: Dizziness, headache, fatigue, tremors, paresthesias, flushing, sweating, anxiety, *lability*, insomnia, carpal tunnel syndrome
CV: Increased B/P
EENT: Conjunctival edema, nasal congestion, voice weakness
ENDO: Abnormal GTT
GI: Nausea, vomiting, constipation, *weight gain*, **cholestatic jaundice**
GU: Hematuria, *amenorrhea*, atrophic

vaginitis, decreased libido, *decreased breast size,* clitoral hypertrophy, testicular atrophy
INTEG: Rash, *acneiform lesions,* oily hair and skin, flushing, sweating, acne vulgaris, alopecia, ***hirsutism***
MS: Cramps, spasms, joint swelling

Contraindications: Severe renal disease, severe cardiac disease, severe hepatic disease, hypersensitivity, genital bleeding (abnormal), pregnancy **X**, children

Precautions: Migraine headaches, seizure disorders

Do Not Confuse:
danazol/Dantrium

Pharmacokinetics

Absorption	GI absorption
Distribution	Unknown
Metabolism	Liver
Excretion	Kidneys
Half-life	4½ hr

Pharmacodynamics

Unknown

Interactions

Individual drugs

Cyclosporine: ↑ risk of nephrotoxicity
Carbamazepine: ↑ carbamazepine level
Insulin: ↑ action

Drug classifications

Anticoagulants: ↑ anticoagulant action
Antidiabetics: ↑ action
Corticosteroids: ↑ action

Lab test interferences

↑ Cholesterol, ↓ cholesterol, ↓ T_4, ↓ T_3, ↓ thyroid ^{131}I uptake test, ↓ 17-KS, ↓ PBI
Interferences: GTT

NURSING CONSIDERATIONS

Assessment

- Assess for pain before and after treatment in endometriosis, fibrocystic breast disease; tenderness, nodules in fibrocystic breast disease
- Monitor potassium, blood sugar, urine glucose while patient is on long-term therapy; liver function tests, periodically; semen volume, sperm count, motility in hereditary angioedema
- Assess breast for fibrocystic nodules; check for pain, tenderness before therapy and throughout to identify if treatment is effective
- Monitor weight daily; notify prescriber if weekly weight gain is >5 lb; I&O ratio; be alert for decreasing urinary output, increasing edema, hypertension, cardiac symptoms, jaundice
- Assess for mental status: affect, mood, behavioral changes, aggression, sleep disorders, depression; change may be extreme
- Assess for signs of virilization: deepening of voice, decreased libido, facial hair (may not be reversible)

Nursing diagnoses

- ✓ Infection, risk for (adverse reactions)
- ✓ Injury, risk for (adverse reactions)
- ✓ Knowledge deficit (teaching)

Implementation

- Start treatment during menstruation in endometriosis, fibrocystic breast disease
- Store in airtight container at room temp
- Provide ROM exercise for patients who are immobile
- Give with food or milk to decrease GI symptoms
- Do not crush, chew caps

Patient/family education

- Teach patient to notify prescriber if therapeutic response decreases; advise that endometriosis tends to recur after drug is discontinued; not to discontinue medication abruptly but to taper over several weeks
- Advise patient that nonhormonal contraceptive measures are needed

during treatment; amenorrhea may occur with higher dosages
- Teach patient to report menstrual irregularities; that amenorrhea usually occurs but menstruation resumes 2-3 mo after termination of therapy; that drug should induce anovulation; reversible within 60-90 days after drug is discontinued
- Teach patient about routine breast self-exam technique, to report any increase in nodule size
- Instruct patient to report masculinization: deepening voice, facial hair growth, body hair growth
- Advise patient to use sunscreen or stay out of the sun to prevent burns

Evaluation

Positive therapeutic outcome
- Decreased pain in endometriosis
- Decreased size, pain in fibrocystic breast disease
- Decreased signs of angioedema (hereditary)

dantrolene (℞)

(dan'troe-leen)

Dantrium

Func. class.: Skeletal muscle relaxant, direct acting

Chem. class.: Hydantoin

Pregnancy category C

Action: Interferes with intracellular release from the sarcoplasmic reticulum of calcium necessary to initiate contraction; slows catabolism in malignant hyperthermia

➔ **Therapeutic Outcome:** Decreased muscle spasticity; absence of malignant hyperthermia

Uses: Spasticity in multiple sclerosis, stroke, spinal cord injury, cerebral palsy, prevention and treatment of malignant hyperthermia

Dosage and routes

Spasticity

Adult: PO 25 mg/day; may increase by 25-100 mg bid-qid, not to exceed 400 mg/day × 1 wk

P ***Child:*** PO 1 mg/kg/day given in divided doses bid-tid; may increase gradually, not to exceed 100 mg qid

Malignant hyperthermia

P ***Adult and child:*** **IV** 1 mg/kg; may repeat to total dose of 10 mg/kg; PO 4-8 mg/kg/day in 4 divided doses × 3 days to prevent further hyperthermia; postcrisis follow-up 4-8 mg/kg/day for 1-3 days

Prevention of malignant hyperthermia

P ***Adult and child:*** PO 4-8 mg/kg/day in 3-4 divided doses × 1-2 days before procedures; give last dose 4 hr preoperatively; **IV** 2.5 mg/kg prior to anesthesia

Available forms: Caps 25, 50, 100 mg; powder for inj 20 mg/vial

Adverse effects

CNS: *Dizziness, weakness, fatigue, drowsiness,* headache, disorientation, insomnia, paresthesias, tremors, **seizures**

CV: Hypotension, chest pain, palpitations

EENT: Nasal congestion, blurred vision, mydriasis

GI: **Hepatic injury,** *nausea,* constipation, vomiting, increased AST and alkaline phosphatase, abdominal pain, dry mouth, anorexia, hepatitis

GU: Urinary frequency, nocturia, impotence, crystalluria

HEMA: **Eosinophilia**

INTEG: Rash, pruritus, photosensitivity

Contraindications: Hypersensitivity, compromised pulmonary function, active hepatic disease, impaired myocardial function

Precautions: Peptic ulcer disease, renal disease, hepatic disease, stroke, seizure disorder, diabetes mellitus, G pregnancy **C,** elderly

Do Not Confuse:
Dantrium/danazol

Pharmacokinetics

Absorption	PO (30%-35%)
Distribution	Unknown
Metabolism	Liver, extensively
Excretion	Kidney
Half-life	9 hr

Pharmacodynamics

	PO	IV
Onset	Unknown	Immediate
Peak	5 hr	5 hr
Duration	Dose related	Dose related

Interactions

Individual drugs

Alcohol: ↑ CNS depression
Clofibrate: ↑ action of dantrolene

Drug classifications

Antidepressants, tricyclic: ↑ CNS depression
Antihistamines: ↑ CNS depression
Barbiturates: ↑ CNS depression
Estrogens: ↑ hepatotoxicity
Hepatotoxic agents: ↑ hepatotoxicity
Opiates: ↑ CNS depression
Sedative/hypnotics: ↑ CNS depression

NURSING CONSIDERATIONS

Assessment

- Monitor I&O ratio; check for urinary retention, frequency, hesitancy, G especially elderly
- Monitor ECG in epileptic patients; poor seizure control has occurred with patients taking this drug; assess for increased seizure activity in epilepsy patient
- Monitor hepatic function by frequent determination of AST, ALT, bilirubin, alkaline phosphatase, GGTP, renal function studies, CBC
- Assess for allergic reactions: rash, fever, respiratory distress
- Monitor for severe weakness, numbness in extremities
- Assess for CNS depression: dizziness, drowsiness, psychiatric symptoms
- ❗ Assess for signs of hepatotoxicity: jaundice, yellow sclera, pain in abdomen, nausea, fever; drug should be discontinued if these signs and symptoms occur

Nursing diagnoses

- ✓ Pain, chronic (uses)
- ✓ Physical mobility, impaired (uses)
- ✓ Injury, risk for (adverse reactions)
- ✓ Knowledge deficit (teaching)

Implementation

PO route

- Give with meals for GI symptoms; capsules may be opened and mixed with liquid; patient should drink after mixing
- Store in airtight container at room temp

IV route

- Administer **IV** after reconstituting 20 mg/60 ml sterile water for inj without bacteriostatic agent (333 μg/ml); shake until clear; give by rapid **IV** push through Y-tube or 3-way stopcock; follow by prescribed doses immediately; may also give by intermittent inf over 1 hr before anesthesia; assess site for extravasation, phlebitis
- Protect diluted sol from light; use reconstituted sol within 6 hr

Patient/family education

- Notify prescriber of abdominal pain, jaundiced sclera, claycolored stools, change in color of urine, rash, itching
- Caution patient not to take with alcohol, other CNS depressants; severe CNS depression can occur; avoid using OTC medication: cough preparations, antihistamines, unless directed by prescriber
- Tell patient that if improvement does not occur within 6 wk, prescriber may discontinue
- Caution patient to avoid hazardous activities if drowsiness, dizziness, blurred vision occurs; wait several days to identify patient response to medication

- Teach patient to use sunscreen, protective clothing for photosensitivity
- Instruct patient to take medication as prescribed; do not double doses; take missed dose within 1 hr of scheduled time

Evaluation

Positive therapeutic outcome

- Decreased pain, spasticity
- Absence or decreased symptoms of malignant hyperthermia

Treatment of overdose: Induce emesis of conscious patient; lavage, dialysis

darbepoetin alfa

See Appendix A, Selected New Drugs

HIGH ALERT

daunorubicin (℞)

(daw-noe-roo'bi-sin)

Cerubidine

daunorubicin citrate liposome (℞)

DaunoXome

Func. class.: Antineoplastic, antibiotic

Chem. class.: Anthracycline glycoside

Pregnancy category D

Action: Inhibits DNA synthesis, primarily; derived from *Streptomyces coeruleorubidus;* replication is decreased by binding to DNA, which causes strand splitting; cell cycle specific (S phase); a vesicant

Therapeutic Outcome: Prevention of rapidly growing malignant cells; immunosuppression

Uses: Myelogenous, monocytic leukemia, acute nonlymphocytic leukemia, Ewing's sarcoma, Wilms' tumor, neuroblastoma, rhabdomyosarcoma; daunorubicin citrate liposome: advanced Kaposi's sarcoma in HIV

Dosage and routes

G Use decreased dose for those >60 yr

Single agent

Adult: **IV** 60 mg/m^2/day × 3-5 day q4 wk

In combination

Adult: **IV** 45 mg/m^2/day × 3 days, then 2 days of subsequent courses in combination

P ***Child:*** **IV** 25-60 mg/m^2 depending on cycle

Daunorubicin citrate liposome

Adult: **IV** 40 mg/m^2 q2 wk

Renal dose

Adult: **IV** serum Cr >3 mg/dl reduce dose by 50%

Hepatic dose

Adult: **IV** serum bilirubin 1.2-3 mg/dl reduce dose by 25%; bilirubin >3 mg/dl reduce dose by 50%

Available forms: Inj 20 mg powder/vial, sol for inj 5 mg/ml; liposome: dispersion for inj 2 mg/ml

Adverse effects

Daunorubicin

CNS: Fever, chills

CV: **Dysrhythmias, CHF, pericarditis, myocarditis,** peripheral edema

GI: Nausea, vomiting, anorexia, mucositis, **hepatotoxicity**

GU: Impotence, sterility, amenorrhea, gynecomastia, hyperuricemia

HEMA: **Thrombocytopenia, leukopenia, anemia**

INTEG: Rash, extravasation, dermatitis, reversible alopecia, cellulitis, thrombophlebitis at inj site

MISC: **Anaphylaxis**

Daunorubicin citrate liposome

CNS: Fatigue, headache, depression, insomnia, dizziness, malaise, neuropathy

CV: Chest pain, edema
GI: Cramps, diarrhea, constipation, stomatitis
INTEG: Sweating, pruritus
MS: Arthralgia, back pain

Contraindications: Hypersensitivity, pregnancy **D,** lactation, systemic infections, cardiac disease

Precautions: Renal, hepatic disease, gout, bone marrow suppression

Do Not Confuse:
daunorubicin/doxorubicin

Pharmacokinetics

Absorption	Complete
Distribution	Widely distributed; crosses placenta
Metabolism	Liver, extensively
Excretion	Biliary (40%-50%)
Half-life	18½ hr, liposome 55½ hr

Pharmacodynamics

Unknown

Interactions

Individual drugs

Cyclophosphamide: ↑ cardiotoxicity, CHF
Radiation: ↑ toxicity, bone marrow suppression

Drug classifications

Antineoplastics: ↑ toxicity, bone marrow suppression
Live virus vaccines: ↓ antibody reaction
NSAIDs: ↑ risk of bleeding
Salicylates: ↑ risk of bleeding

Lab test interferences

↑ Uric acid

NURSING CONSIDERATIONS

Assessment

- Assess buccal cavity q8h for dryness, sores or ulceration, white patches, pain, bleeding, dysphagia; obtain prescription for viscous lidocaine (Xylocaine)
- Assess symptoms indicating severe allergic reaction: rash, pruritus, urticaria, purpuric skin lesions, itching, flushing; drug should be discontinued
- Assess chest x-ray, echocardiography, radionuclide angiography, ECG; watch for ST-T wave changes, low QRS and T, possible dysrhythmias (sinus tachycardia, heart block, PVCs); watch for CHF (jugular vein distention, weight gain, edema, rales or crackles), may occur after 2-6 mo of treatment
- Monitor CBC, differential, platelet count weekly, leukocyte nadir within 2 wk after administration, recovery within 3 wk; do not administer if absoluate granulocyte count is <750/mm^3 (liposome)
- Assess for increased uric acid levels, swelling, joint pain primarily in extremities; patient should be well hydrated to prevent urate deposits
- Monitor renal function studies: BUN, creatinine, serum uric acid, urine CrCl baseline and before each dose; I&O ratio; report fall in urine output to <30 ml/hr
- Monitor temp q4h (may indicate beginning of infection)
- Monitor liver function tests baseline and before each dose (bilirubin, AST, ALT, LDH) as needed or monthly; note jaundice of skin or sclera, dark urine, clay-colored stools, itchy skin, abdominal pain, fever, diarrhea; hepatoxicity can be severe
- Assess for bleeding: hematuria, stool guaiac, bruising or petechiae, mucosa or orifices q8h; check for inflammation of mucosa, breaks in skin
- Identify effects of alopecia on body image; discuss feelings about body changes

Nursing diagnoses

- ✓ Injury, risk for (adverse reactions)
- ✓ Cardiac output, decreased (adverse reactions)
- ✓ Body image disturbance (adverse reactions)

✓ Infection, risk for (adverse reactions)
✓ Knowledge deficit (teaching)

Implementation

- Avoid contact with skin; very irritating; wash completely to remove
- Give fluids **IV** or PO before chemotherapy to hydrate patient; give antiemetic 30-60 min before giving drug to prevent vomiting, and prn; antibiotics for prophylaxis of infection
- Provide liquid diet: carbonated beverages; gelatin may be added if patient is not nauseated or vomiting
- Help patient rinse mouth tid-qid with water, club soda, brush teeth bid-qid with soft brush or cotton-tipped applicators for stomatitis, use unwaxed dental floss
- Drug should be prepared by experienced personnel using proper precautions

IV **IV route: Cerubidine**

- Give after diluting 20 mg/4 ml sterile water for inj (5 mg/ml); rotate; further dilute in 10-15 ml 0.9% NaCl; give over 3-5 min by direct **IV** through Y-tube or 3-way stopcock of inf of D_5W or 0.9% NaCl

Intermittent infusion

- Dilute further in 50-100 ml 0.9% NaCl, LR, D_5W; give over 15 min (50 ml), 30 min (100 ml)

Y-site compatibilities: Amifostine, filgrastim, granisetron, melphalan, methotrexate, ondansetron, sodium bicarbonate, teniposide, thiotepa, vinorelbine

Y-site incompatibilities: Fludarabine

Additive compatibilities: Cytarabine with etoposide, hydrocortisone; not recommended for admixing

Additive incompatibilities: Dexamethasone, heparin

Solution compatibilities: $D_{3.3}$/0.3% NaCl, D_5W, Normosol-R, Ringer's, 0.9% NaCl

IV **IV route: DaunoXome**

- Dilute with D_5W (1 mg/ml), give over 60 min, do not use in-line filter, reconstituted sol may be stored ≤6 hr refrigerated; do not admix

Patient/family education

- Teach patient to avoid use of products containing aspirin or ibuprofen, razors, commercial mouthwash, since bleeding may occur; to report symptoms of bleeding (hematuria, tarry stools)
- Instruct patient to report signs of anemia (fatigue, headache, irritability, faintness, shortness of breath); signs of infection; bleeding, bruising, shortness of breath, swelling, change in heart rate; to avoid crowds, those with known infections
- Advise patient that hair may be lost during treatment; a wig or hairpiece may make patient feel better; new hair may be different in color, texture
- Caution patient not to have any vaccinations without the advice of the prescriber; serious reactions can occur
- Advise patient that contraception is needed during treatment and for 4 mo after the completion of therapy
- Advise patient to avoid alcohol, aspirin, NSAIDs

Evaluation

Positive therapeutic outcome

- Prevention of rapid division of malignant cells

delavirdine (℞)

(de-la-veer'deen)

Rescriptor

Func. class.: Nonnucleoside reverse transcriptase inhibitor (NNRII)

Pregnancy category C

Action: Binds directly to reverse transcriptase and blocks RNA, DNA causing a disruption of the enzyme's site

Therapeutic Outcome: Improvement of HIV-1 infection

Uses: HIV-1 in combination with zidovudine or didanosine

Dosage and routes

P *Adult and child ≥16 yr:* 400 mg tid

Available forms: Tabs 100 mg

Adverse effects

CNS: Headache, fatigue
GI: Diarrhea, anorexia, abdominal pain, nausea, vomiting, dyspepsia, **hepatotoxicity**
GU: **Nephrotoxicity**
HEMA: **Neutropenia, leukopenia, thrombocytopenia, anemia, granulocytopenia**
INTEG: Rash
MS: Pain myalgia

Contraindications: Hypersensitivity to this drug or atevirdine

Precautions: Liver disease, pregnancy **C**, lactation, children, renal disease, myelosuppression

Pharmacokinetics

Absorption	Well
Distribution	Highly protein bound
Metabolism	Liver, extensively
Excretion	Kidneys, feces
Half-life	6 hr

Pharmacodynamics

Onset	Unknown
Peak	1 hr
Duration	8 hr

Interactions

Individual drugs

Alprazolam: ↑ level of alprazolam
Clarithromycin: ↑ level of clarithromycin and delavirdine
Dapsone: ↑ level of dapsone
Felodipine: ↑ level of felodipine
Fluoxetine: ↑ level of fluoxetine
Indinavir: ↑ level of indinavir
Ketoconazole: ↑ level of delavirdine
Midazolam: ↑ level of midazolam
Nifidepine: ↑ level of nifidepine
Pimozide: life-threatening reactions; do not combine
Quinidine: ↑ level of quinidine
Warfarin: ↑ level of warfarin

Drug classifications

Antacids: ↓ delavirdine levels
Anticonvulsants: ↓ delavirdine levels
Antidysrhythmics: life-threatening reactions; do not combine
Ergots: ↑ ergotism
Oral contraceptives: ↓ action of oral contraceptives
Protease inhibitors: ↑ action of protease inhibitors
Sedative/hypnotics: life-threatening reactions; do not combine

NURSING CONSIDERATIONS

Assessment

- Assess signs of infection, anemia
- Assess liver studies: ALT, AST; renal studies
- Assess C&S before drug therapy; drug may be taken as soon as culture is taken; repeat C&S after treatment; determine the presence of other sexually transmitted disease
- Assess bowel pattern before, during teatment; if severe abdominal pain with bleeding occurs, drug should be discontinued; monitor hydration
- Assess skin eruptions; rash, urticaria, itching
- Assess allergies before treatment, reaction to each medication; place allergies on chart
- Assess plasma delavirdine concentrations (trough 10 μm)
- Assess CBC, blood chemistry, plasma HIV RNA, absolute $CD4^+$/$CD8^+$/cell counts/%, serum β_2 microglobulin, serum ICD+24 antigen levels
- Assess for signs of delavirdine toxicity: severe nausea, vomiting, maculopapular rash

Nursing diagnoses

- ✓ Infection (risk for uses)
- ✓ Diarrhea (side effects)
- ✓ Knowledge deficit (teaching)

Implementation

- Add 4 tabs/3-4 oz of water, let stand, stir, swallow, rinse glass, swallow

Patient/family education

- Advise patient to take as prescribed; if dose is missed, take as soon as remembered up to 1 hr before next dose; do not double dose
- Advise patient that drug must be taken in equal intervals around the clock to maintain blood levels for duration of therapy
- Advise patient that tabs may be dissolved, drink right away, rinse cup with water, and drink that to get all medication
- Instruct patient to make sure health care provider knows of all the medications being taken
- Advise patient that if severe rash, mouth sores, swelling, aching muscles/joints, or eye redness occur, stop taking and notify health care provider
- Advise patient not to breastfeed if taking this drug

Evaluation

Positive therapeutic outcome

- Increased $CD4^+$ cell count
- Decreased viral load
- Improvement in symptoms of HIV

denileukin diftitox (℞)

(den-ih-loo′kin dif′tih-tox)

Ontak

Func. class.: Antineoplastic misc agent

Pregnancy category C

Action: A recombinant DNA-derived cytotoxic protein. Inhibits cellular protein synthesis

➔ **Therapeutic Outcome:** Prevention of rapidly growing malignant cells

Uses: Cutaneous T-cell lymphoma that express CD25 component of the IL-2 receptor

Dosage and routes

Adult: **IV** 9-18 μg/kg/day given for 5 days q21 days, give over ≥15 mins

Available forms: Sol for inj, frozen 150 μg/ml

Adverse effects

CNS: *Dizziness, paresthesia, nervousness, confusion, insomnia*

CV: Hypotension, vasodilation, tachycardia, thrombosis, hypertension, dysrhythmia

GI: *Nausea, anorexia, vomiting, diarrhea, constipation, dyspepsia, dysphagia*

GU: *Hematuria,* albuminuria, pyuria, creatinine increase

HEMA: **Thrombocytopenia, leukopenia,** anemia

INTEG: *Rash, pruritus, sweating*

META: Hypoalbuminemia, edema, hypocalcemia, weight decrease, dehydration, hypokalemia

MISC: Fever, chills, asthenia, infection, pain, headache, chest pain, flu-like symptoms

MS: Myalgia, arthralgia

RESP: Dyspnea, cough, pharyngitis, rhinitis

Contraindications: Hypersensitivity to denileukin, diphtheria toxin, interleukin-2

Precautions: Radiation therapy, G pregnancy **C,** elderly, lactation, P children

Pharmacokinetics

Absorption	Complete bioavailability (**IV**)
Distribution	Widely distributed; concentrates in liver/kidneys
Metabolism	Proteolytic degradation
Excretion	Unknown
Half-life	Unknown

Pharmacodynamics

Unknown

Interactions

Individual drugs

Radiation: ↑ toxicity, bone marrow suppression

Drug classifications

Antineoplastics: ↑ toxicity, bone marrow suppression
Bone marrow-suppressing drugs: ↑ bone marrow suppression
Live virus vaccines: ↑ adverse reactions, ↓ antibody reaction

NURSING CONSIDERATIONS

Assessment

- Assess symptoms indicating severe allergic reaction: rash, pruritus, urticaria, purpuric skin lesions, itching, flushing; drug should be discontinued
- Assess for vascular leak syndrome after 2 wk of treatment: hypotension, edema, hypoalbuminemia; monitor weight, B/P, serum albumin, edema
- Obtain CD25 expression on skin biopsy samples
- Monitor CBC, differential, platelet count weekly; withhold drug if WBC count is <4000/mm^3 or platelet count is <100,000/mm^3
- Monitor renal function studies: BUN, creatinine, urine CrCl before and during therapy; I&O ratio; report fall in urine output to <30 ml/hr
- Monitor temp q4h (may indicate beginning of infection)
- Monitor liver function tests before and during therapy (bilirubin, AST, ALT, LDH) as needed or monthly; note jaundice skin or sclera, dark urine, clay-colored stools, itchy skin, abdominal pain, fever, diarrhea; hepatoxicity can be serious and fatal
- Assess for bleeding: hematuria, stool guaiac, bruising or petechiae, mucosa or orifices q8h; check for inflammation of mucosa, breaks in skin

Nursing diagnoses

✓ Injury, risk for (adverse reactions)
✓ Body image disturbance (adverse reactions)
✓ Infection, risk for (adverse reactions)
✓ Knowledge deficit (teaching)

Implementation

- Give fluids **IV** or PO before chemotherapy to hydrate patient
- Give antiemetic 30-60 min before giving drug to prevent vomiting, and prn; antibiotics for prophylaxis of infection
- Provide liquid diet: carbonated beverages; gelatin may be added if patient is not nauseated or vomiting
- Prepare and hold sol in plastic syringes or soft plastic **IV** bags only
- Draw calculated dose from vial, inject into empty **IV** infusion bag, for each 1 ml of drug removed from vial, no more than 9 ml of sterile saline without preservative should be added to **IV** bag; infuse over ≥15 min; do not give by bolus; do not admix with other drugs; do not use a filter
- Use within 6 hr, discard unused portions
- Watch for extravasation; give 3-5 ml of mixture of 4 ml sodium thiosulfate 10% plus 5 ml sterile water SC as prescribed

Patient/family education

- Teach patient to avoid use of products containing aspirin or NSAIDs, razors, commercial mouthwash, since bleeding may occur; to report symptoms of bleeding (hematuria, tarry stools)
- Instruct patient to report signs of anemia (fatigue, headache, irritability, faintness, shortness of breath)
- Caution patient not to have any vaccinations without the advice of prescriber; serious reactions can occur
- Advise patient contraception is needed during treatment and for several months after the completion of therapy; drug has teratogenic properties

Evaluation

Positive therapeutic outcome

- Prevention of rapid division of malignant cells

deslortadine

See Appendix A, Selected New Drugs

desmopressin (℞)

(des-moe-press'in)

DDAVP, Stimate

Func. class.: Pituitary hormone

Chem. class.: Synthetic antidiuretic hormone

Pregnancy category B

Action: Promotes reabsorption of water by action on renal tubular epithelium in the kidney; causes smooth muscle constriction and increase in plasma factor VIII levels, which increases platelet aggregation resulting in vasopressor effect; similar to vasopressor

Therapeutic Outcome: Prevention of nocturnal enuresis, decreased bleeding in hemophilia A, von Willebrand's disease type 1, control and stabilization of water in diabetes insipidus

Uses: Hemophilia A, von Willebrand's disease type 1, nonnephrogenic diabetes insipidus, symptoms of polyuria/polydipsia caused by pituitary dysfunction, nocturnal enuresis

Dosage and routes

Primary nocturnal enuresis

P ***Adult and Child ≥6 yr:*** Intranasal 20 μg (10 μg in each nostril) hs, may increase to 40 μg; PO 0.2 mg hs, may be increased to max 0.6 mg hs

Diabetes insipidus

Adult: Intranasal 0.1-0.4 ml qd in divided doses (1-4 sprays with pump); **IV**/SC 0.5-1 ml qd in divided doses

P ***Child 3 mo-12 yr:*** Intranasal 0.05-0.3 ml qd in divided doses

Hemophilia/von Willebrand's disease

P ***Adult and child >3 mo:*** **IV** 0.3 μg/kg in NaCl over 15-30 min; may repeat if needed

Antihemorrhagic

P ***Adult and child >3 mo:*** **IV** 0.3 μg/kg

P ***Adult and child <50 kg:*** Intranasal 1 spray in one nostril

P ***Adult and child >50 kg:*** 1 spray each nostril

Available forms: Inj 4, 15 μg/ml, Rhinal Tube del 2.5 mg/vial (0.1 mg/ml); tabs 0.1, 0.2 mg; nasal spray pump 10 μg/spray (0.1 mg/ml); nasal sol 1.5 mg/ml (150 μg/dose)

Adverse effects

CNS: Drowsiness, headache, lethargy, flushing

CV: Increased B/P

EENT: Nasal irritation, congestion, rhinitis

GI: Nausea, heartburn, cramps

GU: *Vulval pain*

SYST: **Anaphylaxis IV**

Contraindications: Hypersensitivity, nephrogenic diabetes insipidus

Precautions: Pregnancy **B**, CAD, lactation, hypertension

Pharmacokinetics

Absorption	Nasal (up to 20%)
Distribution	Unknown
Metabolism	Unknown
Excretion	Unknown; breast milk
Half-life	8 min (initial), 76 min (terminal)

Pharmacodynamics

	PO	INTRANASAL	IV/SC
Onset	1 hr	1 hr	Rapid
Peak	4-7 hr	1-4 hr	15-30 min
Duration	Unknown	8-20 hr	3 hr

Interactions
Individual drugs
Alcohol: ↑ antidiuretic action
Carbamazepine: ↑ antidiuretic action
Chlorpropamide: ↑ antidiuretic action
Clofibrate: ↑ antidiuretic action
Demeclocycline: ↑ antidiuretic action
Epinephrine (large doses): ↑ antidiuretic action
Heparin: ↑ antidiuretic action
Lithium: ↑ antidiuretic action
Norepinephrine: ↑ antidiuretic action

NURSING CONSIDERATIONS
Assessment
- Monitor I&O ratio, urine osmolality, sp gr, weight daily; check for edema in extremities; if water retention is severe, diuretic may be prescribed; check pulse, B/P when giving drug **IV** or SC
- Assess for water intoxication: lethargy, behavioral changes, disorientation, neuromuscular excitability, dehydration, poor skin turgor, severe thirst, dry skin, tachycardia
- Assess intranasal use: nausea, congestion, cramps, headache; usually decreased with decreased dosage
- Monitor for enuresis during treatment (nocturnal enuresis)
- Assess for allergic reaction including anaphylaxsis (**IV** route)
- Assess for nasal mucosa changes: congestion, edema, discharge, scarring (nasal route)
- Monitor urine volume osmolality and plasma osmolality (diabetes insipidus)
- Monitor factor VIII coagulant activity before using for hemostasis

Nursing diagnoses
✓ Fluid volume deficit (uses)
✓ Fluid volume excess (side effects)
✓ Knowledge deficit (teaching)

Implementation
- Store in refrigerator or cool environment

IV **IV route**
Direct IV
- Give undiluted over 1 min in diabetes insipidus or **IV** for hemophilia

Intermittent infusion
- Give single dose diluted in 50 ml of P 0.9% NaCl (adult and child >10 kg); a single dose/10 ml as an **IV** inf over 15-30 min in von Willebrand's disease or hemophilia A

Patient/family education
- Use demonstration, return demonstration to teach technique for nasal instillation: draw medication into tube, insert tube into nostril to instill drug and blow on other end to deliver sol into nasal cavity; rinse after use
- Teach patient to notify prescriber of dyspnea, vomiting, cramping, drowsiness, headache, nasal congestion
- Caution patient to avoid OTC products (cough, hay fever), since these preparations may contain epinephrine and decrease drug response; do not use with alcohol
- Advise patient to wear Medic Alert ID or other identification specifying disease and medication used
- Advise patient if dose is missed, take when remembered up to 1 hr before next dose; do not double doses

Evaluation
Positive therapeutic outcome
- Absence of severe thirst
- Decreased urine output, osmolality
- Absence of bleeding (hemophilia)

desoxyribonuclease
See fibrinolysin/desoxyribonuclease

dexamethasone (℞)
(dex-ah-meth'ah-sone)
Decadron, Deronil ♣, Dexasone ♣, Dexon, Hexadrol, Mymethasone

dexamethasone acetate (℞)
Dalalone DP, Dalalone LA, Decadron-LA, Decaject-LA, Dexacen LA-8, Dexasone-LA, Dexone LA, Solurex-LA

dexamethasone sodium phosphate (℞)
Dalalone, Decadron Phosphate, Decaject, Dexacen-4, Dexone, Hexadrol Phosphate, Solurex

Func. class.: Corticosteroid
Chem. class.: Glucocorticoid, long-acting

Pregnancy category C

Action: Decreases inflammation by suppression of migration of polymorphonuclear leukocytes, fibroblasts, reversal of increased capillary permeability and lysosomal stabilization

Uses: Inflammation, allergies, neoplasms, cerebral edema, septic shock, collagen disorders

Dosage and routes

Inflammation

Adult: PO 0.75-9 mg/day or phosphate IM 0.5-9 mg/day; or acetate IM 4-16 mg q1-3 wk

P ***Child:*** PO 0.08-0.3 mg/kg/day in divided doses q6-12h

Shock

Adult: **IV** (phosphate) single dose 1-6 mg/kg or **IV** 40 mg q2-6h as needed up to 72 hr

Cerebral edema

Adult: **IV** (phosphate) 10 mg, then 4-6 mg IM q6h × 2-4 days, then taper over 1 wk

P ***Child:*** PO 0.2 mg/kg/day in divided doses

Adrenocortical insufficiency

P ***Child:*** 23.3 μg/kg/day in 3 divided doses

Suppression test

Adult: PO 1 mg at 11 pm or 0.5 mg q6h × 48 hr

Available forms: Dexamethasone: tabs 0.25, 0.5, 0.75, 1, 1.5, 2, 4, 6 mg; 20, 24 phosphate; elix 0.5 mg/5 ml; oral sol 0.5 mg/5 ml, 0.5 mg/1 ml; inj acetate 8, 16 mg/ml; inj phosphate 4, 10 mg/ml

Adverse effects

CNS: Depression, flushing, sweating, headache, mood changes, euphoria, psychosis, **seizures**

CV: Hypertension, **circulatory collapse, thrombophlebitis, embolism,** tachycardia, edema

EENT: Fungal infections, increased intraocular pressure, blurred vision

ENDO: Hypothalmic-pituitary-adrenal axis suppression

GI: Diarrhea, nausea, abdominal distention, **GI hemorrhage,** *increased appetite,* **pancreatitis**

HEMA: **Thrombocytopenia**

INTEG: Acne, poor wound healing, ecchymosis, petechiae

META: Hypokalemia

MS: Fractures, osteoporosis, weakness

Contraindications: Psychosis, hypersensitivity, idiopathic thrombocytopenia, acute glomerulonephritis, amebiasis, fungal infections, nonasthmatic bronchial disease, P child <2 yr, AIDS, TB

Precautions: Pregnancy **C**, lactation, diabetes mellitus, glaucoma, osteoporosis, seizure disorders, ulcerative colitis, CHF, myasthenia gravis, renal disease, peptic ulcer, esophagitis

Do Not Confuse:
Decadron/Percodan

Pharmacokinetics

Absorption	Unknown
Distribution	Unknown
Metabolism	Liver
Excretion	Kidneys
Half-life	3-4½ hr

Pharmacodynamics

	PO	IM
Onset	1 hr	Unknown
Peak	1-2 hr	8 hr
Duration	2½ days	6 days

Interactions

Individual drugs

Alcohol: ↑ side effects
Amphotericin B: ↑ side effects
Cholestyramine: ↓ action of dexamethasone
Colestipol: ↓ action of dexamethasone
Cyclosporine: ↑ side effects
Digoxin: ↑ side effects
Ephedrine: ↓ action of dexamethasone
Indomethacin: ↑ side effects
Isoniazid: ↓ effects of isoniazid
Ketoconazole: ↑ side effects
Neostigmine: ↓ effects of neostigmine
Phenytoin: ↓ action of dexamethasone
Rifampin: ↓ action of dexamethasone
Sometrem: ↓ effects of sometrem
Theophylline: ↓ action of dexamethasone

Drug classifications

Antacids: ↓ action of dexamethasone
Antibiotics, macrolide: ↑ action of dexamethasone
Anticholinesterases: ↓ effects of anticholinesterases
Anticoagulants: ↓ effects of anticoagulants
Anticonvulsants: ↓ effects of anticonvulsants
Antidiabetics: ↓ effects of antidiabetics
Barbiturates: ↓ action of dexamethasone
Contraceptives, oral: ↑ action of dexamethasone
Diuretics: ↑ side effects
Estrogens: ↑ action of dexamethasone
Salicylates: ↓ effects of salicylates
Toxoids/Vaccines: ↓ effects of toxoids/vaccines

Herb/drug

Aloe: ↑ hypokalemia
Buckthorn bark/berry: ↑ hypokalemia
Cascara sagrada: ↑ hypokalemia
Ephedra: ↑ hypokalemia
Senna pod/leaf: ↑ hypokalemia

Lab test interferences

↑ Cholesterol, ↑ Na, ↑ blood glucose, ↑ uric acid, ↑ Ca, ↑ urine glucose
↓ Ca, ↓ K, ↓ T_4, ↓ T_3, ↓ thyroid ^{131}I uptake test, ↓ urine 17-OHCS, ↓ 17-KS, ↓ PBI
False negative: Skin allergy tests

NURSING CONSIDERATIONS

Assessment

- Monitor K, blood glucose, urine glucose while on long-term therapy; hypokalemia and hyperglycemia
- Monitor weight daily; notify prescriber of weekly gain >5 lb
- Monitor B/P q4h, pulse; notify prescriber of chest pain
- Monitor I&O ratio; be alert for decreasing urinary output, increasing edema
- Monitor plasma cortisol levels during long-term therapy (normal: 138-635 nmol/L SI units when assessed at 8 AM)
- Assess infection: fever, WBC even after withdrawal of medication; drug masks infection
- Assess potassium depletion: paresthesias, fatigue, nausea, vomiting, depression, polyuria, dysrhythmias, weakness
- Assess edema, hypertension, cardiac symptoms
- Assess mental status: affect, mood, behavioral changes, aggression

Nursing diagnoses

- ✓ Infection, risk for (adverse reaction)
- ✓ Knowledge deficit (teaching)
- ✓ Mobility, impaired (uses)

Implementation

IV route

- **IV** undiluted direct over 1 min or less or diluted with 0.9% NaCl or D_5W and give as an **IV** inf at prescribed rate
- After shaking susp (parenteral); do not give susp **IV**
- Titrated dose; use lowest effective dose

Dexamethasone sodium phosphate

Syringe compatibilities:

Granisetron, metoclopramide, ranitidine, sufentanil

Y-site compatibilities:

Acyclovir, allopurinol, amifostine, amikacin, amphotericin B cholesteryl, amsacrine, aztreonam, cefepime, cisatracurium, cisplatin, cladribine, cyclophosphamide, cytarabine, doxorubicin, doxorubicin liposome, famotidine, filgrastim, fluconazole, fludarabine, foscarnet, heparin, melphalan, meperidine, meropenem, morphine, ondansetron, paclitaxel, piperacillin/tazobactam, potassium chloride, propofol, remifentanil, sargramostim, sodium bicarbonate, sufentanil, tacrolimus, teniposide, theophylline, vinorelbine, vit B/C, zidovudine

Additive compatibilities:

Aminophylline, bleomycin, cimetidine, floxacillin, furosemide, lidocaine, meropenem, nafcillin, netilmicin, ondansetron, prochlorperazine, ranitidine, verapamil

IM route

- IM inj deeply in large muscle mass; rotate sites; avoid deltoid; use 21 G needle
- In one dose in AM to prevent adrenal suppression; avoid SC administration, may damage tissue

PO route

- Give with food or milk to decrease GI symptoms
- Provide assistance with ambulation in patient with bone tissue disease to prevent fractures

Patient/family education

- Advise that ID as steroid user should be carried
- Teach to notify prescriber if therapeutic response decreases; dosage adjustment may be needed
- Teach not to discontinue abruptly or adrenal crisis can result
- Teach to avoid OTC products: salicylates, alcohol in cough products, cold preparations unless directed by prescriber
- Teach patient all aspects of drug usage, including cushingoid symptoms
- Instruct patient to notify prescriber of infection
- Teach symptoms of adrenal insufficiency: nausea, anorexia, fatigue, dizziness, dyspnea, weakness, joint pain

Evaluation

Positive therapeutic outcome

Ease of respirations, decreased inflammation

dexmedetomidine (℞)

(deks-med-ee-tome′a-dine)

Precedex

Func. class.: Sedative, α_2-adrenoceptor agonist

Pregnancy category C

Action: Produces α_2 activity as seen at low and moderate doses; also, α_1 at high doses

Uses: Sedation in mechanically ventilated, intubated patients in ICU

Dosage and routes

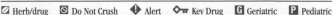

Adult: **IV** Loading dose of 1 μg/kg over 10 min, then 0.2-0.7 μg/kg/hr, do not use for more than 24 hr

Available forms: Inj 100 μg/ml

Adverse effects

CV: Bradycardia, hypotension, hypertension, **atrial fibrillation, infarction**

GI: Nausea, thirst

GU: Oliguria

HEMA: Leukocytosis, anemia

***RESP:* Pulmonary edema, pleural effusion, hypoxia**

Contraindications: Hypersensitivity

G **Precautions:** Elderly, renal disease, respiratory depression, severe respiratory disorders, cardiac dysrhythmias,
P pregnancy **C**, lactation, children

Pharmacokinetics	
Half-life	8 min

Interactions

Drug classifications

Anesthetics: ↑ CNS depression

Antipsychotics: ↑ CNS depression

Opiates: ↑ CNS depression

Sedative/hypnotics: ↑ CNS depression

Skeletal muscle relaxants: ↑ CNS depression

NURSING CONSIDERATIONS

Assessment

- Assess injection site: phlebitis, burning, stinging
- Monitor ECG for changes: atrial fibrillation
- Assess CNS changes: movement, jerking, tremors, dizziness, LOC, pupil reaction
- Assess respiratory dysfunction: respiratory depression, character, rate, rhythm; notify prescriber if respirations are <10/min

Implementation

IV **IV route**

- Give after diluting with D_5W, 0.9% NaCl, withdraw 2 ml of drug and add to 48 ml of 0.9% NaCl to a total of 50 ml, shake to mix well
- Give only with resuscitative equipment available
- Give only by qualified persons trained in management of ICU sedation

Solution compatibilities: LR, D_5W, 0.9% NaCl, 20% mannitol

Additive compatibilities: Atracurium, atropine, etomidate, fentanyl, glycopyrrolate, midazolam, mivacurium, morphine, pancuronium, phenylephrine, succinylcholine, thiopental, vecuronium

- Provide safety measures: side rails, nightlight, call bell within easy reach

Evaluation

- Therapeutic response: induction of sedation

dexmethylphenidate

See Appendix A, Selected New Drugs

dextroamphetamine (℞)

(dex-troe-am-fet′a-meen)

Dexedrine

dextroamphetamine sulfate

Dextrostat

Func. class.: Cerebral stimulant

Chem. class.: Amphetamine

Pregnancy category C

Controlled substance schedule II

Action: Increases release of norepinephrine, dopamine in cerebral cortex to reticular activating system

➡ **Therapeutic Outcome:** Increased alertness, decreased fatigue, ability to stay awake (narcolepsy); increased attention span, decreased hyperactivity (ADHD)

Uses: Narcolepsy, attention deficit disorder with hyperactivity

Dosage and routes

Narcolepsy

Adult: PO 5-60 mg qd in divided doses

P ***Child >12 yr:*** PO 10 mg qd increasing by 10 mg/day at weekly intervals

P ***Child 6-12 yr:*** PO 5 mg qd increasing by 5 mg/wk (max 60 mg/day)

ADHD

Adult: PO 5-60 mg/day in divided doses

P ***Child >6 yr:*** PO 5 mg qd-bid increasing by 5 mg/day at weekly intervals

P ***Child 3-6 yr:*** PO 2.5 mg qd increasing by 2.5 mg/day at weekly intervals

Available forms: Tabs 5, 10 mg; sus rel caps 5, 10, 15 mg

Adverse effects

CNS: Hyperactivity, insomnia, restlessness, talkativeness, dizziness, headache, chills, stimulation, dysphoria, irritability, aggressiveness, tremor, dependence, addiction

CV: Palpitations, **tachycardia,** hypertension, decrease in heart rate, **dysrhythmias**

GI: Anorexia, dry mouth, diarrhea, constipation, weight loss, metallic taste

GU: Impotence, change in libido

INTEG: Urticaria

Contraindications: Hypersensitivity to sympathomimetic amines, hyperthyroidism, hypertension, glaucoma, severe arteriosclerosis, drug abuse, cardiovascular disease, anxiety

Precautions: Gilles de la Tourette's P disorder, pregnancy **C**, lactation, child <3 yr

Pharmacokinetics

Absorption	Well absorbed
Distribution	Widely distributed; crosses placenta
Metabolism	Liver
Excretion	Kidneys, pH dependent: increased pH, increased reabsorption
Half-life	10-30 hr; increased when urine is alkaline

Pharmacodynamics

Onset	½ hr
Peak	1-3 hr
Duration	4-10 hr

Interactions

Individual drugs

Acetazolamide: ↓ excretion, ↑ effect
Ammonium chloride: ↓ effect
Ascorbic acid: ↓ effect
Haloperidol: ↑ CNS effect
Meperidine: Hypertensive crisis
Sodium bicarbonate: ↓ excretion, ↑ effect
Thyroid hormones: ↑ effects

Drug classifications

Adrenergic blockers: ↓ adrenergic blocking effect
Antidepressants, tricyclic: ↑ dysrhythmias
Antidiabetics: ↓ antidiabetic effect
β-Adrenergic blockers: ↑ hypertension
Barbiturates: ↓ absorption of barbiturate
Cardiac glycosides: ↑ dysrhythmias
MAOIs: Hypertensive crisis
Phenothiazines: ↑ CNS effect
Sympathomimetics: ↑ effect

Food/drug

Caffeine: ↑ amine effect

NURSING CONSIDERATIONS

Assessment

- Monitor VS, B/P, since this drug may reverse antihypertensives; check patients with cardiac disease more often for increased B/P
- Monitor CBC, urinalysis; for diabetic

patients monitor blood glucose, urine glucose; insulin changes may be required, since eating will decrease

- Monitor height and weight q3 mo since growth rate in children may be decreased; appetite is suppressed so weight loss is common during the first few months of treatment
- Monitor mental status: mood, sensorium, affect, stimulation, insomnia; aggressiveness may occur; depression with crying spells may occur after drug has worn off
- Assess for physical dependency; should not be used for extended time except in ADHD; dosage should be decreased gradually to prevent withdrawal symptoms
- Assess for narcoleptic symptoms before medication and after; ability to stay awake should increase significantly
- In children or adults with ADHD, monitor for improved organizational skills, attention span, attending to tasks, impulse control, socialization, and ability to get along better with others
- Assess for withdrawal symptoms: headache, nausea, vomiting, muscle pain, weakness; drug tolerance develops after long-term use; dosage should not be increased if tolerance develops; this medication has a high abuse potential

Nursing diagnoses

- ✓ Thought processes, altered (uses, adverse reactions)
- ✓ Coping, impaired individual (uses)
- ✓ Family coping, impaired individual (uses)
- ✓ Knowledge deficit (teaching)

Implementation

- Give at least 6 hr before hs to avoid sleeplessness; titrate to patient's response; lowest dosage should be used to control symptoms
- Give gum, hard candy, frequent sips of water for dry mouth at beginning of treatment; these symptoms tend to lessen with time
- Do not crush, chew sus rel forms

Patient/family education

- Advise patient to decrease caffeine consumption (coffee, tea, cola, chocolate), which may increase irritability and stimulation; to avoid OTC preparations unless approved by prescriber; to avoid alcohol ingestion; these may cause serious drug interactions
- Caution patient to taper off drug over several weeks, or depression, increased sleeping, lethargy may occur
- Caution patient to avoid hazardous activities until patient is stabilized on medication
- Instruct patient not to double doses if medication is missed; prescriber may suggest drug holidays (ADHD) during the school year to assess progress and determine continued drug necessity
- Instruct patient/family to notify prescriber if significant side effects occur: tremors, insomnia, palpitations, restlessness, drug changes may be needed
- Inform patient that if dry mouth occurs to use frequent sips of water, sugarless gum, hard candy during beginning therapy; dry mouth lessens with continued treatment
- Advise patient to get needed rest; patients will feel more tired at end of day; to give last dose at least 6 hr before hs to avoid insomnia

Evaluation

Positive therapeutic outcome

- Decreased activity in ADHD
- Absence of sleeping during day in narcolepsy

Treatment of overdose:

Administer fluids, hemodialysis, peritoneal dialysis, antihypertensives for increased B/P; ammonium chloride for increased excretion

D

dextromethorphan (OTC)

(dex-troe-meth-or'fan)

Balminil DM ♣, Benylin DM, Broncho-Grippol-DM ♣, Children's Hold, Creo-Terpin, Delsym, dextromethorphan, DM Syrup ♣, Hold DM, Koffex ♣, Neo-DM ♣, Ornex-DM ♣, Pertussin, Pertussin ES, Robidex ♣, Robitussin Cough Calmers, Robitussin Pediatric, Sedatuss ♣, St. Joseph Cough Suppressant, Scot-Tussin DM, Sucrets Cough Control, Suppress, Vicks Formula 44

Func. class.: Antitussive, nonnarcotic

Chem. class.: Levorphanol derivative

Pregnancy category C

Action: Depresses cough center in medulla by direct effect related to levorphanol

➡ **Therapeutic Outcome:** Absence of cough

Uses: Nonproductive cough carried by minor respiratory tract infections or irritants that might be inhaled

Investigational uses: Neuropathy

Dosage and routes

P ***Adult and Child ≥12 yr:*** PO 10-20 mg q4h, or 30 mg q6-8h, not to exceed 120 mg/day; sus rel liq 60 mg q12h, not to exceed 120 mg/day

P ***Child 6-12 yr:*** PO 5-10 mg q4h; sus rel liq 30 mg bid, not to exceed 60 mg/day

P ***Child 2-6 yr:*** PO 2.5-5 mg q4h, or 7.5 mg q6-8h, not to exceed 30 mg/day

Neuropathy

Adult: PO doses vary widely

Available forms: Loz 2.5, 5, 7.5, 15 mg; sol; liq 3.5 mg, 7.5, 15 mg/5 ml, 3.5, 5, 7.5, 10, 15 mg/5 ml; syrup 15 mg/15 ml, 10 mg/5 ml; sus action liq equivalent to 30 mg/5 ml; caps 30 mg; ext rel susp 30 mg/5 ml

Adverse effects

CNS: Dizziness, sedation

GI: Nausea

Contraindications: Hypersensitivity, asthma/emphysema, productive cough

Precautions: Nausea/vomiting, increased temp, persistent headache, pregnancy **C**

Pharmacokinetics

Absorption	Rapid (PO); slow (sus rel)
Distribution	Unknown
Metabolism	Liver
Excretion	Kidneys
Half-life	Unknown

Pharmacodynamics

	PO	PO-SUS
Onset	15-30 min	Unknown
Peak	Unknown	Unknown
Duration	3-6 hr	12 hr

Interactions

Individual drugs

Alcohol: ↑ CNS depression

Amiodarone: ↑ adverse reactions

Fluoxetine: ↑ adverse reactions

Quinidine: ↑ adverse reactions

Drug classifications

Analgesics: ↑ CNS depression

Antihistamines: ↑ CNS depression

Antidepressants: ↑ CNS depression

MAOIs: ↑ hypotension, hyperpyrexia

Opiates: ↑ CNS depression

Sedative/hypnotics: ↑ CNS depression

NURSING CONSIDERATIONS

Assessment

- Assess cough: type, frequency, character including sputum; provide adequate hydration to 2 L/day to decrease viscosity of secretions

Nursing diagnoses
- ✓ Airway clearance, ineffective (uses)
- ✓ Knowledge deficit (teaching)

Implementation
- Administer decreased dosage to G elderly patients; their metabolism may be slowed; do not provide water within 30 min of administration because it dilutes drug
- Shake susp before administration

Patient/family education
- Caution patient to avoid driving or other hazardous activities until stabilized on this medication; may cause drowsiness, dizziness in some individuals
- Advise patient to avoid smoking, smoke-filled rooms, perfumes, dust, environmental pollutants, cleaners, which increase cough; may use gum, hard candy to prevent dry mouth
- Advise patient to avoid alcohol or other CNS depressants while taking this medication; drowsiness will be increased
- Caution patient that any cough lasting over a few days should be assessed by prescriber

Evaluation
Positive therapeutic outcome
- Absence of dry, irritating cough

dextrose (D-glucose) (℞)
Glucose, Glutose, Insta-Glucose
Func. class.: Caloric agent

Pregnancy category D

Action: Needed for adequate utilization of amino acids; decreases protein, nitrogen loss; prevents ketosis

Therapeutic Outcome: Provides calories, prevents severe hypoglycemia

Uses: Increases intake of calories; increases fluids in patients unable to take adequate fluids, calories orally; 2.5%-11.5% forms provide calories, increased hydration; 20%-70% forms used to treat severe hypoglycemia

Dosage and routes
P ***Adult and child:*** **IV**, depends on individual requirements

Available forms: Inj **IV** 2.5%, 5%, 10%, 20%, 30%, 40%, 50%, 60%, 70%; oral gel 40%; chewable tabs 5 g

Adverse effects
CNS: Confusion, **loss of consciousness,** dizziness
CV: Hypertension, **CHF, pulmonary edema**
ENDO: Hyperglycemia, rebound hypoglycemia, hyperosmolar syndrome, hyperglycemic nonketolytic syndrome
GU: Glycosuria, osmotic diuresis
INTEG: Chills, flushing, warm feeling, rash, urticaria, extravasation necrosis

Contraindications: Hyperglycemia, delirium tremens, hemorrhage (cranial/spinal), CHF, pregnancy **D**

Precautions: Renal, liver, cardiac disease, diabetes mellitus

Pharmacokinetics

Absorption	Well absorbed (PO); completely absorbed (**IV**)
Distribution	Widely distributed
Metabolism	Unknown
Excretion	Unknown
Half-life	Unknown

Pharmacodynamics

	IV	PO
Onset	Immediate	Rapid
Peak	Immediate	Rapid
Duration	Immediate	Rapid

Interactions
Individual drugs
Insulin: ↑ need for insulin
Drug classifications
Corticosteroids: ↑ fluid retention/electrolyte excretion
Hypoglycemics, oral: ↑ need for hypoglycemic

NURSING CONSIDERATIONS

Assessment

- Assess I&O, skin turgor, edema, electrolytes (potassium, sodium, calcium, chloride, magnesium), blood glucose, ammonia, phosphate
- Monitor inj site for extravasation: redness along vein, edema at site, necrosis, pain, hard tender area; site should be changed immediately
- Monitor temp q4h for increased fever, indicating infection; if infection suspected, inf is discontinued and tubing, bottle, catheter tip cultured
- Monitor serum glucose in patients receiving hypertonic glucose 5% and over
- Assess nutritional status: calorie count by dietician; GI system function

Nursing diagnoses

- ✓ Nutrition: less than body requirements (uses)
- ✓ Fluid volume excess (adverse reactions)
- ✓ Knowledge deficit (teaching)

Implementation

PO route

- Oral glucose preparations (gel, chewable tabs) are to be used for conscious patients only; serum blood glucose should be monitored after first oral dose; if glucose has not increased by 20 mg/100 ml in 20-30 min, dose should be repeated and serum glucose checked again

IV IV route

- Give only protein (4%) and dextrose (up to 12.5%) via peripheral vein; stronger sol requires central **IV** administration
- May be given undiluted via prepared sol; give 10% sol (5 ml/15 sec), 20% sol (1000 ml/3 hr or more), 50% sol (500 ml/30-60 min); too rapid **IV** administration may cause fluid overload and hyperglycemia
- After changing **IV** catheter, change dressing q24h with aseptic technique

Patient/family education

- Teach patient reason for dextrose infusion
- Provide literature and information on when and how to use oral products for hypoglycemia
- Review hypoglycemia/hyperglycemia symptoms
- Review blood glucose monitoring procedure

Evaluation

Positive therapeutic outcome

- Increased weight
- Blood glucose level at normal limits for patient
- Adequate hydration

HIGH ALERT

dezocine (Rx)

(dez'oh-seen)

Dalgan

Func. class.: Narcotic agonist-antagonist analgesic

Chem. class.: Opioid, synthetic

Pregnancy category C

Action: Inhibits ascending pain pathways in limbic system, thalamus, midbrain, hypothalamus by binding to opiate receptor sites, which alters pain perception and response

➔ **Therapeutic Outcome:** Relief of moderate, severe pain

Uses: Moderate to severe pain

Dosage and routes

Adult: IM 5-20 mg q3-6h, not to exceed 120 mg/day; **IV** 2.5-10 mg q2-4h

Available forms: Inj 5, 10, 15 mg single-dose vials, multiple dose 10 mg/ml

Adverse effects

CNS: Drowsiness, dizziness, confusion, sedation, anxiety, headache, depression, delirium, sleep disturbances, dependency, euphoria

CV: Hypotension, pulse irregularity, hypertension, chest pain, pallor, edema, thrombophlebitis, bradycardia
EENT: Blurred vision, slurred speech, diplopia, miosis
GI: Nausea, vomiting, anorexia, constipation, cramps, abdominal pain, dry mouth, diarrhea
GU: Urinary frequency, hesitancy, retention
INTEG: Inj site reactions, pruritus, rash, swelling, chills
RESP: **Respiratory depression,** hiccups

Contraindications: Hypersensitivity

Precautions: Addictive personality, pregnancy **C,** lactation, increased intracranial pressure, respiratory depression, hepatic disease, renal disease, child <18 yr, elderly, biliary surgery, COPD, sulfite sensitivity

P G

Pharmacokinetics

Absorption	Completely absorbed (IM, **IV**)
Distribution	Not known
Metabolism	Liver, extensively
Excretion	Kidneys
Half-life	1½-7 hr

Pharmacodynamics

	IM	IV
Onset	½ hr	10 min
Peak	1-2 hr	30 min
Duration	2-4 hr	2-4 hr

Interactions

Individual drugs

Alcohol: ↑ respiratory depression, hypotension, sedation
Cimetidine: ↑ recovery
Erythromycin: ↑ recovery
Nalbuphine: ↓ analgesia
Pentazocine: ↓ analgesia

Drug classifications

Antihistamines: ↑ respiratory depression, hypotension
CNS depressants: ↑ respiratory depression, hypotension
MAOIs: Do not use 2 wk before dezocine
Phenothiazines: ↑ respiratory depression, hypotension
Sedative/hypnotics: ↑ respiratory depression, hypotension

NURSING CONSIDERATIONS

Assessment

- Assess respiratory status: respiratory depression, character, rate, rhythm; notify prescriber if respirations are <12/min; note CV status, bradycardia, syncope; monitor ECG continuously
- Assess pain: location, intensity, duration, alleviating factors

Nursing diagnoses

✓ Pain (uses)
✓ Sensory-perceptual alteration: visual, auditory (adverse reactions)
✓ Breathing pattern, ineffective (adverse reactions)
✓ Knowledge deficit (teaching) (preoperatively)

Implementation

IM route

- Give deeply in large muscle mass; rotate sites; do not give SC

IV **IV route**

- Give undiluted ≤5 mg over 2-3 min

Patient/family education

- Caution patients to avoid CNS depressants: alcohol, sedative/hypnotics for at least 24 hr after taking this drug
- Discuss with patient that dizziness, drowsiness, and confusion are common; to avoid getting up without assistance
- Advise patient to make position changes to lessen orthostatic hypotension

Evaluation

Positive therapeutic outcome

- Decreased pain perception

Treatment of overdose:

Naloxone 0.2-0.8 **IV**, O_2, **IV** fluids, vasopressors

diazepam 🗝 (℞)
(dye-az'e-pam)

Apo-Diazepam ✤, Diastat, diazepam, Novo-Diapam ✤, PMS-Diazepam ✤, Valium, Valrelease, Vivol ✤

Func. class.: Antianxiety, anticonvulsant, skeletal muscle relaxant, central acting

Chem. class.: Benzodiazepine

Pregnancy category D

Controlled substance schedule IV

Action: Potentiates the actions of GABA, especially in limbic system, reticular formation; enhances presympathetic inhibition, inhibits spinal polysynaptic afferent paths

➔ **Therapeutic Outcome:** Decreased anxiety, restlessness, insomnia

Uses: Anxiety, acute alcohol withdrawal, adjunct in seizure disorders; preoperative skeletal muscle relaxation; rectally for acute repetitive seizures

Investigational uses: Panic attacks

Dosage and routes

Anxiety/convulsive disorders

Adult: PO 2-10 mg bid-qid; ext rel 15-30 mg qd

G ***Elderly:*** PO 1-2 mg qd-bid, increase slowly as needed

P ***Child >6 mo:*** PO 1-2.5 mg tid-qid

Muscle relaxation

Adult: PO 2-10 mg tid-qid or ext rel 15-30 mg qd; **IV**/IM 5-10 mg repeat in 2-4 hr

G ***Elderly:*** PO 2-5 mg bid-qid; **IV**/IM 2-5 mg, may repeat in 2-4 hr

Tetanic muscle spasms

P ***Child <5 yr:*** IM/**IV** 5-10 mg q3-4h prn

P ***Infants >30 days:*** IM/**IV** 1-2 mg q3-4h prn

Status epilepticus

Adult: **IV** bol 5, 20 mg, 2 mg/min, may repeat q5-10 min, not to exceed 60 mg; may repeat in 30 min if seizures reappear

P ***Child:*** **IV** bol 0.1-0.3 mg/kg (1 mg/min over 3 min); may repeat q15 min × 2 doses

Adult: REC 0.2 mg/kg, may repeat 4-12 hr later

P ***Child 6-11 yr:*** REC 0.3 mg/kg, may repeat 4-12 hr later

P ***Child 2-5 yr:*** REC 0.5 mg/kg, may repeat 4-12 hr later

Alcohol withdrawal

Adult: PO 10 mg tid-qid in 1st 24 hr, then 5 mg tid-qid; IM/**IV** 10 mg, then 5-10 mg after 3 hr

Available forms: Tabs 2, 5, 10 mg; caps ext rel 15 mg; inj emulsified 5 mg/ml; oral sol 5 mg/5 ml; gel, rectal delivery system 2.5, 10, 15, 20 mg, twin packs; sterile emulsion for inj 5 mg/ml

Adverse effects

CNS: *Dizziness, drowsiness,* confusion, headache, anxiety, tremors, stimulation, fatigue, depression, insomnia, hallucinations

CV: *Orthostatic hypotension,* **ECG changes, tachycardia,** hypotension

EENT: *Blurred vision,* tinnitus, mydriasis

GI: Constipation, dry mouth, nausea, vomiting, anorexia, diarrhea

HEMA: **Neutropenia**

INTEG: Rash, dermatitis, itching

RESP: **Respiratory depression**

Contraindications: Hypersensitivity to benzodiazepines, narrow-angle glaucoma, psychosis, pregnancy **D,** coma, respiratory depression

G **Precautions:** Elderly, debilitated, hepatic disease, renal disease, addiction

Do Not Confuse:
diazepam/Ditropan

Pharmacokinetics

Absorption	Rapid (PO); erratic (IM)
Distribution	Widely distributed; crosses blood-brain barrier, placenta
Metabolism	Liver, extensively
Excretion	Kidneys, breast milk
Half-life	20-80 hr

Pharmacodynamics

	PO	IM	IV
Onset	½ hr	15 min	Immediate
Peak	1-2 hr	½-1½ hr	15 min
Duration	2-3 hr	1-1½ hr	15 min

Interactions

Individual drugs

Alcohol: ↑ CNS depression
Cimetidine: ↑ toxicity
Digoxin: ↑ digoxin level
Disulfiram: ↓ metabolism of diazepam
Isoniazid: ↓ metabolism of diazepam
Propranolol: ↓ metabolism of diazepam
Valproic acid: ↓ toxicity

Drug classifications

Barbiturates: ↑ toxicity
CNS depressants: ↑ toxicity
Opiates: ↓ diazepam effects
Oral contraceptives: ↓ metabolism of diazepam
SSRIs: ↑ toxicity

Herb/drug

Kava: ↑ diazepam effect

Lab test interferences

↑ AST/ALT, ↑ serum bilirubin
↓ Radioactive iodine uptake
False: ↑ 17-OHCS

NURSING CONSIDERATIONS

Assessment

- Assess degree of anxiety; what precipitates anxiety and whether drug controls symptoms; other signs of anxiety: dilated pupils, inability to sleep, restlessness, inability to focus
- Assess for alcohol withdrawal symptoms, including hallucinations (visual, auditory), delirium, irritability, agitation, fine to coarse tremors
- Monitor B/P (with patient lying, standing), pulse, respiratory rate; if systolic B/P drops 20 mm Hg, hold drug, notify prescriber; monitor respirations q5-15 min if given **IV**
- Monitor blood studies: CBC during long-term therapy; blood dyscrasias have occurred (rarely)
- Monitor for seizure control; type, duration, and intensity of convulsions; what precipitates seizures
- Monitor hepatic studies: AST, ALT, bilirubin, creatinine, LDH, alkaline phosphatase
- Assess mental status: mood, sensorium, affect, sleeping pattern, drowsiness, dizziness, suicidal tendencies, and ability of drug to control these symptoms; check for tolerance, withdrawal symptoms: headache, nausea, vomiting, muscle pain, weakness after long-term use

Nursing diagnoses

- ✓ Anxiety (uses)
- ✓ Injury, risk of (uses, adverse reactions)
- ✓ Coping, ineffective individual (uses)
- ✓ Knowledge deficit (teaching)
- ✓ Noncompliance (teaching)

Implementation

PO route

- Give with food or milk for GI symptoms; crush tab if patient is unable to swallow medication whole; do not crush ext rel caps; use sugarless gum, hard candy, frequent sips of water for dry mouth
- Reduce narcotic dosage by ⅓ if given concomitantly with diazepam
- Check to see PO medication has been swallowed

IV route

- Administer **IV** into large vein; do not dilute or mix with any other drug;

give **IV** 5 mg or less/1 min or total P dose over 3 min or more (children, infants); cont inf is not recommended
- Check **IV** site for thrombosis or phlebitis, which may occur rapidly

Syringe compatibilities: Cimetidine

Syringe incompatibilities: Benzquinamide, doxapram, glycopyrrolate, heparin, nalbuphine

Y-site compatibilities: Cefmetazole, dobutamine, nafcillin, quinidine, sufentanil

Y-site incompatibilities: Hydromorphone, fluconazole, foscarnet, heparin, pancuronium, potassium chloride, vecuronium, vit B with C

Additive compatibilities: Netilmicin, verapamil

Sterile emulsion for injection
- Use **IV** only, within 6 hr, flush line after use and after 6 hr

Rectal route
- Do not use more than 5 ×/mo or for an episode q5 days

Patient/family education
- Advise patient that drug may be taken with food; that drug is not to be used for everyday stress or used longer than 4 mo unless directed by prescriber; take no more than prescribed amount; may be habit forming
- Caution patient to avoid OTC preparations unless approved by a prescriber; to avoid alcohol, other psychotropic medications unless prescribed; that smoking may decrease diazepam effect; not to discontinue medication abruptly after long-term use
- Inform patient to avoid driving, activities that require alertness; drowsiness may occur; to rise slowly or fainting may occur, especially in G elderly
- Advise patient not to become pregnant while using this drug
- Inform patient that drowsiness may worsen at beginning of treatment

Evaluation

Positive therapeutic outcome
- Decreased anxiety, restlessness, insomnia

Treatment of overdose: Lavage, VS, supportive care, flumazenil

diazoxide (℞)

(dye-az-ox'ide)

Hyperstat IV, Proglycem

Func. class.: Antihypertensive

Chem. class.: Vasodilator

Pregnancy category C

Action: Decreases release of insulin from β-cells in pancreas, resulting in an increase in blood glucose; relaxes vascular smooth muscle (peripheral arterioles)

➔ **Therapeutic Outcome:** Decreased B/P, increased blood glucose

Uses: Hypoglycemia caused by hyperinsulinism; emergency treatment of hypertension

Dosage and routes

Hypoglycemia

P ***Adult and child:*** PO 3-8 mg/kg/day in 2-3 divided doses q8-12h

P ***Infants and neonates:*** PO 8-15 mg/kg/day in 2-3 divided doses 8-12h

Hypertension

P ***Adult and child:*** **IV** 1-3 mg/kg q5-15 min, max 150 mg/dose

Available forms: Caps 50 mg; oral susp 50 mg/ml; inj 15 mg/ml, 300 mg/20 ml

Adverse effects

CNS: Headache, weakness, malaise, anxiety, dizziness, insomnia, paresthesia, **seizures, cerebral ischemia, paralysis**

CV: **Tachycardia,** palpitations, hypotension, transient hypertension, **shock, MI**

EENT: Diplopia, cataracts, ring scotoma, subconjunctival hemorrhage, lacrimation
GI: Nausea, vomiting, anorexia, abdominal pain, transient loss of taste, diarrhea
GU: Reversible nephrotic syndrome, decreased urinary output, hematuria
HEMA: **Thrombocytopenia, leukopenia,** eosinophilia, decreased Hgb, Hct
INTEG: Increased hair growth or loss of scalp hair, rash, dermatitis, herpes
META: Hyperuricemia, sodium/fluid retention, ketoacidosis, hyperglycemia, azotemia

Contraindications: Hypersensitivity to this drug or thiazides, functional hypoglycemia

Precautions: Pregnancy **C,** lactation, renal disease, diabetes mellitus, CV disease, gout

Pharmacokinetics

Absorption	Well absorbed (PO); completely absorbed (**IV**)
Distribution	Crosses blood-brain barrier, placenta
Metabolism	Liver (50%)
Excretion	Kidney, unchanged (50%)
Half-life	20-36 hr

Pharmacodynamics

	PO	IV
Onset	1 hr	1-2 min
Peak	8-12 hr	5 min
Duration	8 hr	3-12 hr

Interactions
Individual drugs
Warfarin: ↑ effects
Drug classifications
Diuretics, thiazides: ↑ hyperglycemia
Hydantoins: ↓ anticonvulsant effect
Sulfonylureas: ↑ hyperglycemia

NURSING CONSIDERATIONS
Assessment
- Assess for allergies to sulfonamide; cross-sensitivity may occur
- Assess B/P q5 min until stabilized
- Monitor electrolytes, blood studies: potassium, sodium, chloride, carbon dioxide, CBC, serum glucose
- Monitor weight daily, I&O; edema in feet, legs daily; check skin turgor, dryness of mucous membranes for hydration status
- Assess for rales, dyspnea, orthopnea; peripheral edema, fatigue, weight gain, jugular vein distention (CHF)
- Assess for signs of hyperglycemia: acetone breath, increased urinary output, severe thirst, lethargy, dizziness

Nursing diagnoses
✓ Cardiac output, decreased (adverse reactions)
✓ Injury, risk for (side effects)
✓ Knowledge deficit (teaching)

Implementation
PO route
- Shake susp before using
- Store protected from light and heat

IV **IV route**
- Give by direct **IV** over 30 sec or less; may repeat q5-15 min until desired response; do not administer dark solution
- Give to patient in recumbent position; keep in that position for 1 hr after

Syringe compatibility:
Heparin

Y-site incompatibilities:
Hydralazine, propranolol

Evaluation
Positive therapeutic outcome
- Decreased B/P in hypertension

Treatment of overdose:
Administer levarterenol, dopamine, or norepinephrine for hypotension, dialysis

diclofenac potassium (℞)
(dye-kloe'fen-ak)
Cataflam, Voltaren Rapide ✦

diclofenac sodium
Apo-Dilo ✦, Novo-Difenac ✦, Nu-Diclo, Voltaren, Voltaren SR

Func. class.: Nonsteroidal antiinflammatory, nonopioid analgesic
Chem. class.: Phenylacetic acid

Pregnancy category B

Action: Inhibits prostaglandin synthesis by decreasing enzyme needed for biosynthesis; analgesic, antiinflammatory, antipyretic properties

Therapeutic Outcome: Decreased pain, inflammation

Uses: Acute, chronic rheumatoid arthritis, osteoarthritis, ankylosing spondylitis, analgesia, primary dysmenorrhea, ophthalmic: to decrease inflammation after cataract extraction

Dosage and routes

Osteoarthritis
Adult: PO 100-150 mg/day in 2-3 divided doses (potassium)

Rheumatoid arthritis
Adult: PO 150-200 mg/day in 2-4 divided doses (potassium); 50 mg tid-qid, then reduce to lowest dose needed (25 mg tid) (sodium)

Ankylosing spondylitis
Adult: PO 100-125 mg/day in 4-5 divided doses; give 25 mg qid and 25 mg hs if needed (potassium)

Postcataract surgery
Adult: Ophth 1 gtt of 0.1% sol qid × 2 wk 24 hr postsurgery

Analgesia/primary dysmenorrhea
Adult: PO 50 mg tid, max 150 mg/day (potassium)

Available forms: Potassium: tabs 50, 75 mg; sodium: tabs delayed rel (enteric-coated) 25, 50, 75 mg; ext rel tabs 75, 100 mg; supp 50, 100 mg

Adverse effects

CNS: *Dizziness,* drowsiness, fatigue, tremors, confusion, insomnia, anxiety, depression, nervousness, paresthesia, muscle weakness
CV: **CHF,** tachycardia, peripheral edema, palpitations, dysrhythmias, hypotension, hypertension, fluid retention
EENT: Tinnitus, hearing loss, blurred vision
GI: Nausea, anorexia, vomiting, diarrhea, jaundice, **cholestatic hepatitis,** constipation, flatulence, cramps, dry mouth, peptic ulcer, GI bleeding
GU: **Nephrotoxicity: dysuria, hematuria, oliguria, azotemia, cystitis, UTI**
HEMA: **Blood dyscrasias,** epistaxis, bruising
INTEG: Purpura, rash, pruritus, sweating, erythema, petechiae, photosensitivity, alopecia
RESP: Dyspnea, hemoptysis, pharyngitis, **bronchospasm, laryngeal edema,** rhinitis, shortness of breath
SYST: **Anaphylaxis**

Contraindications: Hypersensitivity to aspirin, iodides, other NSAIDs, asthma, pregnancy (3rd trimester)

Precautions: Pregnancy **B** (1st trimester), lactation, children, bleeding disorders, GI disorders, cardiac disorders, hypersensitivity to other antiinflammatory agents, CrCl <30 ml/min

Do Not Confuse:
Cataflam/Catapres

Pharmacokinetics

Absorption	Well absorbed (PO, ophth)
Distribution	Crosses placenta; 90% bound to plasma proteins
Metabolism	Liver (50%)
Excretion	Breast milk
Half-life	1-2 hr

Pharmacodynamics

	PO	OPHTH
Onset	Unknown	Unknown
Peak	2-3 hr	Unknown
Duration	Unknown	Unknown

Interactions

Individual drugs

Acetaminophen (long-term use): ↑ renal reactions
Alcohol: ↑ adverse reactions, ↑ GI side effects
Aspirin: ↓ effectiveness, ↑ adverse reactions, ↑ GI side effects
Colchicine: ↑ GI side effects
Cyclosporine: ↑ toxicity
Digoxin: ↑ toxicity, ↑ levels
Insulin: ↓ insulin effect
Lithium: ↑ toxicity
Methotrexate: ↑ toxicity
Phenytoin: ↑ toxicity

Drug classifications

Anticoagulants: ↑ risk of bleeding
Antidiabetics: ↑ need for dosage adjustment
Antihypertensives: ↓ effect of antihypertensives
Antineoplastics: ↑ risk of hematologic toxicity
β-Adrenergic blockers: ↑ antihypertension
Cephalosporins: ↑ risk of bleeding
Diuretics: ↓ effectiveness of diuretics
Glucocorticoids: ↑ adverse reactions
NSAIDs: ↑ adverse reactions
Potassium supplements: ↑ adverse reactions
Radiation: ↑ risk of hematologic toxicity

NURSING CONSIDERATIONS

Assessment

- Assess for pain of rheumatoid arthritis, osteoarthritis, ankylosing spondylitis; check ROM, inflammation of joints, characteristics of pain
- Assess ophth patients for pain, inflammation, redness, swelling
- Monitor blood counts during therapy; watch for decreasing platelets; if low, therapy may need to be discontinued, restarted after hematologic recovery
- Assess for asthma, aspirin hypersensitivity, nasal polyps; may develop hypersensitivity
- Monitor LFTs (may be elevated) and uric acid (may be decreased—serum; increased—urine) periodically; also BUN, creatinine, electrolytes (may be elevated)
- Monitor for blood dyscrasias (thrombocytopenia): bruising, fatigue, bleeding, poor healing

Nursing diagnoses

- ✓ Pain (uses)
- ✓ Mobility, impaired physical (uses)
- ✓ Injury, risk for (side effects)
- ✓ Knowledge deficit (teaching)

Implementation

PO route

- Administer with food or milk to decrease gastric symptoms;
- Do not crush, dissolve, or chew enteric coated or sus rel caps

Ophthalmic route

- Administer with patient recumbent or tilting head back; pull down on lower lid; when conjunctival sac is exposed, instill 1 drop; wait a few minutes before instilling other drops

Patient/family education

- Teach patient that drug must be continued for prescribed time to be effective; to avoid aspirin, NSAIDs, acetaminophen, or other OTC medications unless approved by prescriber, alcoholic beverages; to contact prescriber before surgery regarding when to discontinue this drug
- Caution patient to report bleeding, bruising, fatigue, malaise, since blood dyscrasias do occur
- Advise patient to report hepatotoxicity: flu symptoms, nausea, vomiting, jaundice, pruritus, lethargy

- Instruct patient to use sunscreen to prevent photosensitivity
- Teach patient to avoid use in 3rd trimester of pregnancy
- Instruct patient to use caution when driving; drowsiness, dizziness may occur
- (Do Not Crush) Teach patient to take with a full glass of water to enhance absorption; remain upright for ½ hr; if dose is missed, take as soon as remembered within 2 hr if taking 1-2 ×/day, do not double doses; do not crush, break, or chew

Evaluation

Positive therapeutic outcome

- Decreased pain in arthritic conditions
- Decreased inflammation in arthritic conditions
- Decreased ocular irritation

dicloxacillin (℞)

(dye-klox-a-sill'in)

dicloxacillin sodium, Dycill, Dynapen, Pathocil

Func. class.: Antiinfective

Chem. class.: Penicillinase-resistant penicillin

Pregnancy category B

Action: Interferes with cell wall replication of susceptible organisms; osmotically unstable cell wall swells, bursts from osmotic pressure

Therapeutic Outcome: Bactericidal effects for the following: gram-positive cocci *Staphylococcus aureus, Streptococcus pyogenes, Streptococcus viridans, Streptococcus faecalis, Streptococcus bovis, Streptococcus pneumoniae;* infections caused by penicillinase-producing *Staphylococcus* organisms

Uses: Penicillinase-producing staphylococci, streptococci; respiratory tract, skin, skin structure infections; sinusitis

Dosage and routes

(P) ***Adult and Child ≥40 kg:*** PO 0.5-4 g/day in divided doses q6h, max 4 g/day

(P) ***Child ≤40 kg:*** PO 12.5-50 mg/kg in divided doses q6h, max 4 g/d

Available forms: Caps 125, 250, 500 mg; powder for oral susp 62.5 mg/5 ml

Adverse effects

CNS: Lethargy, hallucinations, anxiety, depression, twitching, **coma, convulsions**

GI: *Nausea, vomiting, diarrhea,* increased AST, ALT, abdominal pain, glossitis, pseudomembranous colitis

GU: **Oliguria, proteinuria, hematuria, vaginitis, moniliasis, glomerulonephritis**

HEMA: Anemia, increased bleeding time, **bone marrow depression, granulocytopenia**

SYST: **Anaphylaxis**

Contraindications: Hypersensitivity to penicillins; neonates

Precautions: Hypersensitivity to cephalosporins, pregnancy **B,** severe renal or hepatic disease

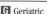

Do Not Confuse:
Pathocil/Bactocil

Pharmacokinetics	
Absorption	Rapid, incomplete (35%-75%)
Distribution	Widely distributed; crosses placenta
Metabolism	Liver (6%-10%)
Excretion	Kidneys, unchanged (60%); breast milk
Half-life	½-1 hr, increased in hepatic renal disease

Pharmacodynamics	
Onset	½ hr
Peak	½-2 hr

Interactions

Individual drugs

Aspirin: ↑ dicloxacillin concentrations

Disulfiram: ↑ dicloxacillin concentrations

Probenecid: ↑ dicloxacillin levels, ↓ renal excretion

Drug classifications

Oral anticoagulants: ↑ anticoagulant effects

Oral contraceptives: ↑ action of oral contraceptives

Food/drug

Food, carbonated drinks, citrus fruit juices: ↓ absorption

Herb/drug

Khat: ↓ absorption

Lab test interferences

False positive: Urine glucose, urine protein

NURSING CONSIDERATIONS

Assessment

- Assess patient for previous sensitivity reaction to penicillins or other cephalosporins; cross-sensitivity between penicillins and cephalosporins is common
- Assess patient for signs and symptoms of infection including characteristics of wounds, sputum, urine, stool, WBC >10,000/mm^3, fever; obtain baseline information and during treatment
- Obtain C&S before beginning drug therapy to identify if correct treatment has been initiated
- Assess for anaphylaxis: rash, urticaria, pruritus, chills, fever, joint pain may occur a few days after therapy begins; epinephrine and resuscitation equipment should be available for anaphylactic reaction
- Identify urine output; if decreasing, notify prescriber (may indicate nephrotoxicity); check for increased BUN, creatinine
- Monitor blood studies: AST, ALT, CBC, Hct, bilirubin, LDH, alkaline phosphatase, Coombs' test monthly if patient is on long-term therapy
- Monitor electrolytes: potassium, sodium, chloride monthly if patient is on long-term therapy
- Assess bowel pattern qd; if severe diarrhea occurs, drug should be discontinued; may indicate pseudomembranous colitis
- Monitor for bleeding: ecchymosis, bleeding gums, hematuria, stool guaiac daily if on long-term therapy
- Assess for overgrowth of infection: perineal itching, fever, malaise, redness, pain, swelling, drainage, rash, diarrhea, change in cough, sputum

Nursing diagnoses

- ✓ Infection, risk for (uses)
- ✓ Diarrhea (side effects)
- ✓ Knowledge deficit (teaching)
- ✓ Noncompliance (teaching)
- ✓ Injury, risk for (side effects)

Implementation

- Give in even doses around the clock; if GI upset occurs, give with food; drug must be given for 10-14 days to ensure organism death and prevent superinfection; store in airtight container
- Do not crush, chew caps
- Shake susp well before each dose; store in refrigerator for 2 wk or 1 wk at room temp

Patient/family education

- Teach patient to report sore throat, bruising, bleeding, joint pain; may indicate blood dyscrasias (rare)
- Advise patient to contact prescriber if vaginal itching, loose, foul-smelling stools, furry tongue occur; may indicate superinfection
- Instruct patient to take all medication prescribed for the length of time ordered
- Advise patient to notify prescriber of diarrhea with blood or pus, which may indicate pseudomembranous colitis

Evaluation

Positive therapeutic outcome

- Absence of signs/symptoms of infection (WBC <10,000/mm^3, temp WNL, absence of red draining wounds)
- Reported improvement in symptoms of infection

Treatment of anaphylaxis: Withdraw drug, maintain airway, administer epinephrine, aminophylline, O_2, **IV** corticosteroids

didanosine (℞)

(dye-dan'oh-seen)

DDL, dideoxyinosine, Videx, Videx EC

Func. class.: Antiretroviral

Chem. class.: Synthetic purine nucleoside reverse transcriptase inhibitor

Pregnancy category B

Action: Nucleoside analog incorporating into cellular DNA by viral reverse transcriptase, thereby terminating the cellular DNA chain that prevents viral replication

Therapeutic Outcome: Antiviral against the retroviruses, primarily HIV

Uses: HIV infection in combination with other antiretrovirals

Dosage and routes

Renal dose

Reduce dosage CrCl <60 ml/min

Adult: PO >60 kg, 200 mg bid tabs, or 250 mg bid buffered powder; caps, del rel 400 mg qd; <60 kg, 125 mg bid tabs, or 167 mg bid buffered powder; caps del rel 250 mg qd

P ***Child:*** PO tabs 90-120 mg/m^2 q12h; buffered powder packets 112.5-150 mg/m^2 q12h; PO (child BSA 1.1-1.4 m^2) tab 100 mg q8-12h; reconstituted pediatric powder 125 mg q8-12h; PO (child BSA 0.8-1 m^2) tabs 75 mg q8-12h; reconstituted pediatric powder 94 mg q8-12h; PO (child BSA 0.5-0.7 m^2) tabs 50 mg q8-12h; reconstituted pediatric powder 62 mg q8-12h; PO (child BSA <0.4 m^2) tabs 25 mg q8-12h; reconstituted pediatric powder 31 mg q8-12h

Available forms: Tabs, buffered, chewable/dispersible 25, 50, 100, 150 mg; powder for oral sol, buffered 100, 167, 250, 375 mg/packet; powder for oral sol, pediatric 10 mg, 20 mg/ml; caps del rel 125, 200, 250, 400

Adverse effects

CNS: **Peripheral neuropathy, seizures,** confusion, *anxiety,* hypertonia, abnormal thinking, asthenia, *insomnia, CNS depression,* pain, dizziness, chills, fever

CV: Hypertension, vasodilatation, **dysrhythmia,** syncope, **CHF,** palpitations

EENT: Ear pain, otitis, photophobia, visual impairment, retinal depigmentation

GI: **Pancreatitis,** *diarrhea, nausea,* vomiting, *abdominal pain,* constipation, stomatitis, dyspepsia, liver abnormalities, flatulence, taste perversion, dry mouth, oral thrush, melena, increased ALT, AST, alkaline phosphatase, amylase, **hepatic failure**

GU: Increased bilirubin, uric acid

HEMA: **Leukopenia, granulocytopenia, thrombocytopenia, anemia**

INTEG: *Rash, pruritus,* alopecia, ecchymosis, hemorrhage, petechiae, sweating

MS: Myalgia, arthritis, myopathy, muscular atrophy

RESP: Cough, pneumonia, dyspnea, asthma, epistaxis, hypoventilation, sinusitis

SYST: **Lactic acidosis, anaphylaxis**

Contraindications: Hypersensitivity

Precautions: Renal, hepatic disease, pregnancy **B,** lactation,

P children, sodium-restricted diets, elevated amylase, preexistent peripheral neuropathy, phenylketonuria, hyperuricemia

Pharmacokinetics

Absorption	Rapidly absorbed (up to 40%)
Distribution	Unknown
Metabolism	Not metabolized
Excretion	Kidneys (55%)
Half-life	0.8-1.6 hr, shorter in children

Pharmacodynamics

Onset	Unknown
Peak	Up to 1 hr, del rel 2 hr
Duration	Unknown

Interactions

Individual drugs

Allopurinol: ↑ didanosine level
Atropine: ↑ anticholinergic effects
Dapsone: ↓ absorption of dapsone
Disopyramide:↑ anticholinergic effects
Itraconazole: ↓ absorption of itraconazole
Ketoconazole: ↓ absorption of ketoconazole
Quinidine: ↑ anticholinergic effects

Drug classifications

Antacids, magnesium, aluminum: ↑ side effects
Antidepressants, tricyclic: ↑ anticholinergic effects
Antihistamines: ↑ anticholinergic effects
Antiretrovirals, other: ↓ concentration
Fluoroquinolones: ↓ absorption of fluoroquinolones
Phenothiazines: ↑ anticholinergic effects
Tetracyclines: ↓ absorption of tetracyclines

Food/drug

↓ Absorption
- Do not use with acidic juices

NURSING CONSIDERATIONS

Assessment

- Assess for peripheral neuropathy: tingling or pain in hands and feet, distal numbness; onset usually occurs 2-6 mo after beginning treatment, if these occur during therapy, drug may be decreased or discontinued
- Assess for pancreatitis: abdominal pain, nausea, vomiting, elevated liver enzymes; drug should be discontinued, since condition can be fatal
- P Assess children by dilated retinal examination q6 mo to rule out retinal depigmentation
- Monitor CBC, differential, platelet count monthly; withhold drug if WBC is <4000/mm^3 or platelet count is <75,000mm^3, viral load, CD4$^+$ count; notify prescriber of results
- Monitor renal function studies: BUN, serum uric acid, urine CrCl before, during therapy; these may be elevated throughout treatment
- Assess for anaphylaxis, lactic acidosis
- Monitor temp q4h; may indicate beginning of infection
- Monitor liver function tests before, during therapy (bilirubin, AST, ALT, amylase, alkaline phosphatase) as needed or monthly

Nursing diagnoses

✓ Infection, risk for (uses)
✓ Injury, risk for (adverse reactions)
✓ Knowledge deficit (teaching)

Implementation

- Give on empty stomach, 1 hr ac or 2 hr pc, q12h; food decreases effectiveness of drug
- Patient should chew tabs; may be crushed and mixed with water
- Pediatric powder for oral sol should be prepared in the pharmacy; shake before using
- Packets for oral sol must be mixed with ½ glass of water; stir until dissolved
- Store tabs, caps in tightly closed

bottle at room temp; store oral sol after dissolving at room temp ≤4 hr

Patient/family education

- Advise patient to take on empty stomach; not to take dapsone at same time as DDL; not to mix powder with fruit juice; to chew tab or crush and dissolve in water; to drink powder immediately after mixing; to use exactly as prescribed
- Instruct patient to report signs of infection: increased temp, sore throat, flu symptoms; to avoid crowds and those with known infections
- Instruct patient to report signs of anemia: fatigue, headache, faintness, shortness of breath, irritability
- Advise patient to report numbness/tingling in extremities
- Instruct patient to report bleeding; avoid use of razors and commercial mouthwash
- Advise patient that hair may be lost during therapy; a wig or hairpiece may make patient feel better
- Caution patient to avoid OTC products and other medications without approval of prescriber; to avoid alcohol
- Teach patient not to have any sexual contact without use of a condom; needles should not be shared; blood from infected individual should not come in contact with another's mucous membranes

Evaluation

Positive therapeutic outcome

- Absence of opportunistic infection, symptoms of HIV

difenoxin with atropine

See diphenoxylate with atropine

HIGH ALERT

digoxin (Key Drug) (℞)

(di-jox'in)

digoxin, Lanoxicaps, Lanoxin

Func. class.: Inotropic antidysrhythmic, cardiac glycoside

Chem. class.: Digitalis preparation

Pregnancy category C

Action: Inhibits sodium-potassium ATPase, which makes more calcium available for contractile proteins, resulting in increased cardiac output; increases force of contraction (positive inotropic effect); decreases heart rate (chronotropic effect); decreases AV conduction speed

Therapeutic Outcome: Decreased edema, pulse, respiration, rales

Uses: Rapid digitalization in acute and chronic CHF, atrial fibrillation, atrial flutter, atrial tachycardia; cardiogenic shock, paroxysmal atrial tachycardia

Dosage and routes

Adult: **IV** *digitalizing dose* 0.6-1.0 mg given as 50% of the dose initially, additional fractions given at 4-8 hr intervals; PO *digitalizing dose* 0.75-1.25 mg given as 50% of the dose initially, additional fractions given at 4-8 hr intervals; *maintenance* 0.063-0.5 mg/day (tabs), or 0.350-0.5 mg/day (gelatin cap)

P ***Child >10 yr:*** **IV** *digitalizing dose* 8-12 µg/kg given as 50% of the dose initially, additional fractions given at 4-8 hr intervals; PO *digitalizing dose* 0.01-0.015 mg/kg given as 50% of the dose initially, additional fractions given at 6-8 hr intervals; maintenance 25%-35% of the loading dose qd as a single dose

P ***Child 5-10 yr:*** **IV** *digitalizing dose* 0.015-0.03 mg/kg given as 50% of the dose initially, additional fractions given at 4-8 hr intervals; PO *digitalizing dose* 0.02-0.035 mg/kg given as 50% of the dose initially, additional fractions given at 6-8 hr intervals; *maintenance* 25%-35% of the loading dose qd in 2 divided doses

P ***Child 2-5 yr:*** **IV** *digitalizing dose* 0.025-0.035 mg/kg given as 50% of the dose initially, additional fractions given at 4-8 hr intervals; PO *digitalizing dose* 0.03-0.04 mg/kg given as 50% of the dosc initially, additional fractions given at 6-8 hr intervals; *maintenance* 25%-35% of the loading dose qd in 2 divided doses

P ***Child 1-2 yr:*** **IV** *digitalizing dose* 0.03-0.05 mg/kg given as 50% of the dose initially, additional fractions given at 4-8 hr intervals; PO *digitalizing dose* 0.035-0.06 mg/kg given as 50% of the dose initially, additional fractions given at 4-8 hr intervals; *maintenance* 25%-35% of the loading dose qd in 2 divided doses

P ***Infants:*** **IV** *digitalizing dose* 0.02-0.03 mg/kg given as 50% of the dose initially, additional fractions given at 4-8 hr intervals; PO *digitalizing dose* 0.025-0.035 mg/kg given as 50% of the dose initially, additional fractions given at 6-8 hr intervals; *maintenance* 25%-35% of the loading dose qd in 2 divided doses

P ***Infants, premature:*** **IV** *digitalizing dose* 0.015-0.025 mg/kg given as 50% of the dose initially, additional fractions given at 4-8 hr intervals; PO *digitalizing dose* 0.02-0.03 mg/kg given as 50% of the dose initially, additional fractions given at 6-8 hr intervals; *maintenance* 20%-30% of the loading dose qd in 2 divided doses

Available forms: Caps 0.05, 0.1, 0.2 mg; elix 0.05 mg/ml; tabs 0.125, 0.25, 0.5 mg; inj 0.05 ✤, 0.25 mg/ml; pediatric inj 0.01 mg/ml

Adverse effects

CNS: *Headache,* drowsiness, apathy, confusion, disorientation, fatigue, depression, hallucinations
CV: **Dysrhythmias, hypotension,** bradycardia, AV **block**
EENT: Blurred vision, yellow-green halos, photophobia, diplopia
GI: Nausea, vomiting, anorexia, abdominal pain, diarrhea

Contraindications: Hypersensitivity to digitalis, ventricular fibrillation, ventricular tachycardia, carotid sinus syndrome, 2nd- or 3rd-degree heart block

Precautions: Renal disease, acute MI, AV block, severe respiratory G disease, hypothyroidism, elderly, pregnancy **C**, sinus nodal disease, lactation, hypokalemia

Do Not Confuse:
Lanoxin/Lasix,
Lanoxin/Lomotil,
Lanoxin/Xanax

Pharmacokinetics

Absorption	Unknown
Distribution	Widely distributed; 20%-25% protein bound
Metabolism	Liver, small amount; also intestinal bacteria
Excretion	Urine
Half-life	1½ days

Pharmacodynamics

	PO	IV
Onset	½-1½ hr	5-30 min
Peak	2-6 hr	1-5 hr
Duration	After steady state	6-8 days

Interactions

Individual drugs

Amiodarone: ↑ digoxin levels, bradycardia
Amphotericin B: ↑ hypokalemia, toxicity
Calcium IV: ↑ risk of fatal dysrhythmias, digoxin toxicity
Carbenicillin: ↑ hypokalemia

Charcoal: ↓ levels of digoxin by absorption
Cholestyramine: ↓ digoxin level
Colestipol: ↓ digoxin level
Diltiazem: ↑ blood levels
Kaolin/pectin: ↓ absorption
Metoclopramide: ↓ digoxin level
Propafenone: ↑ digoxin levels, toxicity
Rifampin: ↓ digoxin effects
Thyroid hormones: ↓ level of digoxin
Ticarcillin: ↑ hypokalemia
Verapamil: ↑ blood levels of digoxin, ↓ positive inotropic effect

Drug classifications
Antacids: ↓ digoxin absorption
Antidysrhythmics: ↑ bradycardia
Barbiturates: ↓ effects of digoxin
β-Adrenergic blockers: ↑ bradycardia
Calcium channel blockers: ↑ digoxin levels, toxicity
Diuretics, thiazide: ↑ hypokalemia, toxicity
Hydantoins: ↓ effects of digoxin

Herb/drug
Aloe: ↑ action of digoxin
Buckthorn bark/berry: ↑ action
Cascara sagrada bark: ↑ action
Castor bean oil: ↑ action of digoxin
Cocoa seeds: ↑ hypokalemia
Cola seeds: ↑ hypokalemia
Ephedra: ↑ dysrhythmia
Guarana seeds: ↑ hypokalemia
Hawthorn: ↑ cardiac toxicity
Horsetail: ↑ hypokalemia
Indian snakeroot: ↑ bradycardia
Licorice: ↑ digoxin toxicity, ↑ hypokalemia
May apple root: ↑ digoxin action
Oleander: ↑ digoxin action
Pheasant's eye: ↑ digoxin action
Phyllium: ↓ absorption of digoxin
Purple foxglove: ↑ digoxin action
Rhubarb root: ↑ digoxin action
Senna pod/leaf: ↑ digoxin action
Squill: ↑ digoxin action
Yellow dock/root: ↑ digoxin action
Yerba maté: ↑ hypokalemia

Lab test interferences
↑ CPK

NURSING CONSIDERATIONS

Assessment

- Assess and document apical pulse for 1 min before giving drug; if pulse P <60 in adult or <90 in an infant or is significantly different, take again in 1 hr; if <60 in adult, call prescriber; note rate, rhythm, character
- Monitor electrolytes: potassium, sodium, chloride, magnesium, calcium; renal function studies: BUN, creatinine; other blood studies: ALT, AST, bilirubin, Hct, Hgb, drug levels (therapeutic level 0.5-2 ng/ml) before initiating treatment and periodically thereafter
- Monitor I&O ratio, daily weights; monitor turgor, lung sounds, edema
- Monitor cardiac status: apical pulse, character, rate, rhythm; resolution of atrial dysrhythmias by ECG; if tachydysrhythmia develops, hold drug; delay cardioversion while drug levels are determined
- Monitor ECG continuously during parenteral loading doses and for patients with suspected toxicity; provide hemodynamic monitoring for patients with heart failure or administer multiple cardiac drugs

Nursing diagnoses

✓ Cardiac output, decreased (uses)
✓ Impaired gas exchange (adverse reactions)
✓ Knowledge deficit (teaching)

Implementation

- Do not give at same time as antacids or other drugs that decrease absorption

PO route

- Give PO with or without food; may crush tabs
- Give potassium supplements if ordered for potassium levels <3, or give foods high in potassium: bananas, orange juice

IV **IV route**

- Give **IV** undiluted or 1 ml of drug/4

ml sterile water, D_5, or 0.9% NaCl; give over >5 min through Y-tube or 3-way stopcock; during digitalization close monitoring is necessary
• Store protected from light

Syringe compatibilities:
Heparin, milrinone

Syringe incompatibility:
Doxapram

Y-site compatibilities:
Amrinone, cefmetazole, ciprofloxacin, cisatracurium, diltiazem, famotidine, meperidine, meropenem, midazolam, milrinone, morphine, potassium chloride, propofol, remifentanil, tacrolimus, vit B/C

Y-site incompatibilities:
Fluconazole, foscarnet

Additive compatibilities:
Bretylium, cimetidine, floxacillin, furosemide, lidocaine, ranitidine, verapamil

Additive incompatibility:
Dobutamine

Patient/family education
• Caution patient to avoid OTC medications including cough, cold, allergy preparations, antacids, since many adverse drug interactions may occur; do not take antacid at same time
• Instruct patient to notify prescriber of any loss of appetite, lower stomach pain, diarrhea, weakness, drowsiness, headache, blurred or yellow-green vision, rash, depression; teach toxic symptoms of this drug and when to notify prescriber
• Advise patient to maintain a sodium-restricted diet as ordered; to take potassium supplements as ordered to prevent toxicity
• Instruct patient to report shortness of breath, difficulty breathing, weight gain, edema, persistent cough
• Teach patient purpose of drug is to regulate the heart's functioning
• Teach patient as outpatient to check and record pulse for 1 min before taking dose; if there is a change of >15 bpm from usual pulse, prescriber should be notified
• Teach patient to take medication at the same time each day, take missed doses within 12 hr; do not double doses; notify prescriber if doses are missed for 2 days or more; how to monitor heart rate
• Advise patient to carry ID describing dosage and reason for digoxin

Evaluation
Positive therapeutic outcome
• Decreased weight, edema, pulse, respiration, rales
• Increased urine output
• Serum digoxin level 0.5-2 ng/ml

Treatment of overdose:
Discontinue drug, administer potassium, monitor ECG, administer an adrenergic blocking agent, digoxin immune Fab

digoxin immune Fab (ovine) (℞)

(di-jox'in)
Digibind
Func. class.: Antidote, digoxin specific

Pregnancy category C

Action: Antibody fragments bind to free digoxin to reverse digoxin or digitoxin toxicity by not allowing digoxin or digitoxin to bind to sites of action

Therapeutic Outcome: Correction of digoxin toxicity

Uses: Reversal of life-threatening digoxin or digitoxin toxicity, including severe bradycardia, ventricular tachycardia/fibrillation, severe hypertension

Dosage and routes
Digoxin toxicity
Adult: **IV** dose (mg) = dose ingested (mg) × serum digoxin conc × 5.6 × wt in kg ÷ 1000; if ingested

amount is unknown, give 800 mg **IV**; if digoxin liquid caps, **IV** or digoxin used, do not multiply ingested dose by 0.8; digitoxin body load in mg = serum digitoxin conc × 0.56 × wt in kg ÷ 1000

Available forms: Inj 38 mg/ vial (binds 0.5 mg of digoxin or digitoxin)

Adverse effects

CV: **Worsening of CHF,** *ventricular rate increase,* **atrial fibrillation,** *low cardiac output*

INTEG: *Hypersensitivity,* allergic reactions, facial swelling, redness

META: *Hypokalemia*

RESP: **Impaired respiratory function, rapid respiratory rate**

Contraindications: Mild digoxin toxicity, hypersensitivity

P **Precautions:** Children, lactation, cardiac disease, renal disease, pregnancy **C,** allergy to ovine proteins

Pharmacokinetics

Absorption	Complete
Distribution	Widely distributed into plasma, interstitial fluids
Metabolism	Unknown
Excretion	Kidneys
Half-life	Biphasic (14-20 hr); increased in renal disease

Pharmacodynamics

Onset	30 min (variable)
Peak	Unknown
Duration	Unknown

Interactions

Individual drugs

Digitoxin: ↓ effect of digitoxin

Digoxin: ↓ effect of digoxin

Lanatoside C: ↓ effect of lanatoside

Lab test interferences

Interference: Immunoassay (digoxin)

NURSING CONSIDERATIONS

Assessment

- Assess for hypokalemia: ST depression, flat T waves, presence of U wave, ventricular dysrhythmias
- Obtain information on previous allergies: previous exposure to sheep (ovine) proteins; scratch test may be performed before use of this product; hypersensitive reactions are more common in persons with previous exposure
- Monitor VS before, during, and after infusion
- Monitor heart rate, B/P q10 min during inf and after completion until stabilized; hemodynamic monitoring is used for unstable or hypotensive patients; check potassium levels until toxicity is resolved
- Assess for oxygen or perfusion deficit: hypotension, chest pain, dizziness, loss of consciousness
- Assess respiratory status: auscultate lung fields for bibasilar crackles in patients with advanced CHF

Nursing diagnoses

✓ Injury, risk for (uses)

✓ Knowledge deficit (teaching)

Implementation

- Give after diluting 40 mg/4 ml of sterile water (10 mg/ml), mix gently; may be further diluted with 0.9% NaCl; sol should be clear, colorless
- Give by bol if cardiac arrest is imminent or **IV** over 30 min using a 0.22 µm filter
- Store reconstituted sol for up to 4 hr in refrigerator

Patient/family education

- Teach that purpose of medication is to bind excess digoxin and reduce high blood levels
- Instruct patients to report fever, chills, itching, sweating, dyspnea
- Advise other prescribers that this medication has been used previously

Evaluation

Positive therapeutic outcome

- Correction of digoxin toxicity
- Digoxin blood levels 0.5-2 ng/ml
- Digitoxin blood level 9-25 ng/ml

dihydroergotamine

See ergotamine

dihydrotachysterol (℞)

(dye-hye-droh-tak-iss′ter-ole)

DHT Intensol ✤, Hytakerol

Func. class.: Parathyroid agent (calcium regulator)

Chem. class.: Vitamin D analog

Pregnancy category C

Action: Increases intestinal absorption of calcium, increases renal tubular absorption of phosphorus; is able to regulate calcium levels by regulation of calcitonin, parathyroid hormone

➔ **Therapeutic Outcome:** Prevention of continued calcium loss in bones

Uses: Renal osteodystrophy, hypoparathyroidism, pseudohypoparathyroidism, familial hypophosphatemia, postoperative tetany

Investigational uses: Renal osteodystrophy

Dosage and routes

Hypophosphatemia

P ***Adult and child:*** PO 0.5-2 mg qd; maintenance 0.3-1.5 mg qd

Hypoparathyroidism/ pseudohypoparathyroidism

Adult: PO 0.8-2.4 mg qd × 4 days, maintenance 0.2-2 mg qd regulated by serum calcium levels

P ***Child:*** PO 1-5 mg qd 1 wk, maintenance 0.2-1 mg qd regulated by serum calcium levels

Renal osteodystrophy

Adult: PO 0.1-0.6 mg qd, then 0.2-1 mg/day

Available forms: Tab 0.125, 0.2, 0.4 mg; cap 0.125 mg; oral sol 0.2, 0.25 mg/5 ml, 0.2 mg/ml ✤ (Intensol)

Adverse effects

CNS: Drowsiness, headache, vertigo, fever, lethargy, depression

CV: **Dysrhythmias**, hypertension

EENT: Tinnitus

GI: Nausea, diarrhea, vomiting, jaundice, anorexia, dry mouth, constipation, cramps, metallic taste

GU: **Polyuria,** hypercalciuria, hyperphosphatemia, **hematuria,** thirst, nocturia, renal calculi

MS: Myalgia, arthralgia, decreased bone development, weakness

Contraindications: Hypersensitivity, renal disease, hyperphosphatemia, hypercalcemia

Precautions: Pregnancy **C,** renal calculi, lactation, CV disease

Pharmacokinetics

Absorption	Well absorbed from small intestine
Distribution	Liver, fat
Metabolism	Liver
Excretion	Feces (inactive, active metabolites)
Half-life	Unknown

Pharmacodynamics

Onset	2 wk
Peak	2 wk
Duration	2 wk

Interactions

Individual drugs

Cholestyramine: ↓ absorption of dihydrotachysterol

Colestipol: ↓ absorption of dihydrotachysterol

Mineral oil: ↓ absorption of dihydrotachysterol

Phenytoin: ↓ effect of dihydrotachysterol

Verapamil: ↑ dysrhythmias

Drug classifications

Barbiturates: ↓ effect of dihydrotachysterol

Calcium supplements: ↑ hypercalcemia

Cardiac glycosides: ↑ dysrhythmias

Corticosteroids: ↓ effect of dihydrotachysterol
Diuretics, thiazide: ↑ hypercalcemia

Lab test interferences

False ↑ cholesterol

NURSING CONSIDERATIONS

Assessment

- Monitor BUN, urinary calcium, AST, ALT, cholesterol, alkaline phosphatase, creatinine, uric acid, chloride, magnesium, electrolytes, urine pH, phosphate; may increase calcium; should be kept at 9-10 mg/dl; keep vit D at 50-135 IU/dl, phosphate at 70 mg/dl; these tests should be checked before and throughout treatment
- Monitor for increased blood level, since toxic reaction may occur rapidly
- Monitor for dry mouth, metallic taste, polyuria, bone pain, muscle weakness, headache, fatigue, tinnitus, change in LOC, irregular pulse, dysrhythmias, increased respirations, anorexia, nausea, vomiting, cramps, diarrhea, constipation; may indicate hypercalcemia; if these occur, discontinue drug, give laxatives, low-calcium diet
- Monitor renal status: decreased urinary output (oliguria, anuria), edema in extremities, weight gain >5 lb, periorbital edema
- Assess nutritional status; check diet for sources of vit D (milk, some seafood), calcium (dairy products, dark green vegetables); phosphates (dairy products) must be avoided

Nursing diagnoses

✓ Nutrition: Less than body requirements (uses)
✓ Knowledge deficit (teaching)

Implementation

- ⊘ Do not crush, chew caps
- May be increased q4 wk depending on blood level; give with meals for GI symptoms
- Store in tight, light-resistant containers at room temp
- Restrict sodium, potassium if required
- Restriction of fluids may be required for chronic renal failure

Patient/family education

- Teach symptoms of hypercalcemia and when to report symptoms to prescriber
- Teach patient about foods rich in calcium, vit D; provide list of calcium-rich foods; renal failure patients are given a renal diet
- Caution patient not to double doses, take exactly as prescribed

Evaluation

Positive therapeutic outcome

- Prevention of bone deficiencies
- Calcium, phosphorus at normal levels

HIGH ALERT

diltiazem (℞)

(dil-tye′a-zem)

Apo-Diltiaz ✦, Cardizem, Cardizem SR, Cardizem CD, diltiazem, Dilacor-XR, Tiazac

Func. class.: Calcium channel blocker, antianginal

Chem. class.: Benzothiazepine

Pregnancy category C

Action: Inhibits calcium ion influx across cell membrane during cardiac depolarization, produces relaxation of coronary vascular smooth muscle, dilates coronary arteries, slows SA/AV node conduction times, dilates peripheral arteries

➡ **Therapeutic Outcome:** Decreased angina pectoris, dysrhythmias, B/P

Uses

Oral: Angina pectoris due to coronary insufficiency, hypertension, vasospasm

Parenteral: Atrial fibrillation, flutter

Investigational use: Raynaud's syndrome

Dosage and routes

Adult: PO 30 mg qid, increasing dose gradually to 180-360 mg/day in divided doses or 60-120 mg bid; may increase to 240-360 mg/day

Adult: **IV** 0.25 mg/kg as bol over 2 min initially, then 0.35 mg/kg may be given after 15 min; if no response, may give cont inf 5-15 mg/hr for up to 24 hr

Adult: PO 180-240 mg qd (Cardizem CD)

Available forms: Tab 30, 60, 90, 120 mg; tab ext rel 120, 180, 240 mg; caps sus rel 60, 90, 120, 180, 240 mg; caps ext rel 120, 180, 240, 300, 360 mg; inj **IV** 5 mg/ml (5, 10 ml)

Adverse effects

CNS: Headache, fatigue, drowsiness, dizziness, depression, weakness, insomnia, tremor, paresthesia

CV: **Dysrhythmia,** *edema,* **CHF,** bradycardia, hypotension, palpitations, **heart block,** peripheral edema, angina

GI: Nausea, vomiting, diarrhea, gastric upset, *constipation,* increased liver function studies

GU: Nocturia, polyuria, **acute renal failure**

INTEG: Rash, pruritus, flushing, photosensitivity

Contraindications: Sick sinus syndrome, 2nd- or 3rd-degree heart block, hypotension less than 90 mm Hg systolic, acute MI, pulmonary congestion

Precautions: CHF, hypotension, hepatic injury, pregnancy **C**, lactation, P children, renal disease

Do Not Confuse:
Cardizem/Cardene, Cardizem CD/Cardizem SR, Cardizem SR/Cardene SR

Pharmacokinetics

Absorption	Well absorbed
Distribution	Not known
Metabolism	Liver, extensively
Excretion	Metabolites (96%)
Half-life	3½-9 hr

Pharmacodynamics

	PO	PO–SUS REL	IV
Onset	½ hr	Unknown	Unknown
Peak	2-3 hr	Unknown	Unknown
Duration	6-8 hr	12 hr	Unknown

Interactions

Individual drugs

Alcohol: ↑ hypotension
Carbamazepine: ↑ toxicity
Cyclosporine: ↑ cyclosporine effect
Digoxin: ↑ digoxin levels, bradycardia, CHF
Phenobarbital: ↓ effectiveness
Phenytoin: ↓ effectiveness
Propranolol: ↑ toxicity

Drug classifications

Antihypertensives: ↑ hypotension
β-Adrenergic blockers: ↑ bradycardia, CHF, ↑ β-blocker effect
Nitrates: ↑ nitrates

Food/drug

Grapefruit juice: ↑ hypotension

NURSING CONSIDERATIONS

Assessment

- Assess fluid volume status: I&O ratio and record, weight, distended red veins, crackles in lung, color, quality, and sp gr of urine, skin turgor, adequacy of pulses, moist mucous membranes, bilateral lung sounds, peripheral pitting edema; dehydration symptoms of decreasing output, thirst, hypotension, dry mouth and mucous membranes should be reported
- Monitor B/P and pulse, respiration, ECG and intervals (PR, QRS, QT); PCWP, CVP often during infusion; if B/P drops 30 mm Hg, stop inf and call prescriber
- Monitor ALT, AST, bilirubin daily; if

these are elevated, hepatotoxicity is suspected

• If platelets are <150,000/mm^3, drug is usually discontinued and another drug started

• Assess for extravasation: change site q48h

Nursing diagnoses

✓ Cardiac output, decreased (uses)

✓ Knowledge deficit (teaching)

Implementation

PO route

• Give with meals for GI symptoms; may be crushed and mixed with food/fluids for swallowing difficulty

⊘ • Do not chew or crush sus rel caps

• Store in airtight container at room temp

IV route

• Give direct **IV** undiluted over 2 min

• For continuous inf dilute 125 mg/100 ml (1.25 mg/ml) or 250 mg/250 ml (1 mg/ml) or 250 mg/500 ml (0.5 mg/ml) of D_5W, 0.9% NaCl, D_5/0.45% NaCl; give 10 mg/hr; may increase by 5 mg/hr to 15 mg/hr; may continue inf up to 24 hr

Y-*site compatibilities:*

Albumin, amikacin, amphotericin B, aztreonam, bretylium, bumetanide, cefazolin, cefotaxime, cefotetan, cefoxitin, ceftazidime, ceftriaxone, cefuroxime, cimetidine, ciprofloxacin, clindamycin, digoxin, dobutamine, dopamine, doxycycline, epinephrine, erythromycin, esmolol, fentanyl, fluconazole, gentamicin, hetastarch, hydromorphone, imipenem-cilastatin, labetalol, lidocaine, lorazepam, meperidine, metoclopramide, metronidazole, midazolam, milrinone, morphine, multivitamins, nicardipine, nitroglycerin, norepinephrine, oxacillin, penicillin G potassium, pentamidine, piperacillin, potassium chloride, potassium phosphates, ranitidine, sodium nitroprusside, theophylline, ticarcillin, ticarcillin/clavulanate, tobramycin, trimethoprim-sulfamethoxazole, vancomycin, vecuronium

Patient/family education

• Caution patient to avoid hazardous activities until stabilized on drug and dizziness is no longer a problem

• Instruct patient to limit caffeine consumption; to avoid alcohol and OTC drugs unless directed by prescriber

• Tell patient to comply in all areas of medical regimen; diet, exercise, stress reduction, drug therapy; to notify prescriber of irregular heart beat, shortness of breath, swelling of feet and hands, pronounced dizziness, constipation, nausea, hypotension

• Teach patient to use as directed even if feeling better; may be taken with other cardiovascular drugs (nitrates, β-blockers)

Evaluation

Positive therapeutic outcome

• Decreased anginal pain

• Decreased B/P

• Absence of dysrhythmias

Treatment of overdose:

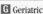

Atropine for AV block, vasopressor for hypotension

dimenhydrinate (OTC, ℞)

(dye-men-hye'dri-nate)

Apo-Dimenhydrinate ♣, Calm-X, Children's Dramamine, dimenhydrinate, Dimentabs, Dinate, Dramamine, Dramanate, Dymenate, Gravol ♣, Gravol L/A ♣, Hydrate, Nauseatol ♣, Novo-Dimenate ♣, PMS-Dimenhydrinate ♣, Travamine ♣, Triptone Caplets

Func. class.: Antiemetic, antihistamine, anticholinergic

Chem. class.: H_1-receptor antagonist, ethanolamine derivative

Pregnancy category B

Action: Vestibular stimulator is decreased; anticholinergic, antiemetic, antihistamine response

➔ **Therapeutic Outcome:** Absence of motion sickness

Uses: Motion sickness, nausea, vomiting

Dosage and routes

Adult: PO 50-100 mg q4h; IM/**IV** 50 mg as needed

P ***Child:*** IM/PO 5 mg/kg divided in 4 equal doses

Available forms: Tab 50 mg; inj 50 mg/ml; elix 15 mg/5 ml ♣, chew tab 50 mg

Adverse effects

CNS: *Drowsiness,* restlessness, headache, dizziness, insomnia, confusion, nervousness, tingling, vertigo; hallucinations and **seizures** in young P children

CV: Hypertension, *hypotension,* palpitations

EENT: Dry mouth, blurred vision, diplopia, nasal congestion, photosensitivity

GI: Nausea, anorexia, vomiting, *constipation*

INTEG: Rash, urticaria, fever, chills, flushing

MISC: **Anaphylaxis**

Contraindications: Hypersensitivity to narcotics, shock

P G **Precautions:** Children, cardiac dysrhythmias, elderly, asthma, pregnancy **B,** prostatic hypertrophy, bladder neck obstruction, narrow-angle glaucoma, stenosing peptic ulcer, pyloroduodenal obstruction

D

Pharmacokinetics

Absorption	Well absorbed (PO, IM)
Distribution	Unknown; crosses placenta
Metabolism	Liver
Excretion	Kidneys, breast milk
Half-life	Unknown

Pharmacodynamics

	PO	IM	IV
Onset	15-60 min	30 min	Immediate
Peak	1-2 hr	1-2 hr	Unknown
Duration	4-6 hr	4-6 hr	4-6 hr

Interactions

Individual drugs

Alcohol: ↑ CNS depression

Atropine: ↑ anticholinergic reactions

Disopyramide: ↑ anticholinergic reactions

Haloperidol: ↑ anticholinergic reactions

Quinidine: ↑ anticholinergic reactions

Drug classifications

Antidepressants: ↑ anticholinergic reactions

Antihistamines: ↑ anticholinergic reactions

CNS depressants: ↑ CNS depression

MAOIs: ↑ anticholinergic effect

Opiates: ↑ CNS depression

Phenothiazines: ↑ anticholinergic reactions

Sedative/hypnotics: ↑ CNS depression

Herb/drug
Henbane leaf: ↑ anticholinergic effect
Lab test interferences
False negative: Skin allergy tests (discontinue antihistamines 3 days before testing)

NURSING CONSIDERATIONS
Assessment
- Assess for signs of toxicity to other drugs or masking of symptoms of disease (brain tumor, intestinal obstruction); monitor GI symptoms including nausea, vomiting, abdominal pain, increased bowel sounds
- Monitor VS, B/P; check patients with cardiac disease more often
- Monitor I&O; check for dehydration (poor skin turgor, increased sp gr, tachycardia, severe thirst) especially in G the elderly

Nursing diagnoses
✓ Injury, risk for (side effects)
✓ Knowledge deficit (teaching)

Implementation
PO route
- Tabs may be swallowed whole, chewed, or allowed to dissolve; give 1-2 hr before activity that may cause motion sickness; use measuring device for liq for correct dosing

IM route
- Give IM inj in large muscle mass; aspirate to avoid **IV** administration; massage

IV **IV route**
- Give **IV** directly after diluting 50 mg/10 ml or NaCl inj; give 50 mg or less over 2 min

Syringe compatibilities: Atropine, diphenhydramine, droperidol, fentanyl, heparin, hydromorphone, meperidine, metoclopramide, morphine, pentazocine, perphenazine, ranitidine, scopolamine

Syringe incompatibilities: Butorphanol, chlorpromazine, glycopyrrolate, hydroxyzine, midazolam, pentobarbital, prochlorperazine, promazine, promethazine, thiopental

Y-site compatibilities: Acyclovir

Y-site incompatibilities: Aminophylline, heparin, hydrocortisone sodium succinate, hydroxyzine, phenobarbital, phenytoin, prednisolone, prochlorperazine, promazine, promethazine

Additive compatibilities: Amikacin, calcium gluconate, chloramphenicol, corticotropin, erythromycin, heparin, hydroxyzine, methicillin, norepinephrine, penicillin G potassium, pentobarbital, phenobarbital, potassium chloride, prochlorperazine, vancomycin, vit B/C

Additive incompatibilities: Tetracycline, thiopental

Patient/family education
- Teach all aspects of drug uses; to notify prescriber if confusion, sedation, hypotension occur; to avoid driving and other hazardous activity if drowsiness occurs; to avoid alcohol and other CNS depressants that may potentiate effect
- Tell patient not to exceed recommended dosage
- Inform patient hard candy, gum, frequent rinsing of mouth may be used for dryness
- Advise patient that a false negative result may occur with skin testing; these procedures should not be scheduled until 4 days after discontinuing use
- Caution patient to avoid hazardous activities, activities requiring alertness; dizziness may occur; instruct patient to request assistance with ambulation
- Caution patient to avoid alcohol, other CNS depressants when taking this medication; response will be increased

Evaluation

Positive therapeutic outcome

- Absence of motion sickness
- Absence of nausea, vomiting

dinoprostone (℞)

(dye-noe-prost′one)

Cervidil Vaginal Insert, Prepidil, Prostin E_2

Func. class.: Oxytocic, abortifacient

Chem. class.: Prostaglandin E_2

Pregnancy category C

Action: Stimulates uterine contractions similar to labor by myometrium stimulation, causing abortion; acts within 30 hr for complete abortion; GI smooth muscle stimulation, effacement, dilatation of the cervix

Therapeutic Outcome: Beginning of labor, fetal expulsion

Uses: Abortion during 2nd trimester, benign hydatidiform mole, expulsion of uterine contents in fetal deaths to 28 wk, missed abortion, cervical effacement and dilatation in term pregnancy when they have not occurred spontaneously

Dosage and routes

Abortifacient

Adult: VAG SUPP 20 mg; repeat q3-5h until abortion occurs; max dose is 240 mg

Cervical ripening

Adult: GEL; warm to room temperature; choose correct length shielded catheter (10 or 20 mm), fill catheter by pushing plunger; have patient recumbent for 15-30 min; insert one 10 mg insert

Available forms: Vag supp 20 mg; gel 0.5 mg/3 g (prefilled syringe); gel 0.5 mg; 10 mg insert

Adverse effects

CNS: *Headache,* dizziness, chills, fever

CV: Hypotension, **dysrhythmias**

EENT: Blurred vision

GI: *Nausea, vomiting, diarrhea*

GU: Vaginitis, vaginal pain, vulvitis, vaginismus

INTEG: Rash, skin color changes

MS: *Leg cramps, joint swelling,* weakness

Insert: Uterine hyperstimulation, fever, nausea, vomiting, diarrhea, abdominal pain

Gel: Uterine contractile abnormality, GI side effects, back pain, fever; **fetal: bradycardia, late deceleration**

Suppository: Uterine rupture, anaphylaxis

Contraindications: Hypersensitivity, uterine fibrosis, cervical stenosis, pelvic surgery, PID, respiratory disease

Precautions: Hepatic, renal, cardiac disease, asthma, anemia, jaundice, diabetes mellitus, convulsive disorders, hypertension, hypotension, pregnancy **C**

Do Not Confuse:
Prepidil/bepridil

Pharmacokinetics

Absorption	Rapidly absorbed
Distribution	Unknown
Metabolism	Enzymes
Excretion	Kidneys
Half-life	Unknown

Pharmacodynamics

	GEL	SUPP
Onset	Rapid	10 min
Peak	30-45 min	Unknown
Duration	Unknown	2-3 hr

Interactions

Individual drugs

Alcohol: ↓ oxytoxic effect

Oxytocin: ↑ effect

NURSING CONSIDERATIONS

Assessment

- Assess dilatation and effacement of the cervix, uterine contractions, fetal heart tones; watch for contractions lasting over 1 min, hypertonus, fetal

distress; drug should be slowed or discontinued
- Assess for fever that occurs approximately 30 min after supp insertion (abortion)
- Monitor for nausea, vomiting, diarrhea; these may require medication
- Assess for hypersensitivity reaction: dyspnea, rash, chest discomfort
- Assess respiratory rate, rhythm, depth; notify prescriber of abnormalities, in pulse, B/P
- Check vaginal discharge; itching, irritation indicates vaginal infection

Nursing diagnoses
✓ Injury, high risk for (side effects)
✓ Knowledge deficit (teaching)

Implementation
Suppository route
- Warm supp by running warm water over package; insert high in vagina, wear gloves to prevent absorption; have patient recumbent for at least 10 min

Gel route
- Do not allow to come in contact with skin; use soap and water to wash after use
- Gel should be at room temp
- Place patient in dorsal or lithotomy position to insert gel into cervical canal; remove catheter; discard all items after use; keep supine 15-30 min

Patient/family education
- Teach patient all aspects of treatment including purpose of medication and expected results
- Tell patient that gel may produce warmth in her vagina
- Caution patient that if contractions are longer than 1 min to notify nurse or prescriber
- Advise patient to notify prescriber of cramping, pain, increased bleeding, chills, increased temp, or foul-smelling discharge; these symptoms may indicate uterine infection
- Advise patient to remain supine 10-15 min after insertion of suppository; 2 hr after insert, 15-30 min after gel

Evaluation
Positive therapeutic outcome
- Progression of labor
- Abortion

diphenhydramine (Key Drug) (OTC, ℞)

(dye-fen-hye'dra-meen)

Allerdryl ✤, AllerMax, Allermed, Banophen, Benadryl, Benadryl 25, Benadryl Kapseals, Benahist 10, Benahist 50, Ben-Allergin-50, Benoject-10, Benoject-50, Benylin Cough, Bydramine, Compoz, Diphenadryl, Diphen Cough, Diphenhist, diphenhydramine HCl, Dormin, Genahist, Hydramine, Hydramyn, Hydril, Hyrexin-50, Insomnal ✤, Nervine, Nidryl, Nighttime Sleep Aid, Nordryl, Nordryl Cough, Nytol, Phendry, Siladril, Sleep-Eze 3, Sominex 2, Tusstat, Twilite, Uni-Bent Cough, Wehdryl

Func. class.: Antihistamine (1st generation, nonselective), antitussive

Chem. class.: Ethanolamine derivative, H_1-receptor antagonist

Pregnancy category B

Action: Acts on blood vessels, GI, respiratory system by competing with histamine for H_1-receptor site; decreases allergic response by blocking histamine; causes increased heart rate, vasodilatation, secretions

➡ Therapeutic Outcome: Absence of allergy symptoms and rhinitis, decreased dystonic symptoms, absence of motion sickness, absence of cough, ability to sleep

Uses: Allergy symptoms, rhinitis, motion sickness, antiparkinsonism, nighttime sedation, infant colic, nonproductive cough, anaphylaxis, nasal allergies, allergic dermatoses, dystonic reactions

Dosage and routes

Adult: PO 25-50 mg q4-6h, not to exceed 400 mg/day; IM/**IV** 10-50 mg, not to exceed 400 mg/day

P ***Child >12 kg:*** PO/IM/**IV** 5 mg/kg/day in 4 divided doses, not to exceed 300 mg/day

Nighttime sleep aid

P ***Adult and child ≥12 yr:*** PO 25-50 mg hs

Antitussive (syrup only)

P ***Adult and child ≥12 yr:*** 25 mg q4h, max 100 mg/24 hr

P ***Child 6-12 yr:*** 12.5 mg q4h, max 50 mg/24 hr

P ***Child 2-6 yr:*** 6.25 mg q4h, max 25-50 mg/24 hr

Renal dose

CrCl 10-50 ml/min dose q6-12h; CrCl <10 ml/min dose q12-18h

Available forms: Caps 25, 50 mg; tabs 25, 50 mg; chew tabs 25 mg; elix 12.5 mg/5 ml; syr 12.5 mg/5 ml; inj 10, 50 mg/ml

Adverse effects

CNS: *Dizziness, drowsiness,* poor coordination, fatigue, anxiety, euphoria, confusion, paresthesia, neuritis, **seizures**

EENT: Blurred vision, dilated pupils, tinnitus, nasal stuffiness, dry nose, throat, mouth

GI: Nausea, anorexia, diarrhea

GU: *Retention,* dysuria, frequency

HEMA: **Thrombocytopenia, agranulocytosis, hemolytic anemia**

INTEG: Photosensitivity

MISC: **Anaphylaxis**

RESP: Increased thick secretions, wheezing, chest tightness

Contraindications: Hypersensitivity to H_1-receptor antagonist, acute asthma attack, lower respiratory tract disease

Precautions: Increased intraocular pressure, renal disease, cardiac disease, hypertension, bronchial asthma, seizure disorder, stenosed peptic ulcers, hyperthyroidism, prostatic hypertrophy, bladder neck obstruction, pregnancy **B**

Do Not Confuse:
diphenhydramine/dicyclomine

Pharmacokinetics

Absorption	Well absorbed (PO, IM); completely absorbed (**IV**)
Distribution	Widely distributed; crosses placenta
Metabolism	Liver (95%)
Excretion	Kidneys, breast milk
Half-life	2½-7 hr

Pharmacodynamics

	PO	IM	IV
Onset	15-60 min	30 min	Immediate
Peak	1-4 hr	1-4 hr	Unknown
Duration	4-8 hr	4-8 hr	4-8 hr

Interactions

Individual drugs

Alcohol: ↑ CNS depression

Disopyramide: ↑ anticholinergic response

Quinidine: ↑ anticholinergic response

Drug classifications

Antidepressants, tricyclic: ↑ anticholinergic response

CNS depressants: ↑ CNS depression

MAOIs: ↑ anticholinergic effect

Opiates: ↑ CNS depression

Sedative/hypnotics: ↑ CNS depression

Herb/drug

Henbane leaf: ↑ anticholinergic effect

Lab test interferences

False negative: Skin allergy tests (discontinue antihistamines 3 days before testing)

NURSING CONSIDERATIONS

Assessment

- Assess respiratory status: rate, rhythm, increase in bronchial secretions, wheezing, chest tightness; provide fluids to 2 L/day to decrease secretion thickness
- Monitor I&O ratio: be alert for urinary retention, frequency, dysuria, G especially elderly; drug should be discontinued if these occur
- Monitor CBC during long-term therapy; blood dyscrasias may occur but are rare
- If giving for dystonic reactions, assess type of involuntary movements and evaluate response to this medication
- Assess cough characteristics including type, frequency, thickness of secretions, and evaluate response to this medication if using for cough

Nursing diagnoses

✓ Injury, risk for (side effects)
✓ Sleep pattern disturbance (uses)
✓ Knowledge deficit (teaching)

Implementation

- Give 20 min before hs if using for sleep aid

PO route

- Give with meals if GI symptoms occur; absorption may be slightly decreased; cap may be opened and drug mixed with food/fluids for patients with swallowing difficulties

IM route

- Give IM injection in large muscle mass; aspirate to avoid **IV** administration; rotate sites

IV **IV route**

- Give **IV** undiluted 25 mg/min; may be diluted with 0.9% NaCl, D_5W, $D_{10}W$, 0.45% NaCl, D_5/0.9% NaCl, D_5/0.45% NaCl, D_5/0.25% NaCl, LR, Ringer's, give 25 mg/min or less

Syringe compatibilities:
Atropine, butorphanol, chlorpromazine, cimetidine, cisatracurium, dimenhydrinate, doxorubicin liposome, droperidol, fentanyl, fluphenazine, glycopyrrolate, hydromorphone, hydroxyzine, meperidine, metoclopramide, midazolam, morphine, nalbuphine, pentazocine, perphenazine, prochlorperazine, promazine, promethazine, ranitidine, remifentanil, scopolamine, sufentanil, thiothixene

Syringe incompatibilities:
Pentobarbital, phenytoin, thiopental

Y-site compatibilities:
Acyclovir, aldesleukin, amifostine, amsacrine, aztreonam, ciprofloxacin, cisplatin, cladribine, cyclophosphamide, cytarabine, doxorubicin, famotidine, filgrastim, fluconazole, fludarabine, gallium, granisetron, heparin, hydrocortisone, idarubicin, melphalan, meperidine, meropenem, methotrexate, ondansetron, paclitaxel, piperacillin/tazobactam, potassium chloride, propofol, sargramostim, sufentanil, tacrolimus, teniposide, thiotepa, vinorelbine, vit B/C

Y-site incompatibilities:
Foscarnet

Additive compatibilities:
Amikacin, aminophylline, ascorbic acid, bleomycin, cephapirin, erythromycin, hydrocortisone, lidocaine, methicillin, methyldopate, nafcillin, netilmicin, penicillin G potassium, penicillin G sodium, polymyxin B, vit B/C

Additive incompatibilities:
Amobarbital, cephalothin, thiopental

Patient/family education

- Tell patient that a false-negative result may occur with skin testing; these procedures should not be scheduled until 3 days after discontinuing use
- Caution patient to avoid hazardous activities and activities requiring alertness, since dizziness may occur; instruct patient to request assistance with ambulation
- Teach patient to use sunscreen to prevent photosensitivity
- Advise patient to avoid alcohol,

other depressants; CNS depression may occur

- Teach all aspects of drug uses; to notify prescriber if confusion, sedation, hypotension occur; to avoid driving and other hazardous activity if drowsiness occurs; to avoid alcohol or other CNS depressants that may potentiate effect

Evaluation

Positive therapeutic outcome

- Absence of motion sickness
- Absence of nausea, vomiting
- Ability to sleep
- Absence of cough
- Decrease in involuntary movements

Treatment of overdose:

- Administer ipecac syrup or lavage, diazepam, vasopressors, barbiturates (short acting)

diphenoxylate with atropine/difenoxin with atropine (℞)

(dye-fen-ox'i-late)

Diphenatol, Lofene, Logen, Lomanate, Lomotil, Lonox, Lo-Trop, Motofen, Nor-mil

Func. class.: Antidiarrheal

Chem. class.: Phenylpiperidine derivative, opiate agonist

Pregnancy category C

Controlled substance schedule V

Action: Inhibits gastric motility by acting on mucosal receptors responsible for peristalsis; related to narcotic analgesics as adjunct

➡ **Therapeutic Outcome:** Decreased loose stools

Uses: Diarrhea (cause undetermined)

Dosage and routes

Adult: PO 2.5-5 mg qid, titrated to patient response

P ***Child 2-12 yr:*** PO 0.3-0.4 mg/kg/day in divided doses

Available forms: Tab 2.5 mg diphenoxylate/0.025 mg atropine; tab 1 mg difenoxin/0.025 mg atropine; liq 2.5 mg diphenoxylate/0.025 mg atropine/5 ml

Adverse effects

CNS: Drowsiness, headache, sedation, depression, weakness, lethargy, flushing, **hyperthermia**

CV: Tachycardia

EENT: Blurred vision, nystagmus, mydriasis

GI: *Nausea, vomiting,* abdominal pain, glossitis, colitis

GU: Urine retention

INTEG: Rash, urticaria, pruritus, **angioneurotic edema**

Contraindications: Hypersensitivity, severe liver disease, pseudomembranous enterocolitis,

P glaucoma, child <2 yr, electrolyte imbalances

Precautions: Hepatic, renal disease, ulcerative colitis, pregnancy

G **C**, lactation, elderly

Do Not Confuse:

Diphenatol/diphenidol, Lomotil/Lamictal, Lomotil/Lanoxin, Lomotil/Lasix

Pharmacokinetics

Absorption	Well absorbed
Distribution	Unknown
Metabolism	Liver, active metabolite
Excretion	Kidneys
Half-life	2½ hr

Pharmacodynamics

Onset	45-60 min
Peak	2 hr
Duration	3-4 hr

Interactions

Individual drugs

Alcohol: ↑ action of alcohol
Disopyramide: ↑ anticholinergic effect

Drug classifications

Anticholinergics: ↑ anticholinergic effect
Antidepressants, tricyclic: ↑ anticholinergic effect
Antihistamines: ↑ CNS depression
Barbiturates: ↑ action of barbiturates
CNS depressants: ↑ action of CNS depressants
MAOIs: Hypertensive crisis; do not use together
Opiates: ↑ action of narcotics
Sedative/hypnotics: ↑ CNS depression

NURSING CONSIDERATIONS

Assessment

- Monitor electrolytes (potassium, sodium, chloride) if on long-term therapy; fluid status, skin turgor
- Assess bowel pattern before, during treatment; check for rebound constipation after termination of medication; check bowel sounds
- Check response after 48 hr; if no response, drug should be discontinued and other treatment initiated
- Assess for abdominal distention and toxic megacolon, which may occur in ulcerative colitis
- Assess hepatic function if on long-term therapy

Nursing diagnoses

✓ Diarrhea (uses)
✓ Constipation (adverse reactions)
✓ Knowledge deficit (teaching)
✓ Noncompliance (teaching)

Implementation

- Give for 48 hr only; tabs may be given with food, crushed and mixed with fluids; liq should be measured accurately

Patient/family education

- Advise patient to avoid alcohol and OTC products unless directed by prescriber; may cause increased CNS depression
- Caution patient not to exceed recommended dosage; that drug may be habit forming
- Advise patient that drug may cause drowsiness; to avoid hazardous activities until response to drug is determined
- Teach patient that dry mouth can be decreased by frequent sips of water, hard candy, sugarless gum

Evaluation

Positive therapeutic outcome

- Decreased diarrhea

dipyridamole (℞)

(dye-peer-id′a-mole)

Apo-Dipyridamole ♣,
dipyridamole, Novo-Dipiradol ♣,
Persantine, Persantine IV

Func. class.: Coronary vasodilator, antiplatelet agent
Chem. class.: Nonnitrate

Pregnancy category B

Action: Inhibits adenosine uptake, which produces coronary vasodilatation; increases oxygen saturation in coronary tissues, coronary blood flow; acts on small vessels with little effect on vascular resistance; may increase development of collateral circulation; decreased platelet aggregation by the inhibition of phosphodiesterases (enzymes)

➔ **Therapeutic Outcome:** Inhibition of platelet aggregation; absence of ischemic attacks, reinfarction

Uses: Prevention of transient ischemic attacks, inhibition of platelet adhesion to prevent myocardial reinfarction, thromboembolism, with warfarin in prosthetic heart valves, prevention of coronary bypass graft occlusion with aspirin; possibly effective for long-term therapy of chronic angina pectoris

Dosage and routes

Transient ischemic attacks

Adult: PO 50 mg tid, 1 hr ac, not to exceed 400 mg qd

Inhibition of platelet adhesion

Adult: PO 50-75 mg qid in combination with aspirin or warfarin

Available forms: Tabs 25, 50, 75 mg; inj 10 mg/2 ml

Adverse effects

CNS: *Headache, dizziness, weakness, fainting, syncope*
CV: *Postural hypotension*
GI: *Nausea, vomiting,* anorexia, diarrhea
INTEG: *Rash,* flushing

Contraindications: Hypersensitivity, hypotension

Precautions: Pregnancy **B**

Pharmacokinetics

Absorption	30%-50% (PO)
Distribution	Widely distributed; crosses placenta
Metabolism	Liver
Excretion	Bile, undergoes enterohepatic recirculation; enters breast milk
Half-life	10 hr

Pharmacodynamics

	PO	IV
Onset	Unknown	Unknown
Peak	2½ hr	6 min
Duration	6 hr	½ hr
Therapeutic effect	Several mo	

Interactions

Individual drugs

Aspirin: ↑ risk of bleeding
Cefamandole: ↑ risk of bleeding
Cefotetan: ↑ risk of bleeding
Cefoperazone: ↑ risk of bleeding
Plicamycin: ↑ risk of bleeding
Sulfinpyrazone: ↑ risk of bleeding
Theophylline: ↓ effects of disopyramide (thallium)
Valproic acid: ↑ risk of bleeding

Drug classifications

Anticoagulants: ↑ risk of bleeding
NSAIDs: ↑ risk of bleeding
Thrombolytics: ↑ risk of bleeding

D

NURSING CONSIDERATIONS

Assessment

- Monitor B/P, pulse baseline and during treatment until stable; take B/P with patient lying, standing; orthostatic hypotension is common
- Assess cardiac status: chest pain, what aggravates or ameliorates condition
- If using by **IV** route, monitor VS before, during, and after infusion; monitor for chest pain, bronchospasm; use ECG for identifying dysrhythmias; use aminophylline up to 250 mg **IV** for bronchospasm and chest pain if chest pain is unrelieved with the 250 mg dose of aminophylline; give SL dose of nitroglycerin

Nursing diagnoses

- ✓ Cardiac output, decreased (uses)
- ✓ Pain (uses)
- ✓ Knowledge deficit (teaching)

Implementation

PO route

- Give with 8 oz of water; to improve absorption give on an empty stomach; if GI symptoms occur may give with meals
- Tabs may be crushed, mixed with food or fluids for swallowing difficulty or swallowed whole
- Store at room temp

IV **IV intermittent infusion**

- Give by **IV** after diluting each 5 mg/2 ml or more in D_5W, 0.45% NaCl, or 0.9% NaCl; 20-50 ml should be given; give over 4 min; do not give undiluted

Patient/family education

- Teach patient that this medication is not a cure; that drug may have to be taken continuously in evenly spaced doses only as directed; if a dose is missed, take one when remembered up to 4 hr; do not double doses

- Inform patient that it is necessary to quit smoking to prevent excessive vasoconstriction
- Advise patient to rise slowly from sitting or lying down to prevent orthostatic hypotension
- Caution patient not to use alcohol or OTC medication unless approved by prescriber
- Caution patient to avoid hazardous activities until stabilized on medication; dizziness may occur

Evaluation

Positive therapeutic outcome

- Absence of reinfarction, ischemic attacks

Treatment of overdose:
Administer **IV** phenylephrine

dirithromycin (℞)
(die-rith-roe-mie'sin)

Dynabac

Func. class.: Antibacterial

Chem. class.: Macrolide

Pregnancy category C

Action: Binds to 50S ribosomal subunits of susceptible bacteria; suppresses protein synthesis

Therapeutic Outcome: Bactericidal action against *Moraxella catarrhalis, Streptococcus pneumoniae, Streptococcus pyogenes, Streptococcus viridans, Legionella pneumophilia, Mycoplasma pneumoniae, Staphylococcus aureus, Staphylococcus agalactiae, Bordetella pertussis, Propionibacterium acnes*

Uses: Infections of upper and lower respiratory tract

Dosage and routes
Adult: PO 500 mg qd, given for 7-14 days depending on infections

Available forms: Tab, enteric coated 250 mg

Adverse effects
CNS: *Headache, dizziness, insomnia*

GI: *Abdominal pain, nausea, diarrhea, vomiting, dyspepsia,* GI disorders, flatulence, abnormal stools, anorexia, constipation, **pseudomembranous colitis**

HEMA: Increased platelet count, increased eosinophils

INTEG: Pruritus, urticaria

RESP: Cough, dyspnea

Contraindications: Hypersensitivity to this drug or any other macrolide or to erythromycin, bacteremias

Precautions: Pregnancy **C**, [P] lactation, children, hepatic, renal disease

Pharmacokinetics	
Absorption	Rapidly absorbed
Distribution	Widely distributed
Metabolism	No hepatic metabolism
Excretion	Bile, feces (up to 97%)
Half-life	Plasma half-life 8 hr, terminal 44 hr

Pharmacodynamics

Unknown

Interactions
Drug classifications

Antacids: Slightly enhanced absorption of dirithromycin

H_2 antagonists: Slightly enhanced absorption of dirithromycin

Xanthines: May alter effect of xanthine

Food/drug

↑ Absorption

NURSING CONSIDERATIONS
Assessment

- Assess I&O ratio; report hematuria, oliguria in renal disease

- Monitor liver function studies: AST, ALT if on long-term therapy
- Monitor renal studies: urinalysis, protein, blood
- Monitor C&S before drug therapy; drug may be given as soon as culture is taken; C&S may be repeated after treatment
- Assess bowel pattern before, during treatment; pseudomembranous colitis may occur
- Assess for skin eruptions, itching
- Assess respiratory status: rate, character, wheezing, tightness in chest; discontinue drug
- Identify allergies before treatment, reaction of each medication; place allergies on chart, notify all people giving drugs

Nursing diagnoses

✓ Infection, risk for (uses)
✓ Diarrhea (side effects)
✓ Knowledge deficit (teaching)
✓ Noncompliance (teaching)

Implementation

- Give adequate intake of fluids (2 L) during diarrhea episodes
- ⊘ Administer whole; do not cut, crush, chew tablets
- Give with food or within 1 hr of food at same time each day
- Store at room temperature in tight container

Patient/family education

- Teach patient to take with full glass of water; give with food
- Instruct patient to report sore throat, fever, fatigue; may indicate superinfection
- Teach patient to notify nurse of diarrhea, dark urine, pale stools, yellow discoloration of eyes or skin, severe abdominal pain
- Instruct patient to take at evenly spaced intervals; complete dosage regimen

Evaluation

Positive therapeutic outcome

- C&S negative for infection

Treatment of hypersensitivity: Withdraw drug, maintain airway, administer epinephrine, aminophylline, O_2, **IV** corticosteroids

D

disopyramide (℞)

(dye-soe-peer′a-mide)

disopyramide, Norpace, Norpace CR, Rhythmodan

Func. class.: Antidysrhythmic (class IA)

Chem. class.: Nonnitrate

Pregnancy category C

Action: Prolongs action potential duration and effective refractory period; reduces disparity in refractory period between normal and infarcted myocardium; prevents increased myocardial excitability and conduction contractility

➔ **Therapeutic Outcome:** Suppression of supraventricular dysrhythmias

Uses: PVCs, ventricular tachycardia, supraventricular tachycardia, atrial flutter, fibrillation

Investigational uses: Supraventricular tachycardia (prevention, treatment)

Dosage and routes

Adult: PO 100-200 mg q6h; in renal dysfunction 100 mg q6h; sus rel cap 200 mg q12h

P ***Child 12-18 yr:*** PO 6-15 mg/kg/day, in divided doses q6h

P ***Child 4-12 yr:*** PO 10-15 mg/kg/day in divided doses q6h

P ***Child 1-4 yr:*** PO 10-20 mg/kg/day in divided doses q6h

P ***Child <1 yr:*** PO 10-30 mg/kg/day, in divided doses q6h

Renal dose

CrCl 30-40 ml/min dose q8h; CrCl

15-30 ml/min dose q12h; CrCl <15 ml/min dose q24h

Available forms: Caps 100, 150 mg (as phosphate); cont rel caps 100, 150 mg; tabs, sus rel 250 mg ✤

Adverse effects

CNS: ***Headache, dizziness,*** psychosis, fatigue, depression, paresthesias, anxiety, insomnia

CV: ***Hypotension, bradycardia,*** angina, PVCs, tachycardia, increases in QRS and QT segments, **cardiac arrest,** edema, weight gain, AV block, ***CHF,*** syncope, chest pain

EENT: ***Blurred vision, dry nose, throat, eyes,*** narrow-angle glaucoma

GI: ***Dry mouth, constipation,*** nausea, anorexia, flatulence, diarrhea, vomiting

GU: ***Retention, hesitancy,*** impotence

HEMA: **Thrombocytopenia, agranulocytosis,** anemia (rare), decreased Hgb, Hct

INTEG: Rash, pruritus, urticaria

META: Hypoglycemia

MS: Weakness, pain in extremities

Contraindications: Hypersensitivity, 2nd- or 3rd-degree heart block, cardiogenic shock, CHF (uncompensated), sick sinus syndrome, QT prolongation

Precautions: Pregnancy **C**, lactation, diabetes mellitus, renal, hepatic disease, children, myasthenia gravis, narrow-angle glaucoma, cardiomyopathy, conduction abnormalities

Pharmacokinetics

Absorption	Well absorbed
Distribution	Widely distributed
Metabolism	Liver
Excretion	Kidneys
Half-life	4-10 hr

Pharmacodynamics

	PO	PO–SUS REL
Onset	½-3½ hr	Unknown
Peak	2 hr	Unknown
Duration	1½-8 hr	12 hr

Interactions

Individual drugs

Erythromycin: ↑ effects of disopyramide

Flecainide: ↑ levels, toxicity

Lidocaine: Bradycardia, cardiac arrest

Mexiletine: ↑ levels, toxicity

Phenobarbital: ↓ effects of disopyramide

Phenytoin: ↑ blood levels, toxicity

Procainamide: ↑ levels, toxicity

Quinidine: ↑ levels, toxicity

Rifampin: ↓ disopyramide levels

Warfarin: ↑ level, bleeding

Drug classifications

Anticoagulants: ↓ prothrombin time

Antidysrhythmics: Widening of QRS or QT

β-Adrenergic blockers: ↑ dysrhythmias, cardiac arrest

Lab test interferences

↑ CPK

NURSING CONSIDERATIONS

Assessment

- Assess respiratory status: auscultate lung fields for bibasilar crackles in patients with advanced CHF
- Monitor I&O ratio and electrolytes: potassium, sodium, chloride; watch for decreasing urinary output, possible retention
- Monitor liver function studies: AST, ALT, bilirubin, alkaline phosphatase
- Monitor ECG to determine drug effectiveness, measure PR, QRS, QT intervals; check for PVCs, other dysrhythmias; monitor B/P for hypotension; check for prolonged widening QT intervals, QRS complex; if QT or QRS increase by 50% or more, withhold next dose, notify prescriber
- Monitor for dehydration or hypovolemia
- Monitor for CNS symptoms: psychosis, numbness, depression; if these occur, drug should be discontinued

Nursing diagnoses

✓ Cardiac output, decreased (uses)
✓ Knowledge deficit (teaching)

Implementation
- Do not crush or break sus rel caps
- Give 1 hr ac or 2 hr pc
- If changing from regular release to sus rel cap, give sus rel 6 hr after last dose of regular release

Patient/family education
- Teach patient to report side effects immediately to prescriber; to take exactly as prescribed; if dose is missed take when remembered if within 3-4 hr of next dose; do not double doses
- Teach patient to complete follow-up appointment with prescriber including pulmonary function studies, chest x-ray
- Instruct patient that dry mouth may be relieved by frequent sips of water, hard candy, sugarless gum
- Caution patient to make position changes from lying to standing slowly to prevent orthostatic hypotension

Evaluation
Positive therapeutic outcome
- Decreased PVCs, ventricular tachycardia

Treatment of overdose: Administer O_2, artificial ventilation, ECG; administer dopamine for circulatory depression; administer diazepam or thiopental for convulsions, isoproterenol

divalproex sodium
See valproate

dobutamine (℞)
(doe-byoo'ta-meen)

dobutamine, Dobutrex

Func. class.: Adrenergic direct-acting β_1-agonist, inotropic agent, cardiac stimulant

Chem. class.: Catecholamine

Pregnancy category B

Action: Causes increased contractility, increased coronary blood flow and heart rate by acting on β_1-receptors in heart; minor α/β_2 effects

Therapeutic Outcome: Cardiac output increased with decreased fatigue and dyspnea

Uses: Cardiac decompensation due to organic heart disease or cardiac surgery

Investigational uses: Cardiogenic shock in children, congenital heart disease in children undergoing cardiac caterization

Dosage and routes
Adult: **IV** inf 2.5-10 μg/kg/min; may increase to 40 μg/kg/min if needed

Child: **IV** inf 5-20 μg/kg/min over 10 min for cardiac cath

Available forms: Inj 12.5 mg/ml

Adverse effects
CNS: *Anxiety,* headache, dizziness

CV: Palpitations, tachycardia, hypertension, PVCs, angina

GI: Heartburn, nausea, vomiting

MS: Muscle cramps (leg)

Contraindications: Hypersensitivity, idiopathic hypertrophic subaortic stenosis

Precautions: Pregnancy **B**, lactation, children, hypertension

Do Not Confuse: dobutamine/dopamine, Dobutrex/Diamox

Pharmacokinetics	
Absorption	Complete
Distribution	Unknown
Metabolism	Liver
Excretion	Kidney
Half-life	2 min

Pharmacodynamics	
Onset	1-5 min
Peak	10 min
Duration	<10 min

Interactions

Individual drugs

Bretylium: ↑ dysrhythmias
Disopyramide: ↑ hypotension
Guanethidine: ↑ pressor response
Oxytocin: ↑ dysrhythmias
Phenytoin: ↑ hypotension, bradycardia

Drug classifications

Anesthetics: ↑ dysrhythmias
Antidepressants, tricyclic: ↑ pressor response
Antihypertensives: ↑ hypotension
β-Adrenergic blockers: ↑ pressor response
Cardiac glycosides: ↑ inotropic effect
MAOIs: ↑ dysrhythmias

NURSING CONSIDERATIONS

Assessment

- Assess for hypovolemia; if present, correct before beginning treatment with dobutamine; avoid use in patients with atrial fibrillation before digitalization
- Monitor ECG for dysrhythmias, ischemia during treatment; some patients may not need continuous ECG moni-toring; also monitor PCWP, CVP, CO_2, urinary output; notify prescriber if <30 ml/hr
- Assess for heart failure: bibasilar crackles, S_3 gallop, dyspnea, neck vein distention in patients with cardiomyopathy or CHF
- Assess for oxygenation or perfusion deficit: decreased B/P, chest pain, dizziness, loss of consciousness
- Monitor B/P and pulse q5 min during inf; if B/P drops 30 mm Hg, stop inf and call prescriber
- Monitor ALT, AST, bilirubin daily
- Monitor for sulfite sensitivity, which may be life threatening

Nursing diagnoses

✓ Cardiac output, decreased (uses)
✓ Knowledge deficit (teaching)

Implementation

IV IV route

- Reconstitute 250 mg/10 ml of D_5W or sterile water for inj; may add another 10 ml to dissolve completely if needed, then dilute in 50 ml or more of D_5W, 0.9% NaCl, 0.45% NaCl, D_5/0.45% NaCl, D_5/0.9% NaCl, D_5/LR, LR; titrate to patient response; use infusion pump for correct dose
- Use a CVP catheter or large peripheral vein, use infusion pump, titrate to patient response
- Change **IV** site q48h

Syringe compatibilities:

Heparin, ranitidine

Syringe incompatibility:

Doxapram

Y-site compatibilities:

Amifostine, amrinone, atracurium, aztreonam, bretylium, calcium chloride, calcium gluconate, ciprofloxacin, cladribine, diazepam, diltiazem, dopamine, enalaprilat, epinephrine, famotidine, fentanyl, fluconazole, granisetron, haloperidol, hydromorphone, regular insulin, labetalol, lidocaine, lorazepam, magnesium sulfate, meperidine, milrinone, morphine, nicardipine, nitroglycerin, norepinephrine, pancuronium, potassium chloride, propofol, ranitidine, sodium nitroprusside, streptokinase, tacrolimus, theophylline, thiotepa, tolazoline, vecuronium, verapamil, zidovudine

Y-site incompatibilities:

Acyclovir, alteplase, aminophylline, foscarnet, phytonadione

Additive compatibilities:

Amiodarone, atracurium, atropine, dopamine, enalaprilat, epinephrine, flumazenil, hydralazine, isoproterenol, lidocaine, meperidine, meropenem, metaraminol, morphine, nitroglycerin, norepinephrine, phentolamine, phenylephrine, procainamide, propranolol, ranitidine, verapamil

Additive incompatibilities: Acyclovir, aminophylline, bumetanide, calcium gluconate, diazepam, digoxin, furosemide, insulin, magnesium sulfate, phenytoin, potassium phosphate, sodium bicarbonate

Patient/family education
- Teach patient reason for medication and expected results, reason for all monitoring and procedures
- Advise patient to report dyspnea, headache, **IV** site discomfort

Evaluation
Positive therapeutic outcome
- Increased cardiac output
- Decreased PCWP, adequate CVP
- Decreased dyspnea, fatigue, edema, ECG
- Increased urine output

Treatment of overdose: Discontinue drug, support circulation

docusate calcium (OTC)
(dok'yoo-sate)
DC Softgels, Pro-Cal-Sof, Sulfalax Calcium, Surfak

docusate sodium (OTC)
Colace, Coloxyl, Diocto, Dioeze, Diosuccin, Disonate, Di-Sosal, DOS, Doxinate, D-S-S, Duosol, Modane, Pro-Sof, Regulex SS, Regulex ✤, Regutol
Func. class.: Laxative, emollient
Chem. class.: Anionic surfactant

Pregnancy category C

Action: Increases water, fat penetration in intestine; allows for easier passage of stool; increases electrolyte, water secretion in colon

➔ **Therapeutic Outcome:** Passage of softened stool, absence of constipation

Uses: To soften stools, prevent constipation, soften fecal impaction (rec route)

Dosage and routes

Adult: PO 50-300 mg qd (docusate sodium) or 240 mg (docusate calcium or docusate potassium) prn; enema 5 ml (docusate sodium)

P ***Child >12 yr:*** Enema 2 ml (docusate sodium)

P ***Child 6-12 yr:*** PO 40-120 mg qd (docusate sodium)

P ***Child 3-6 yr:*** PO 20-60 mg qd (docusate sodium)

P ***Child <3 yr:*** PO 10-40 mg qd (docusate sodium)

Available forms: Caps 50, 100, 240, 250, 300 mg; tabs 50, 100 mg; oral sol 10, 50 mg/ml, 16.7, 20 mg/ml; enema conc 18 g/100 ml
Docusate calcium: Caps 50, 240 mg
Docusate sodium: Caps 50, 100, 240, 250 mg; tabs 50, 100 mg; syr 50, 60 mg/15 ml; liq 150 mg/15 ml; oral sol 10, 50 mg/ml; enema 283 mg/3.9 g cap

Adverse effects
EENT: Bitter taste, throat irritation
GI: Nausea, anorexia, cramps, diarrhea
INTEG: Rash

Contraindications: Hypersensitivity, obstruction, fecal impaction, nausea/vomiting

Precautions: Pregnancy **C**

Pharmacokinetics

Absorption	Minimal (PO)
Distribution	Unknown
Metabolism	Not metabolized
Excretion	Bile
Half-life	Unknown

Pharmacodynamics

	PO	REC
Onset	24-72 hr	4-6 hr
Peak	Unknown	Unknown
Duration	Unknown	Unknown

Interactions: None

NURSING CONSIDERATIONS

Assessment

- Assess cramping, rectal bleeding, nausea, vomiting; if these symptoms occur, drug should be discontinued; identify cause of constipation; identify whether fluids, bulk, or exercise is missing from lifestyle

Nursing diagnoses

✓ Bowel elimination, altered: constipation (uses)
✓ Bowel elimination, altered: diarrhea (side effects)
✓ Knowledge deficit (teaching)
✓ Noncompliance (teaching)

Implementation

PO route

- Dilute oral sol in juice or other fluid to disguise taste
- Give tabs or caps with 8 oz of liq; give on empty stomach for increased absorption, results

Patient/family education

- Discuss with patient that adequate fluid consumption is as necessary as bulk, exercise for adequate bowel function
- Teach patient that normal bowel movements do not always occur daily
- Advise patient not to use in presence of abdominal pain, nausea, vomiting; tell patient to notify prescriber if unrelieved constipation or if symptoms of electrolyte imbalance occur: muscle cramps, pain, weakness, dizziness, excessive thirst
- Advise patient that drug may take up to 3 days to soften stools
- Instruct patient to take oral preparation with a full glass of water and increase fluid intake unless on fluid restrictions
- Caution patients with heart disease to avoid using the Valsalva maneuver to expedite evacuation

Evaluation

Positive therapeutic outcome

- Decreased constipation within 3 days

dofetilide

(doff-ee-till'-lide)

Tikosyn

Func. class.: Antidysrhythmic (Class III)

Pregnancy category C

Action: Blocks cardiac ion channel carrying the rapid component of delayed potassium current, no effect on sodium channels

➔ **Therapeutic Outcome:** Absence of atrial fibrillation

Uses: Atrial fibrillation, flutter

Dosage and routes

Adult: PO initial dose for CrCl > 60 mg/ml 500 μg bid; CrCl 40-60 mg/min 250 μg bid; CrCl 20-39 mg/min 125 μg bid; CrCl <20 mg/min do not use 2-3 hr after initial dose; measure QTc, if >15% compared with baseline, then give ½ initial dose except 125 μg bid, give same dose

Available forms: Caps 125, 250, 500 μg

Adverse effects

CNS: *Syncope, dizziness,* headache
CV: *Hypotension, postural hypotension, bradycardia,* chest pain, angina, PVCs, substernal pressure, precipitation of angina
GI: *Nausea, vomiting,* severe diarrhea, anorexia

Contraindications: Hypersensitivity, digitalis toxicity, aortic stenosis, **P** pulmonary hypertension, children

Precautions: Renal disease, pregnancy **C,** lactation

Pharmacokinetics

Absorption	>90%
Distribution	Unknown
Metabolism	Not metabolized
Excretion	Kidneys 80%
Half-life	Unknown

Pharmacodynamics

Unknown

Interactions
Individual drugs
Cimetidine: Do not use together
Ketoconazole: Do not use together
Prochlorperazine: Do not use together
Trimethoprim/sulfamethoxazole: Do not use together
Verapamil: Do not use together

NURSING CONSIDERATIONS
Assessment
- Monitor ECG continuously to determine drug effectiveness; measure PR, QRS, QT intervals; check for PVCs, other dysrhythmias; monitor B/P continuously; this drug is available only to facilities that have been educated in its administration; patient must be hospitalized
- Before administration, QTc must be determined using an average of 5-10 beats, if the QTc >440 msec or 500 msec in ventricular conduction abnormalities, do not use; do not use if heart rate <60 bpm
- Before dosing, identify CrCl, using CrCl to determine dosing

Nursing diagnoses
✓ Cardiac output, decreased (uses)
✓ Gas exchange, impaired (adverse reactions)
✓ Knowledge deficit (teaching)

Implementation
PO route
- Give for 3 days with patient hospitalized

Patient/family education
- Notify prescriber if fast heartbeats with fainting or dizziness occur
- Notify all prescribers of all medications and supplements taken

Evaluation
Positive therapeutic outcome
- Increased control in atrial fibrillation

D

dolasetron (℞)
(do-la'se-tron)
Anzemet
Func. class.: Antiemetic
Chem. class.: 5-HT receptor antagonist

Pregnancy category C

Action Prevents nausea, vomiting by blocking serotonin peripherally, centrally, and in the small intestine

➔ **Therapeutic Outcome:** Control of nausea, vomiting

Uses: Prevention of nausea, vomiting associated with cancer chemotherapy and prevention of postoperative nausea, vomiting

Investigational uses: Radiotherapy-induced nausea/vomiting

Dosage and routes
Prevention of nausea/vomiting associated with cancer chemotherapy
Adult: **IV** 1.8 mg/kg as a single dose ½ hr before chemotherapy; PO 100 mg 1 hr before chemotherapy

P ***Child 2-16 yr:*** PO 1.8 mg/kg 1 hr before chemotherapy, max 100 mg

Prevention of postoperative nausea/vomiting
Adult: **IV** 12.5 mg as a single dose 15 min before cessation of anesthesia; PO 100 mg 2 hr before surgery (prevention only)

P ***Child 2-16 yr:*** **IV** 0.35 mg/kg as a single dose 15 min before cessation of anesthesia; PO 1.2 mg/kg within 2 hr before surgery (prevention only)

Available forms: Tabs 50, 100 mg; inj 20 mg/ml (12.5 mg/0.625 ml)

Adverse effects

CNS: Headache, dizziness, fatigue, drowsiness

CV: **Dysrhythmias,** ECG changes, hypotension, tachycardia, hypertension, bradycardia

GI: Diarrhea, constipation, increased AST, ALT, abdominal pain, anorexia

GU: Urinary retention, oliguria

MISC: Rash, **bronchospasm**

Contraindications: Hypersensitivity

P G **Precautions:** Pregnancy **C,** lactation, children, elderly

Pharmacokinetics

Absorption	Completely absorbed
Distribution	Unknown
Metabolism	Liver, extensively
Excretion	Kidneys
Half-life	Unknown

Pharmacodynamics

Unknown

Interactions

Individual drugs

Cimetidine: ↑ dolasetron levels

Rifampin: ↓ dolasetron levels

Drug classifications

Antidysrhythmics: ↑ dysrhythmias

NURSING CONSIDERATIONS

Assessment

- Assess for absence of nausea, vomiting during chemotherapy
- Assess for hypersensitivity reaction: rash, bronchospasm
- Assess for cardiac conditions, electrolyte imbalances or dysrhythmias

Nursing diagnoses

✓ Knowledge deficit (teaching)
✓ Noncompliance (teaching)

Implementation

IV **IV route**

- Administer by inj 100 mg/30 sec or less or diluted in 50 ml of compatible sol; give over 15 sec
- Store at room temp for 24 hr after dilution

Patient/family education

- Instruct patient to report diarrhea, constipation, rash, or changes in respirations; may cause headache, use analgesic
- Teach patient reason for medication and expected results

Evaluation

Positive therapeutic outcome

- Absence of nausea, vomiting during cancer chemotherapy

donepezil (℞)

(don-ep-ee'zill)

Aricept

Func. class.: Reversible cholinesterase inhibitor

Pregnancy category C

Action: Elevates acetylcholine concentrations (cerebral cortex) by slowing degradation of acetylcholine released in cholinergic neurons; does not alter underlying dementia

➔ **Therapeutic Outcome:** Decreased symptoms of Alzheimer's disease

Uses: Treatment of mild to moderate dementia in Alzheimer's disease

Dosage and routes

Adult: PO 5 mg qd; may increase to 10 mg qd after 4-6 wk

Available forms: Tabs 5, 10 mg

Adverse effects

CNS: Dizziness, insomnia, somnolence, headache, fatigue, abnormal dreams, syncope, **seizures**

CV: **Atrial fibrillation,** hypotension or hypertension

GI: Nausea, vomiting, anorexia, *diarrhea*
GU: Frequency, UTI, incontinence
INTEG: Rash, flushing
MS: Cramps, arthritis
RESP: Rhinitis, URI, cough, pharyngitis

Contraindications: Hypersensitivity to this drug or piperidine derivatives

Precautions: Sick sinus syndrome, history of ulcers, GI bleeding, hepatic disease, bladder obstruction, asthma, P pregnancy **C**, lactation, children, seizures, asthma, COPD

Pharmacokinetics

Absorption	Well
Distribution	Unknown
Metabolism	Liver to metabolities
Excretion	Unknown
Half-life	10 hr (single dose)

Pharmacodynamics

Unknown

Interactions

Individual drugs

Carbamazepine: ↓ donepezil effect
Dexamethasone: ↓ donepezil effect
Phenobarbital: ↓ donepezil effect
Phenytoin: ↓ donepezil effect
Rifampin: ↓ donepezil effect

Drug classification

Anticholinergics: ↓ activity
Cholinergic agonists: Synergistic effects
Cholinesterase inhibitors: Synergistic effects
NSAIDs: ↑ gastric acid secretions

NURSING CONSIDERATIONS

Assessment

- Monitor B/P: hypotension, hypertension
- Assess mental status: affect, mood, behavioral changes, depression, complete suicide assessment
- Assess GI status: nausea, vomiting, anorexia, diarrhea
- Assess GU status: urinary frequency, incontinence

Nursing diagnoses

✓ Confusion, chronic (uses)
✓ Memory, impaired (uses)

Implementation

- Give between meals; may be given with meals for GI symptoms
- Administer dosage adjusted to response no more than q6 wk
- Provide assistance with ambulation during beginning therapy; dizziness, ataxia may occur

Patient/family education

- Advise patient to report side effects: twitching, nausea, vomiting, sweating; indicates overdose
- Advise patient to use drug exactly as prescribed; at regular intervals, preferably between meals; may be taken with meals for GI upset
- Advise patient to notify prescriber of nausea, vomiting, diarrhea (dose increase or beginning treatment), or rash
- Advise patient not to increase or abruptly decrease dose, serious consequences may result
- Instruct patient that drug is not a cure

Evaluation

Positive therapeutic outcome

- Decrease in confusion; improved mood

Treatment of overdose:

Withdraw drug, administer tertiary anticholinergics, provide supportive care

HIGH ALERT

dopamine (℞)
(doe'pa-meen)
dopamine HCl, Intropin,
Revimine ✦
Func. class.: Agonist, vasopressor, inotropic agent
Chem. class.: Catecholamine

Pregnancy category C

Action: Causes increased cardiac output; acts on β_1- and α-receptors, causing vasoconstriction in blood vessels; when low doses are administered, causes renal and mesenteric vasodilatation; β_1 stimulation produces inotropic effects with increased cardiac output

➔ **Therapeutic Outcome:** Increased B/P, cardiac output

Uses: Shock; to increase perfusion; hypotension

Investigational uses: COPD,
P RDS in infants

Dosage and routes
Shock
Adult: **IV** inf 2-5 μg/kg/min, not to exceed 50 μg/kg/min; titrate to patient's response

P ***Child:*** **IV** 5-20 μg/kg/min adjust depending on response

COPD
Adult: **IV** 4 μg/kg/min

CHF
Adult: **IV** 2-5 μg/kg/min

RDS
P ***Infants:*** **IV** 5 μg/kg/min

Available forms: Inj 40, 160 mg/ml; conc for **IV** inf 0.8, 1.6, 3.2 mg/ml in D_5W

Adverse effects
CNS: *Headache*
CV: *Palpitations,* **tachycardia,** *hypertension,* **ectopic beats,** *angina,* **wide QRS complex,** peripheral vasoconstriction
GI: *Nausea, vomiting, diarrhea*
INTEG: Necrosis, tissue sloughing with extravasation, **gangrene**
RESP: Dyspnea

Contraindications: Hypersensitivity, ventricular fibrillation, tachydysrhythmias, pheochromocytoma

Precautions: Pregnancy **C,** lactation, arterial embolism, peripheral vascular disease

Do Not Confuse:
dopamine/dobutamine

Pharmacokinetics	
Absorption	Complete
Distribution	Widely
Metabolism	Liver
Excretion	Kidney, plasma
Half-life	2 min

Pharmacodynamics	
Onset	2-5 min
Peak	Unknown
Duration	<10 min

Interactions
Individual drugs
Phenytoin: ↑ hypotension, bradycardia
Drug classifications
α-Adrenergic blockers: ↓ action of dopamine
Anesthetics: ↑ dysrhythmias
Antidepressants, tricyclic: ↑ pressor response
β-Adrenergic blockers: ↓ cardiac response
Cardiac glycosides: ↑ inotropic effect
Ergots: Severe hypertension
MAOIs: ↑ hypertension (severe)

NURSING CONSIDERATIONS
Assessment
- Monitor ECG for dysrhythmias, ischemia during treatment; some patients may not need continuous ECG monitoring; also monitor PCWP, CVP,

CO_2, urinary output; notify prescriber if <30 ml/hr
- Assess for heart failure: bibasilar crackles, S_3 gallop, dyspnea, neck vein distention in patients with cardiomyopathy or CHF
- Assess for oxygenation or perfusion deficit: decreased B/P, chest pain, dizziness, loss of consciousness
- Monitor B/P and pulse q5 min during inf; if B/P drops 30 mm Hg, stop inf and call prescriber
- Check for extravasation: change site q48h

Nursing diagnoses

- ✓ Cardiac output, decreased (uses)
- ✓ Tissue perfusion, altered (uses)
- ✓ Fluid volume excess (uses)
- ✓ Knowledge deficit (teaching)

Implementation

- Give by continuous inf; dilute 200-400 mg/250-500 ml of D_5W, 0.9% NaCl, D_5/LR, D_5/0.45% NaCl, D_5/0.9% NaCl, LR; do not use discolored sol; sol is stable for 24 hr; give 0.5-5 μg/kg/min; may increase by 1-4 μg/kg/min q15-30 min until desired patient response; use infusion pump

Syringe compatibilities: Doxapram, heparin, ranitidine

Y-*site compatibilities:* Aldesleukin, amifostine, amiodarone, amrinone, atracurium, aztreonam, cefmetazole, cefpirome, ciprofloxacin, cladribine, diltiazem, dobutamine, enalaprilat, epinephrine, esmolol, famotidine, fentanyl, fluconazole, foscarnet, granisetron, haloperidol, heparin, hydrocortisone, hydromorphone, labetalol, lidocaine, lorazepam, meperidine, methylprednisolone, metronidazole, midazolam, milrinone, morphine, nicardipine, nitroglycerin, norepinephrine, ondansetron, pancuronium, piperacillin/tazobactam, potassium chloride, propofol, ranitidine, sargramostim, sodium nitroprusside, streptokinase, tacrolimus, theophylline, thiotepa, tolazoline, vecuronium, verapamil, vit B/C, warfarin, zidovudine

Additive compatibilities: Aminophylline, atracurium, bretylium, calcium chloride, cephalothin, chloramphenicol, dobutamine, enalaprilat, flumazenil, heparin, hydrocortisone, kanamycin, lidocaine, meropenem, methylprednisolone, nitroglycerin, oxacillin, potassium chloride, ranitidine, verapamil

Patient/family education

- Teach patient reason for medication, expected results, reason for all monitoring, and procedures
- Advise patient to report all side effects

Evaluation

Positive therapeutic outcome
- Increased cardiac output

Treatment of overdose:

Discontinue drug, support circulation; give a short-acting α-blocker

---

HIGH ALERT

doxacurium (℞)

(dox'a-cure-ee-yum)

Nuromax

Func. class.: Neuromuscular blocker (nondepolarizing)

Pregnancy category C

Action: Inhibits transmission of nerve impulses by binding with cholinergic receptor sites, antagonizing action of acetylcholine; no analgesic response

➔ **Therapeutic Outcome:** Paralysis of all skeletal muscles

Uses: Facilitation of endotracheal intubation, skeletal muscle relaxation during mechanical ventilation, surgery, or general anesthesia

Dosage and routes

Adult: **IV** 0.05 mg/kg; 0.08 mg/kg

is used for prolonged neuromuscular blockade; maintenance 0.025 mg/kg

P *Child 2-12 yr:* **IV** 0.03-0.05 mg/kg; may decrease for maintenance dose

Available forms: Inj 1 mg/ml

Adverse effects

CV: *Decreased B/P,* **ventricular fibrillation, MI, cardiovascular accident**

EENT: Diplopia

INTEG: Rash, urticaria

MS: *Weakness,* prolonged skeletal muscle relaxation, *paralysis*

RESP: **Prolonged apnea, bronchospasm,** *wheezing,* **respiratory depression**

Contraindications: Hypersensitivity, P neonates

Precautions: Pregnancy **C**, renal, P hepatic disease, lactation, children <3 mo, fluid and electrolyte imbalances, neuromuscular disease, respiratory G disease, obesity, elderly, severe burns

Pharmacokinetics	
Absorption	Complete
Distribution	Unknown
Metabolism	Unknown
Excretion	Kidneys, bile, unchanged
Half-life	½-2 hr; increased in renal transplant patient

Pharmacodynamics	
Onset	Up to 5 min
Peak	Unknown
Duration	1½ hr

Interactions

Individual drugs

Clindamycin: ↑ paralysis length and intensity

Colistin: ↑ paralysis length and intensity

Lidocaine: ↑ paralysis length and intensity

Lithium: ↑ paralysis length and intensity

Magnesium: ↑ paralysis length and intensity

Polymyxin B: ↑ paralysis length and intensity

Procainamide: ↑ paralysis length and intensity

Quinidine: ↑ paralysis length and intensity

Succinylcholine: ↑ paralysis length and intensity

Drug classifications

Aminoglycosides: ↑ paralysis length and intensity

β-Adrenergic blockers: ↑ paralysis length and intensity

Diuretics, potassium-losing: ↑ paralysis length and intensity

General anesthesia: ↑ paralysis length and intensity

NURSING CONSIDERATIONS

Assessment

- Monitor for electrolyte imbalances (potassium, magnesium) before drug is used; electrolyte imbalances may lead to increased action of this drug
- Monitor VS (B/P, pulse, respirations, airway) until fully recovered; rate, depth, pattern of respirations, strength of hand grip; patient should be intubated before use
- Monitor recovery: decreased paralysis of face, diaphragm, leg, arm, rest of body; residual weakness and respiratory problems may occur during recovery period
- Monitor allergic reactions: rash, fever, respiratory distress, pruritus; drug should be discontinued

Nursing diagnoses

✓ Breathing pattern, ineffective (uses)
✓ Communication, impaired verbal (adverse reactions)
✓ Anxiety (adverse reactions)
✓ Knowledge deficit (teaching)

Implementation

- Anesthesiologist uses peripheral nerve stimulator to determine neuromuscular blockade; deep tendon reflexes should be monitored during extended periods

- Give direct **IV** undiluted over 1 min, or diluted in 1050 ml of D_5W, 0.9% NaCl or NS and give as an inf at prescribed rate (only by qualified person, usually an anesthesiologist); do not administer IM
- Further dilute in D_5W, 0.9% NaCl, D_5/0.9% NaCl q15-25 min (intermittent inf)
- Maintenance is given q20-45 min after 1st dose (cont inf); titrate to patient response
- Store in light-resistant area, at room temp; do not freeze; stable for 24 hr

Y-site compatibilities: Etomidate, thiopental

Solution compatibilities: LR, D_5/LR, D_5/0.9% NaCl, 0.9% NaCl

Patient/family education

- Provide reassurance if communication is difficult during recovery from neuromuscular blockade
- Provide explanation to patients regarding all procedures or treatments; patient will remain conscious if anesthesia is not given also

Evaluation

Positive therapeutic outcome

- Paralysis of jaw, eyelid, head, neck, rest of body as evaluated by peripheral nerve stimulator

Treatment of overdose: Administer edrophonium or neostigmine, atropine; monitor VS; may require mechanical ventilation

doxapram (℞)

(dox'a-pram)

Dopram

Func. class.: Analeptic (respiratory/cerebral stimulant)

Pregnancy category B

D

Action: Respiratory stimulation through activation of peripheral carotid chemoreceptor in low dosages; with higher dosages medullary respiratory centers are stimulated, with progressive general CNS stimulation

➔ **Therapeutic Outcome:** Ease of breathing, ABGs at normal limits

Uses: COPD, postanesthesia CNS and respiratory depression, prevention of acute hypercapnia, drug-induced CNS depression

Investigational uses: Treatment of apnea in premature infants when methylxanthines have failed

Dosage and routes

Postanesthesia stimulation

Adult: **IV** inj 0.5-1 mg/kg, not to exceed 1.5 mg/kg total as a single inj; **IV** inf 250 mg in 250 ml sol, not to exceed 4 mg/kg; run at 1-3 mg/min

Drug-induced CNS depression

Adult: **IV** priming dose of 2 mg/kg, repeated in 5 min; repeat q1-2h until patient awakens; **IV** inf priming dose 2 mg/kg at 1-3 mg/min, not to exceed 3 g/day

COPD (hypercapnia)

Adult: **IV** inf 1-2 mg/min, not to exceed 3 mg/min for no longer than 2 hr

Apnea of premature infant

P ***Infant:*** **IV** 1-1.5 mg/kg/hr loading dose followed by inf of 0.5-2.5 mg/kg/hr

Available forms: Inj **IV** 20 mg/ml

Adverse effects

CNS: **Seizures** (clonus/generalized), *headache,* restlessness, dizziness, confusion, paresthesias, flushing, sweating, bilateral Babinski's sign, rigidity, depression
CV: Chest pain, hypertension, change in heart rate, lowered T waves, tachycardia, arrhythmias
EENT: Pupil dilation, sneezing
GI: Nausea, vomiting, diarrhea, hiccups, desire to defecate
GU: Retention, incontinence, elevation of BUN, albuminuria
INTEG: Pruritus, irritation at inj site
RESP: **Laryngospasm, bronchospasm,** rebound hypoventilation, dyspnea, cough, tachypnea, hiccups

Contraindications: Hypersensitivity, seizure disorders, severe hypertension, severe bronchial asthma, severe dyspnea, severe cardiac disorders, pneumothorax, pulmonary embolism, severe respiratory disease

Precautions: Bronchial asthma, pheochromocytoma, severe tachycardia, dysrhythmias, pregnancy **B**, P hypertension, lactation, children

Pharmacokinetics	
Absorption	Complete
Distribution	Unknown
Metabolism	Liver
Excretion	Kidneys, metabolites
Half-life	2.5-4 hr

Pharmacodynamics	
Onset	20-40 sec
Peak	1-2 min
Duration	5-10 min

Interactions

Individual drugs

Enflurane: ↑ dysrhythmias; delay use of doxapram for 10 min
Halothane: ↑ dysrhythmias; delay use of doxapram for 10 min

Drug classifications

MAOIs: ↑ hypertension
Skeletal muscle relaxants: May mask the effects of skeletal muscle relaxants
Sympathomimetics: Synergistic pressor effect

NURSING CONSIDERATIONS

Assessment

- Monitor B/P, heart rate, deep tendon reflexes, level of consciousness, ABGs before administration q30 min; check for Po_2, Pco_2, O_2 saturation during treatment
- Monitor ECG; watch for hypertension, increased pulse, increased pulmonary artery pressures
- Monitor for hypertension: dysrhythmias, tachycardia, dyspnea, skeletal muscle hyperactivity; may indicate overdosage; discontinue if these occur
- Assess for respiratory stimulation: increased respiratory rate, depth, abnormal rhythm; check for patent airway; elevate head of bed to 45 degrees or higher, position patient on side
- Check for extravasation: redness, inflammation, pain; may cause phlebitis; change **IV** site q48h

Nursing diagnoses

✓ Breathing pattern, ineffective (uses)
✓ Impaired gas exchange (uses)
✓ Knowledge deficit (teaching)

Implementation

- May give **IV** diluted with equal parts of sterile water for inj; may be diluted 250 mg/250 ml (1 mg/ml) of D_5W, $D_{10}W$ (dilute 400 mg/180 ml of compatible **IV** sol [2 mg/ml] and run as inf over 2 hr)
- Give **IV** undiluted over 5 min; **IV** inf at 1-3 mg/min; adjust for desired respiratory response, using infusion pump **IV**; if an inf is used after initial dose, start at 1-3 mg/min; adjust for desired respiratory response, using infusion pump **IV**; if an inf is used after initial dose, start at 1-3 mg/min depending on patient response; discontinue after 2 hr; wait 1-2 hr and repeat

- Give only after adequate airway is established; ensure O_2, **IV** barbiturates, resuscitative equipment available
- Discontinue inf if side effects occur; narrow margin of safety

Syringe compatibilities: Amikacin, bumetadine, chlorpromazine, cimetidine, cisplatin, cyclophosphamide, dopamine, doxycycline, epinephrine, hydroxyzine, imipramine, isoniazid, lincomycin, methotrexate, netilmicin, phytonadione, pyridoxine, terbutaline, thiamine, tobramycin, vincristine

Syringe incompatibilities: Aminophylline, ascorbic acid, cefoperazone, cefotaxime, cefotetan, cefuroxime, dexamethasone, diazepam, digoxin, dobutamine, folic acid, furosemide, hydrocortisone, ketamine, methylprednisolone, minocycline, thiopental, ticarcillin

Patient/family education
- Teach all aspects of drug, purpose, expected reactions
- Caution patient if difficulty breathing or shortness of breath occurs to notify nurse or prescriber

Evaluation
Positive therapeutic outcome
- Increased breathing capacity
- ABGs WNL for patient

doxazosin (℞)
(dox-ay'zoe-sin)
Cardura
Func. class.: Peripheral α-adrenergic blocker, antihypertensive
Chem. class.: Quinazoline
Pregnancy category B

Action: Peripheral blood vessels are dilated, peripheral resistance lowered; reduction in B/P results from α-adrenergic receptors being blocked

Therapeutic Outcome: Decreased B/P, decreased symptoms of benign prostatic hypertrophy (BPH)

Uses: Hypertension alone or as an adjunct, urinary outflow obstruction, symptoms of benign prostatic hyperplasia

Investigational uses: CHF with digoxin and diuretics

Dosage and routes
BPH
Adult: PO 1 mg qd, increase in stepwise manner to 2, 4, 8 mg qd as needed, max 8 mg
Hypertension
Adult: PO 1 mg qd, increasing up to 16 mg qd if required; usual range 4-16 mg/day
G ***Elderly:*** PO 0.5 mg qhs, gradually increase

Available forms: Tabs 1, 2, 4, 8 mg

Adverse effects
CNS: *Dizziness,* headache, drowsiness, anxiety, depression, vertigo, weakness, fatigue, asthenia
CV: Palpitations, *orthostatic hypotension,* **tachycardia,** edema, **dysrhythmias,** chest pain
EENT: Epistaxis, tinnitus, dry mouth, red sclera, pharyngitis, rhinitis
GI: Nausea, vomiting, diarrhea, constipation, abdominal pain
GU: Incontinence, polyuria

Contraindications: Hypersensitivity to quinazolines

Precautions: Pregnancy **B,** P children, lactation, hepatic disease

Do Not Confuse:
Cardura/Coumadin, Cardura/Ridaura

Pharmacokinetics

Absorption	Well absorbed
Distribution	Not known; 98% plasma protein bound
Metabolism	Liver, extensively (<63%)
Excretion	Kidneys
Half-life	22 hr

Pharmacodynamics

Onset	2 hr
Peak	2-6 hr
Duration	6-12 hr

Interactions
Individual drugs
Clonidine: ↓ effects of clonidine
Indomethacin: ↓ hypotensive effects
Verapamil: ↑ hypotensive effects
Drug classifications
β-Adrenergic blockers: ↑ postural hypotension
NSAIDs: ↓ hypotensive effects
Herb/drug
Angelica: ↑ doxazosin effect
Lab test interferences
False positive: Urine acetone

NURSING CONSIDERATIONS
Assessment
- Monitor B/P (lying, standing) and pulse, syncope; check for edema in feet, legs daily; I&O; monitor for weight daily; notify prescriber of changes
- Assess skin turgor, dryness of mucous membranes for hydration status
- Assess for orthostatic hypotension; tell patient to rise slowly from sitting or lying position; assess pulse, jugular venous distention q4h, rales, dyspnea, orthopnea with B/P

Nursing diagnoses
- ✓ Cardiac output, decreased (uses)
- ✓ Injury, potential for physical (side effects)
- ✓ Knowledge deficit (teaching)
- ✓ Noncompliance (teaching)

Implementation
- Store in tight container at 86° F (30° C) or less
- May be used in combination with other antihypertensives
- May be given with food to prevent GI symptoms

Patient/family education
- Teach patient not to discontinue drug abruptly; emphasize the importance of complying with dosage schedule, even if feeling better; if dose is missed take as soon as remembered; take at same time each day
- Instruct patient to take 1st dose at hs to decrease orthostatic B/P changes
- Teach patient not to use OTC products (cough, cold, allergy) unless directed by prescriber; also to avoid large amounts of caffeine
- Emphasize the need to rise slowly to sitting or standing position to minimize orthostatic hypotension
- Teach patient to notify prescriber of mouth sores, sore throat, fever, swelling of hands or feet, irregular heartbeat, chest pain
- Caution patient to report excessive perspiration, dehydration, vomiting, diarrhea; may lead to fall in B/P
- Caution patient that drug may cause dizziness, fainting, lightheadedness; may occur during 1st few days of therapy; to avoid hazardous activities
- Teach patient how to take B/P, and normal readings for age group; to take B/P q7 days

Evaluation
Positive therapeutic outcome
- Decreased B/P in hypertension
- Decreased symptoms of BPH

Treatment of overdose:
Administer volume expanders or vasopressors; discontinue drug; place in supine position

doxepin (℞)

(dox′e-pin)

Adepin, doxepin HCl, Novo-Doxepin ✱, Sinequan, Sinequan Concentrate, Triadapin ✱, Zonolon Topical Cream

Func. class.: Antidepressant, tricyclic; antianxiety

Chem. class.: Dibenzoxepin, tertiary amine

Pregnancy category C

Action: Blocks reuptake of norepinephrine, serotonin into nerve endings, increasing action of norepinephrine, serotonin in nerve cells; has anticholinergic effects

➔ **Therapeutic Outcome:** Decreased symptoms of depression after 2-3 wk

Uses: Major depression, anxiety

Investigational uses: Chronic pain management; topical—pruritus

Dosage and routes

Oral conc should be diluted with 120 ml of water, milk, or orange, grapefuit, tomato, prune, pineapple juice; do not mix with grape juice.

Depression/anxiety

Adult: PO 75 mg/day, may increase to 300 mg/day for severely ill

G ***Elderly:*** PO 10-25 mg hs, increase qwk by 10-25 mg to desired dose

Pruritus

Adult: PO 10 mg hs, may increase to 25 mg hs; top apply a thin film qid ≥3 hr apart

Available forms: Caps 10, 25, 50, 75, 100, 150 mg; oral conc 10 mg/ml; cream 5%

Adverse effects

CNS: *Dizziness, drowsiness,* confusion, headache, anxiety, tremors, stimulation, weakness, insomnia, G nightmares, EPS (elderly), increased psychiatric symptoms, paresthesia

CV: *Orthostatic hypotension, ECG changes,* **tachycardia,** *hypertension,* palpitations, **dysrhythmias**

EENT: *Blurred vision,* tinnitus, mydriasis, ophthalmoplegia, glossitis

GI: *Diarrhea, dry mouth,* nausea, vomiting, **paralytic ileus,** increased appetite, cramps, epigastric distress, jaundice, **hepatitis,** stomatitis, constipation

GU: *Retention,* **acute renal failure**

HEMA: **Agranulocytosis, thrombocytopenia, eosinophilia, leukopenia**

INTEG: Rash, urticaria, sweating, pruritus, photosensitivity

Contraindications: Hypersensitivity to tricyclic antidepressants, urinary retention, narrow-angle glaucoma, prostatic hypertrophy

Precautions: Suicidal patients, G elderly, pregnancy **C** (PO), seizures

Do Not Confuse:
Sinequan/Serentil

Pharmacokinetics

Absorption	Well absorbed
Distribution	Widely distributed; crosses placenta
Metabolism	Liver, extensively
Excretion	Kidneys, breast milk
Half-life	8-24 hr

Pharmacodynamics

Unknown

Interactions

Individual drugs

Alcohol: ↑ CNS depression
Cimetidine: ↑ levels, toxicity
Clonidine: Severe hypotension; avoid use
Disulfiram: Organic brain syndrome
Fluoxetine: ↑ levels, toxicity
Guanethidine: ↓ effects of guanethidine
Sertraline: ↑ doxepin effect

Drug classifications

Analgesics: ↑ CNS depression
Anticholinergics: ↑ side effects

Antihistamines: ↑ CNS depression
Antihypertensives: May block antihypertensive effect
Barbiturates: ↑ CNS depression
Benzodiazepines: ↑ CNS depression
CNS depressants: ↑ CNS depression
MAOIs: Hypertensive crisis, convulsions
Oral contraceptives: ↑ effects, toxicity
Phenothiazines: ↑ toxicity
Sedative/hypnotics: ↑ CNS depression
Sympathomimetics, indirect acting: ↓ effects

Smoking

↑ Metabolism, ↓ effects

Lab test interferences

↑ Serum bilirubin, ↑ blood glucose, ↑ alkaline phosphatase
↓ Blood glucose

NURSING CONSIDERATIONS

Assessment

- Monitor B/P (with patient lying, standing), pulse q4h; if systolic B/P drops 20 mm Hg, hold drug, notify prescriber; take VS q4h in patients with CV disease
- Monitor blood studies: CBC, leukocytes, differential, cardiac enzymes if patient is receiving long-term therapy
- Monitor hepatic studies: AST, ALT, bilirubin
- Check weight weekly; appetite may increase with drug
- Assess ECG for flattening of T wave, bundle branch block, AV block, dysrhythmias in cardiac patients; drug should be discontinued gradually several days before surgery
- Assess for extrapyramidal symptoms G primarily in elderly: rigidity, dystonia, akathisia
- Assess mental status: mood, sensorium, affect, suicidal tendencies; increase in psychiatric symptoms: depression, panic
- Monitor urinary retention, P constipation; constipation is more G likely to occur in children or elderly
- Assess for withdrawal symptoms: headache, nausea, vomiting, muscle pain, weakness; do not usually occur unless drug was discontinued abruptly
- Identify alcohol consumption; if alcohol is consumed, hold dose until AM

Nursing diagnoses

✓ Coping, ineffective individual (uses)
✓ Injury, risk for (side effects)
✓ Knowledge deficit (teaching)

Implementation

- Give with food or milk for GI symptoms; do not give with carbonated beverages
- Give dosage hs if oversedation occurs during day; may take entire G dose hs; elderly may not tolerate once/day dosing
- Store at room temp; do not freeze
- Provide safety measures, primarily G for elderly

Patient/family education

- Tell patient that therapeutic effects of decreased depression may take 2-3 wk, antianxiety effects sooner; to use caution in driving and other activities requiring alertness because of drowsiness, dizziness, blurred vision
- Advise patient to avoid rising quickly from sitting to standing, G especially elderly
- Teach patient to avoid alcohol ingestion, other CNS depressants; not to discontinue medication quickly after long-term use: may cause nausea, headache, malaise
- Teach patient to wear sunscreen or large hat, since photosensitivity occurs
- Teach patient to increase fluids, bulk in diet if constipation occurs, G especially elderly; to take gum, hard sugarless candy, or frequent sips of water for dry mouth

Evaluation

Positive therapeutic outcome

- Decrease in depression
- Absence of suicidal thoughts

Treatment of overdose: ECG monitoring, induce emesis, lavage, activated charcoal, administer anticonvulsant

doxercalciferol (℞)
(dox-er-kal'-cif-er-ol)

Hectorol

Func. class.: Parathyroid agent (calcium regulator)

Chem. class.: Vitamin D hormone

Pregnancy category C

Therapeutic Outcome: Calcium at normal level

Uses: To lower high parathyroid hormone levels in patients undergoing chronic kidney dialysis

Dosage and routes
Adult: PO 10 μg 3×/wk at dialysis

Available forms: Caps 2.5 μg

Adverse effects
CNS: Drowsiness, headache, lethargy

GI: Nausea, diarrhea, vomiting, anorexia, dry mouth, constipation, cramps, metallic taste

GU: Polyuria, hypercalciuria, hyperphosphatemia, hematuria

MS: Myalgia, arthralgia, decreased bone development

RESP: Shortness of breath

Contraindications: Hypersensitivity, hyperphosphatemia, hypercalcemia, vit D toxicity

Precautions: Pregnancy **C**, renal calculi, lactation, CV disease

Pharmacokinetics

Absorption	Unknown
Distribution	Unknown
Metabolism	Unknown
Excretion	Unknown
Half-life	Unknown

Pharmacodynamics
Unknown

Interactions
Individual drugs

Cholestyramine: ↓ doxercalciferol levels, do not use together

Magnesium antacids: Do not use together

Mineral oil: ↓ doxercalciferol levels, do not use together

NURSING CONSIDERATIONS
Assessment
- Assess GI symptoms, polyuria, flushing, head swelling, tingling, headache; may indicate hypercalcemia
- Identify nutritional status; check diet for sources of vit D (milk, some seafood), calcium (dairy products, dark green vegetables), phosphates
- Monitor BUN, creatinine, uric acid, chloride electrolytes, urine pH, urinary calcium, magnesium, phosphate, urinalysis (calcium should be kept at 9-10 mg/dl; vit D 50-135 IU/dl), alkaline phosphatase baseline and q3-6 mo
- Assess for increased drug level, since toxic reactions occur rapidly; have calcium chloride on hand if calcium level drops too low; check for tetany

Nursing diagnoses
- ✓ Injury, risk for (adverse reactions)
- ✓ Pain, chronic (uses)
- ✓ Knowledge deficit (teaching)

Implementation
- Give with meals for GI symptoms
- Do not crush or chew caps

Patient/family education
- Teach patient the symptoms of hypercalcemia and about foods rich in calcium
- Advise patient to avoid products with sodium: cured meats, dairy products, cold cuts, olives, beets, pickles, soups, meat tenderizers in chronic renal failure
- Advise patient to avoid products with potassium: oranges, bananas, dried fruit, peas, dark green leafy

D

vegetables, milk, melons, beans in chronic renal failure

- Advise patient to avoid OTC products containing calcium, potassium, or sodium in chronic renal failure
- Instruct patient to avoid all preparations containing vit D
- Instruct patient to monitor weight weekly

Evaluation

Positive therapeutic outcome

- Calcium levels 9-10 mg/dl

HIGH ALERT

doxorubicin (℞)

(dox-oh-roo'bi-sin)

Adriamycin PFS, Adriamycin RDF, Rubex

doxorubicin liposome (℞)

Doxil

Func. class.: Antineoplastic, antibiotic

Chem. class.: Anthracycline glycoside

Pregnancy category D

Action: Inhibits DNA synthesis primarily; derived from *Streptomyces peucetius;* replication is decreased by binding to DNA, which causes strand splitting; active throughout entire cell cycle; a vesicant

Therapeutic Outcome: Prevention of rapidly growing malignant cells

Uses: Wilms' tumor; bladder, breast, cervical, head, neck, liver, lung, ovarian, prostatic, stomach, testicular, thyroid cancer; Hodgkin's disease; acute lymphoblastic leukemia; myeloblastic leukemia; neuroblastomas; lymphomas; sarcomas

Dosage and routes

Doxorubicin

Adult: **IV** 60-75 mg/m^2 q3 wk, or 30 mg/m^2 on days 1-3 of 4-wk cycle, not to exceed 550 mg/m^2 cumulative dose

P ***Child:*** **IV** 30 mg/m^2/day × 3 days, may repeat q4 wk

Doxorubicin liposome

Adult: **IV** 20 mg/m^2 q3 wk

Available forms: Inj 10, 20, 50 mg

Adverse effects

CV: Increased B/P, **sinus tachycardia, PVCs,** chest pain, **bradycardia, extrasystole**

GI: Nausea, vomiting, anorexia, mucositis, **hepatotoxicity**

GU: Impotence, sterility, amenorrhea, gynecomastia, hyperuricemia

HEMA: **Thrombocytopenia, leukopenia, anemia**

INTEG: Rash, necrosis at inj site, dermatitis, reversible alopecia, cellulitis, thrombophlebitis at inj site

Contraindications: Hypersensitivity, pregnancy **D** (1st trimester), lactation, systemic infections

Precautions: Renal, hepatic, cardiac disease, gout, bone marrow suppression (severe)

Do Not Confuse:
Adriamycin/Aredia, Adriamycin/Idamycin, doxorubicin/daunorubicin, doxorubicin/idarubicin

Pharmacokinetics

Absorption	Complete bioavailability
Distribution	Widely distributed; crosses placenta
Metabolism	Liver, extensively
Excretion	Bile (40%-50%)
Half-life	12 min; 3½ hr; 29⅔ hr

Pharmacodynamics

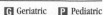

Unknown

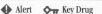

Interactions

Individual drugs

Cyclophosphamide: ↑ cardiotoxicity, CHF
Mercaptopurine: ↑ liver disorders, hepatitis
Radiation: ↑ toxicity, bone marrow suppression

Drug classifications

Antineoplastics: ↑ toxicity, bone marrow suppression
Live virus vaccines: ↑ adverse reactions, ↓ antibody response

Lab test interferences

↑ Uric acid

NURSING CONSIDERATIONS

Assessment

- Monitor ECG; watch for ST-T wave changes, low QRS and T; possible dysrhythmias (sinus tachycardia, heart block, PVCs) may occur
- Assess buccal cavity q8h for dryness, sores or ulceration, white patches, pain, bleeding, dysphagia; obtain prescription for viscous lidocaine (Xylocaine)
- Assess symptoms indicating severe allergic reaction: rash, pruritus, urticaria, purpuric skin lesions, itching, flushing; drug should be discontinued
- Assess tachypnea, ECG changes, dyspnea, edema, fatigue
- Monitor CBC, differential, platelet count weekly; withhold drug if WBC is $<4000/mm^3$ or platelet count is $<100,000/mm^3$; notify prescriber of results if WBC $<20,000/mm^3$, platelets $<150,000/mm^3$
- Assess for increased uric acid levels, swelling, joint pain, primarily extremities; patient should be well hydrated to prevent urate deposits
- Monitor renal function studies: BUN, creatinine, serum uric acid, urine CrCl before and during therapy; I&O ratio; report fall in urine output to <30 ml/hr
- Monitor temp q4h (may indicate beginning of infection)
- Monitor liver function tests before and during therapy (bilirubin, AST, ALT, LDH) as needed or monthly; note jaundice of skin or sclera, dark urine, clay-colored stools, itchy skin, abdominal pain, fever, diarrhea
- Assess for bleeding: hematuria, stool guaiac, bruising or petechiae, mucosa or orifices q8h; inflammation of mucosa, breaks in skin
- Identify effects of alopecia on body image; discuss feelings about body changes

Nursing diagnoses

- ✓ Injury, risk for (adverse reactions)
- ✓ Body image disturbance (adverse reactions)
- ✓ Infection, risk for (adverse reactions)
- ✓ Knowledge deficit (teaching)

Implementation

- Avoid contact with skin; very irritating; wash completely to remove; give fluids **IV** or PO before chemotherapy to hydrate patient
- Give antiemetic 30-60 min before giving drug to prevent vomiting and prn; give antibiotics for prophylaxis of infection
- Provide liq diet: carbonated beverages; gelatin may be added if patient is not nauseated or vomiting
- Help patient to rinse mouth tid-qid with water or club soda, brush teeth bid-qid with soft brush or cotton-tipped applicators for stomatitis, use unwaxed dental floss
- Drug should be prepared by experienced personnel using proper precautions
- Do not interchange doxorubicin with doxorubicin liposome
- Give **IV** after diluting 10 mg/5 ml of NaCl for inj; another 5 ml of diluent/10 mg is recommended; shake; give over 3-5 min; give through Y-tube or 3-way stopcock through free-flowing D_5 inf or 0.9% NaCl
- **IV** liposome inj (Doxil): dilute dose up to 90 mg/250 ml of D_5W, give

over ½ hr; do not admix with other solution medications
- Use hydrocortisone, dexamethasone, or sodium bicarbonate (1 mEq/1 ml) for extravasation: apply ice compress

Syringe compatibilities: Bleomycin, cisplatin, cyclophosphamide, droperidol, fluorouracil, leucovorin, methotrexate, metoclopramide, mitomycin, vincristine

Syringe incompatibilities: Furosemide, heparin

Y-site compatibilities: Amifostine, aztreonam, bleomycin, chlorpromazine, cimetidine, cisplatin, cladribine, cyclophosphamide, dexamethasone, diphenhydramine, droperidol, famotidine, filgrastim, fludarabine, fluorouracil, granisetron, hydromorphone, leucovorin calcium, lorazepam, melphalan, methotrexate, methylprednisolone, metoclopramide, mitomycin, morphine, ondansetron, paclitaxel, prochlorperazine, promethazine, propofol, ranitidine, sargramostim, sodium bicarbonate, teniposide, thiotepa, vinblastine, vincristine, vinorelbine

Y-site incompatibilities: Furosemide, heparin

Additive compatibilities: Ondansetron

Additive incompatibilities: Aminophylline, cephalothin, dexamethasone, diazepam, fluorouracil, hydrocortisone

Patient/family education
- Tell patient that urine and other body fluids may be red-orange for 48 hr; contraceptive measures are recommended during and 4 mo after therapy; drug is teratogenic to fetus
- Advise patient to avoid use of products containing aspirin or ibuprofen, razors, commercial mouthwash, since bleeding may occur; to report symptoms of bleeding (hematuria, tarry stools)
- Instruct patient to report signs of anemia (fatigue, headache, irritability, faintness, shortness of breath)
- Inform patient that hair may be lost during treatment; a wig or hairpiece may make patient feel better; new hair may be different in color, texture
- Caution patient not to have any vaccinations without the advice of the prescriber; serious reactions can occur

Evaluation

Positive therapeutic outcome
- Prevention of rapid division of malignant cells

doxycycline (℞)

(dox-i-sye′kleen)

Apo-Doxy ✦, Doryx, Doxy, Doxy-Caps, Doxycin ✦, doxycycline, Monodox, Novodoxyclin ✦, Periostat, Vibramycin, Vibramycin **IV**, Vibra-Tabs

Func. class.: Antiinfective

Chem. class.: Tetracycline

Pregnancy category D

Action: Inhibits protein synthesis, phosphorylation in microorganisms by binding to 30S ribosomal subunits, reversibly binding to 50S ribosomal subunits; bacteriostatic

➔ **Therapeutic Outcome:** Bactericidal action against the following: gram-positive pathogens *Bacillus anthracis, Clostridium perfringens, Clostridium tetani, Listeria monocytogenes, Nocardia, Propionibacterium acnes, Actinomyces israelii;* gram-negative pathogens *Hamophilus influenzae, Legionella pneumophila, Yersinia enterocolitica, Yersinia pestis, Neisseria gonorrhoeae, Neisseria meningitidis, Mycoplasma, Chlamydia, Rickettsia*

Uses: Syphilis, gonorrhea, *Chla-*

mydia, lymphogranuloma venereum, uncommon gram-negative or -positive organisms, malaria prophylaxis, acne

Investigational uses: Traveler's diarrhea, Lyme disease, prevention of chronic bronchitis

Dosage and routes

Adult: PO/**IV** 100 mg q12h on day 1, then 100 mg/day; **IV** 200 mg in 1-2 inf on day 1, then 100-200 mg/day

P ***Child >8 yr (>45 kg):*** PO/**IV** 2.2-4.4 mg/kg/day in divided doses q12h

Gonorrhea (patients allergic to penicillin)

Adult: Uncomplicated, PO 200 mg, then 100 mg hs and 100 mg bid × 3 days or 300 mg, then 300 mg in 1 hr; disseminated, 100 mg PO bid × at least 7 days

Chlamydia trachomatis

Adult: PO 100 mg bid × 7days

Syphilis

Adult: PO 300 mg/day in divided doses × 10 days

Periodontitis

Adult: 20 mg after sealing and root planing for ≤9 mo; give ≥1 hr before meal AM or PM

Available forms: Tabs 20, 100 mg; caps 50, 100 mg; syr 25, 50 mg/5 ml; powder for inj 100, 200 mg; powder for oral susp 25 mg/5 ml

Adverse effects

CNS: Fever

CV: Pericarditis

EENT: Dysphagia, glossitis, decreased calcification of deciduous teeth, oral candidiasis

GI: *Nausea, abdominal pain, vomiting, diarrhea,* anorexia, enterocolitis, **hepatotoxicity,** flatulence, abdominal cramps, gastric burning, stomatitis

GU: *Increased BUN*

HEMA: **Eosinophilia, neutropenia, thrombocytopenia, hemolytic anemia**

INTEG: Rash, urticaria, photosensitivity, increased pigmentation, **exfoliative dermatitis**, pruritus, **angioedema**

Contraindications: Hypersensitivity to tetracyclines, P children <8 yr, pregnancy **D**

Precautions: Hepatic disease, lactation

Pharmacokinetics

Absorption	Well absorbed
Distribution	Widely distributed, crosses placenta
Metabolism	Some hepatic recycling
Excretion	Bile, feces; kidneys unchanged (20%-40%), enters breast milk
Half-life	14-17 hr; increased in severe renal disease

Pharmacodynamics

	PO	IV
Onset	1½-4 hr	Immediate
Peak	1½-4 hr	Infusion's end

Interactions

Individual drugs

Calcium: Forms chelates, ↓ absorption

Carbamazepine: ↑ effect of carbamazepine

Cholestyramine: ↓ doxycycline effect

Colestipol: ↓ doxycycline effect

Iron: Forms chelates, ↓ absorption

Magnesium: Forms chelates, ↓ absorption

Phenytoin: ↓ effect of doxycycline

Sucralfate: ↓ doxycycline effect

Warfarin: ↑ effect of warfarin

Drug classifications

Anticoagulants, oral: ↑ effect of anticoagulants

Barbiturates: ↓ effect of doxycycline

Contraceptives, oral: ↓ effect of oral contraceptive

Food/drug

↓ Absorption with dairy products

Lab test interferences

False ↑ Urinary catecholamines, ↑ ALT, ↑ AST

NURSING CONSIDERATIONS
Assessment
- Assess patient for previous sensitivity reaction
- Assess patient for signs and symptoms of infection including characteristics of wounds, sputum, urine, stool, WBC >10,000/mm^3, fever; obtain baseline information before and during treatment
- Obtain C&S before beginning drug therapy to identify if correct treatment has been initiated
- Assess for allergic reactions: rash, urticaria, pruritus, chills, fever, joint pain; angioedema may occur a few days after therapy begins
- Assess bowel pattern daily; if severe diarrhea occurs, drug should be discontinued
- Monitor for bleeding: ecchymosis, bleeding gums, hematuria, stool guaiac daily if on long-term therapy; blood dyscrasias may occur
- Assess for overgrowth of infection: perineal itching, fever, malaise, redness, pain, swelling, drainage, rash, diarrhea, change in cough, sputum

Nursing diagnoses
✓ Infection, risk for (uses)
✓ Diarrhea (side effects)
✓ Injury, risk for (side effects)
✓ Knowledge deficit (teaching)
✓ Noncompliance (teaching)

Implementation
PO route
- ⃠ Do not crush, chew caps
- Give around the clock to maintain proper blood levels; give with food to increase absorption of drug; do not give within 3 hr of other agents; drug reactions may occur
- Give with 8 oz of water, 1 hr before hs to prevent ulceration
- Shake liq preparation well before giving; use calibrated device for proper dosing
- Do not give with iron, calcium, magnesium products or antacids, which decrease absorption and form insoluble chelate

IV IV route
- Check for irritation, extravasation, phlebitis daily; change site q72h
- For intermittent inf, dilute each 100 mg/10 ml of 0.9% NaCl, sterile water for inj; further dilute in at least 100 ml of 0.9% NaCl, D_5W, Ringer's, LR, D_5/LR; protect from direct light; keep at room temp; give over 1-4 hr; **IV** sol stable for 12 hr at room temp, 72 hr refrigerated, discard if precipitate forms

Syringe compatibilities:
Doxapram

Y-site compatibilities:
Acyclovir, amifostine, amiodarone, aztreonam, cyclophosphamide, diltiazem, filgrastim, fludarabine, granisetron, hydromorphone, magnesium sulfate, melphalan, meperidine, morphine, ondansetron, perphenazine, propofol, sargramostim, tacrolimus, teniposide, theophylline, thiotepa, vinorelbine

Y-site incompatibilities:
Hetastarch

Additive compatibilities:
Ranitidine

Patient/family education
- Teach patient to report sore throat, bruising, bleeding, joint pain; may indicate blood dyscrasias (rare)
- Advise patient to contact prescriber if vaginal itching, loose, foul-smelling stools, furry tongue occur; may indicate superinfection; report itching, rash, pruritus, urticaria
- Instruct patient to take all medication prescribed for the length of time ordered; drug must be taken around the clock to maintain blood levels; do not give medication to others
- Advise patient to notify prescriber of diarrhea with blood or pus

Evaluation
Positive therapeutic outcome
- Absence of signs/symptoms of

infection (WBC <10,000/mm^3, temp WNL, absence of red draining wounds)

• Reported improvement in symptoms of infection

HIGH ALERT

droperidol (℞)

(droe-per'i-dole)

droperidol, Inapsine

Func. class.: Neuroleptic, tranquilizer, antiemetic

Chem. class.: Butyrophenone derivative

Pregnancy category C

Action: Acts on CNS at subcortical levels, producing tranquilization, sleep; antiemetic

Therapeutic Outcome: Maintenance of anesthesia

Uses: Premedication for surgery; induction, maintenance in general anesthesia; postoperatively for nausea and vomiting

Dosage and routes

Induction

Adult: **IV**/IM 0.22-0.275 mg/kg given with analgesic or general anesthetic; may give 1.25-2.5 mg additionally

P ***Child 2-12 yr:*** **IV**/IM 88-165 µg/kg, titrated to response needed

Premedication

Adult: IM/**IV** 2.5-10 mg ½-1 hr before surgery, may give 1.25-2.5 mg additionally

P ***Child 2-12 yr:*** IM/**IV** 88-165 µg/kg

Maintaining general anesthesia

Adult: **IV** 1.25-2.5 mg

Regional anesthesia adjunct

Adult: IM/**IV** 2.5-5 mg

Diagnostic procedures without general anesthesia

Adult: IM 2.5-10 mg ½-1 hr before procedure; 1.25-2.5 mg may be needed additionally

Antiemetic

Adult: **IV** 0.5-1.25 mg q4h prn (unlabeled)

Available forms: Inj 2.5 mg/ml

Adverse effects

CNS: Dystonia, akathisia, flexion of arms, fine tremors, dizziness, anxiety, drowsiness, restlessness, hallucinations, depression, **seizures**

CV: **Tachycardia,** *hypotension*

EENT: Upward rotation of eyes, oculogyric crisis

INTEG: *Chills, facial sweating, shivering*

RESP: **Laryngospasm, bronchospasm**

Contraindications: Hypersensitivity, P child <2 yr

G **Precautions:** Elderly, CV disease (hypotension, bradydysrhythmias), renal, liver disease, Parkinson's disease, pregnancy **C**

Pharmacokinetics	
Absorption	Well absorbed (IM)
Distribution	Crosses blood-brain barrier, placenta
Metabolism	Liver
Excretion	Kidneys, unchanged (10%)
Half-life	2-3 hr

Pharmacodynamics	IM/IV
Onset	3-10 min
Peak	30 min
Duration	3-6 hr

Interactions

Individual drugs

Alcohol: ↑ CNS depression

Lithium: ↑ side effects of lithium

Drug classifications

Amphetamines: ↓ effects of amphetamines

Anticholinergics: ↓ effects of anticholinergics
Anticoagulants: ↓ effects of anticoagulants
Anticonvulsants: ↓ effects of anticonvulsants
Antihistamines: ↑ CNS depression
Antihypertensives: ↑ hypotension
Antiparkinsonian agents: ↓ effects of antiparkinsonian agents
Antipsychotics: ↑ CNS depression
Barbiturates: ↑ CNS depression
CNS depressants: ↑ CNS depression
Nitrates: ↑ hypotension
Opiates: ↑ CNS depression

Herb/drug

Kava: ↑ action

NURSING CONSIDERATIONS

Assessment

- Check VS q10 min during **IV** administration, q30 min after IM dose; for increasing heart rate or decreasing B/P, notify prescriber at once; do not place patient in Trendelenburg's position, sympathetic blockade may occur, causing respiratory arrest
- Assess extrapyramidal reactions: dystonia, akathisia, extended neck, restlessness, tremors; if these occur, an anticholinergic should be given
- If given for nausea or vomiting, monitor for significant loss of fluids, bowel sounds before and during administration

Nursing diagnoses

- ✓ Injury, risk for (adverse reactions)
- ✓ Knowledge deficit (teaching)

Implementation

IM route

- Give deeply in large muscle mass

IV route

- Give direct **IV** undiluted; give through Y-tube or 3-way stopcock at 10 mg or less/min; titrate to patient response
- Intermittent inf may be given by adding dose to 250 ml of LR, D_5W, 0.9% NaCl; give slowly, titrate to patient response
- Give anticholinergics (benztropine, diphenhydramine) for extrapyramidal reaction
- Give only with resuscitative equipment nearby

Syringe compatibilities:

Atropine, bleomycin, butorphanol, chlorpromazine, cimetidine, cisplatin, cyclophosphamide, dimenhydrinate, diphenhydramine, doxorubicin, fentanyl, glycopyrrolate, hydroxyzine, meperidine, metoclopramide, midazolam, mitomycin, morphine, nalbuphine, pentazocine, perphenazine, prochlorperazine, promazine, promethazine, scopolamine, vinblastine, vincristine

Syringe incompatibilities:

Fluorouracil, furosemide, heparin, leucovorin, methotrexate, pentobarbital

Y-site compatibilities:

Amifostine, aztrenonam, bleomycin, cisatracurium, cisplatin, cladribine, cyclophosphamide, cytarabine, doxorubicin, doxorubicin liposome, famotidine, filgrastim, fluconazole, fludarabine, granisetron, hydrocortisone sodium succinate, idarubicin, melphalen, meperidine, metoclopramide, mitomycin, ondansetron, paclitaxel, potassium chloride, propofol, remifentanil, sargramostim, teniposide, thiotepa, vinblastine, vincristine, vinorelbine, vit B/C

Y-site incompatibilities:

Fluorouracil, foscarnet, furosemide, leucovorin, methotrexate, nafcillin

Additive incompatibilities:

Barbiturates

Patient/family education

- Advise patient that orthostatic hypotension is common; to rise from lying or sitting position slowly; to avoid ambulation without assistance
- Caution patient that drowsiness may occur; to call for assistance for ambulation

Evaluation

Positive therapeutic outcome

- Decreased anxiety
- Absence of vomiting during and after surgery

drotrecogin alfa

See Appendix A, Selected New Drugs

dutasteride

See Appendix A, Selected New Drugs

dyphylline (℞)

(dye'fi-lin)

Dilor, Dyflex-200, Dylline, dyphylline, Lufyllin, Neothylline

Func. class.: Bronchodilator, phosphodiesterase inhibitor

Chem. class.: Xanthine, theophylline derivative

Pregnancy category B

Action: Relaxes smooth muscle of respiratory system by blocking phosphodiesterase, which increases cyclic AMP; cyclic AMP results in positive inotropic, chronotropic effects, bronchodilatation, stimulation of CNS

Therapeutic Outcome: Bronchodilatation with ease of breathing

Uses: Bronchial asthma, bronchospasm in chronic bronchitis and emphysema, COPD

Dosage and routes

Adult: PO 200-800 mg q6h; IM 250-500 mg q6h injected slowly, max 15 mg/kg/dose

Available forms: Tabs 200, 400 mg; elix 33.3, 53.3 mg/5 ml; inj 250 mg/ml

Adverse effects

CNS: *Anxiety, restlessness, insomnia, dizziness,* **convulsions,** headache, lightheadedness, muscle twitching

CV: *Palpitations, sinus tachycardia,* hypotension, flushing, **dysrhythmias, circulatory failure**

GI: *Nausea, vomiting, anorexia,* dyspepsia, epigastric pain, rectal irritation, bleeding

INTEG: Flushing, urticaria

OTHER: Fever, dehydration, **albuminuria,** hyperglycemia

RESP: Tachypnea, **respiratory arrest**

Contraindications: Hypersensitivity to xanthines, tachydysrhythmias, hyperthyroidism, active peptic ulcer disease

G **Precautions:** Elderly, CHF, cor pulmonale, hepatic disease, diabetes
P mellitus, hypertension, children, renal disease, pregnancy **B,** glaucoma

Pharmacokinetics

Absorption	Well absorbed (PO)
Distribution	Unknown
Metabolism	Liver
Excretion	Kidneys (85%), breast milk
Half-life	2 hr; increased in renal disease

Pharmacodynamics

	PO	IM
Onset	Unknown	Unknown
Peak	1 hr	Unknown
Duration	6 hr	Unknown

Interactions

Individual drugs

Cimetidine: ↓ metabolism, ↑ toxicity

Ketamine: Do not use together; seizures may occur

Phenytoin: ↓ levels of phenytoin

Drug classifications

Barbiturates: ↓ effect of dyphylline

β-Adrenergic blockers: ↓ metabolism, ↑ toxicity

Benzodiazepines: ↓ sedative effect

Sympathomimetics: ↑ CNS, CV adverse reactions

Smoking

↑ Metabolism, ↓ effect

Food/drug

Caffeinated foods (cola, coffee, tea, chocolate): ↑ CNS, CV, adverse reactions

NURSING CONSIDERATIONS

Assessment

- Monitor dyphylline blood levels (therapeutic level is <20 μg/ml); toxicity (dysrhythmias, seizures, diuresis, flushing, headache) may occur with small increase above 20 μg/ml, especially elderly; determine whether theophylline was given recently (24 hr)
- Monitor I&O; an increase in diuresis occurs; dehydration may result in elderly or children
- Assess respiratory rate, rhythm, depth; before and during treatment auscultate lung fields bilaterally; notify prescriber of abnormalities
- Assess for allergic reactions: rash, urticaria; if these occur, drug should be discontinued
- Assess for drug toxicity: nausea, vomiting, anorexia, cramping, diarrhea, confusion

Nursing diagnoses

- ✓ Injury, high risk for (uses, adverse reactions)
- ✓ Airway clearance, ineffective (uses)
- ✓ Activity intolerance (uses)
- ✓ Knowledge deficit (teaching)

Implementation

PO route

- Give around the clock to maintain blood levels, qd dose each AM
- Give 1 hr ac and 2 hr pc to increase absorption; elix should be measured accurately

IM route

- Inject slowly; do not give by **IV** route; do not administer if cloudy or a precipitate occurs, avoid this route

Patient/family education

- Teach patient to take doses as prescribed, not to skip doses or double dose; patient should check OTC medications and current prescription medications for ephedrine, which increases CNS stimulation; tell patient not to drink alcohol or caffeine products (tea, coffee, chocolate, colas) or CV effects may occur, not to change brands
- Advise patient to avoid hazardous activities; dizziness may occur
- Caution patient if GI upset occurs, to take drug with 8 oz of water and food
- Teach patient to notify prescriber of change in smoking habit; a change in dosage may be required
- Instruct patient to report nausea, vomiting, insomnia, tachycardia, dysrhythmias, convulsions, or restlessness; can indicate toxicity
- Teach patient to increase fluids to 2 L/day to decrease viscosity of secretions
- Advise patient to obtain drug level q6-12 mo

Evaluation

Positive therapeutic outcome

- Decreased dyspnea
- Clear lung fields bilaterally

edrophonium (℞)

(ed-roe-fone'ee-yum)

Enlon, Reversol, Tensilon

Func. class.: Cholinergics, anticholinesterase

Chem. class.: Quaternary ammonium compound

Pregnancy category C

Action: Inhibits destruction of acetylcholine, which increases concentration at sites where acetylcholine is released; this facilitates transmission of impulses across myoneural junction

Therapeutic Outcome: Reversal of nondepolarizing neuromuscular blockers; absence of difficulty with muscular function in myasthenia gravis

Uses: Diagnosis of myasthenia gravis; curare antagonist; differentiation of myasthenic crisis from cholinergic crisis; reversal of nondepolarizing neuromuscular blockers

Dosage and routes

Tensilon test (myasthenia gravis diagnosis)

Adult: **IV** 1-2 mg over 15-30 sec, then 8 mg if no response; IM 10 mg; if cholinergic reaction occurs, retest after ½ hr with 2 mg IM

P ***Child >34 kg:*** **IV** 2 mg; if no response in 45 sec, then 1 mg q45 sec, not to exceed 10 mg; IM 5 mg

P ***Child <34 kg:*** **IV** 1 mg; if no response in 45 sec, then 1 mg q45 sec, not to exceed 5 mg; IM 2 mg

P ***Infant:*** **IV** 0.5 mg

Reversal of nondepolarizing neuromuscular blockers

Adult: **IV** 10 mg over 30-45 sec, may repeat, not to exceed 40 mg

Differentiation of myasthenic crisis from cholinergic crisis

Adult: **IV** 1 mg, if no response in 1 min, may repeat

Available forms: Inj 10 mg/ml

Adverse effects

CNS: Dizziness, headache, sweating, weakness, **seizures,** uncoordination, **paralysis,** drowsiness, **loss of consciousness**

CV: Dysrhythmias, bradycardia, hypotension, **AV block,** ECG changes, **cardiac arrest,** syncope

EENT: Miosis, blurred vision, lacrimation, visual changes

GI: Nausea, diarrhea, vomiting, cramps, increased salivary and gastric secretions, dysphagia, increased peristalsis

GU: Frequency, incontinence, urgency

INTEG: Rash, urticaria

RESP: **Respiratory depression, bronchospasm, constriction, laryngospasm, respiratory arrest,** dyspnea, increased bronchial secretions

Contraindications: Obstruction of intestine, renal system, hypersensitivity

Precautions: Seizure disorders, bronchial asthma, coronary occlusion, hyperthyroidism, dysrhythmias, peptic ulcer, megacolon, poor GI motility, pregnancy **C**, bradycardia, hypotension

Pharmacokinetics

Absorption	Unknown
Distribution	Unknown
Metabolism	Unknown
Excretion	Unknown
Half-life	Unknown

Pharmacodynamics

	IM	IV
Onset	2-10 min	30-60 sec
Peak	Unknown	Unknown
Duration	12-45 min	6-25 min

Interactions

Individual drugs

Atropine: ↓ action of edrophonium
Digitalis: ↑ bradycardia
Magnesium: ↓ action of edrophonium
Polymixin: ↓ action of edrophonium
Procainamide: ↓ action of edrophonium
Quinidine: ↓ action of edrophonium

Drug classifications

Anesthetics: ↓ action of edrophonium
Anticholinergics: ↓ effect of edrophonium
Antidysrhythmics: ↓ action of edrophonium
Antihistamines: ↓ action of edrophonium

Corticosteroids: ↓ action of edrophonium
Muscle relaxants, depolarizing: ↑ action of muscle relaxant
Phenothiazines: ↓ edrophonium action

NURSING CONSIDERATIONS
Assessment
- Assess vital signs, respiration during test
- Monitor diabetic patient carefully, this drug lowers blood glucose

Nursing diagnoses
✓ Breathing pattern, ineffective (uses)
✓ Knowledge deficit (teaching)

Implementation
IV route
- Administer undiluted 2 mg or less over 15-30 sec, or give as continuous inf in myasthenia crisis
- Give only after ensuring that atropine sulfate is available for cholinergic crisis
- Give only after all other cholinergics have been discontinued
- Store at room temp

Y-site compatibilities: Heparin, hydrocortisone, potassium chloride, vit B/C

Patient/family education
- Instruct patient to wear Medic Alert ID specifying myasthenia gravis and drugs taken

Evaluation
Positive therapeutic outcome
- Increased muscle strength, hand grasp; improved gait; absence of labored breathing (if severe)

Treatment of overdose: Respiratory support, atropine 1-4 mg (**IV**)

efavirenz (℞)
(ef-ah-veer'enz)
Sustiva
Func. class.: Antiretroviral
Chem. class.: Nonnucleoside reverse transcriptase inhibitor (NNRTI)

Pregnancy category C

Action: Binds directly to reverse transcriptase and blocks RNA, DNA causing a disruption of the enzyme's site

Therapeutic Outcome: Improvement of HIV-1 infection

Uses: HIV-1 in combination with other antiretrovirals

Dosage and routes
Given in combination with protease inhibitor or nucleoside analog reverse transcriptase inhibitors (NRTIs)

P ***Adult and child >40 kg:*** PO 600 mg qd hs

P ***Child:***
10-15 kg: PO 200 mg qd hs
15-20 kg: PO 250 mg qd hs
20-25 kg: PO 300 mg qd hs
25-32.5 kg: PO 350 mg qd hs
32.5-40 kg: PO 400 mg qd hs

Available forms: Caps 50, 100, 200 mg

Adverse effects
CNS: Headache, dizziness, fatigue, impaired concentration, insomnia, abnormal dreams, depression
GI: *Diarrhea,* abdominal pain, *nausea*, hyperlipidemia
GU: Hematuria, kidney stones
INTEG: *Rash,* **erythema multiforme, Stevens-Johnson syndrome, toxic epidermal necrolysis**

Contraindiations Hypersensitivity

Precautions: Liver disease, pregnancy **C,** lactation, children <3 yr, renal disease, myelosuppression

Pharmacokinetics

Absorption	Well
Distribution	Highly protein bound (99%)
Metabolism	Liver
Excretion	Kidneys, feces
Half-life	Terminal 52-76 hr

Pharmacodynamics

Unknown

Interactions

Individual drugs

Biaxin: ↓ level of biaxin
Indinavir: ↑ level of indinavir
Midazolam: Do not give together
Ritonavir: ↑ levels of both drugs
Saquinavir: ↓ level of saquinavir
Triazolam: Do not give together
Warfarin: ↑ level of warfarin

Drug classifications

Benzodiazepines: Do not give together
Ergots: Do not give together
Estrogens: ↑ levels of both drugs

Food/drug

↑ Absorption of high fat foods

Lab test interferences

↑ ALT
False positive: Cannabinoids

NURSING CONSIDERATIONS

Assessment

- Assess signs of infection, anemia
- Assess liver studies: ALT, AST; renal studies
- Assess bowel pattern before, during treatment; if severe abdominal pain with bleeding occurs, drug should be discontinued; monitor hydration
- Assess skin eruptions; rash, urticaria, itching
- Assess allergies before treatment, reaction to each medication
- Assess CBC, blood chemistry, plasma HIV RNA, absolute $CD4^+$/$CD8^+$/cell counts/%, serum β_2 microglobulin, serum ICD+24 antigen levels, cholesterol, hepatic enzymes
- Assess for signs of toxicity: severe nausea/vomiting, maculopapular rash

Nursing diagnoses

- ✓ Infection, risk for (uses)
- ✓ Diarrhea (side effects)
- ✓ Knowledge deficit (teaching)

Implementation

- Give hs to decrease CNS side effects, may be given without regard to food, avoid high-fat foods

Patient/family education

- Inform patient that drug does not cure disease but controls symptoms, HIV still can be transmitted to others
- Advise patient to take as prescribed; if dose is missed, take as soon as remembered; do not double dose, take with water/juice; may be taken with or without food
- Instruct patient to make sure health care provider knows of all the medications being taken, supplements, herbs, OTC drugs
- Advise patient that if severe rash occurs, stop taking and notify health care provider
- Advise patient not to breast-feed or become pregnant if taking this drug
- Advise patient that adverse reactions: rash, dizziness, abnormal dreams, insomnia, lessen after a month
- Teach patient to avoid hazardous activities if dizziness, drowsiness occurs

Evaluation

Positive therapeutic outcome

- Increased CD4, cell counts
- Decreased viral load
- Improvement in symptoms and progression of HIV-1 infection

E

enalapril/ enalaprilat (℞)

(e-nal′april/e-nal′a-pril-at)

Vasotec, Vasotec IV

Func. class.: Antihypertensive

Chem. class.: Angiotensin-converting enzyme inhibitor

Pregnancy category
D (2nd/3rd trimesters), C (1st trimester)

Action: Selectively suppresses renin-angiotensin-aldosterone system; inhibits ACE; prevents conversion of angiotensin I to angiotensin II, resulting in dilatation of arterial and venous vessels

Therapeutic Outcome: Decreased B/P in hypertension; decreased preload, afterload in CHF

Uses: Hypertension, systolic CHF, diabetic neuropathy, after MI, left ventricular dysfunction

Dosage and routes

Adult: PO 5 mg/day, may increase or decrease to desired response; range 10-40 mg/day

Hypertension

Adult: **IV** 1.25 mg q6h over 5 min

P ***Child:*** PO 0.1 mg/kg/day in 1-2 divided doses, max 0.5 mg/kg/day

P ***Child:*** **IV** 5-10 μg/kg/dose q8-24h

Patients on diuretics

Adult: **IV** 0.625 mg over 5 min, may give additional doses of 1.25 mg q6h

Renal dose

Adult: PO 2.5 mg qd (CrCl <30 ml/min) increase gradually; **IV** CrCl >30 ml/min 1.25 mg q6h; CrCl <30 ml/min 0.625 mg as one-time dose, increase as per B/P

CHF

Adult: PO 5-20 mg/day in 2 divided doses

Available forms: Enalapril: tabs 2.5, 5, 10, 20 mg; enalaprilat: inj 1.25 mg/ml

Adverse effects

CNS: *Insomnia, dizziness,* paresthesias, headache, fatigue, anxiety

CV: *Hypotension,* chest pain, tachycardia, **dysrhythmias,** syncope

EENT: *Tinnitus,* visual changes, sore throat, double vision, dry burning eyes

GI: Nausea, vomiting, colitis, cramps, diarrhea, constipation, flatulence, dry mouth, loss of taste

GU: **Proteinuria, renal failure,** increased frequency of polyuria or oliguria

HEMA: **Agranulocytosis, neutropenia**

INTEG: Rash, purpura, alopecia, hyperhidrosis

META: Hyperkalemia

RESP: Dyspnea, dry cough, rales, angioedema

Contraindications: Hypersensitivity, history of angioedema, pregnancy **D** (2nd/3rd trimesters), lactation

Precautions: Renal disease, hyperkalemia, hepatic failure, dehydration, bilateral renal artery stenosis, pregnancy **C** (1st trimester)

Do Not Confuse:
enalapril/Eldepryl, enalapril/ramipril

Pharmacokinetics	
Absorption	Well absorbed (PO), complete (**IV**)
Distribution	Unknown
Metabolism	Liver (active metabolite—enalaprilat)
Excretion	Kidneys (60%—enalaprilat, 20%—enalapril)
Half-life	Enalaprilat 11 hr, increased in renal disease

Pharmacodynamics

	PO	IV
Onset	1 hr	15 min
Peak	4-6 hr	1-4 hr
Duration	24 hr	6 hr

Interactions

Individual drugs

Alcohol: ↑ hypotension (large amounts)
Allopurinol: ↑ hypersensitivity
Digoxin: ↑ serum levels
Hydralazine: ↑ toxicity
Indomethacin: ↓ antihypertensive effect
Lithium: ↑ serum levels
Prazosin: ↑ toxicity

Drug classifications

α-Adrenergic blockers: ↑ hypotension
Antacids: ↓ absorption
Diuretics: ↑ hypotension
Diuretics, potassium-sparing: ↑ toxicity
Nitrates: ↑ hypotension
Phenothiazines: ↑ hypotension
Potassium supplements: ↑ toxicity
Sympathomimetics: ↑ toxicity

Lab test interferences

↑ ALT, ↑ AST, ↑ bilirubin, ↑ alkaline phosphatase, ↑ glucose, ↑ uric acid
False positive: ANA titer

NURSING CONSIDERATIONS

Assessment

- Monitor blood studies: neutrophils, decreased platelets with differential baseline and q3 mo if neutrophils <1000/mm^3, discontinue treatment
- Monitor B/P, orthostatic hypotension, syncope; if changes occur dosage change may be required; obtain peak/trough levels
- Monitor electrolytes: K, Na, Cl during 1st 2 wk of therapy
- Monitor renal studies: protein, BUN, creatinine; increased levels may indicate nephrotic syndrome and renal failure
- Monitor renal symptoms: polyuria, oliguria, frequency, dysuria
- Establish baselines in renal, liver function tests before therapy begins and 1 wk into therapy
- Check potassium levels throughout treatment, although hyperkalemia rarely occurs
- Check for edema in feet, legs daily
- Assess for allergic reactions: rash, fever, pruritus, urticaria; drug should be discontinued if antihistamines fail to help

Nursing diagnoses

✓ Cardiac output, decreased (uses)
✓ Injury, potential for (adverse reactions)
✓ Knowledge deficit (teaching)
✓ Noncompliance (teaching)

Implementation

PO route

- Store in air-tight container at 86° F (30° C) or less
- Severe hypotension may occur after 1st dose of this medication; decreased hypotension may be prevented by reducing or discontinuing diuretic therapy 3 days before beginning benazepril therapy
- Give by **IV** inf of 0.9% NaCl (as ordered) to expand fluid volume if severe hypotension occurs

IV **IV route**

- Give **IV** direct over 5 min
- Dilute in 50 ml of 0.9% NaCl, D_5W, D_5/0.9% NaCl, D_5/LR; diluted solution may be used for 24 hr

Y-site compatibilities:

Allopurinol, amifostine, amikacin, aminophylline, ampicillin, ampicillin/sulbactam, aztreonam, butorphanol, calcium gluconate, cefazolin, cefoperazone, ceftazidime, ceftizoxime, chloramphenicol, cimetidine, cladribine, clindamycin, dextran 40, dobutamine, dopamine, erythromycin lactobionate, esmolol, famotidine, fentanyl, filgrastim, ganciclovir, gentamicin, granisetron, heparin, hetastarch, hydrocortisone, labetalol, lidocaine, magnesium sulfate, melphalan, meropenem, methylprednisolone, metronidazole, morphine, nafcillin, nicardipine, penicillin G potassium, phenobarbital, piperacillin, piperacillin/tazobactam, potassium chloride, potassium phosphate, propofol, ranitidine, teniposide, thiotepa, tobramycin, trimethoprim/sulfamethoxazole, vancomycin, vinorelbine

Y-site incompatibilities: Amphotericin B, phenytoin

Additive compatibilities: Dobutamine, dopamine, heparin, meropenem, nitroglycerin, nitroprusside, potassium chloride

Patient/family education

- Advise patient not to discontinue drug abruptly; advise patient to tell all persons associated with health care that drug is being taken
- Teach patient not to use OTC products (cough, cold, allergy medications) unless directed by physician, to avoid salt substitutes; serious side effects can occur; xanthines, such as coffee, tea, chocolate, cola can prevent action of drug
- Instruct patient on the importance of complying with dosage schedule, even if feeling better; to continue with medical regimen to decrease B/P: exercise, cessation of smoking, decreasing stress, diet modifications
- Emphasize the need to rise slowly to sitting or standing position to minimize orthostatic hypotension; not to exercise in hot weather, which can cause increased hypotension
- Advise patient to notify prescriber of mouth sores, sore throat, fever, swelling of hands or feet, irregular heartbeat, chest pain, coughing, shortness of breath
- Caution patient to report excessive perspiration, dehydration, vomiting, diarrhea; may lead to fall in B/P
- Caution patient that drug may cause skin rash or impaired perspiration; that angioedema may occur and to discontinue if it occurs
- Caution patient that drug may cause dizziness, fainting, light-headedness; may occur during 1st few days of therapy; to avoid activities that may be hazardous
- Teach patient how to take B/P, and normal readings for age group

Evaluation

Positive therapeutic outcome

- Decreased B/P in hypertension

Treatment of overdose:

Lavage, **IV** atropine for bradycardia; **IV** theophylline for bronchospasm, digitalis, O_2; diuretic for cardiac failure, hemodialysis

enoxacin (℞)

(en-ox'a-sin)

Penetrex

Func. class.: Antiinfective

Chem. class.: Fluoroquinolone

Pregnancy category C

Action: Interferes with conversion of intermediate DNA fragments into high–molecular-weight DNA in bacteria; DNA gyrase inhibitor

➡ **Therapeutic Outcome:** Bactericidal against the following organisms: staphylococci, *Enterobacter* sp, *Escherichia coli, Klebsiella* sp, *Neisseria gonorrhea, Pseudomonas aeruginosa*

Uses: Uncomplicated urethral or cervical gonorrhea, uncomplicated and complicated UTI

Dosage and routes

Gonorrhea

Adult: PO 400 mg as a single dose

Uncomplicated UTI

Adult: PO 200 mg q12h × 7 days

Complicated UTI

Adult: PO 400 mg q12h × 14 days

Renal dose
CrCl <30 ml/min give initial dose, then give 50% of dose q12h

Available forms: Tabs 200, 400 mg

Adverse effects
CNS: *Dizziness, headache,* fatigue, somnolence, depression, insomnia, anxiety, **seizures**
EENT: Visual disturbances, dizziness
GI: *Diarrhea, nausea, vomiting,* anorexia, flatulence, heartburn, abdominal pain, dry mouth, increased AST, ALT
INTEG: Rash, pruritus, photosensitivity
SYST: **Anaphylaxis, Stevens-Johnson syndrome**

Contraindications: Hypersensitivity to quinolones

P G **Precautions:** Pregnancy **C,** lactation, children, elderly, renal disease, seizure disorders

Do Not Confuse:
enoxacin/enoxaparin

Pharmacokinetics	
Absorption	Well absorbed
Distribution	Widely
Metabolism	Liver 20%
Excretion	Kidneys 50%-80%
Half-life	3-6 hr, increased in renal disease

Pharmacodynamics	
Onset	Unknown
Peak	Unknown

Interactions
Individual drugs
Aminophylline: ↑ level of aminophylline
Bismuth subsalicylate: ↓ enoxacin level, ↓ effects of enoxacin
Caffeine: ↓ effect of enoxacin
Cimetidine: ↑ action of enoxacin
Cyclosporine: ↑ nephrotoxicity
Digoxin: ↑ digoxin levels
Nitrofurantoin: ↓ effectiveness
Probenecid: ↑ blood levels
Sucralfate: ↓ absorption of enoxacin
Theophylline: ↑ toxicity
Warfarin: ↑ warfarin effect, ↑ toxicity
Zinc sulfate: ↓ absorption of enoxacin, ↓ effects of enoxacin
Drug classifications
Oral anticoagulants:
Food/drug
↓ Absorption, dairy products

NURSING CONSIDERATIONS

Assessment
- Assess patient for previous sensitivity reaction to quinolones
- Assess patient for signs and symptoms of infection including WBC >10,000/mm^3, hematuria, foul-smelling urine; obtain baseline information before and during treatment
- Complete C&S testing before beginning drug therapy; this will identify if correct treatment has been initiated
- Assess for anaphylaxis: rash, urticaria, pruritus; may occur a few days after therapy begins, emergency equipment should be available
- Identify urine output; also monitor increases in BUN, creatinine
- Monitor blood studies: AST, ALT, alkaline phosphatase

Nursing diagnoses
- ✓ Infection, risk for (uses)
- ✓ Diarrhea (adverse reactions)
- ✓ Knowledge deficit (teaching)
- ✓ Noncompliance (teaching)

Implementation
- Give 1 hr ac or 2 hr pc to maintain proper blood levels
- Give with 8 oz of water, 1 hr before hs to prevent ulceration
- Do not give 4 hr before or 2 hr after medication
- Give 2 hr before or 2 hr after antacids, zinc, iron, or calcium

Patient/family education
- Instruct patient to increase fluids to 2 L/day to prevent crystallization in the kidney

- Instruct patient to report itching, rash, pruritus, urticaria
- Instruct patient to contact prescriber if adverse reactions occur or if inflammation or pain of tendon occurs
- Instruct patient to take all medication prescribed for the length of time ordered; drug must be taken as ordered
- Advise patient to limit intake of alkaline foods and drugs: milk, dairy products, peanuts, vegetables, alkaline antacids, sodium bicarbonate, not to double or miss doses
- Advise patient to ambulate, perform activities with assistance, do not perform hazardous activities
- Advise to avoid OTC medications unless approved by prescriber

Evaluation

Positive therapeutic outcome

- Reported improvement in symptoms of infection
- Negative C&S test results

HIGH ALERT

enoxaparin (℞)

(ee-nox'a-par-in)

Lovenox

Func. class.: Anticoagulant, antithrombotic

Chem. class.: Unfractionated porcine heparin (low-molecular heparin)

Pregnancy category B

Action: Prevents conversion of fibrinogen to fibrin and prothrombin to thrombin by enhancing inhibitory effects of antithrombin III; produces higher ratio of anti-factor Xa to anti-factor IIa

➡ **Therapeutic Outcome:** Prevention of deep vein thrombosis

Uses: Prevention of deep vein thrombosis, pulmonary emboli in hip and knee replacement

Dosage and routes

Hip/knee replacement

Adult: SC 30 mg bid given 12-24 hr postoperatively for 7-10 days, provided that hemostasis has been established

Abdominal surgery

Adult: SC 40 mg qd × 7-10 days to prevent thromboembolic complications, start 2 hr before surgery

Prevention of ischemic complications in unstable angina/non-Q-wave MI with aspirin

Adult: SC 1 mg/kg q12h until stable with aspirin 100-325 mg qd

Available forms: Inj 30 mg/0.3 ml, 40 mg/0.4 ml, 60 mg/0.6 ml, 80 mg/0.8 ml, 100 mg/1 ml

Adverse effects

CNS: Fever, confusion

CV: **Cardiac toxicity**

GI: Nausea

GU: Edema, peripheral edema

HEMA: **Hypochromic anemia, thrombocytopenia,** bleeding

INTEG: Ecchymosis

Contraindications: Hypersensitivity to this drug, heparin, or pork; hemophilia; leukemia with bleeding; peptic ulcer disease; thrombocytopenic purpura, heparin-induced thrombocytoparia

G **Precautions:** Alcoholism, elderly, pregnancy **B,** hepatic disease (severe), renal disease (severe), blood dyscrasias, severe hypertension, subacute bacterial endocarditis, acute nephritis,
P lactation, children

Do Not Confuse: enoxaparin/enoxacin

Pharmacokinetics

Absorption	Well absorbed (90%)
Distribution	Unknown
Metabolism	Unknown
Excretion	Kidneys
Half-life	4½ hr

Pharmacodynamics	
Onset	Unknown
Peak	3-5 hr
Duration	Unknown

Interactions
Drug classifications
Anticoagulants: ↑ bleeding
Antiplatelets: ↑ bleeding
NSAIDs: ↑ bleeding
Salicylates: ↑ bleeding
Herb/drug
Bromelain: ↑ risk of bleeding
Cinchona bark: ↑ risk of bleeding
Lab test interferences
↑ T_3 uptake, AST/ALT
↓ Uric acid, platelets

NURSING CONSIDERATIONS
Assessment
- Monitor blood studies (Hct, CBC, coagulation studies, occult blood in stools), anti-Xa levels q3 mo; platelet count q2-3 days; thrombocytopenia may occur
- Assess patient for bleeding gums, petechiae, ecchymosis, black tarry stools, hematuria, epistaxis, decrease in B/P; indicate bleeding and possible hemorrhage; notify prescriber immediately
- Assess for neurosymptoms in patients that have received spinal anesthesia

Nursing diagnoses
- ✓ Injury, risk for (uses, adverse reactions)
- ✓ Tissue perfusion, altered (uses)
- ✓ Knowledge deficit (teaching)

Implementation
- Give at same time each day to maintain steady blood levels
- Administer SC deeply; do not give IM, begin 2 hr before surgery, do not aspirate, do not expel bubble from syringe before administration; sol is clear to yellow; do not use sol with precipitate; apply gentle pressure for 1 min
- Leave vascular access sheath in place for 6 hr after dose, then give next dose, 6 hr after sheath removed
- Give to recumbent patient, rotate sites (left/right anterolateral, left/right posterolateral abdominal wall)

Patient/family education
- Warn patient to avoid OTC preparations unless directed by prescriber because they could cause serious drug interactions
- Instruct patient to use soft-bristled toothbrush to avoid bleeding gums; to avoid contact sports; to use electric razor; to avoid IM inj
- Advise patient to report any signs of bleeding, bruising: gums, under skin, urine, stools

Evaluation
Positive therapeutic outcome
- Absence of deep vein thrombosis

entacapone (℞)
(en-ta'-ka-pone)
Comtan
Func. class.: Antiparkinsonian agent
Chem. class.: COMT

Pregnancy category C

Action: Inhibits COMT (catechol-O-methyltransferase) and alters the plasma pharmacokinetics of levodopa; given with levodopa/carbidopa

Therapeutic Outcome: Decreased symptoms of Parkinson's disease (involuntary movements)

Uses: Parkinsonism in those experiencing end of dose, decreased effect as an adjunct to levodopa/carbidopa

Dosage and routes
Adult: PO 200 mg given with carbidopa/levodopa, max 1600 mg/day

Available forms: Tabs 200 mg film coated

Adverse effects
CNS: *Involuntary choreiform movements, dyskinesia, hypokinesia,*

hyperkinesia, hand tremors, fatigue, headache, anxiety, twitching, numbness, weakness, confusion, agitation, nightmares, psychosis, hallucinations, hypomania, severe depression, dizziness
CV: *Orthostatic hypotension*
GI: *Nausea, vomiting, anorexia, abdominal distress, dry mouth, flatulence, dyspepsia,* gastritis, GI disorder, *diarrhea, constipation*
INTEG: Rash, sweating, alopecia
MISC: Dark urine, back pain, taste perversion, dyspnea, purpura, fatigue, asthenia, infection-bacterial

Contraindications: Hypersensitivity

Precautions: Renal, hepatic disease, pregnancy **C,** affective disorders, psychosis, lactation, children P

Pharmacokinetics	
Absorption	Well absorbed
Distribution	Protein binding 98%
Metabolism	Liver extensively
Excretion	Kidneys, feces; breast milk
Half-life	0.5 hr initial, 2.5 hr second

Pharmacodynamics	
Onset	Unknown
Peak	Unknown
Duration	≤8 hr

Interactions

Individual drugs

Ampicillin: ↓ excretion of entacapone
Apomorphine: ↑ CV reactions, avoid use
Bitolterol: ↑ CV reactions, avoid use
Chloramphenicol: ↓ excretion of entacapone
Cholestyramine: ↓ excretion
Dobutamine: ↑ CV reactions, avoid use
Dopamine: ↑ CV reactions, avoid use
Epinephrine: ↑ CV reactions, avoid use
Erythromycin: ↓ excretion of entacapone
Isoetharine: ↑ CV reactions, avoid use
Methyldopa: ↑ CV reactions, avoid use
Norepinephrine: ↑ CV reactions, avoid use
Probenecid: May decrease excretion of entacapone
Rifampin: ↓ excretion of entacapone

Drug classifications

MAOIs: Prevents catecholamine metabolism, do not use together

NURSING CONSIDERATIONS

Assessment

- Assess for neuroleptic malignant syndrome: high temp, increased CPK, rigidity, change in consciousness
- Monitor B/P, respiration during initial treatment; hypotension should be reported
- Assess mental status: affect, mood, behavioral changes, depression; complete suicide assessment
- Monitor liver function enzymes: AST, ALT, alkaline phosphatase; also check LDH, bilirubin, CBC
- Assess for involuntary movements in parkinsonism: akinesia, tremors, staggering gait, muscle rigidity, drooling; these symptoms should improve with therapy when given with levodopa/carbidopa

Nursing diagnoses

- ✓ Mobility, impaired (uses)
- ✓ Injury, risk for (uses)
- ✓ Knowledge deficit (teaching)
- ✓ Noncompliance (teaching)

Implementation

- Adjust dosage to patient response
- Give with meals to decrease GI upset; limit protein taken with drug
- Give only after MAOIs have been discontinued for 2 wk

Patient/family education

- Advise patient that hallucinations, mental changes, nausea, dyskinesia can occur
- Caution patient to change positions slowly to prevent orthostatic

hypotension; not to drive or operate machinery until stabilized on medication and mental performance is not affected

- Instruct patient to use drug exactly as prescribed
- Inform patient that urine, sweat may darken
- Inform patient to notify prescriber if pregnancy is suspected; if lactating, drug is excreted in breast milk

Evaluation

Positive therapeutic outcome

- Decreased akathisia, other involuntary movements when used with levodopa/carbidopa
- Increased mood when used with levodopa/carbidopa

HIGH ALERT

ephedrine (℞, OTC)

(e-fed'rin)

ephedrine, ephedrine sulfate, Neorespin, Kondon's Nasal Jelly, Pretz-D, Vicks Vatronel

Func. class.: Bronchodilator, nonselective, adrenergic, mixed direct and indirect effects; bronchodilator, nasal decongestant, vasopressor

Chem. class.: Phenylisopropylamine

Pregnancy category C

Action: Increases contractility and heart rate by acting on β-receptors in the heart; also acts on α-receptors, causing vasoconstriction in blood vessels

➔ **Therapeutic Outcome:** Decreased nasal congestion, bronchodilatation, stimulation, increased B/P

Uses: Shock; increased perfusion; hypotension, bronchodilatation; nasal congestion; orthostatic hypotension, depression, narcolepsy; vasopressor

Dosage and routes

Adult: IM/SC 25-50 mg, not to exceed 150 mg/24 hr; **IV** 10-25 mg, not to exceed 150 mg/24 hr

P ***Child:*** SC/**IV** 3 mg/kg/day or 100 mg/m²/day in divided doses q4-6h or 16.7 mg/m² q4-6h

Bronchodilator

P ***Adult and child ≥12 yr:*** PO 25-50 mg bid-qid, not to exceed 400 mg/day; IM/SC 12½-25 mg

P ***Child 6-12 yr:*** 6.25-12.5 mg q4h, max 75 mg/24 hr

P ***Child >2 yr:*** PO 2-3 mg/kg/day or 100 mg/m²/day in 4-6 divided doses

Nasal decongestant

P ***Adult and child >6 yr:*** Nasal i-ii sprays in each nostril prn q4h for <3-4 days

Stimulation

Adult: PO 25-50 mg q3-4h prn

P ***Child:*** PO 3 mg/kg/day or 100 mg/m²/day in 4-6 divided doses

Orthostatic hypotension

Adult: PO 25 mg qd-qid

P ***Child:*** PO 3 mg/kg/day in 4-6 divided doses

Labor

Adult: Administer dose to maintain B/P at or <130/80 mm Hg

Available forms: Inj 25, 30, 50 mg/ml; caps 25, 50 mg; nasal spray 0.25%; nasal drops 0.5%; nasal jelly 1%

Adverse effects

CNS: *Tremors, anxiety,* insomnia, sweating, headache, dizziness, confusion, hallucinations, **seizures, CNS depression, cerebral hemorrhage**

CV: Palpitations, tachycardia, hypertension, chest pain, **dysrhythmias**

EENT: Rebound congestion (nasal)

GI: *Anorexia, nausea, vomiting*

GU: Dysuria, urinary retention

RESP: *Dyspnea*

Contraindications: Hypersensitivity to sympathomimetics, angle-closure glaucoma, nonanaphylactic shock during general anesthesia

Precautions: Pregnancy **C,** cardiac disorders, hyperthyroidism, diabetes mellitus, prostatic hypertrophy, hypertension

Pharmacokinetics

Absorption	Well absorbed (PO/IM/SC) complete (**IV**)
Distribution	Unknown
Metabolism	Liver
Excretion	Kidneys—unchanged
Half-life	3-5 hr

Pharmacodynamics

	PO	SC	IM	IV	NASAL
Onset	¼-1 hr	Unkn	15-30 min	5 min	Unkn
Peak	Unkn	Unkn	Unkn	Unkn	Unkn
Duration	2-4 hr	1 hr	1 hr	2 hr	6 hr

Interactions

Drug classifications

α-Adrenergic blockers: ↓ effect of ephedrine
Anesthetics, halothane: Increased dysrhythmias
Antidepressants, tricyclic: ↓ effect of vasopressor
β-Adrenergic blockers: Blocks therapeutic effect
Bronchodilators, aerosol: ↑ action of bronchodilator
Cardiac glycosides: ↑ dysrhythmia
Diuretics: ↓ effect of ephedrine
MAOIs: ↑ chance of hypertensive crisis, do not use together
Oxytoxics: ↑ severe hypertension
Sympathomimetics: ↑ adrenergic side effects

NURSING CONSIDERATIONS

Assessment

- Monitor respiratory function: vital capacity, forced expiratory volume, ABGs, lung sounds, heart rate, baseline rhythm (bronchodilator)
- Monitor for evidence of allergic reactions; paradoxical bronchospasm; withhold dose; notify prescriber
- Monitor ECG, B/P, pulse, q5 min when using **IV** route (shock)
- Assess for paresthesias and coldness of extremities; peripheral blood flow may decrease; long-term use may produce pseudo anxiety state requiring sedatives, increased lactic acid with severe metabolic acidosis
- Assess nasal congestion to identify factors contributing to ongoing congestion (nasal use)
- Assess mental status and sleeping patterns; mood, sensorium, ability to stay awake

Nursing diagnoses

- ☑ Airway clearance, ineffective (uses)
- ☑ Gas exchange impaired (uses)
- ☑ Sleep pattern disturbance (uses)
- ☑ Knowledge deficit (teaching)

Implementation

PO route

- Administer several hr (up to 6 hr) before hs to prevent sleeplessness

IV route

- Give **IV** directly undiluted using 3-way stopcock or Y-site; give 10-25 mg slowly, may repeat in 5-10 min
- Use clear sol without precipitate; unused sol should be discarded, protect from light

Syringe compatibilities:
Pentobarbital

Y-site compatibilities:
Etomidate, propofol

Additive compatibilities:
Chloramphenicol, lidocaine, metaraminol, nafcillin, penicillin G potassium

Solution compatibilities:
0.9% NaCl, 0.45% NaCl, D_5W, $D_{10}W$, Ringer's, LR

Patient/family education

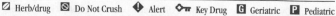

- Advise patient to avoid use of OTC

medications; extra stimulation may occur, and not to use alcohol

Evaluation

Positive therapeutic outcome

- Increased B/P (vasopressor)
- Ability to stay awake (absence of narcolepsy) or improved mood (absence of depression)
- Absence of bronchospasm
- Decreased nasal congestion

HIGH ALERT

epinephrine (℞, OTC)

(ep-i-nef'rin)

Ana-Guard, AsthmaHaler, AsthmaNefrin (racepinephrine), Bronitin Mist, Bronkaid Mist, Dysne-Inhal, epinephrine, Epinal, Epitrate, Eppy/N, Glaucon, Epinephrine Pediatric, EpiPen, EpiPen Jr., Medihaler-Epi, microNefrin, Nephron Inhalant, Primatene Mist, S-2 Inhalant, Sus-Phrine, Vaponefrin

Func. class.: Bronchodilator, nonselective adrenergic agonist, cardiac stimulant, vasopressor

Chem. class.: Catecholamine

Pregnancy category C

Action: β_1- and β_2-agonist causing increased levels of cyclic AMP producing bronchodilatation, cardiac and CNS stimulation; large doses cause vasoconstriction via α-receptors; small doses can cause vasodilation via β_2-vascular receptors

Therapeutic Outcome: Vasoconstrictor, cardiac stimulator, bronchodilator, decreased aqueous humor

Uses: Acute asthmatic attacks, hemostasis, bronchospasm, anaphylaxis, allergic reactions, cardiac arrest, adjunct in anesthesia, shock

Dosage and routes

Asthma

P ***Adult and child:*** INH 1-2 puffs of 1:100 or 2.25% racemic q15 min

Bronchodilator (parenteral epinephrine solution)

Adult: SC 0.2-0.5 mg, q20 min-4 hr max 1 mg/dose

Anaphylactic shock/ vasopressor

Adult: SC/IM 0.1-0.5 mg, repeat q5 min if needed, then **IV** 0.1-0.25 mg, repeat q5-15 min or inf 1 mg/min, increase to 4 mg/min

P ***Child <30 kg:*** SC/IM/**IV** 10 μg/ kg, repeat q5-15 min, up to 0.3 mg

Anaphylactic reaction/ asthma

Adult: SC/IM 0.2-0.5 mg, repeat q10-15 min, not to exceed 1 mg/dose; epinephrine susp 0.5 mg SC, may repeat 0.5-1.5 mg q6h

P ***Child:*** SC 0.01 mg/kg, repeat q15 min × 2 doses, then q4h as needed, up to 0.5 mg/dose; epinephrine susp 0.025 mg/kg SC, may repeat q6h, max 0.75 mg in child ≤30 kg

Bronchodilator

P ***Adult and child:*** INH 1-2 puffs of 1:100 or 2.25% racepineprine, 0.2 mg/dose, may repeat q3h

Adult: OPHTH: 1 gtt qd or bid

Cardiac arrest

Adult: IC, **IV**, endotracheal 0.1-1 mg repeat q5 min prn

P ***Child:*** IC, **IV**, endotracheal 5-10 μg q5 min, may use 0.1 μg/kg/min **IV** inf after initial dose

Available forms: Aerosol 0.16, 0.2, 0.25 mg/spray, inj 1:1000 (1 mg/ml), 1:200 (5 mg/ml), 0.01 mg/ml (1:100,000), 0.1 mg/ml (1:10,000), 0.5 mg/ml (1:2,000); IM, **IV**, SC; sol for nebulization 1:100, 1.25% 2.25% (base)

Adverse effects

CNS: *Tremors, anxiety,* insomnia,

headache, dizziness, weakness, drowsiness, headache, confusion, hallucinations, **cerebral hemorrhage**
CV: Palpitations, tachycardia, hypertension, *dysrhythmias,* increased T-wave
GI: Anorexia, nausea, vomiting
RESP: Dyspnea

Contraindications: Hypersensitivity to sympathomimetics, narrow-angle glaucoma, nonanaphylactic shock during general anesthesia, organic brain syndrome, cardiac dilatation, coronary insufficiency, cerebral arteriosclerosis, organic heart disease

Precautions: Pregnancy **C**, cardiac disorders, hyperthyroidism, diabetes mellitus, prostatic hypertrophy, G elderly, lactation, hypertension

Pharmacokinetics

Absorption	Well absorbed (PO), complete (**IV**)
Distribution	Unknown, crosses placenta
Metabolism	Liver
Excretion	Breast milk
Half-life	Unknown

Pharmacodynamics

	SC	IM	IV	INH
Onset	3-5 min	5-10 min	Immediate	1 min
Peak	Unknown	Unknown	Unknown	Unknown
Duration	1-4 hr	1-4 hr	Unknown	1-4 hr

Interactions
Individual drugs
Insulin: ↑ need for insulin in diabetics
Lithium: ↓ effect of epinephrine
Methyldopa: ↑ pressor response
Drug classifications
α-Adrenergic blockers: ↓ hypertensive effects
Anesthetics, general: ↑ dysrythmias
Antidepressants, tricyclic: ↑ pressor response
Antihistamines: ↑ pressor response
β-Adrenergic blockers: Block therapeutic effect
Bronchodilators, aerosol: ↑ action of bronchodilator
Cardiac glycosides: ↑ dysrhythmias
Diuretics: ↓ vascular response
Ergots: ↓ vascular response
MAOIs: ↑ chance of hypertensive crisis
Other sympathomimetics: ↑ adrenergic side effects, additive effects
Phenothiazines: ↓ vascular response

NURSING CONSIDERATIONS
Assessment
- Monitor respiratory function: vital capacity, forced expiratory volume, ABGs, lung sounds, heart rate, rhythm (baseline); amount, color of sputum
- Monitor ECG during administration continuously; if B/P increases, drug should be decreased; check B/P, pulse q5 min after parenteral route; CVP, PCWP, SVR; inadvertent high arterial B/P can result in angina, aortic rupture, cerebral hemorrhage
- Check inj site for tissue sloughing; if this occurs, administer phentolamine mixed with 0.9% NaCl
- Monitor for evidence of allergic reactions, paradoxical bronchospasm, withhold dose, notify prescriber; sulfite sensitivity, which may be life threatening

Nursing diagnoses
- ✓ Airway clearance, ineffective (uses)
- ✓ Gas exchange impaired (uses)
- ✓ Cardiac output, decreased (uses)
- ✓ Sensory-perceptual alteration, visual (uses) (ophth)
- ✓ Knowledge deficit (teaching)

Implementation
- Check for correct concentration, route, dosage before administration

IV IV route
- Give after diluting 1 mg of 1:1000

sol/10 ml or more; 0.9% NaCl yields 1:10,000 sol, give l mg/min

- Give by continuous inf after further diluting in 0.9% NaCl, D_5W, $D_{10}W$, D_5/LR, LR via 3-way stopcock; for Y-site, use infusion pump, protect from light; increase dose of insulin in diabetic patients

Syringe compatibilities:
Doxapram, heparin, milrinone

Y-site compatibilities:
Amrinone, atracurium, calcium chloride, calcium gluconate, diltiazem, dobutamine, dopamine, famotidine, fentanyl, furosemide, heparin, hydrocortisone sodium succinate, hydromorphone, labetalol, lorazepam, midazolam, milrinone, morphine, nicardipine, nitroglycerin, norepinephrine, pancuronium, phytonadione, potassium chloride, propofol, ranitidine, vecuronium, vit B/C

Y-site incompatibilities:
Ampicillin

Additive compatibilities:
Amikacin, cimetidine, dobutamine, floxacillin, furosemide, metaraminol, ranitidine, verapamil

Additive incompatibilities:
Aminophylline, mephentermine, sodium bicarbonate, warfarin

SC/IM route

- Rotate inj sites, massage well, do not use gluteal (IM) site
- Shake susp before using

Inhalation route

- Use 2.25% sol diluted in nebulizer/respirator
- 10 gtt of a 1% sol should be placed in nebulizer
- Dilute racepinephrine 2.25% sol

Endotracheal route

- Only used in intubated patient; use **IV** dose that should be injected by endotracheal tube into bronchi

Patient/family education

- Tell patient not to use OTC medications; extra stimulation may occur; to use this medication before other medications and allow at least 5 min between each, to prevent overstimulation
- Teach patient that paradoxical bronchospasm may occur and to stop drug immediately and notify prescriber; to limit caffeine products such as chocolate, coffee, tea, and colas
- Patient should rinse mouth after inh
- Patient should report blurred vision, irritation with ophth preparations

Evaluation

Positive therapeutic outcome

- Absence of dyspnea, wheezing
- Improved airway exchange, improved ABGs
- Decreased aqueous humor
- Stabilization of heart rate and cardiac output

Treatment of overdose:
Administer a β_2-adrenergic blocker, vasodilators, α-blocker

HIGH ALERT

epirubicin (℞)
(ep-i-roo′-bi-sin)
Ellence
Func. class.: Antineoplastic, antibiotic
Chem. class.: Anthracycline
Pregnancy category D

Action: Inhibits DNA synthesis primarily; replication is decreased by binding to DNA, which causes strand splitting; maximum cytotoxic effects at S and G_2 phases; a vesicant

➔ Therapeutic Outcome: Prevention of rapidly growing malignant cells

Uses: Breast cancer as an adjuvant therapy, with axillary node involvement, after resection

Dosage and routes

Adult: **IV** inf 100-120 mg/m²

initially given with other antineoplastics; given in repeated cycles; 3-4 wk cycles

Hepatic Dose

Adult: **IV**, bilirubin 1.2-3 mg/dl or AST 2-4 × normal upper limit, 50% of starting dose; bilirubin >3 mg/dl or AST >4 × normal upper limit, 25% of starting dose

Available forms: Inj 2 mg/ml

Adverse effects

CV: Increased B/P, **sinus tachycardia, PVCs,** chest pain, **bradycardia, extrasystole, CHF**

GI: Nausea, vomiting, diarrhea, anorexia, mucositis

GU: Hot flashes, amenorrhea, hyperuricemia

HEMA: **Thrombocytopenia, leukopenia, anemia, neutropenia, secondary AML**

INTEG: Rash, necrosis at inj site, alopecia

MISC: Infection, febrile neutropenia, lethargy, fever, conjunctivitis

Contraindications: Hypersensitivity to this drug, anthracyclines, anthracenediones, pregnancy **D,** lactation, systemic infections, severe hepatic disease, baseline neutrophil count <1500 cell/mm^3, severe myocardial insufficiency, recent MI

Precautions: Renal, hepatic, cardiac disease, gout, bone marrow suppression (severe), elderly [G], children [P]

Pharmacokinetics

Absorption	Complete bioavailability
Distribution	Widely distributed, crosses placenta
Metabolism	Liver, extensively
Excretion	Bile (60%)
Half-life	3 min; 2.5 hr; 33 hrs

Pharmacodynamics

Unknown

Interactions

Individual drugs

Cimetidine: ↑ epirubicin level, stop cimetidine before giving epirubicin

Radiation: ↑ toxicity, bone marrow suppression

Drug classifications

Antineoplastics: ↑ toxicity, bone marrow suppression

Live virus vaccines: ↑ adverse reactions, ↓ antibody response

NURSING CONSIDERATIONS

Assessment

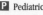

- Monitor left ventricular ejection fraction, multigated acquisition scan or echocardiogram, ECG; watch for ST-T wave changes, low QRS and T; possible dysrhythmias (sinus tachycardia, heart block, PVCs) may occur; assess tachypnea, ECG changes, dyspnea, edema, fatigue; cardiac status: B/P, pulse, character, rhythm, rate, ABGs
- Assess for bone marrow depression, infection
- Assess symptoms indicating severe allergic reaction: rash, pruritus, urticaria, purpuric skin lesions, itching, flushing; drug should be discontinued
- Monitor CBC, differential, platelet count weekly; withhold drug if baseline neutrophil count is <1500/mm^3; notify prescriber of results if WBC <20,000/mm^3, platelets <150,000/mm^3; leukocyte nadir occurs 10-14 days after administration, recovery by 21st day
- Assess for increased uric acid levels, swelling, joint pain, primarily extremities; patient should be well hydrated to prevent urate deposits
- Monitor renal function studies: BUN, creatinine, serum uric acid, urine CrCl before and during therapy; I&O ratio; report fall in urine output to <30 ml/hr; dosage adjustment is needed if serum creatinine >5 mg/dl
- Monitor liver function tests before and during therapy (bilirubin, AST,

ALT, LDH) as needed or monthly; note jaundice of skin or sclera, dark urine, clay-colored stools, itchy skin, abdominal pain, fever, diarrhea
- Assess for bleeding: hematuria, stool guaiac, bruising or petechiae, mucosa or orifices q8h; inflammation of mucosa, breaks in skin
- Identify effects of alopecia on body image; discuss feeling about body changes

Nursing diagnoses

- ✓ Injury, risk for (adverse reactions)
- ✓ Body image disturbance (adverse reactions)
- ✓ Infection, risk for (adverse reactions)
- ✓ Knowledge deficit (teaching)

Implementation

- Avoid contact with skin; very irritating; wash completely to remove; give fluids **IV** or PO before chemotherapy to hydrate patient
- Give antiemetic 30-60 min before giving drug to prevent vomiting and prn
- Administer prophylactic antibiotic with a fluoroquinolone or trimethoprim/sulfamethoxazole if dose of epirubicin is 120 mg/m^2
- Provide liq diet: carbonated beverages; gelatin may be added if patient is not nauseated or vomiting
- Drug should be prepared by experienced personnel using proper precautions
- Give into tubing of free flowing **IV** inf 0.9% NaCl or D_5 over 3-5 min; do not admix with other drugs in syringe
- Use hydrocortisone, dexamethasone, or sodium bicarbonate (1 mEq/1 ml) for extravasation: apply ice compress

Patient/family education

- Advise patient to avoid use of products containing aspirin or NSAIDs, razors, commercial mouthwash, since bleeding may occur; to report symptoms of bleeding (hematuria, tarry stools)
- Instruct patient to report signs of anemia (fatigue, headache, irritability, faintness, shortness of breath)
- Inform patient that hair may be lost during treatment; a wig or hairpiece may make patient feel better; new hair may be different in color, texture
- Caution patient not to have any vaccinations without the advice of the prescriber; serious reactions can occur
- Advise patient to use contraception during treatment and 4 mo afterwards
- Advise patient that urine may appear red for 2 days
- Instruct patient to avoid crowds, persons with known infection
- Caution patient to avoid OTC medications, supplements unless approved by prescriber

Evaluation

Positive therapeutic outcome

- Prevention of rapid division of malignant cells

epoetin (℞)

(ee-poe'e-tin)

Epogen, rHU-EPO, Eprex ✦, Erythropoietin, Procrit

Func. class.: Antianemic, biologic modifier, hormone

Chem. class.: Amino acid polypeptide

Pregnancy category C

Action: Erythropoietin is one factor controlling rate of red cell production; drug is developed by recombinant DNA technology

Therapeutic Outcome: Decreased anemia with increased RBCs

Uses: Anemia caused by reduced endogenous erythropoietin production, primarily end-stage renal disease; to correct hemostatic defect in uremia; anemia caused by AZT (zidovudine) treatment in HIV-positive patients; anemia caused by chemotherapy;

reduction of allogeneic blood transfusion in surgery patients

Dosage and routes

Anemia secondary to chemotherapy

Adult: SC 150 U/kg 3×/wk, may increase after 2 mo up to 300 U/kg 3×/wk

Anemia in chronic renal failure

Adult: SC/**IV** 50-100 U/kg 3×/wk, then adjust dose by 25 U/kg/dose to maintain appropriate Hct; maintenance 12.5-25 U/kg, titrate to target Hct

Anemia secondary to zidovudine treatment

Adult: SC/**IV** 100 U/kg 3×/wk × 2 mo; may increase by 50-100 U/kg q1-2 mo, up to 300 U/kg 3×/wk

Surgery

Adult: SC 300 U/kg/day × 10 days before surgery, the day of surgery and for 4 days postsurgery or 600 U/kg 3, 2, 1 wk before and on day of surgery

Available forms: Inj 2000, 3000, 4000, 10,000, 20,000 U/ml

Adverse effects

CNS: **Seizures,** coldness, sweating, headache

CV: *Hypertension,* **hypertensive encephalopathy**

MS: Bone pain

Contraindications: Hypersensitivity to mammalian cell-derived products, or human albumin, severe hypertension, erythropoietin levels of >200 mU/ml, uncontrolled hypertension

Precautions: Seizure disorder, porphyria, pregnancy **C**

Pharmacokinetics

Absorption	Well absorbed (SC), completely absorbed (**IV**)
Distribution	Unknown
Metabolism	Unknown
Excretion	Unknown
Half-life	5-14 hr

Pharmacodynamics

	SC/IV
Onset	Unknown
Peak	Unknown
Duration	Unknown
Increased RBC count	1-6 wk

Interactions

Drug classifications

Anticoagulants: Need for ↑ anticoagulants during hemodialysis

NURSING CONSIDERATIONS

Assessment

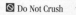

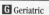

- Monitor renal studies: urinalysis, protein, blood, BUN, creatinine; I&O; report drop in output to <50 ml/hr
- Monitor blood studies: ferritin, transferrin monthly, transferrin sat ≥20%; ferritin ≥100 ng/ml; Hct 2×/wk until stabilized in target range (30%-33%) then at regular intervals; those with endogenous erythropoietin levels of <500 U/L respond to this agent; check for symptoms of anemia: fatigue, pallor, dyspnea
- Assess for CNS symptoms: coldness, sweating, pain in long bones
- Assess CV status: B/P before and during treatment; hypertension may occur rapidly leading to hypertension encephalopathy, antihypertensives may be needed
- Assess patient during hemodialysis for bruits, thrills, or shunts; drug prevents severe anemia in chronic renal failure; clotting may need to be treated with increased anticoagulant
- Assess for seizures if Hct is increased within 2 wk by 4 points
- Monitor serum iron levels, ferritin, transferrin levels; iron therapy may be

needed to prevent recurring anemia
- Monitor B/P, check for rising B/P as Hct rises
- Monitor blood studies: BUN, creatinine, uric acid, platelets, WBC, phosphorus, potassium, bleeding time; Hct, Hgb, RBCs, reticulocytes should be checked in chronic renal failure

Nursing diagnoses

✓ Fatigue (uses)
✓ Activity intolerance (uses)
✓ Knowledge deficit (teaching)

Implementation

IV **IV route**

- Administer by direct route at end of dialysis by venous line, do not shake vial
- If Hct increases by 4% in 2 wk, decrease dose by 25 U/kg
- Give additional heparin to lower chance of clots

Solution compatibilities: NaCl 0.9%, $D_{10}W$, $D_{10}W$/albumin, sterile water for inj, TPN

SC route

- Give by SC route in patients not using dialysis, admix before giving, using 0.9% NaCl with benzyl alcohol 0.9% 1:1

Patient/family education

- Teach patient how to take B/P
- Advise patients to take iron supplements, vit B_{12}, folic acid as directed
- Teach patient to avoid driving or hazardous activity during treatment
- Teach patients with renal disease to include high-iron and low-potassium foods in their diets (meat, dark green leafy vegetables, eggs, enriched breads)
- Teach patient the reason for treatment, expected results
- Advise patient to use contraception (pregnancy may occur)

Evaluation

Positive therapeutic outcome

- Increased appetite
- Enhanced sense of well-being
- Increase in reticulocyte count in 1-2 wk, Hgb, Hct

eprosartan mesylate/ hydrochlorothiazide

See Appendix A, Selected New Drugs

E

HIGH ALERT

eptifibatide (℞)

(ep-tih-fib'ah-tide)

Integrilin

Func. class.: Antiplatelet agent

Chem. class.: Glycoprotein IIb/IIIa inhibitor

Pregnancy category B

Action: Platelet glycoprotein antagonist; reversibly prevents fibrinogen, von Willebrand's factor from binding to the glycoprotein IIb/IIIa receptor, inhibiting platelet aggregation

➔ **Therapeutic Outcome:** Decreased platelets

Uses: Acute coronary syndrome including those with percutaneous coronary intervention (PCI)

Dosage and routes

Acute coronary syndrome

Adult: **IV** BOL 180 μg/kg as soon as diagnosed, then **IV** cont inf 2 μg/kg/min until discharge or coronary artery bypass graft (CABG) up to 72 hr; may decrease inf rate to 0.5 μg/kg/min if undergoing PCI; continue inf for 20-24 hr postprocedure, allowing up to 96 hr of treatment

PCI in patients without acute coronary syndrome

Adult: **IV** BOL 135 μg/kg given immediately before PCI; then 0.5 μg/kg/min × 20-24 hr

Available forms: Sol for inj 2 mg/ml (10 ml), 0.75 mg/ml (100 ml)

Adverse effects

CV: **Stroke**, hypotension
SYST: **Bleeding, anaphylaxis**

Contraindications: Hypersensitivity, active internal bleeding; history of bleeding, stroke within 1 mo; major surgery with severe trauma, severe hypotension, history of intracranial bleeding, intracranial neoplasm, arteriovenous malformation/aneurysm, aortic dissection, dependence on renal dialysis

P **Precautions:** Bleeding, pregnancy
G **B**, lactation, children, elderly, renal function impairment

Pharmacokinetics	
Absorption	Unknown
Distribution	Unknown
Metabolism	Limited
Excretion	Kidneys
Half-life	2.5 hr

Pharmacodynamics	
Onset	Unknown
Peak	Unknown
Duration	Unknown

Interactions

Individual drugs

Abciximab: ↑ bleeding
Aspirin: ↑ bleeding
Clopidogrel: ↑ bleeding
Dipyridamole: ↑ bleeding
Heparin: ↑ bleeding
Plicamycin: ↑ bleeding
Ticlopidine: ↑ bleeding
Valproate: ↑ bleeding

Drug classifications

Anticoagulants: ↑ bleeding
NSAIDs: ↑ bleeding
Platelet receptor inhibitors IIb, IIIa: Do not give together
Thrombolytics: ↑ bleeding

NURSING CONSIDERATIONS

Assessment

- Monitor platelets, Hgb, Hct, creatinine, PT/APTT baseline, INR, within 6 hr of loading dose and qd thereafter; patients undergoing PCI should have ACT monitored; maintain APTT 50-70 sec unless PCI is to be performed; during PCI, ACT should be 300-350 sec; if platelets drop <100,000/mm^3, obtain additional platelet counts; if thrombocytopenia is confirmed, discontinue drug; also draw Hct, Hgb, serum creatinine
- Assess for bleeding: gums, bruising, ecchymosis, petechiae; from GI, GU tract, cardiac catheter sites, IM inj sites

Nursing diagnoses

✓ Tissue perfusion, altered (uses)
✓ Knowledge deficit (teaching)

Implementation

- Aspirin and heparin may be given with this drug
- Discontinue heparin before removing femoral artery sheath after PCI

IV **IV route**

- After withdrawing the bolus dose from 10-ml vial, give **IV** push over 1-2 min; follow bolus dose with cont inf using infusion pump, give drug undiluted directly from the 100-ml vial, spike the 100-ml vial with a vented infusion set, use caution when centering the spike on the circle of the stopper top
- Do not use discolored sol or those with particulate

Y-site compatibilities: Alteplase, atropine, dobutamine, heparin, lidocaine, meperidine, metoprolol, midazolam, morphine, nitroglycerin, verapamil

Solution compatibilities: 0.9% NaCl, D_5/0.9% NaCl

- Discontinuing drug before CABG
- Give all medications PO if possible, avoid IM inj and catheters

Patient/family education

- Teach patient to report bruising, bleeding, chest pain immediately
- Inform patient of reason for medication and expected results

Evaluation

Positive therapeutic outcome

- Decreased platelets

ergocalciferol

See vitamin D

ergonovine (℞)

(er-goe-noe'veen)

Ergometrine, ergotrate

Func. class.: Oxytocic

Chem. class.: Ergot alkaloid

Pregnancy category N/A

Action: Stimulates uterine and vascular smooth muscle contractions, decreases bleeding

Therapeutic Outcome: Uterine contraction, decreases bleeding

Uses: Treatment of postpartum or postabortion hemorrhage

Investigational uses: To induce a coronary artery spasm for diagnostic purposes

Dosage and routes

Oxytoxic

Adult: PO/SL 0.2-0.4 mg q6-12h; IM 0.2 mg q2-4h, not to exceed 5 doses; **IV** 0.2 mg given over 1 min

Induced coronary artery spasm

Adult: **IV** 50 mg q5 min up to 400 µg or until chest pain occurs

Available forms: Inj 0.2, 0.25 mg/ml

Adverse effects

CNS: *Headache, dizziness,* fainting

CV: Hypertension, chest pain

EENT: Tinnitus

GI: *Nausea, vomiting,* diarrhea

GU: Cramping

INTEG: Sweating

RESP: Dyspnea

Contraindications: Hypersensitivity to ergot medication, augmentation of labor, before delivery of placenta, spontaneous abortion (threatened), PID

Precautions: Hepatic, renal, cardiac disease, asthma, anemia, seizure disorders, hypertension, glaucoma, obliterative vascular disease

Pharmacokinetics

Absorption	Well absorbed (IM), completely absorbed (**IV**)
Distribution	Unknown
Metabolism	Liver
Excretion	Kidneys
Half-life	Unknown

Pharmacodynamics

	IM	IV
Onset	2-5 min	Immediate
Peak	Unknown	Unknown
Duration	3 hr	45 min

Interactions

Drug classifications

Ergots: ↑ hypertension

Sympathomimetics: ↑ hypertension

NURSING CONSIDERATIONS

Assessment

- Monitor B/P, pulse; watch for change that may indicate hemorrhage; check respiratory rate, rhythm, depth; notify prescriber of abnormalities
- Assess fundal tone, nonphasic contractions; check for relaxation or severe cramping
- Assess for ergotism or overdose: nausea, vomiting, weakness, muscular pain, insensitivity to cold, paresthesia of extremities; drug should be decreased or inf discontinued
- Before administering ergonovine, calcium levels should be checked; if hypocalcemia is present, correction should be made to increase effectiveness of this drug
- Monitor prolactin levels and decreased breast milk production

Nursing diagnoses

- ✓ Tissue perfusion, decreased (uses)
- ✓ Injury, risk for (adverse reactions)
- ✓ Knowledge deficit (teaching)

Implementation

IM route

- Contractions begin in 2-5 min, drug is given q2-4h for contractions to continue; give deeply in large muscle mass; rotate inj sites if additional doses are given

IV **IV route**

- Give **IV** directly after dilution with 5 ml of 0.9% NaCl, give over >1 min through Y-site of free-running **IV** of 0.9% NaCl or D_5W

Additive compatibilities: Amikacin, cephapirin, sodium bicarbonate

Patient/family education

- Advise patient to report increased blood loss, increased temp or foul-smelling lochia; need for pad count
- Inform patient that cramping is normal; pad count should be done to determine amount of bleeding
- Tell patient not to smoke during treatment to prevent excessive vasoconstriction

Evaluation

Positive therapeutic outcome

- Absence of severe bleeding

Treatment of overdose: Stop drug; give vasodilators, heparin, dextran

ergotamine (℞)

(er-got′a-meen)

Ergostat, Ergomar ✤, Gynergen, Medihaler Ergotamine

dihydroergotamine

(dy-hy′droh-er-got′ah-meen)

DHE 45, Dihydroergotamine Sandoz ✤, Migranal

Func. class.: α-Adrenergic blocker, vascular headache suppressant

Chem. class.: Ergot alkaloid-amino acid

Pregnancy category X

Action: Constricts smooth muscle in peripheral, cranial blood vessels; relaxes uterine muscle; blocks serotonin release

➔ **Therapeutic Outcome:** Absence of headache

Uses: Vascular headache (migraine, histamine, cluster)

Dosage and routes

Ergotamine

Adult: 2 mg, then 1-2 mg qh or q½h for SL, not to exceed 6 mg/day or 10 mg/wk; inh 1 puff, may repeat in 5 min, not to exceed 6/24 hr

Dihydroergotamine

Adult: SC/IM 1 mg, may repeat in 1 hr to 3 mg, max 3 mg/day or 6 mg/wk; **IV** 0.5 mg, may repeat in 1 hr, max 2 mg/day or 6 mg/wk

P ***Child ≥6 yr:*** SC/IM 0.5 mg, may repeat in 1 hr; **IV** 0.25 mg, may repeat in 1 hr

Severe acute migraine

P ***Child 12-16 yr:*** **IV** 0.25-0.5 mg, may repeat q20 min for 1-2 doses

Available forms: SL tab 2 mg; tab 1 mg; oral inh 360 μg/dose

Adverse effects

CNS: ***Numbness in fingers, toes,*** headache, weakness

CV: Transient tachycardia, chest pain,

bradycardia, edema, claudication, increase or decrease in B/P, **MI**
GI: Nausea, vomiting
MS: Muscle pain

Contraindications: Hypersensitivity to ergot preparations, occlusion (peripheral, vascular), CAD, hepatic, renal disease, peptic ulcer, hypertension, Raynaud's disease, peripheral vascular disease, intermittent claudication, pregnancy **X**

G P **Precautions:** Lactation, elderly, children, anemia

Pharmacokinetics

Absorption	Erratic (PO), poor (SL), rapidly (SC, IM)
Distribution	Crosses blood-brain barrier
Metabolism	Liver—extensively
Excretion	Kidneys (metabolites)
Half-life	Biphasic 2.7 hr, 21 hr

Pharmacodynamics

	PO	SL	IM/SC	IV
Onset	1-2 hr	Unknown	Unknown	Unknown
Peak	½-3 hr	Unknown	Unknown	¼-2 hr
Duration	Unknown	Unknown	8 hr	8 hr

Interactions
Individual drugs
Methysergide: ↑ effect
Sumatriptan: ↑ vasoconstriction
Drug classifications
Antiinfectives (macrolide): ↑ vasoconstriction, ↑ ergot toxicity
Ergots: ↑ hypertension
Oral contraceptives: ↑ vasoconstriction
Sympathomimetics: ↑ hypertension

NURSING CONSIDERATIONS
Assessment
• Assess characteristics of pain: duration, intensity, location, frequency, alleviating factors; also identify if halos, nausea, vomiting, blurred vision occur with headache; assess before and during treatment
• Assess for ergotism or overdose: nausea, vomiting, weakness, muscular pain, insensitivity to cold, paresthesia of extremities; drug should be decreased or infusion discontinued
• Check for hypertension: B/P, pulse, monitor all peripheral pulses; if hypertension occurs, notify prescriber; also check for tachycardia or bradycardia

Nursing diagnoses
✓ Pain, acute (uses)
✓ Injury, risk for (adverse reactions)
✓ Knowledge deficit (teaching)

Implementation
SL route
• Have patient place tab under tongue; patient should not chew, crush, or swallow SL tab
• Patient should not drink, eat, or smoke until tab has dissolved

Inhalation route
• Teach patient how to use inhaler, protect ampules from heat/light

IV **IV route**
• Give dihydroergotamine undiluted over 1 min

Patient/family education
• Caution patient not to smoke during treatment to prevent excessive vasoconstriction
• Advise patient to avoid alcohol or OTC medications unless approved by prescriber
• Tell patient to inform prescriber if pregnancy occurs

Treatment of overdose: Stop drug, give vasodilators, heparin, dextran

ertapenem
See Appendix A, Selected New Drugs

erythromycin base (℞)
(eh-rith-roh-my'sin)
Apo Erythro ♣, E-Mycin, Eramycin, Erybid ♣, Ery C, Erythromid ♣, Erythromycin Base Filmtab, Erythromycin Delayed-Release, Novo-Rythro Encap ♣, Robimycin

erythromycin estolate (℞)
Ilosone, Ilosone Pulvules, Novo-Rythro ♣

erythromycin ethylsuccinate (℞)
Apo-Erythro-ES ♣, EES, Ery Ped, Novo-Rythro ♣

erythromycin gluceptate (℞)

erythromycin lactobionate (℞)
Erythrocin, erythromycin lactobionate

erythromycin stearate (℞)
Apo-Erythro-s ♣, erythromycin stearate, Novo-Rythro ♣

Func. class.: Antiinfective
Chem. class.: Macrolide

Pregnancy category C

Action: Binds to 50S ribosomal subunits of susceptible bacteria and suppresses protein synthesis

Therapeutic Outcome: Bactericidal action against the following organisms: *Neisseria gonorrhoeae, Streptococcus pneumoniae, Mycoplasma pneumoniae, Corynebacterium diphtheriae, Bordetella pertussis, Borrelia burgdorferi, Listeria monocytogenes;* syphilis, Legionnaire's disease; streptococci, staphylocci; gram-positive bacilli: *Clostridium, Corynebacterium;* gram-negative pathogens: *Neisseria, Haemophilus influenzae, Legionella pneumophila, Mycoplasma, Chlamydia trachomatis, Entamoeba histolytica*

Uses: Mild to moderate respiratory tract, skin, soft tissue infections

Dosage and routes

Soft tissue infections

Adult: PO 250-500 mg q6-12h (base, estolate, stearate); PO 400-800 mg q6-12h (ethylsuccinate); **IV** inf 15-20 mg/kg/day (lactobionate) divided q6h

P ***Child:*** PO 30-50 mg/kg/day in divided doses q6h (salts); **IV** 20-40 mg/kg/day in divided doses q6h (lactobionate)

N. gonorrhoeae/PID

Adult: **IV** 500 mg q6h × 3 days (gluceptate, lactobionate), then PO 250 mg (base, estolate, stearate) or 400 mg (ethylsuccinate) q6h × 1 wk

Syphilis

Adult: PO 20 g in divided doses over 15 days (base, estolate, stearate)

Chlamydia

Adult: PO 500 mg q6h × 1 wk or 250 mg qid × 2 wk

P ***Infant:*** PO 50 mg/kg/day in 4 divided doses × 3 wk or more

P ***Newborn:*** PO 50 mg/kg/day in 4 divided doses × 2 wk or more

Intestinal amebiasis

Adult: PO 250 mg q6h × 10-14 days (base, estolate, stearate)

P ***Child:*** PO 30-50 mg/kg/day in divided doses q6h × 10-14 days (base, estolate, stearate)

Available forms: Base: tab, enteric-coated 250, 333 mg; tabs, film-coated 250, 500 mg; caps, enteric-coated 125, 250 mg; estolate: tabs, chewable 125, 250 mg; tab 500 mg; caps 125, 250 mg; drops 100 mg/ml; susp 125, 250 mg/5 ml; stearate: tabs, film-coated 250, 500 mg; ethylsuccinate: tabs, chewable 100, 200 mg/2.5 ml, 200, 400 mg/5 ml; susp 200, 400 mg; powder for susp 100 mg/2.5 ml, 200, 400 mg/

5 ml; powder for inj 500 mg, 1 g (lactobionate); 250 mg, 500 mg, 1 g (as gluceptate)

Adverse effects

***CV:* Dysrhythmias**
EENT: Hearing loss, tinnitus
GI: *Nausea, vomiting, diarrhea,* ***hepatotoxicity,*** abdominal pain, stomatitis, heartburn, anorexia, pruritus ani
GU: *Vaginitis, moniliasis*
INTEG: Rash, urticaria, pruritus, thrombophlebitis (**IV** site)
***SYST:* Anaphylaxis**

Contraindications: Hypersensitivity, preexisting liver disease (estolate), hepatic disease

Precautions: Pregnancy **B,** hepatic disease, lactation

Pharmacokinetics

Absorption	Well absorbed (PO),
Distribution	Widely distributed; minimally distributed (CSF); crosses placenta
Metabolism	Liver, partially
Excretion	Bile, unchanged; kidneys (minimal), unchanged
Half-life	1-3 hr

Pharmacodynamics

	PO	IV
Onset	1 hr	Rapid
Peak	4 hr	Infusion's end

Interactions

Individual drugs

Alfentanil: ↑ toxicity
Bromocriptine: ↑ toxicity
Carbamazepine: ↑ toxicity, from ↑ levels
Clindamycin: ↑ action of clindamycin
Cyclosporine: ↑ toxicity
Digoxin: ↑ blood levels of digoxin, ↑ action of digoxin
Dihydropyridine: ↑ action of dihydropyridine
Disopyramide: ↑ toxicity
Lovastatin: ↑ action of lovastatin
Methylprednisolone: ↑ toxicity
Midazolam: ↑ action of midazolam
Pimozide: ↑ serious dysrhythmias, do not use together
Simvastatin: ↑ action of simvastatin
Sparfloxacin: ↑ serious dysrhythmias; do not use together
Theophylline: ↑ toxicity from ↑ levels
Triazolam: ↑ effects of triazolam

Drug classifications

Antihistamines: ↑ levels of antihistamine
Calcium antagonists: ↑ action of calcium antagonists
Ergots: ↑ ergotism
Oral anticoagulants: ↑ effects of oral anticoagulants
Penicillins: ↑ or ↓ action of penicillins

Lab test interferences

↑ AST/ALT
↓ Folate assay
False ↑ 17-OHCS/17-KS

NURSING CONSIDERATIONS

Assessment

- Assess patient for previous sensitivity reaction
- Assess patient for signs and symptoms of infection including characteristics of wounds, sputum, urine, stool, WBC >10,000/mm^3, earache, fever; obtain baseline information before and during treatment
- Obtain C&S test results before beginning drug therapy to identify if correct treatment has been initiated
- Assess for allergic reactions: rash, urticaria may occur a few days after therapy begins
- Identify urine output; if decreasing, notify prescriber (may indicate nephrotoxicity); also monitor increases in BUN, creatinine
- Monitor blood studies: AST, ALT, CBC, Hct, bilirubin, LDH, alkaline phosphatase, Coombs' test monthly if patient is on long-term therapy

- Monitor electrolytes: potassium, sodium, chloride monthly if patient is on long-term therapy
- Assess bowel pattern qd; if severe diarrhea occurs, drug should be discontinued
- Assess for overgrowth of infection: perineal itching, fever, malaise, redness, pain, swelling, drainage, rash, diarrhea, change in cough, sputum

Nursing diagnoses

- ✓ Infection, risk for (uses)
- ✓ Diarrhea (adverse reactions)
- ✓ Knowledge deficit (teaching)
- ✓ Noncompliance (teaching)
- ✓ Injury, risk for (adverse reactions)

Implementation

PO route

- Give around the clock on an empty stomach, at least 1 hr ac or 2 hr pc; may be taken with food if GI upset occurs; do not take with juices; take dose with a full glass of water: use calibrated measuring device for drops or susp; shake well
- Store susp in refrigerator
- Chewable tab may be crushed or chewed, not swallowed whole
- (Do Not Crush) Do not open, crush, or chew time-release cap or tab, enteric-coated tab may be given

IV route

- Add 10 ml of sterile water for inj without preservatives to 250- or 500-mg vials and 20 ml to 1-g vial; sol is stable for 1 wk after reconstitution if refrigerated
- Intermittent inf: dilute further in 100-250 ml of 0.9% NaCl or D_5W
- Give over 20-60 min to avoid phlebitis; assess for pain along vein; slow inf if pain occurs; apply ice to site and notify prescriber if unable to relieve pain
- Cont inf: may also be administered as an infusion in a dilution of 1 g/L of 0.9% NaCl, D_5W, over 4 hr

Syringe incompatibilities:
Heparin

Additive compatibilities:
Calcium gluconate, hydrocortisone, lidocaine, methicillin, penicillin G potassium, potassium chloride, sodium bicarbonate

Additive incompatibilities:
Aminophylline, cephapirin, pentobarbital, secobarbital, streptomycin, tetracycline

Erythromycin lactobionate
Syringe compatibilities:
Methicillin

Syringe incompatibilities:
Ampicillin, heparin

Y-site compatibilities:
Acyclovir, amiodarone, cyclophosphamide, enalaprilat, esmolol, famotidine, foscarnet, hydromorphone, idarubicin, labetalol, lorazepam, magnesium sulfate, merperidine, midazolam, morphine, multivitamins, perphenazine, vit B/C, zidovudine

Y-site incompatibilities:
Fluconazole

Additive compatibilities:
Aminophylline, ampicillin, cimetidine, diphenhydramine, hydrocortisone, lidocaine, methicillin, penicillin G potassium, penicillin G sodium, pentobarbital, polymyxin B, potassium chloride, prednisolone, prochlorperazine, promazine, ranitidine, sodium bicarbonate, verapamil

Additive incompatibilities:
Cephalothin, colistimethate, floxacillin, furosemide, heparin, metaraminol, metoclopramide, tetracycline, vit B/C

Patient/family education

- Teach patient to report sore throat, bruising, bleeding, joint pain; may indicate blood dyscrasias (rare)
- Advise patient to contact prescriber if vaginal itching, loose, foul-smelling stools, furry tongue occur; may indicate superimposed infection
- Instruct patient to take all medication prescribed for the length of time ordered

Evaluation

Positive therapeutic outcome

- Absence of signs/symptoms of infection (WBC <10,000/mm^3, temp WNL, absence of red, draining wounds, earache)
- Reported improvement in symptoms of infection

Treatment of overdose: Withdraw drug, maintain airway, administer epinephrine, aminophylline, O_2, **IV** corticosteroids

esmolol (℞)

(ez′moe-lole)

Brevibloc

Func. class.: β-Adrenergic blocker (antidysrhythmic II)

Pregnancy category C

Action: Competitively blocks stimulation of β_1-adrenergic receptors in the myocardium; produces negative chronotropic, inotropic activity (decreases rate of SA node discharge, increases recovery time), slows conduction of AV node, decreases heart rate, decreases O_2 consumption in myocardium; also decreases renin-aldosterone-angiotensin system at high doses; inhibits β_2-receptors in bronchial system slightly

➔ **Therapeutic Outcome:** Decreased supraventricular tachycardia

Uses: Supraventricular tachycardias, noncompensatory tachycardia, hypertensive crisis

Dosage and routes

Adult: **IV** loading dose 500 µg/kg/min over 1 min; maintenance 50 µg/kg/min for 4 min; may repeat q5 min, increasing maintenance inf by 50 µg/kg/min (max of 200 µg/kg/min); titrate to patient response

Available forms: Inj 10 mg, 250 mg/ml

Adverse effects

CNS: Confusion, light-headedness, paresthesia, somnolence, fever, dizziness, fatigue, headache, depression, anxiety, **seizures**

CV: Hypotension, bradycardia, chest pain, peripheral ischemia, shortness of breath, CHF, conduction disturbances

GI: *Nausea,* vomiting, anorexia, gastric pain, flatulence, constipation, heartburn, bloating

GU: Urinary retention, impotence, dysuria

INTEG: *Induration, inflammation at inj site,* discoloration, edema, erythema, burning pallor, flushing, rash, pruritus, dry skin, alopecia

RESP: **Bronchospasm,** dyspnea, cough, wheezing, nasal stuffiness

Contraindications: Heart block (2nd- or 3rd-degree), cardiogenic shock, CHF, cardiac failure, hypersensitivity

Precautions: Hypotension, pregnancy **C,** peripheral vascular disease, diabetes, hypoglycemia, thyrotoxicosis, renal disease, lactation

Do Not Confuse: Brevibloc/Brevital

Pharmacokinetics	
Absorption	Complete
Distribution	Unknown
Metabolism	Liver
Excretion	Kidneys
Half-life	9 min

Pharmacodynamics	
Onset	Rapid
Peak	Unknown
Duration	1-2 min

Interactions

Individual drugs

Alcohol: ↑ hypotension (large amounts)

Dobutamine: ↓ action of dobutamine

Dopamine: ↓ action of dopamine
Ephedrine: ↑ α-Adrenergic stimulation
Epinephrine: α-Adrenergic
Hydralazine: ↑ hypotension, bradycardia
Norepinephrine: ↑ α-Adrenergic stimulation
Phenylephrine: ↑ α-Adrenergic stimulation
Prazosin: ↑ hypotension, bradycardia
Pseudoepedrine: ↑ α-Adrenergic stimulation
Thyroid hormones: ↓ effect of thyroid
Verapamil: ↑ myocardial depression

Drug classifications
Antihypertensives: ↑ hypertension
β_2-Agonists: ↓ bronchodilatation
Cardiac glycosides: ↑ bradycardia
Nitrates: ↑ hypotension
Theophyllines: ↓ bronchodilatation

Smoking
↑ Tachycardia

Herb/drug
Aloe: ↑ hypokalemia
Buckthorn bark/berry: ↑ hypokalemia
Cascara sagrada bark: ↑ hypokalemia
Senna pod/leaf: ↑ hypokalemia

Lab test interferences
↑ Liver function tests

NURSING CONSIDERATIONS

Assessment

- Monitor B/P during beginning treatment, periodically thereafter; pulse q4h; note rate, rhythm, quality; apical/radial pulse before administration; notify prescriber of any significant changes (pulse <50 bpm)
- Check for baselines in renal, liver function tests before therapy begins
- Assess for edema in feet, legs daily, monitor I&O, daily weight; check for jugular vein distention, rales bilaterally, dyspnea (CHF)
- Monitor skin turgor, dryness of mucous membranes for hydration status, especially elderly

Nursing diagnoses

- ✓ Cardiac output, decreased (uses)
- ✓ Injury, risk for (adverse reactions)
- ✓ Knowledge deficit (teaching)
- ✓ Noncompliance (teaching)

Implementation

- Give by intermittent inf after diluting 5 g/500 ml of D_5W, 0.9% NaCl, D_5/0.45% NaCl, D_5/LR, D_5/0.9% NaCl, 0.45% NaCl, LR (10 mg/ml)
- Give loading dose over 1 min, then maintenance dose over 4 min, may repeat loading dose q5 min with increased maintenance dose; maintenance dose should not be >200 μg/kg/min and be administered up to 48 hr; dosage should be tapered at a rate of 25 μg/kg/min
- Store at room temp for 24 hr; sol should be clear

Y-site compatibilities:
Amikacin, aminophylline, ampicillin, amiodarone, atracurium, butorphanol, calcium chloride, cefazolin, cefmetazole, cefoperazone, ceftazidime, ceftizoxime, chloramphenicol, cimetidine, cisatracurium, clindamycin, diltiazem, dopamine, enalaprilat, erythromycin, famotidine, fentanyl, gentamicin, heparin, hydrocortisone, regular insulin, labetalol, magnesium sulfate, methyldopate, metronidazole, midazolam, morphine, nafcillin, nitroglycerin, norepinephrine, nitroprusside, pancuronium, penicillin G potassium, phenytoin, piperacillin, polymyxin B, potassium chloride, potassium phosphate, propofol, ranitidine, remifentanil, streptomycin, tacrolimus, tobramycin, trimethoprim-sulfamethoxazole, vancomycin, vecuronium

Y-site incompatibilities:
Furosemide

Additive compatibilities:
Aminophylline, atracurium, bretylium, heparin

Additive incompatibilities: Diazepam, procainamide, sodium bicarbonate, thiopental

Patient/family education

- Teach patient need for medication and expected results
- Caution patient to rise slowly to prevent orthostatic hypotension
- Advise patient to notify if pain, swelling occurs at **IV** site

Evaluation

Positive therapeutic outcome

- Absence of dysrhythmias

Treatment of overdose: Defibrillation, vasopressor for hypotension

esomeprazole

See Appendix A, Selected New Drugs

estradiol (℞)

(ess-tra-dye'ole)

Estrace

estradiol cypionate

depGynogen, Depo-Estradiol, Depogen, Dura-Estrin, E-Cypionate, Estragyn LAS, Estro-Cyp, Estrofem, Estroject-LA, Estro-L.A.

estradiol valerate

Clinagen LA, Delestrogen, Dioval, Duragan, Estra-L, Estro-span, Femogex ♣, Gynogen LA, Menaval, Valergen

estradiol transdermal system

Alora, Climera, Esclim, Estraderm, FemPatch, Vivelle

estradiol vaginal tablet

Vagifem

estradiol vaginal ring

Estring

Func. class.: Estrogen, progestin

Chem. class.: Nonsteroidal synthetic estrogen

Pregnancy category X

Action: Needed for adequate functioning of female reproductive system; affects release of pituitary gonadatropins, inhibits ovulation, promotes adequate calcium use in bone structure

➔ **Therapeutic Outcome:** Decreased tumor size in prostatic cancer; increased estrogen levels in menopause, female hypogonadism

Uses: Menopause, breast cancer, prostatic cancer, atrophic vaginitis, kraurosis vulvae, hypogonadism, castration, primary ovarian failure, prevention of osteoporosis

Dosage and routes

Menopause/hypogonadism/castration/ovarian failure

Adult: PO 1-2 mg qd 3 wk on, 1 wk off or 5 days on, 2 days off; IM 1-5 mg q3-4 wk (cypionate), 10-20 mg q4 wk (valerate); top Estraderm 0.05 mg/24 hr applied 2×/wk, Climera 0.05 mg/hr applied 1×/wk in a cyclic regimen, women with hysterectomy may use continuously

Prostatic cancer

Adult: PO 1-2 mg qd 3 wk on, 1 wk off or 5 days on, 2 days off; IM 0.2-1 mg qwk

Breast cancer

Adult: PO 10 mg tid × 3 mo or longer

Atropic vaginitis/kraurosis vulvae

Adult: Vag cream 2-4 g qd × 1-2 wk, then 1 g 1-3 ×/wk cycled

Available forms: Estradiol tabs 0.5, 1, 2 mg; cypionate inj IM 5 mg/ml; valerate inj IM 10, 20, 40 mg/ml; TD 0.1 mg/24-hr release rate; vag cream 100 μg/g; vag ring 2 mg/90 days

Adverse effects

CNS: Dizziness, headache, migraine, depression, **seizures**

CV: Hypotension, thrombophlebitis, edema, **thromboembolism, stroke, pulmonary embolism, MI**

EENT: Contact lens intolerance, increased myopia, astigmatism

GI: *Nausea,* vomiting, diarrhea, anorexia, pancreatitis, cramps, constipation, increased appetite, increased weight, **cholestatic jaundice, hepatic adenoma**

GU: Amenorrhea, cervical erosion, breakthrough bleeding, dysmenorrhea, vaginal candidiasis, breast changes, *gynecomastia, testicular atrophy, impotence,* **increased risk of breast, endometrial cancer**

INTEG: Rash, urticaria, acne, hirsutism, alopecia, oily skin, seborrhea, purpura, melasma

META: Folic acid deficiency, hypercalcemia, hyperglycemia

Contraindications: Breast cancer, thromboembolic disorders, reproductive cancer, genital bleeding (abnormal, undiagnosed), pregnancy **X**

Precautions: Hypertension, asthma, blood dyscrasias, gallbladder disease, CHF, diabetes mellitus, bone disease, depression, migraine headache, convulsive disorders, hepatic, renal disease, family history of cancer of breast or reproductive tract

Pharmacokinetics

Absorption	Well absorbed
Distribution	Widely distributed, crosses placenta
Metabolism	Unknown
Excretion	Unknown
Half-life	Unknown

Pharmacodynamics

	PO	IM	IV
Onset	Rapid	Slow	Rapid
Peak	Unknown	Unknown	Unknown
Duration	Unknown	Unknown	Unknown

Interactions

Individual drugs

Cyclosporine: ↑ toxicity

Dantrolene: ↑ toxicity

Tamoxifen: ↓ tamoxifen action

Drug classifications

Anticoagulants: ↓ action of anticoagulants

Antidepressants, tricyclic: ↑ toxicity

Barbiturates: ↓ action of chlorotrianisene

Corticosteroids: ↑ action of corticosteroids

Oral hypoglycemics: ↓ action of hypoglycemics

Food/drug

Grapefruit juice: ↑ estrogen level

Lab test interferences

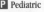

↑ BSP retention test; ↑ PBI; ↑ T_4; ↑ serum sodium; ↑ platelet aggregation; ↑ thyroxine-binding globulin (TBS); ↑ prothrombin; ↑ factors VII, VIII, IX, X; ↑ triglycerides

↓ Serum folate, ↓ serum triglyceride, ↓ T_3 resin uptake test, ↓ glucose tolerance test, ↓ antithrombin III, ↓ pregnanediol, ↓ metyrapone test
False positive: LE prep, ANA titer

NURSING CONSIDERATIONS

Assessment

- Monitor blood glucose in patient with diabetes; increased urine glucose may occur
- Monitor B/P q4h; watch for increase caused by water and sodium retention
- Monitor I&O ratio; be alert for decreasing urinary output and increasing edema; monitor weight daily; notify prescriber if weekly weight gain is >5 lb; if increased, diuretic may be ordered
- Obtain liver function studies baseline, periodically, including AST, ALT, bilirubin, alkaline phosphatase
- Assess edema, hypertension, cardiac symptoms, jaundice
- Assess mental status: affect, mood, behavioral changes, aggression; depression may occur, drug may need to be discontinued
- Assess female patient for intact uterus, if so, progesterone should be added to estrogen therapy to decrease risk of endometrial cancer

Nursing diagnoses

✓ Sexual dysfunction (uses)
✓ Injury, risk for (adverse reactions)

Implementation

PO route

- Give titrated dose, use lowest effective dose
- Give with food or milk to decrease GI symptoms

IM route

- Administer deeply in large muscle mass; drug is painful
- Rotate syringe to mix oil and medication

TD route

- Apply to area free of hair to ensure adhesion
- Start TD dose 7 days before last PO dose if routes are to be changed

Vaginal route

- Place cream in applicator by attaching tube to applicator; squeeze cream into tube to mark; insert with patient reclining
- Applicator should be washed after each use

Patient/family education

- Tell patient to take exactly as prescribed; do not double doses
- ❗ Advise patient that increased weight gain and symptoms of fluid retention should be reported to prescriber: edema of feet, ankles, sacral area; abnormal vaginal bleeding; breast lumps; hepatic disease (dark urine, clay-colored stools, jaundice of skin, sclera, pruritus)
- ❗ Caution patient that thromboembolic symptoms should be reported: tenderness in legs, chest pain, dyspnea, headaches, blurred vision
- Inform patient to use sunscreen and protective clothing because sunburns may occur
- Advise patient to stop smoking; smokers have a greater chance of thromboembolic disorder
- Tell patient to use nonhormonal birth control, and to notify prescriber if pregnancy is suspected

Evaluation

Positive therapeutic outcome

- Reversal of menopausal symptoms
- Decrease in tumor size in prostatic or breast cancer
- Decrease in itching, inflammation of vagina
- Absence of symptoms of osteoporosis

estrogens, conjugated 🔑 (℞)

Cenestin, C.E.S ♣, Congest ♣, conjugated estrogens, Premarin, Premarin Intravenous

estrogens, conjugated synthetic A

Cenestin

Func. class.: Estrogen hormone
Chem. class.: Nonsteroidal synthetic estrogen

Pregnancy category X

Action: Needed for adequate functioning of female reproductive system; affects release of pituitary gonadotropins; inhibits ovulation; promotes adequate calcium use in bone structures

Therapeutic Outcome: Decreased tumor size in prostatic cancer; increased estrogen levels in menopause, female hypogonadism

Uses: Menopause, breast cancer, prostatic cancer, abnormal uterine bleeding, hypogonadism, castration, primary ovarian failure, osteoporosis

Dosage and routes

Menopause
Adult: PO 0.3-1.25 mg qd 3 wk on, 1 wk off

Osteoporosis
Adult: PO 0.625 mg qd or in a cycle

Atrophic vaginitis
Adult: Vag 2-4 g cream qd × 21 days, off 7 days, repeat

Prostatic cancer
Adult: PO 1.25-2.5 mg tid

Breast cancer
Adult: PO 10 mg tid × 3 mo or longer

Abnormal uterine bleeding
Adult: **IV**/IM 25 mg, repeat in 6-12 hr

Ovariectomy/primary ovarian failure
Adult: PO 1.25 mg qd 3 wk on, 1 wk off

Hypogonadism
Adult: PO 2.5 mg bid-tid × 20 days/mo

Available forms: Tabs 0.3, 0.625, 0.9, 1.25, 2.5 mg; inj 25 mg/vial; vag cream 0.625 mg/g

Adverse effects

CNS: Dizziness, headache, migraine, depression, **seizures**
CV: Hypotension, thrombophlebitis, edema, **thromboembolism, stroke, pulmonary embolism, MI**
EENT: Contact lens intolerance, increased myopia, astigmatism
GI: *Nausea,* vomiting, diarrhea, anorexia, pancreatitis, cramps, constipation, increased appetite, increased weight, **cholestatic jaundice, hepatic adenoma**
GU: Amenorrhea, cervical erosion, breakthrough bleeding, dysmenorrhea, vaginal candidiasis, breast changes, *gynecomastia, testicular atrophy, impotence,* **increased risk of breast, endometrial cancer**
INTEG: Rash, urticaria, acne, hirsutism, alopecia, oily skin, seborrhea, purpura, melasma
META: Folic acid deficiency, hypercalcemia, hyperglycemia

Contraindications: Breast cancer, thromboembolic disorders, reproductive cancer, genital bleeding (abnormal, undiagnosed), pregnancy **X,** lactation

Precautions: Hypertension, asthma, blood dyscrasias, gallbladder disease, CHF, diabetes mellitus, bone disease, depression, migraine headache, convulsive disorders, hepatic, renal disease, family history of cancer of breast or reproductive tract

Do Not Confuse:
Premarin/Provera

Pharmacokinetics

Absorption	Well absorbed (PO), completely absorbed **(IV)**
Distribution	Widely distributed, crosses placenta
Metabolism	Liver—exclusively; hepatic recirculation
Excretion	Kidney
Half-life	Unknown

Pharmacodynamics

	PO	IM	IV
Onset	Rapid	Slow	Immediate
Peak	Unknown	Unknown	Unknown
Duration	Unknown	Unknown	Unknown

Interactions
Individual drugs
Cyclosporine: ↑ toxicity
Dantrolene: ↑ toxicity
Phenylbutazone: ↓ action of phenylbutazone
Rifampin: ↓ action of phenylbutazone
Tamoxifen: ↓ tamoxifen action
Drug classifications
Anticoagulants: ↓ action of anticoagulants
Anticonvulsants: ↓ action of chlorotrianisene
Antidepressants, tricyclic: ↑ toxicity
Barbiturates: ↓ action of chlorotrianisene
Corticosteroids: ↑ action of corticosteroids
Oral hypoglycemics: ↓ action of hypoglycemics
Food/drug
Grapefruit juice: ↑ estrogen level
Lab test interferences
↑ BSP retention test; ↑ PBI, ↑ T_4; ↑ serum sodium; ↑ platelet aggressability; ↑ thyroxine-binding globulin (TBG); ↑ prothrombin; ↑ factors VII, VIII, IX, X; ↑ triglycerides
↓ Serum folate, ↓ serum triglyceride, ↓ T_3 resin uptake test, ↓ glucose tolerance test, ↓ antithrombin III, ↓ pregnanediol, ↓ metyrapone test
False positive: LE prep, ANA titer

NURSING CONSIDERATIONS
Assessment
- Monitor blood glucose in patient with diabetes; increased urine glucose may occur
- Monitor B/P q4h; watch for increase caused by water and sodium retention
- Monitor I&O ratio; be alert for decreasing urinary output and increasing edema; monitor weight daily; notify prescriber if weekly weight gain is >5 lb; if increased, diuretic may be ordered
- Obtain liver function studies, including AST, ALT, bilirubin, alkaline phosphatase
- Assess edema, hypertension, cardiac symptoms, jaundice
- Assess mental status: affect, mood, behavioral changes, aggression; depression may occur, drug may need to be discontinued
- Assess female patient for intact uterus; if so, progesterone should be added to estrogen therapy to decrease risk of endometrial cancer

Nursing diagnoses
✓ Sexual dysfunction (uses)
✓ Injury, risk for (adverse reactions)

Implementation
PO route
- Give titrated dose, use lowest effective dose
- Give in one dose in AM for prostatic cancer, vaginitis, hypogonadism
- Give with food or milk to decrease GI symptoms

IM route
- Reconstitute after withdrawing at least 5 ml of air from container and inject sterile diluent on vial side, rotate to dissolve

• Give IM injection deeply in large muscle

IV **IV route**

• Direct **IV**: reconstitute as for IM, inject into distal port of running **IV** line of D_5W, 0.9% NaCl, LR, at a rate of 5 mg/min or less

Y-site compatibilities: Heparin/hydrocortisone, potassium chloride, vit B/C

Vaginal route

• Place cream in applicator by attaching tube to applicator, squeeze cream into tube to mark, insert with patient recumbent

• Applicator should be washed after each use

Patient/family education

• Caution patient to take exactly as prescribed and not to double doses

• Advise patient that increased weight gain and symptoms of fluid retention should be reported to prescriber: edema of feet, ankles, sacral area; abnormal vaginal bleeding; breast lumps; hepatic disease (dark urine, clay-colored stools, jaundice of skin, sclera, pruritus)

• Caution patient that thromboembolic symptoms should be reported: pain, redness, tenderness in legs; chest pain, dyspnea, headaches, blurred vision

• Inform patient that sunburns may occur and to use sunscreen and protective clothing

• Advise patient to stop smoking; smokers have a greater chance of thromboembolic disorder

• Tell patient to use nonhormonal birth control, and to notify prescriber if pregnancy is suspected

Evaluation

Positive therapeutic outcome

• Reversal of menopause symptoms

• Decrease in tumor size in prostatic, breast cancer

• Decrease in itching, inflammation of vagina

• Absence of symptoms of osteoporosis

etanercept (℞)

(eh-tan′er-sept)

Enbrel

Func. class.: Antirheumatic agent (disease-modifying)

Pregnancy category B

Action: Binds to tumor necrosis factor (TNF), which decreases inflammation and immune response

Therapeutic Outcome: Decreased pain, inflammation

Uses: Acute, chronic rheumatoid arthritis that has not responded to other disease-modifying agents; polyarticular course juvenile rheumatoid arthritis (JRA)

Investigational uses: CHF, psoriasis/psoriatic arthritis

Dosage and routes

Osteoarthritis

Adult: SC 25 mg 2×/wk, may be given with other drugs for rheumatoid arthritis

P ***Child 4-17 yr:*** SC 0.4 mg/kg 2×/wk, max 25 mg/dose

CHF

Adult: SC 5-12 mg/m^2 2×/wk × 3 mo

Psoriasis/psoriatic arthritis

Adult: SC 25 mg 2×/wk × 12 wk

Available forms: Powder for inj: 25 mg

Adverse effects

CNS: Headache, asthenia, dizziness
GI: Abdominal pain, dyspepsia
INTEG: Rash, *inj site reaction*
RESP: Pharyngitis, rhinitis, *cough*, *URI*, non-URI sinusitis

Contraindications: Hypersensitivity, sepsis

Precautions: Pregnancy **B,** lactation, children <4 yr, elderly

Pharmacokinetics

Absorption	Rapidly (60%)
Distribution	Unknown
Metabolism	Unknown
Excretion	Unknown
Half-life	115 hr

Pharmacodynamics

Onset	Unknown
Peak	Unknown
Duration	Unknown

Interactions

Drug classifications

Immunizations: Do not give concurrently

Vaccines: Do not give concurrently

NURSING CONSIDERATIONS

Assessment

- Assess for pain of rheumatoid arthritis; check ROM, inflammation of joints, characteristics of pain
- Assess inj site for pain, swelling, usually occurs after 2 inj (4-5 days)

Nursing diagnoses

- ✓ Pain (uses)
- ✓ Mobility, impaired physical (uses)
- ✓ Injury, risk for (side effects)
- ✓ Knowledge deficit (teaching)

Implementation

SC route

- Administer after reconstituting 1 ml of supplied diluent, slowly inject diluent into vial, swirl contents, do not shake, sol should be clear/colorless, do not use if cloudy or discolored
- Do not admix with other sol or medications; do not use filter
- May be injected SC into upper arm, abdomen, thigh; rotate inj sites

Patient/family education

- Teach patient that drug must be continued for prescribed time to be effective; to avoid aspirin, alcoholic beverages
- Instruct patient to use caution when driving; dizziness may occur
- Teach patient about self-administration, if appropriate: inj should be made in thigh, abdomen, upper arm; rotate sites at least 1 in from old site

Evaluation

Positive therapeutic outcome

- Decreased pain in arthritic conditions
- Decreased inflammation in arthritic conditions

ethambutol (℞)

(e-tham′byoo-tole)

Etibi ✤, Myambutol

Func. class.: Antitubercular

Chem. class.: Diisopropylethylene diamide derivative

Pregnancy category B

Action: Inhibits RNA synthesis, decreases tubercle bacilli replication

Therapeutic Outcome: Resolution of TB infection

Uses: Pulmonary TB, as an adjunct, other mycobacterial infections

Dosage and routes

Adult and child >13 yr: PO 15-25 mg/kg/day as a single dose or 50 mg/kg 2×/wk or 25-30 mg/kg 3×/wk

Renal dose

CrCl 10-50 ml/min dose q24-36h; CrCl <10 ml/min dose q48h

Retreatment

Adult: PO 25 mg/kg/day as single dose × 2 mo with at least 1 other drug, then decrease to 15 mg/kg/day as single dose, max 2.5 g/day

Child: PO 15 mg/kg/day

Available forms: Tabs 100, 400 mg

Adverse effects

CNS: *Headache, confusion,* fever,

malaise, dizziness, *disorientation,* hallucinations
EENT: Blurred vision, optic neuritis, photophobia, decreased visual acuity
GI: *Abdominal distress, anorexia, nausea, vomiting*
INTEG: Dermatitis, pruritus, **toxic epidermal necrolysis**
META: *Elevated uric acid, acute gout,* liver function impairment
MISC: **Thrombocytopenia,** joint pain, bloody sputum, **anaphylaxis**

Contraindications: Hypersensitivity, optic neuritis, P child <13 yr

Precautions: Renal disease, diabetic retinopathy, cataracts, ocular defects, hepatic and hematopoietic disorders, pregnancy **B**

Pharmacokinetics

Absorption	Rapidly absorbed
Distribution	Widely distributed, crosses blood-brain barrier, placenta
Metabolism	Liver
Excretion	Kidneys— unchanged
Half-life	3 hr, increased in liver, kidney disease

Pharmacodynamics

Onset	Rapid
Peak	2-4 hr

Interactions

Individual drugs

Cisplatin: ↑ renal toxicity

Drug classifications

Antacids, aluminum: ↓ absorption
Neurotoxic agents, other: ↑ neurotoxicity

NURSING CONSIDERATIONS

Assessment

- Obtain C&S tests including sputum tests before initiating treatment; monitor qmo to detect resistance
- Monitor liver function studies qwk × 2 wk, then q2 mo: ALT, AST, bilirubin; renal studies: before, qmo: BUN, creatinine, output, sp gr, urinalysis, uric acid
- Assess patient's mental status often: affect, mood, behavioral changes; psychosis may occur with hallucinations, confusion
- Assess patient's hepatic status: decreased appetite, jaundice, dark urine, fatigue
- Assess patient for visual disturbance that may indicate optic neuritis: blurred vision, change in color perception; may lead to blindness

Nursing diagnoses

- ✓ Infection, risk for (uses)
- ✓ Diarrhea (adverse reactions)
- ✓ Sensory-perceptual alterations (adverse reactions)
- ✓ Knowledge deficit (teaching)
- ✓ Noncompliance (teaching)

Implementation

- Give with meals to decrease GI symptoms, at same time each day to maintain blood level
- Give 2 hr before antacids
- Give antiemetic if vomiting occurs

Patient/family education

- Advise patient that compliance with dosage schedule and duration is necessary to eradicate disease; to keep scheduled appointments including ophthalmic appointments or relapse may occur
- Caution patient to report weakness, fatigue, loss of appetite, nausea, vomiting, yellowing of skin or eyes, tingling/numbness of hands/feet, weight gain, or decreased urine output
- Instruct patient to report any visual changes; rash; hot, swollen, painful joints; numbness or tingling of extremities to physician
- Caution patient to inform prescriber if pregnancy is suspected

Evaluation

Positive therapeutic outcome

- Decreased symptoms of TB
- Decrease in acid-fast bacteria

etidronate (℞)

(eh-tih-droe′nate)

Didronel, Didronel IV

Func. class.: Parathyroid agent (calcium regulator)

Chem. class.: Diphosphate

Pregnancy category C

Action: Decreases bone resorption and new bone development (accretion)

Therapeutic Outcome: Decreased bone reabsorption, calcium levels WNL

Uses: Paget's disease, heterotopic ossification, hypercalcemia of malignancy

Dosage and routes

Paget's disease

Adult: PO 5-10 mg/kg/day, 2 hr ac with water, not to exceed 20 mg/kg/day, max 6 mo or 11-20 mg/kg/day for max of 3 mo

Heterotopic ossification

Adult: PO 20 mg/kg qd × 2 wk, then 10 mg/kg/day for 10 wk, total 12 wk

Hypercalcemia

Adult: **IV** 7.5 mg/kg/day × 3 days, then 20 mg/kg/day (PO)

Heterotopic ossification/hip replacement

Adult: PO 20 mg/kg/day × 4 wk before and 3 mo after surgery

Available forms: Tabs 200, 400 mg; inj 300 mg/6 ml

Adverse effects

CNS: **Seizures**

GI: *Nausea, diarrhea,* metallic taste (**IV**)

GU: **Nephrotoxicity**

MS: *Bone pain,* hypocalcemia, decreased mineralization of nonaffected bones

Contraindications: Pathologic fractures, children, colitis, severe renal disease with creatinine >5 mg/dl

Precautions: Pregnancy **C**, renal disease, lactation, restricted vit D/Ca

Do Not Confuse:
etidronate/etomidate, etidronate/etretinate

Pharmacokinetics

Absorption	Poorly absorbed (PO), completely absorbed (**IV**)
Distribution	50% bond to crystals in osteogenesis
Metabolism	None
Excretion	Feces (unabsorbed), kidney (unchanged)
Half-life	5-7 hr; in bone >3 mo

Pharmacodynamics

	PO	IV
Onset	4 wk	24 hr
Peak	Unknown	3-4 days
Duration	Up to 1 yr	10-12 days

Interactions

Individual drugs

Didanosine: ↓ absorption of etidronate

Calcitonin: ↑ effect of calcitonin

Drug classifications

Antacids: ↓ absorption of etidronate

Mineral supplements with magnesium, calcium, or aluminum: ↓ absorption of etidronate

Food/drug

Dairy products: ↓ absorption of etidronate

NURSING CONSIDERATIONS

Assessment

- Assess for GI symptoms, polyuria, flushing, head swelling, tingling, headache, may indicate hypercalcemia; nervousness, irritability, twitching, seizures, spasm, paresthesia indicates hypocalcemia at start of treatment
- Identify nutritional status; evaluate diet for sources of vit D (milk, some seafood), calcium (dairy products, dark green vegetables), phosphates
- Monitor BUN, creatinine, uric acid,

chloride, electrolytes, urine pH, urinary calcium, magnesium, phosphate, urinalysis (calcium should be kept at 9-10 mg/dl), albumin, alkaline phosphatase baseline and q3-6 mo; check urine sediment for casts throughout treatment
- Assess for increased drug level; toxic reactions occur rapidly; have calcium chloride or gluconate on hand if calcium level drops too low; check for tetany

Nursing diagnoses
- ✓ Injury, risk for (adverse reactions)
- ✓ Pain, chronic (uses)
- ✓ Knowledge deficit (teaching)

Implementation
PO route
- Administer on empty stomach to improve absorption (2 hr ac)

IV **IV route**
- Used in hypercalcemias; give by intermittent inf after diluting 300 mg/250 ml or more 0.9% NaCl; run over 2-3 hr, therapy should not last >6 mo

Patient/family education
- Teach method of inj if patient will be responsible for self-medication
- Caution patient to notify prescriber if hypercalcemia recurs: renal calculi, nausea, vomiting, thirst, lethargy, deep bone or flank pain, heat over bone, restricted mobility
- Teach patient that warmth and flushing occur and last 1 hr
- Teach patient to follow a low-calcium diet as prescribed (Paget's disease, hypercalcemia)
- Advise patient to notify prescriber of diarrhea, nausea; dose may be divided to lessen these symptoms
- Inform patient that metallic taste may occur with **IV** dosing

Evaluation
Positive therapeutic outcome
- Calcium levels 9-10 mg/dl
- Decreasing symptoms of Paget's disease including pain
- Decreased bone loss in osteoporosis

etodolac (℞)
(ee-toe-doe'lak)

Lodine, Lodine XL

Func. class.: Nonsteroidal antiinflammatory, nonopioid analgesic

Pregnancy category C

Action: Inhibits prostaglandin synthesis by decreasing enzyme needed for biosynthesis; analgesic, antiinflammatory properties

➔ **Therapeutic Outcome:** Decreased pain, inflammation

Uses: Mild to moderate pain, osteoarthritis

Dosage and routes
Osteoarthritis
Adult: PO 800-1200 mg/day in divided doses q6-8h initially, then adjust to 600-1200 mg/day in divided doses; do not exceed 1200 mg/day; patients <60 kg not to exceed 20 mg/kg

Analgesia
Adult: PO 200-400 mg q6-8h prn for acute pain; do not exceed 1200 mg/day; patients <60 kg not to exceed 20 mg/kg

Available forms: Caps 200, 300 mg; tabs 400, 500 mg; ext rel tabs 400, 600 mg

Adverse effects
CNS: Dizziness, headache, drowsiness, fatigue, tremors, confusion, insomnia, anxiety, depression, light-headedness, vertigo
CV: Tachycardia, peripheral edema, fluid retention, palpitations, dysrhythmias, CHF
EENT: Tinnitus, hearing loss, blurred vision, photophobia
GI: *Nausea, anorexia,* vomiting, diarrhea, jaundice, **cholestatic hepatitis,** constipation, flatulence,

cramps, dry mouth, peptic ulcer, dyspepsia, **GI bleeding**
GU: **Nephrotoxicity: dysuria, hematuria, oliguria, azotemia, cystitis, UTI**
HEMA: **Blood dyscrasias**, epistaxis, bruising
INTEG: Erythema, urticaria, purpura, rash, pruritus, sweating, **Stevens-Johnson syndrome**
SYST: **Angioedema, anaphylaxis**

Contraindications:
Hypersensitivity; patients in whom aspirin, iodides, or other NSAIDs have produced asthma, rhinitis, urticaria, nasal polyps, angioedema, bronchospasm

Precautions: Pregnancy **C**, lactation, children, bleeding, GI, cardiac disorders, elderly; renal, hepatic disorders

P G

Do Not Confuse:
Lodine/codeine

Pharmacokinetics

Absorption	Well absorbed
Distribution	Highly bound to plasma protein
Metabolism	Unknown
Excretion	Unknown
Half-life	7 hr

Pharmacodynamics

Onset	½ hr
Peak	1-2 hr
Duration	4-12 hr

Interactions
Individual drugs
Acetaminophen (long-term use): ↑ renal reactions
Alcohol: ↑ adverse reactions
Aspirin: ↓ effectiveness, ↑ adverse reactions
Cyclosporine: ↑ toxicity
Digoxin: ↑ toxicity, ↑ levels
Insulin: ↓ insulin effect
Lithium: ↑ toxicity
Methotrexate: ↑ toxicity
Phenytoin: ↑ toxicity
Probenecid: ↑ toxicity
Sulfonylurea: ↑ toxicity
Warfarin: ↑ anticoagulant effects

Drug classifications
Antacids: ↓ etodolac effect
Anticoagulants: ↑ risk of bleeding
Antihypertensives: ↓ effect of antihypertensives
Antineoplastics: ↑ risk of hematologic toxicity
β-Adrenergic blockers: ↓ effect
Cephalosporins: ↑ risk of bleeding
Diuretics: ↓ effectiveness of diuretics, ↓ antihypertensive effects
Glucocorticoids: ↑ adverse reactions
Hypoglycemics: ↓ hypoglycemic effect
Nonsteroidal antiinflammatories: ↑ adverse reactions
Potassium supplements: ↑ adverse reactions
Radiation: ↑ risk of hematologic toxicity
Sulfonamides: ↑ toxicity

NURSING CONSIDERATIONS
Assessment
- Assess pain: location, frequency, characteristics; relief after medication
- Assess for GI bleeding: black stools, hematemesis
- Assess for asthma, aspirin hypersensitivity, nasal polyps that may be hypersensitive to etodolac
- Monitor blood counts during therapy; watch for decreasing platelets; if low, therapy may need to be discontinued, then restarted after hematologic recovery; watch for blood dyscrasia (thrombocytopenia): bruising, fatigue, bleeding, poor healing

Nursing diagnoses
- ✓ Pain (uses)
- ✓ Mobility, impaired physical (uses)
- ✓ Knowledge deficit (teaching)
- ✓ Injury, risk for (adverse reactions)

Implementation
- Administer with food or milk to decrease gastric symptoms; food will

E

slow absorption slightly, will not decrease absorption.

- Do not crush, chew ext rel tabs

Patient/family education

- Inform patient that drug must be continued for prescribed time to be effective; to avoid aspirin, alcoholic beverages, NSAIDs
- Caution patient to report bleeding, bruising, fatigue, malaise because blood dyscrasias can occur
- Instruct patient to use caution when driving; drowsiness, dizziness may occur
- Teach patient to take with a full glass of water to enhance absorption; do not crush, break, or chew medication

Evaluation

Positive therapeutic outcome

- Decreased pain
- Decreased inflammation
- Increased mobility

HIGH ALERT

etoposide (VP-16) (℞)

(e-toe′poe-side)

Etopophos, VePesid

Func. class.: Antineoplastic—misc.

Chem. class.: Semisynthetic podophyllotoxin

Pregnancy category D

Action: Inhibits mitotic activity through metaphase to mitosis; also inhibits cells from entering mitosis, depresses DNA, RNA synthesis, cell cycle specific S and G_2

Therapeutic Outcome: Prevention of rapid growth of malignant cells

Uses: Leukemias, lung, testicular cancer, lymphomas, neuroblastoma, melanoma, ovarian cancer; being investigated for use in leukemia, lymphoma

Dosage and routes

Testicular cancer

Adult: **IV** 50-100 mg/m^2/day × 3-5 days given q3-5 wk or 200-250 mg/m^2/wk, or 125-140 mg/m^2/day 3 × wk, q5 wk

Lung cancer

Adult: PO 35 mg/m^2/day × 4 days, repeated q3-4 wk; **IV** 35 mg/m^2/day × 4 days

Available forms: Inj 20 mg/ml; 113.6 etoposide phosphate = 100 etoposide; caps 50, 100 mg

Adverse effects

CNS: Headache, *fever,* peripheral neuropathy, paresthesia, confusion

CV: *Hypotension,* **MI,** dysrhythmia, radiation recall

GI: *Nausea, vomiting, anorexia,* **hepatotoxicity,** dyspepsia, diarrhea, constipation

GU: **Nephrotoxicity**

HEMA: **Thrombocytopenia, leukopenia, myelosuppression, anemia**

INTEG: *Rash, alopecia,* phlebitis at **IV** site

RESP: **Bronchospasm,** pleural effusion

SYST: Anaphylaxis

Contraindications: Hypersensitivity, bone marrow depression, severe hepatic disease, severe renal disease, bacterial infection, pregnancy **D**, viral infection

Precautions: Renal, hepatic disease, lactation, children, gout

Do Not Confuse:
VePesid/Versed

Pharmacokinetics	
Absorption	Variably absorbed
Distribution	Rapidly absorbed, 97% protein binding, crosses placenta
Metabolism	Liver—some
Excretion	Kidneys, unchanged 50%, breast milk
Half-life	3 hr initially, 15 hr terminally

Pharmacodynamics
Unknown

Interactions
Individual drugs
Radiation: ↑ toxicity, bone marrow suppression
Drug classifications
Antineoplastics: ↑ toxicity, bone marrow suppression
Live virus vaccines: ↑ adverse reactions

NURSING CONSIDERATIONS
Assessment
- Monitor B/P, (baseline and q15 min) during administration
- Monitor CBC, differential, platelet count weekly; withhold drug if WBC is <4000/mm^3 or platelet count is <75,000/mm^3; notify prescriber of results; recovery will take 3 wk
- Monitor renal function studies: BUN, urine CrCl before, during therapy; I&O ratio; report fall in urine output of 30 ml/hr; for decreased hyperuricemia
- Monitor for cold, fever, sore throat (may indicate beginning of infection); notify prescriber if these occur
- Assess for bleeding: hematuria, guaiac, bruising or petechiae, mucosa or orifices q8h: no rectal temp; avoid IM inj; use pressure to venipuncture sites
- Identify nutritional status: an antiemetic may need to be prescribed
- ❗ Assess for symptoms indicating severe allergic reactions: rash, pruritus, urticaria, itching, flushing, bronchospasm, hypotension; epinephrine and crash cart should be nearby

Nursing diagnoses
- ✓ Injury, risk for (adverse reactions)
- ✓ Body image disturbance (adverse reactions)
- ✓ Infection, risk for (adverse reactions)
- ✓ Knowledge deficit (teaching)

Implementation
PO route
- Caps need to be refrigerated

IV **IV route**
- Give by intermittent inf
- Sol should be prepared by qualified personnel and only under controlled conditions
- Use Luer Loc tubing to prevent leakage; do not let sol come in contact with skin; if contact occurs, wash well with soap and water
- Give after diluting 100 mg/250 ml or more D_5W or NaCl to a concentration of 0.2-0.4 mg/ml; infuse over 30-60 min; phosphate may be given over 5 min-3½ hr; may dilute further to 0.1 mg/ml in 0.9% NaCl, D_5W
- Give hyaluronidase 150 U/ml to 1 ml NaCl to infiltration area; ice compress for treatment of vesicant activity

Y-site compatibilities:
Allopurinol, amifostine, aztreonam, cladribine, fludarabine, granisetron, melphalan, ondansetron, paclitaxel, piperacillin/tazobactam, sargramostim, sodium bicarbonate, teniposide, thiotepa, vinorelbine

Y-site incompatibility:
Idarubicin

Additive compatibilities:
Carboplatin, cisplatin, cytarabine, floxuridine, fluorouracil, hydroxyzine, ifosfamide, ondansetron

Patient/family education
- Teach patient to avoid use of products containing aspirin or ibuprofen, razors, commercial mouthwash because bleeding may occur; to report symptoms of bleeding (hematuria, tarry stools)
- Instruct patient to report signs of anemia (fatigue, headache, irritability, faintness, shortness of breath)
- Teach patient to report any changes in breathing or coughing even several months after treatment
- Advise patient that contraception will be necessary during treatment

because teratogenesis may occur
• Caution patient that hair loss may occur during treatment; a wig or hairpiece may make patient feel better; new hair will be different in color, texture
• Advise patient to avoid vaccinations during treatment because serious reactions may occur
• Teach patient to report signs/symptoms of infection; fever, chills, sore throat; patient should avoid crowds and persons with known infections

Evaluation

Positive therapeutic outcome
• Decreased spread of malignant, leukemic cells

exemestane (℞)

(x-ee-mes′-tane)
Aromasin
Func. class.: Antineoplastic
Chem. class.: Aromatase inhibitor

Pregnancy category D

Action: Lowers serum estradiol concentrations; many breast cancers have strong estrogen receptors

Therapeutic Outcome: Prevention of rapidly growing malignant cells

Uses: Advanced breast carcinoma that has not responded to other therapy in estrogen receptor–positive patients (postmenopausal)

Dosage and routes

Adult: PO 25 mg qd pc

Available forms: Tabs 25 mg

Adverse effects

CNS: Hot flashes, headache, fatigue, depression, insomnia, anxiety
CV: Hypertension
GI: Nausea, vomiting, increased appetite, diarrhea, constipation, abdominal pain
RESP: Cough, dyspnea

Contraindications: Hypersensitivity, premenopausal women, pregnancy **D**

P G **Precautions:** Lactation, children, elderly, hepatic, renal disease

Pharmacokinetics

Absorption	Rapidly absorbed
Distribution	Unknown
Metabolism	Liver
Excretion	Feces, urine
Half-life	24 hr

Pharmacodynamics

Unknown

NURSING CONSIDERATIONS

Assessment

• Assess B/P, hypertension may occur

Nursing diagnoses

✓ Injury, risk for (adverse reactions)
✓ Knowledge deficit (teaching)

Implementation

• Give with food or fluids for GI upset
• Store in light-resistant container at room temp

Patient/family education

• Instruct patient to report any complaints, side effects to prescriber; if dose is missed, do not double next dose
• Advise patient that hot flashes can occur, and are reversible after discontinuing treatment
• Inform patient about who should be told about therapy

Evaluation

Positive therapeutic outcome
• Decreased spread of malignant cells in breast cancer

HIGH ALERT

factor IX complex (human)/factor IX (℞)

Konyne 80, Proplex T, Proplex SX-T, Profilnine Heat-Treated/ Alphanine, Alpha Nine SD, Mononine

Func. class.: Hemostatic

Chem. class.: Factors II, VII, IX, X

Pregnancy category C

Action: Causes an increase in blood levels of clotting factors II, VII, IX, X; factor IX (human) has IX activity only

➔ **Therapeutic Outcome:** Replacement of factors II, VII, IX, X

Uses: Hemophilia B (Christmas disease), factor IX deficiency, anticoagulant reversal, control of bleeding in patients with factor VIII inhibitors; reversal of overdose of anticoagulants in emergencies

Dosage and routes

Bleeding in hemophilia A and inhibitors of factor VIII

P ***Adult and child:*** 75 U/kg, repeat in 12 hr

Bleeding in hemophilia B

P ***Adult and child:*** Give to establish 25% of normal factor IX activity or 60-75 U/kg/day then 10-20 U/kg/ day × 1 wk

Prophylaxis of bleeding in hemophilia B

P ***Adult and child:*** 10-20 U/kg/ day × 1 wk

Reversal of oral anticoagulant

P ***Adult and child:*** 15 U/kg

Factor VII deficiency (use Proplex T)

P ***Adult and child:*** 0.5 U/kg × body weight (kg) × desired factor IX increase (in % of normal); repeat q4-6h if needed

Factor IX AlphaNine, AlphaNine SD (minor to moderate hemorrhage)

P ***Adult and child:*** Give amount to increase plasma factor IX level to 20%-30%

Serious hemorrhage

P ***Adult and child:*** Give amount to increase plasma factor IX level to 30%-50% given as daily inf

Mononine

Minor hemorrhage

P ***Adult and child:*** Give amount to increase plasma factor IX level to 15%-25% (20-30 U/kg), may repeat in 24 hr

Major trauma

P ***Adult and child:*** Give amount to increase plasma factor IX level to 25%-50% (75 U/kg) q1830h for up to 10 days

Available forms: Inj (number of units noted on label)

Adverse effects

CNS: Headache, dizziness, malaise, paresthesia, *lethargy, chills, fever, flushing*

CV: Hypotension, tachycardia, **MI, venous thrombosis, pulmonary embolism**

EENT: Tinnitus, eyelid swelling

GI: Nausea, vomiting, abdominal cramps, jaundice, **viral hepatitis**

HEMA: **Thrombosis, hemolysis, AIDS, disseminated intravascular coagulation (DIC)**

INTEG: Rash, flushing, *urticaria*

RESP: **Bronchospasm**

Contraindications: Hypersensitivity to mouse protein, hepatic disease, DIC, elective surgery, mild factor IX deficiency

Precautions: Neonates/infants, P pregnancy **C**

F

Pharmacokinetics

Absorption	40% (PO), complete (**IV**)
Distribution	Unknown
Metabolism	Rapidly cleared from plasma, liver 30%
Excretion	Kidneys—70% unchanged
Half-life	24 hr

Pharmacodynamics

Unknown

Interactions

Individual drugs

Aminocaproic acid: ↑ risk of thrombosis; do not use together

NURSING CONSIDERATIONS

Assesment

- Monitor blood studies (coagulation factor assays by % normal: 5% prevents spontaneous hemorrhage, 30%-50% for surgery, 80%-100% for severe hemorrhage); check for bleeding q15-30 min, immobilize and apply ice to affected joints
- Monitor for increased B/P, pulse
- Monitor I&O; if urine becomes orange or red, notify prescriber
- Assess for allergic or pyrogenic reaction: fever, chills, rash, itching; slow inf rate if not severe
- ◆ Assess for DIC: bleeding, ecchymosis, hypersensitivity, changes in coagulation tests

Nursing diagnoses

- ✓ Injury, risk for (uses)
- ✓ Tissue perfusion, altered (uses)
- ✓ Knowledge deficit (teaching)

Implementation

IV IV route

- Give hepatitis B vaccine before administration
- Give **IV** after warming to room temp 3 ml/min or less, with plastic syringe only; do not admix
- Give after dilution with provided diluent, 50 or 25 U/ml; give so as not to exceed 10 ml/min; decrease rate if fever, headache, flushing, tingling occur
- Give after crossmatch is completed if patient has blood type A, B, AB, to determine incompatibility with factor
- Store reconstituted sol for 3 hr at room temp or up to 2 yr if refrigerated (powder); check expiration date

Patient/family education

- Advise patient to report any signs of bleeding: gums, under skin, urine, stools, emesis
- Caution patient about risk of viral hepatitis, AIDS; that immunization for hepatitis B may be given first; to be tested q2-3 mo for HIV, even though the risk is low
- Tell patient to carry ID identifying disease and treatment; avoid salicylates, NSAIDs, to inform other health professionals about condition

Evaluation

Positive therapeutic outcome

- Prevention of hemorrhage

famciclovir (℞)

(fam-sye-klo'vir)

Famvir

Func. class.: Antiviral

Chem. class.: Guanosine nucleoside

Pregnancy category B

Action: Inhibits DNA polymerase and viral DNA synthesis by the conversion of this guanosine nucleoside to penciclovir

➔ Therapeutic Outcome: Decreasing size and number of lesions

Uses: Treatment of acute herpes zoster (shingles), genital herpes, recurrent mucocutaneous herpes simplex virus (HSV) in HIV patients

Dosage and routes

Herpes zoster

Adult: PO 500 mg q8h

Renal dose

CrCl ≥ 60 ml/min 500 mg q8h; 40-59

ml/min 500 mg q12h; 20-39 ml/min 500 mg q24h

Recurrent mucocutaneous herpes simplex

Adult: PO 500 mg q12h × 1 wk

Recurrent HSV

Adult: PO 125 mg q12h × 5 days

Suppression of recurrent HSV

Adult: PO 250 mg q12h up to 1 yr

Available forms: Tabs 125, 250, 500 mg

Adverse effects

CNS: *Headache, fatigue, dizziness,* paresthesia, somnolence, fever

GI: Nausea, vomiting, diarrhea, constipation, abdominal pain, anorexia

GU: Decreased sperm count

INTEG: *Pruritus*

MS: Back pain, arthralgia

RESP: Pharyngitis, sinusitis

Contraindications: Hypersensitivity to this drug or penciclovir

Precautions: Renal disease, pregnancy **B,** hypersensitivity to acyclovir, ganciclovir

Pharmacokinetics	
Absorption	Well absorbed
Distribution	Unknown
Metabolism	Intestinal tissue, blood, liver
Excretion	Breast milk, kidney, bile
Half-life	3 hr

Pharmacodynamics	
Onset	Unknown
Peak	1 hr
Duration	8 hr

Interactions

Individual drugs

Cimetidine: ↓ metabolism

Digoxin: ↓ renal excretion

Probenecid: ↓ renal excretion

Theophylline: ↓ renal excretion

NURSING CONSIDERATIONS

Assessment

- Assess amount and distribution of lesions; also burning, itching, or pain (early symptoms of herpes infection); posttherapeutic neuralgia during and after treatment
- Monitor renal function studies: urine CrCl, BUN before and during treatment if patient has decreased renal function; dose may need to be lowered
- Monitor bowel pattern before, during treatment; diarrhea may occur

Nursing diagnoses

✓ Infection, risk for (uses)

✓ Knowledge deficit (teaching)

Implementation

- Give with or without meals; absorption does not appear to be lowered when taken with food
- Give within 72 hr of the appearance of rash in herpes zoster

Patient/family education

- Teach patient how to recognize signs of beginning of infection
- Teach patient how to prevent the spread of infection to others
- Teach patient reason for medication and expected results
- Advise patient that this medication does not prevent spread of disease to others, that condoms should be used
- Advise women with genital herpes to have yearly Pap smears, cervical cancer is more likely

Evaluation

Positive therapeutic outcome

- Decreased size and spread of lesions

F

famotidine (℞, OTC)

(fa-moe'to-deen)

Pepcid AC, Pepcid, Pepcid IV, Pepcid RPD ✱

Func. class.: H_2-histamine receptor antagonist, antiulcer agent

Pregnancy category B

Action: Inhibits histamine at H_2-receptor site in gastric parietal cells, which inhibits gastric acid secretion

➔ **Therapeutic Outcome:** Healing of duodenal ulcers or gastric ulcers; prevention of duodenal ulcers; decreases symptoms of gastroesophageal reflux disease or Zollinger-Ellison syndrome, heartburn

Uses: Short-term treatment of active duodenal ulcer, maintenance therapy for duodenal ulcer, Zollinger-Ellison syndrome, multiple endocrine adenomas, gastric ulcers, heartburn

Investigational uses: GI disorders in those taking NSAIDs, urticaria, prevention of stress ulcers, aspiration pneumonitis, inactivation of oral pancreatic enzymes in pancreatic disorders, prevention of paclitaxel hypersensitivity reactions

Dosage and routes

Active ulcer

Adult: PO 40 mg qd hs × 4-8 wk, then 20 mg qd hs if needed (maintenance); **IV** 20 mg q12h if unable to take PO

P ***Child 1-16 yr:*** PO 0.5 mg/kg/day hs or divided bid, max 40 mg qd

Hypersecretory conditions

Adult: PO 20 mg q6h; may give 160 mg q6h if needed; **IV** 20 mg q12h if unable to take PO

P ***Child 1-16 yr:*** PO 1 mg/kg/day divided bid, max 40 mg bid

Paclitaxel hypersensitivity reactions

Adult: **IV** 20 mg ½ hr before inf

Heartburn relief/prevention

Adult: PO 10 mg with water or 1 hr before eating

Renal dose

CrCl <10 ml/min 20 mg hs or dose q36-48h

Available forms: Tabs 10 (OTC), 20, 40 mg; powder for oral susp 40 mg/5 ml; inj 10 mg/ml, 20 mg/50 ml 0.9% NaCl; orally disintegrating tabs (RPD) 20, 40 mg; chew tabs 10 mg

Adverse effects

CNS: *Headache, dizziness,* paresthesia, **seizures,** depression, anxiety, somnolence, insomnia, fever

CV: **Dysrhythmias**

EENT: Taste change, tinnitus, orbital edema

GI: *Constipation,* nausea, vomiting, anorexia, cramps, abnormal liver enzymes

HEMA: **Thrombocytopenia, aplastic anemia**

INTEG: Rash, diarrhea

MS: Myalgia, arthralgia

Contraindications: Hypersensitivity

Precautions: Pregnancy **B,** P lactation, children <12 yr, severe renal disease, severe hepatic disease, G elderly

Pharmacokinetics

Absorption	50% absorbed (PO)
Distribution	Plasma, protein binding (15%-20%)
Metabolism	Liver (30% active metabolizing)
Excretion	Kidneys (70%)
Half-life	2½-3½ hr

Pharmacodynamics

	PO	IV
Onset	30-60 min	Immediate
Peak	1-3 hr	½-3 hr
Duration	6-12 hr	8-15 hr

Interactions

Individual drugs

Ketoconazole: ↓ absorption of ketoconazole

Drug classifications

Antacids: ↓ absorption of famotidine

NURSING CONSIDERATIONS

Assessment

- Assess patient with ulcers or suspected ulcers: epigastric, abdominal pain, hematemesis, occult blood in stools, blood in gastric, aspirate before treatment; throughout treatment, monitor gastric pH (5 should be maintained)
- Monitor I&O ratio, BUN, creatinine, CBC with differential monthly

Nursing diagnoses

✓ Pain (uses)
✓ Knowledge deficit (teaching)

Implementation

PO route

- Give antacids 1 hr before or 2 hr after famotidine; may be given with foods or liq
- Administer oral susp after shaking well; discard unused sol after 1 mo

IV **IV route**

- Give **IV** direct after diluting 2 ml of drug (10 mg/ml) in 0.9% NaCl to total volume of 5-10 ml; inject over 2 min to prevent hypotension
- Administer **IV** intermittent inf after diluting 20 mg of drug in 100 ml of LR, 0.9% NaCl, D_5W, $D_{10}W$; run over 15-30 min
- Store in cool environment (oral); **IV** solution is stable for 48 hr at room temp; do not use discolored sol

Y-site compatibilities:

Acyclovir, allopurinol, amifostine, aminophylline, amphotericin, ampicillin, ampicillin/sulbactam, amrinone, amsacrine, atropine, aztreonam, bretylium, calcium gluconate, cefazolin, cefoperazone, cefotaxime, cefotetan, cefoxitin, ceftazidime, ceftizoxime, ceftriaxone, cefuroxime, cephalothin, cephapirin, chlorpromazine, cisplatin, cladribine, cyclophosphamide, cytarabine, dexamethasone, dextran 40, digoxin, diphenhydramine, dobutamine, dopamine, doxorubicin, droperidol, enalaprilat, epinephrine, erythromycin lactobionate, esmolol, filgrastim, fluconazole, fludarabine, folic acid, gentamicin, granisetron, haloperidol, heparin, hydrocortisone, hydromorphone, hydroxyzine, imipenem/cilastatin, regular insulin, isoproterenol, labetalol, lidocaine, lorazepam, magnesium sulfate, melphalan, meperidine, methotrexate, methylprednisolone, metoclopramide, mezlocillin, midazolam, morphine, nafcillin, nitroglycerin, nitroprusside, norepinephrine, ondansetron, oxacillin, paclitaxel, perphenazine, phenylephrine, phenytoin, phytonadione, piperacillin, potassium chloride, potassium phosphate, procainamide, propofol, sargramostim, sodium bicarbonate, teniposide, theophylline, thiamine, thiotepa, ticarcillin, ticarcillin/clavulanate, verapamil, vinorelbine

Additive compatibilities:

Cefazolin, cefmetazole, flumazenil

Patient/family education

- Caution patient to avoid driving, other hazardous activities until stabilized on this medication; dizziness may occur
- Advise patient to avoid black pepper, caffeine, alcohol, harsh spices, extremes in temperature of food; tell patient to avoid OTC preparations: aspirin, cough, cold preparations; condition may worsen
- Tell patient that smoking decreases the effectiveness of the drug; that smoking cessation should be considered
- Instruct patient that drug must be continued for prescribed time to be effective and taken exactly as prescribed; doses are not to be doubled; not to use OTC and prescription products at the same time; to take

missed dose when remembered up to 1 hr before next dose
- Tell patient to report bruising, fatigue, malaise; blood dyscrasias may occur
- Tell patient to report diarrhea, black tarry stools, sore throat, rash, dizziness, confusion, rash, or delirium to prescriber immediately

Evaluation

Positive therapeutic outcome
- Decreased pain in abdomen
- Healing of ulcers

fat emulsions (℞)

(fat ee-mul'shuns)

Intralipid 10%, Intralipid 20%, Liposyn II 10%, Liposyn II 20%, Liposyn III 10%, Liposyn III 20%, Soyacal 20%

Func. class.: Caloric

Chem. class.: Fatty acid, long chain

Pregnancy category C

Action: Needed for energy, heat production; consists of neutral triglycerides, primarily unsaturated fatty acids

Therapeutic Outcome: Increased available calories and fatty acids

Uses: Increase calorie intake, prevent fatty acid deficiency

Dosage and routes

Deficiency

P ***Adult and child:*** **IV** 8%-10% of required calorie intake (intralipid)

Adjunct to TPN

Adult: **IV** 1 ml/min over 15-30 min (10%) or 0.5 ml/min over 15-30 min (20%); may increase to 500 ml over 4-8 hr if no adverse reactions occur; not to exceed 2.5 g/kg

P ***Child:*** **IV** 0.1 ml/min over 10-15 min (10%) or 0.05 ml/ min over 10-15 min (20%); may increase to 1 g/kg over 4 hr if no adverse reactions occur; not to exceed 4 g/kg

Prevention of deficiency

Adult: **IV** 500 ml 2 × wk (10%), given 1 ml/min for 30 min, not to exceed 500 ml over 6 hr

P ***Child:*** **IV** 5-10 ml/kg/day (10%), given 0.1 ml/min for 30 min, not to exceed 100 ml/hr

Available forms: Sol 10% (50, 100, 200, 250, 500 ml), 20% (50, 100, 200, 250, 500 ml)

Adverse effects

CNS: Dizziness, headache, drowsiness, focal seizures

CV: **Shock**

GI: Nausea, vomiting, **hepatomegaly**

HEMA: **Hyperlipemia, hypercoagulation, thrombocytopenia, leukopenia, leukocytosis**

RESP: Dyspnea, **fat in lung tissue**

Contraindications: Hypersensitivity, hyperlipemia, lipid necrosis, acute pancreatitis accompanied by hyperlipemia, hyperbilirubinemia of P the newborn

Precautions: Severe liver disease, diabetes mellitus, thrombocytopenia, gastric ulcers, premature, term P newborns, pregnancy **C**, sepsis

Pharmacokinetics

Absorption	Completely absorbed
Distribution	Intravascular space
Metabolism	Conversion to triglycerides, to free fatty acids
Excretion	Unknown
Half-life	Unknown

Pharmacodynamics

Unknown

Interactions: None

NURSING CONSIDERATIONS

Assessment

- Monitor triglycerides, free fatty acid levels, platelet counts daily to prevent fat overload, thrombocytopenia

- Monitor liver function studies: AST, ALT, Hct, Hgb; notify prescriber if abnormal
- Assess nutritional status: calorie count by dietitian; monitor weight daily

Nursing diagnoses

✓ Nutrition, less than body requirements (uses)
✓ Knowledge deficit (teaching)

Implementation

- Administer using infusion pump at prescribed rate; do not use in-line filter sized for lipid emulsion; clogging will occur
- Do not use mixed sol that looks oily or is not separated; discard unused sol
- Change **IV** tubing at each inf: infection may occur with old tubing
- Give by intermittent inf at a rate of 10% sol (1 ml/min); 20% sol (0.5 ml/min) initially for 15-30 min; may be increased to 10% sol (120 ml/hr) or 20% sol (62.5 ml/hr) if no adverse reactions occur; do not give more than **P** 500 ml during the first day; children should be given 10% (0.1 mg/ ml) or 20% (0.05 ml/min) initially for 15-30 min, may be increased 1 g/kg/4 hr, do not give more than 10% (100 ml/hr) or 20% (50 ml/hr)

Y-site compatibilities: Ampicillin, cefamandole, cefazolin, cefoxitin, cephapirin, clindamycin, digoxin, dopamine, erythromycin, furosemide, gentamicin, IL-2, isoproterenol, lidocaine, kanamycin, norepinephrine, oxacillin, penicillin G potassium, ticarcillin, tobramycin

Y-site incompatibilities: Amikacin, tetracycline

Additive compatibilities: Cefamandole, chloramphenicol, cimetidine, cyclosporine, diphenhydramine, famotidine, heparin, hydrocortisone, multivitamins, nizatidine, penicillin G potassium

Patient/family education

- Teach patient reason for use of lipids and expected results

Evaluation

Positive therapeutic outcome

- Increased weight
- Fatty acids at adequate levels

felodipine (℞)

(feh-loh'dih-peen)

Plendil, Renedil ♣

Func. class.: Calcium-channel blocker, antihypertensive, antianginal

Chem. class.: Dihydropyridine

Pregnancy category C

Action: Inhibits calcium ion influx across cell membrane, resulting in inhibition of excitation/contraction

➡ **Therapeutic Outcome:** Decreased B/P in hypertension

Uses: Essential hypertension, alone or with other antihypertensives, angina pectoris, Prinzmetal's angina (vasospastic)

Dosage and routes

Adult: PO 5 mg qd initially, usual range 5-10 mg qd; max 20 mg qd; do not adjust dosage at intervals of <2 wk

G ***Elderly:*** PO 2.5 mg qd

Hepatic dose

PO 2.5-5 mg qd, max 10 mg/day

Available forms: Ext rel tabs 2.5, 5, 10 mg

Adverse effects

CNS: Headache, fatigue, drowsiness, dizziness, anxiety, depression, nervousness, insomnia, light-headedness, paresthesia, tinnitus, psychosis, somnolence

CV: **Dysrhythmias**, edema, **CHF**, hypotension, palpitations, **MI, pulmonary edema**, tachycardia, syncope, AV block, angina

GI: Nausea, vomiting, diarrhea, gastric

upset, constipation, increased liver function studies, dry mouth
HEMA: Anemia
INTEG: Rash, pruritus
MISC: Flushing, sexual difficulties, cough, nasal congestion, shortness of breath, wheezing, epistaxis, respiratory infection, chest pain, **Stevens-Johnson syndrome,** gingival hyperplasia

Contraindications: Hypersensitivity, sick sinus syndrome, 2nd- or 3rd-degree heart block

Precautions: CHF, hypotension <90 mm Hg systolic, hepatic injury, P pregnancy **C,** lactation, children, renal G disease, elderly

Do Not Confuse:
Plendil/pindolol, Plendil/Prinivil

Pharmacokinetics

Absorption	Well absorbed
Distribution	Unknown; protein binding >99%
Metabolism	Liver, extensively
Excretion	Kidneys
Half-life	11-16 hr

Pharmacodynamics

Onset	2-3 hr
Peak	2½-5 hr
Duration	<24 hr

Interactions
Individual drugs
Alcohol: ↑ hypotension
Carbamazepine: ↑ toxicity
Digoxin: ↑ digoxin levels, ↑ bradycardia, CHF
Phenobarbital: ↓ effectiveness
Phenytoin: ↓ effectiveness
Propranolol: ↑ toxicity
Theophylline: ↓ theophylline level
Drug classifications
Antihypertensives: ↑ hypotension
β-Adrenergic blockers: ↑ bradycardia, CHF
Nitrates: ↑ nitrates
Food/drug
Grapefruit juice: ↑ felodipine level

NURSING CONSIDERATIONS
Assessment
- Assess fluid volume status: I&O ratio and record; weight; skin turgor; adequacy of pulses; moist mucous membranes; bilateral lung sounds; peripheral pitting edema; dehydration symptoms of decreasing output, thirst, hypotension, dry mouth, and mucous membranes should be reported; for CHF: weight gain, rales/crackles, dyspnea, edema, jugular venous distention
- Monitor ALT, AST, bilirubin daily if these are elevated
- Monitor cardiac status: B/P, pulse, respiration, ECG, periodically
- Assess for anginal pain: duration, intensity, ameliorating, aggravating factors

Nursing diagnoses
- ✓ Cardiac output, decreased (uses)
- ✓ Knowledge deficit (teaching)

Implementation
- Give once a day, with food for GI symptoms
- Do not crush, chew tabs, sus rel products

Patient/family education
- Caution patient to avoid hazardous activities until stabilized on drug, and dizziness is no longer a problem
- Instruct patient to limit caffeine consumption; to avoid alcohol and OTC drugs unless directed by prescriber
- Urge patient to comply in all areas of medical regimen: diet, exercise, stress reduction, drug therapy; to notify prescriber of irregular heart beat, shortness of breath, swelling of feet and hands, pronounced dizziness, constipation, nausea, hypotension
- Teach patient to use as directed even if feeling better; may be taken with other CV drugs (nitrates,

β-blockers), that capsules may appear in stools, but are insignificant

Evaluation

Positive therapeutic outcome

- Decreased B/P

fenofibrate (℞)

(fen-oh-fee' brate)

Tricor

Func. class.: Antilipemic

Chem. class.: Fibric acid derivative

Pregnancy category C

Action: Inhibits biosynthesis of low-density and very low-density lipoproteins, which are responsible for triglyceride development; mobilizes triglycerides from tissue; increases excretion of neutral sterols

Therapeutic Outcome: Decreasing cholesterol levels and low-density lipoproteins, decreased pruritus

Uses: Patients with Types IV, V hyperlipidemia who do not respond to other treatment and who are at risk for pancreatitis

Investigational uses: Polymetabolic syndrome X

Dosage and routes

Hypertriglyceridemia

Adult: PO 67-200 mg/day, may increase q4-8 wk, max 201 mg/day

Primary hypercholesterolemia/mixed hyperlipidemia

Adult: PO 200 mg/day

Renal dose/elderly

G ***Adult:*** PO 67 mg/day (CrCl <50 ml/min)

Available forms: Micronized caps 67, 134, 200 mg

Adverse effects

CNS: Fatigue, weakness, drowsiness, dizziness

CV: Angina, **dysrhythmias**

GI: Nausea, vomiting, dyspepsia, increased liver enzymes, flatulence, hepatomegaly, gastritis

GU: Dysuria, proteinuria, oliguria

INTEG: *Rash,* urticaria, pruritus

MISC: Polyphagia, weight gain

MS: Myalgias, arthralgias

Contraindications: Severe hepatic disease, severe renal disease, primary biliary cirrhosis

Precautions: Peptic ulcer, pregnancy **C**, lactation, pancreatitis

Pharmacokinetics	
Absorption	Unknown
Distribution	Protein binding 99%
Metabolism	Liver
Excretion	Urine 60%
Half-life	20 hr

Pharmacodynamics	
Peak	6-8 hr

Interactions

Drug classifications

Anticoagulants, oral: ↑ effect of anticoagulants

Bile acid sequestrants: ↓ absorption

Diuretics, thiazide: ↓ action of fenofibrate

Estrogens: ↓ action of fenofibrate

HMG-CoA reductase inhibitors: Do not use together, rhabdomyolysis may occur

Immunosuppressants: ↓ fenofibrate elimination

Nephrotoxics: ↓ fenofibrate elimination

Food/drug

↑ Absorption

NURSING CONSIDERATIONS

Assessment

- Assess lipid levels, liver function tests, baseline and periodically during treatment; CPK if muscle pain occurs, CBC, Hct, Hgh, pro-time with anticoagulant therapy
- Assess for pancreatitis, cholelithia-

F

sis, renal failure, rhabdomyolysis, myositis, drug should be discontinued
- Assess nutrition: fat, protein, carbohydrates, nutritional analysis should be completed by dietician
- Assess skin integrity after patient has been receiving drug; itching, pruritus often occur from bile deposits on skin
- Monitor cardiac glycoside level if both drugs are being administered; cardiac glycoside levels will be decreased
- Monitor for signs of vit A, D, K deficiency; serum cholesterol, triglyceride levels, electrolytes if on extended therapy
- Monitor bowel pattern daily; increase bulk, water in diet if constipation develops

Nursing diagnoses

✓ Knowledge deficit (teaching)
✓ Noncompliance (teaching)

Implementation

- Give with evening meal; if dose is increased, take with breakfast and evening meal
- Do not chew, crush caps
- Store in cool environment in tight, light-resistant container

Patient/family education

- Inform patient that compliance is needed
- Teach patient that risk factors—high-fat diet, smoking, alcohol consumption, absence of exercise—should be decreased
- Caution patient to notify prescriber if pregnancy is planned or suspected
- Teach patient to notify prescriber if the GI symptoms of diarrhea, abdominal or epigastric pain, nausea, or vomiting occur
- Instruct patient to report GU symptoms: dysuria, proteinuria, oliguria, decreased libido, impotence
- Advise patient to notify prescriber of muscle pain, weakness, fever, fatigue, epigastric pain

Evaluation

Positive therapeutic outcome
- Decrease in cholesterol to desired level after 8 wk

fenoldopam (℞)
(fen-nahl'doh-pam)
Corlopam
Func. class.: Antihypertensive, vasodilator

Pregnancy category B

Action: Antagonizes D_1-like dopamine receptors; binds to α_2-adrenoreceptors; increases renal blood flow

Therapeutic Outcome: B/P, decreased

Uses: Hypertensive crisis, malignant hypertension

Dosage and routes

Adult: **IV** 0.01-1.6 µg/kg/min titrated slowly result in less reflex tachycardia

Available forms: Inj conc 10 mg/ml

Adverse effects

CNS: ***Headache,*** anxiety, dizziness
CV: ***Hypotension,*** ST-T-wave changes, angina pectoris, palpitations, **MI, ischemic heart disease**
GI: Nausea, vomiting, constipation, diarrhea
HEMA: **Leukocytosis, bleeding**
META: Increased BUN, glucose, LDH, creatinine, hypokalemia

Contraindications: Hypersensitivity, sulfite sensitivity

Precautions: Tachycardia, pregnancy **B,** lactation, children, intraocular pressure, hypokalemia

Pharmacokinetics

Absorption	Unknown
Distribution	Steady state 20 min
Metabolism	Unknown
Excretion	Unknown
Half-life	5 min (elimination)

Pharmacodynamics

Onset	Unknown
Peak	Unknown
Duration	Unknown

Interactions
Drug classifications
β-Adrenergic blockers: ↑ hypotension

NURSING CONSIDERATIONS
Assessment
- Monitor B/P q5 min until stabilized, then q1h × 2 hr, then q4h; pulse, jugular venous distention q4h
- Monitor electrolytes, blood studies: K, Na, Cl, CO_2, CBC, serum glucose
- Assess skin turgor, dryness of mucous membranes for hydration status
- Assess **IV** site for extravasation, rate

Nursing diagnoses
✓ Tissue perfusion, altered (uses)
✓ Knowledge deficit (teaching)
✓ Noncompliance (teaching)

Implementation
IV **IV route**
- Administer after diluting contents of ampules in 0.9% NaCl, or 5% dextrose inj (40 µg/ml); then add 4 ml of conc (40 mg of drug/1000 ml); 2 ml of conc (20 mg of drug/500 ml); 1 ml of conc (10 mg of drug/250 ml); do not admix
- Give to patient in recumbent position; keep in that position for 1 hr after administration
- Diluted sol is stable in normal light/temp for 24 hr

Patient/family education
- Teach patient reason for medication and expected results
- Instruct patient to report dyspnea, chest pain, bleeding

Evaluation
Positive therapeutic outcome
- Decreased B/P

HIGH ALERT

fentanyl (℞)
(fen′ta-nill)
fentanyl, Sublimaze, Fentanyl Oralet, Actiq
Func. class.: Opioid analgesic
Chem. class.: Synthetic phenylpiperidine derivative

Pregnancy category C

Controlled substance schedule II

Action: Inhibits ascending pain pathways in CNS, increases pain threshold, alters pain perception by binding to opiate receptors

➡ **Therapeutic Outcome:** Relief of pain, supplement to anesthesia

Uses: Preoperatively, postoperatively; adjunct to general anesthetic, when combined with droperidol; Fentanyl Oralet for anesthesia as premedication, conscious sedation; Actiq for breakthrough cancer pain

Dosage and routes
Anesthetic
Adult: **IV** 0.05-0.1 mg q2-3 min prn

Preoperatively
Adult: IM 0.05-0.1 mg q30-60 min before surgery

Postoperatively
Adult: IM 0.05-0.1 mg q1-2hr prn

P ***Child:*** IM 0.02-0.03 mg/9 kg

Fentanyl Oralet
Adult: Transmucosal: 5 μg/kg = fentanyl IM 0.75-1.25 μg/kg, do not exceed 5 μg/kg

P ***Child:*** Transmucosal may need doses of 5-15 μg/kg; must be watched continuously for hypoventilation

Actiq
Adult: Transmucosal 200 μg, redose if needed 15 min after completion of 1st dose, do not give more than 2 doses during titration period

Available forms: Inj 0.05 mg/ml; lozenges 100, 200, 300, 400 μg; lozenges on a stick 200, 400, 600, 800, 1200, 1600 μg

Adverse effects
CNS: Dizziness, delirium, euphoria, light-headedness, sedation, dysphoria, agitation, anxiety
CV: **Bradycardia, cardiac arrest,** hypotension or hypertension, facial flushing, chills
EENT: Blurred vision, miosis
GI: Nausea, vomiting, diarrhea, cramps
GU: Urinary retention
INTEG: Rash, diaphoresis
MS: Muscle rigidity
RESP: **Respiratory depression, arrest, laryngospasm**

Contraindications: Hypersensitivity to opiates, myasthenia gravis

G **Precautions:** Elderly, respiratory depression, increased ICP, seizure disorders, severe respiratory disorders, cardiac dysrhythmias, pregnancy **C**

Pharmacokinetics

Absorption	Well absorbed (IM), completely absorbed (**IV**)
Distribution	Unknown, crosses placenta
Metabolism	Extensively—liver, 80% bound to plasma proteins
Excretion	Kidneys—up to 25% unchanged, breast milk
Half-life	1½-6 hr

Pharmacodynamics

	IM	IV
Onset	7-8 min	Rapid
Peak	30 min	3-5 min
Duration	1-2 hr	½-1 hr

Interactions
Individual drugs
Alcohol: ↑ respiratory depression, hypotension, ↑ sedation
Cimetidine: ↑ recovery
Erythromycin: ↑ recovery
Nalbuphine: ↓ analgesia
Pentazocine: ↓ analgesia
Drug classifications
Antihistamines: ↑ respiratory depression, hypotension
CNS depressants: ↑ respiratory depression, hypotension
MAOIs: Do not use 2 wk before fentanyl
Phenothiazines: ↑ respiratory depression, hypotension
Sedative/hypnotics: ↑ respiratory depression, hypotension
Herb/drug
Kava: ↑ fentanyl action
Lab test interferences
↑ Amylase, ↑ lipase

NURSING CONSIDERATIONS
Assessment
- Monitor VS after parenteral route (B/P, pulse, respiration); note muscle rigidity; take drug history before administering drug; check liver, kidney function tests; assess for respiratory dysfunction: respiratory depression, character, rate, rhythm; notify prescriber if respirations are <10/min
- Monitor CNS changes: dizziness, drowsiness, hallucinations, euphoria, LOC, pupil reaction
- Monitor allergic reactions: rash, urticaria; drug should be discontinued
- Assess for pain: intensity, location, duration, type, before and 15 min after IM route or 3-5 min after **IV** route

Nursing diagnoses

- ✓ Pain (uses)
- ✓ Sensory-perceptual alteration: visual, auditory (adverse reactions)
- ✓ Breathing pattern, ineffective (adverse reactions)
- ✓ Knowledge deficit (teaching)

Implementation

- Give by inj (IM, **IV**), only with resuscitative equipment available; give slowly to prevent rigidity
- Give **IV** undiluted by anesthesiologist or diluted with 5 ml or more sterile water or 0.9% NaCl given through Y-tube or 3-way stopcock given at 0.1 mg or less/ 1.2 min
- Store in light-resistant area at room temp

Transmucosal route

- Remove foil just before administration, instruct patient to place under tongue and suck, not chew (Oralet); place between cheek and lower gum, moving it back and forth and suck, not chew (Actiq); all products not used or partially used should be flushed down the toilet

Syringe compatibilities: Atracurium, atropine, bupivacaine/ketamine, butorphanol, chlorpromazine, cimetidine, clonidine/lidocaine, dimenhydrinate, diphenhydramine, droperidol, heparin, hydromorphone, hydroxyzine, meperidine, metoclopramide, midazolam, morphine, pentazocine, perphenazine, prochlorperazine, promazine, promethazine, ranitidine, scopolamine

Syringe incompatibilities: Pentobarbital

Y-site compatibilities: Amphotericin B cholesteryl, atracurium, cisatracurium, diltiazem, dobutamine, dopamine, enalaprilat, epinephrine, esmolol, etomidate, furosemide, heparin, hydrocortisone, hydromorphone, labetalol, lorazepam, midazolam, milrinone, morphine, nafcillin, nicardipine, nitroglycerin, norepinephrine, pancuronium, potassium chloride, propofol, ranitidine, remifentanil, sargramostim, thiopental, vecuronium, vit B/C

Additive compatibilities: Bupivacaine, sodium bicarbonate

Additive incompatibilities: Methohexital, pentobarbital, thiopental

Solution compatibilities: D_5W, 0.9% NaCl

Patient/family education

- Advise patient to report any symptoms of CNS changes, allergic reactions
- Instruct patient to avoid CNS depressants: alcohol, sedative/hypnotics for at least 24 hr after taking this drug
- Teach patient that dizziness, drowsiness, confusion are common, and to avoid getting up without assistance
- Discuss in detail with patient all aspects of the drug

Evaluation

Positive therapeutic outcome

- Maintenance of anesthesia
- Decreased pain

Treatment of overdose:

Naloxone 0.2-0.8 **IV**, O_2, **IV** fluids, vasopressors

fentanyl transdermal (℞)

(fen'ta-nill)

Duragesic-25, Duragesic-50, Duragesic-75, Duragesic-100

Func. class.: Opioid, analgesic

Chem. class.: Synthetic phenylpiperidine

Pregnancy category C

Controlled substance schedule II

Action: Inhibits ascending pain pathways in CNS, increases pain threshold, alters pain perception by binding to opiate receptors

Therapeutic Outcome: Relief of chronic pain

Uses: Management of chronic pain for those requiring opioid analgesia

Dosage and routes

Adult: TD 25 μg/hr; may increase until pain relief occurs; apply patch to flat surface on upper torso and wear for 72 hr; apply new patch on different site for continued relief

Available forms: Patches 2.5, 5, 7.5, 10 mg

Adverse effects

CNS: Dizziness, delirium, euphoria, light-headedness, sedation, dysphoria, agitation, anxiety, confusion, headache, depression
CV: Bradycardia, **cardiac arrest,** hypotension or hypertension, facial flushing, chills, chest pain, dysrhythmia
EENT: Blurred vision, miosis
GI: Nausea, vomiting, diarrhea, cramps, anorexia, constipation, dyspepsia
GU: Urinary retention, urgency, dysuria, frequency, oliguria
INTEG: Sweating pruritus, rash, erythema, papules
MS: Asthenia
RESP: **Respiratory depression, laryngospasm, bronchospasm;** depresses cough; hypoventilation, dyspnea, hiccups, **apnea**

Contraindications: Hypersensitivity to opiates, myasthenia gravis

Precautions: Elderly, respiratory depression, increased ICP, seizure disorders, severe respiratory disorders, cardiac dysrhythmias, pregnancy **C**, fever

Pharmacokinetics	
Absorption	92% (skin), continuously for 72 hr
Distribution	Crosses placenta
Metabolism	Extensively—liver
Excretion	Up to 25%—kidneys unchanged
Half-life	17 hr after removal of patch

Pharmacodynamics	
Onset	6 hr
Peak	12-24 hr
Duration	72 hr

Interactions

Individual drugs

Alcohol: ↑ respiratory depression, hypotension, ↑ sedation
Cimetidine: ↑ recovery
Erythromycin: ↑ recovery
Nalbuphine: ↓ analgesia
Pentazocine: ↓ analgesia

Drug classifications

Antihistamines: ↑ respiratory depression, hypotension
CNS depressants: ↑ respiratory depression, hypotension
MAOIs: Do not use 2 wk before fentanyl
Phenothiazines: ↑ respiratory depression, hypotension
Sedative/hypnotics: ↑ respiratory depression, hypotension

Herb/drug

Kava: ↑ fentanyl level

Lab test interferences

↑ Amylase, ↑ lipase

NURSING CONSIDERATIONS

Assessment

- Assess for respiratory dysfunction: respiratory depression, character, rate, rhythm; notify prescriber if respirations are <10/min
- Monitor CNS changes: dizziness, drowsiness, hallucinations, euphoria, LOC, pupil reaction
- Monitor allergic reactions: rash, urticaria; drug should be discontinued
- Assess for pain: intensity, location,

duration, type, before and after administration

Nursing diagnoses

- ✓ Pain (uses)
- ✓ Sensory-perceptual alteration: visual, auditory (adverse reactions)
- ✓ Breathing pattern, ineffective (adverse reactions)
- ✓ Knowledge deficit (teaching)

Implementation

- Opioids should be used to control pain until relief is obtained with TD patch; patients may continue to require other narcotics for breakthrough pain; if >100 μg/hr is required, use multiple systems
- Apply patch to chest on a flat area with skin intact; for skin preparation, use clear water with no soap; clip hair, skin should be dry before applying patch; apply immediately after removing from package and press firmly in place with palm of hand; flush old patch down toilet immediately upon removal

Use pain dosing

- Dosage is titrated based on patient's report of pain; dosage is determined by calculating the previous 24-hr requirement and converting to equianalgesic morphine dose
- To convert to another narcotic analgesic, remove TD patch and begin treatment with half the equal pain-controlling dose of the new analgesic in 12-18 hr
- Medication should be tapered gradually after long-term use to prevent withdrawal symptoms

Patient/family education

- Advise patient to report any symptoms of CNS changes, allergic reactions
- Instruct patients to avoid CNS depressants: alcohol, sedative/hypnotics for at least 24 hr after this drug
- Discuss with patient that dizziness, drowsiness, and confusion are common and to avoid getting up without assistance
- Discuss with patient that excessive heat may increase absorption; excessive perspiration may alter adhesiveness

Evaluation

Positive therapeutic outcome

- Decreased pain

Treatment of overdose:

Naloxone 0.2-0.8 **IV**, O_2, **IV** fluids, vasopressors

F

ferrous fumarate
(℞, OTC)
(fer'us)
Femiron, Feostat, Feostat Drops, Hemocyte, Ircon, Nephro-Fer, Novofumar ♣, Palafer ♣, Span-FF

ferrous gluconate
(℞, OTC)
Fergon, Fertinic ♣, Novoferrogluc ♣

ferric gluconate complex (℞, OTC)
Ferrlecit

ferrous sulfate
(℞, OTC)
Apo-Ferrous Sulfate ♣, Feosol, Fer-gen-sol, Fer-Iron Drops, Fero-Grad, Mol-Iron

ferrous sulfate, dried (℞, OTC)
Fe^{50}, Feosol, Feratab, Novoferrosulfa ♣, PMS-Ferrous Sulfate, Slow Fe

iron, carbonyl
(kar'boh-nil)
Feosol

iron polysaccharide
(pah-lee-sack'ah-ride)
Hytinic, Niferex, Nu-Iron, Nu-Iron 150

Func. class.: Hematinic
Chem. class.: Iron preparation

Pregnancy category A

Action: Replaces iron stores needed for red blood cell development, energy and O_2 transport, utilization; fumarate contains 33% elemental iron; gluconate, 12%; sulfate, 20%; iron, 30%; ferrous sulfate exsiccated

➔ **Therapeutic Outcome:** Prevention and correction of iron deficiency

Uses: Iron deficiency anemia, prophylaxis for iron deficiency in pregnancy

Dosage and routes

Fumarate
Adult: PO 200 mg tid-qid
P ***Child 2-12 yr:*** PO 3 mg/kg/day (elemental iron) tid-qid
P ***Child 6 mo-2 yr:*** PO up to 6 mg/kg/day (elemental iron) tid-qid
P ***Child 6 mo-2 yr:*** PO 6 mg/kg/day in 3-4 divided doses
P ***Infants:*** PO 10-25 mg/day (elemental iron) in 3-4 divided doses

Gluconate
Adult: PO 200-600 mg tid
P ***Child 6-12 yr:*** PO 300-900 mg qd
P ***Child <6 yr:*** PO 100-300 mg qd

Sulfate
Adult: PO 0.750-1.5 g/day in divided doses tid
P ***Child 6-12 yr:*** 600 mg/day in divided doses

Pregnancy
Adult: PO 300-600 mg/day in divided doses

Complex
Adult: **IV** inf (125 mg) 10 ml/100 ml of NaCl for inj given over 1 hr

Iron polysaccharide
Adult: 100-200 mg tid
P ***Child:*** PO 4-6 mg/kg/day in 3 divided doses

Available forms

Fumarate: Tabs 63, 195, 200, 324, 325 mg; tabs, chewable 100 mg; tabs, controlled-release 300 mg; oral susp 100 mg/5 ml, 45 mg/0.6 ml

Gluconate: Tabs 300, 320, 325, mg; caps 86, 325, 435 mg; tabs, film-coated 300 mg; elix 300 mg/5 ml

Sulfate: Tabs 195, 300, 325, mg; tabs, enteric-coated 325 mg; tabs, ext rel, time-release caps 525 mg

Dried: Tabs, 200 mg; tabs ext rel 160 mg; caplets ext rel 160 mg

Complex: Inj 62.5 mg/5 ml (12.5 mg/ml)

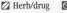

Iron polysaccharide: Tabs 50 mg; caps 150 mg; sol 100 mg/5 ml

Adverse effects

GI: *Nausea, constipation, epigastric pain, black and red tarry stools,* vomiting, diarrhea

INTEG: Temporarily discolored tooth enamel and eyes

Contraindications: Hypersensitivity, ulcerative colitis/regional enteritis, hemosiderosis/hemochromatosis, peptic ulcer disease, hemolytic anemia, cirrhosis

Precautions: Anemia (long-term), pregnancy **B** (ferric gluconate complex), **C** (iron dextran, oral products)

Pharmacokinetics

Absorption	Up to 30%
Distribution	Bound to transferrin, crosses placenta
Metabolism	Recycled
Excretion	Feces, urine, skin, breast milk
Half-life	Unknown

Pharmacodynamics

Unknown

Interactions

Individual drugs

Chloramphenicol: ↑ absorption of iron products
Cholestyramine: ↓ absorption of iron
Cimetidine: ↓ absorption of iron
L-Thyroxine: ↓ L-thyroxine absorption
Levodopa: ↓ absorption of levodopa
Methyldopa: ↓ absorption of methyldopa
Penicillamine: ↓ absorption of penicillamine
Quinolone: ↓ absorption of quinolone
Tetracycline: ↓ absorption of iron products
Vit C: ↑ absorption of iron products

Drug classifications

Fluoroquinolones: ↓ absorption of fluoroquinolone

Food/drug

Caffeine: ↓ absorption
Dairy products: ↓ absorption

Lab test interferences

False positive: Occult blood

NURSING CONSIDERATIONS

Assessment

- Monitor blood studies: Hct, Hgb, reticulocytes, bilirubin before treatment, at least monthly
- Assess for toxicity: nausea, vomiting, diarrhea (green, then tarry stools,) hematemesis, pallor, cyanosis, shock, coma
- Assess bowel elimination; if constipation occurs, increase water, bulk, activity before laxatives are required
- Assess nutrition: amount of iron in diet (meat, dark green leafy vegetables, dried beans, dried fruits, eggs); provide referral to dietitian if indicated
- Identify cause of iron loss or anemia, including salicylates, sulfonamides, antimalarials, quinidine

Nursing diagnoses

✓ Nutrition, less than body requirements (uses)
✓ Fatigue (uses)
✓ Knowledge deficit (teaching)

Implementation

- Give between meals for best absorption; may give with juice; do not give with antacids or milk, delay at least 1 hr; if GI symptoms occur, give pc even if absorption is decreased; eggs, milk products, chocolate, caffeine interfere with absorption
- ⊘ Do not crush, chew tabs
- Give liq preparations through plastic straw to avoid discoloration of tooth enamel; dilute thoroughly
- Give at least 1 hr before bedtime because corrosion may occur in stomach
- Give for <6 mo for anemia

- Store in air-tight, light-resistant container

Patient/family education

- Advise patient that iron will make stools black or dark green; that iron poisoning may occur if increased beyond recommended level
- Tell patient not to crush; swallow tab whole; to keep out of reach of **P** children
- Caution patient not to substitute one iron salt for another; elemental iron content differs (e.g., 300 mg ferrous fumarate contains about 100 mg elemental iron, whereas 300 mg ferrous gluconate contains only about 30 mg elemental iron)
- Caution patient to avoid reclining position for 15-30 min after taking drug to avoid esophageal corrosion; to follow diet high in iron

Evaluation

Positive therapeutic outcome

- Decreased fatigue, weakness
- Improvement in Hct, Hgb, reticulocytes

Treatment of overdose: Induce vomiting; give eggs, milk until lavage can be done

fexofenadine (℞)

(fex-oh-fin'a-deen)

Allegra

Func. class.: H_1-histamine antagonist

Chem. class: Piperidine, peripherally selective

Pregnancy category C

Action: Acts on blood vessels, GI, respiratory system by competing with histamine for H_1-receptor site; decreases allergic response by blocking pharmacologic effects of histamine; less sedation rate than with other antihistamines; causes increased heart rate, vasodilation, increased secretions

➔ Therapeutic Outcome: Absence of allergy symptoms and rhinitis

Uses: Rhinitis, allergy symptoms, chronic idiopathic urticaria

Dosage and routes

P ***Adult and child >12 yr:*** 60 mg bid

P ***Child 6-11 yr:*** PO 30 mg bid

Renal dose

CrCl <80 ml/min 60 mg qd

Available forms: Caps 60 mg; ext rel tabs 180 mg; tabs 30 mg

Adverse effects

CNS: Headache, stimulation, drowsiness, sedation, fatigue, confusion, blurred vision, tinnitus, restlessness, **P** tremors, paradoxical excitation in **G** children or elderly

CV: Hypotension, palpitations, bradycardia, tachycardia, **dysrhythmias (rare)**

GI: Nausea, diarrhea, abdominal pain, vomiting, constipation

GU: Frequency, dysuria, urinary retention, impotence

HEMA: **Hemolytic anemia, thrombocytopenia, leukopenia, agranulocytosis, pancytopenia**

INTEG: Rash, eczema, photosensitivity, urticaria

RESP: Thickening of bronchial secretions; dry nose, throat

Contraindications: Hypersen- **P** sitivity, newborn or premature infants, lactation, severe hepatic disease

Precautions: Pregnancy **C**, **G** elderly, children, respiratory **P** disease, narrow-angle glaucoma, prostatic hypertrophy, bladder neck obstruction, asthma

Pharmacokinetics	
Absorption	Well absorbed
Distribution	Unknown
Metabolism	Liver
Excretion	Kidneys

Pharmacodynamics

Onset	15-30 min
Peak	1-2 hr
Duration	8-12 hr

Interactions

Individual drugs

Alcohol: ↑ CNS depression
Procarbazine: ↑ CNS depression

Drug classifications

Anticoagulants, oral: ↓ action
CNS depressants: ↑ CNS depression
MAOIs: ↑ anticholinergic effect
Opiates: ↑ CNS depression
Sedative/hypnotics: ↑ CNS depression

Food/drug

↓ Absorption

Lab test interferences

False negative: Skin allergy tests (discontinue antihistamine 3 days before testing)

NURSING CONSIDERATIONS

Assessment

- Assess respiratory status: rate, rhythm, increase in bronchial secretions, wheezing, chest tightness; provide fluids to 2 L/day to decrease secretion thickness
- Monitor I&O ratio: be alert for urinary retention, frequency, dysuria, G especially elderly; drug should be discontinued if these occur

Nursing diagnoses

✓ Airway clearance, ineffective (uses)
✓ Injury, risk for (side effects)
✓ Knowledge deficit (teaching)
✓ Noncompliance (teaching, overuse)

Implementation

- Give on an empty stomach 1 hr before or 2 hr pc to facilitate absorption
- Store in tight, light-resistant container

Patient/family education

- Teach all aspects of drug uses; to notify prescriber if confusion, sedation, hypotension occur; to avoid driving or other hazardous activity if drowsiness occurs; to avoid alcohol or other CNS depressants that may potentiate effect
- Instruct patient to take 1 hr before or 2 hr pc to facilitate absorption
- Instruct patient not to exceed recommended dose; dysrhythmias may occur
- Teach patient that hard candy, gum, frequent rinsing of mouth may be used for dryness

Evaluation

Positive therapeutic outcome

- Absence of running or congested nose, rashes

Treatment of overdose:

Administer ipecac syrup or lavage, diazepam, vasopressors, barbiturates (short acting)

fibrinolysin/ desoxyribonuclease

(℞)
(fye-brin-oe-lye'sin/dez-ox-ee-rye-boe-nuke'lee-ase)
Elase
Func. class.: Enzyme
Chem. class.: Proteolytic, bovine

Pregnancy category C

Action: Dissolves fibrin in clots and fibrinous exudates, attacks DNA in areas of disintegrating cells

➡ **Therapeutic Outcome:** A clean wound

Uses: Debridement of wounds, vaginitis, cervicitis, ulcerative colitis, 2nd-, 3rd-degree burns; irrigating wounds, topically

Dosage and routes

Debridement/intravaginally

Adult: Oint 5 g × 5 applications

Irrigating

Adult: Irrigating dilution depends on type of wound

Available forms: Fibrinolysin with desoxyribonuclease 666.6 U/g; powder for reconstitution fibrinolysin 25 U/desoxyribonuclease 15,000 U

Adverse effects

INTEG: Hyperemia

Contraindications: Hypersensitivity to bovine or mercury products, hematoma

Precautions: Pregnancy **C**

Pharmacokinetics

Absorption	Not absorbed
Distribution	Unknown
Metabolism	Unknown
Excretion	Unknown
Half-life	Unknown

Pharmacodynamics

Unknown

Interactions: None

NURSING CONSIDERATIONS

Assessment

- Assess for signs of irritation and inflammation around wound; drug should be discontinued
- Assess wound for drainage, color, odor, size, depth before and during therapy

Nursing diagnoses

✓ Skin integrity, altered (uses)
✓ Knowledge deficit (teaching)

Implementation

Top route

- Apply after reconstituting top sol with 10-50 ml of sterile NaCl sol; use only fresh sol; reconstituted sol is stable for 24 hr; remove necrotic debris, dry eschar
- Saturate gauze with sol; pack area; remove in 6-8 hr and clean; repeat tid-qid
- Apply top oint after flushing wound with saline, water, or let dry or pat dry, then apply a small amount of oint to area and cover with a nonadhesive dressing; change qd or bid

Vaginal route

- Place 5 ml in applicator, apply with patient recumbent

Patient/family education

- Teach patient reason for treatment and expected results

Evaluation

Positive therapeutic outcome

- Decrease in wound scarring, tissue necrosis

filgrastim (℞)

(fill-gras′stim)

Neupogen

Func. class.: Biologic modifier

Chem. class.: Granulocyte colony-stimulating factor

Pregnancy category C

Action: Stimulates proliferation and differentiation of neutrophils; a glycoprotein

➔ **Therapeutic Outcome:** Absence of infection

Uses: To decrease infection in patients receiving antineoplastics that are myelosuppressive; to increase WBC in patients with drug-induced neutropenia

Investigational uses: Neutropenia in HIV infection

Dosage and routes

After myelosuppressive chemotherapy

P ***Adult and child:*** **IV**/SC 5 μg/kg/day in a single dose × 14 days; may increase by 5 μg/kg in each chemotherapy cycle; give qd for up to 2 wk until ANC has reached 10,000/mm^3; response to G-CSF is much greater with SC than **IV** therapy

After bone marrow transplantation

IV/SC 10 μg/kg as an inf (**IV**) over 4 or 24 hr, begin 24 hr after chemotherapy and 24 hr after bone marrow transplantation

Peripheral blood progenitor cell collection/therapy
Adult: 10 μg/kg/day as a bol or cont inf × 4 days or more before leukapheresis, continue to last leukapheresis, may alter dose if WBC >100,000/mm^3

Severe neutropenia (chronic)
Adult: SC 5 μg/kg as single SC inj qd

Available forms: Inj 300 μg/ml

Adverse effects
CNS: Fever
GI: Nausea, vomiting, diarrhea, mucositis, anorexia
HEMA: **Thrombocytopenia**
INTEG: Alopecia, exacerbation of skin conditions
MS: Osteoporosis, skeletal pain
RESP: **Respiratory distress syndrome**

Contraindications: Hypersensitivity to proteins of *Escherichia coli*

Precautions: Pregnancy **C**, lactation, cardiac conditions, children, myeloid malignancies

P

Pharmacokinetics

Absorption	Well absorbed (SC), completely absorbed (**IV**)
Distribution	Unknown
Metabolism	Unknown
Excretion	Unknown
Half-life	Unknown

Pharmacodynamics

	IV	SC
Onset	5-60 min	5-60 min
Peak	24 hr	2-8 hr
Duration	up to 1 wk	up to 1 wk

Interactions
Drug classifications
Antineoplastics: ↑ neutrophils, do not use together 24 hr before or after antineoplastics
Lab test interferences
↑ Uric acid, ↑ lactate dehydrogenase, ↑ alkaline phosphatase

NURSING CONSIDERATIONS
Assessment
- Monitor blood studies: CBC, platelet count before treatment and twice weekly; neutrophil counts (ANC) may be increased for 2 days after therapy, but treatment should continue until ANC >10,000/mm^3
- Assess for bone pain: frequency, intensity, duration; analgesics may be given; opiates should not be used
- Check B/P, heart rate, respiration, baseline and during treatment

Nursing diagnoses
✓ Infection, risk for (uses)
✓ Pain, acute (adverse reaction)
✓ Knowledge deficit (teaching)

Implementation
IV **IV route**
- Give 300 μg/ml or 480 μg/1.6 ml; allow to warm to room temp; give single dose over 1 min or less through Y-tube or medport
- Use single-use vials; after dose is withdrawn, do not reenter vial
- Give for 2 wk or until ANC = 10,000/mm^3 after the expected chemotherapy neutrophil nadir
- Store in refrigerator; do not freeze; may store at room temp for up to 6 hr; avoid shaking

Y-site compatibilities:
Acyclovir, allopurinol, amikacin, aminophylline, ampicillin, ampicillin/sulbactam, aztreonam, bleomycin, bumetanide, buprenorphine, butorphanol, calcium gluconate, carboplatin, carmustine, cefazolin, cefotetan, ceftazidime, chlorpromazine, cimetidine, cisplatin, cyclophosphamide, cytarabine, dacarbazine, daunorubicin, dexamethasone, diphenhydramine, doxorubicin, doxycycline, droperidol, enalaprilat, famotidine, floxuridine, fluconazole, fludarabine, gallium, ganciclovir, granisetron, haloperidol, hydrocortisone, hydromorphone, hydroxyzine, idarubicin, ifosfamide, leucovorin, lorazepam, mechlorethamine, melphalan, meperi-

F

dine, mesna, methotrexate, metoclopramide, miconazole, minocycline, mitoxantrone, morphine, nalbuphine, netilmicin, ondansetron, plicamycin, potassium chloride, promethazine, ranitidine, sodium bicarbonate, streptozocin, ticarcillin, ticarcillin/clavulanate, tobramycin, trimethoprim-sulfamethoxazole, vancomycin, vinblastine, vincristine, vinorelbine, zidovudine

Patient/family education

- Teach patient technique for self-administration: dose, side effects, disposal of containers and needles; provide instruction sheet

Evaluation

Positive therapeutic outcome

- Absence of infection

finasteride (℞)

(fin-ass'te-ride)

Propecia, Proscar

Func. class.: Androgen hormone inhibitor, hair stimulant

Chem. class.: 5-α-reductase inhibitor

Pregnancy category X

Action: Inhibits 5-α-reductase and reduction in dihydrotestosterone (DHT); DHT induces androgenic effects by binding to androgen receptors in the cell nuclei of the prostate gland, liver, skin; prevents development of benign prostatic hypertrophy (BPH)

Therapeutic Outcome: Reduced prostate size

Uses: Symptomatic BPH; male-pattern baldness (Propecia)

Dosage and routes

BPH

Adult: PO 5 mg qd × 6-12 mo

Male pattern baldness

Adult: PO 1 mg qd

Available forms: Tabs 1, 5 mg

Adverse effects

GU: Impotence, decreased libido, decreased volume of ejaculate

Contraindications: Hypersensitivity, pregnancy **X**, children, women who are pregnant or may become pregnant should not handle tabs

Precautions: Large residual urinary volume, severely diminished urinary flow, liver function abnormalities

Do Not Confuse:
Proscar/Prosom, Proscar/Prozac

Pharmacokinetics	
Absorption	63%, readily
Distribution	Plasma protein binding, crosses blood-brain barrier
Metabolism	Liver
Excretion	Kidneys—metabolites (39%), feces (57%)
Half-life	6-15 hr

Pharmacodynamics	
Onset	Immediate
Peak	1-2 hr
Duration	14 days

Interactions

Drug classifications

Anticholinergics: ↓ effect of finasteride

Bronchodilators, adrenergic: ↓ effect of finasteride

Theophylline: ↓ effect of finasteride

NURSING CONSIDERATIONS

Assessment

- Assess urinary patterns, residual urinary volume, severely diminished urinary flow; prostate-specific antigen (PSA) levels and digital rectal exam results before initiating therapy and periodically thereafter
- Monitor liver function studies before initiating treatment; extensively metabolized in liver

Nursing diagnoses

✓ Urinary elimination, altered (uses)
✓ Knowledge deficit (teaching)

Implementation

- Administer without regard to meals; give for a minimum of 6 mo; not all patients will respond
- Store at temp <86° F (30° C); protect from light; keep container tightly closed

Patient/family education

- Advise patient that pregnant women or women who may become pregnant should not touch crushed tab or come into contact with semen of a patient taking this drug; may adversely affect development of male fetus
- Inform patient that volume of ejaculate may be decreased during treatment; impotence and decreased libido may also occur
- Inform patient that Propecia results may not occur for 3 mo
- Inform patient that Proscar results may not occur for 6-12 mo

Evaluation

Positive therapeutic outcome

- Decreased postvoiding dribbling, frequency, nocturia
- Increased urinary flow
- Hair growth within 3-6 mo

flecainide (℞)

(flek'a-nide)

Tambocor

Func. class.: Antidysrhythmic (Class IC)

Pregnancy category C

Action: Decreases conduction in all parts of the heart, with greatest effect on the His-Purkinje system, which stabilizes the cardiac membrane

➔ **Therapeutic Outcome:** Absence of dysrhythmias

Uses: Life-threatening ventricular dysrhythmias, sustained ventricular tachycardia; supraventricular tachydysrhythmias

Dosage and routes

Adult: PO 50-100 mg q12h; may increase every 4 days by 50 mg q12h to desired response, not to exceed 400 mg/day

Renal dose

CrCl <35 ml/min dose 50%-75%

Available forms: Tabs 50, 100, 150 mg

Adverse effects

CNS: *Headache, dizziness,* involuntary movement, confusion, psychosis, restlessness, irritability, paresthesias, ataxia, flushing, somnolence, depression, anxiety, malaise

CV: *Hypotension,* **bradycardia,** angina, PVCs, **heart block, cardiovascular collapse, arrest, dysrhythmias, CHF, fatal ventricular tachycardia**

EENT: Tinnitus, *blurred vision,* hearing loss

GI: Nausea, vomiting, anorexia, constipation, abdominal pain, flatulence, change in taste

GU: Impotence, decreased libido, polyuria, urinary retention

HEMA: **Leukopenia, thrombocytopenia**

INTEG: Rash, urticaria, edema, swelling

RESP: Dyspnea, **respiratory depression**

Contraindications: Hypersensitivity, severe heart block, cardiogenic shock, nonsustained ventricular dysrhythmias, frequent PVCs, non–life-threatening dysrhythmias

Precautions: Pregnancy **C,** lactation, [P] children, renal disease, liver disease, CHF, respiratory depression, myasthenia gravis

F

Pharmacokinetics

Absorption	Well absorbed
Distribution	Widely distributed
Metabolism	Liver
Excretion	30% kidneys, unchanged
Half-life	14 hr

Pharmacodynamics

Onset	Unknown
Peak	3 hr
Duration	Unknown

Interactions
Individual drugs
Amiodarone: ↑ blood levels, ↑ toxicity
Digoxin: ↑ blood levels, ↑ toxicity
Disopyramide: ↑ CV depressant action
Flecainide: ↑ levels, ↑ toxicity
Lidocaine: bradycardia, arrest
Mexiletine: ↑ levels, ↑ toxicity
Phenytoin: ↑ blood levels
Procainamide: ↑ levels, ↑ toxicity
Quinidine: ↑ levels, ↑ toxicity
Verapamil: ↑ CV depressant action
Warfarin: ↑ level, ↑ bleeding
Drug classifications
β-Adrenergic blockers: ↑ dysrhythmias, cardiac arrest
Calcium channel blockers: ↑ dysrhythmias, cardiac arrest

NURSING CONSIDERATIONS
Assessment
- Monitor ECG continuously to determine drug effectiveness; measure PR, QRS, QT intervals; check for PVCs, other dysrhythmias; monitor B/P continuously for hypotension, hypertension, and rebound hypertension (after 1-2 hr); check for dehydration or hypovolemia
- Monitor I&O ratio; electrolytes: (K [potassium], Na [sodium]), Cl (chloride); check weight daily and for signs of CHF or pulmonary toxicity: dyspnea, fatigue, cough, fever, chest pain, jugular vein distention, rales, crackles; if these occur, drug should be discontinued
- Monitor liver function studies: AST, ALT, bilirubin, alk phosphatase
- Assess patient for CNS symptoms: confusion, psychosis, numbness, depression, involuntary movements; if these occur, drug should be discontinued
- Assess patient for hypothyroidism: lethargy, dizziness, constipation, enlarged thyroid gland, edema of extremities, cool, pale skin; assess patient for hyperthyroidism: restlessness; tachycardia; eyelid puffiness; weight loss; frequent urination; menstrual irregularities; dyspnea; warm, moist skin
- Monitor cardiac rate, respiration: rate, rhythm, character, chest pain; watch for ventricular tachycardia, supraventricular tachycardia, or fibrillation

Nursing diagnoses
☑ Cardiac output, decreased (uses)
☑ Knowledge deficit (teaching)

Implementation
- Give reduced dosage slowly with ECG monitoring; do not increase dose fewer than 4 days apart
- Give with meals if GI upset occurs

Patient/family education
- Instruct patient to report side effects immediately to prescriber
- Instruct patient to complete follow-up appointment with health care provider including pulmonary function studies, chest x-ray

Evaluation
Positive therapeutic outcome
- Absence of dysrythmias

fluconazole (℞)
(floo-kon'a-zole)
Diflucan
Func. class.: Antifungal
Pregnancy category C

Action: Inhibits ergosterol biosynthesis, causes direct damage to membrane phospholipids in the cell wall of fungi

Therapeutic Outcome: Fungistatic fungicidal against the following susceptible organisms: *Candida, Cryptococcus neoformans*

Uses: Oropharyngeal esophageal candidiasis in AIDS patients, chronic mucocutaneous candidiasis, urinary candidiasis, cryptococcal meningitis, peritonitis

Dosage and routes
Renal dose
CrCl 11-50 ml/min dose 50%

Vaginal candidiasis
Adult: PO 150 mg as a single dose

Serious fungal infections
Adult: PO/**IV** 50-400 mg initially, then 200 mg once daily for 4 wk

P ***Child:*** 6-12 mg/kg/day

Oropharyngeal candidiasis in AIDS patients
Adult: PO 200 mg initially, then 100 mg daily for at least 2 wk

P ***Child:*** 3 mg/kg/day

Available forms: Tabs 50, 100, 150, 200 mg; inj 2 mg/ml; powder for oral susp 50, 200 mg/ml

Adverse effects
CNS: Headache
GI: Nausea, vomiting, diarrhea, cramping, flatus, increased AST, ALT, **hepatotoxicity**
INTEG: **Stevens-Johnson syndrome**

Contraindications: Hypersensitivity

Precautions: Renal disease, pregnancy **C**

Do Not Confuse:
Diflucan/Diprivan

Pharmacokinetics

Absorption	Well absorbed (PO)
Distribution	Widely distributed (peritoneum, CSF)
Metabolism	<10%—liver
Excretion	80% kidneys (unchanged)
Half-life	30 hr, increased in renal disease

Pharmacodynamics

	PO	IV
Onset	Unknown	Immediate
Peak	2-4 hr	Infusion's end
Duration	Unknown	Unknown

Interactions
Individual drugs
Cimetidine: ↓ effect of fluconazole
Phenytoin: ↑ effect
Rifampin: ↑ effect
Tacrolimus: ↑ effect
Theophylline: ↑ effect
Warfarin: ↑ anticoagulation
Zidovudine: ↑ effect
Drug classification
Cyclosporines: ↑ renal dysfunction
Oral contraceptives: ↓ effect
Sulfonylureas: ↑ effect

NURSING CONSIDERATIONS
Assessment
- Assess for signs and symptoms of infection: clearing of CSF culture during treatment, obtain C&S baseline and during treatment, drug may be started as soon as culture is taken
- Monitor for hepatotoxicity: increased AST, ALT, alkaline phosphatase, bilirubin; drug will be discontinued if hepatotoxicity occurs

F

Nursing diagnoses
- ✓ Infection, risk for (uses)
- ✓ Injury, risk for (adverse reactions)
- ✓ Knowledge deficit (teaching)

Implementation
PO route
- Shake oral susp before each use

IV route
- Give after diluting according to package directions; run at 200 mg/hr or less; do not use plastic containers in connections
- Do not admix
- Administer **IV** using an in-line filter, using distal veins; check for extravasation and necrosis q2h
- Give drug only after C&S confirms organism, drug needed to treat condition
- Store protected from moisture and light, diluted sol is stable for 24 hr

Y-site compatibilities: Acyclovir, aldesleukin, allopurinol, amifostine, amikacin, aminophylline, ampicillin/sulbactam, aztreonam, benztropine, cefazolin, cefepime, cefotetan, cefoxitin, chlorpromazine, cimetidine, dexamethasone, diphenhydramine, dobutamine, dopamine, droperidol, famotidine, filgrastim, fludarabine, foscarnet, gallium, ganciclovir, gentamicin, granisetron, heparin, hydrocortisone, immune globulin, leucovorin, lorazepam, melphalan, meperidine, meropenem, metoclopramide, metronidazole, midazolam, morphine, nafcillin, nitroglycerin, ondansetron, oxacillin, paclitaxel, pancuronium, penicillin G, potassium, phenytoin, piperacillin/tazobactam, prochlorperazine, promethazine, propofol, ranitidine, sargramostim, sulfamethoxazole, tacrolimus, teniposide, theophylline, thiotepa, ticarcillin/clavulanate, tobramycin, vancomycin, vecuronium, vinorelbine, zidovudine

Y-site incompatibilities: Amphotericin B, ampicillin, calcium gluconate, cefotaxime, ceftriaxone, ceftazidime, cefuroxime, chloramphenicol, clindamycin, diazepam, digoxin, erythromycin lactobionate, furosemide, haloperidol, hydroxyzine, imipenem/cilastatin, pentamidine, ticarcillin, trimethoprim/sulfamethoxazole

Additive compatibilities: Acyclovir, amikacin, amphotericin B, cefazolin, ceftazidime, clindamycin, gentamicin, heparin, meropenem, metronidazole, morphine, piperacillin, potassium chloride, theophylline

Patient/family education
- Caution patient that long-term therapy may be needed to clear infection; to take entire course of medication; take in equal intervals (PO)
- Teach patient the signs and symptoms of hepatotoxicity: nausea, vomiting, clay-colored stools, dark urine, anorexia, fatigue, jaundice; prescriber should be notified immediately
- Inform patient that medication may be taken with food to reduce GI effects
- Advise patient to consider using alternative contraception if using oral contraceptives

Evaluation
Positive therapeutic outcome
- Decreasing oral candidiasis, fever, malaise, rash
- Negative C&S for infecting organism

fludrocortisone (℞)
(floo-droe-kor'ti-sone)
Florinef
Func. class.: Corticosteroid
Chem. class.: Mineralocorticoid
Pregnancy category C

Action: Promotes increased reabsorption of sodium and loss of potassium, water, hydrogen from the distal renal tubules

Therapeutic Outcome: Treatment of adrenal insufficiency symptoms

Uses: Adrenal insufficiency, salt-losing adrenogenital syndrome

Investigational uses: Renal tubular acidosis (type IV), idiopathic orthostatic hypertension

Dosage and routes
Adult: PO 0.1-0.2 mg qd
Child: PO 0.05-0.1 mg/day

Available forms: Tabs 0.1 mg

Adverse effects
CNS: *Flushing, sweating,* headache, paralysis
CV: *Hypertension,* **circulatory collapse, thrombophlebitis, embolism,** tachycardia, **CHF**
ENDO: Weight gain, adrenal suppression
META: *Hypokalemia*
MISC: Hypersensitivity
MS: Fractures, osteoporosis, weakness

Contraindications: Hypersensitivity, acute glomerulonephritis, amebiasis psychoses, Cushing's syndrome

Precautions: Pregnancy **C,** osteoporosis, CHF, lactation

Pharmacokinetics

Absorption	Well absorbed
Distribution	Widely
Metabolism	Liver
Excretion	Kidneys, breast milk
Half-life	3½ hr

Pharmacodynamics

Unknown

Interactions
Individual drugs
Amphotericin B: ↑ hypokalemia
Mezlocillin: ↑ hypokalemia
Phenobarbital: ↓ effect of fludrocortisone
Piperacillin: ↑ hypokalemia
Rifampin: ↓ effect of fludrocortisone
Drug classifications
Diuretics, loop: ↑ hypokalemia
Nondepolarizing neuromuscular blocking agents: ↑ neuromuscular blockade
Food/drug
↑ **Salt/sodium ingestion:** ↑ hypokalemia, ↑ hypernatremia
Herb/drug
Aloe: ↑ hypokalemia
Buckthorn: ↑ hypokalemia
Cascara sagrada: ↑ hypokalemia
Senna: ↑ hypokalemia
Lab test interferences
↑ Potassium, ↑ chloride
↓ Hematocrit

NURSING CONSIDERATIONS

Assessment

- Monitor patient for fluid retention: weigh daily, notify prescriber of weekly gain >5 lb; B/P q4h, pulse; notify prescriber if chest pain occurs; I&O ratio; be alert for decreasing urinary output and increasing edema
- Check for potassium depletion: paresthesias, fatigue, nausea, vomiting, depression, polyuria, dysrhythmias, weakness; also sodium, chloride

Nursing diagnoses

✓ Fluid volume deficit (uses)
✓ Fluid volume excess (adverse reactions)
✓ Knowledge deficit (teaching)

Implementation

- Administer titrated dose; use lowest effective dose; scored tab may be broken if lower dose is necessary
- Give with food or milk to decrease GI symptoms

Patient/family education

- Advise patient to carry ID as steroid user at all times during diagnosis and treatment
- Caution patient not to discontinue this medication abruptly; Addisonian crisis may occur
- Counsel patient to follow dietary regimen recommended by prescriber;

should include high potassium and, possibly, low sodium

- Advise patient to report weight gain >5 lb; edema in legs, hands; abdominal cramping; muscle cramps; nausea; vomiting; anorexia; dizziness or weakness

Evaluation

Positive therapeutic outcome

- Correction of adrenal insufficiency
- Electrolytes and fluids in normal range

flumazenil (℞)

(flu-maz'e-nil)

Mazicon, Ronazicon

Func. class.: Benzodiazepine receptor antagonist

Chem. class.: Imidazobenzodiazepine derivative

Pregnancy category C

Action: Antagonizes the actions of benzodiazepines on the CNS, competitively inhibits the activity at the benzodiazepine receptor complex

Therapeutic Outcome: Reversed benzodiazepine toxic effects

Uses: Reversal of the sedative effects of benzodiazepines

Dosage and routes

Reversal of conscious sedation or in general anesthesia

Adult: **IV** 0.2 mg (2 ml) given over 15 sec; wait 45 sec, then give 0.2 mg (2 ml) if consciousness does not occur; may be repeated at 60-sec intervals as needed, up to 4 additional times (max total dose 1 mg); dose is to be individualized

Management of suspected benzodiazepine overdose

Adult: **IV** 0.2 mg (2 ml) given over 30 sec; wait 30 sec, then give 0.3 mg (3 ml) over 30 sec if consciousness does not occur; further doses of 0.5 mg (5 ml) can be given over 30 sec at intervals of 1 min up to cumulative dose of 3 mg

Available forms: Inj 0.1 mg/ml

Adverse effects

CNS: Dizziness, agitation, emotional lability, confusion, **seizures,** somnolence

CV: Hypertension, palpitations, cutaneous vasodilation, **dysrhythmias,** bradycardia, tachycardia, chest pain

EENT: Abnormal vision, blurred vision, tinnitus

GI: Nausea, vomiting, hiccups

SYST: Headache, injection site pain, increased sweating, fatigue, rigors

Contraindications: Hypersensitivity to this drug or benzodiazepines, serous tricyclic antidepressant overdose, patients given benzodiazepine for control of life-threatening condition

P G **Precautions:** Pregnancy **C,** lactation, children, elderly, renal disease, seizures, head injury, labor and delivery, hepatic disease, hypoventilation, panic disorder, drug and alcohol dependency, ambulatory patients

Do Not Confuse:
Mazicon/Mivacron

Pharmacokinetics	
Absorption	Complete
Distribution	Unknown
Metabolism	Liver
Excretion	Unknown
Half-life	41-79 min

Pharmacodynamics	
Onset	1 min
Peak	10 min
Duration	Unknown

Interactions: None

NURSING CONSIDERATIONS

Assessment

- Assess cardiac status using continuous monitoring

- Assess for seizures, protect patient from injury; most likely in those who usually experience withdrawal from sedatives
- Assess for GI symptoms: nausea, vomiting; place in side-lying position to prevent aspiration
- Assess for allergic reactions: flushing, rash, urticaria, pruritus

Nursing diagnoses

✓ Injury, risk for (uses)
✓ Poisoning (uses)

Implementation

- Give directly undiluted or diluted in 0.9% NaCl, D_5W, or LR; give over 15 sec into running **IV**
- Check airway and **IV** access before administration

Additive compatibilities:
Aminophylline, cimetidine, dobutamine, dopamine, famotidine, heparin, lidocaine, procainamide, ranitidine

Patient/family education

- Caution patient that amnesia may continue
- Instruct patient to avoid any hazardous activities for 18-24 hr after discharge
- Inform patient not to take any alcohol or nonprescription drugs for 18-24 hr; serious reactions may occur

Evaluation

Positive therapeutic outcome

- Decreased sedation, respiratory depression
- Absence of toxicity

HIGH ALERT

fluorouracil (℞)

(flure-oh-yoor′a-sil)
Adrucil, Efudex, 5-FU
Func. class.: Antineoplastic, antimetabolite
Chem. class.: Pyrimidine antagonist
Pregnancy category D

F

Action: Inhibits DNA, RNA synthesis; interferes with cell replication by competitively inhibiting thymidylate synthesis, cell cycle–specific (S phase), a vesicant

➡ **Therapeutic Outcome:** Prevention of rapidly growing malignant cells

Uses: *Systemic:* cancer of breast, colon, rectum, stomach, pancreas; multiple active keratoses; *Topical:* basal cell carcinoma

Dosage and routes

Adult: **IV** 12 mg/kg/day × 4 days, not to exceed 800 mg/day; may repeat with 6 mg/kg on day 6, 8, 10, 12; maintenance is 10-15 mg/kg/wk as a single dose, not to exceed 1 g/wk

Adult: TOP 1, 2% sol apply to lesion on head, neck, or on other areas 5% bid

Available forms: Inj 50 mg/ml; cream 1, 5%; sol 1, 2, 5%

Adverse effects

Systemic use

CNS: Lethargy, malaise, weakness, acute cerebellar dysfunction
CV: Myocardial ischemia, angina
EENT: Epistaxis
GI: *Anorexia, stomatitis,* diarrhea, nausea, vomiting, **hemorrhage, enteritis glossitis**
HEMA: **Thrombocytopenia, leukopenia, myelosuppression, anemia, agranulocytosis**
INTEG: *Rash,* fever, photosensitivity

Contraindications: Hypersensitivity, myelosuppression, pregnancy **D,**

poor nutritional status, serious infections

Precautions: Renal disease, hepatic disease, bone marrow depression, angina, lactation, children

Do Not Confuse:
fluorouracil/flucytosine

Pharmacokinetics

Absorption	Completely bioavailable (**IV**), minimal (top)
Distribution	Widely distributed, concentration in tumor
Metabolism	Liver—converted to active metabolite
Excretion	Lungs (60%-80%), kidneys (up to 15%)
Half-life	20 hr terminal

Pharmacodynamics

Unknown

Interactions

Individual drugs

Radiation: ↑ toxicity, bone marrow suppression

Drug classifications

Antineoplastics: ↑ toxicity, bone marrow depression

Live virus vaccines: ↓ antibody response

Lab test interferences

↑ Liver function studies, ↑ 6-HIAA
↓ Albumin

NURSING CONSIDERATIONS

Assessment

- Monitor ECG; watch for ST-T wave changes, low QRS and T, possible dysrhythmias (sinus tachycardia, heart block, PVCs)
- Assess buccal cavity q8h for dryness, sores or ulceration, white patches, oral pain, bleeding, dysphagia; obtain prescription for viscous lidocaine (Xylocaine)
- Assess tachypnea, ECG changes, dyspnea, edema, fatigue; identify dyspnea, rales, unproductive cough, chest pain, tachypnea
- Monitor CBC, differential, platelet count qd (**IV**); withhold drug if WBC is <4000/mm^3 or platelet count is <100,000/mm^3; notify prescriber of results if WBC <20,000/mm^3, platelets <50,000/mm^3; nadir of leukopenia within 2 wk, recovery 1 mo
- Monitor renal function studies: BUN, creatinine, serum uric acid, urine CrCl before and during therapy; I&O ratio; report fall in urine output to <30 ml/hr
- Monitor temp q4h (may indicate beginning of infection)
- Monitor liver function tests before and during therapy (bilirubin, AST, ALT, LDH) as needed or monthly; jaundice of skin, sclera, dark urine, clay-colored stools, itchy skin, abdominal pain, fever, diarrhea
- Assess for bleeding: hematuria, stool guaiac, bruising or petechiae, mucosa or orifices q8h; inflammation of mucosa, breaks in skin

Nursing diagnoses

- ✓ Injury, risk for (adverse reactions)
- ✓ Body image disturbance (adverse reactions)
- ✓ Infection, risk for (adverse reactions)
- ✓ Knowledge deficit (teaching)

Implementation

- Avoid contact with skin (very irritating); wash completely to remove
- Give fluids **IV** or PO before chemotherapy to hydrate patient
- Give antiemetic 30-60 min before giving drug to prevent vomiting, and prn for several days thereafter; antibiotics for prophylaxis of infection
- Provide liq diet: carbonated beverages; gelatin may be added if patient is not nauseated or vomiting
- Provide rinsing of mouth tid-qid with water, club soda; brushing of teeth bid-qid with soft brush or cotton-tipped applicators for stomatitis; use unwaxed dental floss

IV route

- Prepare in biologic cabinet using gloves, gown, mask
- **IV** undiluted; may inject through Y-tube or 3-way stopcock; give over 1-3 min
- May be diluted in 0.9% NaCl, D_5W, given over 2-8 hr as an **IV** inf

Topical route

- Wear gloves when applying; may use with a loose dressing, use a plastic or wooden applicator

Syringe compatibilities:
Bleomycin, cisplatin, cyclophosphamide, furosemide, heparin, leucovorin, methotrexate, metoclopramide, mitomycin, vinblastine, vincristine

Syringe incompatibilities:
Droperidol

Y-site compatibilities:
Allopurinol, amifostine, aztreonam, bleomycin, cefepime, cisplatin, cyclophosphamide, doxorubicin, fludarabine, furosemide, granisetron, heparin, hydrocortisone, leucovorin, mannitol, melphalan, methotrexate, metoclopramide, mitomycin, paclitaxel, piperacillin/tazobactam, potassium chloride, propofol, sargramostin, thiotepa, thiposide, vinblastine, vincristine, vit B/C

Y-site incompatibilities:
Droperidol, vinorelbine

Additive compatibilities:
Bleomycin, cephalothin, cyclophosphamide, etoposides, floxuridine, hydromorphone, ifosfamide, leucovorin, methotrexate, mitoxantrone, prednisolone, vincristine

Additive incompatibilities:
Carboplatin, cisplatin, cytarabine, diazepam, doxorubicin

Solution compatibilities:
Amino acids 4.25%/D_{25}, D_5/LR, $D_{3.3}$/0.3% NaCl, D_5W, 0.9% NaCl, TPN #23

Patient/family education

- Caution patient that contraceptive measures are recommended during therapy
- Teach patient to avoid using aspirin, NSAIDs, or ibuprofen-containing products, razors, commercial mouthwash because bleeding may occur; to report symptoms of bleeding (hematuria, tarry stools)
- Instruct patient to report signs of anemia (fatigue, headache, irritability, faintness, shortness of breath)
- Instruct patient to report signs of stomatitis (bleeding, white spots, ulcerations in the mouth); tell patient to examine mouth qd, to report symptoms; viscous lidocaine (Xylocaine) may be used
- Teach patient to avoid crowds, persons with known infections
- Advise patient to avoid vaccinations during therapy, to use sunscreen or stay out of the sun to prevent burns; about hair loss, explore use of wigs or other products

Evaluation

Positive therapeutic outcome

- Prevention of rapid division of malignant cells

fluoxetine (℞)

(floo-ox'uh-teen)

Prozac, Prozac Weekly

Func. class.: Antidepressant, SSRI (selective serotonin reuptake inhibitor)

Pregnancy category B

Action: Inhibits CNS neuron uptake of serotonin, but not of norepinephrine

Therapeutic Outcome: Decreased symptoms of depression after 2-3 wk

Uses: Major depressive disorder, obsessive-compulsive disorder (OCD), bulimia nervosa

Investigational uses: Alcoholism, anorexia nervosa, attention deficit hyperactivity disorder, bipolar II affective disorder, borderline personality disorder, cataplexy, narcolepsy, kleptomania, migraine, obesity, posttraumatic stress disorder, schizophrenia, Gilles de la Tourette's syndrome, trichotillomania, levodopa-induced dyskinesia, social phobia

Dosage and routes

Depression/OCD

Adult: PO 20 mg qd AM; after 4 wk if no clinical improvement is noted, dose may be increased to 20 mg bid in AM, afternoon, not to exceed 80 mg/day; PO weekly

G ***Elderly:*** PO 10 mg/day, increase as needed

P ***Child 5-18 yr:*** PO 5-10 mg/kg/day, max 20 mg/day

Bulimia nervosa

Adult: PO 60 mg/day in AM

Available forms: Pulvules 10, 20, 40 mg; tabs 10 mg; Prozac Weekly liq 20 mg/5 ml

Adverse effects

CNS: *Headache, nervousness, insomnia, drowsiness, anxiety, tremor, dizziness, fatigue, sedation, poor concentration, abnormal dreams, agitation,* **seizures**

CV: *Hot flashes, palpitations,* angina pectoris, **hemorrhage,** hypertension, first-degree tachycardia

EENT: Visual changes, ear/eye pain, photophobia, tinnitus

GI: *Nausea, diarrhea, dry mouth, anorexia, dyspepsia, constipation, cramps, vomiting, taste changes, flatulence, decreased appetite*

GU: *Dysmenorrhea, decreased libido, urinary frequency, urinary tract infection,* amenorrhea, cystitis, impotence

INTEG: *Sweating, rash, pruritus,* acne, alopecia, urticaria

MS: *Pain,* arthritis, twitching

RESP: *Infection, pharyngitis, nasal congestion, sinus headache, sinusitis, cough dyspnea, bronchitis,* asthma, hyperventilation, pneumonia

SYST: *Asthenia, viral infection, fever, allergy, chills*

Contraindications: Hypersensitivity

P G **Precautions:** Pregnancy **B,** lactation, children, elderly

Do Not Confuse:
Prozac/Proscar, Prozac/Prilosec, Prozac/Prosom

Pharmacokinetics	
Absorption	Well absorbed
Distribution	Crosses blood-brain barrier
Metabolism	Liver, extensively to norfluoxetine
Excretion	Kidneys, unchanged (12%), metabolite (7%); steady state 28-35 days, protein binding 94%
Half-life	1-3 days metabolite up to 1 wk

Pharmacodynamics	
Onset	Unknown
Peak	6-8 hr
Duration	Unknown

Interactions

Individual drugs

Alcohol: ↑ CNS depression
Buspirone: ↑ worsening of OCD
Carbamazepine: ↑ toxicity
Clozapine: ↑ clozapine levels
Dextromethorphan: ↑ hallucinations
Digoxin: ↑ toxicity
Haloperidol: ↑ haloperidol effect
Lithium: ↑ toxicity
L-Tryptophan: ↑ toxicity
Phenytoin: ↑ hydantoin levels

Drug classifications

Barbiturates: ↑ CNS depression
Benzodiazepines: ↑ CNS depression
CNS depressants: ↑ CNS depression
MAOIs: Hypertensive crisis, convulsions

Oral anticoagulants: ↑ effects, toxicity
Sedative/hypnotics: ↑ CNS depression

Herb/drug

Kava: ↑ action
St. John's wort: Do not use together

Lab test interferences

↑ Serum bilirubin, ↑ blood glucose, ↑ alkaline phosphatase
↓ VMA, ↓ 5-HIAA, ↓ blood glucose
False: ↑ Urinary catecholamines

NURSING CONSIDERATIONS

Assessment

- Monitor B/P (lying, standing), pulse q4h; if systolic B/P drops 20 mm hg, hold drug and notify prescriber; take VS q4h in patients with CV disease
- Monitor blood studies: CBC, leukocytes, differential, cardiac enzymes if patient is receiving long-term therapy; check platelets, bleeding can occur
- Monitor hepatic studies: AST, ALT, bilirubin
- Check weight qwk; appetite may increase with drug
- Assess ECG for flattening of T wave, bundle branch block, AV block, dysrhythmias in cardiac patients
- Assess mental status: mood, sensorium, affect, suicidal tendencies; increase in psychiatric symptoms: depression, panic
- Monitor urinary retention, P constipation; constipation is more G likely to occur in children or elderly
- Identify patient's alcohol consumption; if alcohol is consumed, hold dose until AM
- Assess appetite in bulimia nervosa, weight qd, increase nutritious foods in diet, watch for bingeing and vomiting
- Assess allergic reactions: itching, rash, urticaria, drug should be discontinued; may need to give antihistamine

Nursing diagnoses

✓ Coping, ineffective individual (uses)
✓ Injury, risk for (side effects)
✓ Knowledge deficit (teaching)
✓ Noncompliance (teaching)

Implementation

- Give with food or milk for GI symptoms
- Give dosage hs if oversedation occurs during day; may take entire G dose hs; elderly may not tolerate once/day dosing, crushed if patient unable to swallow whole (tabs only)
- Store at room temp; do not freeze

Patient/family education

- Teach patient that therapeutic effects may take 1-4 wk
- Instruct patient to use caution in driving or other activities requiring alertness because of drowsiness, dizziness, blurred vision; to avoid rising quickly from sitting to standing, G especially elderly; to use sunscreen to prevent photosensitivity
- Caution patient to avoid alcohol ingestion, other CNS depressants
- Advise patient not to discontinue medication quickly after long-term use: may cause nausea, headache, malaise
- Instruct patient to increase fluids, bulk in diet if constipation, urinary G retention occur, especially elderly
- Advise patient to take gum, hard sugarless candy, or frequent sips of water for dry mouth
- Teach patient to avoid all OTC drugs unless approved by prescriber
- Advise patient to change positions slowly, orthostatic hypotension may occur

Evaluation

Positive therapeutic outcome

- Decrease in depression
- Absence of suicidal thoughts
- Decreased symptoms of OCD

F

fluphenazine decanoate (℞)
(floo-fen'ah-zeen)
Modecate ♣, Modecate Concentrate, Prolixin Decanoate
fluphenazine enanthate (℞)
Moditen Enanthate ♣, Prolixin Enanthate
fluphenazine hydrochloride (℞)
Apo-Fluphenazine ♣, Moditen HCL ♣, Moditen HCl-H.P. ♣, Permitil ♣, Prolixin
Func. class.: Antipsychotic/neuroleptic
Chem. class.: Phenothiazine, piperazine
Pregnancy category C

Action: Depresses cerebral cortex, hypothalamus, limbic system, which control activity and aggression; blocks neurotransmission produced by dopamine at synapse; exhibits strong α-adrenergic and anticholinergic blocking action; mechanism for antipsychotic effects is unclear

➔ **Therapeutic Outcome:** Decreased signs and symptoms of psychosis

Uses: Psychotic disorders, schizophrenia

Dosage and routes
Decanoate
P ***Adult and child >6 yr:*** IM/SC 12.5-25 mg q1-3 wk, may increase slowly

P ***Child 12-16 yr:*** IM/SC 6.25-18.75 mg, then repeat q1-3 wk, then increase slowly, max 25 mg

P ***Child 5-12 yr:*** IM/SC 3.125-12.5 mg, then repeat q1-3 wk, increase slowly

HCl
Adult: PO 2.5-10 mg, in divided doses q6-8h, not to exceed 20 mg qd; IM initially 1.25 mg then 2.5-10 mg in divided doses q6-8h

P ***Child:*** PO 0.25-3.5 mg qd in divided doses q4-6h, max 10 mg/qd

Enanthate
Adult: IM/SC 25 mg q1-3 wk, may increase slowly, max 100 mg/dose

Available forms: HCl tabs 1, 2.5, 5, 10 mg; elixir 2.5 mg/5 ml; conc 5 mg/ml; inj 2.5, 10 mg/ml, enanthate, decanoate depot inj 25 mg/ml

Adverse effects
CNS: *Extrapyramidal symptoms: pseudoparkinsonism, akathisia, dystonia, tardive dyskinesia, drowsiness, headache,* **seizures, neuroleptic malignant syndrome**
CV: *Orthostatic hypotension,* hypertension, **cardiac arrest,** ECG changes, **tachycardia**
EENT: Blurred vision, glaucoma, dry eyes
GI: *Dry mouth, nausea, vomiting, anorexia, constipation,* diarrhea, jaundice, weight gain, **paralytic ileus, hepatitis**
GU: Urinary retention, urinary frequency, enuresis, impotence, amenorrhea, gynecomastia
HEMA: Anemia, **leukopenia, leukocytosis, agranulocytosis, aplastic anemia, thrombocytopenia**
INTEG: *Rash,* photosensitivity, dermatitis
RESP: **Laryngospasm,** dyspnea, **respiratory depression**

Contraindications: Hypersensitivity, circulatory collapse, liver damage, cerebral arteriosclerosis, coronary disease, severe hypertension/hypotension, blood dyscrasias, coma, P child <12 yr, brain damage, bone marrow depression, alcohol and barbiturate withdrawal, narrow-angle glaucoma

Precautions: Pregnancy **C,** lactation, seizure disorders, hypertension, hepatic disease, cardiac disease, G elderly

Do Not Confuse:
Prolixin/Proloid

Pharmacokinetics

Absorption	Well absorbed (PO, IM)
Distribution	Widely absorbed, crosses blood-brain barrier, placenta
Metabolism	Liver, extensively
Excretion	Kidneys (metabolites)
Half-life	HCl-4.7-15.3 hr, enanthate 3½-4 days, decanoate 6.8-14.3 days

Pharmacodynamics

	PO/IM	IM	IM
	HCl	Enanthate	Decanoate
Onset	1 hr	1-2 days	1-3 days
Peak	1½-2 hr	2-3 days	1-2 days
Duration	6-8 hr	1-3 wk	>4 wk

Interactions
Individual drugs
Alcohol: ↑ effects of both drugs, oversedation
Bromocriptine: ↓ antiparkinson activity
Disopyramide: ↑ anticholinergic effects
Epinephrine: ↑ toxicity
Guanethidine: ↓ antihypertensive response
Levodopa: ↓ antiparkinson activity
Lithium: ↓ fluphenazine levels, ↑ extrapyramidal symptoms, masking of lithium toxicity
Magnesium hydroxide: ↓ absorption of fluphenazine
Norepinephrine: ↓ vasoresponse, ↑ toxicity
Drug classifications
Antacids: ↓ absorption of fluphenazine
Anticholinergics: ↑ anticholinergic effects
Antidepressants: ↑ CNS depression
Antidiarrheals, adsorbent: ↓ absorption
Antihistamines: ↑ CNS depression
Antihypertensives: ↑ hypotension
Antithyroid agents: ↑ agranulocytosis
Barbiturates: ↑ CNS depression
β-Adrenergic blockers: ↑ effects of both drugs
General anesthetics: ↑ CNS depression
MAOIs: ↑ CNS depression
Opiates: ↑ CNS depression
Sedative/hypnotics: ↑ CNS depression
Lab test interferences
↑ Liver function tests, ↑ cardiac enzymes, ↑ cholesterol, ↑ blood glucose, ↑ prolactin, ↑ bilirubin, ↑ PBI, ↑ cholinesterase I, ↑ alkaline phosphatase, ↑ leukocytes, ↑ granulocytes, ↑ platelets
↓ Hormones (blood and urine)
False positive: Pregnancy tests, PKU, urine bilirubin
False negative: Urinary steroids, 17-OHCS

NURSING CONSIDERATIONS
Assessment
- Assess mental status: orientation, mood, behavior, presence of hallucinations, and type before initial administration and monthly; this drug should significantly reduce psychotic behavior
- Check for swallowing of PO medication; check for hoarding or giving of medication to other patients
- Monitor I&O ratio, palpate bladder if low urinary output occurs, G especially in elderly; urinalysis recommended before, during prolonged therapy
- Monitor bilirubin, CBC, liver function studies monthly
- Assess affect, orientation, LOC, reflexes, gait, coordination, sleep pattern disturbances
- Monitor B/P with patient sitting, standing, and lying down; take pulse and respirations q4h during initial treatment; establish baseline before starting treatment; report drops of 30

mm Hg; obtain baseline ECG, Q-wave and T-wave changes
- Check for dizziness, faintness, palpitations, tachycardia on rising; severe orthostatic hypotension is common
- ◆ Assess for neuroleptic malignant syndrome: hyperpyrexia, muscle rigidity, increased CPK, altered mental status; drug should be discontinued
- Assess for extrapyramidal symptoms including akathisia (inability to sit still, no pattern to movements), tardive dyskinesia (bizarre movements of the jaw, mouth, tongue, extremities), pseudoparkinsonism (rigidity, tremors, pill rolling, shuffling gate), an antiparkinson drug should be prescribed
- Assess for constipation, urinary retention daily; if these occur, increase bulk, water in diet

Nursing diagnoses
- ✓ Thought processes, altered (uses)
- ✓ Coping, ineffective individual (uses)
- ✓ Knowledge deficit (teaching)
- ✓ Noncompliance (teaching)

Implementation
PO route
- Give drug in liq form mixed in glass of juice or cola if hoarding is suspected; do not mix in caffeine drinks, tannics, or pectinates; G decrease dose in elderly
- Give PO with full glass of water, milk; or give with food to decrease GI upset
- Store in tight, light-resistant container, oral sol in amber bottle

SC route
- May be given by this route; however, it is painful

IM route
- Inject in deep muscle mass, use a 21-G needle into dorsal gluteal site, keep patient recumbent for ½ hr to prevent orthostatic hypotension

Syringe compatibilities:
Benztropine, diphenhydramine, hydroxyzine

Patient/family education
- Teach patient to use good oral hygiene; frequent rinsing of mouth, sugarless gum for dry mouth
- Caution patient to avoid hazardous activities until drug response is determined; dizziness, blurred vision may occur
- Inform patient that orthostatic hypotension occurs often and to rise from sitting or lying position gradually, to remain lying down after IM inj for at least 30 min; tell patient to avoid hot tubs, hot showers, tub baths because hypotension may occur; tell patient that in hot weather, heat stroke may occur; extra precautions are necessary to stay cool
- Instruct patient to avoid abrupt withdrawal of this drug, or extrapyramidal symptoms may result; drug should be withdrawn slowly
- Teach patient to avoid OTC preparations (cough, hay fever, cold) unless approved by physician because serious drug interactions may occur; avoid use with alcohol, CNS depressants; increased drowsiness may occur
- Instruct patient to use a sunscreen and sunglasses to prevent burns
- Teach patient about extrapyramidal symptoms and necessity of meticulous oral hygiene beause oral candidiasis may occur
- Instruct patient to take antacids 2 hr before or after this drug
- Advise patient to report sore throat, malaise, fever, bleeding, mouth sores; if these occur, CBC should be performed and drug discontinued

Evaluation
Positive therapeutic outcome
- Decrease in emotional excitement, hallucinations, delusions, paranoia
- Reorganization of patterns of thought, speech

Treatment of overdose:
Lavage if orally ingested; provide airway; *do not induce vomiting or use epinephrine*

flurazepam (℞)
(flure-az'e-pam)

Apo-flurazepam ♣, Dalmane, Durapam, flurazepam, Novoflupam ♣, Somnol ♣, Som-Pam ♣

Func. class.: Sedative-hypnotic
Chem. class.: Benzodiazepine derivative

Pregnancy category UK

Controlled substance schedule IV (USA), **schedule** F (Canada)

Action: Produces CNS depression at the limbic, thalamic, hypothalamic levels of CNS; may be mediated by neurotransmitter γ-aminobutyric acid (GABA); results are sedation, hypnosis, skeletal muscle relaxation, anticonvulsant activity, anxiolytic action

➔ **Therapeutic Outcome:** Ability to sleep, relaxation

Uses: Insomnia

Dosage and routes
Adult: PO 15-30 mg hs; may repeat dose once if needed

G ***Elderly:*** PO 15 mg hs; may increase if needed

Available forms: Caps 15, 30 mg

Adverse effects
CNS: *Lethargy, drowsiness, daytime sedation,* dizziness, confusion, lightheadedness, headache, anxiety, irritability
CV: Chest pain, pulse changes, palpitations
GI: Nausea, vomiting, diarrhea, heartburn, abdominal pain, constipation
HEMA: **Leukopenia, granulocytopenia (rare)**
MISC: Physical, psychologic dependence

Contraindications: Hypersensitivity to benzodiazepines, pregnancy **UK,** lactation, intermittent porphyria, uncontrolled pain

Precautions: Anemia, hepatic disease, renal disease, suicidal individuals, drug abuse, elderly G, psychosis, child <15 yr P

Pharmacokinetics

Absorption	Well absorbed
Distribution	Widely absorbed, crosses blood-brain barrier, crosses placenta
Metabolism	Liver to active, inactive metabolites
Excretion	Kidneys, breast milk
Half-life	2½ hr, 30-200 hr active metabolites

Pharmacodynamics

Onset	15-30 min
Peak	½-1 hr
Duration	7-8 hr

Interactions
Individual drugs
Alcohol: ↑ CNS depression
Cimetidine: ↑ action of flurazepam
Disulfiram: ↑ action of flurazepam
Fluoxetine: ↑ action of flurazepam
Isoniazid: ↑ action of flurazepam
Ketoconazole: ↑ action of flurazepam
Levodopa: ↓ action of levodopa
Metoprolol: ↑ action of flurazepam
Propoxyphene: ↑ action of flurazepam
Propranolol: ↑ action of flurazepam
Rifampin: ↓ action of flurazepam
Theophylline: ↓ sedative effects
Valproic acid: ↑ action of flurazepam
Drug classifications
Analgesics, opioid: ↑ CNS depression
Antidepressants: ↑ CNS depression
Antihistamines: ↑ CNS depression
Barbiturates: ↓ effect of flurazepam
Oral contraceptives: ↑ effect
Herb/drug
Kava: ↑ effect

Lab test interferences
↑ AST/ALT, ↑ serum bilirubin
False: ↑ urinary 17-OHCS, ↓ radioactive iodine uptake

NURSING CONSIDERATIONS

Assessment

- Assess anxiety reaction: inability to sleep, apprehension, dread, foreboding, or uneasiness related to unidentified source of danger
- Assess for previous drug dependence or tolerance; if drug dependent or tolerant, amount of medication should be restricted
- Monitor B/P (lying, standing), pulse; if systolic B/P drops 20 mm Hg, hold drug, notify prescriber; I&O, may indicate renal dysfunction
- Monitor blood studies: CBC during long-term therapy; blood dyscrasias have occurred rarely
- Monitor hepatic studies: AST, ALT, bilirubin, creatinine, LDH, alkaline phosphatase
- Monitor patient's mental status: mood, sensorium, affect, sleeping patterns, drowsiness, dizziness, suicidal tendencies

Nursing diagnoses

✓ Sleep pattern disturbance (uses)
✓ Knowledge deficit (teaching)
✓ Noncompliance (teaching)

Implementation

- Give after removing cigarettes to prevent fires
- Give after trying conservative measures for insomnia
- Give ½-1 hr before hs for sleeplessness; caps may be opened and mixed with food; give pc to decrease GI symptoms if used for sedation
- Provide assistance with ambulation after receiving dose
- Provide safety measures: nightlight, call bell within easy reach
- Check to see if PO medication has been swallowed
- Store in tight container in cool environment

Patient/family education

- Inform patient that drug may be taken with food; if dose is missed take as soon as remembered; do not double doses
- Advise patient to avoid OTC preparations unless approved by a physician, to avoid alcohol ingestion or other psychotropic medications unless approved by prescriber, that 1-2 wk of therapy may be required before therapeutic effects occur
- Caution patient to avoid driving, activities requiring alertness, drowsiness may occur; until medication response is known, tell patient that drowsiness may worsen at beginning of treatment
- Instruct patient not to discontinue medication abruptly after long-term use
- G Caution patient to rise slowly or fainting may occur, especially in elderly
- G Inform patient that hangover is common in elderly

Evaluation

Positive therapeutic outcome

- Increased well-being
- Decreased anxiety, restlessness, sleeplessness, dread

Treatment of overdose: Lavage, activated charcoal; monitor electrolytes, VS

flurbiprofen (℞)

(flure-bi'proe-fen)
Ansaid, Froben ✦, Ocufen
Func. class.: Nonsteroidal antiinflammatory
Chem. class.: Phenylalkanoic acid
Pregnancy category C

Action: Inhibits prostaglandin synthesis by decreasing enzyme needed for biosynthesis; analgesic, antiinflammatory, antipyretic; inhibits enzyme system necessary for biosynthesis of prostaglandins; inhibits miosis

Therapeutic Outcome: Decreased pain, inflammation

Uses: Mild-to-moderate pain, osteoarthritis, rheumatoid arthritis, acute gout, arthritis, ankylosing spondylitis, inflammation, dysmenorrhea; inhibition of intraoperative miosis, corneal edema

Dosage and routes

Adult: PO 200-300 mg qd in 2-4 divided doses, max 300 mg/day or 100 mg/dose; ophth 1 gtt q½-2h before surgery (4 gtt total)

Available forms: Sol 0.03%; tabs 50, 100 mg

Adverse effects

CNS: Depression, flushing, sweating, headache, mood changes
CV: Hypertension, **circulatory collapse,** thrombophlebitis, embolism, tachycardia, edema
EENT: Burning, stinging in the eye, irritation, bleeding or redness; fungal infections, increased intraocular pressure, blurred vision
GI: Diarrhea, nausea, abdominal distention, **GI hemorrhage,** increased appetite, pancreatitis
INTEG: Acne, poor wound healing, ecchymosis, petechiae
MS: Fractures, osteoporosis, weakness

Contraindications: Hypersensitivity, epithelial herpes simplex keratitis

Precautions: Pregnancy **C**, lactation, child, aspirin or NSAID hypersensitivity, allergy, bleeding disorder

Do Not Confuse:
Ansaid/Asacol, Ocufen/Ocuflox, Ocufen/Ocupress

Pharmacokinetics	
Absorption	Well absorbed (PO)
Distribution	Widely distributed (PO)
Metabolism	Liver—extensively
Excretion	Kidneys
Half-life	3-6 hr

Pharmacodynamics
Unknown

Interactions

Individual drugs
Alcohol: ↑ GI upset
Aspirin: ↓ effect of flurbiprofen
Carbachol: ↓ effect when used with other ophthalmics
Epinephrine: ↓ effect of epinephrine
Heparin: ↑ bleeding
Radiation: ↑ effects

Drug classifications
Antihypertensives: ↓ antihypertensive effect
Cephalosporins: ↑ bleeding
Hypoglycemics, oral: ↑ hypoglycemic effect
NSAIDs: ↑ GI upset

NURSING CONSIDERATIONS

Assessment

- Assess for pain: joint pain (duration, intensity, ROM); baseline and during treatment

Implementation

Ophthalmic route
- Excess sol must be wiped away promptly to prevent its flow into lacrimal system, producing systemic symptoms
- Protect sol from sun

PO route
- Give ½ hr ac or 2 hr pc

Patient/family education

- Advise patient to report change in vision, blurring, or loss of sight during miosis; rash, tinnitus, black stools, headache, chills, fever (systemic)
- Caution patient not to use for any other condition than prescribed
- Inform patient to avoid use with

OTC medications for pain or with alcohol unless approved by prescriber
- Advise patient to avoid hazardous activities because dizziness or drowsiness occurs

Evaluation
Positive therapeutic outcome
- Absence of corneal edema, intraoperative miosis (ophth)
- Decreased pain, inflammation

flutamide (℞)
(floo'ta-mide)
Eulexin
Func. class.: Antineoplastic hormone
Chem. class.: Antiandrogen

Pregnancy category D

Action: Interferes with testosterone uptake in the nucleus or testosterone activity in target tissues; arrests tumor growth in androgen-sensitive tissue, i.e., prostate gland

➔ Therapeutic Outcome: Prevention of rapidly growing malignant cells

Uses: Metastatic prostatic carcinoma, stage D_2 in combination with LHRH agonistic analogs (leuprolide)

Dosage and routes
Adult: PO 250 mg q8h tid, for a daily dosage of 750 mg

Stage B_2-C prostatic carcinoma
Start 8 wk before radiation therapy and continue during radiation therapy; give with goserelin

Stage D_2 metastatic carcinoma
Adult: Give with LHRH agonist and continue until progression

Available forms: Caps 125, 250 mg

Adverse effects
CNS: *Hot flashes,* drowsiness, confusion, depression, anxiety, paresthesia
GI: *Diarrhea, nausea, vomiting,* increased liver function studies, **hepatitis,** anorexia
GU: *Decreased libido, impotence, gynecomastia*
HEMA: Leukopenia, thrombocytopenia, hemolytic anemia
INTEG: Irritation at site, rash, photosensitivity
MISC: Edema, neuromuscular and pulmonary symptoms, hypertension

Do Not Confuse:
Eulexin/Edecrin

Contraindications: Hypersensitivity, pregnancy **D**

Pharmacokinetics

Absorption	Well absorbed
Distribution	Unknown
Metabolism	Liver
Excretion	Unknown
Half-life	6 hr

Pharmacodynamics
Unknown

Interactions
Individual drugs
Leuprolide: ↑ synergistic effect

NURSING CONSIDERATIONS
Assessment
- Monitor CBC, bilirubin, creatinine, AST, ALT, alkaline phosphatase, which may be elevated, drug may need to be discontinued
- Identify CNS symptoms: drowsiness, confusion, depression, anxiety

Nursing diagnoses
- ✓ Injury, risk for (adverse reactions)
- ✓ Sexual dysfunction (adverse reactions)
- ✓ Body image disturbance (adverse reactions)
- ✓ Infection, risk for (adverse reactions)
- ✓ Knowledge deficit (teaching)

Implementation
- Used in combination with LHRH agonist (leuprolide)
- May be given with food or fluids

Patient/family education

- Tell the patient to report side effects: decreased libido, impotence, breast enlargement, hot flashes, diarrhea, which occur when the two drugs are given together; also nausea, vomiting; jaundice in eyes, skin; dark urine, clay-colored stools, hepatotoxicity may occur
- Inform patient that this drug is taken with leuprolide for medical castration, do not change dosing

Evaluation

Positive therapeutic outcome

- Prevention of rapid division of malignant cells

fluvastatin (℞)

(flu'vah-stay-tin)

Lescol

Func. class.: Antilipidemic

Chem. class.: HMG-CoA reductase inhibitor

Pregnancy category X

Action: Inhibits HMG-CoA reductase enzyme, which reduces cholesterol synthesis

➔ Therapeutic Outcome: Decreased cholsterol levels and LDLs, increased HDLs

Uses: As an adjunct in primary hypercholesterolemia (types Ia, Iib), coronary atherosclerosis in CAD

Dosage and routes

Adult: PO 20-40 mg qd in PM initially, usual range 20-80, not to exceed 80 mg; should be given in 2 doses (40 mg AM, 40 mg PM); dosage adjustments may be made in 4 wk intervals or more

Available forms: Caps 20, 40 mg

Adverse effects

CNS: Headache, dizziness, insomnia
EENT: Lens opacities
GI: Nausea, constipation, diarrhea, dyspepsia, flatus, liver dysfunction, pancreatitis
HEMA: **Thrombocytopenia, hemolytic anemia, leukopenia**
INTEG: Rash, pruritus
MISC: Fatigue, influenza
MS: Myalgia, myositis, rhabdomyolysis
RESP: Upper respiratory infection, rhinitis, cough, pharyngitis, sinusitis

Contraindications: Hypersensitivity, pregnancy **X,** lactation, active liver disease

Precautions: Past liver disease, alcoholism, severe acute infections, trauma, hypotension, uncontrolled seizure disorders, severe metabolic disorders, electrolyte imbalance

Pharmacokinetics

Absorption	Unknown
Distribution	Unknown
Metabolism	Liver
Excretion	Feces, kidneys
Half-life	14 hr

Pharmacodynamics

Unknown

Interactions

Individual drugs

Cholestyramine: ↓ action of fluvastin
Clofibrate: ↑ myalgia, myositis
Colestipol: ↓ action of fluvastin
Cyclosporine: ↑ risk of myopathy
Digoxin: ↑ action
Erthyromycin: ↑ risk of myopathy
Gemfibrozil: ↑ risk of myopathy
Niacin: ↑ risk of myopathy
Rifampin: ↓ effects of fluvastin
Warfarin: ↑ action

Drug classifications:

Azole antiinfectives given with clofibrate: ↑ myalgia, ↑ myositis

NURSING CONSIDERATIONS

Assessment

- Assess nutrition: fat, protein, carbohydrates; nutritional analysis should be completed by dietitian before treatment

- Monitor bowel pattern daily; diarrhea may be a problem
- Assess fasting lipid profile (cholesterol, LDL, HDL, triglycerides) q8 wk, then q3-6 mo when stable
- Monitor liver function studies q1-2 mo during the first 1½ yr of treatment; AST, ALT, liver function test results may be increased
- Monitor renal studies in patients with compromised renal system: BUN, I&O ratio, creatinine
- Obtain ophth exam before, 1 mo after treatment begins, annually; lens opacities may occur

Nursing diagnoses

✓ Diarrhea (adverse reactions)
✓ Knowledge deficit (teaching)
✓ Noncompliance (teaching)

Implementation

- Give with evening meal; if dosage is increased, take with breakfast and evening meal
- Store in cool environment in airtight, light-resistant container

Patient/family education

- Inform patient that compliance is needed for positive results to occur, not to double doses
- Advise patient to notify prescriber if GI symptoms of diarrhea, abdominal or epigastric pain, nausea, vomiting, or if chills, fever, sore throat occur; also muscle pain, weakness, tenderness
- Advise patient that treatment is chronic
- Advise patient that blood studies and eye exam will be necessary during treatment
- Instruct patient to report suspected pregnancy, not to use during pregnancy
- Advise patient that previously prescribed regimen will continue, including diet, exercise, smoking cessation
- Advise patient to use sunscreen or stay out of the sun to prevent burns
- Instruct patient to notify all health care providers of drugs taken

Evaluation

Positive therapeutic outcome

- Decreased LDL, VLDL, total cholesterol levels
- Improved ratio of HDLs

folic acid (vitamin B_9)

(PO, OTC; IM/IV, Ph)
(foe-lik a'sid)
Apo-Folic ♣, Folate, Folvite, Novofolacid ♣, Vitamin B_9
Func. class.: Vitamin B-complex group
Chem. class.: Supplement
Pregnancy category A

Action: Needed for erythropoiesis; increases RBC, WBC, and platelet formation in megaloblastic anemias

➔ Therapeutic Outcome: Absence of macrocytic, megaloblastic anemias

Uses: Megaloblastic or macrocytic anemia caused by folic acid deficiency; liver disease; alcoholism; hemolysis; intestinal obstruction; pregnancy

Dosage and routes

Supplement

Adult: PO/IM/SC/**IV** 0.1 mg qd

P ***Child:*** PO/IM/SC/**IV** 0.05 mg qd

Megaloblastic/macrocytic anemia

P ***Adult and child >4 yr:*** PO/SC/IM/**IV** 1 mg qd × 4-5 days

P ***Child <4 yr:*** PO/SC/IM/**IV** 0.3 mg or less qd

Pregnancy/lactation: PO/SC/IM/**IV** 0.8 mg qd

Prevention of megaloblastic/macrocytic anemia

Pregnancy: PO/SC/IM/**IV** 1 mg qd

Available forms: Tabs 0.4, 0.8, 1 mg; inj 5, 10 mg/ml

Adverse effects

INTEG: Flushing
***RESP:* Bronchospasm**

Contraindications: Hypersensitivity, anemias other than megaloblastic/macrocytic anemia, vit B_{12} deficiency anemia, uncorrected pernicious anemia

Precautions: Pregnancy **A**

Pharmacokinetics

Absorption	Well absorbed
Distribution	Liver, crosses placenta
Metabolism	Liver (converted to active metabolite)
Excretion	Kidneys (unchanged)
Half-life	Unknown

Pharmacodynamics

Onset	Unknown
Peak	½-1 hr
Duration	Unknown

Interactions

Individual drugs

Aspirin: ↓ folate level
Carbamazepine: ↑ need for folic acid
Methotrexate: ↓ action of folic acid
Phenytoin: ↑ need for folic acid
Sulfasalazine: ↓ action of folic acid
Triamterene: ↓ action of folic acid

Drug classifications

Estrogens: ↑ need for folic acid
Glucocorticoids: ↑ need for folic acid
Hydantoins: ↑ need for folic acid
Sulfonamides: ↓ action of folic acid

NURSING CONSIDERATIONS

Assessment

- Assess patient for fatigue, dyspnea, weakness, shortness of breath, activity intolerance (signs of megaloblastic anemia)
- Monitor Hgb, Hct, and reticulocyte count; folate levels: 6-15 µg/ml baseline and throughout treatment
- Assess nutritional status: bran, yeast, dried beans, nuts, fruits, fresh vegetables, asparagus; if high folic acid foods are missing from the diet, a referral to a dietitian may be indicated
- Identify drugs currently taken: alcohol, oral contraceptives, estrogens, glucocorticoids, carbamazepine, hydantoins, trimethoprim; these drugs may cause increased folic acid use by the body and contribute to deficiency

Nursing diagnoses

✓ Nutrition, less than body requirements (uses)
✓ Fatigue (uses)
✓ Activity intolerance (uses)
✓ Knowledge deficit (teaching)

Implementation

IV IV route

- Give **IV** directly, undiluted 5 mg or less over 1 min or more, or may be added to most **IV** sol or TPN
- Store in light-resistant container

Y-site compatibilities:

Famotidine

Solution compatibilities:

$D_{20}W$

Solution incompatibilities:

$D_{40}W$, $D_{50}W$, calcium gluconate

Patient/family education

- Advise patient to take drug exactly as prescribed; not to double doses, toxicity may occur
- Instruct patient to notify prescriber of side effects; rash or fever may indicate hypersensitivity
- Advise patient that urine may become more yellow
- Instruct patient to increase intake of foods rich in folic acid in diet as recommended by dietitian or health care provider

Evaluation

Positive therapeutic outcome

- Absence of fatigue, weakness, dyspnea
- Absence of symptoms of megaloblastic anemia
- Increase in reticulocyte count within 5 days

F

fondaparinux sodium

See Appendix A, Selected New Drugs

formoterol fumarate

See Appendix A, Selected New Drugs

foscarnet (℞)

(foss-kar'net)

Foscavir

Func. class.: Antiviral

Chem. class.: Inorganic pyrophosphate organic analog

Pregnancy category C

Action: Antiviral activity is produced by selective inhibition at the pyrophosphate binding site on virus-specific DNA polymerases and reverse transcriptases at concentrations that do not affect cellular DNA polymerases

➔ **Therapeutic Outcome:** Virostatic agents against cytomegalovirus (CMV) retinitis

Uses: Treatment of CMV, retinitis, herpes simplex virus (HSV) infections; used with ganciclovir for relapsing patients

Dosage and routes

CMV retinitis

Adult: **IV** inf 60 mg/kg given over at least 1 hr, q8h × 2-3 wk initially, then 90-120 mg/kg/day over 2 hr, usually give with at least 750-1000 ml of 0.9% NaCl qd

HSV

Adult: **IV** 40 mg/kg q8-12h × 2-3 wk

Renal dose

Adult: **IV**

Male:

$$\frac{\text{weight (kg)} \times (140 - \text{age})}{72 \times \text{serum creatinine (mg/dl)}} = \text{CrCl}$$

Female: 0.85 × above value; dose based on table provided in package insert

Available forms: Inj 24 mg/ml

Adverse effects

CNS: *Fever,* dizziness, ***headache,*** **seizures,** *fatigue,* neuropathy, tremor, ataxia, dementia, stupor, EEG abnormalities, vertigo, **coma,** abnormal gait, hypertonia, extrapyramidal disorders, hemiparesis, **paralysis,** hyperreflexia, paraplegia, **tetany,** hyporeflexia, neuralgia, neuritis, celebral edema, ***paresthesia,*** depression, *confusion, anxiety,* insomnia, somnolence, amnesia, hallucinations, agitation

CV: Hypertension, palpitations, ECG abnormalities, 1st degree AV block, nonspecific ST-T segment changes, hypotension, cerebrovascular disorder, cardiomyopathy, **cardiac arrest,** bradycardia, **dysrhythmias**

EENT: Visual field defects, vocal cord paralysis, speech disorders, taste perversion, eye pain, conjunctivitis, tinnitus, otitis

GI: *Nausea, vomiting, diarrhea, anorexia,* abdominal pain, constipation, dysphagia, rectal hemorrhage, dry mouth, melena, flatulence, ulcerative stomatitis, pancreatitis, enteritis, enterocolitis, glossitis, proctitis, stomatitis, increased amylases, gastroenteritis, **pseudomembranous colitis,** duodenal ulcer, **paralytic ileus, esophageal ulceration,** abnormal A-G ratio, increased AST, ALT, cholecystitis, **hepatitis,** dyspepsia, tenesmus, hepatosplenomegaly, jaundice

GU: **Acute renal failure,** decreased CrCl and increased serum creatinine, **glomerulonephritis, toxic nephropathy, nephrosis, renal tubular disorders, pyelonephritis, uremia, hematuria, albuminuria,** dysuria, polyuria

HEMA: Anemia, *granulocytopenia, leukopenia, thrombocytopenia,* platelet abnormalities, **thrombosis,**

pulmonary embolism, coagulation disorders, decreased prothrombin, hypochromic anemia, pancytopenia, hemolysis, leukocytosis, lymphadenopathy, epistaxis, lymphopenia
INTEG: *Rash,* sweating, pruritus, skin ulceration, seborrhea, skin discoloration, alopecia, acne, dermatitis, pain/inflammation at injection site, facial edema, dry skin, urticaria
MS: Arthralgia, myalgia
RESP: *Coughing, dyspnea,* pneumonia, sinusitis, pharyngitis, **pulmonary infiltration,** stridor, **pneumothorax, hemoptysis, bronchospasm,** bronchitis, **respiratory depression, pleural effusion, pulmonary hemorrhage,** rhinitis
SYST: *Hypokalemia, hypocalcemia, hypomagnesemia,* increased alkaline phosphatase, LDH, BUN, acidosis, hypophosphatemia, hyperphosphatemia, dehydration, glycosuria, increased creatine phosphokinase, hypervolemia, infection, **sepsis, death, ascites,** hyponatremia, hypochloremia, hypercalcemia

Contraindications: Hypersensitivity, CrCl <0.4 ml/min/kg

P G **Precautions:** Pregnancy **C**, lactation, children, elderly, renal disease, seizure disorders, electrolyte/mineral imbalances, severe anemia

Pharmacokinetics

Absorption	Complete (**IV**)
Distribution	14%-17% plasma protein binding
Metabolism	Not metabolized
Excretion	Kidneys (90%) unchanged, breast milk
Half-life	2-8 hr; ↑ in renal disease

Pharmacodynamics

Onset	48 hr
Peak	2 wk
Duration	Unknown

Interactions
Individual drugs
Amphotericin B: ↑ nephrotoxicity
Ciprofloxacin: Seizures
Pentamide: ↑ nephrotoxicity
Zidovudine: ↑ anemia
Drug classification
Aminoglycosides: ↑ nephrotoxicity

NURSING CONSIDERATIONS
Assessment
- Culture should be done before treatment with foscarnet is begun; cultures of blood, urine, and throat may all be taken; CMV is not confirmed by this method; the diagnosis is made by an ophth exam
- Assess kidney and liver function; increased hemopoietic studies: BUN, serum creatinine, creatinine clearance, if CrCl <0.4 ml/min/kg, discontinue drug; AST, ALT, A-G ratio, baseline and during treatment; blood counts should be done q2wk; watch for decreasing granulocytes, Hgb; if low, therapy may have to be discontinued and restarted after hematologic recovery; blood transfusions may be required
- Assess for GI symptoms: severe nausea, vomiting, diarrhea; severe symptoms may necessitate discontinuing drug
- Monitor electrolytes and minerals: calcium, phosphorous, magnesium, sodium, potassium; watch closely for tetany during first administration
- Assess for symptoms of blood dyscrasias (anemia, granulocytopenia); bruising, fatigue, bleeding, poor healing
- Assess for symptoms of allergic reactions: flushing, rash, urticaria, pruritus

Nursing diagnoses
✓ Infection, risk for (uses)
✓ Injury, risk for (adverse reactions)
✓ Knowledge deficit (teaching)

Implementation

IV route

- Administer increased fluids before and during drug administration to induce diuresis and minimize renal toxicity
- Administer via infusion pump, at no more than 1 mg/kg/min; do not give by rapid or bolus **IV**; give by central venous line or peripheral vein; standard 24 mg/ml sol may be used without dilution if using by central line; dilute the 24 mg/ml sol to 12 mg/ml with D_5W or 0.9% NaCl if using peripheral vein
- Monitor patient closely during therapy; if tingling, numbness, paresthesias occur, stop inf and obtain lab sample for electrolytes

Y-site compatibilities: Aldesleukin, aminophylline, amikacin, ampicillin, aztreonam, benzquinamide, cefazolin, cefoperazone, cefoxitin, ceftazidime, ceftizoxime, ceftriaxone, cefuroxime, chloramphenicol, cimetidine, clindamycin, dexamethasone, dopamine, erythromycin, fluconazole, flucytosine, furosemide, gentamicin, heparin, hydrocortisone, hydromorphone, hydroxyzine, imipenem-cilastatin, metoclopramide, metronidazole, miconazole, morphine, nafcillin, oxacillin, penicillin G potassium, phenytoin, piperacillin, ranitidine, ticarcillin/clavulanate, tobramycin

Y-site incompatibilities: Acyclovir, amphotericin B, calcium, cotrimoxazole, diazepam, digoxin, gancyclovir, haloperidol, leucovorin, midazolam, pentamidine, phenytoin, prochlorperazine, vancomycin

Patient/family education

- Advise patient to notify prescriber if sore throat, swollen lymph nodes, malaise, fever occur, may indicate presence of other infections
- Advise patient to report perioral tingling, numbness in extremities, and paresthesias; inf should be stopped and electrolytes should be requested
- Caution patient that serious drug interactions may occur if OTC products are ingested; check first with prescriber
- Inform patient that drug is not a cure, but will control symptoms
- Advise patient that ophth exams must be continued

Evaluation

Positive therapeutic outcome

- Improvement in CMV retinitis

fosinopril (℞)

(foss-in-o'pril)

Monopril

Func. class.: Antihypertensive

Chem. class.: Angiotensin-converting enzyme (ACE) inhibitor

Pregnancy category
C (1st trimester),
D (2nd/3rd trimesters)

Action: Selectively suppresses renin-angiotensin-aldosterone system; inhibits ACE; prevents conversion of angiotensin I to angiotensin II; results in dilation of arterial, venous vessels

Therapeutic Outcome: Decreased B/P in hypertension

Uses: Hypertension, alone or in combination with thiazide diuretics, systolic CHF

Dosage and routes

Hypertension

Adult: PO 10 mg qd initially, then 20-40 mg/day divided bid or qd

CHF

Adult: PO 10 mg qd, then up to 40 mg/day, increased over several weeks, use lower dose in those undergoing diuresis before fosinopril

Renal dose

Adult: 5 mg qd

Available forms: Tabs 10, 20, 40 mg

Adverse effects

CNS: *Insomnia, paresthesia, headache, dizziness,* fatigue, memory disturbance, tremor, mood change
CV: *Hypotension,* chest pain, palpitations, angina, orthostatic hypotension
GI: *Nausea,* constipation, vomiting, diarrhea
GU: **Proteinuria,** increased BUN, creatinine, decreased libido
HEMA: Decreased Hct, Hgb, **eosinophilia, leukopenia, neutropenia**
INTEG: **Angioedema,** rash, flushing, sweating, photosensitivity, pruritus
META: Hyperkalemia
MS: Arthralgia, myalgia
RESP: Cough, sinusitis, dyspnea, **bronchospasm**

Contraindications: Hypersensitivity to ACE inhibitors, lactation, P children, pregnancy **D** (2nd/3rd trimesters)

Precautions: Impaired liver function, hypovolemia, blood dyscrasias, CHF, COPD, asthma, G elderly, pregnancy **C** (1st trimester)

Do Not Confuse:
Monopril/minoxidil

Pharmacokinetics

Absorption	30%
Distribution	Crosses placenta
Metabolism	Liver—converted to fosinoprilate
Excretion	50% kidneys (metabolities), 50% feces
Half-life	12 hr—fosinoprilat

Pharmacodynamics

Onset	1 hr
Peak	2-6 hr
Duration	24 hr

Interactions

Individual drugs

Alcohol, acute ingestion: ↑ hypotension (large amounts)
Allopurinol: ↑ hypersensitivity
Digoxin: ↑ toxicity
Hydralazine: ↑ toxicity
Indomethacin: ↓ antihypertensive effect
Lithium: ↑ toxicity
Prazosin: ↑ toxicity

Drug classifications

Adrenergic blockers: ↑ hypotension
Antacids: ↓ absorption
Antihypertensives: ↑ hypotension
Diuretics: ↑ hypotension
Diuretics, potassium-sparing: ↑ toxicity
Ganglionic blockers: ↑ hypotension
Nitrates: ↑ hypotension
Phenothiazines: ↑ hypotension
Potassium supplements: ↑ toxicity
Sympathomimetics: ↑ toxicity

Lab test interferences

↑ AST, ↑ ALT, ↑ alkaline phosphatase, ↑ glucose, ↑ bilirubin, ↑ uric acid
Positive: ANA titer
False positive: Urine acetone

NURSING CONSIDERATIONS

Assessment

- Monitor blood studies: neutrophils, decreased platelets; obtain WBC with differential baseline and qmo × 6 mo, then q2-3 mo × 1 yr; if neutrophils <1000/mm^3, discontinue
- Monitor B/P, check for orthostatic hypotension, syncope; if changes occur, dosage change may be required
- Monitor renal studies: protein, BUN, creatinine; watch for increased levels that may indicate nephrotic syndrome and renal failure; monitor urine daily for protein; monitor renal symptoms: polyuria, oliguria, frequency, dysuria
- Establish baselines in renal, liver function tests before therapy begins
- Check potassium levels throughout treatment although hyperkalemia rarely occurs
- Check for edema in feet, legs daily, monitor weight daily
- Assess for allergic reactions: rash, fever, pruritus, urticaria; drug should be discontinued if antihistamines fail to help

F

Nursing diagnoses

- ✓ Cardiac output, decreased (uses)
- ✓ Injury, risk for (side effects)
- ✓ Knowledge deficit (teaching)
- ✓ Noncompliance (teaching)

Implementation

- Store in air-tight container at 86° F (30° C) or less
- Severe hypotension may occur after 1st dose of this medication; hypotension may be prevented by reducing or discontinuing diuretic therapy 3 days before beginning benzapril therapy

Patient/family education

- Advise patient not to discontinue drug abruptly; warn patient to tell all persons associated with his or her care
- Teach patient not to use OTC products (cough, cold, allergy) unless directed by prescriber because serious side effects can occur; xanthines such as coffee, tea, chocolate, cola can prevent action of drug
- Teach patient the importance of complying with dosage schedule, even if feeling better; to continue with medical regimen to decrease B/P: exercise, smoking cessation, decreasing stress, diet modifications
- Emphasize the need to rise slowly to sitting or standing position to minimize orthostatic hypotension; not to exercise in hot weather or increased hypotension can occur
- Teach patient to notify prescriber of mouth sores, sore throat, fever, swelling of hands or feet, irregular heartbeat, chest pain, coughing, shortness of breath
- Instruct patient to report excessive perspiration, dehydration, vomiting, diarrhea; may lead to fall in B/P
- Caution patient that drug may cause dizziness, fainting, light-headedness; may occur during 1st few days of therapy; to avoid activities that may be hazardous
- Teach patient how to take B/P, and normal readings for age group
- Advise patient to notify prescriber if pregnancy is planned or suspected

Evaluation

Positive therapeutic outcome

- Decreased B/P in hypertension

Treatment of overdose: 0.9% NaCl **IV** inf, hemodialysis

fosphenytoin (℞)

(foss-fen'i-toy-in)

Cerebyx

Func. class.: Anticonvulsant

Chem. class.: Hydantoin

Pregnancy category D

Action: Inhibits spread of seizure activity in motor cortex by altering ion transport; increases AV conduction

➔ **Therapeutic Outcome:** Decreased seizures, absence of dysrhythmias

Uses: Generalized tonic-clonic seizures, status epilepticus

Dosage and routes

Status epilepticus

P ***Adult and child:*** **IV** loading dose 15-20 mg PE/kg given at 100-150 mg PE/min

Nonemergency/ maintenance dosing

P ***Adult and child:*** IM/**IV** loading dose 10-20 mg PE/kg; maintenance dosing 4-6 mg PE/kg/day given at a rate of <150 mg PE/min

Available forms: Inj 150 mg (100 mg phenytoin), 750 mg (500 mg phenytoin)

Adverse effects

CNS: Drowsiness, dizziness, insomnia, paresthesias, depression, suicidal tendencies, aggression, headache, confusion

CV: Hypotension, **ventricular fibrillation**

EENT: Nystagmus, diplopia, blurred vision

GI: Nausea, vomiting, constipation, anorexia, weight loss, hepatitis, jaundice, gingival hyperplasia
GU: **Nephritis**, urine discoloration
HEMA: **Agranulocytosis, leukopenia, aplastic anemia, thrombocytopenia, megaloblastic anemia**
INTEG: Rash, lupus erythematosus, *Stevens-Johnson syndrome,* hirsutism
SYST: Hypocalcemia, hypokalemia, hyperglycemia

Contraindications: Hypersensitivity, psychiatric conditions, pregnancy **D**, bradycardia, SA and AV block, Stokes-Adams syndrome

Precautions: Allergies, hepatic disease, renal disease

Pharmacokinetics

Absorption	Unknown
Distribution	Unknown
Metabolism	Liver
Excretion	Kidneys
Half-life	Unknown

Pharmacodynamics

Unknown

Interactions

Individual drugs

Alcohol: ↑ CNS depression
Amiodarone: ↑ fosphenytoin level
Carbamazepine: ↓ effectiveness
Chloramphenicol: ↑ fosphenytoin level
Cimetidine: ↑ fosphenytoin level
Isoniazid: ↓ metabolism, ↑ action
Methylphenidate: ↑ fosphenytoin level
Trazodone: ↑ fosphenytoin
Valproic acid: ↑ seizures

Drug classifications

Anticonvulsants: ↑ CNS depression
Antidepressants: ↑ CNS depression
Antihistamines: ↑ CNS depression
Azole antiinfectives: ↑ fosphenytoin level
Barbiturates: ↑ CNS depression, ↓ effect of fosphonytoin
Benzodiazepines: ↑ fosphenytoin level
Estrogens: ↑ fosphenytoin level
General anesthetics: ↑ CNS depression
H_2-receptor antagonists: ↑ fosphenytoin level
Hypnotics: ↑ CNS depression
Opiates: ↑ CNS depression
Phenothiazines: ↑ fosphenytoin level
Salicylates: ↑ fosphenytoin level
Sedatives: ↑ CNS depression
Sulfonamides: ↑ fosphenytoin level

Food/drug

↓ Folic acid absorption

Lab test interferences

↓ Dexamethasone, ↓ metyrapone test serum, ↓ PBI, ↓ urinary steroids
↑ Glucose, ↑ alkaline phosphatase, ↑ BSP

NURSING CONSIDERATIONS

Assessment

- Assess seizure activity including type, location, duration, and character; provide seizure precaution
- Assess renal studies: urinalysis, BUN, urine creatinine
- Monitor hepatic studies: ALT, AST, bilirubin, creatinine
- Assess allergic reaction: red raised rash; if this occurs, drug should be discontinued
- Monitor for toxicity: bone marrow depression, nausea, vomiting, ataxia, diplopia, cardiovascular collapse, slurred speech, confusion
- Assess drug level: toxic level 30-50 μg/ml
- ❗ Assess for rash, discontinue as soon as rash develops, serious adverse reactions such as Stevens-Johnson syndrome can occur
- Assess mental status: mood, sensorium, affect, memory (long, short), G especially elderly
- Assess for blood dyscrasias: fever, sore throat, bruising, rash, jaundice, epistaxis (long-term treatment only)
- Monitor blood studies: RBC, Hct,

F

Hgb, reticulocyte counts weekly for 4 wk then monthly; also check thyroid function tests, serum calcium

Nursing diagnoses

- ✓ Injury, risk for (uses, adverse reactions)
- ✓ Knowledge deficit (teaching)
- ✓ Noncompliance (teaching)

Implementation

IV IV route

- Administer by direct **IV** after diluting with D_5 or 0.9% NaCl 1.5-25 mg PE/ml

Solution compatibilities: D_5W, $D_{10}W$, amino acid inj 10%, D_5LR, D_5/0.9% NaCl, Plasmalyte A, LR, per sterile water for inj

Additive compatibilities: Potassium chloride

Patient/family education

- Teach patient the reason for and expected outcome of treatment
- Instruct patient not to use machinery or engage in hazardous activity; drowsiness, dizziness may occur
- Advise patient to carry ID identifying drug used, name of prescriber
- Advise patient to notify prescriber of rash, bleeding, bruising, slurred speech, jaundice of skin or eyes, joint pain, nausea, vomiting, severe headache
- Advise patient to keep all medical appointments, including lab work, physical assessment
- Advise patient to notify prescriber if pregnancy is planned or suspected; to use contraception with this product

Evaluation

Positive therapeutic outcome

- Decreased seizure activity

frovatriptan

See Appendix A, Selected New Drugs

furosemide (Key Drug) (℞)

(fur-oh'se-mide)

Apo-Furosemide ♣, Furoside ♣, Lasix, Lasix Special ♣, Myrosemide, Novosemide ♣, Uritol ♣

Func. class.: Loop diuretic
Chem. class.: Sulfonamide derivative

Pregnancy category C

Action: Acts on the ascending loop of Henle in the kidney, inhibiting reabsorption of electrolytes sodium and chloride, causing excretion of sodium, calcium, magnesium, chloride, water, and some potassium; decreases reabsorption of sodium and chloride and increases excretion of potassium in the distal tubule of the kidney; responsible for slight antihypertensive effect and peripheral vasodilation

→ **Therapeutic Outcome:** Decreased edema in lung tissue, peripherally; decreased B/P

Uses: Edema in CHF, nephrotic syndrome, ascites, caused by hepatic disease, hepatic cirrhosis; may be used alone or as adjunct with antihypertensives such as spironolactone, triamterene; should not be used with ethacrynic acid

Investigational uses: Hypercalcemia in malignancy

Dosage and routes

Adult: PO 20-80 mg/day in AM, may give another dose in 6 hr, up to 600 mg/day; IM/**IV** 20-40 mg, increased by 20 mg q2h until desired response

P ***Child:*** PO/IM/**IV** 2 mg/kg, may increase by 1-2 mg/kg/q6-8h up to 6 mg/kg

Pulmonary edema

Adult: **IV** 40 mg given over several min, repeated in 1 hr; increase to 80 mg if needed

Antihypercalcemia
Adult: IM/**IV** 80-100 mg q1-4h or PO 120 mg qd or divided bid

P ***Child:*** IM/**IV** 25-50 mg, repeat q4h if needed

Available forms: Tabs 20, 40, 80 mg; oral sol 10 mg/ml, 40 mg/5 ml; inj IM, **IV** 10 mg/ml

Adverse effects
CNS: Headache, fatigue, weakness, vertigo, paresthesias
CV: Orthostatic hypotension, chest pain, ECG changes, **circulatory collapse**
EENT: *Loss of hearing,* ear pain, tinnitus, blurred vision
ELECT: *Hypokalemia, hypochloremic alkalosis, hypomagnesemia, hyperuricemia, hypocalcemia, hyponatremia,* metabolic alkalosis
GI: *Nausea,* diarrhea, dry mouth, vomiting, anorexia, cramps, oral or gastric irritations, pancreatitis
GU: *Polyuria,* **renal failure,** *glycosuria*
HEMA: **Thrombocytopenia, agranulocytosis, leukopenia, neutropenia, anemia**
INTEG: *Rash, pruritus, purpura,* **Stevens-Johnson syndrome,** sweating, photosensitivity, urticaria
MS: Cramps, stiffness

Contraindications: Hypersensitivity to sulfonamides, anuria, hypovolemia, infants, lactation, electrolyte depletion

Precautions: Diabetes mellitus, dehydration, severe renal disease, pregnancy **C**, cirrhosis, ascites

Do Not Confuse:
furosemide/torsemide, Lasix/Lanoxin, Lasix/Lomotil, Lasix/Luvox

Pharmacokinetics

	PO
Absorption	GI tract (60%-70%)
	PO/IM/**IV**
Distribution	Crosses placenta
Metabolism	Liver (30%-40%)
Excretion	Breast milk, urine, feces
Half-life	½-1 hr

Pharmacodynamics

	PO	IM	IV
Onset	1 hr	½ hr	5 min
Peak	1-2 hrs	Unknown	½ hr
Duration	6-8 hr	4-8 hr	2 hr

Interactions
Individual drugs
Alcohol: ↑ orthostatic hypotension
Chloral hydrate: ↑ sweating, flushing when given with **IV** furosemide
Cisplatin: ↑ risk of ototoxicity
Clofibrate: ↑ furosemide effects
Ethacrynic acid: Combination with furosemide may cause ↑ chance of dysrhythmias (do not use together)
Lithium: ↓ renal clearance, causing increased toxicity
Phenytoin: ↓ diuretic effect caused by ↓ absorption
Probenecid: ↓ effects of furosemide
Succinylcholine: Action of succinylcholine is ↑ by low doses and ↓ by high doses of furosemide
Theophylline: May ↑ or ↓ the effect of theophylline
Vancomycin: ↑ risk of ototoxicity
Drug classifications
Adrenergic blockers: ↑ effects
Aminoglycosides: ↑ ototoxicity, nephrotoxicity
Antidiabetics: ↓ hypoglycemic effect
Antihypertensives: ↑ antihypertensive effect
Cephalosporins: ↑ nephrotoxicity
Corticosteroids: ↑ potassium loss caused by potassium depletion effects of both drugs
Digitalis glycosides: ↑ potassium and magnesium loss with relating dysrhythmias

Opiates: ↑ orthostatic hypotension
Salicylates: ↓ diuretic effect
Food/drug
↓ Diuresis

NURSING CONSIDERATIONS
Assessment

- Assess patient for tinnitus, hearing loss, ear pain; periodic testing of hearing is needed when high doses of this drug are given by **IV** route
- Monitor for renal, cardiac, neurologic, GI, pulmonary manifestations of hypokalemia: acidic urine, reduced urine osmolality, nocturia, polyuria and polydipsia; hypotension, broad T-wave, U-wave, ectopy, tachycardia, weak pulse; muscle weakness, altered LOC, drowsiness, apathy, lethargy, confusion, depression; anorexia, nausea, cramps, constipation, distension, paralytic ileus; hypoventilation, respiratory muscle weakness
- Monitor for CNS, GI, cardiovascular, integumentary, neurologic manifestations of hypocalcemia: personality changes, anxiety, disturbances, depression and psychosis; nausea, vomiting, constipation, abdominal pain from muscle spasm; decreased contractility, decreased cardiac output, hypotension, lengthened ST segment, prolonged QT interval; scaling eczema, alopecia, hyperpigmentation; tetany, muscle twitching, cramping grimacing, seizure, altered deep tendon reflexes, spasm
- Monitor for CNS, neuromuscular, GI, cardiac manifestations of hypomagnesemia, agitation; muscle twitching, paresthesias, hyperactive reflexes, positive Babinski reflex, dysphagia, nystagmus seizures, tetnany; nausea, vomiting, diarrhea, anorexia, abdominal distention; ectopy, tachycardia, broad, flat or inverted T-waves, depressed ST segment, prolonged QT, decreased cardiac output, hypotension
- Monitor for CV, GI, neurologic manifestations of hyponatremia: increased B/P, cold, clammy skin, hypovolemia or hypervolemia; anorexia, nausea, vomiting, diarrhea, abdominal cramps; lethargy, increased ICP, confusion, headache, seizures, coma, fatigue, tremors, hyperreflexia
- Monitor for neurologic, respiratory manifestations of hyperchloremia: weakness, lethargy, coma; deep rapid breathing
- Assess fluid volume status: I&O ratios and record, count or weigh diapers as appropriate, weight, distended red veins, crackles in lung, color, quality and sp gr of urine, skin turgor, adequacy of pulses, moist mucous membranes, bilateral lung sounds, peripheral pitting edema; dehydration symptoms of decreasing output, thirst, hypotension, dry mouth and mucous membranes should be reported
- Monitor electrolytes: potassium, sodium, calcium, magnesium; also include BUN, blood pH, ABGs, uric acid, CBC, blood sugar
- Assess B/P before and during therapy lying, standing and sitting as appropriate; orthostatic hypotension can occur rapidly

Nursing diagnoses

✓ Fluid volume deficit (side effects)
✓ Fluid volume excess (uses)
✓ Knowledge deficit (teaching)

Implementation

- Give in AM to avoid interference with sleep
- Potassium replacement if potassium level is <3.0 mg/dl whole, or use oral sol slightly, drug may be crushed if patient is unable to swallow

PO route

- With food, if nausea occurs, absorption may be reduced

IV **IV route**

- Do not use sol that is yellow, has a precipitate, or crystals

Implementation

IV **Direct IV**

- Give undiluted through Y-tube on

3-way stopcock; give 20 mg or less/min

Intermittent Infusion

- May be added to NS, D_5W, $D_{10}W$, $D_{20}W$; invert sugar 10% in electrolyte #1, LR, sodium lactate y_6m, use within 24 hr to assure compatibility; give through Y-tube or 3-way stopcock; give at 4 mg/min or less, use infusion pump

Syringe compatibilities:

Bleomycin, cisplatin, cyclophosphamide, fluorouracil, heparin, leucovorin, methotrexate, mitomycin

Syringe incompatibilities:

Doxapram, doxorubicin, droperidol, metaclopramide, milrinone

Y-site compatibilities:

Allopurinol, amifostine, amikacin, aztrenom, bleomycin, cefepime, cefmetazole, cisplatin, cladribine, cyclophosphamide, cytarabine, dexamethasone, epinephrine, fentanyl, fludarabine, fluorouracil, foscarnet, gallium, granisetron, heparin, hydrocortisone, hydromorphone, indomethacin, kanamycin, leucovorin, lorazepam, melphalan, meropenem, methotrexate, mitomycin, morphine, nitroglycerin, norepinephrine, paclitaxel, piperacillin/tazobactam, potassium chloride, propofol, ranitidine, sargramostim, tacrolimus, teniposide, thiotepa, tobramycin, tolazoline, vit B complex with C

Y-site incompatibilities:

Amsacrine, bleomycin, doxorubicin, droperidol, esmolol, fluconazole, gentamicin, idarubicin, metoclopramide, milrinone, netilmicin, ondansetron, quinidine, vinblastine, vincristine

Additive compatibilities:

Amikacin, aminophylline, ampicillin, atropine, bumetanide, calcium gluconate, cefamandole, cefoperazone, cefuroxime, cimetidine, cloxacillin, dexamethasone, diamorphine, digoxin, epinephrine, heparin, isosorbide, kanamycin, lidocaine, meropenem, morphine, nitroglycerin, penicillin G, potassium chloride, ranitidine, scopolamine, sodium bicarbonate, theophylline, tobramycin, verapamil

Additive incompatibilities:

Bleomycin, dobutamine, gentamicin, chlorpromazine, diazepam, erythromycin, isoproterenol, meperidine, metoclopramide, netilmicin, opium alkaloids, prochlorperazine, tetracycline

F

Patient/family education

General

- Teach patient to take the medication early in the day to prevent nocturia
- Instruct the patient to take with food or milk if GI symptoms of nausea and anorexia occur
- Teach patient to maintain a record of weight on a weekly basis and notify physician of weight loss of >5 lb
- Caution the patient that this drug causes a loss of potassium, that food rich in potassium should be added to the diet; refer to a dietitian for assistance in planning
- Caution the patient not to exercise in hot weather or stand for prolonged periods of time because orthostatic hypotension will be enhanced
- Advise patient to wear protective clothing and sunscreen to prevent photosensitivity
- Teach patient not to use alcohol or any OTC medications without physician's approval, serious drug reactions may occur
- Emphasize the need to contact physician immediately if muscle cramps, weakness, nausea, dizziness, or numbness occurs
- Teach patient to take and record own B/P and pulse
- Caution the patient that orthostatic hypotension may occur and to rise slowly from sitting or reclining positions and lie down if dizziness occurs
- Teach patient to continue taking

medication even if feeling better, this drug controls symptoms but does not cure the condition

- Advise the patient with hypertension to continue other medical treatment (exercise, weight loss, relaxation techniques, cessation of smoking)

Evaluation

Positive therapeutic outcome

- Decreased edema
- Decreased B/P
- Lowered calcium level in malignancy
- Increased diuresis

gabapentin (℞)

(gab′a-pen-tin)

Neurontin

Func. class.: Anticonvulsant

Pregnancy category C

Action: Mechanism unknown; may increase seizure threshold; structurally similar to GABA; gabapentin binding sites in neocortex, hippocampus

➔ **Therapeutic Outcome:** Decreased seizure activity

Uses: Adjunct treatment of partial seizures, with or without generalization in patients >12 yr; adjunct in P partial seizures in children 3-12 yr

Investigational uses: Tremors in multiple sclerosis, neuropathic pain, bipolar disorder, migraine prophylaxis, alcohol/cocaine withdrawal, diabetic neuropathy

Dosage and routes

P ***Adult and child >12 yr:*** PO 900-1800 mg/day in 3 divided doses; may titrate by giving 300 mg on the first day, 300 mg bid on second day, 300 mg tid on third day; may increase to 1800 mg/day by adding 300 mg on subsequent days

P ***Child 3-12 yr:*** PO 10-15 mg/kg/day in 3 divided doses, initially, titrate dose upward over approximately 3 days; 25-35 mg/kg/day in children ≥5 yr; 40 mg/kg/day in children 3-4 yr; all given in 3 divided doses; rec 200 mg as a single dose

Renal dose

P ***Adult and child >12 yr:*** CrCl 30-60 ml/min 300 mg bid; CrCl 15-30 ml/min 300 mg qd; CrCl <15 ml/min 300 mg qod

Available forms: Caps 100, 300, 400 mg; tabs 600, 800 mg; oral sol 250 mg/5 ml

Adverse effects

CNS: Dizziness, fatigue, anxiety, somnolence, ataxia, amnesia, abnormal thinking, unsteady gait, depression

CV: Vasodilation, peripheral edema

EENT: Dry mouth, blurred vision, diplopia

GI: Constipation, increased appetite, dental abnormalities

GU: Impotence, bleeding, *UTI*

HEMA: **Leukopenia,** decreased WBC

INTEG: Pruritus, abrasion

MS: Myalgia

RESP: Rhinitis, pharyngitis, coughing

Contraindications: Hypersensitivity to this drug

Precautions: Hepatic disease, P renal disease, pregnancy **C,** lactation, G child <12 yr, elderly

Pharmacokinetics	
Absorption	Unknown
Distribution	Unknown
Metabolism	None
Excretion	Urine unchanged
Half-life	5-7 hr

Pharmacodynamics	
Onset	Unknown
Peak	Unknown
Duration	Unknown

Interactions

Drug classifications

Antacids: ↓ gabapentin levels

NURSING CONSIDERATIONS
- Assess renal studies: urinalysis, BUN, urine creatinine q3 mo
- Hepatic studies: ALT, AST, bilirubin
- Assess description of seizures
- Assess mental status: mood, sensorium, affect, behavioral changes; if mental status changes, notify prescriber
- Assess eye problems, need for ophth exam before, during, after treatment (slit lamp, fundoscopy, tonometry)
- Monitor for allergic reaction: purpura, red raised rash; if these occur, drug should be discontinued

Nursing diagnoses
✓ Knowledge deficit (teaching)
✓ Noncompliance (teaching)

Implementation
- Give at least 2 hr pc with antacids
- Store at room temp away from heat and light
- Give hard candy, frequent rinsing of mouth, gum for dry mouth
- Provide assistance with ambulation during early part of treatment; dizziness occurs
- Provide seizure precautions: padded side rails; move objects that may harm patient
- Provide increased fluids, bulk in diet for constipation

Evaluation
Positive therapeutic outcome
- Decreased seizure activity; document on patient's chart

Patient/family education
- Advise patient to carry ID stating patient's name, drugs taken, condition, prescriber's name and phone number
- Teach patient to avoid driving, other activities that require alertness
- Teach patient not to discontinue medication quickly after long-term use, withdrawal-precipitated seizures may occur
- Teach patient not to break, crush, or chew caps
- Advise patient to notify prescriber if pregnancy is planned or suspected, avoid breast-feeding

Treatment of overdose:
Lavage, VS

galantamine
See Appendix A, Selected New Drugs

HIGH ALERT

gallamine (℞)
(gal'a-meen)
Flaxedil
Func. class.: Neuromuscular blocker (nondepolarizing)
Pregnancy category C

Action: Inhibits transmission of nerve impulses by binding with cholinergic receptor sites, antagonizing action of acetylcholine; no analgesic response

Therapeutic Outcome: Paralysis of all skeletal muscles

Uses: Facilitation of endotracheal intubation, skeletal muscle relaxation during mechanical ventilation, surgery, or general anesthesia

Dosage and routes
P ***Adult and child >1 mo:*** **IV** 1 mg/kg, not to exceed 100 mg, then 0.5-1 mg/kg q30-40 min

P ***Child <1 mo, >5 kg:*** **IV** 0.25-0.75 mg/kg, then 0.01-0.05 mg/kg q30-40 min

Available forms: Inj 20 mg/ml

Adverse effects
CNS: **Malignant hyperthermia**
CV: Bradycardia, tachycardia, increased, decreased B/P
EENT: Increased secretions

GI: Decreased motility
INTEG: Rash, flushing, pruritus, urticaria
RESP: **Prolonged apnea, bronchospasm, cyanosis, respiratory depression**

Contraindications: Hypersensitivity to iodides

Precautions: Pregnancy **C,** thyroid disease, collagen disease, cardiac disease, lactation, P children <2 yr, electrolyte imbalances, dehydration, neuromuscular disease (myasthenia gravis), respiratory disease, renal disease

Pharmacokinetics

Absorption	Complete bioavailability
Distribution	Extracellular space, crosses placenta
Metabolism	Plasma
Excretion	Kidneys—unchanged
Half-life	2½ hr

Pharmacodynamics

Onset	2 min
Peak	5 min
Duration	30 min

Interactions

Individual drugs

Clindamycin: ↑ paralysis, length, and intensity
Colistin: ↑ paralysis, length, and intensity
Lidocaine: ↑ paralysis, length, and intensity
Lithium: ↑ paralysis, length, and intensity
Magnesium: ↑ paralysis, length, and intensity
Polymyxin B: ↑ paralysis, length, and intensity
Procainamide: ↑ paralysis, length, and intensity
Quinidine: ↑ paralysis, length, and intensity
Succinylcholine: ↑ paralysis, length, and intensity

Drug classifications

Aminoglycosides: ↑ paralysis, length, and intensity
β-Adrenergic blockers: ↑ paralysis, length, and intensity
Diuretics, potassium-losing: ↑ paralysis, length, and intensity
General anesthetics: ↑ paralysis, length, and intensity

NURSING CONSIDERATIONS

Assessment

- Monitor for electrolyte imbalances (potassium, magnesium), before drug is used; electrolyte imbalances may lead to increased action of this drug
- Monitor vital signs (B/P, pulse, respirations, airway) until fully recovered; rate, depth, pattern of respirations, strength of hand grip; patient should be intubated before use
- Monitor recovery: decreased paralysis of face, diaphragm, leg, arm, rest of body; residual weakness and respiratory problems may occur during recovery period
- Monitor allergic reactions: rash, fever, respiratory distress, pruritus; if present, drug should be discontinued

Nursing diagnoses

✓ Breathing pattern, ineffective (uses)
✓ Communication, impaired verbal (adverse reactions)
✓ Fear (adverse reactions)
✓ Knowledge deficit (teaching)

Implementation

- Use peripheral nerve stimulator by anesthesiologist to determine neuromuscular blockade; deep tendon reflexes should be monitored during extended use
- Give **IV** undiluted by direct **IV** over 1 min, or diluted in 10-50 ml of D_5W, ½ NaCl or NS and give as inf at prescribed rate (only by qualified person, usually an anesthesiologist); do not administer IM
- Further dilute in D_5W, 0.9% NaCl, D_5/0.9% NaCl q15-25 min (intermittent inf)

• Maintenance dose is given q20-45 min after 1st dose (cont inf); titrate to patient response
• Store in light-resistant area

Patient/family education
• Provide reassurance if communication is difficult during recovery from neuromuscular blockade
• Provide explanation regarding all procedures or treatments; patient will remain conscious if anesthetic is not given also

Evaluation
Positive therapeutic outcome
• Paralysis of jaw, eyelid, head, neck, rest of body as evaluated by peripheral nerve stimulator

Treatment of overdose: Administer edrophonium or neostigmine, atropine, monitor VS; may require mechanical ventilation

gallium (℞)
(gal′ee-yum)
Ganite
Func. class.: Electrolyte modifier
Chem. class.: Hypocalcemic drug
Pregnancy category C

Action: Lowers serum calcium levels by inhibiting calcium resorption from bone

→ **Therapeutic Outcome:** Decrease calcium level to 5-9 mg/dl

Uses: Cancer-related hypercalcemia

Dosage and routes
Adult: **IV** 100-200 mg/m^2 qd × 5 days; inf over 24 hr, rest period of 2-4 wk between courses

Available forms: Inj 25 mg/ml

Adverse effects
CV: Tachycardia, hypotension
EENT: Blurred vision, optic neuritis, hearing loss
GI: Nausea, vomiting, diarrhea, constipation, mucositis, metallic taste
GU: **Nephrotoxicity**, increased BUN, creatinine
HEMA: **Anemia, leukopenia, thrombocytopenia**
META: Hypophosphatemia, hypocalcemia, decreased serum bicarbonate

Contraindications: Hypersensitivity, severe renal disease

Precautions: Pregnancy **C**, lactation, children, mild renal disease

Pharmacokinetics	
Absorption	Completely absorbed
Distribution	Unknown
Metabolism	Unknown
Excretion	Kidneys (unchanged)
Half-life	Unknown

Pharmacodynamics	
Onset	12-48 hr
Peak	Unknown
Duration	4-14 days

Interactions
Individual drugs
Amphotericin B: ↑ nephrotoxicity
Drug classifications
Aminoglycosides: ↑ nephrotoxicity

NURSING CONSIDERATIONS
Assessment
• Renal status: BUN, creatinine, urine output; if creatinine level is 2.5 mg/dl or more, drug should be discontinued
• Monitor calcium, phosphate, bicarbonate; all levels may be decreased and supplements of phosphate may be needed; calcium daily, phosphate 2-3 ×/wk
• Assess for hypercalcemia: nausea, vomiting, fatigue, weakness, thirst, dehydration, dysrhythmias, headache, confusion, coma, decreased reflexes
• For hypocalcemia: dysrhythmias, hypotension, paresthesia; twitching, colic, laryngospasm; hypercalcemia: poor coordination, myalgia, hypotonia, shortened ST segment and QT interval, prolonged PR interval, cone-shaped T wave, sinus

bradycardia; Trousseau's, Chvostek's sign: tremors, tetany, cramping, grimacing, seizures, altered deep tendon reflexes and spasms, personality changes including irritability, depression, psychosis

- Monitor for indications of hypophosphatemia: weakness, malaise, tremors, memory loss, inattention, confusion, decreased reflexes, aching bone pain, joint stiffness, rapid, shallow respiration, decreased tidal volume, nausea, vomiting, anorexia, portal hypertension

Nursing diagnoses

✓ Injury, risk for (uses)
✓ Knowledge deficit (teaching)

Implementation

- Provide adequate hydration with **IV** saline, 2 L/day during treatment; saline increases the extracellular calcium
- Give by cont **IV** inf after dilution of dose/1 L of 0.9% NaCl or D_5W, run over 24 hr, use infusion pump
- Store solution for 48 hr at room temp or 1 wk in refrigerator

Y-site compatibilities: Acyclovir, allopurinol, aminophylline, ampicillin/sulbactam, amifostine, aztreonam, cefazolin, ceftazidime, ceftriaxone, cimetidine, ciprofloxacin, cladribine, cyclophosphamide, dexamethasone, diphenhydramine, filgrastim, fluconazole, furosemide, granisetron, heparin, hydrocortisone, fosfamide, magnesium sulfate, mannitol, melphalan, meperidine, mesna, methotrexate, metoclopramide, ondansetron, piperacillin, piperacillin/tazobactam, potassium chloride, ranitidine, sodium bicarbonate, teniposide, thiotepa, ticarcillin/clavulanate, trimethoprim, sulfamethoxazole, vancomycin, vinorelbine

Patient/family education

- Instruct patient to follow dietary guidelines given by prescriber, including avoiding calcium (dietary products, broccoli) and vit D (fortified milk, grain products, fish oil)
- Explain purpose of drug and expected results

Evaluation

Positive therapeutic outcome

- Decreased serum calcium levels to 5-9 mg/dl

ganciclovir (℞)

(gan-sye'kloe-vir)

Cytovene, Vitrasert

Func. class.: Antiviral

Chem. class.: Synthetic nucleoside analog

Pregnancy category C

Action: Inhibits replication of herpes viruses in vitro, in vivo by selective inhibition of the human cytomegalovirus (CMV) DNA polymerase and by direct incorporation into viral DNA

➔ **Therapeutic Outcome:** Decreased proliferation of virus responsible for CMV retinitis

Uses: CMV retinitis in immunocompromised persons, including those with AIDS, after indirect ophthalmoscopy confirms diagnosis

Investigational uses: CMV pneumonia in organ transplant patients, CMV gastroenteritis in patients with irritable bowel syndrome, CMV pneumonitis

Dosage and routes

Induction treatment

Adult: **IV** 5 mg/kg given over 1 hr q12h × 2-3 wk

Maintenance treatment

Adult: **IV** inf 5 mg/kg given over 1 hr, qd × 7 days/wk; or 6 mg/kg qd × 5 days/wk; dosage must be reduced in renal impairment; **IV** 200 µg every week; intravitreal: 4.5-mg implant

Prevention of CMV infection
Adult: **IV** 5 mg/kg q12h × 1-2 wk, then 5 mg/kg/day × 7 days/wk or 6 mg/kg × 5 days/wk; PO 1000 mg tid
Renal dose
CrCl <70 ml/min reduce dose

Available forms: Powder for inj 500 mg/vial, caps 250, 500 mg; implant, intravitreal 4.5 mg/5-8 wk

Adverse effects
CNS: *Fever,* chills, **coma,** *confusion,* abnormal thoughts, dizziness, bizarre dreams, *headache,* psychosis, tremors, somnolence, *paresthesia, weakness,* **seizures**
CV: Dysrhythmia, hypertension/hypotension
EENT: Retinal detachment in CMV retinitis
GI: *Abnormal LFTs, nausea, vomiting, anorexia, diarrhea, abdominal pain,* **hemorrhage**
GU: **Hematuria,** increased creatinine, BUN
HEMA: **Granulocytopenia, thrombocytopenia, irreversible neutropenia, anemia, eosinophilia**
INTEG: *Rash,* alopecia, *pruritus,* urticaria, pain at inj site, phlebitis
RESP: Dyspnea

Contraindications: Hypersensitivity to acyclovir or ganciclovir, ANC <500/mm^3, platelet count <25,000/mm^3

Precautions: Preexisting cytopenias, renal function impairment, P pregnancy **C**, lactation, children <6 G mo, elderly

Do Not Confuse:
Cytovene/Cytosar

Pharmacokinetics

Absorption	Completely absorbed
Distribution	Crosses blood-brain barrier, CSF
Metabolism	Not metabolized
Excretion	Kidneys (90%) unchanged, breast milk
Half-life	3 hr

Pharmacodynamics
Unknown

Interactions
Individual drugs
Cyclosporine: ↑ toxicity
Imipenem with cilastatin: ↑ chance of seizures
Probenecid: ↑ toxicity
Radiation: ↑ bone marrow depression
Zidovudine: ↑ bone marrow depression
Drug classifications
Antineoplastics: ↑ bone marrow depression

NURSING CONSIDERATIONS
Assessment
- Culture should be done before treatment with ganciclovir is initiated; cultures of blood, urine, and throat may all be taken; CMV is not confirmed by this method; the diagnosis is made by an ophth exam
- Assess kidney, liver function; increases in hemopoietic studies: BUN, serum creatinine, AST creatinine clearance, ALT, A-G ratio, baseline, and drip treatment; blood counts should be done q2 wk; watch for decreasing granulocytes, Hgb; if low, therapy may have to be discontinued and restarted after hematologic recovery; blood transfusions may be required
- Assess for GI symptoms: severe nausea, vomiting, diarrhea; severe symptoms may necessitate discontinuing drug
- Monitor electrolytes and minerals: calcium, phosphorus, magnesium, sodium, potassium; watch closely for tetany during 1st administration
- Assess for symptoms of blood dyscrasias (anemia, granulocytopenia); bruising, fatigue, bleeding, poor healing
- Assess for symptoms of allergic reactions: flushing, rash, urticaria, pruritus

• Monitor for leukopenia/neutropenia/thrombocytopenia: WBCs, platelets q2 days during 2 ×/day dosing and q1 wk thereafter; check for leukopenia with qd WBC count in patients with prior leukopenia with other nucleoside analogs or for whom leukopenia counts are <1000 cells/mm^3 at start of treatment
• Monitor serum creatinine or creatinine clearance at least q2 wk

Nursing diagnoses
✓ Infection, risk for (uses)
✓ Injury, risk for (uses, adverse reactions)
✓ Knowledge deficit (teaching)

Implementation
PO route
• Give with food

IV **IV route**
• Medicine should be mixed under strict aseptic conditions using gloves, gown, and mask, and using precautions for antineoplastics
• Administer **IV** after diluting 500 mg/10 ml of sterile water for inj (50 mg/ml); shake; further dilute in 100 ml of D_5W, 0.9% NaCl, LR and run over 1 hr; use infusion pump, in-line filter
• Give slowly; do not give by bolus

IV, IM, SC inj
• Use diluted sol within 12 hr, do not refrigerate or freeze; do not use sol with particulate matter or discoloration, fludarabine, sargramostim

Y-site compatibilities: Allopurinol, cisplatin, cyclophosphamide, enalaprilat, filgrastim, fluconazole, granisetron, melphalan, methotrexate, paclitaxel, propofol, tacrolimus, teniposide, thiotepa

Y-site incompatibilities: Amsacrine, fludarabine, foscarnet, ondansetron, sargramostim, vinorelbine

Patient/family education
• Advise patient to notify prescriber if sore throat, swollen lymph nodes, malaise, fever occur; may indicate other infections
• Advise patient to report perioral tingling, numbness in extremities, and paresthesias
• Caution patient that serious drug interactions may occur if OTC products are ingested; check first with prescriber
• Inform patient that drug is not a cure, but will control symptoms
• Advise patient that regular ophth exams must be continued
• Inform patient that major toxicities may necessitate discontinuing drug
• Instruct patient to use contraception during treatment and that infertility may occur; men should use barrier contraception for 90 days after treatment
• Teach patient to take PO with food
• Teach patient to report infection: fever, chills, sore throat; blood dyscrasias: bruising, bleeding, petechiae
• Tell patient to avoid crowds, persons with respiratory infection
• Advise patient to use sunscreen to prevent burns

Evaluation
Positive therapeutic outcome
• Decreased symptoms of CMV infection

ganirelix (℞)
(gan-i-rell′-ex)
Antagon
Func. class.: Gonadotropin-releasing hormone antagonist
Chem. class.: Synthetic decapeptide
Pregnancy category X

Action: Inhibitor of pituitary gonadotropin secretion; initially increases LH and FSH, induces a rapid suppression of gonadotropin secretion

Therapeutic Outcome: Pregnancy

Uses: For inhibition of premature LH surges in women undergoing controlled ovarian hyperstimulation

Dosage and routes

Adult: SC 250 µg qd during early to mid follicular phase, continue until day of hCG administration

Available forms: Inj 250 µg/ 0.5 ml

Adverse effects

CNS: Headache

ENDO: Ovarian hyperstimulation syndrome, abdominal pain (gyn)

GI: Nausea

INTEG: Pain on inj

SYST: **Fetal death**

Contraindications: Hypersensitivity, pregnancy **X,** latex allergy, lactation

Pharmacokinetics	
Absorption	Unknown
Distribution	Unknown
Metabolism	To metabolites
Excretion	Unknown
Half-life	13-16 hr

Pharmacodynamics	
Onset	Unknown
Peak	Unknown
Duration	Treatment length

Interactions: None

NURSING CONSIDERATIONS

Assessment

- Assess for suspected pregnancy, drug should not be used
- Assess for latex allergy, drug should not be used

Nursing diagnoses

✓ Sexual dysfunction (uses)
✓ Knowledge deficit (teaching)

Implementation

- Administer SC using abdomen, around navel or upper thigh, swab inj area with disinfectant, clean a 2 in circle and allow to dry, pinch up area between thumb and finger, insert needle at 45-90° to surface, if positioned correctly, no blood will be drawn back into syringe, if blood is drawn into syringe, reposition needle without removing it
- Protect from light

Patient/family education

- Teach patient to report abdominal pain, vaginal bleeding

Evaluation

Positive therapeutic outcome

- Pregnancy

G

gatifloxacin (℞)

(gat-i-floks'-a-sin)

Tequin

Func. class.: Urinary antiinfective

Chem. class.: Fluoroquinolone antibacterial

Pregnancy category C

Action: Interferes with conversion of intermediate DNA fragments into high-molecular-weight DNA in bacteria; DNA gyrase inhibitor

➔ **Therapeutic Outcome:** Bactericidal action against the following: gram-positive organisms methicillin-resistant strains of *Staphylococcus aureus, Streptococcus pneumoniae;* gram-negative organisms *Escherichia coli, Haemophilus influenzae, Haemophilus parainfluenzae, Klebsiella pneumoniae, Moraxella catarrhalis, Neisseria gonorrhoeae, Proteus mirabilis;* and other microorganisms: *Chlamydia pneumoniae, Legionella pneumophilia, Mycoplasma pneumoniae*

Uses: Adult urinary tract infections (including complicated); lower respiratory, skin, bone, joint infections, acute bacterial exacerbation of chronic bronchitis, acute sinusitis, community-acquired respiratory tract infections, gonorrhea

Investigational uses:
Multidrug-resistant *S. pneumoniae,* in children with acute otitis media; sinusitis; *Mycobacterium leprae*

Dosage and routes
Renal dose
CrCl ≥40 ml/min 400 mg qd; CrCl <40 ml/min 200 mg qd after 400 mg initially; hemodialysis 200 mg qd after 400 mg initially

Uncomplicated urinary tract infections
Adult: PO/**IV** 400 mg single dose

Complicated/severe urinary tract infections
Adult: PO/**IV** 400 mg × 7-10 days

Chronic bronchitis
Adult: PO/**IV** 400 mg × 7-10 days

Acute sinusitis
Adult: PO/**IV** 400 mg × 10 days

Community acquired pneumonia
Adult: PO/**IV** 400 mg × 7-14 days

Gonorrhea
Adult: PO/**IV** 400 mg single dose

Available forms: Tabs 200, 400; inj 20 ml (200 mg), 40 ml (400 mg)

Adverse effects
CNS: Headache, dizziness, insomnia, paresthesia, tremor, vasodilation
ENDO: Increased blood glucose
GI: Nausea, constipation, increased ALT, AST, diarrhea, **pseudomembranous colitis**
INTEG: Rash, pruritus, urticaria, photosensitivity, flushing, fever, chills
RESP: Dyspnea, pharyngitis
SYST: **Anaphylaxis, Stevens-Johnson syndrome**

Contraindications: Hypersensitivity to quinolones

Precautions: Pregnancy **C**, lactation, children, renal disease [P]

Pharmacokinetics

Absorption	Well absorbed (PO); complete (**IV**)
Distribution	Protein binding 20%
Metabolism	Liver
Excretion	Kidneys unchanged (70%)
Half-life	1 hr

Pharmacodynamics

	PO	IV
Onset	Rapid	Immediate
Peak	2-5 hr	Infusion's end

Interactions
Individual drugs
Cyclosporine: ↑ nephrotoxicity
Probenecid: ↑ blood levels of gatifloxacin
Sucralfate: ↓ absorption of gatifloxacin
Theophylline: ↑ levels, toxicity
Warfarin: ↑ warfarin level

Drug classifications
Antacids: ↓ absorption of gatifloxacin

NURSING CONSIDERATIONS
Assessment
- Assess patient for previous sensitivity reaction
- Assess patient for signs and symptoms of infection including characteristics of wounds, sputum, urine, stool, WBC >10,000/mm^3, fever; obtain baseline information before and during treatment
- Obtain C&S before beginning drug therapy to identify if correct treatment has been initiated
- Assess for allergic reactions and anaphylaxis: rash, urticaria, pruritus, chills, fever, joint pain; may occur a few days after therapy begins; epinephrine and resuscitation equipment should be available for anaphylactic reaction
- Identify urine output; if decreasing, notify prescriber (may indicate nephrotoxicity); also check for increased BUN, creatinine
- Monitor blood studies: AST, ALT,

CBC, Hct, bilirubin, LDH, alkaline phosphatase, blood glucose, Coombs' test monthly if patient is on long-term therapy
- Monitor electrolytes: potassium, sodium, chloride monthly if patient is on long-term therapy
- Assess bowel pattern qd; if severe diarrhea occurs, drug should be discontinued
- Monitor for bleeding: ecchymosis, bleeding gums, hematuria, stool guaiac daily if on long-term therapy
- Assess for overgrowth of infection: perineal itching, fever, malaise, redness, pain, swelling, drainage, rash, diarrhea, change in cough, sputum

Nursing diagnoses
- ✓ Infection, risk for (uses)
- ✓ Diarrhea (side effects)
- ✓ Injury, risk for (side effects)
- ✓ Knowledge deficit (teaching)
- ✓ Noncompliance (teaching)

Implementation
PO route
- Give 2 hr before or 2 hr after antacids, zinc, iron, calcium

IV **IV route**
- Check for irritation, extravasation, phlebitis daily
- Do not use flexible containers in series connections, air embolism may occur
- Do not use if particulate matter is present
- Do not admix with other drugs
- Dilute with compatible sol to 2 mg/ml before administration

Solution compatibilities: D_5, 0.9% NaCl, D_5/0.9% NaCl LR/D_5, water for inj

Patient/family education
- Teach patient to report sore throat, bruising, bleeding, joint pain; may indicate blood dyscrasias (rare)
- Instruct patient to increase fluid intake to 2 L/day to prevent crystalluria
- Advise patient to contact prescriber if vaginal itching, loose, foul-smelling stools, furry tongue occur; may indicate superinfection; report itching, rash, pruritus, urticaria
- Instruct patient to take all medication prescribed for the length of time ordered; drug must be taken around the clock to maintain blood levels: do not give medication to others
- Advise patient to notify prescriber of diarrhea with blood or pus
- Advise patient to notify prescriber if theophylline is also being taken

G

Evaluation
Positive therapeutic outcome
- Absence of signs/symptoms of infection (WBC <10,000/mm^3, temp WNL, absence of pain on urination, urgency)
- Reported improvement in symptoms of infection

gemcitabine (℞)
(gem-sit'a-been)

Gemzar

Func. class.: Misc. antineoplastic

Chem. class.: Nucleoside analog

Pregnancy category D

Action: Exhibits antitumor activity by killing cells undergoing DNA synthesis (S phase) and blocking G_1/S-phase boundary

➔ **Therapeutic Outcome:** Prevention of growth of tumor

Uses: Adenocarcinoma of the pancreas: nonresectable stage II, III, or metastatic stage IV; in combination with cisplatin for inoperable, advanced, or metastatic non-small cell lung cancer

Dosage and routes
Pancreatic carcinoma

Adult: **IV** 100 mg/m^2 given over ½ hr qwk × 7 wk, then 1 wk rest period; subsequent cycles should be infused once qwk × 3 wk out of every 4 wk

3 wk schedule

Adult: **IV** 1250 mg/m^2 given over ½ hr on days 1, 8 of each 21-day cycle; give cisplatin 100 mg/m^2 after the inf of gemcitabine on day 1

Non-small cell lung cancer

4 wk schedule

Adult: **IV** 1000 mg/m^2 given over ½ hr on days 1, 8, 15 of each 28-day cycle; give cisplatin **IV** 100 mg/m^2 on day 1 after gemcitabine

Available forms: Lyophilized powder for inj 20 mg/ml

Adverse effects

GI: Diarrhea, nausea, vomiting, anorexia, constipation, stomatitis

GU: Proteinuria, hematuria

HEMA: **Leukopenia, anemia, neutropenia, thrombocytopenia**

INTEG: Irritation at site, rash, alopecia

MISC: Dyspnea, fever, ***hemorrhage,*** infection, flulike syndrome, paresthesia

Contraindications: Hypersensitivity, pregnancy **D**

P G **Precautions:** Lactation, children, elderly, myelosuppression, irradiation

Pharmacokinetics

Absorption	Unknown
Distribution	Crosses placenta
Metabolism	Unknown
Excretion	Unknown
Half-life	42-79 min

Pharmacodynamics

Unknown

Interactions

Drug classifications

Antineoplastics: ↑ myelosuppression, diarrhea

Live virus vaccines: ↓ antibody response

NSAIDs: ↑ bleeding

Salicylates: ↑ bleeding

Radiation: ↑ myelosuppression

NURSING CONSIDERATIONS

Assessment

- Monitor CBC, differential, platelet count before each dose; absolute granulocyte count >1000/mm^3, platelets >100,000/mm^3, give complete dose; absolute granulocyte count 500-1000/mm^3, platelets 50,000-100,000/mm^3, give 75%; absolute granulocyte count <500/mm^3, platelets <50,000/mm^3, do not give
- Assess for blood dyscrasias, bruising, bleeding, petechiae
- Monitor I&O, nutritional intake
- Monitor hepatic/renal studies
- Assess food preferences: list likes, dislikes
- Assess buccal cavity q8h for dryness, sores or ulceration, white patches, oral pain, bleeding, dysphagia
- Assess GI symptoms: frequency of stools; cramping
- Assess signs of dehydration: rapid respirations, poor skin turgor, decreased urine output, dry skin, restlessness, weakness

Nursing diagnoses

✓ Infection, risk for (adverse reactions)

✓ Nutrition, altered: less than body requirements (adverse reaction)

Implementation

- Provide for rinsing of mouth tid-qid with water, club soda; brushing of teeth bid-tid with soft brush or cotton-tipped applicator for stomatitis; use unwaxed dental floss
- Give nutritious diet with iron, vitamin supplement, low fiber, few dairy products
- Give increased fluid intake to 2-3 L/day to prevent dehydration, unless contraindicated

IV **IV route**

- Prepare in biologic cabinet using gown, mask, gloves
- After reconstituting with 0.9% NaCl 5 ml/200 mg vial of drug or 25 ml/1 g of drug, shake (40 mg/ml); may be further diluted with 0.9% NaCl to concentrate as low as 0.1 mg/ml;

discard unused portion, give over ½ hr, do not admix
- Change **IV** site q48h

Patient/family education
- Advise patient to avoid foods with citric acid or hot or rough texture if stomatitis is present; to drink adequate fluids
- Advise patient to report stomatitis; any bleeding, white spots, ulcerations in mouth; tell patient to examine mouth qd, report symptoms
- Advise patient to report signs of anemia: fatigue, headache, faintness, shortness of breath, irritability; hematuria, dysuria
- Advise patient to use contraception during therapy
- Instruct patient to avoid use with NSAIDs, salicylates, alcohol; not to receive vaccinations during treatment

Evaluation
Positive therapeutic outcome
- Decrease in tumor size, decrease in spread of cancer

Treatment of overdose:
Induce vomiting, provide supportive care

gemfibrozil (℞)
(gem-fye'broe-zil)
gemfibrozil, Lopid
Func. class.: Antilipemic
Chem. class.: Fibric acid derivative
Pregnancy category C

Action: Inhibits biosynthesis of VLDL, decreases triglycerides, increases HDLs

➔ Therapeutic Outcome: Decreased hepatic triglyceride production, VLDL; accelerates removal of cholesterol from liver

Uses: Type IIb, III, IV, V hyperlipidemia as adjunct with diet therapy

Dosage and routes
Adult: PO 1200 mg in divided doses bid 30 min ac

Available forms: Caps 300 mg, Tabs 600 mg

Adverse effects
CNS: Dizziness, blurred vision
GI: Nausea, vomiting, *dyspepsia, diarrhea, abdominal pain, flatulence*
HEMA: **Leukopenia, anemia, eosinophilia, thrombocytopenia**
INTEG: Rash, urticaria, pruritus
MISC: Task perversion

Contraindications: Severe hepatic disease, preexisting gallbladder disease, severe renal disease, primary biliary cirrhosis, hypersensitivity

Precautions: Monitor hematologic and hepatic function, pregnancy **C**, lactation

Pharmacokinetics	
Absorption	Well absorbed
Distribution	Unknown, plasma protein binding >90%
Metabolism	Liver—minimal
Excretion	Kidney—unchanged (70%), feces (6%)
Half-life	1½ hr

Pharmacodynamics	
Onset	1-2 hr
Peak	1-2 hr
Duration	2-4 months

Interactions
Individual drugs
Cyclosporine: ↓ gemifibrozil effect
Lovastatin: ↑ rhabdomyolysis
Simivastatin: ↑ rhabdomyolysis
Drug classifications
Anticoagulants, oral: ↑ effect of anticoagulants
HMG-CoA reductase inhibitors: ↑ risk of myositis, myalgia
Sulfonylureas: ↑ hypoglycemic effect
Lab test interferences
↑ Liver function studies, ↑ CPK,

↑ BSP, ↑ thymol turbidity, ↑ glucose
↓ Hgb, ↓ Hct, ↓ WBC

NURSING CONSIDERATIONS

Assessment

• Assess nutrition: fat, protein, carbohydrates; nutritional analysis should be performed by dietitian before treatment is initiated
• Assess renal function studies, LFTs, CBC, blood glucose if patient is on long-term therapy; if LFT results increase, drug should be discontinued
• Monitor bowel pattern daily; diarrhea may be a problem
• Monitor triglycerides, cholesterol, lipids baseline and during treatment; LDL and VLDL should be watched closely and if increased, drug should be discontinued

Nursing diagnoses

✓ Diarrhea (adverse reactions)
✓ Knowledge deficit (teaching)
✓ Noncompliance (teaching)

Implementation

• Give 30 min before AM and PM meals
⊘ • Do not crush, chew caps

Patient/family education

• Inform patient that compliance is needed for positive results to occur; not to double doses; that drug may be discontinued if no improvement in 3 mo
• Caution patient to decrease risk factors: high-fat diet, smoking, alcohol consumption, lack of exercise
• Advise patient to notify prescriber if GI symptoms of diarrhea, abdominal or epigastric pain, nausea, vomiting occur; or if chills, fever, sore throat occur; also occurrence of muscle cramps, abdominal cramps, severe flatulence

Evaluation

Positive therapeutic outcome
• Decreased cholesterol levels, serum triglyceride and improved ratio with HDLs

HIGH ALERT

gemtuzumab (℞)

(gem-tue-zue′mab)
Mylotarg
Func. class.: Misc. antineoplastic
Chem. class.: Monoclonal antibody

Pregnancy category D

Action: Composed of recombinant humanized IgG_4 κ antibody, binds to CD33 antigen that is released in myeloid cells

➔ **Therapeutic Outcome:** Decreasing signs/symptoms of leukemia

Uses: Acute myeloid leukemia (AML)

Dosage and routes

Adult: **IV** 9 m/m^2 as a 2 hr inf; before giving inf, give diphenhydramine 50 mg PO, acetaminophen 650-1000 mg PO 1 hr before inf; then use acetaminophen 650-1000 mg q1-4h prn

Available forms: Powder for inj, lyophilized 5 mg

Adverse effects

CNS: *Dizziness,* insomnia, depression
CV: Hypertension, **hemorrhage,** tachycardia, hypotension
INTEG: *Rash,* herpes simplex, local reaction, petechiae
GI: Anorexia, diarrhea, constipation, nausea, stomatitis, vomiting
GU: Hematuria, **vaginal hemorrhage**
MISC: *Fever, myalgias, headache, chills*
RESP: Cough, pneumonia, epistaxis, rhinitis
META: Hypokalemia, hypomagnesemia

Contraindications: Hypersensitivity, pregnancy **D,** severe myelosuppression

P **Precautions:** Lactation, children, severe renal or hepatic disease

Pharmacokinetics

Absorption	Unknown
Distribution	Unknown
Metabolism	Unknown
Excretion	Unknown
Half-life	45, 100 hr, respectively

Pharmacodynamics

Unknown

Interactions
None known

NURSING CONSIDERATIONS
Assessment
- Assess for symptoms of infection; chills, fever, headache, may be masked by drug fever
- Assess CNS reaction: LOC, mental status, dizziness, confusion
- Assess cardiac status: lung sounds; ECG before and during treatment, especially in those with cardiac disease
- Assess bone marrow depression: bruising, bleeding, blood in stools, urine, sputum, emesis

Nursing diagnoses
✓ Risk for infection (adverse reactions)
✓ Altered nutrition: less than body requirements (adverse reactions)
✓ Altered oral mucous membrane (adverse reactions)

Implementation
- Do not give **IV** push or bolus
- Protect from light, use biologic safety hood, allow to come to room temp
- Reconstitute each vial with 5 ml of sterile water for inj using sterile syringes, swirl each vial, check for discoloration or particulate matter, give over 2 hr, use a separate line with 1.2 μ terminal filter
- Store reconstituted sol for ≤8 hr in refrigerator

Patient/family education
- Advise patient to take acetaminophen for fever
- Instruct patient to avoid hazardous tasks, since confusion, dizziness may occur; avoid prolonged sunlight, use sunscreen
- Instruct patient to report signs of infection: sore throat, fever, diarrhea, vomiting

Evaluation
Positive therapeutic outcome
- Decrease in size, number of lesions

G

gentamicin (℞)
(jen-ta-mye'sin)
Cidomycin ✤, G-mycin, Jenamicin, Gentamicin Sulfate
Func. class.: Antiinfective
Chem. class.: Aminoglycoside
Pregnancy category C

Action: Interferes with protein synthesis in bacterial cell by binding to ribosomal subunit, causing misreading of genetic code; inaccurate peptide sequence forms in protein chain, causing bacterial death

➔ **Therapeutic Outcome:** Bactericidal effects for the following organisms: *Proteus aeruginosa, Proteus, Klebsiella, Serratia, Escherichia coli, Enterobacter, Citrobacter, Staphylococcus, Shigella, Salmonella, Acinetobacter*

Uses: Severe systemic infections of CNS; respiratory, GI, and urinary tracts; bone; skin; soft tissues; acute PID caused by susceptible strains

Dosage and routes
Severe systemic infections
Adult: **IV** inf 3-5 mg/kg/day in 3 divided doses q8h; dilute in 50-200 ml 0.9% NaCl or D_5W given over 30 min-1 hr; IM 3 mg/kg/day in divided doses q8h

P ***Child:*** **IV**/IM 2-2.5 mg/ kg q8h

P ***Neonates and infants:*** **IV**/IM 2.5 mg/kg q8-12h

P ***Neonates <1 wk:*** 2.5 mg/kg q12-24h

Once-daily dosing/extended interval dosing (unlabeled)
Adult: **IV** 4-7 mg/kg q24h adjust according to levels

Renal dose
Adult: IM/**IV** 1-1.7 mg/kg initially, then adjust according to CrCl levels

Available forms: Inj 10, 40 mg/ml; premixed inj 40, 60, 70, 80, 100 mg/50 ml; 40, 60, 80, 90, 100, 120, 160, 180 mg/ml

Adverse effects
CNS: Confusion, depression, numbness, tremors, **convulsions,** muscle twitching, **neurotoxicity,** dizziness, vertigo
CV: Hypotension, hypertension, palpitations
EENT: *Ototoxicity, deafness,* visual disturbances, tinnitus
GI: *Nausea, vomiting, anorexia,* increased ALT, AST, bilirubin, hepatomegaly, **hepatic necrosis,** splenomegaly
GU: **Oliguria, hematuria, renal damage, azotemia, renal failure, nephrotoxicity**
HEMA: **Agranulocytosis, thrombocytopenia, leukopenia, eosinophilia,** anemia
INTEG: *Rash,* burning, urticaria, dermatitis, alopecia

Contraindications: Severe renal disease, hypersensitivity

P **Precautions:** Neonates, mild renal disease, pregnancy **C,** hearing deficits, G myasthenia gravis, lactation, elderly, Parkinson's disease

Do Not Confuse:
Garamycin/kanamycin

Pharmacokinetics

Absorption	Well absorbed (IM)
Distribution	Distributed in extracellular fluids, poorly distributed in CSF; crosses placenta
Metabolism	Liver, minimal
Excretion	Mostly unchanged (79%) kidneys
Half-life	1-2 hr, infants 6-7 hr, increased in renal disease

Pharmacodynamics

	IM	IV
Onset	Rapid	Rapid
Peak	½-1½ hr	Infusion's end

Interactions
Individual drugs
Amphotericin B: ↑ ototoxicity, neurotoxicity, nephrotoxicity
Cisplatin: ↑ ototoxicity, neurotoxicity, nephrotoxicity
Ethacrynic acid: ↑ ototoxicity, neurotoxicity, nephrotoxicity
Furosemide: ↑ ototoxicity, neurotoxicity, nephrotoxicity
Mannitol: ↑ ototoxicity, neurotoxicity, nephrotoxicity
Methoxyflurane: ↑ ototoxicity, neurotoxicity, nephrotoxicity
Polymyxin: ↑ ototoxicity, neurotoxicity, nephrotoxicity
Succinylcholine: ↑ neuromuscular blockade, respiratory depression
Vancomycin: ↑ ototoxicity, neurotoxicity, nephrotoxicity
Drug classifications
Anesthetics: ↑ neuromuscular blockade, respiratory depression
Aminoglycosides: ↑ otoxicity, neurotoxicity
Nondepolarizing neuromuscular blockers: ↑ neuromuscular blockade, respiratory depression
Penicillins: ↑ ototoxicity, neurotoxicity, nephrotoxicity

NURSING CONSIDERATIONS

Assessment

- Assess patient for previous sensitivity reaction
- Assess patient for signs and symptoms of infection including characteristics of wounds, sputum, urine, stool, WBC >10,000/mm^3, fever; obtain baseline information and during treatment
- Complete culture and sensitivity before beginning drug therapy; this will ensure that correct treatment has been initiated
- Assess for allergic reactions: rash, urticaria, pruritus, chills, fever, joint pain may occur a few days after therapy begins
- Identify urine output; if decreasing, notify prescriber (may indicate nephrotoxicity); also, increased BUN, creatinine, urine CrCl <80 ml/min
- Monitor blood studies: AST, ALT, CBC, Hct, bilirubin, LDH, alkaline phosphatase, Coombs' test monthly if patient is on long-term therapy
- Monitor electrolytes: potassium, sodium, chloride, magnesium monthly if patient is on long-term therapy
- Monitor for bleeding: ecchymosis, bleeding gums, hematuria; assess stool guaiac daily if on long-term therapy
- Assess for overgrowth of infection: perineal itching, fever, malaise, redness, pain, swelling, drainage, rash, diarrhea, change in cough, sputum
- Obtain weight before treatment; calculation of dosage is usually based on ideal body weight, but may be calculated on actual body weight
- Monitor I&O ratio; urinalysis daily for proteinuria, cells, casts; report sudden change in urine output
- Monitor VS during inf, watch for hypotension, change in pulse
- Assess **IV** site for thrombophlebitis including pain, redness, swelling q30 min, change site if needed; apply warm compresses to discontinued site
- Obtain serum peak, measured at 30-60 min after **IV** inf or 60 min after IM inj, trough level measured just before next dose; blood level should be 2-4 times bacteriostatic level
- Assess urine pH if drug is used for UTI; urine should be kept alkaline
- Assess for deafness by audiometric testing, ringing, roaring in ears, vertigo; assess hearing before, during, after treatment
- Assess for dehydration: high sp gr, decrease in skin turgor, dry mucous membranes, dark urine

Nursing diagnoses

- ✓ Infection, risk for (uses)
- ✓ Diarrhea (side effects)
- ✓ Knowledge deficit (teaching)
- ✓ Noncompliance (teaching)
- ✓ Injury, risk for (side effects)

Implementation

IM route

- Give deeply in large muscle mass; rotate sites

Topical route

- Wash hands, wear gloves, clean skin before applying

IV IV route

- Give in even doses around the clock; drug must be given for 10-14 days to ensure organism death and prevent superimposed infection
- Give by intermittent inf over ½-1 hr, flush with 0.9% NaCl or D_5W after inf
- Separate aminoglycosides and penicillins by ≥1 hr
- Store in tight container

Syringe compatibilities:
Clindamycin, methicillin, penicillin G sodium

Y-site compatibilities:
Acyclovir, amifostine, amiodarone, amsacrine, atracurium, aztreonam, cefpirome, ciprofloxacin, cyclophosphamide, cytarabine, diltiazem, enalaprilat, esmolol, famotidine, fluconazole, fludarabine, foscarnet, granisetron, hydromorphone, IL-2, insulin, labetalol, lorazepam, magnesium sulfate, melphalan, meperidine, meropenem, midazolam, morphine,

G

multivitamins, ondansetron, paclitaxel, pancuronium, perphenazine, sargramostim, tacrolimus, teniposide, theophylline, thiotepa, tolazine, vecuronium, vinorelbine, vit B with C, zidovudine

Y-site incompatibilities: Idarubicin, indomethacin, zidovudine

Additive compatibilities: Atracurium, aztreonam, bleomycin, cefoxitin, cimetidine, ciprofloxacin, fluconazole, meropenem, methicillin, metronidazole, ofloxacin, penicillin G sodium, ranitidine, verapamil

Patient/family education

- Teach patient to report sore throat, bruising, bleeding, joint pain; may indicate blood dyscrasias (rare)
- Advise patient to contact prescriber if vaginal itching, loose, foul-smelling stools, furry tongue occur; may indicate superimposed infection

Evaluation

Positive therapeutic outcome

- Absence of signs/symptoms of infection (WBC <10,000/mm^3, temp WNL, absence of red, draining wounds)
- Reported improvement in symptoms of infection

Treatment of overdose: Withdraw drug, hemodialysis

glatiramer (℞)

(glah-teer'a-mer)

Copaxone

Func. class.: Multiple sclerosis agent

Pregnancy category B

Action: Unknown; may modify the immune responses responsible for multiple sclerosis

Therapeutic outcome: Decreased symptoms of multiple sclerosis

Uses: Reduction of the frequency of relapses in patients with relapsing-remitting multiple sclerosis

Dosage and routes

Adult: SC 20 mg/day

Available forms: Inj 20 mg/ml

Adverse effects

CNS: Anxiety, hypertonia, tremor, vertigo, speech disorder, agitation, confusion
CV: Migraine, palpitations, syncope, tachycardia, vasodilation
EENT: Ear pain
GI: Nausea, vomiting, diarrhea, anorexia, gastroenteritis
GU: Urgency, dysmenorrhea, vaginal moniliasis
HEMA: Ecchymosis, lymphadenopathy
INTEG: Pruritus, rash, sweating, urticaria, erythema
META: Edema, weight gain
MS: Arthralgia
RESP: Bronchitis, dyspnea

Contraindications: Hypersensitivity to this drug or mannitol

Precautions: Immune disorders, renal disease, pregnancy **B,** lactation

Pharmacokinetics

Absorption	Unknown
Distribution	Unknown
Metabolism	Unknown
Excretion	Unknown
Half-life	Unknown

Pharmacodynamics

Unknown

NURSING CONSIDERATIONS

Assessment

- Monitor blood, renal, hepatic studies; before treatment
- Assess for CNS symptoms: anxiety, confusion, vertigo
- Assess GI status: diarrhea, vomiting, abdominal pain, gastroenteritis
- Assess cardiac status: tachycardia, palpitations, vasodilation, chest pain

Nursing diagnoses
- ✓ Knowledge deficit (teaching)
- ✓ Noncompliance (teaching)

Implementation
SC route
- Use a sterile syringe/needle to transfer the supplied diluent into the vial, rotate vial gently, do not shake; withdraw medication using a syringe with 27-G needle; administer SC into hip, thigh, arm; discard unused portion
- Use SC route only; do not give IM or **IV**
- Do not use sol that contains precipitate or is discolored

Patient/family education
- Give written, detailed instructions about the drug; provide initial and return demonstrations on inj procedure; give information on use and disposal of drug
- Advise patient that blurred vision, sweating may occur
- Advise patient that irregular menses, dysmenorrhea, or metorrhagia as well as breast pain may occur; use contraception during treatment
- Advise patient that if pregnancy is suspected or if nursing to notify prescriber
- Advise patient not to change dosing or to stop taking drug without advice of prescriber

Evaluation
Positive therapeutic outcome
- Decreased symptoms of multiple sclerosis

glipizide (℞)
(glip-i'zide)
Glucotrol, Glucotrol **XL**

glimepiride (℞)
(gly-meh'pih-ride)
Amaride

Func. class.: Antidiabetic
Chem. class.: Sulfonylurea (2nd generation)

Pregnancy category C

G

Action: Causes functioning β-cells in pancreas to release insulin, leading to drop in blood glucose levels; may improve insulin binding to insulin receptors or increase the number of insulin receptors with prolonged administration; may also reduce basal hepatic glucose secretion; not effective if patient lacks functioning β-cells

➔ **Therapeutic Outcome:** Decrease in polyuria, polydipsia, polyphagia, clear sensorium, absence of dizziness, stable gait

Uses: Stable adult-onset diabetes mellitus (type II) NIDDM

Dosage and routes
Glipizide

Adult: PO 5 mg initially, then increase to desired response; max 40 mg/day in divided doses or 15 mg/dose

G ***Elderly/hepatic dose:*** PO 2.5 mg initially, then increase to desired response; max 40 mg/day in divided doses or 15 mg/dose

Glimepiride

Adult: PO 1-2 mg qd, then increase q1-2 wk up to 8 mg/day

Renal dose

Adult: CrCl <22 ml/min; PO 1 mg qd with breakfast, may titrate upward as needed

Available forms: *glipizide* tabs 5, 10 mg scored; ext rel tab 5, 10 mg; *glimepiride* tabs 1, 2, 4 mg

Adverse effects

CNS: Headache, weakness, dizziness, drowsiness, tinnitus, fatigue, vertigo
ENDO: **Hypoglycemia**
GI: **Hepatotoxicity, cholestatic jaundice,** nausea, vomiting, diarrhea, heartburn
HEMA: **Leukopenia, thrombocytopenia, agranulocytosis, aplastic anemia,** increased AST, ALT, alkaline phosphatase, **pancytopenia, hemolytic anemia**
INTEG: Rash, allergic reactions, pruritus, urticaria, eczema, photosensitivity, erythema

Contraindications: Hypersensitivity to sulfonylureas, juvenile or type I PM diabetes

G **Precautions:** Pregnancy **C,** elderly, cardiac disease, severe renal disease, severe hepatic disease, thyroid disease

Do Not Confuse:
Glucotrol/glyburide

Pharmacokinetics

Absorption	Completely absorbed GI tract
Distribution	Unknown
Metabolism	Liver
Excretion	Via kidneys
Half-life	2-4 hr

Pharmacodynamics

Onset	1-1½ hr
Peak	1-3 hr
Duration	10-24 hr

Interactions

Individual drugs

Alcohol: Disulfiram-like reaction
Chloramphenicol: ↑ hypoglycemia
Cimetidine: ↑ hypoglycemia
Diazoxide: Both drugs may have action decreased
Digoxin: ↓ action of glipizide
Guanethidine: ↑ hypoglycemia
Insulin: ↑ hypoglycemia
Isoniazid: Possible ↓ action of glipizide
Methyldopa: ↑ hypoglycemia
Phenobarbital: Possible ↓ action of glipizide
Phenytoin: Possible ↓ action of glipizide
Probenecid: ↑ hypoglycemia
Rifampin: Possible ↓ action of glipizide

Drug classifications

Anticoagulants: ↑ hypoglycemia
Calcium channel blockers: Possible ↓ action of glipizide
Corticosteroids: Possible ↓ action of glipizide
Diuretics, thiazide: Possible ↓ action of glipizide
Estrogens: Possible ↓ action of glipizide
MAOIs: ↑ hypoglycemia
NSAIDs: ↑ hypoglycemia
Oral contraceptives: Possible ↓ action of glipizide
Phenothiazine: Possible ↓ action of glipizide
Salicylates: ↑ hypoglycemia
Sympathomimetics: Possible ↓ action of glipizide
Thyroid preparations: Possible ↓ action of glipizide

Herb/drug

Broom: ↓ hyperglycemic effect
Buchu: ↓ hyperglycemic effect
Chromium: ↑ or ↓ hypoglycemic effect
Dandelion: ↓ hyperglycemic effect
Fenugreek: ↑ or ↓ hypoglycemic effect
Ginseng: ↑ or ↓ hypoglycemic effect
Karela: ↑ glucose tolerance
Juniper: ↓ hyperglycemic effect

NURSING CONSIDERATIONS

Assessment

- Assess for hypoglycemic/hyperglycemic reactions that can occur soon pc; hypoglycemic reactions (sweating, weakness, dizziness, anxiety, tremors, hunger); hyperglycemic reactions
- Monitor CBC, glycosylated Hgb (baseline, q3 mo) during treatment;

check liver function tests periodically: AST, LDH, and renal studies: BUN, creatinine during treatment

Nursing diagnoses

✓ Nutrition, altered: more than body requirements (uses)
✓ Nutrition altered: less than body requirements (adverse reactions)
✓ Injury, risk for (adverse reactions)
✓ Knowledge deficit (teaching)
✓ Noncompliance (teaching)

Implementation

- Convert from other oral hypoglycemic agents or insulin dosage of <40 U/day; change may be made without gradual dosage change.
- Patients taking >40 U/day of insulin convert gradually by receiving oral hypoglycemic agents and 50% of previous insulin dosage for 3-5 days
- Monitor serum or urine glucose and ketones 3 ×/day during conversion
- Give drug 30 min before breakfast; if large dose is required, may be divided into 2 doses; give with meals to decrease GI upset and provide best absorption; if patient is NPO, may need to hold dose to prevent hypoglycemia
- Give tab crushed and mixed with meal or fluids for patients with difficulty swallowing
- For severe hypoglycemia give **IV** $D_{50}W$, then **IV** dextrose solution
- Store in tight container in cool environment

Patient/family education

- Teach patient to check for symptoms of cholestatic jaundice: dark urine, pruritus, yellow sclera; if these occur, prescriber should be notified
- Teach patient to use capillary blood glucose test or Chemstrip 3 ×/day
- Teach patient symptoms of hypo/hyperglycemia, what to do about each
- Instruct patient that drug must be continued on daily basis; explain consequence of discontinuing drug abruptly
- Teach patient to take drug in AM to prevent hypoglycemic reactions at night
- Caution patient to avoid OTC medications unless approved by a prescriber
- Teach patient that diabetes is a lifelong illness; that this drug is not a cure
- Teach patient to avoid alcohol; inform about disulfiram reaction (nausea, headache, cramps, flushing, hypoglycemia)
- Instruct patient that all food included in diet plan must be eaten to prevent hypoglycemia
- Advise patient to use sunscreen or stay out of the sun to prevent burns
- Advise patient to carry ID and a glucagon emergency kit for emergency purposes; also prescriber name, phone number, and medications taken

Evaluation

Positive therapeutic outcome

- Decrease in polyuria, polydipsia, polyphagia, clear sensorium, absence of dizziness, stable gait

glyburide (℞)

(glye'byoor-ide)

DiaBeta ♣, Euglucon ♣, Glynase PresTab, Micronase

Func. class.: Antidiabetic

Chem. class.: Sulfonylurea (2nd generation)

Pregnancy category C

Action: Causes functioning β-cells in pancreas to release insulin, leading to drop in blood glucose levels; may improve insulin binding to insulin receptors and increase number of insulin receptors with prolonged administration; may also reduce basal hepatic glucose secretion; not effective if patient lacks functioning β-cells

➡ **Therapeutic Outcome:** Decrease in polyuria, polydipsia, polyphagia, clear sensorium, absence of dizziness, stable gait

Uses: Stable adult-onset diabetes mellitus (type II) NIDDM

Dosage and routes

DiaBeta/Micronase

Adult: PO 1.25-5 mg initially, then increased to desired response at weekly intervals up to 20 mg/day

G ***Elderly:*** PO 1.25 mg initially, then increased to desired response; max 20 mg/day, maintenance 1.25-20 mg/qd

Glynase PresTab (micronized)

Adult: PO 1.5-3 mg/day initially, may increase by 1.5 mg/wk, max 12 mg/day

G ***Elderly:*** PO 0.75-3 mg/day, may increase by 1.5 mg/wk

Available forms: Tabs 1.25, 2.5, 5 mg; tabs micronized (Glynase PresTab) 1.5, 3, 6 mg

Adverse effects

CNS: ***Headache, weakness,*** paresthesia, tinnitus, fatigue, vertigo

ENDO: **Hypoglycemia**

GI: Nausea, fullness, heartburn, **hepatoxicity, cholestatic jaundice,** vomiting, diarrhea

HEMA: **Leukopenia, thrombocytopenia, agranulocytosis, aplastic anemia,** increased AST, ALT, alkaline phosphatase

INTEG: Rash, allergic reactions, pruritus, urticaria, eczema, photosensitivity, erythema

MS: Joint pains

Contraindications: Hypersensitivity to sulfonylureas, juvenile or type I diabetes

G **Precautions:** Pregnancy **C,** elderly, cardiac disease, severe renal disease, severe hepatic disease, thyroid disease, severe hypoglycemic reactions

Do Not Confuse:
DiaBeta/Zebeta, glyburide/Glucotrol

Pharmacokinetics	
Absorption	Completely absorbed GI tract
Distribution	99% plasma protein binding
Metabolism	Liver
Excretion	Urine, feces (metabolites), crosses placenta
Half-life	10 hr

Pharmacodynamics	
Onset	2-4 hr
Peak	4 hr
Duration	24 hr

Interactions

Individual drugs

Alcohol: Disulfiram-like reaction
Charcoal: ↓ glyburide action
Chloramphenicol: ↑ hypoglycemia
Cholestyramine: ↓ glyburide action
Diazoxide: Both drugs may have action decreased
Digoxin: ↓ digoxin level
Fenfluramine: ↑ glyburide action
Gemfibrozil: ↑ glyburide
Guanethidine: ↑ hypoglycemia
Insulin: ↑ hypoglycemia
Isoniazid: ↓ action of glyburide
Methyldopa: ↑ hypoglycemia
Phenobarbital: ↓ action of glyburide
Phenylbutazone: ↑ glyburide
Phenytoin: ↓ action of glyburide
Probenecid: ↑ hypoglycemia
Rifampin: ↓ action of glyburide
Sulfinpyrazone: ↑ glyburide

Drug classifications

Androgens: ↑ glyburide action
Anticoagulants: ↑ hypoglycemia
Antidepressants, tricyclics: ↑ glyburide action
β-Adrenergic blockers: ↑ masking of symptoms of hypoglycemia
Diuretics, thiazide: ↓ action of glyburide
Estrogens: ↓ action of glyburide
Histamine H_2-antagonists: ↑ glyburide action
Magnesium salts: ↑ glyburide action
MAOIs: ↑ hypoglycemia

NSAIDs: ↑ hypoglycemia
Salicylates: ↑ hypoglycemia
Sulfonamides: ↑ glyburide action
Urinary acidifers: ↑ glyburide acid
Urinary alkalinizers: ↓ glyburide action

Herb/drug
Broom: ↓ glyburide action
Buchu: ↓ glyburide action
Chromium: ↑ or ↓ glyburide effect
Dandelion: ↓ glyburide action
Fenugreek: ↑ or ↓ glyburide effect
Ginseng: ↑ or ↓ glyburide effect
Karela: ↑ glucose tolerance
Juniper: ↓ glyburide action

NURSING CONSIDERATIONS

Assessment

- Assess for hypoglycemic/hyperglycemic reactions that can occur soon pc; hypoglycemic reactions (sweating, weakness, dizziness, anxiety, tremors, hunger); hyperglycemic reactions
- Monitor CBC, glycosylated Hgb (baseline, q3 mo) during treatment; check liver function tests periodically, AST, LDH and renal studies: BUN, creatinine during treatment

Nursing diagnoses

- ✓ Nutrition, altered: more than body requirements (uses)
- ✓ Nutrition altered: less than body requirements (adverse reactions)
- ✓ Injury, risk for (adverse reactions)
- ✓ Knowledge deficit (teaching)
- ✓ Noncompliance (teaching)

Implementation

- Conversion from other oral hypoglycemic agents or insulin dosage of <40 U/day; change may be made without gradual dosage change
- Patients taking >40 U/day of insulin convert gradually by receiving oral hypoglycemic agents and 50% of previous insulin dosage for 3-5 days
- Monitor serum or urine glucose and ketones 3 ×/day during conversion
- Give drug 30 min before breakfast; if large dose is required, may be divided into two; give with meals to decrease GI upset and provide best absorption, if patient is NPO, may need to hold dose to avoid hypoglycemia
- Give tab crushed and mixed with meal or fluids for patients with difficulty swallowing
- For severe hypoglycemia, give **IV** $D_{50}W$, then **IV** dextrose sol
- Store in tight container in cool environment

Patient/family education

- Teach patient to check for symptoms of cholestatic jaundice: dark urine, pruritus, yellow sclera; if these occur, prescriber should be notified
- Teach patient to use capillary blood glucose test or Chemstrip 3 ×/day
- Teach patient symptoms of hypo/hyperglycemia, what to do about each
- Instruct patient that drug must be continued on daily basis; explain consequence of discontinuing drug abruptly
- Teach patient to take drug in AM to prevent hypoglycemic reactions at night
- Caution patient to avoid OTC medications unless approved by a prescriber
- Teach patient that diabetes is a lifelong illness; that this drug is not a cure
- Instruct patient that all food included in diet plan must be eaten to prevent hypoglycemia
- Advise patient to carry ID and a glucagon emergency kit for emergency purposes; also prescriber name, phone number, and medications
- Advise patient to use sunscreen or stay out of the sun to prevent burns

Evaluation

Positive therapeutic outcome

- Decrease in polyuria, polydipsia, polyphagia, clear sensorium, absence of dizziness, stable gait

G

glycerin (OTC)

(gli'ser-in)

Fleet Babylax, glycerin USP, Glycerol, Ophthalgan, Osmoglyn, Sani-Supp

Func. class.: Laxative, hyperosmotic, antiglaucoma agent

Chem. class.: Trihydric alcohol

Pregnancy category C

Action: Increases osmotic pressure by drawing fluid into colon lumen from extravascular spaces to intravascular

→ Therapeutic Outcome: Absence of constipation, intraocular pressure, ICP, absence of edema in the cornea

Uses: Constipation, intraocular pressure in glaucoma; ICP, edema in the superficial layers of the cornea

Dosage and routes

P ***Adult and child >6 yr:*** REC SUPP 3 g; enema 5-15 ml

P ***Child <6 yr:*** REC SUPP 1-1.5 g; enema 2-5 ml

Corneal edema

Adult: OPHTH 1-2 gtt q3-4 h

Intraocular pressure reduction

Adult: PO 1-1.5 g/kg once, then 500 mg/kg q6h

P ***Child:*** PO 1-1.5 g/kg qd once, then 500 mg/kg 4-8 hr after first dose

Available forms: Rec sol 4 ml/applicator; supp; oral sol 0.6/ml; ophth sol 7.5 ml/container

Adverse effects

CNS: Headache, confusion, **convulsions**

GI: Nausea, vomiting, diarrhea

META: Dehydration

Contraindications: Hypersensitivity

Precautions: Pregnancy **C**

Pharmacokinetics

Absorption	Well absorbed (PO), not absorbed (rec)
Distribution	To intravascular space
Metabolism	Liver—80%, kidneys—20%
Excretion	Kidneys
Half-life	30 min

Pharmacodynamics

	PO	REC	OPHTH
Onset	10-30 min	Unknown	Unknown
Peak	30-120 min	30 min	Unknown
Duration	6-8 hr	Unknown	Up to 4 hr

Interactions

Drug classifications

Diuretics: ↓ effect of glycerin (ophth)

NURSING CONSIDERATIONS

Assessment

- Assess patient for cause of constipation; identify whether fluids, bulk, or exercise is missing from lifestyle; check for distention, bowel sounds
- After administration, check for cramping, rectal bleeding, nausea, vomiting; if these symptoms occur, drug should be discontinued
- Identify stool characteristics: consistency, color, amount, shape, volume

Nursing diagnoses

✓ Constipation (uses)

✓ Knowledge deficit (teaching)

Implementation

Rectal route

- Insert glycerin supp after removing wrapper; may cause evacuation in ½ hr
- For evening use 4-ml applications of fluid, have patient in side-lying position, have patient retain for a few min

Ophthalmic route

- Instill 1-2 gtt in one or both eyes by

pulling down on conjunctival sac
- Do not use ophth sol that is discolored, has a precipitate, or is cloudy

PO route
- Pour over cracked ice and sip through a straw
- To prevent severe cerebral dehydration headache have patient recumbent during and after administration
- Give by mixing 50% glycerin sol with 0.9% NaCl with flavoring, or use oral sol that is already flavored; flavoring improves taste and prevents GI symptoms
- Store in cool environment; do not freeze

Patient/family education
- Caution patient not to use laxatives for long-term therapy; normal bowel tone will be lost; that normal bowel movements do not always occur daily
- Advise patient not to use in presence of abdominal pain, nausea, vomiting
- Instruct patient to notify prescriber if constipation is unrelieved or if weakness, dizziness, excessive thirst occur

Evaluation
Positive therapeutic outcome
- Decreased constipation
- Decreased intraocular pressure

glycopyrrolate (℞)
(glye-koe-pye'roe-late)
glycopyrrolate, Robinul, Robinul-Forte
Func. class.: Cholinergic blocker
Chem. class.: Quaternary ammonium compound

Pregnancy category B

Action: Inhibits action of acetylcholine at receptor sites in autonomic nervous system, which controls secretions, free acids in stomach

Therapeutic Outcome: Decreased secretions in the respiratory tract, GI system

Uses: Decreased secretions before surgery, reversal of neuromuscular blockade, peptic ulcer disease, irritable bowel syndrome

Investigational uses: Drooling

Dosage and routes
Preoperatively
Adult: IM 4.4 μg mg/lb ½-1 hr before surgery, max 0.1 mg
P ***Child:*** IM 4.4-8.8 μg

Reversal of neuromuscular blockage
P ***Adult and child:*** **IV** 200 μg for each mg of neostigmine or 5 mg **IV** of pyridostigmine simultaneously

Drooling
Adult: PO doses vary widely

GI disorders
Adult: PO 1-2 mg bid-tid; IM/**IV** 100-200 μg tid-qid, titrated to patient response

Antidysrhythmic
Adult: **IV** 100 μg, may repeat q2 min
P ***Child:*** **IV** 4.4 μg/kg, may repeat q2 min, max 100 μg

Available forms: Tabs 1, 2 mg; inj 200 μg 0.2 mg/ml

Adverse effects
CNS: Confusion, anxiety, restlessness, irritability, delusions, hallucinations, headache, sedation, depression, incoherence, dizziness, lethargy, flushing, weakness
CV: Palpitations, tachycardia, postural hypotension, paradoxical bradycardia
EENT: Blurred vision, photophobia, dilated pupils, difficulty swallowing, increased intraocular pressure, mydriasis, cycloplegia
GI: *Dryness of mouth, constipation,* nausea, vomiting, abdominal distress, paralytic ileus, altered taste perception
GU: Hesitancy, retention, impotence

G

INTEG: Urticaria, allergic reactions
MISC: Suppression of lactation, nasal congestion, decreased sweating, **anaphylaxis**

Contraindications: Hypersensitivity, narrow-angle glaucoma, myasthenia gravis, GI/GU obstruction, child <3 yr, tachycardia, myocardial ischemia, hepatic disease, ulcerative colitis, toxic megacolon

Precautions: Pregnancy **B**, elderly, lactation, prostatic hypertrophy, renal disease, CHF, pulmonary disease, hyperthyroidism

Pharmacokinetics

Absorption	Well absorbed (PO, SC, IM)
Distribution	Unknown
Metabolism	Not metabolized
Excretion	Unchanged feces
Half-life	2 hr

Pharmacodynamics

	PO	IM	IV
Onset	Unknown	15-30 min	Immediate
Peak	1 hr	30-45 min	10-15 min
Duration	8-12 hr	2-7 hr	2-7 hr

Interactions
Individual drugs
Amantadine: ↑ anticholinergic effect
Disopyramide: ↑ anticholinergic effect
Potassium chloride, oral: ↑ GI lesions
Quinidine: ↑ anticholinergic effect
Drug classifications
Antacids: ↓ absorption of glycopyrrolate
Anticholinergics: ↑ anticholinergic effect
Antidepressants, tricyclic: ↑ anticholinergic effect
Antidiarrheals: ↓ absorption of glycopyrrolate
Antihistamines: ↑ anticholinergic effect

NURSING CONSIDERATIONS
Assessment
- Monitor I&O ratio; retention commonly causes decreased urinary output; check for urinary hesitation; palpate bladder if retention occurs
- Monitor ECG for ectopic ventricular beats, PVC, tachycardia
- Monitor for bowel sounds; check for constipation; increase fluids, bulk, exercise if constipation occurs
- Assess mental status: affect, mood, CNS depression, worsening of psychiatric symptoms during early therapy

Nursing diagnoses
✓ Knowledge deficit (teaching)

Implementation
IV route
- Administer **IV** undiluted, give at a rate of 0.2 mg or less over 5-15 min through Y-tube or 3-way stopcock; do not add to **IV** sol
- Administer parenteral dose with patient recumbent to prevent postural hypotension

Syringe compatibilities:
Atropine, benzquinamide, chlorpromazine, cimetidine, codeine, diphenhydramine, droperidol, droperidol/fentanyl, hydromorphone, hydroxyzine, levorphanol, lidocaine, meperidine, meperidine/promethazine, midazolam, morphine, nalbuphine, neostigmine, oxymorphone, procaine, prochlorperazine, promazine, promethazine, pyridostigmine, ranitidine, scopolamine, triflupromazine, trimethobenzamide

Y-site compatibilities:
Propofol

Solution compatibilities:
D_5W, 0.9% NaCl, Ringer's D_5/0.45% NaCl

PO route
- Give PO with or after meals to

prevent GI upset; may give with fluids other than water

IM route

- Give IM deeply in large muscle mass

Patient/family education

- Caution patient not to operate machinery or engage in hazardous activities if drowsiness, blurred vision occurs
- Advise patient not to take OTC products, cough, cold preparations with alcohol, antihistamines without approval of prescriber
- Teach patient to avoid hot temperatures; since sweating is decreased, heat stroke is possible
- Advise patient to notify prescriber of eye pain, blurred vision, light sensitivity
- Caution patient not to discontinue this drug abruptly; tapering should be done over 1 wk

Evaluation

Positive therapeutic outcome

- Decreased secretions, bronchial, GI
- Decreased pain in GI disorders
- Reversal of neuromuscular blockade

goserelin (℞)

(goe'se-rel-lin)

Zoladex

Func. class.: Gonado- tropin-releasing hormone, antineoplastic

Chem. class.: Synthetic decapeptide analog of LHRH

Pregnancy category X

Action: Inhibitor of pituitary gonadotropin secretion; initially increases LH and FSH, with increases in testosterone, reduction in sex steroid levels

Therapeutic Outcome: Decrease in tumor size and spread of malignant cells

Uses: Advanced prostate cancer (10.8 mg); endometriosis, advanced breast cancer, endometrial thinning (3.6 mg)

Dosage and routes

Adult: SC 3.6 mg q4 wk (implant) or 10.8 mg q12 wk

Endometrial thinning

Adult: SC 1-2 depot inj; usually 1 depot, surgery performed at 4 wk; if 2 depots, surgery performed 2-4 wk after 2nd depot

Available forms: Depot inj 3.6, 10.8 mg

G

Adverse effects

CNS: Headaches, **spinal cord compression,** anxiety, depression

CV: **Dysrhythmia, cerebrovascular accident,** hypertension, **MI,** chest pain

ENDO: Gynecomastia, breast tenderness, hot flashes

GI: Nausea, vomiting, constipation, diarrhea, ulcer

GU: *Spotting, breakthrough bleeding, decreased libido,* renal insufficiency, urinary obstruction, urinary tract infection

INTEG: Rash, pain on inj

MS: Osteoneuralgia

Contraindications: Hypersensitivity to LHRH, LHRH-agonist analogs, lactation, nondiagnosed vaginal bleeding, pregnancy **X,** breast cancer (**D**)

P **Precautions:** Children, lactation

Pharmacokinetics	
Absorption	Well absorbed
Distribution	Unknown
Metabolism	Unknown
Excretion	Unknown
Half-life	4½ hr

Pharmacodynamics	
Onset	Unknown
Peak	14-28 days
Duration	Treatment length

Interactions: None

Lab test interferences
↑ Alkaline phosphatase, ↑ estradiol, ↑ FSH, ↑ LH, ↑ testosterone levels
↓ Testosterone levels, ↓ progesterone

NURSING CONSIDERATIONS

Assessment

- Assess for relief of bone pain (back pain), change in motor function
- Monitor I&O ratios, palpate bladder for distention (urinary obstruction) at beginning of treatment; renal insufficiency and obstruction may occur
- Monitor acid phosphatase, prostate-specific antigen baseline and periodically

Nursing diagnoses

✓ Sexual dysfunction (uses)
✓ Knowledge deficit (teaching)

Implementation

- Administer via implant inserted by qualified persons into upper subcutaneous tissue in abdominal wall q28 days or q12 wk (10.8 mg)

Patient/family education

- Caution patient that gynecomastia and postmenopausal symptoms may occur but will decrease after treatment is discontinued; that bone pain may increase, then decrease
- Teach patient to contact prescriber if difficulty urinating, hot flashes occur during treatment

Evaluation

Positive therapeutic outcome

- More normal levels of PSA, acid phosphatase, alkaline phosphatase; testosterone level of <25 mg/dl

granisetron (℞)

(grane-iss'e-tron)
Kytril
Func. class.: Antiemetic
Chem. class.: 5-HT_3 receptor antagonist

Pregnancy category C

Action: Prevents nausea, vomiting by blocking serotinin peripherally, centrally, and in the small intestine

➔ **Therapeutic Outcome:** Absence of nausea and vomiting

Uses: Prevention of nausea, vomiting associated with cancer chemotherapy including high-dose cisplatin

Investigational uses: Acute nausea, vomiting after surgery

Dosage and routes

Nausea, vomiting in chemotherapy

P ***Adult and child:*** **IV** 10 μg/kg over 5 min, 30 min before the start of cancer chemotherapy

Adult: PO 1 mg bid, give 1st dose 1 hr before chemotherapy and next dose 12 hr after 1st

Available forms: Inj 1 mg/ml; tabs 1 mg

Adverse effects

CNS: *Headache, asthenia,* anxiety, dizziness
CV: Hypertension
GI: Diarrhea, *constipation,* increased AST, ALT, *nausea*
HEMA: **Leukopenia,** anemia, **thrombocytopenia**
MISC: Rash, **bronchospasm**

Contraindications: Hypersensitivity

P G **Precautions:** Pregnancy lactation, children, elderly

Pharmacokinetics

Absorption	Unknown
Distribution	Unknown
Metabolism	Liver
Excretion	Unknown
Half-life	10-12 hr

Pharmacodynamics

Unknown

Interactions: None

NURSING CONSIDERATIONS
Assessment
- Assess patient for absence of nausea, vomiting during chemotherapy
- Assess patient for hypersensitive reaction: rash, bronchospasm

Nursing diagnoses
✓ Fluid deficit (uses)
✓ Knowledge deficit (teaching)

Implementation
- Administer **IV**
- Dilute in 0.9% NaCl for inj or D_5W (20-50 ml), give over 5-15 min
- Store at room temp for 24-hr dilution

Y-site compatibilities: Acyclovir, allopurinol, amifostine, amikacin, aminophylline, amphotericin B cholesteryl, ampicillin, ampicillin/sulbactam, amsacrine, aztreonam, bleomycin, bumetanide, buprenorphine, butorphanol, calcium gluconate, carboplatin, carmustine, cefazolin, cefepime, cefonicid, cefoperazone, cefotaxime, cefotetan, cefoxitin, ceftazidime, ceftizoxime, ceftriaxone, cefuroxime, chlorpromazine, cimetidine, ciprofloxacin, cisplatin, cladribine, clindamycin, cyclophosphamide, cytarabine, dacarbazine, dactinomycin, daunorubicin, dexamethasone, diphenhydramine, dobutamine, dopamine, doxorubicin, doxorubicin liposome, doxycycline, droperidol, enalaprilat, etoposide, famotidine, filgrastim, floxuridine, fluconazole, fluorouracil, fludarabine, furosemide, gallium, ganciclovir, gentamicin, haloperidol, heparin, hydrocortisone, hydromorphone, hydroxyzine, idarubicin, ifosfamide, imipenem-cilastatin, leucovorin, lorazepam, magnesium sulfate, melphalan, meperidine, mesna, methotrexate, methylprednisolone, metoclopramide, metronidazole, mezlocillin, miconazole, minocycline, mitomycin, mitoxantrone, morphine, nalbuphine, netilmicin, ofloxacin, paclitaxel, piperacillin, piperacillin/tazobactam, plicamycin, potassium chloride, prochlorperazine, promethazine, propofol, ranitidine, sargramostim, sodium bicarbonate, streptozocin, teniposide, thiotepa, ticarcillin, ticarcillin/clavulanate, tobramycin, trimethoprim-sulfamethoxazole, vancomycin, vinblastine, vincristine, vinorelbine, zidovudine

Y-site incompatibilities: Fluorouracil, furosemide, sodium bicarbonate

Additive compatibilities: Dexamethasone, methylprednisolone

Solution compatibilities: D_5W, 0.9% NaCl

Patient/family education
- Advise patient to report diarrhea, constipation, rash, or changes in respirations

Evaluation
Positive therapeutic outcome
- Absence of nausea, vomiting during cancer chemotherapy

griseofulvin microsize (℞)
(gris-ee-oh-ful'vin)
Fulvicin-U/F, Grifulvin V, Grisactin, Grisovin-FP ✤

griseofulvin ultramicrosize (℞)
Fulvicin-P/G, Grisactin Ultra, Gris-PEG

Func. class.: Antifungal
Chem. class.: Penicillium griseofulvum derivative

Pregnancy category C

Action: Arrests fungal cell division at metaphase (mitosis); binds to human keratin, making it resistant to disease

Therapeutic Outcome: Absence of fungicidal infection

Uses: Mycotic infections: tinea corporis, tinea pedis, tinea cruris, tinea barbae, tinea capitis, tinea unguium if caused by *Epidermophyton, Microsporum, Trichophyton*

Dosage and routes
Adult: PO 500-1000 mg qd in single or divided doses (microsize), 125-165 mg bid (ultramicrosize), or 250-330 mg qd; may need 500-660 mg in divided doses for severe infections

P ***Child:*** PO 10 mg/kg/day or 30 mg/m^2/day (microsize) or 5 mg/kg/day (ultramicrosize)

Available forms: Microcaps 125, 250 mg; tabs 250, 500 mg; oral susp 125 mg/5 ml; ultratabs 125, 165, 250, 330 mg

Adverse effects
CNS: *Headache,* peripheral neuritis, paresthesias, confusion, dizziness, fatigue
EENT: Transient hearing loss
GU: Proteinuria, cylinduria, precipitate porphyria, increased thirst
GI: *Nausea, vomiting, anorexia,* diarrhea, cramps, dry mouth, flatulence, **bleeding**
HEMA: **Leukopenia, granulocytopenia, neutropenia, monocytosis**
INTEG: *Rash, urticaria,* photosensitivity, lichen planus
SYST: **Serum sickness**

Contraindications: Hypersensitivity, porphyria, hepatic disease, lupus erythematosus

Precautions: Penicillin sensitivity, pregnancy **C**

Pharmacokinetics
Absorption	Ultra products (completely absorbed), others (variably absorbed)
Distribution	Keratin in skin; liver, muscle, fat
Metabolism	Liver
Excretion	Feces
Half-life	10-24 hr

Pharmacodynamics
Onset	4 hr
Peak	1 day
Duration	2 day

Interactions
Individual drugs
Alcohol: ↑ CNS depression, tachycardia
Cyclosporine: ↓ action of warfarin
Phenobarbital: ↓ action of griseofulvin
Drug classifications
Contraceptives, oral: ↓ effect of contraceptive
Salicylates: ↓ action of warfarin
Food/drug
Fat (meat, dairy products): ↑ absorption

NURSING CONSIDERATIONS
Assessment
- Assess patient's skin for fungal infections: peeling, dryness, itching before and throughout treatment
- Monitor blood studies: leukocytes,

CBC, platelets, although blood dyscrasias are rare

- Monitor for renal toxicity: increased BUN, serum creatinine; if serum creatinine >1.7 mg/100 dl, dosage may be reduced (rare)
- Monitor for hepatotoxicity: increasing AST, ALT, alkaline phosphatase
- Monitor for allergic reaction: dermatitis, rash; drug should be discontinued, give antihistamines for mild reaction or epinephrine for severe reaction; if patient is allergic to penicillin a cross-sensitivity may exist with this medication

Nursing diagnoses

- ✓ Skin integrity, impaired (uses)
- ✓ Infection, risk for (uses)
- ✓ Knowledge deficit (teaching)

Implementation

- Give with meals (fatty) to prevent GI upset
- Administer drug carefully, making sure there is no confusion with dosage form (microsize vs ultrasize); with meals to decrease GI symptoms; store in tight, light-resistant container at room temp
- Administer drug until three separate cultures are negative for infective organism; use PO only when topical drug is ineffective

Patient/family education

- Teach patient that long-term therapy may be needed to clear infection (2 wk-6 mo depending on organism); compliance is needed even after feeling better
- Instruct patient in proper hygiene: hand-washing technique, nail care, use of concomitant top agents if prescribed to clear infection
- Advise patient to avoid alcohol because nausea, vomiting, hypertension may occur
- Advise patient to use sunscreen or avoid direct sunlight to prevent photosensitivity
- Caution patient to notify prescriber of sore throat, fever, skin rash, which may indicate overgrowth of organisms
- Advise patient to use a nonhormonal form of contraception during treatment and to notify prescriber if pregnancy is anticipated

Evaluation

Positive therapeutic outcome

- Decrease in itching, peeling, dryness

guaifenesin (℞, OTC)

(gwye-fen′e-sin)

Anti-tuss, Benylin-E ♣, Breonesin, Calmylin Expectorant ♣, Diabetic Tussin EX, Duratuss-G, Fenesin, Gee-Gee, Genatuss, GG-Cen, Glyate, Glycotuss, Glytuss, guaifenesin, Guaifenex LA, Guiatuss, Halotussin, Humibid, Humibid L.A., Hytuss, Hytuss 2X, Liquibid, Malotuss, Monafed, Muco-Fen LA, Mytussin, Naldecon Senior EX, Organidin NR, Pneumomist, Respa-GF, Resyl ♣, Robitussin, Scot-Tussin Expectorant, Sinumist-SR, Uni-Tussin

Func. class.: Expectorant

Pregnancy category C

Action: Acts as an expectorant by stimulating a gastric mucosal reflex to increase the production of lung mucus

Therapeutic Outcome: Decreased cough

Uses: Dry, nonproductive cough

Dosage and routes

Adult: PO 200-400 mg q4-6h, or 600-1200 mg q12h (ext rel) not to exceed 2.4 g/day

P ***Child 6-12 yr:*** PO 100-200 mg q4h or 600 mg q12h (ext rel); not to exceed 1.2 g/day

P ***Child 2-6 yr:*** PO: 50-100 mg q4h; not to exceed 600 mg/day

Available forms: Tabs 100, 200 mg; tabs, ext rel 600, 1200 mg; caps 200 mg; syr 100 mg, 200/5 ml; liq 200 mg/5 ml; ext rel caps 300 mg

Adverse effects

CNS: Drowsiness

GI: Nausea, anorexia, vomiting

Contraindications: Hypersensitivity, persistent cough

Precautions: Pregnancy **C**

Pharmacokinetics

Absorption	Well absorbed
Distribution	Unknown
Metabolism	Unknown
Excretion	Unknown
Half-life	Unknown

Pharmacodynamics

	PO	PO ER
Onset	½ hr	Unknown
Peak	Unknown	Unknown
Duration	4-6 hr	12 hr

Interactions: None

NURSING CONSIDERATIONS

Assessment

- Assess cough: type, frequency, character, including characteristics of sputum; lung sounds bilaterally; fluids should be increased to 2 L/day to decrease secretion viscosity (thickness)

Nursing diagnoses

✓ Airway clearance, ineffective (uses)
✓ Knowledge deficit (teaching)

Implementation

- Store at room temp; provide room humidification to assist with liquefying secretions
- Avoid fluids for ½ hr after administration

Patient/family education

- Caution patient to avoid driving, other hazardous activities if drowsiness occurs (rare)
- Advise patient to avoid smoking, smoke-filled rooms, perfumes, dust, environmental pollutants, cleansers
- Instruct patient to notify prescriber if dry, nonproductive cough lasts over 7 days

Evaluation

Positive therapeutic outcome

- Absence of dry cough
- Thinner, more productive cough that raises secretions

haloperidol (Rx)

(hal-oh-pehr'ih-dol)

Apo-Haloperidol ♣, Haldol, Novo-Peridol ♣, Peridol ♣

haloperidol decanoate (Rx)

Haldol Decanoate, Haldol LA ♣

haloperidol lactate (Rx)

Haldol, Haloperidol Injection, Haloperidol Intensol

Func. class.: Antipsychotic/neuroleptic

Chem. class.: Butyrophenone

Pregnancy category C

Action: Depresses cerebral cortex, hypothalamus, limbic system, which control activity and aggression; blocks neurotransmission produced by dopamine at synapse; exhibits strong α-adrenergic, anticholinergic blocking action; mechanism for antipsychotic effects unclear

➡ **Therapeutic Outcome:** Decreased signs and symptoms of psychosis

Uses: Psychotic disorders, control of tics, vocal utterances in Gilles de la Tourette syndrome, short-term treatment of hyperactive children showing excessive motor activity, prolonged parenteral therapy in chronic schizophrenia, control of severe nausea and vomiting in chemotherapy, organic mental syndrome with psychotic features, hiccups (short-term)

Investigational uses: Nausea, vomiting in chemotherapy, surgery

Dosage and routes

Psychosis

Adult: PO 0.5-5 mg bid or tid initially depending on severity of condition; increase to desired dosage, max 100 mg/day; IM 2-5 mg q4-8h or bid-tid

G ***Elderly:*** 0.25-0.5 mg qd-bid, titrate q3-4 days by 0.25-0.5 mg/dose

P ***Child 3-12 yr:*** PO/IM 0.05-0.15 mg/kg/day

Chronic schizophrenia

Adult: IM 50-100 mg q4 wk (decanoate)

P ***Child 3-12 yr:*** PO/IM 0.05-0.15 mg/kg/day

Tics/vocal utterances

Adult: PO 0.5-5 mg bid or tid, increased until desired response occurs

P ***Child 3-12 yr:*** PO 0.05-0.075 mg/kg/day

Hyperactive children

P ***Child 3-12 yr:*** PO 0.05-0.075 mg/kg/day

Available forms: Tabs 0.5, 1, 2, 5, 10, 20 mg; lactate: conc 2 mg/ml; inj 5 mg/ml, 50, 100 mg base/ml

Adverse effects

CNS: *Extrapyramidal symptoms: pseudoparkinsonism, akathisia, dystonia, tardive dyskinesia, drowsiness, headache,* **seizures, neuroleptic malignant syndrome,** confusion

CV: *Orthostatic hypotension,* hypertension, **cardiac arrest,** ECG changes, **tachycardia**

EENT: Blurred vision, glaucoma, dry eyes

GI: *Dry mouth, nausea, vomiting, anorexia, constipation,* diarrhea, jaundice, weight gain, **ileus, hepatitis**

GU: Urinary retention, urinary frequency, enuresis, impotence, amenorrhea, gynecomastia

INTEG: *Rash,* photosensitivity, dermatitis

RESP: **Laryngospasm,** dys pnea, **respiratory depression**

Contraindications: Hypersensitivity, blood dyscrasias, coma, P child <3 yr, brain damage, bone marrow depression, alcohol and barbiturate withdrawal states, Parkinson's disease, angina, epilepsy, urinary retention, narrow-angle glaucoma

Precautions: Pregnancy **C,** lactation, seizure disorders, hypertension, hepatic disease, cardiac disease, G elderly

Do Not Confuse:
Haldol/Stadol, haloperidol/Halotestin

H

Pharmacokinetics

Absorption	Well absorbed (PO, IM); decanoate (IM) absorbed slowly
Distribution	High concentrations in liver, crosses placenta
Metabolism	Liver, extensively
Excretion	Kidneys, breast milk
Half-life	21-24 hr

Pharmacodynamics

	PO	IM	IM (decanoate)
Onset	Erratic	½ hr	3-9 days
Peak	2-6 hr	30-45 min	4-11 days
Duration	8-12 hr	4-8 hr	3 wk

Interactions

Individual drugs

Alcohol: ↑ effects of both drugs, oversedation

Aluminum hydroxide: ↓ absorption

Bromocriptine: ↓ antiparkinson activity

Disopyramide: ↑ anticholinergic effects

Epinephrine: ↑ toxicity

Guanethidine: ↓ antihypertensive response
Levodopa: ↓ antiparkinsonian activity
Lithium: ↓ haloperidol levels, ↑ extrapyramidal symptoms, masking of lithium toxicity
Magnesium hydroxide: ↓ absorption
Norepinephrine: ↓ vasoresponse, ↑ toxicity
Phenobarbital: ↓ effectiveness, ↑ metabolism

Drug classifications
Antacids: ↓ absorption
Anticholinergics: ↑ anticholinergic effects
Antidepressants: ↑ CNS depression
Antidiarrheals, adsorbent: ↓ absorption
Antihistamines: ↑ CNS depression
Antihypertensives: ↑ hypotension
Antithyroid agents: ↑ agranulocytosis
Barbiturate anesthetics: ↑ CNS depression
β-Adrenergic blockers: ↑ effects of both drugs
General anesthetics: ↑ CNS depression
MAOIs: ↑ CNS depression
Opiates: ↑ CNS depression
Sedative/hypnotics: ↑ CNS depression

Herb/drug
Kava: ↑ action

Lab test interferences
↑ Liver function tests, ↑ cardiac enzymes, ↑ cholesterol, ↑ blood glucose, ↑ prolactin, ↑ bilirubin, ↑ PBI, ↑ cholinesterase, ↑ alkaline phosphatase
↓ Hormones (blood and urine), ↓ pro-time
False positive: Pregnancy tests, PKU, urine bilirubin
False negative: Urinary steroids, 17-OHCS

NURSING CONSIDERATIONS

Assessment

- Assess mental status: orientation, mood, behavior, presence and type of hallucinations before initial administration and monthly; this drug should significantly reduce psychotic behavior
- Check for swallowing of PO medication; check for hoarding or giving of medication to other patients
- Monitor I&O ratio; palpate bladder if low urinary output occurs, especially in elderly; urinalysis is recommended before, during prolonged therapy
- Monitor bilirubin, CBC, liver function studies monthly
- Assess affect, orientation, LOC, reflexes, gait, coordination, sleep pattern disturbances
- Monitor B/P with patient sitting, standing, and lying; take pulse and respirations q4h during initial treatment; establish baseline before starting treatment; report drops of 30 mm Hg; obtain baseline ECG, Q-wave and T-wave changes
- Check for dizziness, faintness, palpitations, tachycardia on rising; severe orthostatic hypotension is common
- Assess for neuroleptic malignant syndrome: hyperpyrexia, muscle rigidity, increased CPK, altered mental status; drug should be discontinued immediately; if seizures, hypertension/hypotension, tachycardia occur, notify prescriber immediately
- Assess for extrapyramidal symptoms including akathisia (inability to sit still, no pattern to movements), tardive dyskinesia (bizarre movements of the jaw, mouth, tongue, extremities), pseudoparkinsonism (ragged tremors, pill rolling, shuffling gate); an antiparkinsonian drug should be prescribed
- Assess for constipation and urinary retention daily; if these occur, increase bulk, water in diet

Nursing diagnoses

- ✓ Thought processes, altered (uses)
- ✓ Coping, ineffective individual (uses)
- ✓ Knowledge deficit (teaching)
- ✓ Noncompliance (teaching)

Implementation

PO route

- Give drug in liquid form mixed in glass of juice or caffeine-free cola if hoarding is suspected; do not mix in caffeine drinks, tannics, pectins
- G • Give decreased dosage in elderly because of slower metabolism
- Give PO with full glass of water, milk; or give with food to decrease GI upset
- Store in tight, light-resistant container, oral sol in amber bottle

IM route

- Inject in deep muscle mass, do not give SC; use 21-G 2-inch needle; do not administer sol with a precipitate; give <3 ml per inj site; give slowly, may be painful

Syringe compatibilities:

Hydromorphone, sufentanil

Y-*site compatibilities:*

Amifostine, amsacrine, aztreonam, cimetidine, cisatracurium, cladribine, dobutamine, dopamine, doxorubicin liposome, famotidine, filgrastim, fludarabine, granisetron, lidocaine, lorazepam, melphalan, midazolam, nitroglycerin, norepinephrine, ondansetron, paclitaxel, phenylephrine, propofol, remifentanil, sufentanil, tacrolimus, teniposide, theophylline, thiotepa, vinorelbine

Y-*site incompatibilities:*

Fluconazole, foscarnet, heparin, sargramostim

Patient/family education

- Teach patient to use good oral hygiene; use frequent rinsing of mouth, sugarless gum for dry mouth
- Advise patient to avoid hazardous activities until drug response is determined; dizziness, blurred vision are common
- Inform patient that orthostatic hypotension occurs often and to rise from sitting or lying position gradually; to remain lying down after IM inj for at least 30 min; tell patient to avoid hot tubs, hot showers, tub baths, since hypotension may occur; tell patient that in hot weather heat stroke may occur; take extra precautions to stay cool
- Instruct patient to avoid abrupt withdrawal of this drug, or extrapyramidal symptoms may result; drug should be withdrawn slowly
- Caution patient to avoid OTC preparations (cough, hay fever, cold) unless approved by prescriber, since serious drug interactions may occur; avoid use with alcohol, CNS depressants since increased drowsiness may occur
- Advise patient to use a sunscreen and sunglasses to prevent burns
- Teach patient about extrapyramidal symptoms and necessity of meticulous oral hygiene, since oral candidiasis may occur
- Instruct patient to take antacids 2 hr before or after this drug
- Tell patient to report sore throat, malaise, fever, bleeding, mouth sores; if these occur, CBC should be obtained and drug discontinued

Evaluation

Positive therapeutic outcome

- Decrease in emotional excitement, hallucinations, delusions, paranoia, reorganization of patterns of thought, speech; improvement in specific behaviors
- Reorganization of patterns of thought, speech

Treatment of overdose:

Lavage if orally ingested; provide airway; *do not induce vomiting*

H

HIGH ALERT

heparin (℞)

(hep'a-rin)

Calcilean ♣, Calciparine, Hepalean ♣, Heparin Sodium and 0.45% Sodium Chloride, Heparin Sodium and 0.9% Sodium Chloride, Heparin Leo ♣, Heparin Lock Flush, Heparin Sodium, Hep-Lock, Hep-Lock U/P, Liquaemin Sodium

Func. class.: Anticoagulant, antithrombotic

Pregnancy category C

Action: Prevents conversion of fibrinogen to fibrin and prothrombin to thrombin by enhancing inhibitory effects of antithrombin III

Therapeutic Outcome: Prevention of thrombi

Uses: Deep vein thrombosis (DVT) and pulmonary emboli (PE) (treatment and prevention), MI, open heart surgery, disseminated intravascular clotting syndrome, atrial fibrillation with embolization, as an anticoagulant in transfusion and dialysis procedures

Dosage and routes

DVT/MI

Adult: **IV** push 5000-7000 U q4h then titrated to PTT or activated coagulation time (ACT) level; **IV** bol 5000-7500 U, then **IV** inf; **IV** inf after bol dose, then 1000 U/hr titrated to PTT or ACT level

P ***Child:*** **IV** inf 50 U/kg, maintenance 100 U/kg q4h or 20,000 U/m^2 qd

Anticoagulation

Adult: SC 5000 U IV then 10,000-20,000 U, then 8,000-10,000 U q8h or 15,000-20,000 U q12h

Pulmonary embolism

Adult: **IV** push 7500-10,000 q4h then titrated to PTT or ACT level; **IV** bol 7500-10,000, then **IV** inf; **IV** inf after bol dose, then 1000 U/hr titrated to PTT or ACT level

P ***Child:*** **IV** inf 50 U/kg; maintenance 100 U/kg q4h or 20,000 U/m^2 qd

CV surgery

Adult: **IV** inf 150-300 U/kg, prophylaxis for DVT/PE; SC 5,000 U q8-12h

Heparin flush

P ***Adult/child:*** **IV** 10-100 U

Available forms: Sodium: carpuject 5000 U/ml; disposable inj 1000, 2500, 5000, 7500, 10,000, 15,000, 20,000, 40,000 U/ml; unit dose 1000, 5000, 10,000, 20,000, 40,000 U/ml; vials 1000, 2000, 2500, 5000, 7500, 10,000, 20,000, 40,000 U/ml; flush, disposable syringes 10, 100 U/ml; vials 10, 100 U/ml; ampules 12,500 U/0.5 ml; 20,000 U/0.8 ml

Adverse effects

CNS: *Fever,* chills

GI: *Diarrhea,* nausea, vomiting, anorexia, stomatitis, abdominal cramps, **hepatitis**

GU: **Hematuria**

HEMA: **Hemorrhage, thrombocytopenia**

INTEG: *Rash,* dermatitis, urticaria, alopecia, pruritus

SYST: **Anaphylaxis**

Contraindications: Hypersensitivity, hemophilia, leukemia with bleeding, peptic ulcer disease, thrombocytopenic purpura, hepatic disease (severe), renal disease (severe), blood dyscrasias, severe hypertension, subacute bacterial endocarditis, acute nephritis

Precautions: Alcoholism, elderly, pregnancy **C**

Pharmacokinetics	
Absorption	Well absorbed (SC)
Distribution	Unknown
Metabolism	Unknown
Excretion	Lymph, spleen
Half-life	1½ hr

Pharmacodynamics

	SC	IV
Onset	½-1 hr	5 min
Peak	2 hr	10 min
Duration	8-12 hr	2-6 hr

Lab test interferences

↓ Uric acid

False: ↑ T_3 uptake, ↑ serum thyroxine, ↑ BSP

False negative: ^{125}I fibrinogen uptake

NURSING CONSIDERATIONS

Assessment

- Assess for blood studies (Hct, occult blood in stools) q3 mo if patient is on long-term therapy
- Monitor PPT, which should be 1½-2 × control, PTT; often done qd, APTT, ACT
- Monitor platelet count q2-3 days; thrombocytopenia may occur on 4th day of treatment and resolve, or continue to 8th day of treatment
- Assess for bleeding gums, petechiae, ecchymosis, black tarry stools, hematuria, epistaxis, decrease in Hct, B/P; may indicate bleeding and possible hemorrhage; notify prescriber immediately
- Monitor for hypersensitivity: fever, skin rash, urticaria; notify prescriber immediately

Nursing diagnoses

✓ Injury, risk for (uses, adverse reactions)

✓ Tissue perfusion, altered (uses)

✓ Knowledge deficit (teaching)

Implementation

IV route

- Give directly; **IV** loading dose over 1 min
- Give **IV** diluted in 0.9% NaCl, dextrose, Ringer's and by intermittent or cont inf; inf may run from 4-24 hr; use infusion pump

Syringe compatibilities:

Aminophylline, amphotericin B, ampicillin, atropine, azlocillin, bleomycin, cefamandole, cefazolin, cefoperazone, cefotaxime, cefoxitin, chloramphenicol, cimetidine, cisplatin, clindamycin, cyclophosphamide, diazoxide, digoxin, dimenhydrinate, dobutamine, dopamine, epinephrine, fentanyl, fluorouracil, furosemide, leucovorin, lidocaine, lincomycin, methotrexate, metoclopramide, mezlocillin, mitomycin, moxalactam, nafcillin, naloxone, neostigmine, nitroglycerin, norepinephrine, pancuronium, penicillin G, phenobarbital, piperacillin, sodium nitroprusside, succinylcholine, trimethoprim-sulfamethoxazole, verapamil, vincristine

Y-site compatibilities:

Acyclovir, aldesleukin, allopurinol, amifostine, aminophylline, ampicillin, ampicillin/sulbactam, atracurium, atropine, aztreonam, betamethasone, bleomycin, calcium gluconate, cefazolin, cefotetan, ceftazidime, ceftriaxone, cephalothin, cephapirin, chlordiazepoxide, chlorpromazine, cimetidine, cisplatin, cladribine, clindamycin, conjugated estrogens, cyanocobalamin, cyclophosphamide, cytarabine, dexamethasone, digoxin, diphenhydramine, dopamine, doxorubicin liposome, edrophonium, enalaprilat, epinephrine, erythromycin, esmolol, ethacrynate, famotidine, fentanyl, fluconazole, fludarabine, fluorouracil, foscarnet, furosemide, gallium, granisetron, hydralazine, hydrocortisone, hydromorphone, regular insulin, isoproterenol, kanamycin, leucovorin, lidocaine, lorazepam, magnesium sulfate, melphalan, menadiol sodium, meperidine, meropenem, methicillin, methotrexate, methoxamine, methyldopate, methylergonovine, metoclopramide, metronidazole, midazolam, milrinone, minocycline, mitomycin, morphine, nafcillin, neostigmine, nitroglycerin, nitroprusside, norepinephrine, ondansetron, oxacillin, oxytocin, paclitaxel, pancuronium, penicillin G potassium, pentazocine, phytonadione, piperacillin, piperacillin/tazobactam, propofol, potassium chloride, prednisolone, procainamide, prochlorperazine, propofol, propranolol, pyridostigmine, ranitidine, remifentanil, sargramostim, scopolamine, sodium bicarbonate, streptokinase, succinylcholine, tacrolimus, teniposide, theophylline, thiopental, thiotepa, ticarcillin, ticarcillin/clavulanate, trimethobenzamide, vecuronium, vinblastine, vincristine, vinorelbine, warfarin, zidovudine

Y-site incompatibilities:
Alteplase, ciprofloxacin, dacarbazine, diazepam, dobutamine, doxorubicin, ergotamine, gentamicin, haloperidol, idarubicin, methotrimeprazine, phenytoin, promethazine, tobramycin, triflupromazine

Additive compatibilities:
Aminophylline, amphotericin, ascorbic acid, bleomycin, calcium gluconate, cefepime, cephapirin, chloramphenicol, clindamycin, colistimethate, dimenhydrinate, doxacillin, dopamine, enalaprilat, erythromycin, esmolol, floxacillin, fluconazole, flumazenil, furosemide, hydrocortisone, isoproterenol, lidocaine, lincomycin, magnesium sulfate, meropenem, methyldopate, methylprednisolone, metronidazole/sodium bicarbonate, nafcillin, norepinephrine, octreotide, penicillin G, potassium chloride, prednisolone, promazine, ranitidine, sodium bicarbonate, verapamil, vit B complex, vit B complex with C

Additive incompatibilities:
Amikacin, erythromycin lactobionate, gentamicin, kanamycin, meperidine, methadone, morphine, polymyxin B, streptomycin

Heparin lock route
- Inject 10-100 U/0.5-1 ml after each inf or q8-12h

SC route
- Give SC with at least 25-G ⅜-in needle; do not massage area or aspirate fluid when giving SC inj; give in abdomen between pelvic bones, rotate sites; do not pull back on plunger, leave in for 10 sec; apply gentle pressure for 1 min
- Give at same time each day to maintain steady blood levels
- Changing needles is not recommended

Patient/family education
- Advise patient to avoid OTC preparations that may cause serious drug interactions unless directed by prescriber; may contain aspirin or other anticoagulants
- Tell patient that drug may be held during active bleeding (menstruation), depending on condition
- Caution patient to use soft-bristle toothbrush to avoid bleeding gums; avoid contact sports; use electric razor; avoid IM inj
- Instruct patient to carry an ID or other identification identifying drug taken and condition treated
- Advise patient to report any signs of bleeding: gums, under skin, urine, stools; or unusual bruising

Evaluation
Positive therapeutic outcome
- Decrease of DVT
- PTT of 1.5-2.5 × control
- Free-flowing **IV**

Treatment of overdose:
Withdraw drug, give protamine sulfate

hepatitis B immune globulin (℞)
(hep-a-tite'iss)
BayHep B, Nabi-HB
Func. class.: Immune globulin
Pregnancy category C

Action: Provides passive immunity to hepatitis B

Therapeutic Outcome: Passive immunity to hepatitis B

Uses: Prevention of hepatitis B virus in exposed patients, including passive P immunity in neonates born to HBsAg-positive mother

Dosage and routes

Acute exposure to blood with HBsAg

Adult: 2 doses, given after exposure and 1 mo later

Perinatal exposure of infants born to HBsAg-positive mothers

P ***Infant:*** 1 dose at birth, then start hepatitis B vaccine series soon after birth

Sexual exposure to HBsAg

Adult: Administer 1 dose within 2 wk of exposure

Available forms: Bay-Hep B: sol for inj 15%-18% protein; Nabi-HB: sol for inj 5% ± 1% protein

Adverse effects

CNS: Headache, dizziness, fever, faintness, weakness

INTEG: Soreness at inj site, urticaria, erythema, swelling, pruritus

MS: Joint pain

SYST: **Anaphylaxis, angioedema**

Contraindications: Hypersensitivity to immune globulins, coagulation disorders

G **Precautions:** Pregnancy **C**, elderly, P lactation, children, active infection, IgA deficiency

Pharmacokinetics	
Absorption	Slowly absorbed
Distribution	Unknown
Metabolism	Unknown
Excretion	Unknown
Half-life	3 wk

Pharmacodynamics	
Onset	1-7 days
Peak	3-10 days
Duration	2-6 mo

Interactions

Drug classifications

Live vaccines: ↓ or ↑ immune response

NURSING CONSIDERATIONS

Assessment

- Assess for history of allergies, skin conditions (eczema, psoriasis, dermatitis), reactions to vaccinations
- Assess for skin reactions: rash, induration, urticaria
- Assess for sneezing, pruritus, angioedema, dysphagia, vomiting, abdominal pain
- ! Assess for anaphylaxis: inability to breathe, bronchospasm, hypotension, wheezing, diaphoresis, fever, flushing; epinephrine and emergency equipment should be available

Nursing diagnoses

✓ Infection, risk for (uses)
✓ Knowledge deficit (teaching)

Implementation

- Give after rotating vial; do not shake
- Give in deltoid (adult) or anterolateral thigh for better protection; give 2-ml dose in two different sites; do not give **IV**
- Refrigerate unused portion; sol should be clear, light amber, and thick

Patient/family education

- Teach patient purpose of medication and expected results
- Give patient a list of adverse reactions that need to be reported immediately: wheezing, vomiting, sneezing, abdominal pain, sweating, tightness in chest
- Advise patient that pain, rash, swelling at inj site can be expected
- Give patient written record of immunization

Evaluation

Positive therapeutic outcome

- Prevention of hepatitis B

hetastarch (℞)
(het'a-starch)
Hespan
Func. class.: Plasma expander
Chem. class.: Synthetic polymer
Pregnancy category C

Action: Similar to human albumin, which expands plasma volume by colloidal osmotic pressure

Therapeutic Outcome: Increased plasma volume

Uses: Plasma volume expander for sepsis, trauma, burns, leukapheresis

Dosage and routes

Adult: **IV** inf 500-1000 ml (30-60 g); total dose not to exceed 1500 ml/day, not to exceed 20 ml/kg/hr (hemorrhagic shock)

Leukapheresis

Adult: **IV** inf 250-700 ml infused at 1:8 ratio with whole blood; may be repeated twice weekly up to 10 treatments

Available forms: 6% hetastarch/ 0.9% NaCl (6 g/100 ml)

Adverse effects

CNS: Headache
GI: Nausea, vomiting
HEMA: Decreased hematocrit, platelet function, increased bleeding/ coagulation times, increased erythrocyte sedimentation rate
INTEG: Rash, urticaria, pruritus, angioedema, chills, fever, flushing, peripheral edema
RESP: Wheezing, dyspnea, **bronchospasm, pulmonary edema**
SYST: **Anaphylaxis**

Contraindications: Hypersensitivity, severe bleeding disorders, renal failure, CHF (severe)

Precautions: Pregnancy **C**, liver disease, pulmonary edema

Pharmacokinetics

Absorption	Completely absorbed
Distribution	Unknown
Metabolism	Degraded
Excretion	Kidneys, unchanged
Half-life	17 days (90%); 48 days (10%)

Pharmacodynamics

Onset	Immediate
Peak	Infusion's end
Duration	Over 24 hr

Interactions: None

Lab test interferences

False: ↑ Bilirubin

NURSING CONSIDERATIONS

Assessment

- Monitor VS q5 min for 30 min; CVP during inf (5-10 cm H_2O normal range); PCWP; urine output q1h: watch for increase which is common; if output does not increase, inf should be decreased or discontinued
- Monitor CBC with differential, Hgb, Hct, pro-time, PTT, platelet count, clotting time during treatment; treatment may increase clotting time, PTT, pro-time, sedimentary rates, Hct may drop due to increase volume and hemodilution; do not allow Hct to be <30% by volume
- Monitor I&O ratio and sp gr, urine osmolarity; if sp gr is very low, renal clearance is low; drug should be discontinued
- Assess for allergy: rash, urticaria, pruritus, wheezing, dyspnea, bronchospasm; drug should be discontinued immediately
- Assess for circulatory overload: increased pulse, respirations, dyspnea, wheezing, chest tightness, chest pain, increased CVP, jugular vein distention
- Assess for dehydration after inf; decreased output, increased temp, poor skin turgor, increased sp gr, dry skin

Nursing diagnoses
- ✓ Fluid volume deficit (uses)
- ✓ Tissue perfusion, altered (uses)
- ✓ Fluid volume excess (adverse reactions)
- ✓ Knowledge deficit (teaching)

Implementation
- Give by **IV** cont inf, undiluted, run at 20 ml/kg/hr; reduced rate in septic shock, burns; rate is calculated by blood volume and response of patient
- Give up to 20 ml kg (1.2 g/ kg)/hr
- Store at room temp; discard unused portions; do not freeze; do not use if turbid or deep brown or precipitate forms

Y-site compatibilities: Cimetidine, diltiazem, doxycycline, enalaprilat

Y-site incompatibilities: Amikacin, cefamandole, cefoperazone, cefotaxime, cefoxitin, gentamicin, theophylline, tobramycin

Additive compatibilities: Cloxacillin, fosphenytoin

Patient/family education
- Teach patient the reason for administration and expected results
- Advise patient to notify prescriber if flulike symptoms or allergic symptoms occur

Evaluation
Positive therapeutic outcome
- Increased plasma volume as evidenced by higher B/P, blood volume, output

hydralazine (℞)
(hye-dral'a-zeen)

Alazine, Apresoline, Dralzine, Novo-Hylazin ♣, hydralazine HCl, Rolzine, Supres ♣

Func. class.: Antihypertensive, direct-acting peripheral vasodilator

Chem. class.: Phthalazine

Pregnancy category C

Action: Vasodilates arterioles in smooth muscle by direct relaxation; reduces B/P with reflex increases in cardiac function

➔ **Therapeutic Outcome:** Decreased B/P in hypertension, decreased afterload in CHF

Uses: Essential hypertension, severe essential hypertension, CHF

Dosage and routes
Adult: PO 10 mg qid 2-4 days, then 25 mg for rest of 1st wk, then 50 mg qid individualized to desired response, not to exceed 300 mg qd; **IV**/IM bol 20-40 mg q4-6h; administer PO as soon as possible; IM 20-40 mg q4-6h

P ***Child:*** PO 0.75-3 mg/kg/day in 4 divided doses; max 7.5 mg/kg/24 hr; **IV** bol 0.10.2 mg/kg q4-6h; IM 0.1-0.2 mg/kg q4-6h

Available forms: Inj 20 mg/ml; tabs 10, 25, 50, 100 mg

Adverse effects
CNS: *Headache, tremors, dizziness, anxiety,* peripheral neuritis, depression

CV: *Palpitations, reflex tachycardia, angina,* **shock,** edema, rebound hypertension

GI: *Nausea, vomiting, anorexia, diarrhea,* constipation

GU: Impotence, urinary retention, Na^+, H_2O retention

HEMA: **Leukopenia, agranulocytosis,** anemia, **thrombocytopenia**

INTEG: Rash, pruritus

MISC: Nasal congestion, muscle cramps, *lupus-like symptoms*

Contraindications: Hypersensitivity to hydralazines, CAD, mitral valvular rheumatic heart disease, rheumatic heart disease

Precautions: Pregnancy **C**, CVA, advanced renal disease, elderly

Do Not Confuse:
Apresoline/allopurinol

Pharmacokinetics

Absorption	Rapidly absorbed (PO); well absorbed (IM); completely absorbed (**IV**)
Distribution	Widely distributed; crosses placenta
Metabolism	GI mucosa, liver extensively
Excretion	Kidneys
Half-life	2-8 hr

Pharmacodynamics

	PO	IM	IV
Onset	½ hr	10-30 min	5-20 min
Peak	1 hr	1 hr	10-80 min
Duration	2-4 hr	4-6 hr	4-6 hr

Interactions
Individual drugs
Alcohol: ↑ hypotension
Drug classifications
Antihypertensives: ↑ hypotension
β-Adrenergic blockers: ↑ bradycardia, CHF
MAOIs: ↑ hypotension
Nitrates: ↑ action of nitrates
NSAIDs: ↓ antihypertensive effect

NURSING CONSIDERATIONS
Assessment
- Assess B/P q5 min for 2 hr, then q1h for 2 hr, then q4h; pulse, jugular venous distention q4h
- Monitor electrolytes, blood studies: potassium, sodium, chloride, carbon dioxide, CBC, serum glucose; LE prep, ANA titer before starting treatment
- Monitor weight daily, I&O; edema in feet, legs daily; check skin turgor, dryness of mucous membranes for hydration status
- Assess for rales, dyspnea, orthopnea; peripheral edema, fatigue, weight gain, jugular vein distention (CHF)
- For fever, joint pain, rash, sore throat (lupus-like symptoms), notify prescriber

Nursing diagnoses
- ✓ Cardiac output, decreased (adverse reactions)
- ✓ Injury, risk for physical (side effects)
- ✓ Knowledge deficit (teaching)

Implementation
PO route
- Give with meals to enhance absorption
- Store protected from light and heat

IV route
- Give by **IV** undiluted through Y-tube or 3-way stopcock ≤10 mg/min
- Administer with patient in recumbent position; keep in that position for 1 hr after administration

Y-site compatibilities: Heparin, hydrocortisone, potassium chloride, verapamil, vit B/C

Y-site incompatibilities: Aminophylline, ampicillin, diazoxide, furosemide, paclitaxel

Additive incompatibilities: Aminophylline, ampicillin, chlorothiazide, edetate calcium disodium, ethacrynate, hydrocortisone, melphalan, mephentermine, methohexital, nitroglycerin, phenobarbital, verapamil, vinorelbine

Additive compatibilities: Dobutamine

Patient/family education
- Teach patient to take with food to increase bioavailability (PO)
- Teach patient to avoid OTC preparations unless directed by prescriber
- Advise patient to notify prescriber if

chest pain, severe fatigue, fever, muscle or joint pain occur

- Advise patient to rise slowly to prevent orthostatic hypertension
- Advise patient to notify prescriber if pregnancy is suspected

Evaluation

Positive therapeutic outcome

- Decreased B/P in hypertension

Treatment of overdose: Administer vasopressors, volume expanders for shock; if PO, lavage or give activated charcoal, digitalization

hydrochlorothiazide (℞)

(hye-droe-klor-oh-thye′a-zide)

Diaqua, Diachlor H ✤, Esidrix, Hydro-Chlor, hydrochlorothiazide, HydroDiuril, Hydromal, Hydro-T, Hydrozide ✤, Microzide, Neo-Codema ✤, Novohydrazide ✤, Oretic, Thiuretic, Urozide ✤

Func. class: Diuretic, antihypertensive

Chem. class: Thiazide, sulfonamide derivative

Pregnancy category B

Action: Acts on the distal tubule in the kidney, increasing excretion of sodium, water, chloride, magnesium, potassium, and bicarbonate

Therapeutic Outcome: Decreased B/P, decreased edema in lung tissues peripherally

Uses: Edema in CHF, nephrotic syndrome; edema in corticosteroid, NSAID therapy; idiopathic lower extremity edema; may be used alone or as adjunct with antihypertensives

Dosage and routes

Adult: PO 25-200 mg/day

G ***Elderly:*** PO 12.5 mg/day, initially

P ***Child >6 mo:*** PO 2 mg/kg/day

P ***Child <6 mo:*** PO up to 4 mg/kg/day in divided doses

Available forms: Tabs 25, 50, 100 mg; sol 50 mg/5 ml, 100 mg/ml

Adverse effects

CNS: Drowsiness, paresthesia, anxiety, depression, headache, *dizziness, fatigue, weakness*

CV: Irregular pulse, orthostatic hypotension, palpitations, volume depletion, allergic myocarditis

EENT: Blurred vision

ELECT: *Hypokalemia,* hypercalcemia, hyponatremia, hypochloremia, hypomagnesemia

GI: *Nausea, vomiting, anorexia,* constipation, diarrhea, cramps, pancreatitis, GI irritation, **hepatitis**

GU: *Frequency,* polyuria, **uremia,** glucosuria

HEMA: **Aplastic anemia, hemolytic anemia, leukopenia, agranulocytosis, thrombocytopenia, neutropenia**

INTEG: *Rash,* urticaria, purpura, photosensitivity, fever, alopecia, erythema multiform

META: *Hyperglycemia, hyperuricemia,* increased creatinine, BUN

Contraindications: Hypersensitivity to thiazides or sulfonamides, anuria, renal decompensation, lactation

Precautions: Hypokalemia, renal disease, hepatic disease, gout, COPD, lupus erythematosus, diabetes mellitus, elderly, hyperlipidemia, CrCl <25 ml/min, pregnancy **B**

Pharmacokinetics

	PO
Absorption	Variable
Distribution	Extracellular spaces; crosses placenta
Metabolism	Excreted unchanged in urine
Excretion	Breast milk
Half-life	6-15 hr

Pharmacodynamics

Onset	2 hr
Peak	4 hr
Duration	6-12 hr

Interactions

Individual drugs

Cholestyramine: ↓ absorption of hydrochlorothiazide
Colestipol: ↓ absorption of hydrochlorothiazide
Diazoxide: ↑ hyperglycemia, hyperuricemia, hypotension
Digitalis: ↑ toxicity
Lithium: ↑ toxicity
Mezlocillin: ↑ hypokalemia
Piperacillin: ↑ hypokalemia
Ticarcillin: ↑ hypokalemia

Drug classifications

Anticoagulants: ↓ effects of anticoagulants
Antidiabetics: ↓ effect of antidiabetic agent
Antihypertensives: ↑ antihypertensive effect
Diuretics, loop: ↑ effects of diuretic
Glucocorticoids: ↑ hypokalemia
NSAIDs: ↑ risk of renal failure
Sulfonylureas: ↓ effect of sulfonylurea

Food/drug

↑ Absorption

Lab test interferences

↑ BSP retention, ↑ calcium, ↑ amylase, ↑ parathyroid test
↓ PBI, ↓ PSP

NURSING CONSIDERATIONS

Assessment

- Monitor glucose in urine if patient is diabetic
- Assess improvement in CVP q8h
- Check for rashes, temp elevation qd
- Assess for confusion, especially in G elderly; take safety precautions if needed
- Monitor manifestations of hypokalemia: acidic urine, reduced urine, osmolality, nocturia; hypotension, broad T wave, U wave, ectopy, tachycardia, weak pulse; muscle weakness, altered LOC, drowsiness, apathy, lethargy, confusion, depression; anorexia, nausea, cramps, constipation, distention, paralytic ileus; hypoventilation, respiratory muscle weakness
- Monitor for manifestations of hypomagnesemia: agitation, muscle twitching, paresthesias, hyperactive reflexes, positive Babinski reflex, dysphagia, nystagmus seizures, tetany; nausea, vomiting, diarrhea, anorexia, abdominal distention; ectopy, tachycardia, broad, flat, or inverted T waves, depressed ST segment, prolonged QT interval, decreased cardiac output, hypotension
- Monitor for manifestations of hyponatremia: increased B/P, cold, clammy skin, hypovolemia or hypervolemia; anorexia, nausea, vomiting, diarrhea, abdominal cramps; lethargy, increased ICP, confusion, headache, seizures, coma, fatigue, tremors, hyperreflexia
- Monitor for manifestations of hyperchloremia: weakness, lethargy, coma, deep rapid breathing
- Assess fluid volume status: I&O ratios, record, count, or weigh diapers as appropriate, weight, distended red veins, crackles in lungs, color, quality, and sp gr of urine, skin turgor, adequacy of pulses, moist mucous membranes, bilateral lung sounds, peripheral pitting edema; assess for dehydration: symptoms of decreasing output, thirst, hypotension; dry mouth and mucous membranes should be reported
- Monitor electrolytes: potassium, sodium, calcium, magnesium; also include BUN, blood pH, ABGs, uric acid, CBC, blood glucose, renal function
- Assess B/P before and during therapy with patient lying, standing, and sitting as appropriate; orthostatic hypotension can occur rapidly

Nursing diagnoses
- ✓ Altered urinary elimination (side effect)
- ✓ Fluid volume deficit (side effects)
- ✓ Fluid volume excess (uses)
- ✓ Knowledge deficit (teaching)

Implementation
- Give in AM to avoid interference with sleep
- Provide potassium replacement if potassium level is ≤3.0 mg/dl; give whole tab or use oral sol lightly; drug may be crushed if patient is unable to swallow
- Administer with food; if nausea occurs, absorption may be increased

Patient/family education
- Teach patient to take the medication early in the day to prevent nocturia
- Instruct patient to take with food or milk if GI symptoms of nausea and anorexia occur
- Teach patient to maintain a weekly record of weight and notify prescriber of weight loss >5 lb
- Caution patient that this drug causes a loss of potassium and that food rich in potassium should be added to the diet; refer to a dietitian for assistance in planning
- Caution patient not to exercise in hot weather or stand for prolonged periods since orthostatic hypotension will be enhanced
- Teach patient not to use alcohol or any OTC medications without prescriber's approval; serious drug reactions may occur
- Emphasize the need to contact prescriber immediately if muscle cramps, weakness, nausea, dizziness, or numbness occurs
- Teach patient to take own B/P and pulse and record findings
- Caution patient that orthostatic hypotension may occur; patient should rise slowly from sitting or reclining positions and lie down if dizziness occurs
- Teach patient to continue taking medication even if feeling better; this drug controls symptoms but does not cure the condition
- Advise patient with hypertension to continue other medical treatment (exercise, weight loss, relaxation techniques, cessation of smoking)

Evaluation
Positive therapeutic outcome
- Decreased edema
- Decreased B/P
- Increased diuresis

Treatment of overdose:
Lavage if taken orally, monitor electrolytes, administer dextrose in saline, monitor hydration, CV, renal status

hydrocodone (℞)
(hye-droe-koe'done)

Hycodan ✤, Robidone ✤, Tussigon

See Combination products section

Func. class.: Narcotic analgesic

Chem. class.: Opioid analgesic, antitussive

Pregnancy category C

Controlled substance schedule III

Action: Acts directly on cough center in medulla to suppress cough; binds to opiate receptors in the CNS to reduce pain

➔ **Therapeutic Outcome:** Pain relief, decreased cough, decreased diarrhea

Uses: Hyperactive and nonproductive cough, mild pain

Dosages and routes
Adult: PO 5-10 mg q4h prn

P ***Child:*** PO 2-12 mg 1.25-5 mg q4h prn or 0.2 mg/kg q3-4h

Available forms: Syrup 5 mg/5 ml; tabs 5 mg

Adverse effects
CNS: *Drowsiness,* dizziness, light-

headedness, confusion, headache, sedation, euphoria, dysphoria, weakness, hallucinations, disorientation, mood changes, dependence, **seizures**
CV: Palpitations, tachycardia, bradycardia, change in B/P, **circulatory depression,** syncope
EENT: Tinnitus, blurred vision, miosis, diplopia
GI: *Nausea, vomiting, anorexia, constipation,* cramps, dry mouth
GU: Increased urinary output, dysuria, urinary retention
INTEG: Rash, urticaria, flushing, pruritus
RESP: **Respiratory depression**

Contraindications: Hypersensitivity, addiction (narcotic)

Precautions: Addictive personality, pregnancy **C**, lactation, increased ICP, MI (acute), severe heart disease, respiratory depression, hepatic disease, renal disease

Do Not Confuse:
Hycodan/Vicodin, hydrocodone/hydrocortisone

Pharmacokinetics

Absorption	Well absorbed
Distribution	Unknown; crosses placenta
Metabolism	Liver, extensively
Excretion	Kidneys
Half-life	3½-4½ hr

Pharmacodynamics

	PO (analgesic)	PO (antitussive)
Onset	10-20 min	Unknown
Peak	30-60 min	Unknown
Duration	4-6 hr	4-6 hr

Interactions
Individual drugs
Alcohol: ↑ respiratory depression, hypotension, sedation
Cimetidine: ↑ recovery
Erythromycin: ↑ recovery
Nalbuphine: ↓ analgesia
Pentazocine: ↓ analgesia

Drug classifications
Antihistamines: ↑ respiratory depression, hypotension
CNS depressants: ↑ respiratory depression, hypotension
MAOIs: Do not use for 2 wk before taking hydrocodone
Phenothiazines: ↑ respiratory depression, hypotension
Sedative/hypnotics: ↑ respiratory depression, hypotension

Lab test interferences
↑ Amylase, ↑ lipase

NURSING CONSIDERATIONS
Assessment
- Assess pain: intensity, type, location, duration, precipitating factor
- Monitor VS after parenteral route; note muscle rigidity, drug history, liver, kidney function tests, cough, and respiratory dysfunction: respiratory depression, character, rate, rhythm; notify prescriber if respirations are <10/min
- Monitor CNS changes: dizziness, drowsiness, hallucinations, euphoria, LOC, pupil reaction
- Monitor allergic reactions: rash, urticaria

Nursing diagnoses
- ✓ Pain (uses)
- ✓ Sensory-perceptual alteration: visual, auditory (adverse reactions)
- ✓ Breathing pattern, ineffective (adverse reactions)
- ✓ Knowledge deficit (teaching)

Implementation
- Give with antiemetic if nausea, vomiting occur
- Give when pain is beginning to return; determine dosage interval by patient response; continuous dosing of medication is more effective given prn
- Medication should be slowly withdrawn after long-term use to prevent withdrawal symptoms

- Store in light-resistant container at room temp
- May be given with food or milk to lessen GI upset
- Do not crush, chew caps

Patient/family education

- Instruct patient to report any symptoms of CNS changes, allergic reactions; to avoid CNS depressants: alcohol, sedative/hypnotics for at least 24 hr after taking this drug
- Teach patient that dizziness, drowsiness, and confusion are common and to avoid getting up without assistance, driving, or other hazardous activities
- Discuss in detail all aspects of the drug

Evaluation

Positive therapeutic outcome

- Decreased pain
- Decreased cough

Treatment of overdose:

Naloxone HCl (Narcan) 0.2-0.8 **IV**, O_2, **IV** fluids, vasopressors

hydrocortisone (℞)
(hy-droh-kor′tih-sone)
Cortef, Cortenema, Hydrocortone

hydrocortisone acetate (℞)
Cortifoam, Hydrocortone Acetate

hydrocortisone cypionate (℞)
Cortef

hydrocortisone sodium phosphate (℞)
Hydrocortone Phosphate

hydrocortisone sodium succinate (℞)
A-hydroCort, Solu-Cortef

Func. class.: Short-acting glucocorticoid

Chem. class.: Natural nonfluorinated, group IV potency (valerate), group VI potency (acetate and plain)

Pregnancy category C

Action: Decreases inflammation by suppressing migration of polymorphonuclear leukocytes and fibroblasts and reversing increased capillary permeability and lysosomal stabilization (systemic); antipruritic, antiinflammatory (top)

Therapeutic Outcome: Decreased inflammation

Uses: Severe inflammation, septic shock, adrenal insufficiency, ulcerative colitis, collagen disorders (systemic), psoriasis, eczema, contact dermatitis, pruritus (top)

Dosage and routes

Adrenal insufficiency/inflammation

Adult: PO 5-30 mg bid-qid; IM/**IV** 100-250 mg (succinate), then 50-100 mg IM as needed; IM/**IV** 15-240 mg q12h (phosphate)

Shock

Adult: 500 mg-2 g q2-6h (succinate)

P **Child:** IM/**IV** 0.186-1 mg/kg bid-tid (succinate)

Colitis

Adult: Enema 100 mg nightly for 21 days

Topical route

P ***Adult and child >2 yr:*** Apply to affected area qd-qid

Available forms: Oint 0.5%, 1%, 2.5%; cream 0.25%, 0.5%, 1%, 2.5%; lotion 0.25%, 0.5%, 1%, 2%, 2.5%; gel 1%; sol 1%; aerosol/pump spray 0.5%; *acetate:* oint 0.5%, 1%, 2.5%; cream 0.5%; lotion 0.05%; aerosol 1%; *valerate:* oint 0.2%; cream 0.2% (many others)

Adverse effects

CNS: Depression, flushing, sweating, headache, mood changes
CV: Hypertension, **circulatory collapse, thrombophlebitis, embolism,** tachycardia, edema
EENT: Fungal infections, increased intraocular pressure, blurred vision
GI: Diarrhea, nausea, abdominal distention, **GI hemorrhage,** increased appetite, pancreatitis
HEMA: **Thrombocytopenia**
INTEG: Acne, poor wound healing, ecchymosis, petechiae (top), burning, dryness, itching, irritation, acne, folliculitis, hypertrichosis, perioral dermatitis, hypopigmentation, atrophy, striae, miliaria, allergic contact dermatitis, secondary infection
MS: Fractures, osteoporosis, weakness

Contraindications: Psychosis, hypersensitivity, idiopathic thrombocytopenia, acute glomerulonephritis, amebiasis, fungal infections, nonasthmatic bronchial disease, P child <2 yr, AIDS, TB, fungal infections (top)

Precautions: Pregnancy **C,** diabetes mellitus, glaucoma, osteoporosis, seizure disorders, ulcerative colitis, CHF, myasthenia gravis, renal disease, esophagitis, peptic ulcer, lactation, (top) viral infections, bacterial infections

Do Not Confuse:
hydrocortisone/hydrocodone

Pharmacokinetics

Absorption	Well absorbed (PO); systemic (top)
Distribution	Crosses placenta
Metabolism	Liver, extensively
Excretion	Kidney
Half-life	3-5 hr, adrenal suppression 3-4 days

Pharmacodynamics

	PO	IM	IV	TOP
Onset	1-2 hr	20 min	Rapid	Min to hr
Peak	1 hr	4-8 hr	Unkn	Hr to days
Duration	1½ days	1½ days	1½ days	Hr to days

Interactions

Individual drugs

Amphotericin B: ↑ hypokalemia
Cholestyramine: ↓ action of hydrocortisone
Colestipol: ↓ action of hydrocortisone
Ephedrine: ↓ action of hydrocortisone
Insulin: ↑ need for insulin
Mezlocillin: ↑ hypokalemia
Phenytoin: ↓ action, ↑ metabolism
Rifampin: ↓ action, ↑ metabolism
Theophylline: ↓ action of hydrocortisone
Ticarcillin: ↑ hypokalemia

Drug classifications

Anticoagulants: ↓ action of anticoagulant
Barbiturates: ↓ action, ↑ metabolism
Diuretics: ↑ hypokalemia
Hypoglycemic agents: ↑ need for hypoglycemic agents
NSAIDs: ↑ risk of GI bleeding

Herb/drug

Aloe: ↑ hypokalemia
Buckthorn: ↑ hypokalemia
Cascara sagrada: ↑ hypokalemia
Senna: ↑ hypokalemia

Lab test interferences

↑ Cholesterol, ↑ sodium, ↑ blood glucose, ↑ uric acid, ↑ calcium, ↑ urine glucose

↓ Calcium, ↓ potassium, ↓ T_4, ↓ T_3, ↓ thyroid ^{131}I uptake test, ↓ urine 17-OHCS, ↓ 17-KS, ↓ PBI

False negative: Skin allergy tests

NURSING CONSIDERATIONS

Assessment

- Monitor potassium, blood glucose, urine glucose while patient is on long-term therapy; hypokalemia and hyperglycemia may occur
- Monitor I&O ratio; be alert for decreasing urinary output and increasing edema; weigh daily; notify prescriber of weekly gain >5 lb or edema, hypertension, cardiac symptoms
- Monitor plasma cortisol levels during long-term therapy (normal level is 138-635 nmol/L when obtained at 8 AM); check adrenal function periodically for hypothalamic-pituitary-adrenal axis suppression
- Assess for infection: increased temp, WBC even after withdrawal of medication; drug masks infection symptoms; if fever develops, drug should be discontinued
- Check for potassium depletion: paresthesias, fatigue, nausea, vomiting, depression, polyuria, dysrhythmias, weakness
- Assess mental status: affect, mood, behavioral changes, aggression
- Check nasal passages during long-term treatment for changes in mucus (nasal)
- Assess for systemic absorption: increased temp, inflammation, irritation (top)

Nursing diagnoses

✓ Infection, risk for (adverse reactions)
✓ Knowledge deficit (teaching)
✓ Noncompliance (teaching) (top/nasal preparation)

Implementation

PO route

- Give with food or milk to decrease GI symptoms

IV **IV route**

- Give only sodium phosphate product **IV**; reconstitute with sol provided; give 100 mg over >1 min
- May be given by intermittent inf in compatible sol
- Give titrated dose; use lowest effective dosage

Sodium phosphate preparations

Syringe compatibilities:
Fluconazole, fludarabine, metoclopramide

Additive compatibilities:
Amikacin, amphotericin B, bleomycin, cephapirin, metaraminol, sodium bicarbonate, verapamil

Y-site compatibilities:
Allopurinol, amifostine, aztreonam, cefepime, cladribine, famotidine, filgrastim, fluconazole, fludarabine, granisetron, melphalan, ondansetron, paclitaxel, piperacillin/tazobactam, teniposide, thiotepa, vinorelbine

Sodium succinate preparations

Syringe compatibilities:
Metoclopramide, thiopental

Y-site compatibilities:
Acyclovir, allopurinol, amifostine, aminophylline, ampicillin, amphotericin B cholesteryl, amrinone, amsacrine, atracurium, atropine, aztreonam, betamethasone, calcium gluconate, cefepime, cefmetazole, cephalothin, cephapirin, chlordiazepoxide, chlorpromazine, cisatracurium, cladribine, cyanocobalamin, cytarabine, dexamethasone, digoxin, diphenhydramine, dopamine, doxorubicin liposome, droperidol, edrophonium, enalaprilat, epinephrine, esmolol, conjugated estrogens, ethacrynate, famotidine, fentanyl, fentanyl/droperidol, filgrastim, flu-

H

darabine, fluorouracil, foscarnet, furosemide, gallium, granisetron, heparin, hydralazine, regular insulin, isoproterenol, kanamycin, lidocaine, lorazepam, magnesium sulfate, melphalan, menadiol, meperidine, methicillin, methoxamine, methylergonovine, minocycline, morphine, neostigmine, norepinephrine, ondansetron, oxacillin, oxytocin, paclitaxel, pancuronium, penicillin G potassium, pentazocine, phytonadione, piperacillin/tazobactam, prednisolone, procainamide, prochlorperazine, propofol, propranolol, pyridostigmine, remifentanil, scopolamine, sodium bicarbonate, succinylcholine, tacrolimus, teniposide, theophylline, thiotepa, trimethaphan, trimethobenzamide, vecuronium, vinorelbine

Y-site incompatibilities:
Diazepam, ergotamine tartrate, idarubicin, phenytoin, sargramostim

Additive compatibilities:
Amikacin, aminophylline, amphotericin B, calcium chloride, calcium gluconate, cephalothin, cephapirin, chloramphenicol, clindamycin, cloxacillin, corticotropin, daunorubicin, diphenhydramine, dopamine, erythromycin, floxacillin, lidocaine, magnesium sulfate, mephentermine, metronidazole/sodium bicarbonate, mitomycin, mitoxantrone, netilmicin, netilmicin/potassium chloride, norepinephrine, penicillin G potassium/sodium, piperacillin, polymyxin B, potassium chloride, sodium bicarbonate, theophylline, thiopental, vancomycin, verapamil, vit B/C

Additive incompatibilities:
Bleomycin, doxorubicin

Rectal route
- Use applicator provided
- Clean applicator after each use

Topical route
- Apply only to affected areas; do not get in eyes
- Cleanse and dry area before applying medication, then cover with occlusive dressing (only if prescribed); seal to normal skin; change q12h; systemic absorption may occur; use only on dermatoses; do not use on weeping, denuded, or infected area
- Use for a few days after area has cleared
- Store at room temp

Nasal route
- Patient should clear nasal passages before administration; use decongestant if needed; shake inhaler, invert, tilt head backward, insert nozzle into nostril, away from septum; hold other nostril closed and depress activator, inhale through nose, exhale through mouth

Patient/family education
- Teach patient all aspects of drug usage, including cushingoid symptoms
- Advise patient that ID as steroid user should be carried; not to discontinue abruptly; adrenal crisis can result
- Instruct patient to notify prescriber if therapeutic response decreases; dosage adjustment may be needed
- Instruct patient to notify prescriber of signs of infection
- Caution patient to avoid OTC products unless directed by perscriber: salicylates, alcohol in cough products, cold preparations
- Teach patient symptoms of adrenal insufficiency: nausea, anorexia, fatigue, dizziness, dyspnea, weakness, joint pain, and when to notify prescriber
- Advise patient that long-term therapy may be needed to resolve infection (1-2 mo depending on type of infection)

Nasal route
- Instruct patient to clear nasal passages if sneezing attack occurs, then repeat dose; to continue using product even if mild nasal bleeding occurs; bleeding is usually transient
- Teach method of instillation after

providing written instruction from manufacturer on instillation

Evaluation

Positive therapeutic outcome

- Decrease in runny nose (nasal)
- Ease of respirations, decreased inflammation
- Absence of severe itching, patches on skin, flaking (top)

HIGH ALERT

hydromorphone (℞)

(hye-droe-mor'fone)

Dihydromorphinone, Dilaudid, Dilaudid-HP, Dilaudid Cough Syrup (combination with guaifenesin/alcohol), PMS Hydromorphone

Func. class.: Antitussive, opioid analgesic agonist

Chem. class.: Phenanthrene derivative, guaifenesin

Pregnancy category C

Controlled substance schedule II

Action: Depresses pain impulse transmission at the spinal cord level by interacting with opioid receptors; increases respiratory tract fluid by decreasing surface tension and adhesiveness, which increases removal of mucus; analgesic, antitussive

Therapeutic Outcome: Decreased cough, decreased pain

Uses: As an antitussive to suppress cough; moderate to severe pain

Dosage and routes

Antitussive

Adult: PO 1 mg q3-4h prn

Child 6-12 yr: PO 0.03-0.08 mg/kg q4-6h, max 5 mg/dose

Analgesic

Adult: PO 2 mg q3-6h prn; may increase to 4 mg q4-6h; SC/IM 1-2 mg q3-6h prn; may increase to 3-4 mg q4-6h; **IV** 0.5-1 mg q3h prn; rec 3 mg q4-8h prn

Available forms: Inj 1, 2, 3, 4, 10 mg/ml; tabs 1, 2, 3, 4, 8 mg; oral sol 5 mg/5 ml; syrup 1 mg/5 ml

Adverse effects

CNS: Dizziness, drowsiness, *sedation, confusion,* headache, euphoria, dreaming, hallucinations, mood changes, **seizures**

CV: *Hypotension, bradycardia,* tachycardia

EENT: Miosis, diplopia, blurred vision

GI: *Nausea, constipation, vomiting, anorexia,* dry mouth

GU: Retention

INTEG: Urticaria, rash, sweating, flushing

RESP: **Respiratory depression**

Contraindications: Hypersensitivity, increased ICP, status asthmaticus, opiate addiction

Precautions: Hypothyroidism, Addison's disease, CNS depression, brain tumor, asthma, hepatic disease, renal disease, COPD, psychosis, alcoholism, seizure disorders, pregnancy **C**

Do Not Confuse:
Dilaudid/Demerol, hydromorphone/meperidine, hydromorphone/morphine

Pharmacokinetics

Absorption	Well absorbed (PO), complete (**IV**)
Distribution	Unknown; crosses placenta
Metabolism	Liver, extensively
Excretion	Kidneys
Half-life	2-3 hr

Pharmacodynamics

	PO/IM/SC	IV	REC
Onset	15-30 min	10-15 min	15-30 min
Peak	30-60 min	15-30 min	30-90 min
Duration	4-5 hr	2-3 hr	4-5 hr

Interactions

Individual drugs

Alcohol: ↑ respiratory depression, hypotension, sedation
Nalbuphine: ↓ analgesia
Pentazocine: ↓ analgesia

Drug classifications

Antidepressants: ↑ respiratory depression, hypotension
Antihistamines: ↑ respiratory depression, hypotension
CNS depressants: ↑ respiratory depression, hypotension
MAOIs: Serious reactions; dosage should be reduced
Phenothiazines: ↑ respiratory depression, hypotension
Sedative/hypnotics: ↑ respiratory depression, hypotension

Herb/drug

Kava: ↑ action

Lab test interferences

↑ Amylase, ↑ lipase

NURSING CONSIDERATIONS

Assessment

- Assess pain control, sedation by scoring on 0-10 scale, around-the-clock dosing is best for pain control
- Monitor VS after parenteral route; note muscle rigidity, drug history, liver, kidney function tests, respiratory dysfunction: respiratory depression, character, rate, rhythm; notify prescriber if respirations are <10/min
- Monitor CNS changes: dizziness, drowsiness, hallucinations, euphoria, LOC, pupil reaction
- Monitor allergic reactions: rash, urticaria; bowel function, constipation

Nursing diagnoses

- ✓ Pain (uses)
- ✓ Sensory-perceptual alteration: visual, auditory (adverse reactions)
- ✓ Breathing pattern, ineffective (adverse reactions)
- ✓ Knowledge deficit (teaching)

Implementation

- Give with antiemetic if nausea, vomiting occur
- Give when pain is beginning to return; determine dosage interval by patient response; continuous dosing of medication is more effective given prn; explain analgesic effect
- Withdraw medication slowly after long-term use to prevent withdrawal symptoms
- Store in light-resistant container at room temp

PO route

- May be given with food or milk to lessen GI upset

IM/SC route

- Do not give if sol is cloudy or a precipitate has formed; rotate inj sites

IV route

- Give by direct **IV** after diluting with 5 ml or more of sterile water or 0.9% NaCl for inj
- Give slowly at 2 mg over 3-5 min or less through Y-connector or 3-way stopcock

Syringe compatibilities:
Atropine, bupivacaine, ceftazidime, chlorpromazine, cimetidine, dimenhydrinate, diphenhydramine, fentanyl, glycopyrrolate, haloperidol, hydroxyzine, lorazepam, midazolam, pentazocaine, pentobarbital, prochlorperazine, promethazine, ranitidine, scopolamine, tetracaine, thiethylperazine, trimethobenzamide

Y-site compatibilities:
Acyclovir, allopurinol, amifostine, amikacin, amsacrine, aztreonam, cefamandole, cefepime, cefmetazole, cefoperazone, cefotaxime, cefoxitin, ceftazidime, ceftizoxime, cefuroxime, cephalothin, cephapirin, chloramphenicol, cisplatin, cladribine, clindamycin, cyclophosphamide, cytarabine, diltiazem, dobutamine, dopamine, doxorubicin, doxycycline, epinephrine, erythromycin lactobionate, famotidine, fentanyl, filgrastim, fludarabine, foscarnet, furosemide, gentamicin, granisetron, heparin, kanamycin, labetalol, lorazepam, magnesium sulfate, melphalan, metho-

trexate, metronidazole, mezlocillin, midazolam, milrinone, morphine, moxalactam, nafcillin, nicardipine, nitroglycerin, norepinephrine, ondansetron, oxacillin, paclitaxel, penicillin G potassium, piperacillin, piperacillin/tazobactam, propofol, ranitidine, teniposide, thiotepa, ticarcillin, tobramycin, trimethoprim/sulfamethoxazole, vancomycin, vecuronium, vinorelbine

Y-site incompatibilities: Ampicillin, diazepam, minocycline, phenobarbital, phenytoin, sargramostim

Additive compatibilities: Bupivacaine, fluorouracil, midazolam, ondansetron, promethazine, verapamil

Additive incompatibilities: Sodium bicarbonate, thiopental

Solution compatibilities: D_5W, D_5/0.45% NaCl, D_5/0.9% NaCl, D_5/LR, D_5/Ringer's, 0.45% NaCl, 0.9% NaCl, Ringer's and lactated Ringer's

Patient/family education

- Instruct patient to report any symptoms of CNS changes, allergic reactions; to avoid CNS depressants: alcohol, sedative/hypnotics for at least 24 hr after taking this drug
- Advise patient that dizziness, drowsiness, and confusion are common and to avoid getting up without assistance, driving, or other hazardous activities
- Discuss in detail all aspects of the drug

Evaluation

Positive therapeutic outcome

- Decreased pain
- Decreased cough

Treatment of overdose: Naloxone HCl (Narcan) 0.2-0.8 **IV**, O_2, **IV** fluids, vasopressors

hydroxyurea (℞)

(hye-drox-ee-yoo-ree'ah)

Droxia, Hydrea

Func. class.: Antineoplastic, antimetabolite

Chem. class.: Synthetic urea analog

Pregnancy category D

Action: Acts by inhibiting DNA synthesis without interfering with RNA or protein synthesis; incorporates thymidine into DNA, causing direct damage to DNA strands; cell cycle specific (S phase)

➔ **Therapeutic Outcome:** Prevention of rapidly growing malignant cells

Uses: Melanoma, chronic myelocytic leukemia, recurrent or metastatic ovarian cancer, squamous cell carcinoma of the head and neck, sickle cell anemia, psoriasis

Dosage and routes

Solid tumors

Adult: PO 80 mg/kg as a single dose q3 days or 20-30 mg/kg as a single dose qd

In combination with radiation

Adult: PO 80 mg/kg as a single dose q3 days; should be started 7 days before irradiation

Resistant chronic myelocytic leukemia

Adult: PO 20-30 mg/kg/day as a single daily dose

Sickle cell anemia

Adult: PO 15 mg/kg/day, may increase by 5 mg/kg/day, max 35 mg/kg/day

Renal dose

CrCl 10-50 ml/min dose 50%; CrCl <10 ml/min dose 20%

Available forms: Caps 200, 300, 400, 500 mg

Adverse effects

CNS: Headache, confusion, hallucinations, dizziness, **seizures**

CV: Angina, ischemia
GI: Nausea, vomiting, anorexia, diarrhea, stomatitis, constipation
GU: Increased BUN, uric acid, creatinine, temporary renal function impairment
***HEMA:* Leukopenia, anemia, thrombocytopenia, megaloblastic erythropoiesis**
INTEG: *Rash,* urticaria, pruritus, dry skin, facial erythema
MISC: Fever, chills, malaise

Contraindications: Hypersensitivity, leukopenia (<2500/mm^3), thrombocytopenia (<100,000/mm^3), anemia (severe), pregnancy **D**

Precautions: Renal disease (severe)

Pharmacokinetics	
Absorption	Well absorbed
Distribution	Crosses blood-brain barrier
Metabolism	Liver (50%)
Excretion	Kidneys, unchanged (50%), eliminated as CO_2
Half-life	4 hr

Pharmacodynamics	
Onset	Unknown
Peak	2 hr
Duration	Unknown

Interactions

Individual drugs

Cyclophosphamide: ↑ cardiotoxicity, CHF
Radiation: ↑ toxicity, bone marrow suppression

Drug classifications

Antineoplastics: ↑ toxicity, bone marrow suppression

Lab test interferences

↑ Renal function studies

NURSING CONSIDERATIONS

Assessment

- Assess buccal cavity q8h for dryness, sores or ulceration, white patches, oral pain, bleeding, dysphagia; obtain prescription for viscous lidocaine (Xylocaine)
- Assess symptoms indicating severe allergic reaction: rash, pruritus, urticaria, purpuric skin lesions, itching, flushing
- Monitor CBC, differential, platelet count weekly; withhold drug if WBC is <2500/mm^3 or platelet count is <100,000/mm^3; notify prescriber of results if WBC <20,000/mm^3, platelets <150,000/mm^3
- Assess for increased uric acid levels, swelling, joint pain primarily in extremities; patient should be well hydrated to prevent urate deposits
- Monitor renal function studies: BUN, creatinine, serum uric acid, urine CrCl before and during therapy; I&O ratio; report fall in urine output to <30 ml/hr
- Monitor temp q4h (may indicate beginning of infection)
- Monitor liver function tests before and during therapy (bilirubin, AST, ALT, LDH) as needed or monthly
- Assess for bleeding: hematuria, stool guaiac, bruising or petechiae, mucosa or orifices q8h; check for inflammation of mucosa, breaks in skin

Nursing diagnoses

☑ Injury, risk for (adverse reactions)
☑ Body image disturbance (adverse reactions)
☑ Infection, risk for (adverse reactions)
☑ Knowledge deficit (teaching)

Implementation

- Avoid contact with skin, very irritating; wash completely to remove
- Give fluids **IV** or PO before chemotherapy to hydrate patient
- Give antiemetic 30-60 min before giving drug and prn to prevent vomiting; antibiotics for prophylaxis of infection
- Provide liq diet: carbonated beverages; gelatin may be added if patient is not nauseated or vomiting
- Provide rinsing of mouth tid-qid

with water, club soda; brushing of teeth bid-qid with soft brush or cotton-tipped applicators for stomatitis; use unwaxed dental floss
- For difficulty swallowing, cap contents may be mixed with water
- Do not crush or chew caps

Patient/family education
- Advise patient that contraceptive measures are recommended during therapy
- Teach patient to avoid use of products containing aspirin or ibuprofen, razors, commercial mouthwash, since bleeding may occur; instruct patient to report symptoms of bleeding (hematuria, tarry stools)
- Instruct patient to report signs of anemia (fatigue, headache, irritability, faintness, shortness of breath)
- Advise patient to report any changes in breathing or coughing even several mo after treatment; to avoid crowds and persons with respiratory tract or other infections
- Caution patient not to have any vaccinations without the advice of the prescriber, serious reactions can occur

Evaluation

Positive therapeutic outcome
- Prevention of rapid division of malignant cells

hydroxyzine (℞)

(hye-drox'i-zeen)

Apo-hydroxyzine ✱, Atarax, Atarax 100, hydroxyzine HCl, hydroxyzine pamoate, Multipax ✱, Novohydroxyzine ✱, Vistaril, Vistazine 50

Func. class.: Antianxiety, sedative, hypnotic, antihistamine, antiemetic

Chem. class.: Piperazine derivative

Pregnancy category C

Action: Depresses subcortical levels of CNS, including limbic system, reticular formation; anticholinergic, antiemetic, antihistaminic responses

Therapeutic Outcome: Absence of allergy symptoms, rhinitis, pruritus, absence of nausea/vomiting, sedation, absence of anxiety

Uses: Anxiety preoperatively, postoperatively to prevent nausea, vomiting; to potentiate narcotic analgesics; sedation; pruritus; prevention of alcohol, drug withdrawal

Dosage and routes

Adult: PO 25-100 mg tid-qid, max 600 mg/day

G ***Elderly:*** PO 10 mg tid-qid (pruritus)

P ***Child >6 yr:*** PO 50-100 mg/day in divided doses

P ***Child <6 yr:*** PO 50 mg/day in divided doses

Preoperatively/ postoperatively

Adult: IM 25-100 mg q4-6h

P ***Child:*** IM 0.5-1.1 mg/kg q4-6h

Pruritus

Adult: PO 25 mg tid-qid

Antiemetic

Adult: IM 25-100 mg/dose q4-6h prn

Available forms: Tabs 10, 25, 50, 100 mg; caps 25, 50, 100 mg; syrup 10 mg/5 ml; oral susp 25 mg/5 ml; inj 25, 50 mg/ml

Adverse effects

CNS: *Dizziness, drowsiness,* confusion, headache, tremors, fatigue, depression, **seizures**

CV: Hypotension

GI: Dry mouth, nausea, diarrhea, increased appetite, weight gain

Contraindications: Hypersensitivity to this drug or cetirizine, early pregnancy, lactation

G **Precautions:** Elderly, debilitated patients, hepatic disease, renal disease, pregnancy **C**

Do Not Confuse:
Vistaril/Versed

Pharmacokinetics	
Absorption	Well absorbed
Distribution	Not known
Metabolism	Liver, completely
Excretion	Feces, urine, bile
Half-life	3 hr

Pharmacodynamics	PO/IM
Onset	15-30 min
Peak	2-4 hr
Duration	4-6 hr

Interactions
Individual drugs
Alcohol: ↑ CNS depression
Atropine: ↑ anticholinergic reactions
Disopyramide: ↑ anticholinergic reactions
Haloperidol: ↑ anticholinergic reactions
Quinidine: ↑ anticholinergic reactions
Drug classifications
Antidepressants: ↑ anticholinergic reactions
Antihistamines: ↑ anticholinergic reactions
CNS depressants: ↑ CNS depression
Opiates: ↑ CNS depression
Phenothiazines: ↑ anticholinergic reactions
Sedative/hypnotics: ↑ CNS depression
Herb/drug
Henbane: ↑ anticholinergic effect
Kava: ↑ action
Lab test interferences
False: ↑ 17-OHCS

NURSING CONSIDERATIONS
Assessment
- Assess respiratory status: rate, rhythm, increase in bronchial secretions, wheezing, chest tightness; provide fluids to 2 L/day to decrease secretion thickness
- Monitor I&O ratio: be alert for urinary retention, frequency, dysuria, **G** especially in the elderly; drug should be discontinued if these occur
- Observe for drowsiness, dizziness
- Assess cough characteristics including type, frequency, thickness of secretions; evaluate response to this medication if using for cough

Nursing diagnoses
✓ Injury, risk for (side effects)
✓ Anxiety (uses)
✓ Knowledge deficit (teaching)

Implementation
PO route
- Give with meals if GI symptoms occur; absorption may be slightly decreased; cap may be opened and drug mixed with food/fluids for patients with swallowing difficulties

IM route
- Give IM inj in large muscle mass; aspirate to prevent **IV** administration; use Z-track method; severe necrosis can result with improper technique; never give **IV**/SC

Syringe compatibilities:
Atropine, atropine/meperidine, benzquinamide, bupivacaine, butorphanol, chlorpromazine, cimetidine, codeine, diphenhydramine, doxapram, droperidol, fentanyl, fluphenazine, glycopyrrolate, hydromorphone, lidocaine, meperidine, meperidine/atropine, methotrimeprazine, metoclopramide, midazolam, morphine, nalbuphine, oxymorphone, pentazocine, perphenazine, procaine, prochlorperazine, promazine, promethazine, remifentanil, scopolamine, sufentanil, thiothixene

Syringe incompatibilities:
Aminophylline, chloramphenicol, dimenhydrinate, heparin, penicillin G potassium, pentobarbital, phenobarbital, phenytoin

Additive compatibilities:
Cisplatin, cyclophosphamide, cytarabine, dimenhydrinate, etoposide,

lidocaine, mesna, methotrexate, nafcillin

Patient/family education

- Caution patient to avoid hazardous activities and activities requiring alertness, since dizziness may occur; instruct patient to request assistance with ambulation
- Advise patient to avoid alcohol, other CNS depressants including cough, cold preparations; CNS depression may occur
- Teach all aspects of drug use; to notify prescriber if confusion, sedation, hypotension occur; to avoid driving and other hazardous activity if drowsiness occurs; to avoid alcohol and other CNS depressants that may potentiate effect
- Instruct patient to take 1 hr pc or 2 hr ac to facilitate absorption
- May crush if patient unable to swallow whole
- Caution patient not to exceed recommended dosage; dysrhythmias may occur
- Tell patient hard candy, gum, frequent rinsing of mouth may be used for dryness

Evaluation

Positive therapeutic outcome

- Absence of nausea, vomiting
- Decreased anxiety

Treatment of overdose:

Lavage if orally ingested, VS, supportive care, **IV** norepinephrine for hypotension

ibuprofen (OTC)

(eye-byoo-proe'fen)

Actiprofen ✤, Advil, Apo-Ibuprofen ✤, Bayer Select Ibuprofen Pain Relief, Children's Advil, Children's Motrin, Cramp End, Dolgesic, Excedrin IB, Genpril, Haltran, Ibren, Ibuprin, ibuprofen, Ibuprohm, I-Tab, Mediphen, Menadol, Midol-200, Motrin, Motrin IB, Motrin Junior Strength, Novoprosen ✤, Nuprin, Pamprin-IB, PediaCare Children's Fever, Q-Profen, Rufen, Saleto-200, Saleto-400, Saleto-600, Saleto-800, Trendar

Func. class.: Nonsteroidal antiinflammatory; nonopiate analgesic, antipyretic

Chem. class.: Propionic acid derivative

Pregnancy category B

Action: Inhibits prostaglandin synthesis by decreasing enzyme needed for biosynthesis; analgesic, antiinflammatory, antipyretic

Therapeutic Outcome: Decreased pain, inflammation, fever

Uses: Rheumatoid arthritis, osteoarthritis, primary dysmenorrhea, gout, dental pain, musculoskeletal disorders, fever

Dosage and routes

Analgesia

Adult: PO 200-400 mg q4-6h, not to exceed 3.2 g/day

P ***Child:*** PO 4-10 mg/kg/dose q6-8h

Antipyretic

P ***Child 6 mo-12 yr:*** PO 5 mg/kg (temp <102.5° F), 10 mg/kg (temp >102.5° F), may repeat q4-6h; max 40 mg/kg/day

Antiinflammatory

Adult: PO 300-800 mg tid-qid; max 3.2 g/day

P ***Child:*** PO 30-40 mg/kg/day in 3-4 divided doses; max 50 mg/kg/day

Available forms: Tabs 100, 200, 300, 400, 600, 800 mg; Caps, liqui-gel 200 mg; oral susp 100 mg/2.5 ml, 100 mg/5 ml; tabs, chew 50, 100 mg; drops 50 mg/1.25 ml

Adverse effects

CNS: Headache, dizziness, drowsiness, fatigue, tremors, confusion, insomnia, anxiety, depression
CV: Tachycardia, peripheral edema, palpitations, dysrhythmias
EENT: Tinnitus, hearing loss, blurred vision
GI: Nausea, anorexia, vomiting, diarrhea, jaundice, **cholestatic hepatitis,** constipation, flatulence, cramps, dry mouth, peptic ulcer, **GI bleeding**
GU: **Nephrotoxicity,** dysuria, hematuria, oliguria, azotemia
HEMA: **Blood dyscrasias,** increased bleeding time
INTEG: Purpura, rash, pruritus, sweating
SYST: **Anaphylaxis**

Contraindications: Hypersensitivity, asthma, severe renal disease, severe hepatic disease

Precautions: Pregnancy **B** (1st and 2nd trimesters), lactation, children (P), bleeding disorders, GI disorders, cardiac disorders, hypersensitivity to other antiinflammatory agents, elderly (G), CHF, CrCl <25 ml/min

Do Not Confuse:
Nuprin/Lupron

Pharmacokinetics

Absorption	Well absorbed
Distribution	Not known; crosses placenta
Metabolism	Liver, extensively
Excretion	Kidneys, unchanged (10%)
Half-life	3½ hr

Pharmacodynamics

Onset	½ hr
Peak	1-2 hr
Duration	4-6 hr

Interactions

Individual drugs

Acetaminophen (long-term use): ↑ renal reactions
Alcohol: ↑ adverse reactions
Aspirin: ↓ effectiveness, ↑ adverse reactions
Cyclosporine: ↑ toxicity
Digoxin: ↑ toxicity, levels
Furosemide: ↓ effect of furosemide
Insulin: ↓ insulin effect
Lithium: ↑ toxicity
Methotrexate: ↑ toxicity
Phenytoin: ↑ toxicity
Probenecid: ↑ toxicity
Radiation: ↑ risk of hematologic toxicity
Sulfonylurea: ↑ toxicity

Drug classifications

Anticoagulants: ↑ risk of bleeding
Antidiabetics, oral: ↑ hypoglycemia
Antihypertensives: ↓ effect of antihypertensives
Antineoplastics: ↑ risk of hematologic toxicity
Antiplatelet agents: ↑ risk of bleeding
β-Adrenergic blockers: ↑ antihypertension
Cephalosporins: ↑ risk of bleeding
Diuretics: ↓ effectiveness of diuretics
Glucocorticoids: ↑ adverse reactions
Hypoglycemics: ↓ hypoglycemic effect
NSAIDs: ↑ adverse reactions
Potassium supplements: ↑ adverse reactions
Sulfonamides: ↑ toxicity
Thrombolytics: ↑ risk of bleeding

Lab test interferences

↑ Bleeding time

NURSING CONSIDERATIONS

Assessment

- Assess pain: location, duration, type, intensity before dose and 1 hr after
- Assess musculoskeletal status: ROM before dose and 1 hr after
- Monitor liver function studies: AST,

ALT, bilirubin, creatinine if patient is on long-term therapy
- Monitor renal function studies: BUN, urine creatinine if patient is on long-term therapy
- Assess cardiac status: edema (peripheral), tachycardia, palpitations; monitor B/P, pulse for character, quality, rhythm
- Monitor blood studies: CBC, Hct, Hgb, pro-time if patient is on long-term therapy
- Check I&O ratio; decreasing output may indicate renal failure if patient is on long-term therapy
- Assess hepatotoxicity: dark urine, clay-colored stools, jaundice of skin and sclera, itching, abdominal pain, fever, diarrhea if patient is on long-term therapy
- Assess for history of peptic ulcer disorder; asthma, aspirin, hypersensitivity, check closely for hypersensitivity reactions
- Assess for allergic reactions: rash, urticaria; if these occur, drug may have to be discontinued
- Assess for ototoxicity: tinnitus, ringing, roaring in ears; audiometric testing needed before, after long-term therapy
- Assess for visual changes: blurring, halos; may indicate corneal, retinal damage
- Identify prior drug history; there are many drug interactions
- Identify fever: length of time in evidence and related symptoms

Nursing diagnoses

- ✓ Pain (uses)
- ✓ Mobility, impaired (uses)
- ✓ Injury, risk for (side effects)
- ✓ Knowledge deficit (teaching)

Implementation

- Administer to patient crushed or whole; 800-mg tab may be dissolved in water
- Give with food or milk to decrease gastric symptoms; give 30 min pc or 2 hr ac; absorption may be slowed

Patient/family education

- Teach patient to report any symptoms of hepatotoxicity, renal toxicity, visual changes, ototoxicity, allergic reactions, bleeding if patient is on long-term therapy
- Caution patient not to exceed recommended dosage; acute poisoning may result
- Advise patient to read label on other OTC drugs
- Inform patient that the therapeutic response takes 1 mo (arthritis)
- Caution patient to avoid alcohol ingestion, salicylates, NSAIDs; GI bleeding may occur
- Advise patient with allergies that allergic reactions may develop
- Advise patient to use sunscreen to prevent photosensitivity

Evaluation

Positive therapeutic outcome

- Decreased pain
- Decreased inflammation
- Decreased fever
- Increased mobility

HIGH ALERT

ibutilide (℞)

(eye-byoo'te-lide)

Corvert

Func. class.: Antidysrhythmic (Class III)

Pregnancy category C

Action: Prolongs duration of action potential and effective refractory period; noncompetitive α- and β-adrenergic inhibition

➡ **Therapeutic Outcome:** Decreased amount and severity of atrial fibrillation/flutter

Uses: Atrial fibrillation/flutter

Dosage and routes

Adult: **IV** inf (≥60 kg) 1 vial (1 mg) given over 10 min; **IV** inf (<60 kg) 0.1 mg/kg given over 10 min

Available forms: Inj 0.1 mg/ml

Adverse effects

CNS: Headache

CV: Hypotension, bradycardia, **sinus arrest, CHF, dysrhythmias,** hypertension, extrasystoles, ventricular tachycardia, bundle branch block, AV block

GI: Nausea

Contraindications: Hypersensitivity

Precautions: Sinus node dysfunction, 2nd- or 3rd-degree AV block, electrolyte imbalances, pregnancy **C,** P bradycardia, lactation, children <18 G yr, renal/hepatic disease, elderly

Pharmacokinetics	
Absorption	Slow, variable
Distribution	Body tissues; crosses placenta
Metabolism	Liver
Excretion	Kidney
Half-life	15-100 days

Pharmacodynamics	
Onset	1-3 wk
Peak	2-10 hr
Duration	Up to months

Interactions

Individual drugs

Amiodarone: ↑ amiodarone level
Digoxin: ↑ blood levels, ↑ toxicity
Disopyramide: ↑ levels, ↑ toxicity
Flecainide: ↑ levels, ↑ toxicity
Phenytoin: ↑ blood levels
Procainamide: ↑ levels, ↑ toxicity
Quinidine: ↑ levels, ↑ toxicity
Sotalol: ↑ solalol level

Drug classifications

Antidepressants, tricyclic/tetracyclic: prodysrhythmia
Antihistamines: ↑ prodysrhythmia
H_1-receptor antagonists: ↑ prodysrhythmia
Phenothiazines: ↑ prodysrhythmia

Herb/drug

Aloe: ↑ action
Buckthorn: ↑ action
Cascara sagrada: ↑ action
Senna: ↑ action

NURSING CONSIDERATIONS

Assessment

- Monitor I&O ratio; monitor electrolytes: potassium, sodium, chloride
- Monitor liver function studies: AST, ALT, bilirubin, alkaline phosphatase
- Monitor ECG continuously to determine drug effectiveness; measure PR, QRS, QT intervals; check for PVCs, other dysrhythmias; monitor B/P continuously for hypotension, hypertension; check for rebound hypertension after 1-2 hr; discontinue drug when atrial fibrillation/flutter ceases
- Monitor for dehydration or hypovolemia
- Assess for CNS symptoms: confusion, psychosis, numbness, depression, involuntary movements; if these occur drug should be discontinued
- Monitor cardiac rate, respiration; rate, rhythm, character, chest pain, ventricular tachycardia, supraventricular tachycardia or fibrillation

Nursing diagnoses

- ✓ Cardiac output, decreased (uses)
- ✓ Gas exchange, impaired (adverse reactions)
- ✓ Knowledge deficit (teaching)

Implementation

IV route

- Give reduced dosage slowly with ECG monitoring only
- Give undiluted or diluted in 50 ml of 0.9% NaCl or D_5W (0.017 mg/ml), give over 10 min
- Solution is stable for 48 hr refrigerated or 24 hr at room temp
- Do not admix with other solution, drugs

Patient/family education
- Instruct patient to report side effects immediately to prescriber

Evaluation
Positive therapeutic outcome
- Decrease in atrial fibrillation/flutter

HIGH ALERT

idarubicin (℞)
(eye-da-roo′bi-sin)
Idamycin, Idamycin PFS
Func. class.: Antineoplastic, antibiotic
Chem. class.: Anthracycline glycoside

Pregnancy category D

Action: Inhibits DNA synthesis derived from daunorubicin by binding to DNA, which causes strand splitting; cell cycle specific (S phase); a vesicant

Therapeutic Outcome: Prevention of rapidly growing malignant cells

Uses: Used in combination with other antineoplastics for acute myelocytic leukemia in adults

Investigational uses: Breast cancer, solid tumors

Dosage and routes
Adult: **IV** 8-12 mg/m²/day × 3 days in combination with cytosine (induction) or 25 mg/m² **IV** bol followed by 200 mg/m²/day × 5 days by cont inf

Available forms: Inj 1 mg/ml; powder for inj, lyophilized 5, 10, 20 mg

Adverse effects
CNS: Fever, chills, headache
CV: **Dysrhythmias, CHF, pericarditis, myocarditis,** peripheral edema, angina, **MI**
GI: Nausea, vomiting, abdominal pain, mucositis, diarrhea, **hepatotoxicity**
GU: **Nephrotoxicity**
HEMA: **Thrombocytopenia, leukopenia, anemia**
INTEG: Rash, extravasation, dermatitis, reversible alopecia, urticaria, thrombophlebitis, tissue necrosis at inj site

Contraindications: Hypersensitivity, pregnancy **D**, myelosuppression

Precautions: Renal and hepatic disease, gout, bone marrow depression, children

Do Not Confuse:
Idamycin/Adriamycin, idarubicin/doxorubicin

Pharmacokinetics	
Absorption	Complete bioavailability
Distribution	Rapidly distributed; high tissue binding
Metabolism	Liver, extensively
Excretion	Bile
Half-life	22 hr

Pharmacodynamics

Unknown

Interactions
Individual drugs
Radiation: ↑ toxicity, bone marrow suppression

Drug classifications
Antineoplastics: ↑ toxicity, bone marrow suppression
Live virus vaccines: ↓ antibody response

Lab test interferences
↑ Uric acid

NURSING CONSIDERATIONS
Assessment
- Assess symptoms indicating severe allergic reaction: rash, pruritus, urticaria, purpuric skin lesions, itching, flushing; drug should be discontinued
- Assess for tachypnea, ECG changes, dyspnea, edema, fatigue
- Assess for cardiac toxicity: CHF, dysrhythmias, cardiomyopathy; cardiac studies should be done before and periodically during treatment; ECG, chest x-ray

- Monitor CBC, differential, platelet count weekly; withhold drug if WBC is <4000/mm³ or platelet count is <100,000/mm³; notify prescriber of results if WBC <20,000/mm³, platelets <150,000/mm³
- Monitor temp q4h (may indicate beginning of infection)
- Monitor liver function tests before and during therapy (bilirubin, AST, ALT, LDH) as needed or monthly; note jaundice of skin and sclera, dark urine, clay-colored stools, itchy skin, abdominal pain, fever, diarrhea; hepatoxicity can be severe
- Assess for bleeding: hematuria, stool guaiac, bruising or petechiae, mucosa or orifices q8h; assess for inflammation of mucosa, breaks in skin
- Identify effects of alopecia on body image; discuss feelings about body changes

Nursing diagnoses

- ✓ Injury, risk for (adverse reactions)
- ✓ Cardiac output, decreased (adverse reactions)
- ✓ Body image disturbance (adverse reactions)
- ✓ Infection, risk for (adverse reactions)
- ✓ Knowledge deficit (teaching)

Implementation

- Avoid contact with skin; very irritating; wash completely to remove
- Give fluids **IV** or PO before chemotherapy to hydrate patient
- Administer antiemetic 30-60 min before giving drug and prn to prevent vomiting; administer antibiotics for prophylaxis of infection
- Give a liq diet: carbonated beverages; gelatin may be added if patient is not nauseated or vomiting
- Provide rinsing of mouth tid-qid with water, club soda; brushing of teeth bid-qid with soft brush or cotton-tipped applicators for stomatitis; use unwaxed dental floss
- Drug should be prepared by experienced personnel using proper precautions (biologic cabinet, wearing gown, gloves, mask)
- Give after reconstituting 5-mg vial with 5 ml of 0.9% NaCl (1 mg/1 ml); give over 10-15 min through Y-tube or 3-way stopcock of inf of D_5 or 0.9% NaCl; discard unused portion
- Inject hydrocortisone for extravasation; apply ice compress after stopping inf
- Store at room temp for 3 days after reconstituting or 7 days refrigerated

Y-site compatibilities:

Amifostine, amikacin, aztreonam, cimetidine, cladribine, cyclophosphamide, cytarabine, diphenhydramine, droperidol, erythromycin, filgrastim, granisetron, imipenem/cilastatin, magnesium sulfate, mannitol, melphalan, metoclopromide, potassium chloride, ranitidine, sargramostim, thiotepa, vinorelbine

Y-site incompatibilities:

Acyclovir, ampicillin/sulbactam, cefazolin, ceftazidine, clindamycin, dexamethasone, etoposide, furosemide, gentamicin, hydrocortisone, lorazepam, meperidine, methotrexate, mezlocillin, sargramostim, sodium bicarbonate, vancomycin, vincristine

Solution compatibilities:

$D_{3.3}$/0.3% NaCl, D_5/0.9% NaCl, D_5W, Ringer's, 0.9% NaCl, LR

Patient/family education

- Teach patient to avoid use of products containing aspirin or ibuprofen, razors, commercial mouthwash, since bleeding may occur; to report symptoms of bleeding (hematuria, tarry stools)
- Instruct patient to report signs of anemia (fatigue, headache, irritability, faintness, shortness of breath)
- Advise patient that hair may be lost during treatment; a wig or hairpiece may make patient feel better; new hair may be different in color, texture
- Tell patient not to have any vaccinations without the advice of the

prescriber; serious reactions can occur

- Advise patient that contraception is needed during treatment and for several mo after the completion of therapy

Evaluation

Positive therapeutic outcome

- Prevention of rapid division of malignant cells

HIGH ALERT

ifosfamide (℞)

(i-foss′fa-mide)

Ifex

Func. class.: Antineoplastic alkylating agent

Chem. class.: Nitrogen mustard

Pregnancy category D

Action: Alkylates DNA, RNA; inhibits enzymes that allow synthesis of amino acids in proteins; also responsible for cross-linking DNA strands; activity is not cell cycle stage specific

Therapeutic Outcome: Prevention of rapidly growing malignant cells

Uses: Testicular cancer, soft-tissue sarcoma, Ewing's sarcoma, non-Hodgkin's lymphoma, lung, pancreatic cancer, sarcoma

Dosage and routes

Adult: **IV** 1.2 g/m^2/day × 5 days; repeat course q3 wk; give with mesna

Available forms: Inj 1, 3 g

Adverse effects

CNS: Facial paresthesia, fever, malaise, somnolence, confusion, depression, hallucinations, dizziness, disorientation, **seizures, coma,** cranial nerve dysfunction

GI: Nausea, vomiting, anorexia, **hepatotoxicity,** stomatitis, constipation, diarrhea

GU: **Hematuria, nephrotoxicity, hemorrhagic cystitis,** dysuria, urinary frequency

HEMA: **Thrombocytopenia, leukopenia, anemia**

INTEG: Dermatitis, alopecia, pain at inj site

Contraindications: Hypersensitivity, bone marrow suppression, pregnancy **D**

Precautions: Renal disease, P lactation, children

Pharmacokinetics	
Absorption	Complete bioavailability
Distribution	Saturation at high dosages
Metabolism	Liver
Excretion	Breast milk
Half-life	15 hr

Pharmacodynamics
Unknown

Interactions

Individual drugs

Allopurinol: ↑ toxicity

Radiation: ↑ toxicity, bone marrow suppression

Drug classifications

Antineoplastics: ↑ toxicity, bone marrow suppression

Barbiturates: ↑ toxicity

Live virus vaccines: ↓ antibody response

NURSING CONSIDERATIONS

Assessment

- Monitor CBC, differential, platelet count weekly; withhold drug if WBC is <2000 or platelet count is <50,000; notify prescriber of results if WBC <10,000/mm^3, platelets <100,000/mm^3
- Monitor renal function studies: BUN, serum uric acid, urine CrCl before, during therapy; I&O ratio; report fall in urine output of 30 ml/hr
- Monitor for cold, fever, sore throat (may indicate beginning of infection); identify edema in feet and joints,

stomach pain, shaking; prescriber should be notified
- Assess for bleeding: hematuria, guaiac, bruising or petechiae, mucosa or orifices q8h; no rec temp
- Monitor liver function studies before and during therapy (ALT, AST, LDH); jaundice of skin, sclera, dark urine, clay-colored stools, itching, abdominal pain, fever, diarrhea that may indicate liver involvement

Nursing diagnoses

- ✓ Injury, risk for (adverse reactions)
- ✓ Body image disturbance (adverse reactions)
- ✓ Infection, risk for (adverse reactions)
- ✓ Knowledge deficit (teaching)

Implementation

- Give fluids **IV** or PO before chemotherapy to hydrate patient
- Give antiemetic 30-60 min before giving drug and prn to prevent vomiting
- Provide liq diet: carbonated beverages; gelatin may be added if patient is not nauseated or vomiting
- Give **IV** after diluting 1 g/ 20 ml of sterile or bacteriostatic water for inj with parabens or benzyl only; shake
- Give by intermittent inf after further diluting with D_5W, LR, 0.9% NaCl, sterile water for inj (1 g/20 ml = 50 mg/ml; 1 g/50 ml = 20 mg/ml; 1 g/ 200 ml = 5 mg/ml); give over ≥30 min; may also give as a cont inf over 72 hr
- Store powder at room temp; always give with mesna, increase fluids to 3 L/day to prevent ifosfamide-induced hemorrhagic cystitis

Syringe compatibilities:
Mesna

Y-site compatibilities:
Allopurinol, amifostine, aztreonam, filgrastim, fludarabine, gallium, granisetron, melphalan, ondansetron, paclitaxel, piperacillin/tazobactam, propofol, sargramostim, teniposide, thiotepa, vinorelbine

Additive compatibilities:
Carboplatin, cisplatin, etoposide, fluorouracil, mesna

Patient/family education

- Teach patient to avoid use of products containing aspirin or NSAIDs, razors, commercial mouthwash, since bleeding may occur; to report symptoms of bleeding (hematuria, tarry stools)
- Instruct patient to report signs of anemia (fatigue, headache, irritability, faintness, shortness of breath)
- Advise patient to report any changes in breathing or coughing even several mo after treatment; to avoid crowds and persons with respiratory tract or other infections
- Teach patient that hair loss is common; discuss the use of wigs or hairpieces; that hair may be a different texture when regrowth occurs
- Caution patient not to have any vaccinations without the advice of the prescriber; serious reactions can occur
- Advise patient that contraception is needed during treatment and for several mo after completion of therapy

Evaluation

Positive therapeutic outcome
- Prevention of rapid division of malignant cells
- Absence of swelling at night
- Increased appetite, increased weight

imatinib

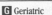

See Appendix A, Selected New Drugs

imipenem/cilastatin (℞)

(i-me-pen'em sye-la-stat'in)

Primaxin IM, Primaxin IV

Func. class.: Antiinfective; miscellaneous penicillin

Chem. class.: Carbapenem

Pregnancy category C

Action: Interferes with cell wall replication of susceptible organisms; osmotically unstable cell wall swells and bursts from osmotic pressure; addition of cilastatin prevents renal inactivation that occurs with high urinary concentrations of imipenem

Therapeutic Outcome: Bactericidal action against the following: *Streptococcus pneumoniae,* group A β-hemolytic streptococci, *Staphylococcus aureus,* enterococcus; gram-negative organisms: *Klebsiella, Proteus, Escherichia coli, Acinetobacter, Serratia, Pseudomonas aeruginosa; Salmonella, Shigella*

Uses: Serious infections caused by gram-positive or gram-negative organisms

Dosage and routes

Adult: **IV** 250-500 mg q6h; severe infections may require 1 g q6h; may give IM q12h (total daily IM dose >1500 mg not recommended); mild to moderate infections

P ***Child:*** **IV** 60-100 mg/kg/day max 4 g/day

Renal dose

CrCl <70 ml/min, reduce dose

Available forms: **IV** inj 250, 500; IM inj 500, 750 mg

Adverse effects

CNS: Fever, somnolence, **seizures,** confusion, dizziness, weakness

CV: Hypotension, palpitations

GI: *Diarrhea, nausea, vomiting,* **pseudomembranous colitis, hepatitis,** glossitis

HEMA: **Eosinophilia, neutropenia,** decreased Hgb, Hct

INTEG: Rash, urticaria, pruritus, pain at inj site, phlebitis, erythema at inj site

RESP: Chest discomfort, dyspnea, hyperventilation

SYST: **Anaphylaxis**

Contraindications: Hypersensitivity, IM hypersensitivity to local anesthetics of the amide type

Precautions: Pregnancy **C,** G lactation, elderly, hypersensitivity to penicillins, seizure disorders, renal P disease, children

Do Not Confuse:
imipenem/Omnipen, Primaxin/Premarin

Pharmacokinetics

Absorption	Complete bioavailability (**IV**)
Distribution	Widely distributed; crosses placenta
Metabolism	Liver
Excretion	Kidneys, unchanged (70%-80%); breast milk
Half-life	1 hr; increased in renal disease

Pharmacodynamics

	IV	IM
Onset	Rapid	Unknown
Peak	½-1 hr	Unknown

Interactions

Individual drugs

Ganciclovir: ↑ risk of seizures

Probenecid: ↓ renal excretion, ↑ blood level

Drug classifications

β-Lactam antibiotics: ↑ toxicity

Cephalosporins: ↓ action

Penicillins: ↓ action

Lab test interferences

False: ↑ Creatinine (serum urine), ↑ urinary 17-KS

False positive: Urinary protein, direct Coombs' test, urine glucose

Interference: Cross-matching

NURSING CONSIDERATIONS

Assessment

- Assess patient for previous sensitivity reaction
- Assess patient for signs and symptoms of infection, including characteristics of wounds, sputum, urine, stool, WBC >10,000/mm^3, fever; obtain baseline information before and during treatment
- Complete C&S tests before beginning drug therapy to identify if correct treatment has been initiated
- Assess for allergic reactions, anaphylaxis: rash, urticaria, pruritus, chills, wheezing, laryngeal edema, fever, joint pain; angioedema may occur a few days after therapy begins; epinephrine, resuscitation equipment should be available for anaphylactic reaction
- Identify urine output; if decreasing, notify prescriber (may indicate nephrotoxicity); also check for increased BUN, creatinine
- Monitor blood studies: AST, ALT, CBC, Hct, bilirubin, LDH, alkaline phosphatase, Coombs' test monthly if patient is on long-term therapy
- Monitor electrolytes: potassium, sodium, chloride monthly if patient is on long-term therapy
- Assess bowel pattern qd; if severe diarrhea occurs, drug should be discontinued; may indicate pseudomembranous colitis
- Monitor for bleeding: ecchymosis, bleeding gums, hematuria, stool guaiac daily if patient is on long-term therapy
- Assess for overgrowth of infection: perineal itching, fever, malaise, redness, pain, swelling, drainage, rash, diarrhea, change in cough, sputum

Nursing diagnoses

- ✓ Infection, risk for (uses)
- ✓ Diarrhea (adverse reactions)
- ✓ Injury, risk for (adverse reactions)
- ✓ Knowledge deficit (teaching)
- ✓ Noncompliance (teaching)

Implementation

IM route

- Reconstitute 500 mg/2 ml or 750 mg/3 ml lidocaine without epinephrine; shake well, withdraw and administer entire vial; give deep in large muscle mass, massage

IV **IV route**

- Reconstitute each 250 or 500 mg/10 ml of compatible diluent; shake well; transfer the resulting susp to not less than 100 ml of compatible diluent; add 10 ml to each previously reconstituted vial and shake to ensure all medication is used; transfer the remaining contents of the vial to the infusion container; do not administer susp by direct inj; reconstitute 120-ml infusion bottles/100 ml of a compatible diluent; shake until clear; may use 0.9% NaCl, D_5W, $D_{10}W$, D_5/0.2% sodium bicarbonate, D_5/0.9% NaCl, D_5/0.45% NaCl, D_5/0.225% NaCl, mannitol 2.5%, 5%, or 10%
- Give by intermittent inf: each 250- or 500-mg dose over 20-30 min, and each 1-g dose over 40-60 min; P administer over 15-20 min for pediatric patients; do not administer direct **IV**; do not admix with other antibiotics

Y-site compatibilities: Acyclovir, amifostine, aztreonam, cefepime, diltiazem, famotidine, fludarabine, foscarnet, granisetron, idarubicin, regular insulin, melphalan, methotrexate, ondansetron, propofol, tacrolimus, teniposide, thiotepa, vinorelbine, zidovudine

Y-site incompatibilities: Fluconazole, meperidine, sargramostim

Additive incompatibilities: Fluconazole, meperidine, sargramostim

Patient/family education

- Teach patient to report sore throat, bruising, bleeding, joint pain; may indicate blood dyscrasias (rare)
- Advise patient to contact prescriber

if vaginal itching, loose, foul-smelling stools, furry tongue occur; may indicate superinfection
- Advise patient to notify prescriber of diarrhea with blood or pus; may indicate pseudomembranous colitis

Evaluation

Positive therapeutic outcome
- Absence of signs/symptoms of infection (WBC <10,000/mm^3, temp WNL, absence of red, draining wounds)
- Reported improvement in symptoms of infection

Treatment of anaphylaxis: Epinephrine, antihistamines, resuscitate if needed

imipramine ⊶ (℞)

(im-ip'ra-meen)

Apo-Imipramine ♣, Imipramine HCl, Impril ♣, Novo Pramine ♣, Tofranil, Tofranil PM

Func. class.: Antidepressant, tricyclic

Chem. class.: Dibenzazepine, tertiary amine

Pregnancy category C

Action: Blocks reuptake of norepinephrine and serotonin into nerve endings, increasing action of norepinephrine and serotonin in nerve cells; has anticholinergic effects

➔ **Therapeutic Outcome:** Decreased symptoms of depression after 2-3 wk; decreased bedwetting in P children

Uses: Depression, enuresis in P children

Investigational uses: Chronic pain, migraine headaches, cluster headaches as adjunct, incontinence

Dosage and routes

Adult: PO/IM 75-100 mg/day in divided doses; may increase by 25-50 mg up to 200 mg, not to exceed 300 mg/day; may give daily dose hs

G ***Elderly:*** PO 25 mg hs, may increase to 100 mg/day in divided doses

P ***Child:*** PO 25-75 mg/day

Enuresis

P ***Child:*** PO 10 mg at hs, max 50 mg

Available forms: Tabs 10, 25, 50 mg; inj 25 mg/2 ml; caps 75, 100, 125, 150 mg

Adverse effects

CV: Orthostatic hypotension, ECG changes, tachycardia, hypertension, palpitations, **dysrhythmias**

CNS: Dizziness, drowsiness, confusion, headache, anxiety, tremors, stimulation, weakness, insomnia, nightmares, extrapyramidal symptoms G (elderly), increased psychiatric symptoms, paresthesia, seizures

EENT: Blurred vision, tinnitus, mydriasis

GI: Diarrhea, dry mouth, nausea, vomiting, **paralytic ileus,** increased appetite, cramps, epigastric distress, jaundice, **hepatitis,** stomatitis

GU: Retention, **acute renal failure**

HEMA: **Agranulocytosis, thrombocytopenia, eosinophilia, leukopenia**

INTEG: Rash, urticaria, sweating, pruritus, photosensitivity

Contraindications: Hypersensitivity to tricyclic antidepressants, recovery phase of MI, convulsive disorders, prostatic hypertrophy

Precautions: Suicidal patients, severe depression, increased intraocular pressure, narrowangle glaucoma, urinary retention, cardiac disease, hepatic disease, hyperthyroidism, electroshock therapy, elective surgery, G elderly, pregnancy **C**

I

Pharmacokinetics

Absorption	Well absorbed
Distribution	Widely distributed; crosses placenta
Metabolism	Liver, extensively
Excretion	Kidneys, breast milk
Half-life	6-20 hr

Pharmacodynamics

	PO	IM
Onset	1 hr	1 hr
Peak	Unknown	Unknown
Duration	Unknown	Unknown

Interactions

Individual drugs

Alcohol: ↑ CNS depression
Cimetidine: ↑ levels, toxicity
Clonidine: Severe hypotension; avoid use
Disulfiram: Organic brain syndrome
Fluoxetine: ↑ levels, toxicity
Guanethidine: ↓ effects

Drug classifications

Analgesics: ↑ CNS depression
Anticholinergics: ↑ side effects
Antihistamines: ↑ CNS depression
Antihypertensives: May block antihypertensive effect
Barbiturates: ↑ effects
Benzodiazepines: ↑ effects
CNS depressants: ↑ effects
MAOIs: Hypertensive crisis, convulsions
Oral contraceptives: ↑ effects, toxicity
Phenothiazines: ↑ toxicity
Sedative/hypnotics: ↑ CNS depression
Selective serotonin reuptake inhibitors: ↑ toxicity
Sympathomimetics, indirect acting: ↓ effects

Herb/drug

Belladonna: ↑ anticholinergic effect
Henbane: ↑ anticholinergic effect
Kava: ↑ imipramine action
Scopolia: ↑ imipramine action

Smoking

↑ Metabolism, ↓ effects

Lab test interferences

↑ Serum bilirubin, ↑ blood glucose, ↑ alkaline phosphatase
↓ VMA, ↓ 5-HIAA, ↓ blood glucose
False: ↑ Urinary catecholamines

NURSING CONSIDERATIONS

Assessment

- Monitor B/P (with patient lying, standing), pulse q4h; if systolic B/P drops 20 mm Hg, hold drug, notify prescriber; take vital signs q4h in patients with CV disease
- Monitor blood studies: CBC, leukocytes, differential, cardiac enzymes if patient is receiving long-term therapy
- Monitor hepatic studies: AST, ALT, bilirubin
- Check weight weekly; appetite may increase with drug
- Assess ECG for flattening of T wave, bundle branch block, AV block, dysrhythmias in cardiac patients
- Assess for extrapyramidal symptoms primarily in elderly: rigidity, dystonia, akathisia (G)
- Assess mental status: mood, sensorium, affect, suicidal tendencies; increase in psychiatric symptoms: depression, panic
- Monitor urinary retention, constipation; constipation is more likely to occur in children or elderly (P) (G)
- (Alert) Assess for withdrawal symptoms: headache, nausea, vomiting, muscle pain, weakness; do not usually occur unless drug was discontinued abruptly
- Identify alcohol consumption; if alcohol is consumed, hold dose until AM

Nursing diagnoses

✓ Coping, ineffective individual (uses)
✓ Injury, risk for physical (side effects)
✓ Knowledge deficit (teaching)
✓ Noncompliance (teaching)

Implementation

PO route

- Give with food or milk
- (Do Not Crush) Do not crush, chew caps
- Store at room temp; do not freeze

IM route

- Put ampule under warm running water for 1 min to dissolve crystals; sol may be yellow or red

Syringe compatibilities: Doxapram

Y-site compatibilities: Cladribine

Patient/family education

- Teach patient that therapeutic effects may take 2-3 wk
- Teach patient to use caution in driving and other activities requiring alertness because of drowsiness, dizziness, blurred vision; to avoid rising quickly from sitting position, G especially elderly
- Teach patient to avoid alcohol ingestion, other CNS depressants
- Teach patient not to discontinue medication quickly after long-term use: may cause nausea, headache, malaise
- Teach patient to wear sunscreen or large hat, since photosensitivity occurs
- Teach patient to increase fluids, bulk in diet if constipation, urinary G retention occur, especially elderly
- Teach patient to take gum, hard sugarless candy, or frequent sips of water for dry mouth

Evaluation

Positive therapeutic outcome

- Decreased depression
- Absence of suicidal thoughts
- P Decreased enuresis in children
- Decreased pain

Treatment of overdose: ECG monitoring, induce emesis, lavage, activated charcoal, administer anticonvulsant

immune globulin (℞)

gamma globulin, Gamimune N, Gammagard S/D, Gammar-P I.V., Iveegam, polygam, polygam S/D, Sandoglobulin, Venoglobulin-I, immune serum globulin

Func. class.: Immune serum

Chem. class.: IgG

Pregnancy category C

Action: Provides passive immunity to hepatitis A, measles, varicella, rubella, immune globulin deficiency; contains γ-globulin antibodies (IgG)

➔ **Therapeutic Outcome:** Absence of infection

Uses: Immunodeficiency syndrome, B-cell chronic lymphocytic leukemia, Kawasaki syndrome, bone marrow transplantation, pediatric HIV infection, agammaglobulinemia, hepatitis A, B exposure, measles exposure, measles vaccine complications, purpura, rubella exposure, chickenpox exposure

Dosage and routes

Adult: IM 30-50 ml qmo; **IV** 100 mg/kg qmo, 0.01-0.02 ml/kg/min over 30 min (Gamimune N); **IV** 200 mg/kg qmo, 0.05-1 ml/min over 15-30 min, then increase to 1.5-2.5 ml/min (Sandoglobulin)

P ***Child:*** IM 20-40 ml qmo

Hepatitis A exposure

P ***Adult and child:*** IM 0.02-0.04 ml/kg or 0.1 mg/kg if treatment is delayed

Hepatitis B exposure

P ***Adult and child:*** IM 0.06 ml/kg within 1 wk, qmo

Measles (postexposure)

P ***Child:*** IM 0.25 ml/kg within 6 days

Immunoglobulin deficiency

P ***Adult and child:*** IM 1.3 ml/kg, then 0.66 ml/kg after 2-4 wk and q2-4 wk thereafter

Idiopathic thrombocytopenic purpura

P ***Adult and child:*** **IV** 0.4 g/kg/day × 5 days or 1g/kg/day × 1-2 days

Kawasaki syndrome

P ***Child:*** PO 2g/kg as a single dose

Available forms: IM inj 2, 10 ml/vial; **IV** inj 5% sol, 0.5, 1, 2.5, 3, 6, 10 g vials

Adverse effects

CNS: Headache, fatigue, malaise

GI: Abdominal pain

INTEG: Pain at inj site, rash, pruritus, chills, chest pain

MS: Arthralgia

SYST: Lymphadenopathy, **anaphylaxis**

Contraindications: Hypersensitivity

Precautions: Pregnancy **C**

Pharmacokinetics

Absorption	Well absorbed (IM); completely absorbed (**IV**)
Distribution	Rapidly
Metabolism	Liver, catabolism
Excretion	Kidneys
Half-life	3-4 wk

Pharmacodynamics

	IM	IV
Onset	Unknown	Rapid
Peak	Unknown	Unknown
Duration	Unknown	Unknown

Interactions

Live virus vaccines: Do not give within 3 mo

NURSING CONSIDERATIONS

Assessment

- Assess for exposure date: this drug should be given within 6 days of measles, 1 wk of hepatitis B, 14 days of hepatitis A; if the date of exposure is outside these limits, immune globulin will not be effective
- Monitor blood studies in leukemia, idiopathic thrombocytopenic purpura: WBCs (leukemia), platelets
- Identify the number of injections of this drug patient has received; multiple injections may lead to sensitization (diaphoresis, fever, chills, malaise)
- Assess for anaphylaxis in patient receiving **IV** immune globulin: diaphoresis, flushing, nausea, vomiting, wheezing, difficulty breathing, hypotension, chest tightness, fever, weakness, sneezing, abdominal pain; VS should be monitored during inf and 1 hr after beginning inf; emergency equipment should be available with epinephrine and antihistamines to treat anaphylaxis

Nursing diagnoses

- ✓ Infection, risk for (uses)
- ✓ Knowledge deficit (teaching)

Implementation

IM route

- Give IM (IGIM) in deltoid or anterolateral thigh in adults or anterolateral thigh in young children; if large amounts are given, several inj may be needed P
- Do not give the IM preparation **IV**, SC, or intradermally
- Sol should be transparent and clear or slightly colored

IV **IV route**

- Warm to room temp before administration (diluent, powder for inj)
- A transfer device is provided by manufacturer; this drug should not be agitated or shaken
- Do not give the **IV** preparation SC, IM, or intradermally
- Check for adverse reaction during inf; stop inf if adverse reactions are present

Y-site compatibilities: Fluconazole, sargramostim

Gamimune N: Dilute **IV** with D_5; give 0.01 ml/kg/min; may increase to 0.02-0.04 ml/kg/min if no adverse reactions are present; may increase to

0.08 ml/kg/hr; sol should be refrigerated; do not freeze

Gammagard S/D: Reconstitute with sterile water for inj (50 mg protein/ml); give within 2 hr of reconstitution; give 0.5 ml/kg/hr; may increase to 4 ml/kg/hr if no adverse reactions occur; use inf set provided

Gammar-IV: Give 0.01 ml/kg/min (50 mg/ml sol) over 15-30 min; may increase to 0.02 ml/kg/min; if adverse reactions are not present, may increase to 0.03-0.06 ml/kg/min; do not freeze; store at room temp

Iveegam (5%): Give 1-2 ml/min; refrigerate, do not freeze

Sandoglobulin: **IV** diluted with provided diluent; give 0.5-1 ml/min over 15-30 min; may increase to 1.5-2.5 ml/min; other inf may be given 2-2.5 ml/min; store at room temp

Venoglobulin-I: Give 50 mg/ml sol 0.01-0.02 ml/kg/min over 30 min if no adverse reactions; increase 0.04 ml/kg/min; store at room temp

Patient/family education

- Advise patient that passive immunity is temporary; explain reason for and expected results of this drug
- Advise patient that pain and tenderness may occur at inj site

Evaluation

Positive therapeutic outcome

- Prevention of infection
- Increased platelets

Treatment of anaphylaxis: Epinephrine, diphenhydramine, O_2, vasopressors, corticosteroids

inamrinone (℞)

(in-am'rih-nohn)

Func. class.: Cardiac inotropic agent
Chem. class.: Bipyrimidine derivative

Pregnancy category C

Action: Positive inotropic agent with vasodilator properties; reduces preload and afterload by direct relaxation of vascular smooth muscle; increases myocardial contractility

➔ **Therapeutic Outcome:** Increased inotropic effect resulting in increased cardiac output

Uses: Short-term management of CHF that has not responded to other medication; can be used with digitalis products

Dosage and routes

P ***Adult and child:*** **IV** bol 0.75 mg/kg given over 2-3 min; start inf of 5-10 µg/kg/min; may give another bol 30 min after start of therapy, max 10 mg/kg total daily dose

P ***Infants:*** **IV** 3-4.5 mg/kg in divided doses, then give by inf 10 µg/kg/min

P ***Neonates:*** **IV** 3-4.5 mg/kg in divided doses, then give by inf 3-5 µg/kg/min

Available forms: Inj 5 mg/ml

Adverse effects

CV: *Dysrhythmias, hypotension,* headache, chest pain
ELECT: Hypokalemia
GI: *Nausea, vomiting, anorexia,* abdominal pain, **hepatotoxicity (rare), ascites,** jaundice, hiccups
HEMA: **Thrombocytopenia**
INTEG: Allergic reactions, burning at inj site
RESP: Pleuritis, **pulmonary densities, hypoxemia,** dyspnea

Contraindications: Hypersensitivity to this drug or bisulfites, severe aortic disease, severe pulmonic valvular disease, acute MI

Precautions: Lactation, pregnancy C, children, renal disease, hepatic disease, atrial flutter/fibrillation, elderly

Do Not Confuse:
amrinone/amiodarone, Inocor/Cordarone

Pharmacokinetics

Absorption	Complete bioavailability
Distribution	Unknown
Metabolism	Liver, 50%
Excretion	Kidney, metabolites (60%-90%)
Half-life	4-6 hr, increased in CHF

Pharmacodynamics

Onset	2-5 min
Peak	10 min
Duration	Variable

Interactions

Individual drugs

Disopyramide: ↑ hypotension

Drug classifications

Antihypertensives: ↑ hypotension
Cardiac glycosides: ↑ inotropic effect

Herb/drug

Aloe: ↑ amrinone action
Buckthorn bark/berry: ↑ amrinone action
Cascara sagrada: ↑ amrinone action
Ephedra: ↑ amrinone action
Senna pod/leaf: ↑ amrinone action

Lab test interferences

↓ Potassium, ↑ hepatic enzymes

NURSING CONSIDERATIONS

Assessment

- Monitor manifestations of hypokalemia: *RENAL:* acidic urine, reduced urine, osmolality, nocturia; *CV:* hypotension, broad T wave, U wave, ectopy, tachycardia, weak pulse; *NEURO:* muscle weakness, altered LOC, drowsiness, apathy, lethargy, confusion, depression; *GI:* anorexia, nausea, cramps, constipation, distention, paralytic ileus; *RESP:* hypoventilation, respiratory muscle weakness
- Assess fluid volume status: CVP in elderly, I&O ratio and record, weight, distended red veins, crackles in lung, color, quality and sp gr of urine, skin turgor, adequacy of pulses, moist mucous membranes, bilateral lung sounds, peripheral pitting edema; dehydration symptoms of decreasing output, thirst, hypotension, dry mouth, and mucous membranes should be reported
- Monitor electrolytes: potassium, sodium, calcium, magnesium; also include BUN, blood pH, ABGs
- Monitor B/P and pulse, PCWP, CVP, index, often during inf; if B/P drops 30 mm Hg, stop infusion and call prescriber
- Monitor ALT, AST, bilirubin daily; if these are elevated, hepatotoxicity is suspected
- If platelets are <150,000/mm^3, drug is usually discontinued and another drug started
- Assess for extravasation: change site q48h

Nursing diagnoses

- Cardiac output, decreased (uses)
- Fluid volume excess (uses)
- Knowledge deficit (teaching)

Implementation

General

- Patients with low potassium levels (hypokalemia) should receive potassium supplements before inamrinone administration
- Administer potassium supplements if ordered for potassium levels <3.0 mg/dl, correct before using inamrinone

IV route

- Do not mix directly with glucose sol; chemical reaction occurs over 24 hr; precipitate forms if inamrinone and furosemide come in contact

Direct IV

- Administer into running dextrose inf through Y-connector or directly into tubing; may give undiluted over 2-3 min or dilute with 0.9%, 0.45% NaCl to concentration of 1-3 mg/ml; run at prescribed rate by cont inf; another loading dose may be given in 30 min

IV **Cont IV**

- Give after diluting with 0.9% or 0.45% NaCl (1-3 mg/ml); do not dilute with dextrose sol; decomposition of drug will occur; use infusion pump; use sol within 24 hr of dilution; titrate to patient response

Syringe compatibilities: Propranolol, verapamil

Y-site compatibilities: Aminophylline, atropine, bretylium, calcium chloride, cimetidine, cisatracurium, digoxin, dobutamine, dopamine, epinephrine, famotidine, hydrocortisone, isoproterenol, lidocaine, metaraminol, methylprednisolone, nitroglycerin, nitroprusside, norepinephrine, phenylephrine, potassium chloride, procainamide, propranolol, remifentanil, verapamil

Y-site incompatibilities: Furosemide, sodium bicarbonate

Patient/family education

- Teach patient reason for medication and expected results
- Instruct patient to make position changes slowly; orthostatic hypotension may occur
- Teach patient signs and symptoms of hypersensitivity reactions and hypokalemia
- Advise patient that burning may occur at **IV** site

Evaluation

Positive therapeutic outcome

- Increased cardiac output
- Decreased PCWP, adequate CVP
- Decreased dyspnea, fatigue, edema, ECG

Treatment of overdose: Discontinue drug, support circulation

indapamide (℞)

(in-dap'a-mide)

indapamide, Lozide ♣, Lozol

Func. class.: Diuretic, thiazide-like, antihypertensive

Chem. class.: Thiazide-like sulfonamide derivative

Pregnancy category B

Action: Acts on the distal tubule and thick ascending loop of Henle in the kidney, increasing excretion of sodium, water, chloride, magnesium, potassium, and bicarbonate

➔ **Therapeutic Outcome:** Decreased B/P, decreased edema in lung tissues, peripherally

Uses: May be used alone or as adjunct with antihypertensives (mild to moderate)

Dosage and routes

Edema

Adult: PO 2.5 mg qd in AM; may be increased to 5 mg qd if needed

Antihypertensive

Adult: PO 1.25-5 mg qd; may increase to 5 mg/day over 8 wks

Available forms: Tabs 1.25, 2.5 mg

Adverse effects

CNS: Depression, *headache, dizziness, fatigue, weakness, nervousness, agitation*

CV: Orthostatic hypotension, palpitations, volume depletion, PVCs

EENT: Blurred vision, nasal congestion, increased intraocular pressure

ELECT: *Hypokalemia, hypercalcemia, hyponatremia, hypochloremia, hypomagnesemia*

GI: *Nausea,* vomiting, anorexia, constipation, diarrhea, cramps, GI irritation, abdominal pain

GU: *Frequency, polyuria, nocturia*

INTEG: Rash, *pruritus,*

META: Hyperglycemia, *hyperuricemia,* increased creatinine, BUN

MS: Cramps

Contraindications: Hypersensitivity to thiazides or sulfonamides, anuria, lactation, hepatic coma

Precautions: Hypokalemia, renal disease, hepatic disease, gout, diabetes mellitus, G elderly, ascites, dehydration, pregnancy **B**, lactation, CrCl <25 ml/min (not effective)

Pharmacokinetics

Absorption	Well absorbed
Distribution	Widely distributed
Metabolism	Liver; 7%
Excretion	Unchanged (urine)
Half-life	14-18 hr

Pharmacodynamics

Onset	1-2 hr
Peak	2 hr
Duration	Up to 36 hr

Interactions

Individual drugs

Alcohol: ↑ hypotension
Amphotericin B: ↓ effects
Lithium: ↑ toxicity
Mezlocillin: ↑ hypokalemia
Piperacillin: ↑ hypokalemia
Ticarcillin: ↑ hypokalemia

Drug classifications

Anticoagulants: ↓ effects
Antigout agents: ↓ effects
Antihypertensives: ↑ antihypertensive effect
Cardiac glycosides: ↑ hypokalemia, ↑ toxicity
Diuretics, other: ↓ potassium
Glucocorticoids: ↑ hypokalemia

Herb/drug

Aloe: ↑ hypokalemia
Buckthorn: ↑ hypokalemia
Licorice: ↑ hypokalemia
Senna: ↑ hypokalemia

Lab test interferences

↑ Calcium, ↑ parathyroid test

NURSING CONSIDERATIONS

Assessment

- Check for rashes, temp elevation qd
- Monitor patients that receive cardiac glycosides for increased hypokalemia, toxicity
- Monitor manifestations of hypokalemia: acidic or reduced urine, osmolality, nocturia; hypotension, broad T wave, U wave, ectopy, tachycardia, weak pulse; muscle weakness, altered LOC, drowsiness, apathy, lethargy, confusion, depression; anorexia, nausea, cramps, constipation, distention, paralytic ileus; hypoventilation, respiratory muscle weakness
- Monitor for manifestations of hypomagnesemia: agitation, muscle twitching, paresthesias, hyperactive reflexes, positive Babinski reflex, dysphagia, nystagmus, seizures, tetany; nausea, vomiting, diarrhea, anorexia, abdominal distention; ectopy, tachycardia, broad, flat or inverted T waves, depressed ST segment, prolonged QT interval, decreased cardiac output, hypotension
- Monitor for manifestations of hyponatremia: increased B/P, cold, clammy skin, hypo/hypervolemia; anorexia, nausea, vomiting, diarrhea, abdominal cramps; lethargy, increased ICP, confusion, headache, seizures, coma, fatigue, tremors, hyperreflexia
- Monitor for manifestations of hyperchloremia: weakness, lethargy, coma, deep rapid breathing
- Assess fluid volume status: I&O ratios and record, weight, distended red veins, crackles in lung, color, quality and sp gr of urine, skin turgor, adequacy of pulses, moist mucous membranes, bilateral lung sounds, peripheral pitting edema; dehydration symptoms of decreasing output, thirst, hypotension, dry mouth and mucous membranes should be reported
- Monitor electrolytes: potassium, sodium, calcium, magnesium; also include BUN, blood pH, ABGs, uric acid, CBC, blood sugar
- Assess B/P before and during therapy with patient lying, standing,

and sitting as appropriate; orthostatic hypotension can occur rapidly

Nursing diagnoses

- ✓ Altered urinary elimination (side effect)
- ✓ Fluid volume deficit (side effects)
- ✓ Fluid volume excess (uses)
- ✓ Knowledge deficit (teaching)

Implementation

- Give in AM to avoid interference with sleep
- Provide potassium replacement if potassium level is <3.0 mg/dl; give whole
- Give with food; if nausea occurs, absorption may be increased

Patient/family education

- Teach patient to take the medication early in the day to prevent nocturia
- Instruct the patient to take with food or milk if GI symptoms of nausea and anorexia occur
- Teach patient to maintain weekly record of weight and notify prescriber of weight loss >5 lb
- Caution the patient that this drug causes a loss of potassium, so food rich in potassium should be added to the diet; refer to a dietitian for assistance in planning
- Caution the patient not to exercise in hot weather or stand for prolonged periods, since orthostatic hypotension will be enhanced
- Teach patient not to use alcohol or any OTC medications without prescriber's approval; serious drug reactions may occur
- Emphasize the need to contact prescriber immediately if muscle cramps, weakness, nausea, dizziness, or numbness occurs
- Teach patient to take own B/P and pulse and record findings
- Caution the patient that orthostatic hypotension may occur and to rise slowly from sitting or reclining positions and lie down if dizziness occurs
- Teach patient to continue taking medication even if feeling better; this drug controls symptoms but does not cure the condition
- Advise the patient with hypertension to continue other medical treatment (exercise, weight loss, relaxation techniques, cessation of smoking)

Evaluation

Positive therapeutic outcome

- Decreased edema
- Decreased B/P
- Increased diuresis

Treatment of overdose:

Lavage, monitor electrolytes, administer **IV** fluids, monitor hydration, CV, renal status

indinavir (℞)

(en-den′a-veer)

Crixivan

Func. class.: Antiviral

Chem. class.: Synthetic peptide-like substrate analog

Pregnancy category C

Action: Inhibits HIV protease; this prevents maturation of the infectious virus

➡ **Therapeutic Outcome:** Decreased signs/symptoms of HIV infection

Uses: HIV infection alone or in combination

Dosage and routes

Reduce dose in mild/moderate hepatic impairment and ketoconazole coadministration

Adult: PO 800 mg q8h; if given with didanosine, given 1 hr apart on empty stomach

Available forms: Caps 200, 400 mg

Adverse effects

CNS: *Headache, insomnia,* dizziness, somnolence

GI: *Diarrhea, abdominal pain, nausea, vomiting,* anorexia, dry mouth

GU: Nephrolithesis
INTEG: Rash
MISC: Asthenia, **insulin-resistant hyperglycemia**, hyperlipidemia, **ketoacidosis**
MS: Pain

Contraindications: Hypersensitivity

Precautions: Liver disease, P pregnancy **C**, lactation, children, renal disease, history of renal stones

Pharmacokinetics

Absorption	Unknown
Distribution	Unknown
Metabolism	Unknown
Excretion	Unknown
Half-life	Unknown

Pharmacodynamics

Unknown

Interactions

Individual drugs

Cerivastatin: ↑ myopathy
Clarithromycin: ↑ levels of both drugs
Delavirdine: ↑ indinavir level
Efavirenz: ↓ indinavir level
Fluconazole: ↓ indinavir level
Isoniazid: ↑ isoniazid level
Itraconazole: ↑ indinavir level
Ketoconazole: ↑ levels of both drugs
Lovastatin: ↑ myopathy
Midazolam: ↑ life-threatening dysrhythmias
Nevirapine: ↓ indinavir level
Simvastatin: ↑ myopathy
Triazolam: ↑ life-threatening dysrhythmias

Drug classifications

Ergots: ↑ life-threatening dysrhythmias
Rifamycins: ↑ life-threatening dysrhythmias

Food/drug

High fat, high protein: ↓ absorption
Grapefruit juice: ↓ absorption

Herb/drug

St. John's wort: ↓ indinavir level, avoid use

NURSING CONSIDERATIONS

Assessment

- Monitor signs of infection, anemia
- Monitor liver studies: ALT, AST
- Determine the presence of other sexually transmitted diseases
- Assess bowel pattern before, during treatment; if severe abdominal pain with bleeding occurs, drug should be discontinued; monitor hydration
- Assess skin eruptions; rash, urticaria, itching
- Assess allergies before treatment, reaction of each medication; place allergies on chart

Nursing diagnoses

✓ Infection, risk for (uses)
✓ Knowledge deficit (teaching)

Implementation

- Give with water, 1 hr ac or 2 hr pc

Patient/family education

- Advise to take as prescribed; if dose is missed, take as soon as remembered up to 1 hr before next dose; do not double dose
- Do not crush, chew caps
- Advise that drug must be taken in equal intervals around the clock to maintain blood levels for duration of therapy
- Instruct patient to increase fluids to prevent kidney stones
- Inform patient that drug does not cure AIDS, controls symptoms only
- Advise patient that hyperglycemia may occur, watch for symptoms (thirst, hunger, dry, itchy skin); notify prescriber

Evaluation

Positive therapeutic outcome

- Decreased signs/symptoms of infection, HIV

indomethacin (℞)

(in-doe-meth'a-sin)

Apo-Indomethacin ✤, Indameth ✤, Indochron E-R, Indocid ✤, Indocin, Indocin IV, Indocin PDA ✤, Indocin SR, indomethacin, Novomethacin ✤, Nu-Indo ✤

Func. class.: NSAID

Chem. class.: Propionic acid derivative

Pregnancy category B

Action: Inhibits prostaglandin synthesis by decreasing enzyme needed for biosynthesis; analgesic, antiinflammatory, antipyretic

→ **Therapeutic Outcome:** Decreased pain, inflammation; or closure of patent ductus arteriosus (premature P infants)

Uses: Rheumatoid arthritis, ankylosing rheumatoid spondylitis, acute gouty arthritis, closure of patent P ductus arteriosus in premature infants

Dosage and routes

Arthritis/antiinflammatory

Adult: PO/REC 25-50 mg bid-tid; may increase by 25 mg/day qwk, not to exceed 200 mg/day; sus rel 75 mg qd; may increase to 75 mg bid

Acute arthritis

Adult: PO/REC 50 mg tid; use only for acute attack, then reduce dosage

Patent ductus arteriosus

Longer or repeated treatment courses may be necessary for very premature P infants

P ***Infant<2 days:*** **IV** 0.2 mg/kg, then 0.1 mg/kg q12-24h

P ***Infant 2-7 days:*** **IV** 0.2 mg/kg, then 0.2 mg/kg × 2 doses after 12, 24 hr

P ***Infant >7 days:*** **IV** 0.2 mg/kg, then 0.25 mg/kg × 2 doses after 12, 24 hr

Available forms: Caps 25, 50 mg; sus rel caps 75 mg; oral susp 25 mg/5 ml; rec supp 50 mg; inj 1-mg vials

Adverse effects

CNS: Dizziness, drowsiness, fatigue, tremors, confusion, insomnia, anxiety, depression, headache

CV: Tachycardia, peripheral edema, palpitations, dysrhythmias, hypertension

EENT: Tinnitus, hearing loss, blurred vision

GI: *Nausea,* anorexia, *vomiting,* diarrhea, jaundice, **cholestatic hepatitis,** *constipation,* flatulence, cramps, dry mouth, peptic ulcer, **ulceration, perforation, GI bleeding**

GU: **Nephrotoxicity (dysuria, hematuria, oliguria, azotemia)**

HEMA: **Blood dyscrasias,** prolonged bleeding

INTEG: Purpura, rash, pruritus, sweating

Contraindications: Hypersensitivity, asthma, severe renal disease, severe hepatic disease, ulcer disease

P **Precautions:** Lactation, children, bleeding disorders, GI disorders, cardiac disorders, hypersensitivity to other antiinflammatory agents, pregnancy **B** (1st trimester), depression

Pharmacokinetics

Absorption	Well absorbed (PO); erratic (rec); complete (**IV**)
Distribution	Crosses blood-brain barrier; placenta, 99% plasma protein binding
Metabolism	Liver, extensively
Excretion	Breast milk
Half-life	2.6-11 hr

Pharmacodynamics

	IV	PO	PO–EXT REL
Onset	2 day	1-2 hr	½ hr
Peak	Unknown	3 hr	Unknown
Duration	Unknown	4-6 hr	4-6 hr

Interactions

Individual drugs

Acetaminophen (long-term use): ↑ renal reactions
Alcohol: ↑ adverse reactions
Aspirin: ↓ effectiveness, ↑ adverse reactions of indomethacin
Cyclosporine: ↑ nephrotoxicity
Digoxin: ↑ toxicity, levels
Insulin: ↓ insulin effect
Lithium: ↑ toxicity, levels
Methotrexate: ↑ toxicity
Phenytoin: ↑ toxicity
Probenecid: ↑ toxicity
Radiation: ↑ risk of hematologic toxicity
Triamterene: ↑ toxicity
Zidovudine: ↑ toxicity, levels

Drug classifications

Aminoglycosides: ↑ toxicity
Anticoagulants: ↑ risk of bleeding
Antihypertensives: ↓ effect of antihypertensives
Antineoplastics: ↑ risk of hematologic toxicity
β-Adrenergic blockers: ↑ antihypertension
Cephalosporins: ↑ risk of bleeding
Diuretics: ↓ effectiveness of diuretics
Glucocorticoids: ↑ adverse reactions
Hypoglycemics: ↓ hypoglycemic effect
NSAIDs: ↑ adverse reactions
Potassium supplements: ↑ adverse reactions
Sulfonamides: ↑ toxicity
Sulfonylureas: ↑ toxicity

NURSING CONSIDERATIONS

Assessment

- Assess for joint pain (duration, intensity, ROM), baseline and during treatment
- Assess for confusion, mood changes, hallucinations, especially in [G] elderly
- Assess renal, liver, blood studies: BUN, creatinine, AST, ALT, Hgb before treatment and periodically thereafter; if renal function decreases, do not give subsequent doses

Nursing diagnoses

- ✓ Pain (uses)
- ✓ Chronic pain (uses)
- ✓ Impaired mobility (uses)
- ✓ Knowledge deficit (teaching)

Implementation

PO route

- [Do Not Crush] Administer to patient whole; do not crush, chew, or break sus rel cap
- Give with food or milk to decrease gastric symptoms, and prevent ulceration

[IV] IV route

- Give after diluting 1 mg/ml or more normal saline or sterile water for inj without preservative; give over ½ hr to avoid dramatic shift in cerebral blood flow; avoid extravasation

Y-site compatibilities:
Furosemide, insulin (regular), potassium chloride, sodium bicarbonate, sodium nitroprusside

Rectal route

- Have patient retain rec supp for 1 hr after insertion

Patient/family education

- Advise patient to report change in vision, blurring, rash, tinnitus, black stools
- Tell patient not to use for any other condition than prescribed
- Advise patient to avoid use with OTC medications for pain unless approved by prescriber
- Advise patient to avoid hazardous activities, since dizziness or drowsiness can occur
- Instruct patient to use sunscreen to prevent photosensitivity

Evaluation

Positive therapeutic outcome

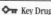

- Decreased stiffness
- Increased joint mobility
- Decreased pain

infliximab (℞)

(in-fliks'ih-mab)

Remicade

Func. class.: Monoclonal antibody

Pregnancy category C

Action: Monoclonal antibody that neutralizes the activity of tumor necrosis factor α (TNFα) that has been found in Crohn's disease; decreased infilitration of inflammatory cells

➡ **Therapeutic Outcome:** Decreased cramping and blood in stools

Uses: Crohn's disease, fistulizing, moderate-severe; rheumatoid arthritis given with methotrexate

Dosage and routes

Crohn's disease (moderate-severe)

Adult: **IV** inf 5 mg/kg × 1

Crohn's disease (fistulizing)

Adult: **IV** inf 5 mg/kg initially, then repeat dose 2, 6 wk after 1st dose

Rheumatoid arthritis

Adult: **IV** 3 mg/kg initially, and 2, 6 wk and q8 wk thereafter, given with methotrexate

Available forms: Powder for inj 100 mg

Adverse effects

CNS: *Headache, dizziness, depression, vertigo, fatigue, anxiety, fever*

CV: Chest pain, hypertension and hypotension, tachycardia

GU: Dysuria, frequency

HEMA: **Anemia**

INTEG: *Rash, dermatitis, urticaria,* dry skin, sweating, flushing, hematoma, pruritus

MS: Myalgia, back pain, arthralgia

RESP: URI, pharyngitis, bronchitis, cough, dyspnea, sinusitis

SYST: **Anaplylaxis**

Contraindications: Hypersensitivity to murines

P G **Precautions:** Pregnancy **C**, lactation, children, elderly

Pharmacokinetics

Absorption	Unknown
Distribution	Vascular compartment
Metabolism	Unknown
Excretion	Unknown
Half-life	9½ days

Pharmacodynamics

Onset	Unknown
Peak	Unknown
Duration	Unknown

Interactions: Unknown

NURSING CONSIDERATIONS

Assessment

- Assess GI symptoms: nausea, vomiting, abdominal pain
- Take periodic blood counts: CBC
- Assess CV status: B/P, pulse, chest pain
- Assess for allergic reaction: rash, dermatitis, urticaria, fever, chills, dyspnea, hypotention; discontinue if severe, administer epinephrine, corticosteroids

Nursing diagnoses

✓ Injury, risk for (uses)
✓ Diarrhea (uses)
✓ Knowledge deficit (teaching)

Implementation

IV infusion route

- Administer immediately after reconstitution; reconstitute with 10 ml of sterile water for inj, further dilute total dose/250 ml of 0.9% NaCl inj to a total conc of between 0.4 and 4 mg/ml; use 21-G or smaller needle for reconstitution, direct sterile water at glass wall of vial, gently swirl
- Give over ≥2 hr, use polyethylene-lined infusion with in-line, sterile, low-protein-bind filter
- Provide refrigerated storage, do not freeze

Patient/family education

- Teach patient not to breastfeed while taking this drug
- Advise patient to notify prescriber of

GI symptoms, hypersensitivity reactions

Evaluation

Positive therapeutic outcome

- Absence of blood in stool
- Reported improvement in comfort
- Weight gain

insulin aspart (℞)

NovoLog

insulin glargine

Lantus

Func. class.: Pancreatic hormone

Pregnancy category C

Action: Decreases blood glucose; by transport of insulin into cells and the conversion of glucose to glycogen, indirectly increases blood pyruvate and lactate, decreases phosphate and potassium; insulin may be beef, pork, human (processed by recombinant DNA technologies)

Therapeutic Outcome: Resolution of signs/symptoms of diabetes

P **Uses:** Adult-onset diabetes, juvenile diabetes, ketoacidosis types I and II, type II (non–insulin-dependent) diabetes mellitus, type I (insulin-dependent) diabetes mellitus

Dosage and routes

Lantus

Adult: SC 10 IU qd, range 2-100 IU/day

P ***Child ≥6 yr:*** Same as adults

Available forms: Lantus (inj 100 IU); NovoLog (inj 100 U/ml human insulin aspart (rDNA)

Adverse effects

EENT: Blurred vision, dry mouth

INTEG: Flushing, rash, urticaria, warmth, *lipodystrophy,* lipohypertrophy, swelling, redness

META: *Hypoglycemia,* rebound hyperglycemia (Somogyi effect 12-72 hr or longer)

SYST: **Anaphylaxis**

Contraindications: Hypersensitivity to protamine

Precautions: Pregnancy **C**

Pharmacokinetics

Absorption	Unknown
Distribution	Unknown
Metabolism	Liver, muscles, kidneys
Excretion	Kidneys
Half-life	Lantus 1½ hr

Pharmacodynamics

	ASPART (NOVOLOG)	GLARGINE (LANTUS)
Onset	0.25 hr	1.1 hr
Peak	1-3 hr	no peak
Duration	3-5 hr	24 hr

Interactions

Individual drugs

Alcohol: ↑ hypoglycemia
Diltiazem: ↑ insulin need
Dobutamine: ↑ insulin need
Fenfluramine: ↓ insulin need
Guanethidine: ↓ insulin need
Phenylbutazone: ↓ insulin need
Rifampin: ↑ insulin need
Sulfinpyrazone: ↓ insulin need
Tetracycline: ↓ insulin need

Drug classifications

Anabolic steroids: ↓ insulin need
β-Adrenergic blockers: Signs/symptoms of hypoglycemia may be masked
Estrogens: ↑ insulin need
Glucocorticoid steroids: ↑ insulin need
MAOIs: ↓ insulin need
Oral anticoagulants: ↓ insulin need
Oral hypoglycemics: ↑ hypoglycemia
Thiazide diuretics: ↑ insulin need
Thyroid hormones: ↑ insulin need

Herb/drug

Broom: ↓ hypoglycemic effect
Buchu: ↓ hypoglycemic effect
Chromium: ↓ or ↑ hypoglycemic effect
Dandelion: ↓ hypoglycemic effect

Fenugreek: ↓ or ↑ hypoglycemic effect
Ginseng: ↓ or ↑ hypoglycemic effect
Juniper: ↓ hypoglycemic effect
Karela: ↑ glucose tolerance

Smoking

↑ Insulin need

Lab test interferences

↑ VMA
↓ Potassium, ↓ magnesium, ↓ inorganic phosphate
Interference: Liver function studies, thyroid function studies

NURSING CONSIDERATIONS

Assessment

- Monitor fasting blood glucose, 2 hr PC (80-150 mg/dl, normal fasting level; 70-130 mg/dl, normal 2-hr level); also glycosylated Hgb may be measured to identify treatment effectiveness
- Monitor urine ketones during illness; insulin requirements may increase during stress, illness, surgery
- Assess for hypoglycemic reaction that can occur during peak time (sweating, weakness, dizziness, chills, confusion, headache, nausea, rapid weak pulse, fatigue, tachycardia, memory lapses, slurred speech, staggering gait, anxiety, tremors, hunger)
- Assess for hyperglycemia: acetone breath, polyuria, fatigue, polydipsia, flushed, dry skin, lethargy

Nursing diagnoses

✓ Injury, risk for (adverse reactions)
✓ Knowledge deficit (teaching)
✓ Noncompliance (teaching)

Implementation

SC route

- Give after warming to room temp by rotating in palms to prevent injecting cold insulin; use only insulin syringes with markings or syringe matching U/ml; rotate inj sites within one area: abdomen, upper back, thighs, upper arm, buttocks; keep record of sites
- Give increased dosages if tolerance occurs; give human insulin to those allergic to beef or pork
- Store at room temp for <1 mo; keep away from heat and sunlight; refrigerate all other supply; do not use if discolored; do not freeze
- Do not mix or add insulin glargine to any other insulin or sol
- Do not mix insulin aspart with crystalline zinc insulin

Patient/family education

- Advise patient that blurred vision occurs; not to change corrective lens until vision is stabilized 1-2 mo
- Advise patient to keep insulin, equipment available at all times
- Teach patient that drug does not cure diabetes, only controls symptoms
- Teach patient to carry ID as diabetic
- Teach patient to recognize hypoglycemic reaction: headache, tremors, fatigue, weakness
- Teach patient the dosage, route, mixing instructions, if any diet restrictions, disease process
- Advise patient to carry candy or lump sugar to treat hypoglycemia
- Advise patient of symptoms of ketoacidosis: nausea, thirst, polyuria, dry mouth, decreased B/P, dry, flushed skin, acetone breath, drowsiness, Kussmaul respirations
- Inform patient that a plan is necessary for diet, exercise; all food on diet should be eaten; exercise routine should not vary
- Teach patient about blood glucose testing; make sure patient is able to determine glucose level
- Advise patient to avoid OTC drugs unless directed by prescriber

Evaluation

Positive therapeutic outcome

- Decrease in polyuria, polydipsia, polyphagia, clear sensorium, absence of dizziness, stable gait

Treatment of overdose:

Glucose 25 g **IV**, via dextrose 50% sol, 50 ml or glucagon 1 mg

HIGH ALERT

INSULINS

insulin, isophane suspension (NPH) Key Drug (℞)

Humulin N, Iletin NPH, Illetin II NPH ✤, Novolin ge NPH ✤, Novolin N, Novolin N PenFill, Novolin N Prefilled, NPH Iletin I, NPH Iletin II, NPH-N

insulin, isophane suspension and insulin injection (℞)

Humalin 50/50, Novolin ge 50/50 ✤,

insulin, isophane suspension and regular insulin (℞)

Humulin 70/30, Humalin 30/70 ✤, Novolin 70/30, Novolin 70/30 PenFill, Novolin 7/30 Prefilled, Novolin ge 30/70 ✤

insulin lispro

Humalog

insulin, regular Key Drug (℞)

Humulin R, Iletin I, Illetin II ✤, Novolin ge Toronto ✤, Novolin R, Novolin R PenFill, Novolin R Prefilled, Novolin R Velosulin, Regular Illetin I, Regular Illetin II, regular purified pork insulin, Velosulin Human BR

insulin, zinc suspension extended (ultralente) (℞)

Humulin U ✤, Humulin U Ultralente, Novolin ge Ultralente

insulin, zinc suspension (lente) (℞)

Humulin L, Iletin ✤, Illetin II ✤, Lente Iletin I, Lente Iletin II, Lente L, Novolin ge Lente ✤, Novolin L

Func. class.: Pancreatic hormone

Chem. class.: Exogenous unmodified insulin

Pregnancy category B

Action: Decreases blood glucose; by transport of insulin into cells and the conversion of glucose to glycogen indirectly increases blood pyruvate and lactate, decreases phosphate and potassium; insulin may be beef, pork, human (processed by recombinant DNA technologies)

Therapeutic Outcome: Decreased blood glucose levels in diabetes mellitus

Uses: Adult-onset diabetes, juvenile diabetes, ketoacidosis types I and II, type II (non–insulin-dependent) diabetes mellitus, type I (insulin-dependent) diabetes mellitus; insulin lispro may be used in combination with sulfonylureas in children >3 yr

Dosage and routes

Insulin lispro

Adult: SC 15 min ac

Human regular

Adult: SC ½-1 ac

Insulin, isophane, suspension

Adult: SC dosage individualized by blood, urine glucose; usual dose 7-26 U; may increase by 2-10 U/day if needed

Regular insulin

Ketoacidosis

Adult: **IV** 5-10 U, then 5-10 U/hr until desired response, then switch to SC dose; **IV**/ inf 2-12 U (50 U/500 ml of normal saline)

P ***Child:*** **IV** 0.1 U/kg

Replacement

P ***Adult and child:*** SC 0.5-1 U/kg/day qid given 30 min pc

Adolescents: SC 0.8-1.2 mg/kg/day; this dosage is used during rapid growth

Available forms: NPH inj 100 U/ml; regular **IV**/IM/SC inj 100 U/ml; insulin analog inj 100 U/ml; insulin zinc susp, ext (ultralente) 100 U/ml; isophane insulin/insulin inj 100 U/ml; zinc susp 100 U/ml; insulin lispro 100 U/ml, 1.5 ml cartridges

Adverse effects

EENT: Blurred vision, dry mouth
INTEG: Flushing, rash, urticaria, warmth, *lipodystrophy,* lipohypertrophy, swelling, redness
META: *Hypoglycemia,* rebound hyperglycemia (Somogyi effect 12-72 hr or longer)
SYST: **Anaphylaxis**

Contraindications: Hypersensitivity to protamine

Precautions: Pregnancy **B**

Do Not Confuse:

Novolin 70/30 Penfill, Novolin 70/30 Prefilled

Pharmacokinetics

Absorption	Rapidly absorbed (SC)
Distribution	Widely distributed
Metabolism	Liver, muscle, kidney
Excretion	Kidneys
Half-life	Regular 3-5 min; NPH 10 min

Interactions

Individual drugs

Alcohol: ↑ hypoglycemia
Diltiazem: ↑ insulin need
Dobutamine: ↑ insulin need
Fenfluramine: ↓ insulin need
Guanethidine: ↓ insulin need
Phenylbutazone: ↓ insulin need
Rifampin: ↑ insulin need
Sulfinpyrazone: ↓ insulin need
Tetracycline: ↓ insulin need

Drug classifications

Anabolic steroids: ↓ insulin need
β-Adrenergic blockers: Signs/symptoms of hypoglycemia may be masked
Estrogens: ↑ insulin need
Glucocorticoid steroids: ↑ insulin need
MAOIs: ↓ insulin need
Oral anticoagulants: ↓ insulin need
Oral hypoglycemics: ↑ hypoglycemia
Thiazide diuretics: ↑ insulin need
Thyroid hormones: ↑ insulin need

Herb/drug

Aceitilla: ↑ hypoglycemia
Adiantam: ↑ hypoglycemia
Agrimony: ↑ hypoglycemia
Aloe gel: ↑ hypoglycemia
Annato: ↓ hypoglycemia
Banana flowers/roots: ↑ hypoglycemia
Banyan stem bark: ↑ hypoglycemia
Bilberry: ↑ hypoglycemia
Bitter melon: ↑ hypoglycemia
Bugleweed: ↑ hypoglycemia
Burdock: ↑ hypoglycemia
Carob: ↑ hypoglycemia
Chromium: ↑ or ↓ hypoglycemia
Cocoa seeds: ↓ hypoglycemia
Coffee beans: ↓ hypoglycemia
Cola seeds: ↓ hypoglycemia
Cumin: ↑ hypoglycemia
Damiana: ↑ hypoglycemia
Dandelion: ↑ hypoglycemia
Eucalyptus: ↑ hypoglycemia
Fenugreek: ↑ hypoglycemia

Pharmacodynamics

	NPH	INSULIN, REGULAR		INSULIN, REGULAR CONC	ZINC SUSP	ZINC SUSP CONC	ZINC SUSP PROMPT	LISPRO
		SC	IV				SC	
Onset	1-2 hr	½-1 hr	10-30 min	½-1 hr	1-2½ hr	4-8 hr	1-1½ hr	Rapid
Peak	4-12 hr	2-4 hr	30-60 min	2-5 hr	7-15 hr	10-30 hr	5-10 hr	½-1 hr
Duration	18-24 hr	5-7 hr	½-1 hr	5-7 hr	12-24 hr	7-36 hr	12-16 hr	3-4 hr

Fo-ti: ↑ hypoglycemia
Garlic: ↑ hypoglycemia
Goat's rue: ↑ hypoglycemia
Guar gum: ↑ hypoglycemia
Guarana: ↓ hypoglycemic effect
Horse chestnut: ↑ hypoglycemia
Jambul: ↑ hypoglycemia
Karela: ↑ glucose tolerance
Konjac: ↑ hypoglycemia
Ma huang: ↓ hypoglycemic effect
Maitake: ↑ hypoglycemia
Masté: ↓ hypoglycemic effect
Onion: ↑ hypoglycemia
Rosemary: ↓ hypoglycemic effect

Smoking
↑ Insulin need

Lab test interferences
↑ VMA
↓ Potassium, ↓ magnesium, ↓ inorganic phosphate
Interference: Liver function studies, thyroid function studies

NURSING CONSIDERATIONS

Assessment

- Monitor fasting blood glucose, 2 hr PC (80-150 mg/dl, normal fasting level; 70-130 mg/dl, normal 2-hr level); also glycosylated Hgb may be measured to identify treatment effectiveness
- Monitor urine ketones during illness; insulin requirements may increase during stress, illness, surgery
- Assess for hypoglycemic reaction that can occur during peak time (sweating, weakness, dizziness, chills, confusion, headache, nausea, rapid weak pulse, fatigue, tachycardia, memory lapses, slurred speech, staggering gait, anxiety, tremors, hunger)
- Assess for hyperglycemia: acetone breath, polyuria, fatigue, polydipsia, flushed, dry skin, lethargy

Nursing diagnoses

✓ Injury, risk for (adverse reactions)
✓ Knowledge deficit (teaching)
✓ Noncompliance (teaching)

Implementation

SC route

- Give after warming to room temp by rotating in palms to prevent injecting cold insulin; use only insulin syringes with markings or syringe matching U/ml; rotate inj sites within one area: abdomen, upper back, thighs, upper arm, buttocks; keep record of sites
- Give increased dosages if tolerance occurs; give human insulin to those allergic to beef or pork
- Give lispro 15 min ac
- Store at room temp for <1 mo; keep away from heat and sunlight; refrigerate all other supply; do not use if discolored; do not freeze

IV **IV route, regular only**

- Do not use if cloudy, thick, or discolored
- Give **IV** direct, undiluted via vein, Y-site, 3-way stopcock; give at 50 U/min or less
- Give by cont inf after diluting with **IV** sol and run at prescribed rate; use **IV** infusion pump for correct dosing; give reduced dose at serum glucose level of 250 mg/100 ml

Syringe compatibilities:
Metoclopramide

Y-site compatibilities:
Amiodarone, ampicillin, ampicillin/sulbactam, aztreonam, cefazolin, cefotetan, dobutamine, esmolol, famotidine, gentamicin, heparin, heparin/hydrocortisone, imipenen/cilastatin, indomethacin sodium trihydrate, magnesium sulfate, meperidine, meropenem, midazolam, morphine, nitroglycerin, nitroprusside, oxytocin, pentobarbital, potassium chloride, propofol, ritodrine, sodium bicarbonate, tacrolimus, terbutaline, ticarcillin, ticarcillin/clavulanate, tobramycin, vancomycin, vit B/C

Y-site incompatibilities:
Nafcillin

Additive compatibilities: Bretylium, cimetidine, lidocaine, meropenem, ranitidine, verapamil

Additive incompatibilities: Aminophylline, amobarbital, chlorothiazide, cytarabine, dobutamine, pentobarbital, phenobarbital, phenytoin, secobarbital, sodium bicarbonate, thiopental

Patient/family education

- Advise patient that blurred vision occurs; not to change corrective lenses until vision is stabilized after 1-2 mo of therapy
- Advise patient to keep insulin and equipment available at all times
- Advise patient to carry ID as diabetic
- Teach patient dosage, route, mixing instructions, disease process; tell patient to continue to use the same brand of insulin and to rotate inj sites
- Instruct patient to carry candy or lump of sugar to treat hypoglycemia; have glucagon emergency kit available; teach how to use these
- Teach patient symptoms of ketoacidosis: nausea, thirst, polyuria, dry mouth, decreased B/P, dry, flushed skin, acetone breath, drowsiness, Kussmaul respirations; to have insulin available at all times
- Advise patient that a plan is necessary for diet, exercise; all food on diet should be eaten, exercise routine should not vary
- Teach patient to avoid OTC drugs and alcohol unless approved by a prescriber
- Instruct patient to notify prescriber if pregnancy is planned
- Caution patient that treatment is lifelong; insulin does not cure condition

Evaluation

Positive therapeutic outcome

- Decrease in polyuria, polydipsia, polyphagia; clear sensorium, absence of dizziness, stable gait
- Blood glucose level under control

Treatment of overdose: Glucose 25 g **IV**, via dextrose 50% sol, 50 ml or glucagon 1 mg

interferon alfa-2a/ interferon alfa-2b (℞)

(in-ter-feer'on)

Roferon-A/Intron-A

Func. class.: Miscellaneous antineoplastic

Chem. class.: Protein product

Pregnancy category C

Action: Antiviral action inhibits viral replication by reprogramming virus; antitumor action suppresses cell proliferation; immunomodulating action phagocytizes target cells; may also inhibit virus replication

➔ **Therapeutic Outcome:** Prevention of rapid growth of malignant cells; treatment of hepatitis non-A, non-B (liver function improvement)

Uses: Hairy cell leukemia in persons >18 yr, condylomata acuminata (alfa 2b), malignant melanoma, AIDS-related Kaposi's sarcoma, chronic hepatitis non-A, non-B (alfa 2b), chronic hepatitis B, C (alfa 2b)

Investigational uses: Bladder tumors, carcinoid tumors, non-Hodgkin's lymphoma, essential thrombocytopenia, cytomegaloviruses, herpes simplex, human papilloma virus–associated diseases

Dosage and routes

Hairy cell leukemia (2a)

Adult: SC/IM 3 million IU/day × 16-24 wk, then 3 million IU 3 ×/wk maintenance

Hairy cell leukemia (2b)

2 million IU/m^2 3 ×/wk; if severe adverse reactions occur, dose should be skipped or reduced by one half

Kaposi's sarcoma (2a)

Adult: SC/IM 36 million IU/

day × 10-12 wk or 3 million IU/day × 3 days, then 9 million IU/day × 3 days, then 18 million IU/day × 3 days, then 36 million IU/day for the rest of the course; if severe reaction occurs reduce dose by one half

Condylomata acuminata (2b)
1 million IU/lesion 3 times a wk × 3 wk

Chronic hepatitis B (2b)
Adult: SC/IM 3 million IU 3 ×/wk × 18-24 mo or 5 million IU/day or 10 million IU 3 ×/wk × 16 wk

Chronic hepatitis C
Adult: SC/IM 36 million IU 3 ×/wk

Available forms: Alfa-2a inj 3, 6, 36 million IU/ml; alfa-2b inj 3, 5, 10, 18, 25 million U/vial, powder for inj 5, 10, 18, 25, 50 million U/vial

Adverse effects

CNS: Dizziness, confusion, numbness, paresthesia, hallucinations, **seizures, coma,** amnesia, anxiety, mood changes, depression, somnolence, paranoia, irritability
CV: Edema, hypotension, hypertension, chest pain, palpitations, dysrhythmias, **CHF, MI, CVA,** tachycardia, syncope
GI: Weight loss, taste changes, nausea, anorexia, diarrhea, xerostomia
GU: Impotence
HEMA: **Neutropenia, thrombocytopenia**
INTEG: Rash, dry skin, itching, alopecia, flushing, photosensitivity
MISC: Flulike syndrome: fever, fatigue, myalgias, headache, chills

Contraindications: Hypersensitivity

Precautions: Severe hypotension, dysrhythmia, tachycardia, pregnancy C, lactation, children, severe renal or hepatic disease, convulsion disorder

Do Not Confuse:
Roferon-A/Imferon

Pharmacokinetics	
Absorption	80%-90% (SC/IM)
Distribution	Unknown
Metabolism	Renal tubular (degraded)
Excretion	Kidneys
Half-life	3.7-8.5 hr (2a); 2-7 hr (2b)

Pharmacodynamics	
Onset	Unknown
Peak	3-8 hr
Duration	Unknown

Interactions

Individual drugs
Aminophylline: ↑ toxicity, blood levels
Radiation: ↑ toxicity, bone marrow suppression
Zidovudine: ↑ neutropenia
Drug classifications
Antineoplastics: ↑ toxicity, bone marrow suppression
Lab test interferences
Interference: AST, ALT, LDH, alkaline phosphatase, WBC, platelets, granulocytes, creatinine

NURSING CONSIDERATIONS

Assessment

- Assess cardiac status: lung sounds, ECG before and during treatment, especially in those with cardiac disease
- Assess bone marrow depression: bruising, bleeding, blood in stools, urine, sputum, emesis
- Assess mental status: depression, suicidal thoughts, hallucinations, amnesia
- Assess for symptoms of infection; may be masked by drug fever; fever, chills, headache, sore throat may occur 6 hr after dose; give acetaminophen for symptoms
- In AIDS patients with Kaposi's sarcoma, assess characteristics of lesions during therapy; symptoms should decrease
- Assess for bleeding: hematuria,

stool guaiac, bruising or petechiae, mucosa or orifices q8h; check for inflammation of mucosa, breaks in skin; avoid IM inj, rec temp, or any other procedures that break the skin
- Assess for CNS reaction: LOC, mental status, dizziness, confusion, poor coordination, difficulty speaking, behavior changes; notify prescriber (alfa-2b)

Nursing diagnoses
- ✓ Injury, risk for (adverse reactions)
- ✓ Body image disturbance (adverse reactions)
- ✓ Infection, risk for (adverse reactions)
- ✓ Knowledge deficit (teaching)

Implementation
- Sol should be prepared by qualified personnel only under controlled conditions in biologic cabinet using gown, gloves, and mask
- Use Luer-Lok tubing to prevent leakage; do not let sol come in contact with skin; if contact occurs, wash well with soap and water
- Give at hs to minimize side effects
- Give acetaminophen as ordered to alleviate fever and headache
- Give by IM/SC after reconstituting 3-5 million IU/1 ml, 10 million IU/2 ml, 25 million IU/5 ml, of diluent provided; mix gently

Alfa-2a
- SC/IM after reconstituting 18 million U/3 ml of diluent provided (6 million U/ml)
- 36 million U/ml is used for Kaposi's sarcoma only
- Store reconstituted sol; must be used within 30 days

Intralesional route (2b)
- Give by intralesional route after reconstituting 10 million IU/1 ml of bacteriostatic water for inj; no more than 5 lesions can safely be treated at a time; using a 25-G needle inject 0.1 ml into base at center

Patient/family education
- Caution patient to avoid hazardous tasks, since confusion, dizziness may occur; fatigue is common; activity may have to be altered; to take hs to minimize flulike symptoms; to take acetaminophen for fever; avoid prolonged sunlight
- Advise patient that brands of this drug should not be changed; each form is different, with different dosages
- Caution patient not to become pregnant while taking drug; possible mutagenic effects; impotence may occur during treatment but is temporary
- Advise patient to report signs of infection: sore throat, fever, diarrhea, vomiting; sores or white patches in mouth
- Advise patient that emotional lability is common; notify prescriber if severe or incapacitating

Evaluation
Positive therapeutic outcome
- Leukocytes, Hgb, platelets, WNL
- Decreased amount of lesions in AIDS patients with Kaposi's sarcoma
- Decreased amount of genital warts

interferon alfa-n 1 lymphoblastoid (℞)
(in-ter-feer'on)

Wellferon

Func. class.: Recombinant type I interferon

Pregnancy category UK

Action: Induces biologic responses and has antiviral, antiproliferative, and immunomodulatory effects; mixture of α interferons isolated from human cells after induction with parainfluenza virus

Uses: Chronic hepatitis C infections

Dosage and routes
Adult: SC/IM 3 million U × 3 ×/wk × 6-12 mo

Available forms: Sol 3 million U/ml

Adverse effects

CNS: *Headache, fever, insomnia, dizziness*
GI: *Abdominal pain, nausea, diarrhea, anorexia, vomiting*
HEMA: **Granulocytopenia, thrombocytopenia, leukopenia, ecchymosis**
INTEG: *Alopecia, pruritus, rash, erythema, dry skin*
MS: *Back pain*
PSYCH: *Nervousness, depression, anxiety, lability, abnormal thinking*
RESP: *Pharyngitis, upper respiratory infection, cough, dyspnea, bronchitis*

Contraindications: Hypersensitivity to α interferons, history of anaphylactic reaction to bovine or ovine immunoglobulins, egg protein, polymyxin B, neomycin sulfate

Precautions: Thyroid disorders, myelosuppression, hepatic, cardiac disease, lactation, P children <18 yr, depression/suicidal tendencies

Pharmacokinetics	
Peak	24-36 hr

Interactions

Individual drugs

Theophylline: Use cautiously

Drug classifications

Myelosuppressive agents: Use together cautiously

NURSING CONSIDERATIONS

Assessment

- Monitor ALT, hepatitis C viral load, patients who show no reduction in ALT, hepatitis C viral load are unlikely to show benefit from treatment after 6 mo
- Monitor platelet counts, heme concentration, ANC, serum creatinine concentration, albumin, bilirubin, TSH, T_4, AFP
- Monitor for myelosuppression, hold dose if neutrophil count is $<500 \times 10^6$/L or if platelets are $<50 \times 10^9$/L
- Assess for hypersensitivity: discontinue immediately if hypersensitivity occurs

Implementation

- Give the same brand of product during the course of treatment

Patient/family education

- Provide patient or family member with written, detailed information about drug
- Teach patient instructions for home use if appropriate
- Advise patient to take in evening to reduce discomfort, sleep through some side effects

Evaluation

Positive therapeutic outcome

- Decrease chronic hepatitis C signs/symptoms
- Undetectable viral load

interferon alfacon-1 (℞)

(in-ter-feer′on al′fa-kon)

Infergen

Func. class.: Recombinant type I interferon

Pregnancy category C

Action: Induces biologic responses and has antiviral, antiproliferative, and immunomodulatory effects

➔ **Therapeutic Outcome:** Decreased signs/symptoms of hepatitis C

Uses: Chronic hepatitis C infections

Investigational uses: Hairy cell leukemia when used with G-CSF

Dosage and routes

Adult: SC 9 μg as a single inj 3×/wk × 24 wk

Available forms: Inj 9 mg/0.3 ml, 15 mg/0.5 ml

Adverse effects

CNS: Headache, fatigue, fever, rigors, insomnia, dizziness
CV: Hypertension, palpitation
EENT: Tinnitus, earache, conjunctivitis, eye pain
GI: Abdominal pain, nausea, diarrhea, anorexia, dyspepsia, vomiting, constipation, flatulence, hemorrhoids, decreased salivation
GU: Dysmenorrhea, vaginitis, menstrual disorders
HEMA: **Granulocytopenia, thrombocytopenia, leukopenia,** ecchymosis
INTEG: Alopecia, pruritus, rash, erythema, dry skin
MS: Back, limb, neck, skeletal pain
PSYCH: Nervousness, depression, anxiety, lability, abnormal thinking
RESP: Pharyngitis, upper respiratory infection, cough, sinusitis, rhinitis, respiratory tract congestion, epistaxis, dyspnea, bronchitis

Contraindications: Hypersensitivity to α-interferons, or products from *Escherichia coli*

Precautions: Thyroid disorders, myelosuppression, hepatic, cardiac disease, lactation, pregnancy **C**, P children <18 yr

Pharmacokinetics

Absorption	Unknown
Distribution	Unknown
Metabolism	Unknown
Excretion	Unknown
Half-life	Unknown

Pharmacodynamics

Onset	Unknown
Peak	24-36 hr
Duration	Unknown

Interactions: None known

NURSING CONSIDERATIONS

Assessment

- Assess platelet counts, heme concentration, ANC, serum creatinine concentration, albumin, bilirubin, TSH, T_4
- Assess for myelosuppression, low dose if neutrophil count is <500 × 10 –6/L or if platelets are <50 × 10 –9/L
- Assess for hypersensitivity; discontinue immediately if hypersensitivity occurs

Nursing diagnoses

✓ Infection, risk for (uses)
✓ Knowledge deficit (teaching)

Patient/family education

- Provide patient or family member with written, detailed instructions about the drug
- Caution patient to use contraception during treatment

Evaluation

Positive therapeutic outcome

- Decreased hepatitis C signs/symptoms

interferon β-1a (℞)

(in-ter-feer′on)

Avonex

interferon β-1b (℞)

Betaseron

Func. class.: Multiple sclerosis agent, immune modifier

Chem. class.: Escherichia coli derivative

Pregnancy category C

Action: Antiviral, immunoregulatory; action not clearly understood; biologic responsemodifying properties mediated through specific receptors on cells, inducing expression of interferon-induced gene products

➔ **Therapeutic Outcome:** Correcting symptoms of multiple sclerosis

Uses: Ambulatory patients with relapsing or remitting multiple sclerosis

Investigational uses: May be useful in treatment of AIDS, AIDS-related Kaposi's sarcoma, malignant melanoma, metastatic renal cell carcinoma, cutaneous T-cell lymphoma, acute non-A, non-B hepatitis

Dosage and routes

Interferon-β-1a

Adult: IM 30 μg qwk

Interferon-β-1b

Relapsing/remitting multiple sclerosis

Adult: SC 0.25 mg (8 IU) qod

Available forms: β-1a 33 μg (6.6 million IU/vial); β-1b powder for inj lyophilized 0.3 mg (9.6 mIU)

Adverse effects

CNS: *Headache, fever, pain, chills, mental changes,* hypertonia, **suicide attempts,** gait disturbances, depression

CV: *Migraine, palpitations, hypertension,* tachycardia, peripheral vascular disorders

EENT: Conjunctivitis, blurred vision, laryngitis

GI: *Diarrhea, constipation, vomiting, abdominal pain*

GU: *Dysmenorrhea, irregular menses, metorrhagia,* cystitis, breast pain, spontaneous abortion

HEMA: **Decreased lymphocytes, WBC;** *lymphadenopathy*

INTEG: *Sweating, inj site reaction,* necrosis

MS: *Myalgia,* **myasthenia,** back pain

RESP: *Sinusitis,* dyspnea

Contraindications: Hypersensitivity to natural or recombinant interferon-β or human albumin

Precautions: Pregnancy **C,** lactation, P child <18 yr, chronic progressive multiple sclerosis, depression, mental disorders

Pharmacokinetics

Absorption	50% is absorbed
Distribution	Unknown
Metabolism	Unknown
Excretion	Unknown
Half-life	8 min-4½ hr

Pharmacodynamics

Onset	Rapid
Peak	Up to 8 hr
Duration	Unknown

Interactions: None

NURSING CONSIDERATIONS

Assessment

- Monitor blood, renal, hepatic studies: CBC, differential, platelet counts, BUN, creatinine, ALT, urinalysis; if neutrophil count is <750/mm^3, or if AST, ALT, is 10 × greater than upper normal limit, or if bilirubin is 5 × greater than upper normal limit; when neutrophil count exceeds 750/mm^3 and liver function or renal studies return to normal, treatment may resume at 50% original dosage
- Assess for CNS symptoms: headache, fatigue, depression; if depression occurs and is severe, drug should be discontinued
- Assess for multiple sclerosis symptoms
- Assess mental status: depression, depersonalization, suicidal thoughts, insomnia
- Monitor GI status: diarrhea or constipation, vomiting, abdominal pain
- Monitor cardiac status: increased B/P, tachycardia

Nursing diagnoses

✓ Physical mobility, impaired (uses)
✓ Knowledge deficit (teaching)

Implementation

- Reconstitute 0.3 mg (9.6 million IU)/1.2 ml of supplied diluent (0.2 mg or 8 million IU concentration); rotate vial gently, do not shake; withdraw 1 ml using a syringe with 27-G needle; administer SC into hip, thigh, arm; discard unused portion

Interferon β-1a

- Reconstitute with 1.1 ml of diluent, swirl, give within 6 hr

Interferon β-1b

- Reconstitute by injecting diluent provided (1.2 ml) into vial, swirl (8 mIU/ml), use 27-G needle for inj
- Give acetaminophen for fever, headache; use SC route only; do not give IM or **IV**
- Store reconstituted sol in refrigerator; do not freeze; do not use sol that contains precipitate or is discolored

Patient/family education

- Provide patient or family member with written, detailed instructions about the drug; provide initial and return demonstrations on inj procedure; give information on use and disposal of drug
- Inform patient that blurred vision, sweating may occur
- Advise women patients that irregular menses, dysmenorrhea, or metorrhagia as well as breast pain may occur; use contraception during treatment; drug may cause spontaneous abortion
- Teach patient to use sunscreen to prevent photosensitivity
- Instruct patient to notify prescriber if pregnancy is suspected
- Teach patient inj technique and care of equipment
- Instruct patient to notify prescriber of increased temp, chills, muscle soreness, fatigue

Evaluation

Positive therapeutic outcome

- Decreased symptoms of multiple sclerosis

interferon gamma-1b (℞)

(in-ter-feer'on)

Actimmune

Func. class.: Biologic response modifier

Chem. class.: Lymphokine, interleukin type

Pregnancy category C

Action: Species-specific protein synthesized in response to viruses; potent phagocyte-activating effects; capable of mediating the killing of *Staphylococcus aureus, Toxoplasma gondii, Leishmania donovani, Listeria monocytogenes, Mycobacterium avium-intracellulare;* enhances oxidative metabolism of macrophages; enhances antibody-dependent cellular cytotoxicity

➔ **Therapeutic Outcome:** Decreased signs/symptoms of infection (serious) in chronic granulomatous disease

Uses: Serious infections associated with chronic granulomatous disease, osteoporosis

Dosage and routes

Adult: SC 50 μg/m^2 (1.5 million U/m^2) for patients with a surface area of >0.5 m^2; 1.5 μg/kg/dose for patient with a surface area of <0.5/m^2; give on Monday, Wednesday, Friday for 3 ×/wk dosing

Available forms: Inj 100 μg (3 million U)/single-dose vial

Adverse effects

CNS: *Headache, fatigue,* depression, fever, chills

GI: *Nausea, anorexia,* abdominal pain, weight loss, diarrhea, vomiting

INTEG: Rash, pain at inj site

MS: Myalgia, arthralgia

Contraindications: Hypersensitivity to interferon γ, *Escherichia coli*–derived products

Precautions: Pregnancy **C**, cardiac disease, seizure disorders, CNS disorders, myelosuppression, lactation, P children

Pharmacokinetics	
Absorption	Slowly absorbed; 89%
Distribution	Unknown
Metabolism	Unknown
Excretion	Unknown
Half-life	5.9 hr

Pharmacodynamics	
Onset	Unknown
Peak	7 hr
Duration	Unknown

Interactions
Individual drugs
Radiation: ↑ toxicity, bone marrow suppression
Drug classifications
Antineoplastics: ↑ toxicity, bone marrow suppression

NURSING CONSIDERATIONS
Assessment
- Monitor blood, renal, hepatic studies: CBC with differential, platelet count, BUN, creatinine, ALT, urinalysis before and q3 mo during treatment
- Assess for infection: headache, fever, chills, fatigue; these are common adverse reactions
- Monitor CNS symptoms: headache, fatigue, depression

Nursing diagnoses
✓ Infection, risk for (uses)
✓ Knowledge deficit (teaching)

Implementation
- Give at hs to minimize adverse reactions; administer acetaminophen for fever, headache; use 50% of the dosage prescribed if severe reactions occur or discontinue treatment until reactions subside
- Give in right or left deltoid and anterior thigh; warm to room temp before use; do not leave at room temp over 12 hr (unopened vial); does not contain preservatives
- Store in refrigerator upon receipt; do not freeze; do not shake

Patient/family education
- Provide patient or family member with written, detailed instructions about the drug; provide initial and return demonstrations on inj procedure; give information on use and disposal of drug
- Caution patient to use contraception during treatment

Evaluation
Positive therapeutic outcome
- Decreased serious infections
- Improvement in existing infections and inflammatory conditions

ipecac syrup (OTC)
(ip'e-kak)

Func. class.: Emetic
Chem. class.: Cephaelis ipecacuanha derivative

Pregnancy category C

Action: Acts on chemoreceptor trigger zone to induce vomiting; irritates gastric mucosa

➔ **Therapeutic Outcome:** Emesis

Uses: In poisoning from noncaustic substances to induce vomiting

Dosage and routes
Adult: PO 15-30 ml, then 200-300 ml of water; may repeat ×1, if vomiting does not occur within 20 min

P ***Child >1 yr:*** PO 15 ml, then 200-300 ml of water; may repeat in 30 min

P ***Child 6-12 mo:*** PO 5-10 ml, then 100-200 ml of water; may repeat dose if needed

Available forms: Syr

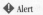

Adverse effects
CNS: **Depression, seizures, coma**
CV: **Circulatory failure, atrial**

fibrillation, fatal myocarditis, dysrhythmias
GI: Nausea, vomiting, bloody diarrhea

Contraindications: Hypersensitivity, unconscious/semiconscious, depressed gag reflex, poisoning with petroleum products or caustic substances, convulsions, shock, alcohol intolerance

Precautions: Lactation, pregnancy P C, child <6 mo

Pharmacokinetics

Absorption	Not absorbed
Distribution	Unknown
Metabolism	Unknown
Excretion	Unknown
Half-life	Unknown

Pharmacodynamics

Onset	15-30 min
Peak	Unknown
Duration	½ hr

Interactions

Individual drugs

Activated charcoal: ↓ effect; do not use together

Drug classifications

Antiemetics: ↓ effect, do not use together

Food/drug

Milk: ↓ effect
Carbonated drinks: ↑ abdominal distention

NURSING CONSIDERATIONS

Assessment

- Assess type of poisoning; do not administer if petroleum products or caustic substances have been ingested: kerosene, gasoline, lye, Drano
- Assess respiratory status before, during, after administration of emetic; check rate, rhythm, character; respiratory depression can occur rapidly with G elderly or debilitated patients
- Monitor LOC; do not give to patients who are semiconscious or unconscious or if gag reflex is not present

Nursing diagnoses

✓ Injury, risk for (uses)
✓ Poisoning (uses)
✓ Knowledge deficit (teaching)

Implementation

PO route

- ! Give **ipecac *syrup*, not ipecac fluid,** which is 14 times stronger, or death may occur
- Give activated charcoal after the patient has finished vomiting; may begin lavage 10-15 min after 2 doses of ipecac syrup without results
- Give with the patient upright; give water immediately after the ipecac syrup (200-300 ml for adults; 100-P 200 ml child <1 yr; 200-300 ml for a child >1 yr)

Patient family education

- Give patient phone number for poison control
- Give patient written guidelines on poisoning and when to induce vomiting; suggest patient keep ipecac P syrup in house if young children are present

Evaluation

Positive therapeutic outcome

- Vomiting within 30 min

ipratropium (℞)

(i-pra-troe'pee-um)
Atrovent
Func. class.: Anticholinergic, bronchodilator
Chem. class.: Synthetic quaternary ammonium compound

Pregnancy category B

Action: Inhibits interaction of acetylcholine at receptor sites on the bronchial smooth muscle, resulting in decreased cyclic guanosine monophosphate (cGMP) and bronchodilatation

Therapeutic Outcome: Bronchodilatation

Uses: Bronchodilatation during bronchospasm for patients with COPD; P rhinorrhea in children 6-11 yr (nasal spray)

Dosage and routes

Adult: INH 2 puffs qid, not to exceed 12 puffs/24 hr; sol 500 μg (1 unit dose) given 3-4 ×1 day

P ***Child 6-11 yr:*** Nasal, 1 spray in each nostril

Available forms: Aerosol 18 μg/actuation; nasal spray 0.03%, 0.06%; sol for inh 0.02%

Adverse effects

CNS: *Anxiety, dizziness, headache,* nervousness
CV: Palpitations
EENT: Dry mouth, blurred vision
GI: *Nausea, vomiting, cramps*
INTEG: Rash
RESP: *Cough, worsening of symptoms,* **bronchospasm**

Contraindications: Hypersensitivity to this drug, atropine, soya lecithin

Precautions: Pregnancy **B,** lactation, P children <12 yr, narrow-angle glaucoma, prostatic hypertrophy, bladder neck obstruction

Do Not Confuse:
Atrovent/Alupent

Pharmacokinetics	
Absorption	Minimal
Distribution	Does not cross blood-brain barrier
Metabolism	Liver, minimal
Excretion	Unknown
Half-life	2 hr

Pharmacodynamics	
Onset	5-15 min
Peak	1-1½ hr
Duration	3-6 hr

Interactions

Drug classifications

Bronchodilators, aerosol: ↑ action of bronchodilator

NURSING CONSIDERATIONS

Assessment

- Monitor respiratory function: vital capacity, FEV, ABGs, lung sounds, heart rate, rhythm (baseline and during treatment); if severe bronchospasm is present, a more rapid medication is required
- Monitor for evidence of allergic reactions, paradoxic bronchospasm; withhold dose and notify prescriber; identify if patient is allergic to belladonna products or atropine; allergy to this drug may occur

Nursing diagnoses

- ✓ Airway clearance, ineffective (uses)
- ✓ Gas exchange, impaired (uses)
- ✓ Knowledge deficit (teaching)

Implementation

- Give after shaking container; have patient exhale, place mouthpiece in mouth, inhale slowly, hold breath, remove, exhale slowly; allow at least 1 min between inhalations

Nebulizer route

- Use solution in nebulizer with a mouthpiece rather than a face mask

Nasal route

- Prime pump, initially requires 7 actuations of the pump, priming again is not necessary if used regularly
- Store in light-resistant container; do not expose to temp over 86° F (30° C)

Patient/family education

- Advise patient not to use OTC medications unless approved by prescriber; extra stimulation may occur; to use this medication before other medications and allow at least 5 min between each to prevent overstimulation
- Teach patient that compliance is necessary with number of inhalations/24 hr, or overdose may occur

• Instruct patient to use spacer device if elderly
• Teach patient the proper use of the inhaler; review package insert with patient; to avoid getting aerosol in eyes; blurring may result; to wash inhaler in warm water qd and dry; to avoid smoking, smoke-filled rooms, persons with respiratory tract infections
• Teach patient if paradoxic bronchospasm occurs to stop drug immediately and notify prescriber; to limit caffeine products such as chocolate, coffee, tea, and colas
• Instruct patient on administration of dose, not to use more than prescribed; serious side effects may occur; if dose is missed, take when remembered; space other doses on new time schedule; do not double doses

Evaluation

Positive therapeutic outcome

• Absence of dyspnea, wheezing after 1 hr
• Improved airway exchange
• Improved ABGs

irbesartan (℞)

(er-be-sar'tan)

Avapro

Func. class.: Antihypertensive

Chem. class.: Angiotensin II receptor (Type AT_1)

Pregnancy category
C (1st trimester);
D (2nd/3rd trimesters)

Action: Blocks the vasoconstrictor and aldosterone-secreting effects of angiotensin II; selectively blocks the binding of angiotensin II to the AT_1 receptor found in tissues

Therapeutic Outcome: Decreased B/P

Uses: Hypertension, alone or in combination

Investigational uses: Heart failure, hypertensive patients with diabetic nephropathy caused by type II diabetes

Dosage and routes

Adult: PO 150 mg qd; may be increased to 300 mg qd

Available forms: Tabs 75, 150, 300 mg

Adverse effects

CNS: Dizziness, anxiety, headache, fatigue

GI: *Diarrhea, dyspepsia*

RESP: *Cough, upper respiratory infection*

Contraindications: Hypersensitivity, pregnancy **D** (2nd, 3rd trimesters)

Precautions: Hypersensitivity to ACE inhibitors; pregnancy **C** (1st trimester), lactation, children, elderly, renal disease

Pharmacokinetics	
Absorption	Well
Distribution	Bound to plasma proteins (90%)
Metabolism	Liver (minimal)
Excretion	Feces, urine
Half-life	11-15 hr

Pharmacodynamics

Unknown

Interactions: None significant

NURSING CONSIDERATIONS

Assessment

• Assess B/P, pulse q4h; note rate, rhythm, quality
• Monitor electrolytes: potassium, sodium, chloride
• Obtain baselines for renal liver function tests before therapy begins
• Monitor for edema in feet, legs daily
• Assess for skin turgor, dryness of mucous membranes for hydration status

Nursing diagnoses

✓ Fluid volume deficit (side effects)

✓ Noncompliance (teaching)
✓ Knowledge deficit (teaching)

Implementation
- Administer without regard to meals
- Give **IV** 0.9% NaCl and place supine for severe hypotension

Patient/family education
- Advise patient to comply with dosage schedule, even if feeling better
- Inform patient that drug may cause dizziness, fainting; lightheadedness may occur
- Caution patient to rise slowly to sitting or standing position to minimize orthostatic hypotension
- Advise patient to notify prescriber if pregnancy is suspected

Evaluation
Positive therapeutic outcome
- Decreased B/P

HIGH ALERT

irinotecan (℞)
(ear-een-oh-tee'kan)

Camptosar, Captothecin-11, CPT-11

Func. class.: Antineoplastic hormone

Chem. class.: Topoisomerase inhibitor

Pregnancy category D

Action: Cytotoxic by producing damage to double-strand DNA during DNA synthesis

➔ **Therapeutic Outcome:** Prevention in growth of tumor size

Uses: Metastatic carcinoma of colon or rectum, or 1st line treatment in combination with fluorouracil (5-FU) and leucovorin for metastatic carcinoma of colon or rectum

Dosage and routes
Adult: **IV** 125 mg/m^2 given over 1½ hr qwk × 4 wk, then 2 wk rest period, may be repeated; 4 wk or 2 wk off, dosage adjustments may be made to 150 mg/m^2 (high) or 50 mg/m^2 (low); adjustments should be made in increments of 25-50 mg/m^2 depending on patient's tolerance

Combination dosage schedule

Regimen 1: Irinotecan 75-125 mg/m^2, leucovorin 20 mg/m^2, 5-FU 300-500 mg/m^2, depending on dosing levels

Hepatic impairment

Adult: 100 mg/m^2 qwk × 4 wk, then 2 wk rest; may repeat cycle or 300 mg/m^2 q3wk, dose may be adjusted up or down

Available forms: Inj 20 mg/ml

Adverse effects
CNS: Fever, headache, chills, dizziness

CV: Vasodilation

GI: **Severe diarrhea,** nausea, vomiting, anorexia, constipation, cramps, flatus, stomatitis, dyspepsia, **hepatotoxicity**

HEMA: **Leukopenia,** anemia, **neutropenia**

INTEG: Irritation at site, rash, sweating, alopecia

RESP: Dyspnea, increased cough, rhinitis

MISC: Edema, asthenia, weight loss

Contraindications: Hypersensitivity, pregnancy **D**

P G **Precautions:** Lactation, children, elderly, myelosuppression, irradiation

Pharmacokinetics	
Absorption	Complete
Distribution	Widely, 30%-68% bond to plasma proteins
Metabolism	Unknown
Excretion	Urine/bile
Half-life	Unknown

Pharmacodynamics

Unknown

Interactions

Individual drugs

Dexamethensone: ↑ lymphocytopenia
Prochlorperazine: ↑ akathisia
Radiation: ↑ myelosuppression

Drug classifications

Antineoplastics: ↑ myelosuppression, diarrhea
Diuretics: ↑ dehydration

NURSING CONSIDERATIONS

Assessment

- Assess for CNS symptoms: fever, headache, chills, dizziness
- Assess CBC, differential, platelet count weekly; withhold drug if WBC is <2000/mm^3, or platelet count is <100,000/mm^3, Hgb ≤ g/dl, neutrophils ≤1000/mm^3; notify prescriber of these results, drug should be discontinued and colony-stimulating factor given
- Assess buccal cavity q8h for dryness, sores or ulceration, white patches, oral pain, bleeding, dysphagia
- Assess GI symptoms: frequency of stools; cramping; severe life-threatening diarrhea may occur with fluid and electrolyte imbalances
- Assess signs of dehydration: rapid respirations, poor skin turgor, decreased urine output; dry skin, restlessness, weakness
- Assess for bone marrow depression: bruising, bleeding, blood in stools, urine, sputum, emesis

Nursing diagnoses

✓ Infection, risk for (adverse reactions)
✓ Knowledge deficit (teaching)

Implementation

- Give antiemetics and dexamethasone 10 mg at least ½ hr before antineoplastics
- Give after preparing in biologic cabinet using gloves, mask, gown

IV route

- Give by intermittent inf after diluting with 0.9% NaCl or D_5W (0.12-1.1 mg/ml); give over 1½ hr
- Do not admix with other solutions or medications
- Provide increased fluid intake to 2-3 L/day to prevent dehydration, unless contraindicated
- Change **IV** site q48h
- Provide rinsing of mouth tid-qid with water, club soda; brushing of teeth bid-tid with soft brush or cotton-tipped applicator for stomatitis; use unwaxed dental floss
- Provide nutritious diet with iron, vitamin supplement, low fiber, few dairy products
- Stable for 24 hr at room temp, 48 hr if refrigerated

Patient/family education

- Advise patient to avoid foods with citric acid or hot or rough texture if stomatitis is present; to drink adequate fluids
- Advise patient to report stomatitis; any bleeding, white spots, ulcerations in mouth; tell patient to examine mouth qd, report symptoms
- Advise patient to report signs of anemia: fatigue, headache, faintness, shortness of breath, irritability
- Advise patient to use contraception during therapy
- Advise patient to avoid vaccinations while taking this drug
- Instruct patient to report diarrhea that occurs 24 hr after administration; severe dehydration can occur rapidly
- Teach patient to avoid salicylates, NSAIDs, alcohol; bleeding may occur

Evaluation

Positive therapeutic outcome

- Decrease in tumor size, decrease in spread of cancer

Treatment of overdose:

Induce vomiting, provide supportive care, prevent dehydration

I

iron, carbonyl

See ferrous fumarate

iron dextran (℞)

DexFerrum, Imferon ♣, InFed

Func. class.: Hematinic

Chem. class.: Ferric hydroxide complex with dextran

Pregnancy category C

Action: Iron is carried by transferrin to the bone marrow, where it is incorporated into hemoglobin

Therapeutic Outcome: Prevention and resolution of iron-deficiency anemia

Uses: Iron-deficiency anemia in patients who cannot take oral preparations

Dosage and routes

P ***Adult and child:*** IM 0.5 ml as a test dose by Z-track, then no more than the following per day:

Adult <50 kg: IM 100 mg

Adult >50 kg: IM 250 mg

P ***Infant <5 kg:*** IM 25 mg

P ***Child 5-9 kg:*** IM 50 mg

Adult: **IV** 0.5 ml (25 mg) test dose, then 100 mg qd after 2-3 days; **IV** 250/1000 ml of NaCl; give 25 mg test dose, wait 5 min, then inf over 6-12 hr or follow equation:

$$\frac{0.3 \times \text{weight (lb)} \times 100\ \text{Hgb (g/dl)} \times 100}{14.8}$$

Patients <30 lb (66 kg) should be given 80% of above formula dose

Available forms: Inj IM/**IV** 50 mg/ml; inj IM only 50 mg/ml

Adverse effects

CNS: Headache, paresthesia, dizziness, shivering, weakness, **seizures**

CV: Chest pain, **shock,** hypotension, tachycardia

GI: *Nausea,* vomiting, metallic taste, abdominal pain

HEMA: **Leukocytosis**

INTEG: Rash, pruritus, urticaria, fever, sweating, chills, brown skin discoloration, pain at inj site, necrosis, sterile abscesses, phlebitis

MISC: **Anaphylaxis**

RESP: Dyspnea

Contraindications: Hypersensitivity, all anemias excluding iron-deficiency anemia, hepatic disease

Precautions: Acute renal disease, P children, asthma, lactation, rheumatoid arthritis (**IV**), P infants <4 mo, pregnancy **C**

Do Not Confuse:
Imferon/Imuran, Imferon/Roferon-A

Pharmacokinetics

Absorption	Well absorbed; lymphatics over wk or mo
Distribution	Crosses placenta
Metabolism	Slow; blood loss, desquamation
Excretion	Breast milk, feces, urine, bile
Half-life	6 hr

Pharmacodynamics

Unknown

Interactions

Individual drugs

Chloramphenicol: ↓ reticulocyte response

Oral iron: Do not use together

Penicillamine: ↓ absorption of penicillamine

Vitamin E: ↓ reticulocyte response

Lab test interferences

False: ↑ Serum bilirubin

False: ↓ Serum calcium

False positive: ^{99m}Tc diphosphate bone scan, iron test (large doses >2 ml)

NURSING CONSIDERATIONS

Assessment

- Monitor blood studies: Hct, Hgb,

reticulocytes, transferrin, plasma iron concentrations, ferritin, total iron-binding bilirubin before treatment, at least monthly

- Assess for allergic reaction and anaphylaxis; rash, pruritus, fever, chills, wheezing, notify prescriber immediately, keep emergency equipment available
- Assess cardiac status: anginal pain, hypotension, tachycardia
- Assess for nutrition: amount of iron in diet (meat, dark green leafy vegetables, dried fruits, eggs); cause of iron loss or anemia, including salicylates, sulfonamides
- Monitor pulse, B/P during **IV** administration
- Assess for toxicity: nausea, vomiting, diarrhea, fever, abdominal pain (early symptoms); cyanotic lips, nailbeds, seizures, CV collapse (late symptoms)

Nursing diagnoses

✓ Fatigue (uses)
✓ Activity intolerance (uses)
✓ Knowledge deficit (teaching)

Implementation

IM route

- Discontinue oral iron before parenteral; give only after test dose of 25 mg by preferred route; wait at least 1 hr before giving remaining portion
- Give IM deep in large muscle mass; use Z-track method and 19-20 G 2-, 3-inch needle; ensure needle is long enough to place drug deep in muscle; change needles after withdrawing medication and injecting to prevent skin and tissue staining

IV **IV route**

- Give **IV** after flushing tubing with 10 ml of 0.9% NaCl; give undiluted; give 1 ml (50 mg) or less over 1 min or more; flush line after use with 10 ml of 0.9% NaCl; patient should remain recumbent for 30-60 min to prevent orthostatic hypotension
- **IV** inj requires single-dose vial without preservative; verify on label **IV** use is approved
- Give by cont inf after diluting in 50-250 ml of 0.9% NaCl for inf; administer over 4-5 hr
- Give only with epinephrine available in case of anaphylactic reaction during dose
- Store at room temp in cool environment

Additive compatibilities:

Netilmicin

Patient/family education

- Caution patient that iron poisoning may occur if increased beyond recommended level; to not take oral iron preparation unless approved by prescriber
- Advise patient that delayed reaction may occur 1-2 days after administration and last 3-4 days (**IV**) or 3-7 days (IM); report fever, chills, malaise, muscle, joint aches, nausea, vomiting, backache

Evaluation

Positive therapeutic outcome

- Increased serum iron levels, Hct, Hgb

Treatment of overdose:

- Discontinue drug, treat allergic reaction, give diphenhydramine or epinephrine as needed for anaphylaxis; give iron-chelating drug in acute poisoning

iron polysaccharide

See ferrous fumarate

iron sucrose (℞)

Venofer

Func. class.: Hematinic

Chem. class.: Ferric hydroxide complex with dextran

Pregnancy category B

Action: Iron is carried by transferrin to the bone marrow, where it is incorporated into hemoglobin

Therapeutic Outcome: Improved signs/symptoms of iron deficiency anemia; iron levels improved

Uses: Iron deficiency anemia

Investigational uses: Dystrophic epidermolysis bullosa (DEB)

Dosage and routes

Adult: **IV** 5 ml (100 mg of elemental iron) given during dialysis, most will need 1000 mg of elemental iron over 10 dialysis sessions

Available forms: Inj 20 mg/ml

Adverse effects

CNS: Headache, dizziness

CV: Chest pain, hypo/hypertension, hypervolemia

GI: *Nausea, vomiting, abdominal pain*

INTEG: Rash, pruritus, urticaria, fever, sweating, chills

MISC: **Anaphylaxis**

RESP: Dyspnea, pneumonia, cough

Contraindications: Hypersensitivity, all anemias excluding iron deficiency anemia, iron overload

G P **Precautions:** Lactation (**IV**), pregnancy **B**, elderly, children

Pharmacokinetics

Absorption	Unknown
Distribution	Unknown
Metabolism	Unknown
Excretion	Urine
Half-life	6 hr

Pharmacodynamics

Unknown

Interactions

Individual drugs

Oral iron: ↑ toxicity, do not use together

NURSING CONSIDERATIONS

Assessment

- Monitor blood studies: Hct, Hgb, reticulocytes, transferrin, plasma iron concentrations, ferritin, total iron binding, bilirubin before treatment, at least monthly
- Assess for allergy: anaphylaxis, rash, pruritus, fever, chills, wheezing; notify prescriber immediately, keep emergency equipment available
- Assess cardiac status: hypotension, hypertension, hypervolemia
- Assess for toxicity: nausea, vomiting, diarrhea, fever, abdominal pain (early symptoms), cyanotic-looking lips and nailbeds, seizures, CV collapse (late symptoms)

Nursing diagnoses

- ✓ Nutrition, less than body requirements (uses)
- ✓ Knowledge deficit (teaching)

Implementation

◆ Give only with epinephrine available in case of anaphylactic reaction during dose

IV IV route

- Give directly in dialysis line by slow inj or inf; give by slow inj at 1 ml/min (5 min/vial); inf dilute each vial exclusively in a maximum of 100 ml of 0.9% NaCl, give at rate of 100 mg of iron/15 min, discard unused portions
- Store at room temp in cool environment, do not freeze

Patient/family education

- Teach patient that iron poisoning may occur if increased beyond recommended level; not to take oral iron preparations

Evaluation

Positive therapeutic outcome

- Increased serum iron levels, Hct, Hgb

Treatment of overdose: Discontinue drug, treat allergic reaction, give diphenhydramine or epinephrine as needed, give iron-chelating drug in acute poisoning

isoniazid (℞)

(eye-soe-nye'a-zid)

INH, isoniazid, Isotamine ♣, Laniazid, Nydrazid, PMS-Isoniazid ♣

Func. class.: Antitubercular

Chem. class.: Isonicotinic acid hydrazide

Pregnancy category C

Action: Inhibits RNA synthesis, decreases tubercle bacilli replication

→ **Therapeutic Outcome:** Resolution of TB infection

Uses: Pulmonary TB as an adjunct; other infections caused by mycobacteria

Dosage and routes

Treatment

Adult: PO/IM 300 mg/day or 15 mg/kg 2-3 ×/wk, max 900 mg 2-3 ×/wk

P ***Child and infant:*** PO/IM 10-20 mg/kg qd in 1-2 divided doses; max 300 mg/day or 20-40 mg/kg, max 900 mg 2-3 ×/wk

Available forms: Tabs 100, 300 mg; inj 100 mg/ml; powder 50 mg/5 ml; syrup 50 mg/5 ml

Adverse effects

Hypersensitivity: fever, skin eruptions, lymphadenopathy, vasculitis

CNS: *Peripheral neuropathy, dizziness,* memory impairment, **toxic encephalopathy, convulsions,** psychosis, dizziness, slurred speech

EENT: Blurred vision, optic neuritis, visual disturbance

GI: *Nausea, vomiting,* epigastric distress, jaundice, **fatal hepatitis**

HEMA: **Agranulocytosis, hemolytic anemia, aplastic anemia, thrombocytopenia, eosinophilia, methemoglobinemia**

MISC: Dyspnea, vit B_6 deficiency, pellagra, hyperglycemia, metabolic acidosis, gynecomastia, rheumatic syndrome, systemic lupus erythematosus–like syndrome

Contraindications: Hypersensitivity, acute liver disease

Precautions: Pregnancy **C,** renal disease, diabetic retinopathy, cataracts, P ocular defects, hepatic disease, child <13 yr

Pharmacokinetics

Absorption	Well
Distribution	Widely
Metabolism	Liver
Excretion	Kidneys
Half-life	1-4 hr

Pharmacodynamics

	PO	IM
Onset	Rapid	Rapid
Peak	1-2 hr	45-60 min
Duration	6-8 hr	6-8 hr

Interactions

Individual drugs

Alcohol: ↑ toxicity

BCG vaccine: ↓ effectiveness of BCG vaccine

Carbamazepine: ↑ toxicity

Cycloserine: ↑ toxicity

Ethionamide: ↑ toxicity

Ketoconazole: ↓ effectiveness of BCG vaccine

Meperidine: ↑ toxicity

Phenytoin: ↓ metabolism of phenytoin

Rifampin: ↑ toxicity

Warfarin: ↑ toxicity

Drug classifications

Antacids, aluminum: ↓ absorption

Benzodiazepines: ↑ toxicity

Food/drug

Tyramine foods: ↑ toxicity

NURSING CONSIDERATIONS

Assessment

- Obtain C&S tests, including sputum tests, before treatment; monitor every mo to detect resistance
- Monitor liver studies weekly: ALT, AST, bilirubin, increased results may

indicate hepatitis; renal studies during treatment and monthly: BUN, creatinine, output, sp gr, urinalysis, uric acid

- Assess mental status often: affect, mood, behavioral changes; psychosis may occur with hallucinations, confusion
- Assess hepatic status: decreased appetite, jaundice, dark urine, fatigue
- Assess for visual disturbance that may indicate optic neuritis: blurred vision, change in color perception; may lead to blindness

Nursing diagnoses

- ✓ Infection, risk for (uses)
- ✓ Diarrhea (adverse reactions)
- ✓ Injury, risk for (adverse reactions)
- ✓ Knowledge deficit (teaching)
- ✓ Noncompliance (teaching)

Implementation

- Give antiemetic for vomiting

PO route

- Give with meals to decrease GI symptoms; absorption is better when taken on empty stomach, 1 hr ac or 2 hr pc

IM route

- Give deep in large muscle mass, massage; rotate inj sites, warm inj to room temp to dissolve crystals

Patient/family education

- Instruct patient that compliance with dosage schedule for duration is necessary; not to skip or double doses; that scheduled appointments must be kept or relapse may occur
- Caution patient to avoid alcohol while taking drug or hepatoxicity may result; to avoid ingestion of aged cheeses, fish or hypertensive crisis may result; give patient written directions on which foods to avoid while taking this medication
- Tell patient to report peripheral neuritis: weakness, tingling/numbness of hands/feet, fatigue; hepatoxicity: loss of appetite, nausea, vomiting, jaundice of skin or eyes

Evaluation

Positive therapeutic outcome

- Decreased symptoms of TB
- Culture negative for TB

Treatment of overdose:

Pyridoxine

isoproterenol (℞)

(eye-soe-proe-ter′e-nole)

Aerolone, Dispos-a-Med, Isoproterenol HCl, Isuprel, Isuprel Glossets, Isuprel Mistometer, Medihaler-Iso, Vapo-Iso

Func. class.: β-Adrenergic-agonist, antidysrhythmic, inotropic

Chem. class.: Catecholamine

Pregnancy category C

Action: Has β_1- and β_2-adrenergic action; relaxes bronchial smooth muscle and dilates the trachea and main bronchi by increasing levels of cAMP, which relaxes smooth muscles; causes increased contractility and heart rate by acting on β-receptors in heart

Therapeutic Outcome: Bronchodilatation, increased heart rate and cardiac output from action on β-receptors in the heart

Uses: Bronchospasm, asthma, heart block, ventricular dysrhythmias, shock

Dosage and routes

Asthma, bronchospasm

Adult: SL tab 10-20 mg q6-8h; inh 1 puff; may repeat in 2-5 min; maintenance 1-2 puffs 4-6 times/day; **IV** 1020 mg during anesthesia

P ***Child:*** SL tab 5-10 mg q6-8h; inh 1 puff; may repeat in 2-5 min; maintenance 1-2 puffs 4-6 times/day

Heart block/ventricular dysrhythmias

Adult: **IV** 0.02-0.06 mg, then 0.01-0.2 mg or 5 μg/min HCl; 0.2 mg, then 0.02-1 mg as needed

Shock

Adult: **IV** inf 0.5-5 μg/min (1 mg/500 ml of D_5W) titrate to B/P, CVP, hourly urine output

Available forms: Sol for nebulization 1:400 (0.25%), 1:200 (0.5%), 1:100 (1%); aerosol 0.25%, 0.2%; powder for inh 0.1 mg/cartridge; inj 1:5000 (0.2 mg/ml) **IV**; glossets (SL) 10, 15 mg

Adverse effects

CNS: ***Tremors, anxiety,*** insomnia, headache, dizziness, stimulation

CV: Palpitations, tachycardia, hypertension, **cardiac arrest**

GI: Nausea, vomiting

META: Hyperglycemia

RESP: Bronchial irritation, edema, dryness of oropharynx, **bronchospasms** (overuse)

Contraindications: Hypersensitivity to sympathomimetics, narrow-angle glaucoma

Precautions: Pregnancy **C**, cardiac disorders, hyperthyroidism, diabetes mellitus, prostatic hypertrophy, G elderly

Pharmacokinetics

Absorption	Erratic (SL, rec), rapid (inh, **IV**)
Distribution	Unknown
Metabolism	Lungs, liver, GI tract
Excretion	Kidneys, unchanged (50%)
Half-life	Unknown

Pharmacodynamics

	SL	INH	IV	REC
Onset	1-2 hr	Rapid	Rapid	2-4 hr
Peak	Unknown	Unknown	Unknown	Unknown
Duration	2 hr	1 hr	10 min	3-4 hr

Interactions

Drug classifications

β-Adrenergic blockers: Block therapeutic effect

Bronchodilators, aerosol: ↑ action of bronchodilator

MAOIs: ↑ chance of hypertensive crisis

Sympathomimetics: ↑ adrenergic side effects

NURSING CONSIDERATIONS

Assessment

- Assess respiratory function: vital capacity, FEV, ABGs, lung sounds, heart rate, rhythm (baseline and during therapy)
- Monitor for evidence of allergic reactions, paradoxic bronchospasm; withhold dose; notify prescriber

Nursing diagnoses

- ✓ Airway clearance, ineffective (uses)
- ✓ Impaired gas exchange (uses)
- ✓ Knowledge deficit (teaching)

Implementation

SL route

- Give ≤q3-4h or no more than tid

Inhalation route

- Give after diluting dose in sterile water or 0.9% NaCl, 0.45% NaCl; give over 15-20 min
- Store in light-resistant container; do not expose to temp over 86° F (30° C)

IV **IV route**

- Give by direct **IV** after diluting 0.2 mg or 1 ml (1:5000 sol)/10 ml of 0.9% NaCl for inj or D_5W (1:50,000 sol); give 1:50,000 sol over 1 min
- Give by cont inf by diluting 2 mg or 10 ml (1:5000 sol)/500 ml of 0.9% NaCl, D_5W, $D_{10}W$, 0.45% NaCl, Ringer's, LR (1:250,000 sol); give at a rate of 1 ml/min by infusion pump; ratio is adjusted according to patient response

Syringe compatibilities: Ranitidine

Y-site compatibilities: Amiodarone, amrinone, atracurium, bretylium, cisatracurium, famotidine, heparin, hydrocortisone, pancuronium, potassium chloride, propofol, remifentanil, tacrolimus, vecuronium, vit B/C

Additive compatibilities: Atracurium, calcium chloride, calcium gluceptate, cephalothin, cimetidine, dobutamine, floxacillin, heparin, magnesium sulfate, multivitamins, netilmicin, potassium chloride, ranitidine, succinylchloride, verapamil, vit B/C

Patient/family education

- Caution patient not to use OTC medications before consulting prescriber; extra stimulation may occur
- Instruct patient to use this medication before other medications and allow at least 5 min between each
- Teach patient use of inhaler; review package insert with patient; advise patient to avoid getting aerosol in eyes, as blurring may result; instruct patient to wash inhaler in warm water qd and dry; to rinse mouth after using; to avoid smoking, smoke-filled rooms, persons with respiratory tract infections
- G Teach elderly patient to use spacer device
- Instruct patient if paradoxic bronchospasm occurs to stop drug immediately and notify prescriber; to limit caffeine products such as chocolate, coffee, tea, and colas
- Instruct patient on administration of dose; not to use more than prescribed; serious side effects may occur; if taking PO regularly and dose is missed, take when remembered; space other doses on new time schedule; do not double doses

Evaluation

Positive therapeutic outcome

- Absence of dyspnea, wheezing
- Improved airway exchange
- Improved ABGs

Treatment of overdose: Administer a β_2-adrenergic blocker

isosorbide dinitrate (℞)

(eye-soe-sor′bide)

Apo-ISDN ✦, Cedocard-SR ✦, Coronex ✦, Dilatrate-SR, ISDN, Iso-Bid, Isonate, Isorbid, Isordil, Isordil Tembids, Isordil Titradose, Isosorbide Dinitrate, Isotrate Timecelles, Novasorbide, Sorbitrate, Sorbitrate SA

isosorbide mononitrate (℞)

Imdur, Ismo, Isotrate ER, Monoket

Func. class.: Antianginal, vasodilator

Chem. class.: Nitrate

Pregnancy category C

Action: Decreases preload, afterload, thus decreasing left ventricular end-diastolic pressure, systemic vascular resistance, and reducing cardiac O_2 demand

➔ **Therapeutic Outcome:** Relief and prevention of angina pectoris

Uses: Chronic stable angina pectoris, prophylaxis of angina pain, CHF

Dosage and routes

Dinitrate

Adult: PO 5-40 mg qid; SL tab 2.5-10 mg; may repeat q2-3h; chew tab 5-10 mg prn or q2-3h as prophylaxis; sus rel cap 40-80 mg q8-12h

Mononitrate

Adult: PO (Ismo, Monoket) 10-20 mg bid, 7 hr apart; (Imdur) initiate at 30-60 mg qd, may increase to 120 mg qd, max 240 mg/day

Available forms: *dinitrate:* sus rel caps 20, 40 mg; ext rel tabs 20, 40, 60 mg; tabs 2.5, 5, 10, 20, 30, 40 mg; chew tabs 5, 10 mg; SL tabs 2.5, 5, 10 mg; *mononitrate:* tabs 10, 20 mg; (Monoket, Ismo) 10, 20 mg; ext rel (Imdur) 30, 60, 120 mg

Adverse effects

CNS: Vascular headache, flushing, dizziness, weakness, faintness
CV: Postural hypotension, tachycardia, **collapse,** syncope
GI: Nausea, vomiting
INTEG: Pallor, sweating, rash
MISC: Twitching, hemolytic anemia, **methemoglobinemia**

Contraindications: Hypersensitivity to this drug or nitrates, severe anemia, increased ICP, cerebral hemorrhage, acute MI

Precautions: Postural hypotension, P pregnancy **C**, lactation, children

Pharmacokinetics

Absorption	Well
Distribution	Unknown
Metabolism	Liver
Excretion	Urine, metabolites
Half-life	Dinitrate 1 hr, mononitrate 5 hr

Pharmacodynamics

	SUS REL	SL	PO
Onset	20-45 min	2-5 min	15-30 min
Peak	Unknown	Unknown	Unknown
Duration	8-12 hr	1-4 hr	4-6 hr

Interactions

Individual drugs

Alcohol: ↑ hypotension

Drug classifications

Antihypertensives: ↑ hypotension
β-Adrenergic blockers: ↑ hypotension
Calcium channel blockers: ↑ hypotension
Phenothiazines: ↑ hypotension

NURSING CONSIDERATIONS

Assessment

- Assess for pain: duration, time started, activity being performed, character, intensity
- Monitor for orthostatic B/P, pulse at baseline and during treatment

Nursing diagnoses

- ✓ Cardiac output, decreased (uses)
- ✓ Tissue perfusion, decreased (uses)
- ✓ Knowledge deficit (teaching)

Implementation

SL route

- Hold SL tab under tongue until dissolved (a few min); do not take anything PO when SL tab is in place

PO route

- Give 1 hr ac or 2 hr pc with 8 oz of water
- ⊘ Sus rel tab should not be chewed, broken, or crushed; chew tab should be chewed thoroughly

Patient/family education

- Instruct patient to swallow sus rel tab whole, do not chew; SL tab should be dissolved under tongue, do not swallow; chew tab should be chewed thoroughly; do not skip or double doses; if dose is missed take when remembered if 2 hr before next dose (dinitrate), 6 hr before next dose (sus rel), or 8 hr before next dose (mononitrate)
- Caution patient to avoid alcohol and OTC medications unless approved by prescriber
- Inform patient that drug may be taken before stressful activity: exercise, sexual activity
- Advise patient that SL tab may sting mucous membranes
- Caution patient to avoid driving and hazardous activities if dizziness occurs
- Advise patient to comply with complete medical regimen
- Caution patient to make position changes slowly to prevent orthostatic hypotension

Evaluation

Positive therapeutic outcome

- Decrease in, prevention of anginal pain

I

isradipine (℞)

(is-ra'di-peen)

DynaCirc, DynaCirc CR

Func. class.: Calcium channel blocker, antihypertensive, antianginal

Chem. class.: Dihydropyridine

Pregnancy category C

Action: Inhibits calcium ion influx across cell membrane during cardiac depolarization; produces relaxation of coronary vascular smooth muscle and peripheral vascular smooth muscle; dilates coronary vascular arteries; increases myocardial oxygen delivery in patients with vasospastic angina

Therapeutic Outcome: Decreased B/P

Uses: Hypertension, pectoris, vasospastic angina

Dosage and routes

Adult: PO 2.5 mg bid; increase at 2-4 wk intervals up to 10 mg bid or 5 mg qd; cont rel, may be increased q2-4wk, max 20 mg/day

Available forms: Caps 2.5, 5 mg; cont rel tabs 5, 10 mg

Adverse effects

CNS: Headache, fatigue, dizziness, fainting, sleep disturbances

CV: Peripheral edema, tachycardia, hypotension, chest pain, **CHF, dysrhythmias**

GI: Nausea, vomiting, diarrhea, gastric upset, constipation, hepatitis

GU: Nocturia, polyuria, **acute renal failure**

HEMA: **Thrombocytopenia, leukopenia, anemia**

INTEG: Rash, pruritus, urticaria, photosensitivity, hair loss, **Stevens-Johnson syndrome**

MISC: Flushing

Contraindications: Sick sinus syndrome, 2nd- or 3rd-degree heart block, hypotension less than 90 mm Hg systolic, hypersensitivity

Precautions: CHF, hypotension, hepatic disease, pregnancy **C**, lactation, children, renal disease, elderly

Pharmacokinetics

Absorption	Well absorbed
Distribution	High plasma protein binding (95%)
Metabolism	Liver, extensively and rapidly
Excretion	Kidney
Half-life	8 hr

Pharmacodynamics

Onset	1-2 hr
Peak	2-3 hr
Duration	12 hr

Interactions

Individual drugs

Alcohol: ↑ hypotension

Digoxin: ↑ bradycardia, conduction defects

Disopyramide: ↑ bradycardia, conduction defects

Fentanyl: ↑ hypotension

Phenytoin: ↑ bradycardia, conduction defects

Quinidine: ↑ hypotension

Drug classifications

Antihypertensives: ↑ hypotension

β-Adrenergic blockers: ↑ bradycardia, conduction defects

Nitrates: ↑ hypotension

NSAIDs: ↓ antihypertensives

NURSING CONSIDERATIONS

Assessment

- Assess fluid volume status: I&O ratio and record, weight, distended red veins, crackles in lung, color, quality and sp gr of urine, skin turgor, adequacy of pulses, moist mucous membranes, bilateral lung sounds, peripheral pitting edema; dehydration symptoms of decreasing output, thirst, hypotension, dry mouth and mucous membranes should be reported
- Monitor ALT, AST, bilirubin; if these are elevated, hepatotoxicity is suspected

- Assess renal, hepatic status, electrolytes before and during treatment
- Monitor cardiac status: B/P, pulse, respiration, ECG; assess anginal pain, precipitating, ameliorating factors

Nursing diagnoses

✓ Cardiac output, decreased (uses)
✓ Knowledge deficit (teaching)

Implementation

- Give once a day, with food for GI symptoms
- Do not crush, chew caps, cont rel tabs

Patient/family education

- Instruct patient to avoid hazardous activities until stabilized on drug and dizziness is no longer a problem
- Instruct patient to limit caffeine consumption; to avoid alcohol and OTC drugs unless directed by prescriber
- Advise patient to comply in all areas of medical regimen: diet, exercise, stress reduction, drug therapy; to notify prescriber of irregular heart beat, shortness of breath, swelling of feet and hands, pronounced dizziness, constipation, nausea, hypotension
- Teach patient to use as directed even if feeling better
- Teach patient to take with a full glass of water

Evaluation

Positive therapeutic outcome

- Decreased B/P

Treatment of overdose: Defibrillation, atropine for AV block, vasopressor for hypotension

itraconazole (℞)

(it-tra-kon′a-zol)

Sporanox

Func. class.: Antifungal (systemic)
Chem. class.: Triazole derivative

Pregnancy category C

Action: Increases cell membrane permeability in susceptible organisms by binding sterols in fungal cell membrane; decreases potassium, sodium, and nutrients in cell

Therapeutic Outcome: Fungistatic against *Histoplasma capsulatum, Blastomyces dermatitis, Cryptococcus neoformans, Aspergillus fumigatus, Candida*

Uses: Systemic candidiasis, chronic mucocandidiasis, oral thrush, candiduria, coccidioidomycosis, histoplasmosis, chromomycosis, paracoccidioidomycosis, blastomycosis (pulmonary and extrapulmonary)

Investigational uses: Dermatophytoses, pityriasis versicolor, sebopsoriasis, vaginal candidiasis, cryptococcal, subcutaneous mycoses, dimorphic infections, leishmaniasis, fungal keratitis, alternariosis, zygomycosis

Dosage and routes

Dose varies with type of infection

Adult: PO 200 mg qd with food; may increase to 400 mg qd if needed; life-threatening infections may require a loading dose of 200 mg tid × 3 days; **IV** 200 mg bid × 4 doses, then 200 mg qd; give each dose over 1 hr, maintenance PO 100 mg/day

P ***Child:*** PO 3-5 mg/kg/day

Available forms: Caps 100 mg; oral sol 10 mg/ml; inj 10 mg/ml

Adverse effects

CNS: Headache, dizziness, insomnia, somnolence, depression
GI: Nausea, vomiting, anorexia, diarrhea, cramps, abdominal pain, flatulence, **GI bleeding, hepatotoxicity**
GU: Gynecomastia, impotence, decreased libido
INTEG: Pruritus, fever, rash
MISC: Edema, fatigue, malaise, hypertension, hypokalemia, tinnitus

Contraindications: Hypersensitivity, lactation, fungal meningitis, onychomycosis or dermatomycosis in cardiac dysfunction

Precautions: Hepatic disease, achlorhydria or hypochlorhydria (drug-induced), children, P pregnancy **C**

Pharmacokinetics

Absorption	Variable
Distribution	Tissue, plasma, CSF
Metabolism	Liver, extensively
Excretion	Feces, breast milk
Half-life	20-21 hr

Pharmacodynamics

Onset	Unknown
Peak	4 hr
Duration	Unknown

Interactions

Individual drugs

Buspirone: ↑ buspirone levels
Busulfan: ↑ toxicity
Carbamazepine: ↑ metabolism, ↓ effect of itraconazole
Clarithromycin: ↑ toxicity
Cyclosporine: ↑ toxicity
Diazepam: ↑ toxicity
Didanosine: ↓ antifungal action
Digoxin: ↑ toxicity
Dofetilide: Life-threatening CV reaction
Felodipine: ↑ toxicity
Indinavir: ↑ toxicity
Isoniazid: ↑ metabolism, ↓ effect of itraconazole
Isradipine: ↑ toxicity
Midazolam: ↑ sedation
Nicardipine: ↑ toxicity
Nifedipine: ↑ toxicity
Nimoldipine: ↑ toxicity
Omeprazole: ↓ action of itraconazole
Phenobarbital: ↑ metabolism, ↓ effect of itraconazole
Phenytoin: ↑ toxicity
Quinidine: ↑ toxicity
Rifampin: ↑ metabolism, ↓ effect of itraconazole
Ritonavir: ↑ toxicity
Saquinavir: ↑ toxicity
Sucralfate: ↓ action of itraconazole
Tacrolimus: ↑ effect of tacrolimus
Triazolam: ↑ sedation
Warfarin: ↑ toxicity

Drug classifications

Antacids: ↓ action of itraconazole
Calcium channel blockers: ↑ edema
Cardiac glycosides: ↑ effects of cardiac glycosides
H_2-receptor antagonists: ↓ action of itraconazole
Oral hypoglycemics: ↑ effects of oral hypoglycemics

Food/drug

↑ Absorption

NURSING CONSIDERATIONS

Assessment

- Assess for infection: WBC, sputum baseline and periodically, may start treatment before obtaining results
- (!) Monitor for hepatotoxicity: increasing AST, ALT, alkaline phosphatase, bilirubin
- Monitor for allergic reaction: dermatitis, rash; drug should be discontinued, antihistamines (mild reaction) or epinephrine (severe reaction) administered; check inj site for thrombophlebitis
- Monitor for hypokalemia, check potassium level: anorexia, drowsiness, weakness, decreased reflexes, dizziness, increased urinary output, increased thirst, paresthesias; if these occur, drug should be decreased or discontinued and potassium administered

Nursing diagnoses

- ✓ Infection, risk for (uses)
- ✓ Injury, risk for physical (adverse reaction)
- ✓ Knowledge deficit (teaching)

Implementation

PO route

- Oral sol: patient should swish in mouth vigorously

- Give with food or milk to prevent nausea and vomiting
- Do not crush, chew caps
- Store in tight container at room temp
- Oral sol and caps are not interchangeable on a mg/mg basis
- Give caps after full meal to ensure absorption, swallow whole

IV route

- **IV** after adding full contents 25 ml to 50 ml of NaCl, mix gently, use flow control device, give over 1 hr; use separate line, flush after use

Patient/family education

- Advise patient that long-term therapy may be needed to clear infection (1 wk-6 mo depending on type of infection)
- Teach patient side effects and when to notify prescriber
- Instruct patient to avoid hazardous activities if dizziness occurs
- Instruct patient to take 2 hr before administration of other drugs that increase gastric pH (antacids, H_2-blockers, omeprazole, sucralfate, anticholinergics)
- Teach patient importance of compliance with drug regimen
- Instruct patient to notify prescriber of GI symptoms, signs of liver dysfunction (fatigue, nausea, anorexia, vomiting, dark urine, pale stools)
- Tell patient not to break, crush, or chew caps

Evaluation

Positive therapeutic outcome

- Decreased fever, malaise, rash
- Negative C&S for infectious organism

kanamycin (℞)

(kan-a-mye'sin)

kanamycin sulfate, Kantrex

Func. class.: Antiinfective

Chem. class.: Aminoglycoside

Pregnancy category C

Action: Interferes with protein synthesis in bacterial cell by binding to the 30S ribosomal subunit, causing inaccurate peptide sequence to form in protein chain, resulting in bacterial death

Therapeutic Outcome: Bactericidal effects for *Escherichia coli, Acinetobacter, Proteus, Serratia, Pseudomonas aeruginosa*

Uses: Severe systemic infections of CNS, respiratory tract, GI tract, urinary tract, bone, skin, soft tissues; peritonitis, preoperatively to sterilize bowel; decreases ammonia-producing bacteria in bowel and IP after fecal spill during surgery

Dosage and routes

Severe systemic infections

Adult and child: **IV** inf 15 mg/kg/day in divided doses q8-12h; diluted 500 mg/200 ml of 0.9% NaCl or D_5W given over 30-60 min, not to exceed 1.5 g/day; IM 15 mg/kg/day in divided doses q8-12h, not to exceed 1.5 g/day; irrigation not to exceed 1.5 g/day; inh 250 mg qid

Preoperative bowel sterilization

Adult: PO 1 g qh × 4 doses, then q6h × 36-72 hr

Available forms: Inj 75, 500 mg/2 ml, 1 g/3 ml; cap 500 mg

Adverse effects

CNS: Confusion, depression, numbness, tremors, **seizures,** muscle twitching, **neurotoxicity**

CV: Hypotension

EENT: *Ototoxicity,* deafness, visual disturbances, dizziness, vertigo, tinnitus

K

GI: *Nausea, vomiting, anorexia,* increased ALT, AST, bilirubin, hepatomegaly, **hepatic necrosis,** splenomegaly
GU: **Oliguria, hematuria, renal damage, azotemia, renal failure, nephrotoxicity**
HEMA: **Agranulocytosis, thrombocytopenia, leukopenia, eosinophilia, anemia**
INTEG: *Rash,* burning, urticaria, dermatitis, alopecia
RESP: Respiratory depression

Contraindications: Bowel obstruction, severe renal disease, hypersensitivity

P **Precautions:** Neonates, myasthenia gravis, hearing deficits, mild renal disease, lactation, Parkinson's disease, pregnancy **C**

Do Not Confuse:
kanamycin/Garamycin

Pharmacokinetics	
Absorption	Well absorbed IM; not absorbed PO
Distribution	Widely distributed in extracellular fluids; crosses placenta
Metabolism	Liver, minimally
Excretion	Kidneys, mostly unchanged (79%)
Half-life	2-3 hr; increased in renal disease

Pharmacodynamics	IM	IV
Onset	Rapid	Rapid
Peak	1-2 hr	1-2 hr

Interactions

Individual drugs

Amphotericin B: ↑ ototoxicity, neurotoxicity, nephrotoxicity
Cisplatin: ↑ ototoxicity, neurotoxicity, nephrotoxicity
Ethacrynic acid: ↑ ototoxicity, neurotoxicity, nephrotoxicity
Furosemide: ↑ ototoxicity, neurotoxicity, nephrotoxicity
Mannitol: ↑ ototoxicity, neurotoxicity, nephrotoxicity
Methoxyflurane: ↑ ototoxicity, neurotoxicity, nephrotoxicity
Polymyxin: ↑ ototoxicity, neurotoxicity, nephrotoxicity
Succinylcholine: ↑ neuromuscular blockade, respiratory depression
Vancomycin: ↑ ototoxicity, neurotoxicity, nephrotoxicity

Drug classifications

Aminoglycosides: ↑ otoxicity, nephrotoxicity, neurotoxicity
Anesthetics: ↑ neuromuscular blockade, respiratory depression
Nondepolarizing neuromuscular blockers: ↑ neuromuscular blockade, respiratory depression
Penicillins: ↑ ototoxicity, neurotoxicity, nephrotoxicity

NURSING CONSIDERATIONS

Assessment

- Assess patient for previous sensitivity reaction
- Assess patient for signs and symptoms of infection including characteristics of wounds, sputum, urine, stool, WBC >10,000/mm^3, fever; obtain baseline information and during treatment
- Obtain C&S tests before beginning drug therapy to identify if correct treatment has been initiated
- Assess for allergic reactions: rash, urticaria, pruritus, chills, fever, joint pain; angioedema may occur a few days after therapy begins
- Identify urine output; if decreasing, notify prescriber (may indicate nephrotoxicity); also check for increased BUN, sp gr, creatinine, urine CrCl <80 ml/min
- Monitor blood studies: AST, ALT, CBC, Hct, bilirubin, LDH, alkaline phosphatase, Coombs' test monthly if patient is on long-term therapy
- Monitor electrolytes: potassium, sodium, chloride, calcium, magnesium monthly if patient is on long-term therapy

- Assess bowel pattern qd; if severe diarrhea occurs, drug should be discontinued; may indicate pseudomembranous colitis
- Monitor for bleeding: ecchymosis, bleeding gums, hematuria, stool guaiac daily if on long-term therapy
- Assess for overgrowth of infection: perineal itching, fever, malaise, redness, pain, swelling, drainage, rash, diarrhea, change in cough, sputum
- Obtain weight before treatment; calculation of dosage is usually based on ideal body weight, but may be calculated on actual body weight
- Monitor I&O ratio; perform urinalysis daily for proteinuria, cells, casts; report sudden change in urine output
- Monitor VS during inf; watch for hypotension, change in pulse
- Assess **IV** site for thrombophlebitis including pain, redness, swelling q30 min; change site if needed; apply warm compresses to discontinued site
- Obtain serum peak, at 30-60 min after **IV** inf or 60 min after IM inj; obtain trough level just before next dose; blood level should be 2-4 times bacteriostatic level
- Assess hearing by audiometric testing, ringing, roaring in ears, vertigo before, during, after treatment
- Assess for dehydration: high sp gr, decrease in skin turgor, dry mucous membranes, dark urine
- Assess vestibular dysfunction: nausea, vomiting, dizziness, headache; drug should be discontinued if severe

Nursing diagnoses

- ✓ Infection, risk for (uses)
- ✓ Diarrhea (adverse reactions)
- ✓ Injury, risk for (adverse reactions)
- ✓ Knowledge deficit (teaching)

Implementation

PO route

- Give in even doses around the clock; if GI upset occurs, give with food; drug must be given for 10-14 days to ensure organism death and prevent superinfection; store in tight container

IM route

- Inject deep in large muscle mass

IV **IV route**

- Dilute 500 mg/100-200 ml; or 1 g/200-400 ml of D_5W, $D_{10}W$, D_5/0.9% NaCl, 0.9% NaCl, LR
- Do not admix; give aminoglycosides and penicillin at least 1 hr apart
- Give by intermittent inf over 30-60 min; flush with 0.9% NaCl or D_5W after inf is complete

Syringe compatibilities: Penicillin G sodium

Syringe incompatibilities: Ampicillin, carbamicillin, heparin

Y-site compatibilities: Cyclophosphamide, furosemide, heparin with hydrocortisone, hydromorphone, magnesium sulfate, meperidine, morphine, perphenazine, potassium chloride

Additive compatibilities: Ascorbic acid, cefoxitin, chloramphenicol, clindamycin, dopamine, furosemide, penicillin G potassium, penicillin G sodium, polymyxin B, sodium bicarbonate, tetracycline, vit B/C; admixing is not recommended

Additive incompatibilities: Amphotericin B, cephalothin, cephapirin, chlorpheniramine, heparin, methohexital

Patient/family education

- Teach patient to report sore throat, bruising, bleeding, joint pain, may indicate blood dyscrasias (rare)
- Advise patient to contact prescriber if vaginal itching, loose, foul-smelling stools, furry tongue occur; may indicate superinfection
- Instruct patient to continue full course of treatment

Evaluation

Positive therapeutic outcome

- Absence of signs/symptoms of infection (WBC <10,000/mm^3, temp

K

WNL, absence of red, draining wounds)
- Reported improvement in symptoms of infection

Treatment of overdose: Withdraw drug, hemodialysis, monitor serum levels of drug

kaolin/pectin (OTC)
(kay'-oh-lin pek'tin)

Donnagel-MB ♣, Kao-Spen, Kapectolin, K-P

Func. class.: Antidiarrheal, adsorbent

Chem. class.: Hydrous magnesium aluminum silicate

Pregnancy category C

Action: Decreases gastric motility, water content of stool; adsorbent, demulcent

➡ **Therapeutic Outcome:** Absence of diarrhea

Uses: Diarrhea (cause undetermined)

Dosage and routes

Adult: PO 60-120 ml (45-90 ml conc) after each loose bowel movement

P ***Child >12 yr:*** PO 60 ml after each loose bowel movement

P ***Child 6-12 yr:*** PO 30-60 ml (15 ml conc) after each loose bowel movement

P ***Child 3-6 yr:*** PO 15-30 ml (7.5 ml conc) after each loose bowel movement

Available forms: Susp kaolin 0.87 g/5 ml, pectin 43 mg/5 ml; kaolin 0.98 g/5 ml, pectin 21.7 mg/5 ml

Adverse effects

GI: Constipation (chronic use)

P **Contraindications:** Child <3 yr, severe abdominal pain

Precautions: Pregnancy **C**

Pharmacokinetics	
Absorption	Not absorbed
Distribution	Unknown
Metabolism	Unknown
Excretion	Unknown
Half-life	Unknown

Pharmacodynamics	
Onset	½ hr
Peak	Unknown
Duration	6 hr

Interactions

All drugs: ↓ action of all other drugs

NURSING CONSIDERATIONS

Assessment
- Assess bowel pattern before, during treatment; for rebound constipation after termination of medication; check bowel sounds
- P Assess for dehydration in children
- Check response after 48 hr; if no response, drug should be discontinued and other treatment initiated

Nursing diagnoses
- ✓ Diarrhea (uses)
- ✓ Constipation (adverse reactions)
- ✓ Knowledge deficit (teaching)
- ✓ Noncompliance (teaching)

Implementation
- Shake susp before use
- Administer for 48 hr only

Patient/family education
- Advise patient not to exceed recommended dosage; to take all other medications ≥2 hr apart

Evaluation

Positive therapeutic outcome
- Decreased diarrhea

ketoconazole (℞)
(kee-toe-koe'na-zole)
Nizoral
Func. class.: Antifungal
Chem. class.: Imidazole derivative

Pregnancy category C

Action: Alters cell membrane and inhibits several fungal enzymes; prevents production of adrenal sterols; prevents fungal metabolism

➔ Therapeutic Outcome: Fungistatic/fungicidal against susceptible organisms: *Blastomycoses, Candida, Coccidioides, Cryptococcus, Histoplasma;* top route: tinea cruris, tinea corporis, tinea versicolor, pityrosporum ovale

Uses: Systemic candidiasis, chronic mucocandidiasis, oral thrush, candiduria, coccidioidomycosis, histoplasmosis, chromomycosis, paracoccidioidomycosis, blastomycosis

Investigational uses: Cushing's syndrome, advanced prostatic cancer, depression

Dosage and routes
Adult: PO 200-400 mg once daily for 1-2 wk (candidiasis), 6 wk (other infections); 400 mg tid (prostate cancer, unlabeled)

P ***Children >2 yr:*** 3.3-6.6 mg/kg/day as single daily dose; <2 yr daily dose not established

P ***Adult and child >2 yr:*** TOP 2% cream applied qd or bid

Adult: Massage shampoo into scalp 1 min, reapply × 3 min, rinse; continue treatment twice/wk × 1 mo, no more than once q3 days

Depression

Adult: PO 200 mg/day, increase by 200 mg q3-4 days for 6 wk

Available forms: Tabs 200 mg; oral susp ✤ 100 mg/5 ml; cream 2%, shampoo 2%

Adverse effects
CNS: Headache, dizziness, somnolence
GI: Nausea, vomiting, anorexia, diarrhea, abdominal pain, **hepatotoxicity**
GU: Gynecomastia, impotence
HEMA: **Thrombocytopenia, leukopenia, hemolytic anemia**
INTEG: Pruritus, fever, chills, photophobia, rash, dermatitis, purpura, urticaria
SYST: **Anaphylaxis**

Contraindications: Hypersensitivity, lactation, fungal meningitis; coadministration with terfenadine

Precautions: Renal, hepatic disease, achlorhydria (drug induced), P pregnancy **C**, children <2 yr, other hepatotoxic agents including terfenadine

K

Pharmacokinetics	
Absorption	pH dependent; ↓ pH ↑ absorption
Distribution	Widely distributed; crosses placenta
Metabolism	Liver, partially
Excretion	Feces, bile, breast milk
Half-life	Biphasic: 2 hr, 8 hr

Pharmacodynamics	
Onset	Unknown
Peak	1-3 hr
Duration	Unknown

Interactions
Individual drugs
Alcohol: ↑ hepatotoxicity
Alfentanil: ↑ toxicity
Alprazolam: ↑ toxicity
Amprenavir: ↑ toxicity
Atorvastatin: ↑ toxicity
Carbamazepine: ↑ metabolism, ↓ effect of ketoconazole
Cimetidine: ↓ absorption
Clarithromycin: ↑ toxicity
Cyclophosphamide: ↑ toxicity
Cyclosporine: ↑ toxicity of cyclosporine

Didanosine: ↓ action of ketoconazole
Digoxin: ↑ effects of digoxin
Erythromycin: ↑ toxicity
Famotidine: ↓ absorption
Fentanyl: ↑ toxicity
Indinavir: ↑ toxicity
Isoniazid: ↑ metabolism, ↓ effect of ketoconazole
Midazolam: ↑ toxicity
Nelfinavir: ↑ toxicity
Nizatidine: ↓ absorption
Omeprazole: ↓ absorption
Paclitaxel: ↓ metabolism
Phenobarbital: ↑ metabolism, ↓ effect of ketoconazole
Phenytoin: ↑ metabolism, ↓ effect of ketoconazole
Ranitidine: ↓ absorption
Rifampin: ↑ metabolism, ↓ effect of ketoconazole
Ritonavir: ↑ toxicity
Saquinavir: ↑ toxicity
Sildenafil: ↑ toxicity
Sufentanil: ↑ toxicity
Theophylline: ↓ effectiveness
Vincristine: ↑ toxicity
Vinblastine: ↑ toxicity
Warfarin: ↑ effects of warfarin

Drug classifications
Anticholinergics: ↓ ketoconazole action
Calcium channel blockers: ↑ toxicity
Cardiac glycosides: ↑ effects of cardiac glycosides
Corticosteroids: ↑ toxicity
Gastric acid pump inhibitors: ↓ ketoconazole action
Oral anticoagulants: ↑ effects of oral anticoagulants
Oral hypoglycemics: ↑ effects of oral hypoglycemics

Food/drug
↑ Absorption

Herb/drug
Yew: ↓ ketoconazole action

NURSING CONSIDERATIONS

Assessment

- Assess for signs and symptoms of infection: drainage, sore throat, urinary pain, hematuria, fever
- Obtain cultures for C&S before beginning treatment; therapy may be started after culture is taken
- Monitor for hepatotoxicity: increased AST, ALT, alkaline phosphatase, bilirubin; drug is discontinued if hepatotoxicity occurs

Nursing diagnoses

- ✓ Infection, risk for (uses)
- ✓ Injury, risk for (adverse reactions)
- ✓ Knowledge deficit (teaching)

Implementation

PO route

- Give in the presence of acid products only; do not use alkaline products, proton pump inhibitors, H_2-antagonists, or antacids within 2 hr of drug; may give coffee, tea, acidic fruit juices, cola; give with food to decrease GI symptoms; dissolve tab/4 ml of aqueous sol 0.2 N HCl, use straw to avoid contact with, rinse with water afterward and swallow
- Give with HCI if achlorhydria is present
- Store in tight container at room temp

Topical route

- Use enough medication to cover fungally infected and surrounding area; rub in; do not use occlusive dressing; do not get in eyes

Shampoo

- Hair should be wet; apply shampoo, lather, rub gently into scalp and hair for 1 min; rinse; reapply × 3 min; continue treatment 2 ×/wk for 1 mo, no more than once q3 days

Patient/family education

- Advise patient that long-term therapy may be needed to clear infection (1 wk-6 mo depending on infection)
- Advise patient to avoid hazardous activities if dizziness occurs
- Instruct patient to take 2 hr before administration of other drugs that increase gastric pH (antacids, H_2-

blockers, omeprazole, sucralfate, anticholinergics)

- Stress the importance of compliance with drug regimen
- Advise patient to notify prescriber of GI symptoms, signs of liver dysfunction (fatigue, nausea, anorexia, vomiting, dark urine, pale stools)
- Teach patient proper hygiene: hand washing, nail care, use of concomitant topical agents if prescribed
- Caution patient to avoid alcohol, since nausea, vomiting, hypertension may occur
- Advise patient to use sunscreen or avoid direct sunlight to prevent photosensitivity
- Advise patient to notify prescriber of sore throat, fever, skin rash, which may indicate superinfection
- Advise patient to use sunglasses to prevent photophobia

Evaluation

Positive therapeutic outcome

- Decreased oral candidiasis, fever, malaise, rash
- Negative C&S for infectious organism
- Absence of dandruff, scaling

ketoprofen (OTC, ℞)

(ke-to-proe'fen)

Actron, Apo-Keto ✦, Apo-Keto-E ✦, Ketoprofen, Orudis, Orudis-E ✦, Orudis-KT, Orudis-SR ✦, Oruvail, Rhodis ✦

Func. class.: NSAID; nonopioid analgesic

Chem. class.: Propionic acid derivative

Pregnancy category B

Action: Inhibits prostaglandin synthesis by decreasing enzyme needed for biosynthesis; analgesic, antiinflammatory

➔ **Therapeutic Outcome:** Decreased pain, inflammation

Uses: Mild to moderate pain, osteoarthritis, rheumatoid arthritis, dysmenorrhea

Dosage and routes

Antiinflammatory

Adult: PO 150-300 mg in divided doses tid-qid, not to exceed 300 mg/day or ext rel 150-200 mg qd

Analgesic

Adult: PO 25-50 mg q6-8h

Available forms: Caps 12.5, 25, 50, 75 mg; ext rel caps 100, 150, 200 mg

Adverse effects

CNS: Dizziness, drowsiness, fatigue, tremors, confusion, insomnia, anxiety, depression, headache

CV: Tachycardia, peripheral edema, palpitations, dysrhythmias, hypertension

EENT: Tinnitus, hearing loss, blurred vision

GI: *Nausea, anorexia, vomiting, diarrhea,* jaundice, **hepatitis,** constipation, flatulence, cramps, dry mouth, peptic ulcer, **GI bleeding**

GU: **Nephrotoxicity: dysuria, hematuria, oliguria, azotemia**

HEMA: **Blood dyscrasias**

INTEG: Purpura, rash, pruritus, sweating

SYST: **Anaphylaxis**

Contraindications: Hypersensitivity, asthma, severe renal disease, severe hepatic disease, ulcer disease

Precautions: Pregnancy **B** (1st trimester) [P], lactation, children, bleeding disorders, GI disorders, cardiac disorders, hypersensitivity to other antiinflammatory agents, elderly [G]

Do Not Confuse:
Oruvail/Clinoril, Oruvail/Elavil

K

Pharmacokinetics	
Absorption	Well absorbed
Distribution	Not known
Metabolism	Liver
Excretion	Kidneys
Half-life	2-4 hr

Pharmacodynamics	
Onset	Unknown
Peak	2 hr
Duration	Unknown

Interactions

Individual drugs

Acetaminophen (long-term use): ↑ renal reactions
Alcohol: ↑ adverse reactions
Aspirin: ↓ effectiveness, ↑ adverse reactions
Clopidogrel: ↑ risk of bleeding
Coumadin: ↑ anticoagulant effects
Cyclosporine: ↑ toxicity
Digoxin: ↑ toxicity, levels
Eptifibatide: ↑ risk of bleeding
Insulin: ↓ insulin effect
Lithium: ↑ toxicity
Methotrexate: ↑ toxicity
Phenytoin: ↑ toxicity
Plicamycin: ↑ risk of bleeding
Probenecid: ↑ toxicity
Radiation: ↑ risk of hematologic toxicity
Sulfonylurea: ↑ toxicity
Ticlopidine: ↑ risk of bleeding
Tirofiban: ↑ risk of bleeding
Valproic acid: ↑ risk of bleeding

Drug classifications

Anticoagulants: ↑ risk of bleeding
Antihypertensives: ↓ effect of antihypertensives
Antineoplastics: ↑ risk of hematologic toxicity
β-Adrenergic blockers: ↑ antihypertension
Cephalosporins: ↑ risk of bleeding
Diuretics: ↓ effectiveness of diuretics
Glucocorticoids: ↑ adverse reactions
Hypoglycemics: ↓ hypoglycemic effect
NSAIDs: ↑ adverse reactions
Potassium supplements: ↑ adverse reactions
Sulfonamides: ↑ toxicity
Thrombolytics: ↑ risk of bleeding

Lab test interferences

↑ Bleeding time, ↑ liver function studies, ↑ serum uric acid, ↑ amylase, ↑ CO_2, ↑ urinary protein
↓ Serum potassium, ↓ PBI, ↓ cholesterol
Interference: Urine catecholamines, pregnancy test, urine glucose tests (Clinistix, Tes-Tape)

NURSING CONSIDERATIONS

Assessment

- Assess for pain: type, location, intensity; ROM before and 1-2 hr after treatment
- Monitor liver function, renal function, studies: AST, ALT, bilirubin, creatinine, BUN, urine creatinine, CBC Hct, Hgb, pro-time if patient is on long-term therapy
- Check I&O ratio; decreasing output may indicate renal failure (long-term therapy)
- Assess hepatotoxicity: dark urine, clay-colored stools, jaundice of skin and sclera, itching, abdominal pain, fever, diarrhea if patient is on long-term therapy
- Assess for allergic reactions: rash, urticaria; if these occur, drug may have to be discontinued
- Assess for ototoxicity: tinnitus, ringing, roaring in ears; audiometric testing needed before, after long-term therapy
- Assess for visual changes: blurring, halos; may indicate corneal, retinal damage
- Assess for GI bleeding: blood in sputum, emesis, stools
- Check edema in feet, ankles, legs
- Identify prior drug history; there are many drug interactions
- Monitor pain: location, duration, type, intensity, before dose and 1 hr after; ROM before dose and after

Nursing diagnoses

- ✓ Pain (uses)
- ✓ Mobility, impaired physical (uses)
- ✓ Injury, risk for (adverse reactions)
- ✓ Knowledge deficit (teaching)

Implementation

- Administer to patient whole; do not crush, break, chew, or open cap
- Give with food or milk to decrease gastric symptoms; give 30 min ac or 2 hr pc; absorption may be slowed

Patient/family education

- Teach patient to report any symptoms of hepatotoxicity, renal toxicity, visual changes, ototoxicity, allergic reactions, bleeding (long-term therapy)
- Advise patient to take with 8 oz of water and sit upright for 30 min after dose to prevent ulceration
- Caution patient not to exceed recommended dosage; acute poisoning may result; to take as prescribed; do not double dose
- Advise patient to read label on other OTC drugs; many contain other antiinflammatories
- Advise patient to use sunscreen to prevent photosensitivity
- Inform patient that the therapeutic response takes 2 wk (arthritis)
- Teach patient to report tinnitus, confusion, diarrhea, sweating, hyperventilation, blurred vision, fever, joint aches
- Caution patient to avoid alcohol ingestion; GI bleeding may occur

Evaluation

Positive therapeutic outcome

- Decreased pain
- Decreased inflammation
- Increased mobility
- Decreased fever

ketorolac (℞)

(kee'toe-role-ak)

Acular, Toradol

Func. class.: NSAID, nonopioid analgesic

Chem. class.: Pyrrolopyrrole

Pregnancy category C

Action: Inhibits prostaglandin synthesis by decreasing an enzyme needed for biosynthesis; analgesic, antiinflammatory, antipyretic effects

→ **Therapeutic Outcome:** Decreased pain, inflammation, ocular itching

Uses: Mild to moderate pain (short term); decreased ocular itching in seasonal allergic conjunctivitis

Dosage and routes

Adult <65 yr: PO 20 mg, then 10 mg q4-6h prn, max 40 mg/day; (single dose) IM 60 mg; **IV** 30 mg; (multiple dosing) IM/**IV** 15 mg q6h, max 60 mg/days × 5 days combined either PO/IM/**IV**

G ***Adult ≥65 yr, renal disease, <50 kg:*** PO 10 mg q4-6h prn, max 40 mg/day; (single dose) IM 30 mg; **IV** 15 mg; (multiple dosing) IM/**IV** 15 mg q6h, max 60 mg/day × 5 days combined either PO/IM/**IV**

Ophthalmic route

Adult: 1 gtt (0.25 mg) qid × 7 days

P ***Child:*** **IV** 1 mg/kg then 0.5 mg/kg q6h

Available forms: Inj 15, 30 mg/ml (prefilled syringes); ophth 0.5% sol; tabs 10 mg

Adverse effects

CV: Hypertension, flushing, syncope, pallor, edema, vasodilation

CNS: Dizziness, *drowsiness,* tremors

EENT: Tinnitus, hearing loss, blurred vision

GI: Nausea, anorexia, vomiting, diarrhea, constipation, flatulence,

cramps, dry mouth, peptic ulcer, **GI bleeding, perforation,** taste change
GU: **Nephrotoxicity: dysuria, hematuria, oliguria, azotemia**
HEMA: **Blood dyscrasias,** prolonged bleeding
INTEG: Purpura, rash, pruritus, sweating

Contraindications: Hypersensitivity, asthma, severe renal disease, severe hepatic disease, peptic ulcer disease

Precautions: Pregnancy **C**, lactation, children, bleeding disorders, GI disorders, cardiac disorders, hypersensitivity to other antiinflammatory agents, elderly, CrCl <25 ml/min

Do Not Confuse:
Toradol/Tegretol, Toradol/Inderal, Toradol/Torecan, Toradol/tramadol

Pharmacokinetics

Absorption	Rapidly, completely absorbed
Distribution	Bound to plasma proteins (99%)
Metabolism	Liver (<50%)
Excretion	Kidney, metabolites (92%); breast milk (6%); feces
Half-life	6 hr (IM); increased in renal disease

Pharmacodynamics

	IM	OPHTH/PO
Onset	Up to 10 min	Unknown
Peak	50 min IM; 2-3 hr PO	Unknown
Duration	4-6 hr PO	Unknown

Interactions

Individual drugs

Alcohol: ↑ GI effects
Aspirin: ↑ ketorolac levels, ↑ GI effects
Clopidogrel: ↑ bleeding risk
Cyclosporine: ↑ toxicity
Eptifibatide: ↑ bleeding risk
Heparin: ↑ bleeding
Lithium: ↑ toxicity
Methotrexate: ↑ effects
Phenytoin: ↑ effects
Plicamycin: ↑ bleeding risk
Probenecid: ↑ ketorolac levels
Sulfinpyrazone: ↓ effects
Ticlopidine: ↑ bleeding risk
Tirofiban: ↑ bleeding risk
Valproic acid: ↑ bleeding risk

Drug classifications

ACE inhibitors: ↑ renal impairment
Anticoagulants: ↑ effects
Cephalosporins, some: ↑ risk of bleeding
Corticosteroids: ↑ GI effects
Diuretics: ↓ antihypertensive effect
NSAIDs: ↑ gastric ulcers
Potassium products: ↑ GI effects
Salicylates: ↓ blood sugar levels
Sulfonamides: ↓ effects
Thrombolytics: ↑ bleeding risk

Lab test interferences

↑ Coagulation studies, ↑ liver function studies, ↑ serum uric acid, ↑ amylase, ↑ CO_2, ↑ urinary protein
↓ Serum potassium, ↓ PBI, ↓ cholesterol
Interference: Urine catecholamines, pregnancy test, urine glucose tests (Clinistix, Tes-Tape)

NURSING CONSIDERATIONS

Assessment

- Monitor blood counts during therapy; watch for decreasing platelets; if low, therapy may need to be discontinued and restarted after hematologic recovery; assess for blood dyscrasia (thrombocytopenia): bruising, fatigue, bleeding, poor healing
- Monitor for aspirin sensitivity, asthma; these patients may be more likely to develop hypersensitivity to NSAIDs
- Assess patient's eyes: redness swelling, tearing, itching
- Monitor for pain: type, location, intensity, ROM before and 1 hr after treatment
- Assess for GI bleeding: blood in sputum, emesis, stools

Nursing diagnoses

- ✓ Pain (uses)
- ✓ Mobility, impaired physical (uses)
- ✓ Injury, risk for (adverse reactions)
- ✓ Knowledge deficit (teaching)

Implementation

PO route

- Administer to patient crushed or whole
- Give with food or milk to decrease gastric symptoms; give 30 min ac or 2 hr pc; absorption may be slowed

IV **IM/IV route**

- **IV** give undiluted ≥15 sec
- Give IM/**IV** for 5 days or less, continue with PO

Y-site compatibilities: Cisatracurium, remifentanil, sufentanil

Syringe incompatibilities: Morphine, meperidine, promethazine, hydroxyzine

Solution compatibilities: D_5W, 0.9% NaCl, LR

Patient/family education

- Teach patient that drug must be continued for prescribed time to be effective; to avoid aspirin, alcoholic beverages, other NSAIDs, acetaminophen
- Caution patient to report bleeding, bruising, fatigue, malaise, since blood dyscrasias do occur
- Instruct patient to use caution when driving; drowsiness, dizziness may occur
- Teach patient to take with a full glass of water to enhance absorption; do not crush, break, or chew tabs
- Caution patient that this drug may cause eye redness, burning if soft contact lenses are worn

Evaluation

Positive therapeutic outcome

- Decreased pain
- Decreased inflammatory response
- Increased mobility
- Decreased ocular itching

labetalol (℞)

(la-bet'a-lole)

Normodyne, Trandate

Func. class.: Antihypertensive, antianginal

Chem. class.: α- and β-blocker

Pregnancy category C

Action: Competitively blocks stimulation of β-adrenergic receptor within vascular smooth muscle; produces chronotropic, inotropic activity (decreases rate of SA node discharge, increases recovery time), slows conduction of AV node, decreases heart rate, which decreases O_2 consumption in myocardium; also has α-adrenergic blocking activity

➡ **Therapeutic Outcome:** Decreased B/P

Uses: Mild to moderate hypertension; treatment of severe hypertension (**IV**)

Investigational uses: Angina pectoris (PO), hypotension during surgery (**IV**)

Dosage and routes

Hypertension

Adult: PO 100 mg bid; may be given with a diuretic; may increase to 200 mg bid after 2 days; may continue to increase q1-3 days; max 400 mg bid

Hypertensive crisis

Adult: **IV** inf 200 mg/160 ml D_5W, run at 2 ml/min; stop inf after desired response obtained; repeat q6-8h as needed; **IV** bol 20 mg over 2 min; may repeat 40-80 mg q10 min, not to exceed 300 mg

Available forms: Tabs 100, 200, 300 mg; inj 5 mg/ml in 20-ml ampules

Adverse effects

CNS: Dizziness, mental changes, drowsiness, fatigue, headache, catatonia, depression, anxiety, nightmares, paresthesias, lethargy

L

CV: *Orthostatic hypotension,* **bradycardia, CHF,** chest pain, **ventricular dysrhythmias,** AV block
EENT: *Tinnitus,* visual changes, sore throat, double vision, dry burning eyes
GI: *Nausea, vomiting, diarrhea*
GU: Impotence, dysuria, ejaculatory failure
HEMA: **Agranulocytosis, thrombocytopenia, purpura** (rare)
INTEG: Rash, alopecia, urticaria, pruritus, fever
RESP: **Bronchospasm,** dyspnea, wheezing

Contraindications: Hypersensitivity to β-blockers, cardiogenic shock, heart block (2nd or 3rd degree), sinus bradycardia, CHF, bronchial asthma

Precautions: Major surgery, pregnancy **C,** lactation, diabetes mellitus, renal disease, thyroid disease, COPD, well-compensated heart failure, CAD, nonallergic bronchospasm, G elderly, hepatic disease

Pharmacokinetics

Absorption	Bioavailability 25% (PO); complete (**IV**)
Distribution	Crosses placenta, CNS
Metabolism	Liver, extensively
Excretion	Breast milk, kidneys, bile
Half-life	6-8 hr

Pharmacodynamics

	PO	IV
Onset	1-2 hr	5 min
Peak	2-4 hr	15 min
Duration	8-12 hr	2-4 hr

Interactions
Individual drugs
Alcohol: ↑ hypotension (large amounts)
Epinephrine: α-Adrenergic stimulation
Glutethimide: ↓ effect of labetolol
Hydralazine: ↑ hypotension, bradycardia
Indomethacin: ↓ antihypertensive effect
Insulin: ↑ hypoglycemia
Methyldopa: ↑ hypotension, bradycardia
Prazosin: ↑ hypotension, bradycardia
Propranolol: ↑ hypotension
Reserpine: ↑ hypotension, bradycardia
Thyroid hormones: ↓ effect of labetolol
Verapamil: ↑ myocardial depression

Drug classifications
Antidiabetics: ↑ hypoglycemia
Antihypertensives: ↑ hypertension
β_2-Adrenergic agonists: ↓ bronchodilatation
Cardiac glycosides: ↑ bradycardia
Hydantoins: ↑ myocardial depression
MAOIs: Do not use within 2 wk
Nitrates: ↑ hypotension
NSAIDs: ↓ antihypertensive effect
Theophyllines: ↓ bronchodilatation

Lab test interferences
False: ↑ urinary catecholamines

NURSING CONSIDERATIONS
Assessment
- Monitor B/P at beginning of treatment, periodically thereafter; pulse q4h; note rate, rhythm, quality: apical/radial pulse before administration; notify prescriber of any significant changes (pulse <50 bpm)
- Check for baselines in renal, liver function tests before therapy begins
- Assess for edema in feet, legs daily, monitor I&O, daily weight; check for jugular vein distention, rales bilaterally, dyspnea (CHF)
- Monitor skin turgor, dryness of mucous membranes for hydration G status, especially elderly

Nursing diagnoses
- ✓ Cardiac output, decreased (uses)
- ✓ Injury, potential for physical (side effects)
- ✓ Knowledge deficit (teaching)
- ✓ Noncompliance (teaching)

Implementation

PO route

- Given ac, hs, tab may be crushed or swallowed whole; give with food to prevent GI upset, increase absorption; reduce dosage in renal dysfunction
- Store protected from light, moisture; place in cool environment

IV route

- Give **IV** undiluted 20 mg/2 min; may increase q10 min 40-80 mg until desired effect
- Give **IV** cont inf by diluting in LR, D_5W, D_5 in 0.2%, 0.9%, 0.33% NaCl or Ringer's; inf is titrated to patient response; 200 mg of drug/160 ml sol (1 mg/ml); 300 mg of drug/ 240 ml sol (1 mg/ml); 200 mg of drug/250 ml sol (2 mg/3ml); use infusion pump
- Keep patient recumbent during and for 3 hr after inf, monitor VS q5-15 min

Y-site compatibilities:

Amikacin, aminophylline, amiodarone, ampicillin, butorphanol, calcium gluconate, cefazolin, ceftazidime, ceftizoxime, chloramphenicol, cimetidine, clindamycin, diltiazem, dobutamine, dopamine, enalaprilat, epinephrine, erythromycin, esmolol, famotidine, fentanyl, gentamicin, hydromorphone, lidocaine, lorazepam, magnesium sulfate, meperidine, metronidazole, midazolam, milrinone, morphine, nicardipine, nitroglycerin, nitroprusside, norepinephrine, oxacillin, penicillin G potassium, piperacillin, potassium chloride, potassium phosphate, propofol, ranitidine, sodium acetate, tobramycin, trimethoprim-sulfamethoxazole, vancomycin, vecuronium

Y-site incompatibilities:

Cefoperazone, nafcillin

Solution compatibilities:

D_5R, D_5LR, $D_{2½}$/0.45% NaCl, D_5/0.2% NaCl, D_5/0.33% NaCl, D_5/0.9% NaCl, D_5W, Ringer's, LR

Solution incompatibilities:

Sodium bicarbonate 5%

Patient/family education

- Teach patient not to discontinue drug abruptly, or precipitate angina might occur; taper over 2 wk
- Teach patient not to use OTC products containing α-adrenergic stimulants (such as nasal decongestants, cold preparations); to avoid alcohol, smoking and to limit sodium intake as prescribed
- Teach patient how to take pulse and B/P at home; advise when to notify prescriber
- Instruct patient to comply with weight control, dietary adjustments, modified exercise program
- Advise patient to carry/wear ID to identify drugs being taken, allergies; that drug controls symptoms but does not cure the condition
- Caution patient to avoid hazardous activities if dizziness, drowsiness are present
- Teach patient to report symptoms of CHF: difficult breathing, especially on exertion or when lying down, night cough, swelling of extremities, bradycardia, dizziness, confusion, depression, fever
- Teach patient to take drug as prescribed, not to double or skip doses; take any missed doses as soon as remembered if at least 4 hr until next dose

Evaluation

Positive therapeutic outcome

- Decreased B/P in hypertension (after 1-2 wk)
- Absence of dysrhythmias

Treatment of overdose:

Lavage, **IV** atropine for bradycardia, **IV** theophylline for bronchospasm, digitalis, O_2, diuretic for cardiac failure, hemodialysis, **IV** glucose for hyperglycemia, **IV** diazepam (or phenytoin) for seizures

L

lactulose (℞)
(lak'tyoo-lose)

Cephulac, Cholac, Chronulac, Constilac, Constulose, Duphalac, Enulose, Heptalac, Lactulax ♣, Lactulose PSE, Portalac

Func. class.: Laxative (hyperosmotic/ammonia detoxicant)

Chem. class.: Lactose synthetic derivative

Pregnancy category B

Action: Increases osmotic pressure; draws fluid into colon; prevents absorption of ammonia in colon; increases water in stool

Therapeutic Outcome: Decreased constipation, decreased blood ammonia level

Uses: Chronic constipation, portal-systemic encephalopathy in patients with hepatic disease

Dosage and routes
Constipation

Adult: PO 15-60 ml qd

P ***Child:*** PO 7.5 ml qd

Encephalopathy

Adult: PO 30-45 ml tid or qid until stools are soft; retention enema 300 ml diluted (unlabeled)

P ***Infant:*** PO 2.5-10 ml/day in divided doses

P ***Child:*** PO 40-90 ml/day in divided doses given 2-4 ×/day

Available forms: Oral sol, rec sol 3.33 g/5 ml; syrup 10 g/15 ml

Adverse effects
GI: ***Nausea, vomiting, anorexia, abdominal cramps, diarrhea,*** flatulence, *distention, belching*

Contraindications: Hypersensitivity, low-galactose diet

Precautions: Pregnancy **B,** lactation, G diabetes mellitus, elderly and debilitated patient

Pharmacokinetics

Absorption	Poorly absorbed
Distribution	Not known
Metabolism	Colonic bacteria to acids
Excretion	Kidneys, unchanged
Half-life	Unknown

Pharmacodynamics
Unknown

Interactions
Individual drugs

Neomycin: ↓ effectiveness (portal-systemic encephalopathy)

Drug classifications

Laxatives: Do not use together (portal-systemic encephalopathy)

NURSING CONSIDERATIONS
Assessment
- Monitor glucose levels in diabetic patients (increases)
- Monitor blood, urine, electrolytes if used often by patient; may cause diarrhea, hypokalemia, hypernatremia; check I&O ratio to identify fluid loss
- Assess cramping, rectal bleeding, nausea, vomiting; if these symptoms occur, drug should be discontinued; identify cause of constipation; identify whether fluids, bulk, or exercise is missing from lifestyle
- Monitor blood ammonia level (30-70 mg/100 ml); monitor for clearing of confusion, lethargy, restlessness, irritability (hepatic encephalopathy); may decrease ammonia level by 50%

Nursing diagnoses
✓ Constipation (uses)
✓ Diarrhea (adverse reactions)
✓ Knowledge deficit (teaching)
✓ Noncompliance (teaching)

Implementation
PO route
- Give with full glass of fruit juice, water, milk to increase palatability of oral form; increase fluids by 2 L/day;

do not give with other laxatives; if diarrhea occurs, reduce dosage

Rectal route

- Administer retention enema by diluting 300 ml of lactulose/700 ml of water or of 0.9% NaCl; administer by rec balloon catheter; retain for 30-60 min; repeat if evacuated too quickly

Patient/family education

- Discuss with patient that adequate fluid consumption is necessary
- Teach patient that normal bowel movements do not always occur daily
- Teach patient not to use in presence of abdominal pain, nausea, vomiting; tell patient to notify prescriber if constipation unrelieved or if symptoms of electrolyte imbalance occur: muscle cramps, pain, weakness, dizziness, excessive thirst
- Teach patient not to use laxatives for long-term therapy; bowel tone will be lost
- Do not give at hs as a laxative; may interfere with sleep
- Notify prescriber if diarrhea occurs; may indicate overdosage

Evaluation

Positive therapeutic outcome

- Decreased constipation
- Decreased blood ammonia level
- Clearing of mental state

lamivudine (3TC) (℞)

(lam-i'vue-dine)

Epivir, Epivir-HBV, 3TC

Func. class.: Antiretroviral

Chem. class.: Nucleoside reverse transcriptase inhibitor

Pregnancy category C

Action: Inhibits replication of HIV virus by incorporating into cellular DNA by viral reverse transcriptase, thereby terminating the cellular DNA chain

➔ **Therapeutic Outcome:** Improved symptoms of HIV infection

Uses: HIV infection in combination with zidovudine (Epivir); chronic hepatitis B (Epivir-HBV)

Investigational uses: Prophylaxis of HIV postexposure with indinavir and zidovudine

Dosage and routes

HIV infection

P ***Adult/child >12 yr:*** PO 150 mg bid with zidovudine; <50 kg: PO 2 mg/kg bid with zidovudine

P ***Child 3 mo-12 yr:*** PO 4 mg/kg bid; may give 150 mg bid with zidovudine

Renal dose

Adult: PO CrCl 30-49 ml/min 150 mg qd; CrCl 15-29 ml/min 150 mg 1st dose, then 10 mg qd; CrCl 5-14 ml/min 150 mg qd, then 50 mg qd; CrCl <5 ml/min 50 mg 1st dose, then 25 mg qd

Chronic hepatitis B

Adult: PO 100 mg qd

Renal dose

Adult: PO CrCl 30-49 ml/min 100 mg 1st dose, then 50 mg qd; CrCl 15-29 ml/min 100 mg 1st dose, then 25 mg qd; CrCl 5-14 ml/min 35 mg 1st dose then 15 mg qd; CrCl <5 ml/min 35 mg 1st dose, then 10 mg qd

Available forms: Tabs 100, 150 mg; oral sol 5, 10 mg/ml

Adverse effects

CNS: *Fever, headache, malaise, dizziness, insomnia, depression, fatigue, chills*

EENT: Taste change, hearing loss, photophobia

GI: *Nausea, vomiting, diarrhea,* anorexia, cramps, dyspepsia, **pancreatitis** (pediatric patients) P

HEMA: **Neutropenia,** anemia, **thrombocytopenia**

INTEG: *Rash*

MS: *Myalgia, arthralgia, pain*

RESP: *Cough*

Contraindications: Hypersensitivity

Precautions: Granulocyte count <1000/mm^3 or Hgb <9.5 g/dl, pregnancy **C**, lactation, children, renal disease, severe hepatic function, pancreatitis, elderly

Pharmacokinetics

Absorption	Rapidly absorbed
Distribution	Extravascular space
Metabolism	Unknown
Excretion	Unchanged in urine
Half-life	Unknown

Pharmacodynamics

Unknown

Interactions

Individual drugs

Trimethoprim-sulfamethoxazole: ↑ level of lamivudine

Zidovudine: ↑ level of zidovudine when given with lamivudine

NURSING CONSIDERATIONS

Assessment

- Monitor blood counts q2 wk; watch for neutropenia, thrombocytopenia, Hgb, CD4, viral load, lipase, triglycerides periodically during treatment; if low, therapy may have to be discontinued and restarted after hematologic recovery; blood transfusions may be required
- Monitor liver function studies: AST, ALT, bilirubin; amylase
- Monitor children for pancreatitis
- Assess for lactic acidosis, severe hepatomegaly with steatosis: obtain baseline LFT; if elevated, discontinue treatment; discontinue even if LFTs are normal and symptoms of lactic acidosis, severe hepatomegaly develop

Nursing diagnoses

✓ Infection, risk for (uses)
✓ Injury, risk for (adverse reactions)
✓ Knowledge deficit (teaching)

Implementation

- Administer PO bid
- Give with other antiretrovirals only
- Store in cool environment; protect from light

Patient/family education

- Teach patient that GI complaints and insomnia resolve after 3-4 wk of treatment
- Tell patient that drug is not a cure for AIDS but will control symptoms
- Teach patient to notify prescriber of sore throat, swollen lymph nodes, malaise, fever; other infections may occur
- Teach patient that virus is still infective, may pass AIDS virus to others
- Encourage patient to continue follow-up visits since serious toxicity may occur; blood counts must be done q2 wk
- Teach patient that drug must be taken tid, even if feeling better
- Tell patient that other drugs may be necessary to prevent other infections
- Teach patient that drug may cause fainting or dizziness

Evaluation

Positive therapeutic outcome

- Absence of infection, symptoms of HIV infection

lamotrigine (℞)

(lam-o-trye'geen)

Lamictal, Lamictal chewable

Func. class.: Anticonvulsant, misc.

Chem. class.: Phenyltriazine

Pregnancy category C

Action: Unknown; may inhibit voltage-sensitive sodium channels

➔ **Therapeutic Outcome:** Decrease in intensity and amount of seizures

Uses: Adjunct in the treatment of partial seizures; children with Lennox-Gastaut syndrome

Investigational uses: Refractory bipolar disorder, generalized tonic-clonic, absence, atypical absence and myoclonic seizures

Dosage and routes

Monotherapy

Adult: PO 50 mg/day for wk 1 and 2, then increase to 100 mg divided bid for wk 3 and 4; maintenance 300-500 mg/day

P ***Child:*** 2 mg/kg/day in 2 divided doses × 2 wk, then 10 mg/kg/day, max 15 mg/kg/day or 400 mg/day

Multiple therapy

Adult: PO 25 mg every other day, wk 1 through 4, then 150 mg/day in divided doses

P ***Child:*** 0.1-0.2 mg/kg/day initially, then increase q2 wk as needed to 2 mg/kg/day or 150 mg/day

Available forms: Tabs 25, 100, 150, 200 mg; chew tabs 2, 5, 25 mg

Adverse effects

CNS: Fever, insomnia, tremor, depression, anxiety, *dizziness*, ataxia, *headache*
EENT: Nystagmus, **diplopia,** *blurred vision*
GI: *Nausea, vomiting, anorexia,* abdominal pain
GU: *Dysmenorrhea*
INTEG: **Rash (potentially life-threatening),** alopecia, photosensitivity
RESP: **Rhinitis,** pharyngitis, cough
SYST: **Stevens-Johnson syndrome**

Contraindications: Hypersensitivity

Precautions: Pregnancy **C,** P lactation, children <16 yr, renal, hepatic disease

Do Not Confuse:
Lamictal/Lamisil,
Lamictal/Lomotil

Pharmacokinetics

Absorption	Well absorbed
Distribution	Unknown
Metabolism	Unknown
Excretion	Unknown
Half-life	Varies, depending on dose

Pharmacodynamics

Unknown

Interactions

Individual drugs

Carbamazepine: ↑ metabolic clearance of lamotrigine
Phenobarbital: ↑ metabolic clearance of lamotrigine
Phenytoin: ↑ metabolic clearance of lamotrigine
Primidone: ↑ metabolic clearance of lamotrigine
Valproic acid: ↓ metabolic clearance of lamotrigine

NURSING CONSIDERATIONS

Assessment

- Assess for rash (Stevens-Johnson syndrome or toxic epidermal necrolysis) in pediatric patients, drug should be discontinued at first sign of rash
- Assess for seizure activity: duration, type, intensity, halo before seizure
- Assess for hypersensitive reactions

Nursing diagnoses

✓ Injury, risk for (uses)
✓ Knowledge deficit (teaching)

Implementation

- May be given with food or fluids
- Dispersible tabs should be swallowed whole, chewed, dispersed in water or diluted fruit juice; if chewed, a small amount of water should be taken

Patient/family education

- Teach patient to take PO in divided doses with or after meals to decrease adverse effects
- Caution patient not to discontinue drug abruptly; seizures may occur

- Caution patient to avoid hazardous activities until stabilized on drug
- Advise patient to notify prescriber of skin rash or increased seizure activity
- Instruct patient to report to prescriber if pregnancy is suspected or planned
- Teach patient to use sunscreen and protective clothing, photosensitivity occurs
- Advise patient to carry ID stating drug use

Evaluation

Positive therapeutic outcome

- Decrease in severity of seizures

lansoprazole (℞)

(lan-soe'prah-zole)

Prevacid

Func. class.: Anti-ulcer–proton pump inhibitor

Chem. class.: Benzimidazole

Pregnancy category B

Action: Suppresses gastric secretion by inhibiting hydrogen/potassium ATPase enzyme system in gastric parietal cell; characterized as gastric acid pump inhibitor since it blocks final step of acid production

➔ **Therapeutic Outcome:** Reduction in gastric pain, swelling, fullness

Uses: Gastroesophageal reflux disease (GERD), severe erosive esophagitis, poorly responsive systemic GERD, pathologic hypersecretory conditions (Zollinger-Ellison syndrome, systemic mastocytosis, multiple endocrine adenomas); possibly effective for treatment of duodenal, gastric ulcers, maintenance of healed duodenal ulcers

Dosage and routes

NG tube

Adult: Use intact granules mixed in 40 ml of apple juice injected through NG tube, then flush with apple juice

Duodenal ulcer

Adult: PO 15 mg qd ac for 4 wk, then 15 mg qd to maintain healing of ulcers; ulcers associated with *Helicobacter:* 30 mg lansoprazole, 500 mg clarithromycin, 1 g amoxicillin bid × 14 days or 30 mg lansoprazole, 1 g amoxicillin tid × 14 days

Erosive esophagitis

Adult: PO 30 mg qd ac for up to 8 wk, may use another 8 wk course if needed

Pathologic hypersecretory conditions

Adult: PO 60 mg qd, may give up to 90 mg bid

Available forms: Caps delayed rel 15, 30 mg

Adverse effects

CNS: Headache, dizziness, confusion, agitation, amnesia, depression

CV: Chest pain, angina, tachycardia, bradycardia, palpitations, **CVA,** hypertension/hypotension, **MI,** shock, vasodilation

EENT: Tinnitus, taste perversion, deafness, eye pain, otitis media

GI: Diarrhea, abdominal pain, vomiting, nausea, constipation, flatulence, acid regurgitation, anorexia, irritable colon

GU: Hematuria, glycosuria, impotence, kidney calculus, breast enlargement

HEMA: **Hemolysis,** anemia

INTEG: Rash, urticaria, pruritus, alopecia

META: Weight gain/loss, gout

RESP: Upper respiratory infections, cough, epistaxis, asthma, bronchitis, dyspnea

Contraindications: Hypersensitivity

Precautions: Pregnancy **B,** lactation, [P] children

Pharmacokinetics

Absorption	Rapid after granules leave stomach
Distribution	Protein binding 97%
Metabolism	Liver extensively
Excretion	Urine, feces; clearance G decreased in elderly, renal, hepatic disease
Half-life	Plasma 1.5 hr

Pharmacodynamics

Unknown

Interactions

Individual drugs

Ampicillin: ↓ absorption of ampicillin
Digoxin: ↓ absorption of digoxin
Iron: ↓ absorption of iron
Ketoconazole: ↓ absorption of ketoconazole
Sucralfate: Delayed absorption of lansoprazole
Theophylline: ↓ clearance of theophylline

NURSING CONSIDERATIONS

Assessment

- Assess GI system; bowel sounds q8h, abdomen for pain, swelling, anorexia
- Monitor hepatic enzymes (AST, ALT, alkaline phosphatase) during treatment

Nursing diagnoses

✓ Pain (uses)
✓ Knowledge deficit (teaching)

Implementation

- Administer before eating; swallow capsule whole
- ⊘ Do not open, chew, crush

Patient/family education

- Instruct patient to report severe diarrhea; drug may have to be discontinued
- Inform diabetic patient that hypoglycemia may occur
- Encourage patient to avoid hazardous activities; dizziness may occur
- Tell patient to avoid alcohol, salicylates, ibuprofen; may cause GI irritation

Evaluation

Positive therapeutic outcome

- Absence of gastric pain, swelling, fullness

leflunomide (℞)

(leh-floo′noh-mide)

Arava

Func. class.: Antirheumatic
Chem. class.: Pyrimidine synthesis inhibitor

Pregnancy category X

Action: Inhibits an enzyme involved in pyrimidine synthesis and has antiproliferative, antiinflammatory effect

➔ **Therapeutic Outcome:** Decreased pain, joint swelling, increased mobility

Uses: Rheumatoid arthritis, to reduce disease process as well as symptoms

Dosage and routes

Adult: **PO** loading dose 100 mg/day × 3 days maintenance 20 mg/day, may be decreased to 10 mg/day if not well tolerated

Available forms: Tabs 10, 20, 100 mg

Adverse effects

CNS: Dizziness, insomnia, depression, paresthesia, anxiety, migraine, neuralgia, headache
CV: Palpitations, hypertension, chest pain, angina pectoris, migraine, peripheral edema
EENT: Pharyngitis, oral candidiasis, stomatitis, dry mouth, blurred vision
HEMA: Anemia, ecchymosis, hyperlipidemia
GI: *Nausea, anorexia, vomiting, constipation, flatulence, diarrhea, ↑ LFTs*

INTEG: Rash, pruritus, alopecia, acne, hematoma, herpes infections
RESP: Pharyngitis, rhinitis, bronchitis, cough, respiratory infection, pneumonia, sinusitis

Contraindications: Hypersensitivity, pregnancy **X,** lactation

Precautions: Hepatic, renal disorders

Pharmacokinetics

Absorption	Unknown
Distribution	Unknown
Metabolism	Liver
Excretion	Kidneys
Half-life	Unknown

Pharmacodynamics

Onset	Unknown
Peak	Unknown
Duration	Unknown

Interactions

Individual drugs

Activated charcoal: ↓ effect of leflunomide
Cholestyramine: ↓ effect of leflunomide
Methotrexate: ↑ side effects

Drug classifications

Live Virus Vaccines: ↓ antibody
NSAIDs: ↑ NSAID effect
Hepatotoxic agents: ↑ side effects of leflunomide

NURSING CONSIDERATIONS

Assessment

- Monitor liver function studies: if ALT elevations are >2-fold ULN, reduce dose to 10 mg/day
- Assess arthritic symptoms: ROM, mobility, swelling of joints, baseline and during treatment

Nursing diagnoses

- ✓ Mobility, impaired (uses)
- ✓ Pain (uses)
- ✓ Knowledge deficit (teaching)

Implementation

PO route

- Give PO with food for GI upset
- To eliminate drug give cholestyramine 8 g tid × 11 days, check levels

Patient/family education

- Teach patient that drug must be continued for prescribed time to be effective
- Instruct patient to take with food, milk, or antacids to avoid GI upset
- Advise patient to use caution when driving; drowsiness, dizziness may occur
- Advise patient to take with a full glass of water to enhance absorption
- Advise patient to avoid pregnancy while taking this drug
- Inform patient that hair may be lost, review alternatives
- Advise patient to avoid live virus vaccinations during treatment

Evaluation

Positive therapeutic outcome

- Increased joint mobility without pain
- Decreased joint swelling

HIGH ALERT

lepirudin (℞)

(lep-ih-roo′din)
Refludan
Func. class.: Anticoagulant
Chem. class.: Hirudin

Pregnancy category B

Action Direct inhibitor of thrombin that is highly specific

➡ **Therapeutic Outcome:** Absence of thrombocytopenia, stroke, MI, or other thromboembolic conditions

Uses: Heparin-induced thrombocytopenia and other thromboembolic conditions

Dosage and routes

Adult: **IV** 0.4 mg/kg (≤110 kg) over 15-20 sec; then 0.15 mg/kg (≤110 kg/hr) as a cont inf for 2-10 days or longer

Available forms: Powder for inj 50 mg

Adverse effects

CNS: *Fever*
CV: **Heart failure, pericardial effusion, ventricular fibrillation**
GI: GI bleeding, abnormal LFTs
GU: **Hematuria,** abnormal kidney function
HEMA: **Hemorrhage, thrombocytopenia**
INTEG: Allergic skin reactions
RESP: Pneumonia
SYST: **Multiorgan failure, sepsis**

Contraindications: Hypersensitivity to hirudins

Precautions: Intracranial bleeding, renal function impairment, lactation, P children, hepatic disease, pregnancy **B**

Pharmacokinetics

Absorption	Unknown
Distribution	Unknown
Metabolism	Possibly by the release of amino acids during catabolism
Excretion	50% unchanged in urine
Half-life	Unknown

Pharmacodynamics

Onset	Unknown
Peak	Unknown
Duration	Unknown

Interactions

Drug classifications

Thrombolytics: ↑ action of lepirudin
Warfarin derivatives: ↑ risk of bleeding

NURSING CONSIDERATIONS

Assessment

- Obtain baseline APTT before treatment; do not start treatment if APTT ratio is ≥2.5, then APTT 4 hr after initiation of treatment and at least qd thereafter; if APTT is above target, stop infusion for 2 hr, then restart at 50%, take APTT in 4 hr; if below target, increase inf rate by 20%, take APTT in 4 hr, do not exceed inf rate of 0.21 mg/kg/hr without checking for coagulation abnormalities
- Monitor APTT, which should be 1.5-2.5 × control
- Assess bleeding gums, petechiae, ecchymosis, black tarry stools, hematuria/epistaxis, B/P, vaginal bleeding, puncture sites; may indicate bleeding and possible hemorrhage
- Assess fever, skin rash, urticaria

Nursing diagnoses

✓ Tissue perfusion, altered (uses)
✓ Injury, risk for (side effects)
✓ Knowledge deficits (teaching)

Implementation

- Administer after reconstitution and further dilution under sterile conditions; use water for inj or 0.9% NaCl; for further dilution 0.9% NaCl or D_5; for rapid and complete reconstitution, inject 1 ml of diluent into vial and shake gently, use immediately, warm to room temp before use
- Avoid all IM injections that may cause bleeding

IV IV route

- Administer **IV** bol: use sol with conc of 5 mg/ml, reconstitute 5 mg (1 vial)/1 ml of water for inj or 0.9% NaCl, use body weight for correct weight calculation
- Administer **IV** inf: use sol with a conc of 0.2 or 0.4 mg/ml; reconstitute 100 mg (2 vials) with 1 ml each (2 ml) water for inj or 0.9% NaCl, transfer to infusion bag with either 500 or 250 ml of 0.9% NaCl or D_5

Patient/family education

- Teach patient to use softbristle toothbrush to avoid bleeding gums, avoid contact sports, use electric razor, avoid IM injection

L

• Teach patient to report any signs of bleeding: gums, under skin, urine, stools

Evaluation

Positive therapeutic outcome

• Absence of thrombocytopenia without significant bleeding

letrozole (℞)

(let'tro-zohl)

Femara

Func. class.: Antineoplastic, nonsteroidal aromatase inhibitor

Pregnancy category D

Action: Binds to the heme group of aromatase; inhibits conversion of androgens to estrogens to reduce plasma estrogen levels; 30% of breast cancers decrease in size when deprived of estrogen

Therapeutic Outcome: Decreased spread of malignancy

Uses: Metastatic breast cancer in postmenopausal women

Dosage and routes

Adult: PO 2.5 mg qd

Available forms: Tabs 2.5 mg

Adverse effects

CNS: Somnolence, dizziness, depression, anxiety, *headache, lethargy*

CV: Hypertension

GI: *Nausea, vomiting, anorexia,* **hepatotoxicity,** constipation, heartburn, diarrhea

INTEG: *Rash, pruritus,* alopecia, sweating, hot flashes

RESP: Dyspnea, cough

Contraindications: Hypersensitivity, pregnancy **D**

Precautions: Hepatic disease, respiratory disease

Pharmacokinetics

Absorption	Well absorbed
Distribution	Widely
Metabolism	Liver
Excretion	Kidneys
Half-life	Unknown

Pharmacodynamics

Unknown

NURSING CONSIDERATIONS

Assessment

• Monitor temperature q4h; may indicate beginning of infection

• Monitor liver function tests before, during therapy (bilirubin, AST, ALT, LDH) as needed or monthly

• Monitor inflammation of mucosa, breaks in skin, yellowing of skin and sclera, dark urine, clay-colored stools, itchy skin, abdominal pain, fever, diarrhea

Nursing diagnoses

☑ Injury, risk for (adverse reactions)

☑ Body image disturbance (adverse reactions)

☑ Infection, risk for (adverse reactions)

☑ Knowledge deficit (teaching)

Implementation

• Give with food or fluids for GI upset

• Give in equal intervals q6h

Patient/family education

• Instruct patient to report side effects

• Advise patient to avoid use of alcohol, which potentiates this drug

• Tell patient that drug may be taken without regard to meals

Evaluation

Positive therapeutic outcome

• Prevention of rapid division of malignant cells, postmenopausal cancer, prostate cancer

Treatment of overdose:

Induce vomiting, provide supportive care

leucovorin (℞)

(loo-koe-vor'in)

Citrovorum Factor, Folinic Acid, leucovorin calcium, Wellcovorin

Func. class.: Vitamin/folic acid antagonist antidote

Chem. class.: Tetrahydrofolic acid derivative

Pregnancy category C

Action: Needed for normal growth patterns; prevents toxicity during antineoplastic therapy by protecting normal cells

➔ **Therapeutic Outcome:** Reversal of severe toxic effects of folic acid antagonists

Uses: Megaloblastic or macrocytic anemia caused by folic acid deficiency, overdose of folic acid antagonist, methotrexate toxicity, toxicity caused by pyrimethamine or trimethoprim, pneumocystosis, toxoplasmosis

Dosage and routes

Megaloblastic anemia caused by enzyme deficiency

P ***Adult and child:*** PO/IM/**IV** up to 16 mg/day

Megaloblastic anemia caused by deficiency of folate

P ***Adult and child:*** IM 1 mg or less qd until adequate response

Advanced colorectal cancer

Adult: **IV** 200 mg/m^2, then 5-fluorouracil 370 mg/m^2; or leucovorin 20 mg/m^2, then 5-fluorouracil 425 mg/m^2; give qd × 5 days q4-5 wk

Methotrexate toxicity

P ***Adult and child:*** PO/IM/**IV** (normal elimination) given 6-36 hr after dose of methotrexate 10 mg/m^2 until methotrexate is <10 M, CrCl has increased 50% above prior level or methotrexate level is 5 × 10 at 24 hr, or at 48 hr level is >9 × 10 M, give leucovorin 100 mg/m^2 q3h until level drops to <10 M

Pyrimethamine toxicity

P ***Adult and child:*** PO/IM 5-15 mg qd

Trimethoprim toxicity

P ***Adult and child:*** PO/IM 400 μg qd

Available forms: Tabs 5, 10, 15, 25 mg; inj 3, 5 mg/ml; powder for inj 10 mg/ml

Adverse effects

HEMA: Thrombocytosis (intraarterial)

INTEG: Rash, pruritus, erythema, thrombocytosis, urticaria

RESP: Wheezing

Contraindications: Hypersensitivity, anemias other than megaloblastic not associated with vit B_{12} deficiency

Precautions: Pregnancy **C**

Do Not Confuse: leucovorin/Leukeran, leucovorin/Leukine

Pharmacokinetics	
Absorption	Rapidly absorbed (PO); completely absorbed (**IV**)
Distribution	Widely distributed
Metabolism	Liver
Excretion	Kidney
Half-life	3½ hr

Pharmacodynamics	PO/IM/IV
Onset	Up to 5 min
Peak	Unknown
Duration	4-6 hr

Interactions

Individual drugs

Chloramphenicol: ↓ folate levels

Phenobarbital: ↑ metabolism of phenobarbital, ↓ effect

L

Drug classifications

Hydantoins: ↑ metabolism of hydantoins, ↓ effect

NURSING CONSIDERATIONS

Assessment

- Obtain CrCl before leucovorin rescue and qd to detect nephrotoxicity
- Monitor I&O; watch for nausea and vomiting; if vomiting occurs IM or **IV** route may be necessary
- Assess diet for inclusion of bran, yeast, dried beans, nuts, fruits, fresh vegetables, asparagus, which have high folic acid levels
- Assess drugs currently taken: alcohol, hydantoins, trimethoprim may cause increased folic acid use by body
- Assess for allergic reactions: rash, dyspnea, wheezing

Nursing diagnoses

- ✓ Injury, risk for (uses)
- ✓ Nutrition, altered: less than body requirements (uses)
- ✓ Knowledge deficit (teaching)

Implementation

PO route

- Use PO route only if patient is not vomiting

IM route

- Give within 1 hr of folic acid antagonist, no reconstitution needed
- Give increased fluid intake if used to treat folic acid inhibitor overdose
- Provide protection from light and heat when storing ampules

IV **IV route**

- Reconstitute 50 mg/5 ml of bacteriostatic water or sterile water for inj (10 mg/ml) or 100 mg/10 ml; use immediately if sterile water for inj is used to reconstitute
- Give by direct **IV** over 160 mg/min or less (16 ml of 10 mg/ml sol/min)
- Give by intermittent inf after diluting in 100-500 ml of 0.9% NaCl, D_5W, $D_{10}W$, LR, Ringer's

Syringe compatibilities:

Bleomycin, cisplatin, cyclophosphamide, doxorubicin, fluorouracil, furosemide, heparin, methotrexate, metoclopramide, mitomycin, vinblastine, vincristine

Y-site compatibilities:

Amifostine, aztreonam, bleomycin, cefepime, cisplatin, cladribine, cyclophosphamide, doxorubicin, filgrastim, fluconazole, fluorouracil, furosemide, granisetron, heparin, methotrexate, metoclopramide, mitomycin, piperacillin/tazobactam, tacrolimus, teniposide, thiotepa, vinblastine, vincristine

Additive compatibilities:

Cisplatin, cisplatin/floxuridine, floxuridine

Patient/family education

- Advise patient to take drug exactly as prescribed; to notify prescriber of side effects immediately
- Advise patient to report signs of hypersensitivity reaction immediately
- Instruct patient about leucovorin rescue; have patient drink 3 L of fluid each day of rescue
- Advise patient with folic acid deficiency to eat folic acid–rich foods: bran, yeast, dried beans, nuts, fruits, fresh green leafy vegetables, asparagus

Evaluation

Positive therapeutic outcome

- Increased weight
- Improved orientation, well-being
- Absence of fatigue

HIGH ALERT

leuprolide (℞)
(loo-proe'lide)

Leupron Depo Ped, Lupron Depot, Lupron, Lupron Depot-3 month, Viadur

Func. class.: Antineoplastic hormone

Chem. class.: Gonadotropin-releasing hormone

Pregnancy category X (depot)

Action: Causes initial increase in circulating levels of LH, FSH; continuous administration results in decreased LH, FSH; in men testosterone is reduced to castration levels; in premenopausal women estrogen is reduced to menopausal levels

➔ **Therapeutic Outcome:** Prevention of rapidly growing malignant cells in prostate cancer, decreased pain in endometriosis, resolution of central precocious puberty (CPP)

Uses: Metastatic prostate cancer, management of endometriosis (depot), CPP

Dosage and routes
Prostate cancer

Adult: SC 1 mg/day; IM 7.5 mg/dose qmo, Viadur implant qyr

Endometriosis

Adult: IM 3.5 mg once a month or 11.25 mg q3 mo

Central precocious puberty

P ***Child:*** SC 50 µg/kg/day; increase as needed by 10 µg/kg/day

P ***Child:*** >37.5 kg: IM 15 mg q4 wk
25-37.5 kg: IM 11.25 mg q4 wk
≤25 kg: 7.5 mg q4 wk

Available forms: Inj (depot) 3.75, 7.5 mg single-dose, multiple-dose vials (5 mg/ml); single-use kit 11.25 mg vial; pediatric depot 7.5, 11.25, 15 mg; 3 mo depot 22.5 mg single use; Viadur once/yr implant

Adverse effects
CV: **MI, pulmonary emboli, dysrhythmias**

GI: Anorexia, diarrhea, **GI bleeding**

GU: Edema, hot flashes, impotence, decreased libido, amenorrhea, vaginal dryness, gynecomastia

Contraindications: Hypersensitivity to GnRH or analogs, thromboembolic disorders, pregnancy **X,** lactation, undiagnosed vaginal bleeding

Precautions: Edema, hepatic disease, CVA, MI, seizures, hypertension, diabetes mellitus

Do Not Confuse:
Lupron/Lopurin, Lupron/Nuprin

Pharmacokinetics

Absorption	Rapidly absorbed (SC); slowly absorbed (IM depot)
Distribution	Unknown
Metabolism	Unknown
Excretion	Unknown
Half-life	3-4 hr

Pharmacodynamics
Unknown

Interactions
Individual drugs

Flutamide: ↑ antineoplastic action
Megestrol: ↑ antineoplastic action

NURSING CONSIDERATIONS
Assessment
- Assess for symptoms of endometriosis/fibroids including lower abdominal pain if drug is given for the diagnosis of endometriosis
- If giving this drug for CPP, the diagnosis should have been confirmed by development of secondary sex P characteristics in child <9 yr; also included to confirm the diagnosis of CPP is estradiol/testosterone, GnRH test, tomography of head, adrenal steroid, chorionic gonadotropin, wrist

x-ray, height, weight; patients diagnosed with CPP display the signs of testicular growth, facial, body hair (males), breast development, menses (females)

- Monitor liver function tests before, during therapy (bilirubin, AST, ALT, LDH) as needed or monthly; prostate-specific antigen in prostate cancer
- Monitor pituitary gonadotropic and gonadal function during therapy and 4-8 wk after therapy is decreased; check LH, FSH, acid phosphate at beginning of treatment
- Monitor worsening of signs and symptoms (normal during beginning therapy): fatigue, increased pulse, pallor, lethargy, edema in feet, joints, stomach pain, shaking
- Monitor renal status: I&O ratio, check for bladder distention daily during beginning therapy (renal obstruction)

Nursing diagnoses

- ✓ Sexual dysfunction (adverse reactions)
- ✓ Injury, risk for (adverse reactions)
- ✓ Knowledge deficit (teaching)

Implementation

- Use syringe and drug packaged together; give deep in large muscle mass; rotate sites
- Use depot only IM; never give SC
- Reconstitute vial (single dose)/1 ml of diluent; shake (appearance should be white); withdraw and use immediately
- Unused vials may be stored at room temp

Patient/family education

- Advise patient to notify prescriber if menstruation continues; menstruation should stop; to use a nonhormonal method of contraception during therapy
- Instruct patient to report any complaints, side effects to nurse or prescriber; hot flashes may occur; record weight, report gain of 2 lb/day
- Teach patient how to prepare, administer; to rotate sites for SC inj; to keep accurate records of dosing (prostate cancer)
- Instruct patient that tumor flare may occur: increase in size of tumor, increased bone pain; tell patient that bone pain disappears after 1 wk; may take analgesics for pain; premenopausal women must use mechanical birth control; ovulation may be induced

Evaluation

Positive therapeutic outcome

- Decreased size, spread of malignancy
- Decreased pain in endometriosis
- Decreased signs of CPP

levalbuterol (℞)

(lev-al-bute'er-ole)

Xopenex

Func. class.: Bronchodilator

Chem. class.: Adrenergic β_2-agonist

Pregnancy category C

Action: Causes bronchodilatation by action on β_2 (pulmonary) receptors by increasing levels of cyclic adenosine monophosphate (cAMP), which relaxes smooth muscle; produces bronchodilatation; CNS, cardiac stimulation, increased diuresis, and increased gastric acid secretion; longer acting than isoproterenol

➔ **Therapeutic Outcome:** Increased ability to breathe because of bronchodilatation

Uses: Treatment or prevention of bronchospasm (reversible obstructive airway disease)

Dosage and routes

P ***Adult and child ≥12 yr:*** INH 0.63 mg tid, q6-8h by nebulization; may increase to 1.25 mg q8h

Available forms: Sol, inh 0.63, 1.25 mg/3 ml

Adverse effects

CNS: *Tremors, anxiety,* insomnia,

headache, dizziness, stimulation, *restlessness,* hallucinations, flushing, irritability
CV: Palpitations, tachycardia, hypertension, angina, hypotension, dysrhythmias
EENT: Dry nose, irritation of nose and throat
GI: Heartburn, nausea, vomiting
MS: Muscle cramps

Contraindications: Hypersensitivity to sympathomimetics, tachydysrhythmias, severe cardiac disease

Precautions: Lactation, pregnancy **C,** cardiac disorders, hyperthyroidism, diabetes mellitus, hypertension, prostatic hypertrophy, narrow-angle glaucoma, seizures

Pharmacokinetics

Absorption	Unknown
Distribution	Unknown
Metabolism	Liver extensively, tissues
Excretion	Unknown, breast milk
Half-life	Unknown

Pharmacodynamics

	INH
Onset	5-15 min
Peak	1-1½ hr
Duration	6-8 hr

Interactions
Drug classifications
β-Adrenergic blockers: Block therapeutic effect
Bronchodilators, aerosol: ↑ action of bronchodilator
MAOIs: ↑ chance of hypertensive crisis
Sympathomimetics: ↑ adrenergic side effects

NURSING CONSIDERATIONS
Assessment
- Assess respiratory function: vital capacity, forced expiratory volume, ABGs, lung sounds, heart rate, rhythm (baseline and during therapy)
- Determine that patient has not received theophylline therapy before giving dose, to prevent additive effect; client's ability to self-medicate
- Monitor for evidence of allergic reactions; paradoxic bronchospasm; withhold dose; notify prescriber

Nursing diagnoses
✓ Airway clearance, ineffective (uses)
✓ Impaired gas exchange (uses)
✓ Knowledge deficit (teaching)

Implementation
- Give by nebulization q6 8h

Patient/family education
- Tell patient not to use OTC medications before consulting prescriber; extra stimulation may occur; instruct patient to use this medication before other medications and allow at least 5 min between each to prevent overstimulation; to limit caffeine products such as chocolate, coffee, tea, and cola
- ❗ Teach patient that if paradoxic bronchospasm occurs to stop drug immediately and notify prescriber

Evaluation
Positive therapeutic outcome
- Absence of dyspnea and wheezing after 1 hr
- Improved airway exchange
- Improved ABGs

Treatment of overdose: Administer a β_1-adrenergic blocker

levetiracetam (℞)
(lev-ee-tye'ra-see-tam)
Keppra
Func. class.: Anticonvulsant
Pregnancy category C

Action: Inhibits nerve impulses by limiting influx of sodium ions across cell membrane in motor cortex

➡ **Therapeutic Outcome:** Absence of seizures

Uses: Partial onset seizures

Dosage and routes
Adult: PO 500 mg bid

Available forms: Tabs 250, 500, 750 mg

Adverse effects
CNS: Dizziness, somnolence, asthenia
HEMA: Decreased Hct, Hgb, infection

Contraindications: Hypersensitivity

Precautions: Hepatic disease, renal disease, cardiac disease, pregnancy **C,** lactation, P children

Pharmacokinetics

Absorption	Rapidly absorbed
Distribution	Widely distributed, not protein bound
Metabolism	Small amount liver
Excretion	Kidneys (66%) unchanged
G **Half-life**	6-8 hr or more in elderly

Pharmacodynamics
Unknown

Interactions
None known

NURSING CONSIDERATIONS
Assessment
- Monitor liver function tests (AST, ALT) and urine function tests (BUN, urine protein) periodically during treatments
- Assess seizure activity including type, location, duration, and character; provide seizure precautions

Nursing diagnoses
✓ Injury, risk for (side effects)
✓ Knowledge deficit (teaching)

Implementation
- Give with food for GI symptoms

Patient/family education
- Teach patient to carry ID stating patient's name, drugs taken, condition, prescriber's name, phone number
- Caution patient to avoid driving, other activities that require alertness until stabilized on medication
- Teach patient not to discontinue medication quickly after long-term use
- Teach patient to use a nonhormonal type of contraception to prevent harm to the fetus
- Teach patient to take exactly as prescribed, do not double or omit doses

Evaluation
Positive therapeutic outcome
- Decreased seizure activity

levobupivacaine (℞)
(lee-voh-bu-piv'ah-kane)
Chirocaine
Func. class.: Local anesthetic
Chem. class.: Amide

Pregnancy category B

Action: Competes with calcium for sites in nerve membrane that control sodium transport across cell membrane; decreases rise of depolarization phase of action potential

➔ **Therapeutic Outcome:** Anesthesia, decreased pain

Uses: Local, regional anesthesia, surgical anesthesia, pain management, continuous epidural analgesia

Dosage and routes
Varies with route of anesthesia

Available forms: Inj 2.5, 5, 7.5 mg/ml

Adverse effects
CNS: Anxiety, restlessness, **seizures, loss of consciousness,** drowsiness, disorientation, tremors, shivering
CV: **Myocardial depression, cardiac arrest, dysrhythmias,** bradycardia, hypotension, hypertension, **fetal bradycardia**
EENT: Blurred vision, tinnitus, pupil constriction
GI: Nausea, vomiting

INTEG: Rash, urticaria, allergic reactions, edema, burning, skin discoloration at injection site, tissue necrosis
RESP: **Status asthmaticus, respiratory arrest, anaphylaxis**

Contraindications: Hypersensitivity, P child <12 yr, G elderly, severe liver disease

Precautions: Severe drug allergies, pregnancy **B**

Pharmacokinetics	
Absorption	Unknown
Distribution	Unknown
Metabolism	Liver
Excretion	Urine (metabolites)
Half-life	Unknown

Pharmacodynamics	
Onset	2-8 min
Peak	Unknown
Duration	3-6 hr

Interactions
Drug classifications
Anesthetics, halothane: ↑ dysrhythmias
Antidepressants, tricyclics: ↑ hypertension
MAOIs: ↑ hypertension
Phenothiazines: ↑ hypertension

NURSING CONSIDERATIONS
Assessment
- Monitor B/P, pulse, respiration during treatment
- Monitor fetal heart tones during labor
- Monitor allergic reactions: rash, urticaria, itching
- Monitor cardiac status: ECG for dysrhythmias, pulse, B/P during anesthesia

Nursing diagnoses
✓ Pain, (uses)
✓ Knowledge deficit (teaching)

Implementation
- Administer only with crash cart, resuscitative equipment nearby
- Administer only drugs without preservatives for epidural or caudal anesthesia
- Discard unused portions

Evaluation
Positive therapeutic outcome
- Anesthesia necessary for procedure

Treatment of overdose: Airway, O_2, vasopressor, **IV** fluids, anticonvulsants for seizures

levodopa (℞)
(lee'voe-doe-pa)
Dopar, Larodopa, L-Dopa
Func. class.: Antiparkinsonian agent
Chem. class.: Catecholamine, dopamine agonist

Pregnancy category C

Action: Decarboxylation to dopamine, which increases dopamine levels in brain

Therapeutic Outcome: Decreased symptoms of Parkinson's disease (involuntary movements)

Uses: Parkinsonism

Dosage and routes
Adult: PO 0.5-1 g qd divided bid-qid with meals; may increase by up to 0.75 g q3-7 days, max 8 g/day unless closely supervised

Available forms: Caps 100, 250, 500 mg; tabs 100, 250, 500 mg

Adverse effects
CNS: *Involuntary choreiform movements, hand tremors, fatigue, headache, anxiety, twitching, numbness, weakness, confusion, agitation, insomnia, nightmares,* psychosis, hallucinations, hypomania, severe depression, dizziness
CV: *Orthostatic hypotension,* tachycardia, hypertension, palpitations

EENT: Blurred vision, diplopia, dilated pupils
GI: *Nausea, vomiting, anorexia, abdominal distress, dry mouth, flatulence, dysphagia,* bitter taste, diarrhea, constipation
HEMA: **Hemolytic anemia, leukopenia, agranulocytosis**
INTEG: Rash, sweating, alopecia
MISC: Urinary retention, incontinence, weight change, dark urine

Contraindications: Hypersensitivity, narrow-angle glaucoma, undiagnosed skin lesions

Precautions: Renal disease, cardiac disease, hepatic disease, respiratory disease, MI with dysrhythmias, convulsions, peptic ulcer, pregnancy **C**, asthma, endocrine disease, affective disorders, psychosis, lactation, children <12 yr peptic ulcer

Do Not Confuse:
L-dopa/methyldopa

Pharmacokinetics

Absorption	Well absorbed
Distribution	Widely distributed
Metabolism	Liver, GI tract, extensively
Excretion	Kidneys to metabolites; breast milk
Half-life	1 hr

Pharmacodynamics

Onset	10-15 min
Peak	1-3 hr
Duration	Up to 24 hr

Interactions
Individual drugs
Haloperidol: ↓ effects of levodopa
Methyldopa: ↑ CNS toxicity
Papaverine: ↓ effects of levodopa
Phenytoin: ↓ effects of levodopa
Pyridoxine: ↓ effects of levodopa
Reserpine: ↓ effects of levodopa
Selegiline: ↑ adverse reaction
Drug classifications
Anticholinergics: ↓ effects of levodopa
Antihypertensives: ↑ hypotension
Hydantoins: ↓ effects of levodopa
MAOIs: Hypertensive crisis
Herb/drug
Kava: ↑ parkinson's symptoms
Food/drug
↑ Pyridoxine will ↓ levodopa effect, ↑ protein food will ↓ absorption
Lab test interferences
↓ VMA
False positive: Urine ketones, urine glucose, Coombs' test, urine, norepinephrine
False negative: Urine glucose (glucose oxidase)
False: ↑ uric acid, ↑ urine protein

NURSING CONSIDERATIONS
Assessment
- Monitor B/P, respiration during initial treatment; hypotension or hypertension should be reported
- Assess mental status: affect, mood, behavioral changes, depression; complete suicide assessment
- Monitor liver function, renal function studies: AST, ALT, alkaline phosphatase; also check LDH, bilirubin, CBC, BUN, PBI
- Assess for involuntary movements in parkinsonism: akinesia, tremors, staggering gait, muscle rigidity, drooling; these symptoms should improve with levodopa therapy
- Assess for levodopa toxicity: mental, personality changes, increased twitching, grimacing, tongue protrusion; these should be reported to prescriber

Nursing diagnoses
- Mobility, impaired (uses)
- Injury, risk for (uses)
- Knowledge deficit (teaching)
- Noncompliance (teaching)

Implementation
- Levodopa/carbidopa should not be started until this drug is withheld for 8 hr; toxicity may result if the two drugs are taken close together
- Give levodopa until NPO before surgery
- Adjust dosage to patient response

• Give with meals to decrease GI upset; limit protein taken with drug
• Give only after MAOIs have been discontinued for 2 wk

Patient/family education

• Advise patient that therapeutic effects may take several wk to a few mo
• Caution patient to change positions slowly to prevent orthostatic hypotension
• Instruct patient to report side effects: twitching, eye spasms; indicate overdose
• Instruct patient to use drug exactly as prescribed; if drug is discontinued abruptly, parkinsonian crisis may occur
• Inform patient that urine, sweat may darken
• Advise patient to avoid vit B_6 preparations, vitamin-fortified foods containing B_6; these foods can reverse effects of levodopa; also OTC preparations should be avoided unless approved by prescriber

Evaluation

Positive therapeutic outcome
• Decreased akathisia, other involuntary movements
• Improved mood

levofloxacin (℞)

(lev-o-floks'a-sin)
Levaquin
Func. class.: Antiinfective
Chem. class.: Fluoroquinolone antibacterial

Pregnancy category C

Action: Interferes with conversion of intermediate DNA fragments into high-molecular- weight DNA in bacteria; DNA gyrase inhibitor

➡ **Therapeutic Outcome:** Bacterial action against the following: *Streptococcus pneumoniae, Haemophilus influenzae, Haemophilus parainfluenzae, Moraxella catarrhalis, Staphylococcus aureus, Klebsiella pneumonia, Mycoplasma pneumoniae*

Uses: Adult urinary tract infections (including complicated); lower respiratory, skin infection

Dosage and routes

Adult: **IV** inf 500 mg by slow inf over 1 hr q24h × 7-14 days depending on infection; PO 500 mg q24h × 7 days depending on infection

Renal dose
CrCl 20-49 ml/min initial 500 mg, then 250 mg q24h; CrCl 10-19 ml/min 250 or 500 mg, depending on condition, then 250 mg q48h

Available forms: Single-use vials (500 mg), 25 mg/ml 20-ml vials, premixed flexible container; tabs 250, 500, 750 mg

Adverse effects:

CNS: *Headache,* dizziness, *insomnia,* anxiety, **seizures,** encephalopathy, paresthesia
CV: Chest pain, palpitations, vasodilation
GI: *Nausea,* flatulence, *vomiting,* diarrhea, abdominal pain, **pseudomembranous colitis**
GU: Vaginitis, crystalluria
HEMA: Eosinophilia, **hemolytic anemia**, lymphophemia
INTEG: Rash, pruritus, urticaria, photosensitivity, **Stevens-Johnson syndrome**
RESP: Pneumonitis

Contraindications: Hypersensitivity to quinolones

Precautions: Pregnancy **C,** lactation, children, renal disease [P]

Pharmacokinetics

Absorption	Unknown
Distribution	Unknown
Metabolism	Liver
Excretion	Kidneys unchanged
Half-life	6-8 hr

Pharmacodynamics	
Onset	Immediate
Peak	Infusion's end

Interactions
Individual drugs
Caffeine: ↑ toxicity
Calcium: ↓ absorption of levofloxacin
Cimetidine: ↑ effect of levofloxacin
Cyclosporine: ↑ nephrotoxicity
Digoxin: ↑ toxicity
Foscarnet: ↑ CNS stimulation, seizures
Iron: ↓ absorption of levofloxacin
Probenecid: ↑ effect of levofloxacin
Sucralfate: ↓ absorption of levofloxacin
Theophylline: ↓ theophylline clearance, ↑ toxicity
Warfarin: ↑ toxicity, bleeding
Zinc: ↓ absorption of levofloxacin
Drug classifications
Antacids: ↓ absorption of levofloxacin
Antidiabetics: Altered blood glucose levels
NSAIDs: ↑ CNS stimulation, seizures
Lab test interferences
↓ Glucose, ↓ lymphocytes

NURSING CONSIDERATIONS
Assessment
- Assess patient for previous sensitivity reaction
- Assess patient for signs and symptoms of infection including characteristics of wounds, sputum, urine, stool, WBC >10,000/mm^3, fever; baseline and during treatment
- Obtain C&S before beginning drug therapy to identify if correct treatment has been initiated
- Assess for allergic reactions and anaphylaxis: rash, urticaria, pruritus, chills, fever, joint pain; may occur a few days after therapy begins; epinephrine and resuscitation equipment should be available for anaphylactic reaction
- Determine urine output; if decreasing, notify prescriber (may indicate nephrotoxicity); also check for increased BUN, creatinine
- Monitor blood studies: AST, ALT, CBC, Hct, bilirubin, LDH, alkaline phosphatase, Coombs' test monthly if patient is on long-term therapy
- Monitor electrolytes: potassium, sodium, chloride monthly if patient is on long-term therapy
- Assess bowel pattern qd; if severe diarrhea occurs, drug should be discontinued
- Monitor for bleeding: ecchymosis, bleeding gums, hematuria, stool guaiac daily if on long-term therapy
- Assess for overgrowth of infection: perineal itching, fever, malaise, redness, pain, swelling, drainage, rash, diarrhea, change in cough, sputum

Nursing diagnoses
✓ Infection, risk for (uses)
✓ Diarrhea (side effects)
✓ Injury, risk for (side effects)
✓ Knowledge deficit (teaching)
✓ Noncompliance (teaching)

Implementation
- Give PO 4 hr before or 2 hr after antacids, iron, calcium, zinc
- Check for irritation, extravasation, phlebitis daily

Patient/family education
- Teach patient to report sore throat, bruising, bleeding, joint pain; may indicate blood dyscrasias (rare)
- Advise patient to contact prescriber if vaginal itching, loose foul-smelling stools, furry tongue occur, may indicate superinfection; report itching, rash, pruritus, urticaria
- Instruct patient to take all medication prescribed for the length of time ordered; drug must be taken around the clock to maintain blood levels; do not give medication to others
- Advise patient to notify prescriber of diarrhea with blood or pus
- Instruct patient to take 4 hr before antacids, iron, calcium, zinc products
- Tell patient to complete full course

of therapy; to increase fluid intake to 2 L/day to prevent crystalluria
- Advise patient to avoid hazardous activities until response to drug is known
- Instruct patient to rinse mouth frequently and use sugarless candy or gum for dry mouth
- Instruct patient to avoid taking other medications unless approved by prescriber
- Advise patient not to use theophylline with this product, as toxicity may result; to contact prescriber if taking theophylline
- Advise patient to avoid sun exposure or use sunscreen to prevent phototoxicity

Evaluation

Positive therapeutic outcome
- Absence of signs/symptoms of infection (WBC <10,000/mm^3, temp WNL)
- Reported improvement in symptoms of infection

levothyroxine (Rx)

(lee-voe-thye-rox'een)

Eltroxin ✤, Levo-T, Levothroid, levothyroxine sodium, Levoxyl, PMS-Levothyroxine Sodium ✤, Synthroid, T_4

Func. class.: Thyroid hormone

Chem. class.: Levoisomer of thyroxine

Pregnancy category A

Action: Controls protein synthesis; increases metabolic rate, cardiac output, renal blood flow, O_2 consumption, body temp, blood volume, growth, development at cellular level

Therapeutic Outcome: Correction of lack of thyroid hormone

Uses: Hypothyroidism, myxedema coma, thyroid hormone replacement, cretinism, thyrotoxicosis, congenital hypothyroidism, some types of thyroid cancer

Dosage and routes

Severe hypothyroidism

Adult: PO 50 μg qd, increased by 0.05-0.1 mg q1-4 wk until desired response; maintenance dosage 75-125 μg qd, IM/**IV** 50-100 μg/day as a single dose

P ***Child >12 yr:*** PO 2-3 μg/kg/day given as a single dose AM

P ***Child 6-12 yr:*** PO 4-5 μg/kg/day given as a single dose AM

P ***Child 1-5 yr:*** PO 5-6 μg/kg/day given as a single dose AM

P ***Child 6-12 mo:*** PO 6-8 μg/kg/day give as a single dose AM

P ***Child to 6 mo:*** PO 8-10 μg/kg/day given as a single dose AM

Myxedema coma

Adult: **IV** 200-500 μg; may increase by 100-300 μg after 24 hr; give oral medication as soon as possible; maintenance 50-100 μg/day

Available forms: Powder for inj 50, 200, 500 μg/vial; tabs 0.025, 0.05, 0.075, 0.088, 0.1, 0.112, 0.125, 0.137, 0.15, 0.175, 0.2, 0.3 mg

Adverse effects

CNS: Anxiety, insomnia, tremors, headache, **thyroid storm**

CV: Tachycardia, palpitations, angina, dysrhythmias, hypertension, **cardiac arrest**

GI: Nausea, diarrhea, increased or decreased appetite, cramps

MISC: Menstrual irregularities, weight loss, sweating, heat intolerance, fever

Contraindications: Adrenal insufficiency, MI, thyrotoxicosis, hypersensitivity to beef, alcohol intolerance (inj only), impaired renal function

G **Precautions:** Elderly, angina pectoris, hypertension, ischemia, cardiac disease, pregnancy **A,** lactation

Do Not Confuse:
Synthroid/Symmetrel

L

Pharmacokinetics

Absorption	Erratic (PO); complete (**IV**)
Distribution	Widely distributed
Metabolism	Liver; enterohepatic recirculation
Excretion	Feces via bile; breast milk (small amounts)
Half-life	6-7 days

Pharmacodynamics

	PO	IV
Onset	Unknown	6-8 hr
Peak	12-48 hr	12-48 hr
Duration	Unknown	Unknown

Interactions

Individual drugs

Cholestyramine: ↓ absorption of thyroid hormone
Colestipol: ↓ absorption of levothyroxine
Digitalis: ↓ effect of digitalis
Insulin: ↑ requirement for insulin
Phenytoin (IV): ↑ release of thyroid hormone

Drug classifications

Amphetamines: ↑ CNS, cardiac stimulation
β-Adrenergic blockers: ↓ effect of β-blockers
Decongestants: ↑ CNS, cardiac stimulation
Oral anticoagulants: ↑ requirements for anticoagulants
Vasopressors: ↑ CNS, cardiac stimulation

Herb/drug

Bugleweed: Do not give together

Lab test interferences

↑ CPK, ↑ LDH, ↑ AST, ↑ PBI, ↑ blood glucose
↓ Thyroid function tests

NURSING CONSIDERATIONS

Assessment

- Determine if the patient is taking anticoagulants, antidiabetic agents; document on chart
- Take B/P, pulse before each dose; monitor I&O ratio and weight every day in same clothing, using same scale, at same time of day
- Monitor height, weight, psychomotor development and growth rate if given to a child (P)
- Monitor T_3, T_4, FTIs, which are decreased; radioimmunoassay of TSH, which is increased; radioactive iodine uptake (RAIU), which is increased if patient is on too low a dosage of medication
- Monitor pro-time (may require decreased anticoagulant); check for bleeding, bruising
- Assess for increased nervousness, excitability, irritability, which may indicate too high a dosage of medication, usually after 1-3 wk of treatment
- Assess cardiac status: angina, palpitations, chest pain, change in VS; (G) the elderly patient may have undetected cardiac problems and baseline ECG should be completed before treatment

Nursing diagnoses

✓ Knowledge deficit (teaching)
✓ Noncompliance (teaching)

Implementation

PO route

- Give in AM if possible as a single dose to decrease sleeplessness; give at same time each day to maintain drug level
- Give crushed and mixed with water, non-soy formula, or breast milk for (P) infants/children
- Give only for hormone imbalances; not to be used for obesity, male infertility, menstrual conditions, lethargy; give lowest dosage that relieves symptoms; lower dosage for (G) the elderly and in cardiac diseases
- Store in tight, light-resistant container
- Remove medication 4 wk before RAIU test

IV route

- Give **IV** after diluting with provided diluent (0.9% NaCl), 0.5 mg/5 ml; shake well; give through Y-tube or

3-way stopcock; give 0.1 mg or less over 1 min; do not add to **IV** inf; 0.1 mg = 1 ml; discard any unused portion

Patient/family education

- Teach patient that drug is not a cure but controls symptoms and treatment is long term
- Instruct patient to report excitability, irritability, anxiety, sweating, heat intolerance, chest pain, palpitations, which indicate overdose
- Advise patient not to switch brands unless approved by prescriber; bioavailability may differ; do not take with food; absorption will be decreased
- Teach patient that drug may be discontinued after giving birth; thyroid panel will be evaluated after 1-2 mo
- Teach patient or parent that hyperthyroid child will show almost immediate behavior/personality change; that hair loss will occur in child but is temporary
- Caution patient that drug is not to be taken to reduce weight
- Caution patient to avoid OTC preparations with iodine; read labels; other medications should not be used unless approved by prescriber
- Teach patient to avoid iodine-rich food: iodized salt, soybeans, tofu, turnips, some seafood, some bread

Evaluation

Positive therapeutic outcome

- Absence of depression
- Weight loss, increased diuresis, pulse, appetite
- Absence of constipation, peripheral edema, cold intolerance, pale, cool dry skin, brittle nails, alopecia, coarse hair, menorrhagia, night blindness, paresthesias, syncope, stupor, coma, rosy cheeks
- Improved levels of T_3, T_4 by laboratory tests
- P Child: age-appropriate weight, height and psychomotor development

Treatment of overdose: Withhold dose for up to 1 wk: acute overdose: gastric lavage or induced emesis, activated charcoal; provide supportive treatment to control symptoms

---

HIGH ALERT

lidocaine, parenteral

(Rx)

(lye'doe-kane)

Lidopen Auto-Injector, Xylocard ✤

Func. class.: Antidysrhythmic (class IB)

Chem. class.: Aminoacyl amide

Pregnancy category B

Action: Increases electrical stimulation threshold of ventricle and His-Purkinje system, which stabilizes cardiac membrane and decreases automaticity; locally produces anesthesia by preventing initiation and conduction of nerve impulses

Therapeutic Outcome: Decreased ventricular dysrhythmia; produces anesthesia locally

Uses: Ventricular tachycardia, ventricular dysrhythmias during cardiac surgery, MI, digitalis toxicity, cardiac catheterization; anesthesia locally

Dosage and routes

Adult: **IV** bol 50-100 mg (1 mg/kg) over 2-3 min; repeat q3-5 min, max 300 mg in 1 hr; begin **IV** inf 20-50 μg/kg/min; IM 200-300 mg (4.3 mg/kg) in deltoid muscle, may repeat in 1-1½ hr if needed

G ***Elderly with CHF, reduced liver function:*** **IV** bol ½ adult dose

P ***Child:*** **IV** bol 1 mg/kg, then **IV** inf 30 μg/kg/min

P ***Adult and child:*** TOP apply as needed to affected areas

Available forms: **IV** inf 0.2% (2 mg/ml), 0.4% (4 mg/ml), 0.8% (8

mg/ml); **IV** admixture 4% (40 mg/ml), 10% (100 mg/ml), 20% (200 mg/ml); **IV** direct 1% (10 mg/ml), 2% (20 mg/ml); IM 300 mg/3 ml; ointment (top) 2.5, 5%; cream (top) 0.5%; spray 10%; jelly 2%; viscous sol 2%; local infiltrative inj 0.5, 1%

Adverse effects

CNS: Headache, dizziness, involuntary movement, confusion, tremor, *drowsiness,* euphoria, **seizures**

CV: Hypotension, bradycardia, **heart block, cardiovascular collapse, arrest**

EENT: Tinnitus, blurred vision

GI: Nausea, vomiting, anorexia

INTEG: Rash, urticaria, edema, swelling, burning, stinging

MISC: Febrile response, phlebitis at inj site

Contraindications: Hypersensitivity to amides, severe heart block, supraventricular dysrhythmias, Adams-Stokes syndrome, Wolff-Parkinson-White syndrome

Precautions: Pregnancy **B**, lactation, children, renal disease, liver disease, CHF, respiratory depression, malignant hyperthermia

P

Pharmacokinetics

Absorption	Complete bioavailability (**IV**)
Distribution	Erythrocytes, cardiovascular endothelium
Metabolism	Liver
Excretion	Kidneys
Half-life	Biphasic 8 min, 1-2 hr

Pharmacodynamics

	IV	IM	TOP
Onset	2 min	5-15 min	Unknown
Peak	Unknown	½ hr	5 min
Duration	20 min	1½ hr	½-1 hr

Interactions

Individual drugs

Cimetidine: ↓ metabolism, ↑ toxicity
Phenytoin: ↑ toxicity
Procainamide: ↑ toxicity
Propranolol: ↑ toxicity
Quinidine: ↑ toxicity

Drug classifications

β-Adrenergic blockers: ↑ toxicity

Herb/drug

Aloe: ↑ action of lidocaine
Buckthorn: ↑ action of lidocaine
Cascara sagrada: ↑ action of lidocaine
Senna: ↑ action of lidocaine

Lab test interferences

↑ LFTs

NURSING CONSIDERATIONS

Assessment

- Assess for oxygenation or perfusion deficit: decreased B/P, chest pain, dizziness, loss of consciousness
- Assess respiratory status: auscultate lung fields for bibasilar crackles in patients with advanced CHF
- Assess for urinary retention: check for pain, abdominal absorption, palpate bladder; check males with benign prostatic hypertrophy; anticholinergic reaction may cause retention
- Monitor I&O ratio, electrolytes (potassium, sodium, chloride); watch for decreasing urinary output, possible retention
- Monitor liver function studies: AST, ALT, bilirubin, alkaline phosphatase
- Monitor ECG continuously to determine drug effectiveness, measure PR, QRS, QT intervals, check for PVCs, other dysrhythmias; monitor B/P continuously for hypotension, hypertension; check for rebound hypertension after 1-2 hr, prolonged PR/QT intervals, QRS complex; if QT or QRS increases by 50% or more, withhold next dose, notify prescriber
- Monitor for CNS symptoms: confusion, numbness, depression, involuntary movements; if these occur, drug should be discontinued
- Monitor blood levels (therapeutic level 1.5-5 μg/ml), notify prescriber of abnormal results

Nursing diagnoses

✓ Cardiac output, decreased (uses)
✓ Impaired gas exchange (adverse reactions)
✓ Knowledge deficit (teaching)

Implementation

IM route

- Administer in deltoid, aspirate to prevent **IV** administration
- Check site daily for extravasation

IV **IV route**

- Give **IV** bolus undiluted (1%, 2% only); give 6 mg or less over 1 min; if using an **IV** line, use port near insertion site, flush with 0.9% NaCl (50 ml)
- Store at room temp; sol should be clear
- Give by cont inf after adding 1 g/250-1000 ml of D_5W; give 1-4 mg/min; use infusion pump for P correct dosage; pediatric inf is 120 mg of lidocaine/100 ml of D_5W; 1-2.5 ml/kg/hr = 20-50 μg/kg/min; use only 1%, 2% sol

Solution compatibilities:

D_5W, D_5/0.9% NaCl, D_5/0.45% NaCl, D_5/LR, LR, 0.9% NaCl, 0.45% NaCl

Syringe compatibilities:

Cloxacillin, glycopyrrolate, heparin, hydroxyzine, methicillin, metoclopramide, milrinone, moxalactam, nalbuphine

Syringe incompatibilities:

Cefazolin

Y-site compatibilities:

Alteplase, amiodarone, amrinone, cefazolin, ciprofloxacin, diltiazem, dobutamine, dopamine, enalaprilat, etomidate, famotidine, haloperidol, heparin, heparin with hydrocortisone, labetalol, meperidine, morphine, nitroglycerin, nitroprusside, potassium chloride, propofol, streptokinase, theophylline, vit B/C, warfarin

Additive compatibilities:

Alteplase, aminophylline, amiodarone, atracurium, bretylium, calcium chloride, calcium gluceptate, calcium gluconate, chloramphenicol, chlorothiazide, cimetidine, dexamethasone, digoxin, diphenhydramine, dobutamine, dopamine, ephedrine, erythromycin, floxacillin, flumazenil, furosemide, heparin, hydrocortisone, nafcillin, hydroxyzine, regular insulin, mephentermine, metaraminol, nafcillin, nitroglycerin, penicillin G potassium, pentobarbital, phenylephrine, potassium chloride, procainamide, prochlorperazine, promazine, ranitidine, sodium bicarbonate, sodium lactate, theophylline, verapamil, vit B/C

Additive incompatibilities:

Methohexital, phenytoin; do not admix with blood transfusions

Infiltration

Physician may order lidocaine with epinephrine to minimize systemic absorption and prolong local anesthesia

Patient/family education

- Teach patient or family reason for use of medication and expected results
- Instruct patient in at-home use of Lidopen Auto-Injector; patient should call prescriber before use if heart attack is imminent

Evaluation

Positive therapeutic outcome

- Decreased B/P, dysrhythmias
- Decreased heart rate
- Normal sinus rhythm

Treatment of overdose:

Oxygen, artificial ventilation, ECG, administer dopamine for circulatory depression, diazepam or thiopental for seizures, decreased drug or discontinuation may be required

L

lindane (OTC)
(lin-dane)
Bio-Well, GBH ♣, G-Well, Hexit ♣, Kwell, Kwellada ♣, Kwildane, lindane, PMS Lindane ♣, Scabene, Thionex
Func. class.: Scabicide/pediculicide
Chem. class.: Chlorinated hydrocarbon (synthetic)

Pregnancy category B

Action: Stimulates nervous system of arthropods, resulting in seizures, death of organism

Therapeutic Outcome: Resolution of infestation

Uses: Scabies, lice (head/pubic/body), nits

Dosage and routes
Lice

P ***Adult and child:*** TOP/cream/lotion: wash area with soap and water 8-12 hr after application; may reapply in 1 wk if needed; shampoo using 30 ml: work into lather, rub for 5 min, rinse, dry with towel; use fine-toothed comb to remove nits

Scabies

P ***Adult and child:*** TOP apply 1% cream/lotion to skin from neck to bottom of feet, toes; repeat in 1 wk if necessary

Available forms: Lotion, shampoo, cream (1%)

Adverse effects
CNS: Tremors, **seizures,** stimulation, dizziness (chronic inhalation of vapors)
CV: **Ventricular fibrillation** (chronic inhalation of vapors)
GI: *Nausea, vomiting, diarrhea,* liver damage (inhalation of vapors)
HEMA: **Aplastic anemia** (chronic inhalation of vapors)
INTEG: ***Pruritus, rash, irritation, contact dermatitis***

Contraindications: Hypersensitivity, P premature neonate, patients with known seizure disorders, inflammation of skin, abrasions, or breaks in skin

Precautions: Pregnancy **B,** P children <10 yr, infants, lactation; avoid contact with eyes

Pharmacokinetics

Absorption	20%
Distribution	Fat
Metabolism	Liver
Excretion	Kidneys
Half-life	18 hr

Pharmacodynamics

Onset	Rapid
Peak	Rapid
Duration	3 hr

Interactions
Oil-based hair dressing:
↑ absorption; wash, rinse, and dry hair before using lindane

NURSING CONSIDERATIONS
Assessment
- Assess head, hair for lice and nits before and after treatment; if scabies are present, check all skin surfaces
- Identify source of infection: school, family members, sexual contacts

Nursing diagnoses
✓ Skin integrity, impaired (uses)
✓ Knowledge deficit (teaching)

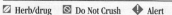

Implementation
- Apply to body areas, scalp only; do not apply to face, lips, mouth, eyes, any mucous membrane, anus, or meatus
- Give top corticosteroids as ordered to decrease contact dermatitis; provide antihistamines
- Apply menthol or phenol lotions to control itching
- Give top antibiotics for infection
- Provide isolation until areas on skin, scalp have cleared and treatment is completed
- Remove nits by using a fine-toothed

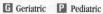

comb rinsed in vinegar after treatment; use gloves

Patient/family education

- Advise patient to wash all inhabitants' clothing, using insecticide; preventive treatment may be required for all persons living in same house, using lotion or shampoo to decrease spread of infection; use rubber gloves when applying drug
- Instruct patient that itching may continue for 4-6 wk; that drug must be reapplied if accidently washed off, or treatment will be ineffective; remove after specified time to prevent toxicity
- Advise patient not to apply to face; if accidental contact with eyes occurs, flush with water
- Advise patient that sexual contacts should be treated simultaneously

Evaluation

Positive therapeutic outcome

- Decreased crusts, nits, brownish trails on skin, itching papules in skinfolds
- Decreased itching after several wk

Treatment of ingestion: Gastric lavage, saline laxatives, **IV** diazepam (Valium) for seizures (if taken orally)

linezolid (℞)

(lih-nee'zoh-lid)

Zyvox

Func. class.: Broad-spectrum antiinfective

Chem. class.: Oxalodinone

Pregnancy category C

Action: Binds to bacterial 235 ribosomal RNA of the 50S subunit preventing formation of the bacterial translation process

➡ **Therapeutic Outcome:** Negative blood cultures, absence of signs/symptoms of infection

Uses: Vancomycin-resistant *Enterococcus faecium* infections, nosocomial pneumonia, uncomplicated or complicated skin and skin structure infections, community-acquired pneumonia

Dosage and routes

Vancomycin-resistant E. faecium infections

Adult: **IV** 600 mg q12h × 14-28 days PO

Nosocomial pneumonia/complicated skin infections/community-acquired pneumonia/concurrent bacterial infection

Adult: **IV**/PO 600 mg q12h × 10-14 days

Uncomplicated skin infections

Adult: **IV**/PO 400 mg q10-14 days

Available forms: Tabs 400, 600 mg; powder for reconstitution 100 mg/5 ml; inj 2 mg/ml

Adverse effects

CNS: *Headache,* dizziness, confusion

GI: *Nausea, diarrhea,* increased ALT, AST, *vomiting,* taste change, tongue color change

HEMA: **Myelosuppression**

MISC: Vaginal moniliasis, fungal infection, oral moniliasis

Contraindications: Hypersensitivity

Precautions: Pregnancy **C,** P lactation, children, thrombocytopenia

Pharmacokinetics

Absorption	Rapidly, excessively
Distribution	Protein binding 31%
Metabolism	Oxidation of the morpholine ring
Excretion	Unknown
Half-life	Unknown

Pharmacodynamics

Unknown

L

Interactions
Drug classifications

Adrenergic blockers: ↑effects of adrenergics
MAOIs: ↓ effects of MAOIs
Serotonergic agents: ↑ effect

NURSING CONSIDERATIONS
Assessment
- Assess CNS symptoms: headache, dizziness
- Monitor liver function studies: AST, ALT
- Monitor allergic reactions: fever, flushing, rash, urticaria, pruritus
- Assess for pseudomembranous colitis: severe diarrhea, cramping
- Monitor CBC weekly, assess for myelosuppression (anemia, leukopenia, pancytopenia, thrombocytopenia)

Nursing diagnoses
✓ Infection, potential for (uses)
✓ Knowledge deficit (teaching)

Implementation
PO route
- Store reconstituted oral suspension at room temperature, use within 3 wk

IV **IV route**
- Give over 30-120 min; do not use **IV** infusion bag in series connections, do not use with additives in sol, do not use with another drug, administer separately

Solution compatibilities: D_5, 0.9% NaCl, LR

Patient/family education
- Advise patient if dizziness occurs, to ambulate, perform activities with assistance
- Advise patient to complete full course of drug therapy
- Advise patient to contact prescriber if adverse reaction occurs
- Advise patient to avoid large amounts of tyramine-containing foods (give list)

Evaluation
Positive therapeutic outcome
- Decreased symptoms of infection, blood cultures negative

liothyronine (T_3) (℞)
(lye-oh-thye'roe-neen)

Cytomel, l-Triiodothyronine, liothyronine sodium, Triostat, T_3

Func. class.: Thyroid hormone
Chem. class.: Synthetic T_3

Pregnancy category A

Action: Controls protein synthesis; increases metabolic rates, cardiac output, renal blood flow, O_2 consumption, body temp, blood volume, growth, development at cellular level

→ **Therapeutic Outcome:** Correction of lack of thyroid hormone

Uses: Hypothyroidism, myxedema coma, thyroid hormone replacement, nontoxic goiter, T_3 suppression test, congenital hypothyroidism

Dosage and routes
Adult: PO 25 µg qd, increased by 12.5-25 µg q1-2 wk until desired response, maintenance dosage 25-75 µg qd

G ***Elderly:*** PO 5 µg/day, increase by 5 µg/day q1-2 wk

Congenital hypothyroidism

P ***Child >3 yr:*** PO 50-100 µg qd

P ***Child <3 yr:*** PO 5 µg qd, increased by 5 µg q3-4 days titrated to response

Myxedema, severe hypothyroidism

Adult: PO 25-50 µg then may increase by 5-10 µg q1-2 wk; maintenance dosage 50-100 µg qd

Myxedema coma/precoma

Adult: **IV** 25-50 µg initially; 5 µg in G elderly; 10-20 µg in cardiac disease; give doses q4-12h

Nontoxic goiter

Adult: PO 5 µg qd, increased by

12.5-25 μg q1-2 wk; maintenance dosage 75 μg qd

Suppression test (T_3)

Adult: PO 75-100 μg qd × 1 wk; ^{131}I is given before and after 1st wk dose

Available forms: Tabs 5, 25, 50 μg; inj 10 μg/ml

Adverse effects

CNS: *Insomnia, tremors,* headache, **thyroid storm**

CV: *Tachycardia, palpitations, angina, dysrhythmias,* hypertension, cardiac arrest

GI: Nausea, diarrhea, increased or decreased appetite, cramps

MISC: Menstrual irregularities, weight loss, sweating, heat intolerance, fever

Contraindications: Adrenal insufficiency, MI, thyrotoxicosis

G **Precautions:** Elderly, angina pectoris, hypertension, ischemia, cardiac disease, pregnancy **A**, lactation

Pharmacokinetics

Absorption	Well (PO); complete (**IV**)
Distribution	Widely distributed; does not cross placenta
Metabolism	Liver
Excretion	Feces via bile, breast milk
Half-life	6-7 days

Pharmacodynamics

	PO/IV
Onset	Unknown
Peak	12-24 hr
Duration	72 hr

Interactions

Individual drugs

Cholestyramine: ↓ absorption of thyroid hormone

Colestipol: ↓ absorption of thyroid hormone

Digitalis: ↓ effect of digitalis

Insulin: ↑ requirement for insulin

Phenytoin (IV): ↑ release of thyroid hormone

Drug classifications

Amphetamines: ↑ CNS, cardiac stimulation

β-Adrenergic blockers: ↓ effect of β-blockers

Decongestants: ↑ CNS, cardiac stimulation

Oral anticoagulants: ↑ requirements for anticoagulants

Vasopressors: ↑ CNS, cardiac stimulation

Herb/drug

Bugleweed: Do not use together

Lab test interferences

↑ CPK, ↑ LDH, ↑ AST, ↑ PBI, ↑ blood glucose

↓ Thyroid function tests

NURSING CONSIDERATIONS

Assessment

- Determine if the patient is taking anticoagulants, antidiabetic agents; document on patient record
- Take B/P, pulse before each dose; monitor I&O ratio and weight every day in same clothing, using same scale, at same time of day
- P Monitor height, weight, psychomotor development, and growth rate if given to a child
- Monitor T_3, T_4, FTIs, which are decreased; radioimmunoassay of TSH, which is increased; radioactive iodine uptake, which is increased if medication dose is too low
- Monitor pro-time; may require decreased anticoagulant; check for bleeding, bruising
- Assess for increased nervousness, excitability, irritability, which may indicate too high a dose, usually after 1-3 wk of treatment
- Assess cardiac status: angina, palpitations, chest pain, change in VS; G elderly patients may have undetected cardiac problems, and baseline ECG should be completed before treatment

Nursing diagnoses

- ☑ Knowledge deficit (teaching)
- ☑ Noncompliance (teaching)

L

Implementation

PO route

- Give in AM if possible as a single dose to decrease sleeplessness; give at same time each day to maintain drug level
- Give only for hormone imbalances; not to be used for obesity, male infertility, menstrual conditions, lethargy; give lowest dose that relieves symptoms; give lower dose to the G elderly and those with cardiac diseases
- Store in air-tight, light-resistant container

IV IV route

- Administer **IV** for myxedema coma and precoma; do not give IM or SC; give q4-12h; use PO dose as soon as feasible

Patient/family education

- Teach patient that drug is not a cure but controls symptoms, and treatment is long term
- Instruct patient to report excitability, irritability, anxiety, sweating, heat intolerance, chest pain, palpitations, which indicate overdose
- Advise patient not to switch brands unless approved by prescriber; bioavailability may differ; do not take with food or absorption will be decreased
- Teach patient that drug may be discontinued after giving birth; thyroid panel will be evaluated after 1-2 mo
- Teach patient that hyperthyroid P child will show almost immediate behavior/personality change; that hair loss will occur in child but is temporary
- Caution patient that drug is not to be taken to reduce weight
- Caution patient to avoid OTC preparations with iodine; read labels; other medications should not be used unless approved by prescriber
- Teach patient to avoid iodine-rich food: iodized salt, soybeans, tofu, turnips, some seafood, some bread

Evaluation

Positive therapeutic outcome

- Absence of depression
- Weight loss
- Increased diuresis, pulse, appetite
- Absence of constipation, peripheral edema, cold intolerance, pale, cool dry skin, brittle nails, alopecia, coarse hair, menorrhagia, night blindness, paresthesias, syncope, stupor, coma, rosy cheeks
- Improved levels of T_3, T_4 by laboratory tests
- P Child: age-appropriate weight, height, and psychomotor development

Treatment of overdose:

Withhold dose for up to 1 wk; for acute overdose: gastric lavage or induce emesis, then activated charcoal; provide supportive treatment to control symptoms

liotrix (℞)

(lye'oh-trix)

T_3/T_4, Thyrolar

Func. class.: Thyroid hormone

Chem. class.: Levothyroxine/liothyronine (synthetic T_4, T_3)

Pregnancy category A

Action: Controls protein synthesis; increases metabolic rates, cardiac output, renal blood flow, O_2 consumption, body temp, blood volume, growth, development at cellular level

→ **Therapeutic Outcome:** Correction of lack of thyroid hormone

Uses: Hypothyroidism, thyroid hormone replacement

Dosage and routes

P ***Adult and child:*** PO 50 μg levothyroxine/12.5 μg liothyronine qd, increased by 50 μg levothyroxine/12.5 μg liothyronine qmo until desired response; may increase by 15-30 mg q2 wk in child

G ***Elderly:*** PO 12.5-25 μg levothyroxine/3.1-6.2 μg liothyronine, may increase by 12.5-25 μg levothyroxine/3.1-6.2 μg liothyronine q6-8 wk until adequate response

Available forms: Tabs 12.5/3.1, 25/6.25, 50/12.5, 100/25, 150 μg levothyroxine/37.5 μg liothyronine

Adverse effects

CNS: *Insomnia, tremors,* headache, **thyroid storm**

CV: *Tachycardia, palpitations, angina, dysrhythmias,* hypertension, cardiac arrest

GI: Nausea, diarrhea, increased or decreased appetite, cramps

MISC: Menstrual irregularities, weight loss, sweating, heat intolerance, fever

Contraindications: Adrenal insufficiency, MI, thyrotoxicosis

G **Precautions:** Elderly, angina pectoris, hypertension, ischemia, cardiac disease, pregnancy **A**, lactation

Do Not Confuse:
Thyrolar/Thyrar

Pharmacokinetics

Absorption	50%-80% (T_4); 95% (T_3)
Distribution	Widely distributed; does not cross placenta
Metabolism	Liver, tissues
Excretion	Feces via bile; breast milk
Half-life	6-7 days (T_4); 2 days (T_3)

Pharmacodynamics

	PO (T_4)	PO (T_3)
Onset	Unknown	Unknown
Peak	Unknown	24-72 hr
Duration	Unknown	72 hr

Interactions

Individual drugs

Cholestyramine: ↓ absorption of thyroid hormone
Colestipol: ↓ absorption of liotrix
Digitalis: ↓ effect of digitalis
Insulin: ↑ requirement for insulin
Phenytoin (IV): ↑ release of thyroid hormone

Drug classifications

Amphetamines: ↑ CNS, cardiac stimulation
β-Adrenergic blockers: ↓ effect of β-blockers
Decongestants: ↑ CNS, cardiac stimulation
Oral anticoagulants: ↑ requirements for anticoagulants
Vasopressors: ↑ CNS, cardiac stimulation

Herb/drug

Bugleweed: Do not use together

Lab test interferences

↑ CPK, ↑ LDH, ↑ AST, ↑ PBI, ↑ blood glucose
↓ Thyroid function tests

NURSING CONSIDERATIONS

Assessment

- Determine if the patient is taking anticoagulants, antidiabetic agents; document on chart
- Take B/P, pulse before each dose; monitor I&O ratio and weight every day in same clothing, using same scale, at same time of day
- Monitor height, weight, psychomotor development, and growth rate if **P** given to a child
- Monitor T_3, T_4, FTIs, which are decreased; radioimmunoassay of TSH, which is increased; radioactive iodine uptake (RAIU), which is increased if medication dose is too low
- Monitor pro-time; may require decreased anticoagulant; check for bleeding, bruising
- Assess for increased nervousness, excitability, irritability, which may indicate too high a dose of medication, usually after 1-3 wk of treatment
- Assess cardiac status: angina, palpitations, chest pain, change in VS; **G** the elderly patient may have undetected cardiac problems, and baseline ECG should be completed before treatment

L

Nursing diagnoses

- ✓ Knowledge deficit (teaching)
- ✓ Noncompliance (teaching)

Implementation

- Give in AM if possible as a single dose to decrease sleeplessness; give at same time each day to maintain drug level
- Give only for hormone imbalances; not to be used for obesity, male infertility, menstrual conditions, lethargy; give lowest dose that relieves symptoms; give lower dose to the G elderly and those with cardiac diseases
- Store in airtight, light-resistant container
- Remove medication 4 wk before RAIU test

Patient/family education

- Teach patient that drug is not a cure but controls symptoms, and treatment is long term
- Instruct patient to report excitability, irritability, anxiety, sweating, heat intolerance, chest pain, palpitations, which indicate overdose
- Advise patient not to switch brands unless approved by prescriber; bioavailability may differ; do not take with food or absorption will be decreased
- Teach patient that drug may be discontinued after giving birth; thyroid panel will be evaluated after 1-2 mo
- Teach patient that hyperthyroid P child will show almost immediate behavior/personality change; that hair loss will occur in child but is temporary
- Caution patient that drug is not to be taken to reduce weight
- Caution patient to avoid OTC preparations with iodine; read labels; other medications should not be used unless approved by prescriber
- Teach patient to avoid iodine-rich food: iodized salt, soybeans, tofu, turnips, some seafood, some bread

Evaluation

Positive therapeutic outcome

- Absence of depression
- Weight loss
- Increased diuresis, pulse, appetite
- Absence of constipation, peripheral edema, cold intolerance, pale, cool dry skin, brittle nails, alopecia, coarse hair, menorrhagia, night blindness, paresthesias, syncope, stupor, coma, rosy cheeks
- Improved levels of T_3, T_4 by laboratory tests
- P Child: age-appropriate weight, height, and psychomotor development

Treatment of overdose:

Withhold dose for up to 1 wk; acute overdose: gastric lavage or induce emesis, then activated charcoal; provide supportive treatment to control symptoms

lisinopril (℞)

(lyse-in'oh-pril)

Prinivil, Zestril

Func. class.: Antihypertensive, angiotensin converting enzyme (ACE) inhibitor

Chem. class.: Enalaprilat lysine analog

Pregnancy category

C (1st trimester),

D (2nd/3rd trimesters)

Action: Selectively suppresses renin-angiotensin-aldosterone system; inhibits ACE; prevents conversion of angiotensin I to angiotensin II; results in dilatation of arterial, venous vessels

→ Therapeutic Outcome: Decreased B/P in hypertension, decreased preload, afterload in CHF

Uses: Mild to moderate hypertension, adjunctive therapy of systolic CHF

Dosage and routes

Hypertension

Adult: PO 10-40 mg qd; may increase to 80 mg qd if required

G ***Elderly:*** PO 2.5-5 mg/day, increase q7 days

CHF
Adult: PO 2.5-5 mg initially with diuretics/digitalis

Available forms: Tabs 5, 10, 20, 40 mg

Adverse effects
CNS: *Vertigo*, depression, stroke, insomnia, paresthesias, *headache*, fatigue, asthenia
EENT: Blurred vision, nasal congestion
GI: Nausea, vomiting, anorexia, constipation, flatulence, GI irritation
GU: **Proteinuria, renal insufficiency,** sexual dysfunction, impotence
HEMA: **Agranulocytopenia,** neutropenia
INTEG: Rash, pruritus
RESP: Dry cough, dyspnea
SYST: **Angioedema**

Contraindications: Hypersensitivity, pregnancy **D** (2nd/3rd trimesters)

Precautions: Pregnancy **C** (1st trimester), lactation, renal disease, hyperkalemia, renal artery stenosis

Do Not Confuse:
Prinivil/Plendil, Prinivil/Prilosec, Prinivil/Proventil

Pharmacokinetics	
Absorption	Variable
Distribution	Unknown
Metabolism	Not metabolized
Excretion	Kidneys, unchanged
Half-life	12 hr

Pharmacodynamics	
Onset	1 hr
Peak	6-8 hr
Duration	24 hr

Interactions
Individual drugs
Alcohol: ↑ hypotension (large amounts)
Allopurinol: ↑ hypersensitivity
Digoxin: ↑ serum levels, toxicity
Hydralazine: ↑ toxicity
Indomethacin: ↓ antihypertensive effect
Lithium: ↑ levels of lithium, toxicity
Prazosin: ↑ toxicity
Drug classifications
Adrenergic blockers: ↑ hypotension
Antacids: ↓ absorption
Antihypertensives: ↑ hypotension
Diuretics: ↑ hypotension
Diuretics, potassium-sparing: ↑ toxicity
Ganglionic blockers: ↑ hypotension
Nitrates: ↑ hypotension
Phenothiazines: ↑ hypotension
Potassium supplements: ↑ toxicity
Sympathomimetics: ↑ toxicity
Food/drug
High-potassium diet (bananas, orange juice, avocados, broccoli, nuts, spinach) should be avoided; hyperkalemia may occur
Lab test interferences
Interference: Glucose/insulin tolerance tests, ANA titer

L

NURSING CONSIDERATIONS
Assessment
- Assess blood studies: platelets, WBC with differential, baseline and periodically q3 mo; if neutrophils <1000/mm^3, discontinue treatment
- Monitor B/P, check for orthostatic hypotension, syncope; if changes occur, dosage change may be required
- Establish baselines in renal, liver function tests before therapy begins
- Monitor renal, liver studies: protein, BUN, creatinine; watch for increased levels that may indicate nephrotic syndrome and renal failure; monitor renal symptoms: polyuria, oliguria, frequency, dysuria; LFTs
- Check potassium levels throughout treatment, although hyperkalemia rarely occurs
- Check for edema in feet, legs daily
- Assess for allergic reactions: rash, fever, pruritus, urticaria; drug should be discontinued if antihistamines fail to help

Nursing diagnoses
✓ Cardiac output, decreased (uses)
✓ Injury, risk for (side effects)
✓ Knowledge deficit (teaching)
✓ Noncompliance (teaching)

Implementation
- Store in airtight container at 86° F (30° C) or less
- Severe hypotension may occur after 1st dose of this medication; may be prevented by reducing or discontinuing diuretic therapy 3 days before beginning lisinopril therapy

Patient/family education
- Caution patient not to discontinue drug abruptly; advise patient to inform all health care providers about taking this drug
- Teach patient not to use OTC products (cough, cold, allergy) unless directed by prescriber; serious side effects can occur
- Teach patient the importance of complying with dosage schedule, even if feeling better; to continue with medical regimen to decrease B/P: exercise, cessation of smoking, decreasing stress, diet modifications
- Teach patient to notify prescriber of mouth sores, sore throat, fever, swelling of hands or feet, irregular heartbeat, chest pain, coughing, shortness of breath
- Caution patient to report excessive perspiration, dehydration, vomiting, diarrhea; may lead to fall in B/P
- Emphasize the need to rise slowly to sitting or standing position to minimize orthostatic hypotension; not to exercise in hot weather or increased hypotension can occur
- Caution patient that drug may cause dizziness, fainting, light-headedness; may occur during 1st few days of therapy; to avoid activities that may be hazardous
- Teach patient how to take B/P, and normal readings for age group; advise patient to take B/P regularly
- Instruct patient to avoid increasing potassium in the diet

Evaluation
Positive therapeutic outcome
- Decreased B/P in hypertension
- Decreased CHF symptoms

Treatment of overdose: 0.9% NaCl **IV** inf, hemodialysis

lithium (℞)
(li'thee-um)

Carbolith ♣, Cibalith-S, Duralith ♣, Eskalith, Eskalith CR, Lithane, lithium carbonate, Lithizine ♣, Lithonate, Lithotabs

Func. class.: Antimanic, antipsychotic

Chem. class.: Alkali metal ion salt

Pregnancy category D

Action: May alter sodium, potassium ion transport across cell membrane in nerve, muscle cells; may balance biogenic amines of norepinephrine, serotonin in CNS areas involved in emotional responses

➔ **Therapeutic Outcome:** Stable mood

Uses: Bipolar disorders (manic phase), prevention of bipolar manic-depressive psychosis

Dosage and routes
Adult: PO 300-600 mg tid; maintenance 300 mg tid or qid; slow rel tab 300 mg bid; dosage should be individualized to maintain blood levels at 0.5-1.5 mEq/L

G ***Elderly:*** PO 300 mg bid, increase q7 days by 300 mg to desired dose

P ***Child:*** PO 15-20 mg (0.4-0.5 mEq)/kg/day in 2-3 divided doses, increase as needed, do not exceed adult doses

Renal dose
PO CrCl 10-50 ml/min 50-75% of dose; CrCl <10 ml/min 25%-50% of dose

Available forms: Caps 150, 300, 600 mg; tabs 300 mg; ext rel tabs 300, 450 mg; syrup 300 mg/5 ml (8 mEq/5 ml); slow rel caps 150, 300 mg ♣

Adverse effects

CNS: *Headache, drowsiness, dizziness, tremors,* twitching, ataxia, **seizures,** slurred speech, restlessness, *confusion,* stupor, memory loss, clonic movements, *fatigue*

CV: *Hypotension,* ECG changes, **dysrhythmias, circulatory collapse, edema**

EENT: Tinnitus, blurred vision, aphasia, dysarthria

ENDO: Hypothyroidism, goiter, hyperglycemia, hyperthyroidism

GI: *Dry mouth, anorexia, nausea, vomiting, diarrhea,* incontinence, abdominal pain, metallic taste

GU: **Polyuria, glycosuria, proteinuria, albuminuria,** urinary incontinence, polydipsia, edema, **renal toxicity**

HEMA: **Leukocytosis**

INTEG: Drying of hair, alopecia, rash, pruritus, hyperkeratosis, *acneiform rash, folliculitis*

MS: *Muscle weakness,* rigidity

SYST: Hyponatremia

Contraindications: Hepatic disease, renal disease, brain trauma, OBS, pregnancy **D,** lactation, schizophrenia, severe cardiac disease, severe renal disease, severe dehydration

G **Precautions:** Elderly, thyroid disease, seizure disorders, diabetes mellitus, systemic infection, urinary retention, children <12 yr P

Pharmacokinetics

Absorption	Completely absorbed
Distribution	Reabsorbed by renal tubules (80%); crosses blood-brain barrier; crosses placenta
Metabolism	Unknown
Excretion	Urine, unchanged
Half-life	18-36 hr depending on age

Pharmacodynamics

Onset	Rapid
Peak	½-4 hr
Duration	Unknown

Interactions

Individual drugs

Acetazolamide: ↑ renal clearance
Aminophylline: ↑ renal clearance
Calcium iodide: ↑ hypothyroid effect
Carbamazepine: ↑ lithium toxicity
Fluoxetine: ↑ lithium toxicity
Haloperidol: ↑ neurotoxicity
Iodinated glycerol: ↑ hypothyroid effect
Indomethacin: ↑ toxicity
Losartan: ↑ toxicity
Mannitol: ↑ renal clearance
Methyldopa: ↑ lithium toxicity
Potassium: ↑ hypothyroid effect
Sodium bicarbonate: ↑ renal clearance
Thioridazine: Brain damage
Urea: ↑ toxicity

Drug classifications

NSAIDs: ↑ lithium toxicity
Phenothiazines: ↑ effect of phenothiazines
Theophyllines: ↓ effect of lithium
Thiazides: ↑ lithium toxicity

Herb/drug

Broom: ↑ lithium effect
Buchu: ↑ lithium effect
Dandelion: ↑ lithium effect
Juniper: ↑ lithium effect

Food/drug

Significant changes in sodium intake will alter lithium excretion

Lab test interferences

↑ Potassium excretion, ↑ urine glucose, ↑ blood glucose, ↑ protein, ↑ BUN
↓ VMA, ↓ T_3, ↓ T_4, ↓ PBI, ↓ ^{131}I

NURSING CONSIDERATIONS

Assessment

- Assess for minor lithium toxicity: vomiting, diarrhea, poor coordination, fine motor tremors, weakness, lassitude; major toxicity: coarse

L

tremors, severe thirst, tinnitus, dilute urine
• Assess weight daily; check for edema in legs, ankles, wrists; report if present; check skin turgor at least daily
• Monitor sodium intake; decreased sodium intake with decreased fluid intake may lead to lithium retention; increased sodium and fluids may decrease lithium retention
• Monitor urine for albuminuria, glycosuria, uric acid during beginning treatment, q2 mo thereafter
• Assess neurologic status: LOC, gait, motor reflexes, hand tremors
• Monitor serum lithium levels weekly initially, then q2 mo (therapeutic level: 0.5-1.5 mEq/L); toxicity and therapeutic levels are very close; toxicity may occur rapidly; blood levels are measured before the AM dose

Nursing diagnoses
- ✓ Ineffective individual coping (uses)
- ✓ Thought processes, altered (uses)
- ✓ Knowledge deficit (teaching)
- ✓ Noncompliance (teaching)

Implementation
• Administer reduced dosage to G elderly; give with meals to avoid GI upset
• Provide adequate fluids (2-3 L/day) to prevent dehydration during initial treatment, 1-2 L/day during maintenance

Patient/family education
• Provide patient with written information on symptoms of minor toxicity: vomiting, diarrhea, poor coordination, fine motor tremors, weakness, lassitude; major toxicity: coarse tremors, severe thirst, tinnitus, dilute urine
• Advise patient to monitor urine sp gr; emphasize need for follow-up care to determine lithium effects
• Advise patient that contraception is necessary, since lithium may harm fetus
• Caution patient not to operate machinery until lithium levels are stable and response determined; that beneficial effects may take 1-3 wk
• Provide to the patient a list of drugs that interact with lithium and discuss need for adequate, stable intake of salt and fluid
⊘ • Advise patient not to crush, chew caps

Evaluation
Positive therapeutic outcome
• Decrease in excitement, poor judgment, insomnia (manic phase)
• Decreased mood swings and lability

Treatment of overdose:
Induce emesis or lavage, maintain airway, respiratory function; dialysis for severe intoxication

lomefloxacin (℞)
(lome-flocks'a-sin)
Maxaquin
Func. class.: Antiinfective
Chem. class.: Fluoroquinolone
Pregnancy category C

Action: Interferes with conversion of intermediate DNA fragments into high-molecular-weight DNA in bacteria; DNA gyrase inhibitor

➔ **Therapeutic Outcome:** Bactericidal for gram-negative organisms *Aeromonas, Citrobacter, Enterobacter, Escherichia coli, Haemophilus influenzae, Klebsiella, Legionella, Moraxella catarrhalis, Morganella morganii, Proteus vulgaris, Proteus mirabilis, Providencia alcalifaciens, Providencia rettgeri, Pseudomonas aeruginosa, Serratia;* gram-positive organisms *Staphylococcus aureus, Staphylococcus epidermidis, Staphylococcus saprophyticus* (methicillin-resistant strains also)

Uses: Treatment of lower respiratory tract infections (pneumonia, bronchitis), genitourinary tract infections (prostatitis, UTIs), preoperatively to reduce UTIs in transurethral surgical procedures

Dosage and routes

Adult: PO 400 mg/day × 7-14 days depending on type of infection

Renal dose

Adult: PO 200 mg/day

Surgical prophylaxis of UTI

Adult: PO 400 mg 2-6 hr before surgery

Available forms: Tabs 400 mg

Adverse effects

CNS: *Dizziness, headache,* somnolence, depression, insomnia, nervousness, confusion, agitation

EENT: Visual disturbances

GI: Diarrhea, *nausea,* vomiting, anorexia, flatulence, heartburn, dry mouth, increased AST, ALT, constipation, abdominal pain, oral thrush, glossitis, stomatitis

INTEG: Rash, pruritus, urticaria, *photosensitivity*

Contraindications: Hypersensitivity to quinolones

P G **Precautions:** Pregnancy **C,** lactation, children, elderly, renal disease, seizure disorders, excessive exposure to sunlight

Pharmacokinetics

Absorption	Well absorbed
Distribution	Widely distributed
Metabolism	Unknown
Excretion	Kidney, unchanged
Half-life	6-8 hr; increased in renal disease

Pharmacodynamics

Onset	Unknown
Peak	1-2 hr

Interactions

Individual drugs

Caffeine: ↑ levels

Calcium: ↓ effects of lomefloxacin

Cimetidine: ↑ lomefloxacin levels, toxicity

Cyclosporine: ↑ levels of cyclosporine, toxicity

Nitrofurantoin: ↓ lomefloxacin levels

NSAIDs: ↑ CNS stimulation, seizures

Probenicid: ↑ lomefloxacin levels, toxicity

Sucralfate: ↓ lomefloxacin levels

Warfarin: ↑ levels of warfarin, toxicity

Drug classifications

Antacids (aluminum, magnesium): ↓ levels of lomefloxacin

Iron sulfate: ↓ levels of lomefloxacin

Zinc sulfate: ↓ levels of lomefloxacin

NURSING CONSIDERATIONS

Assessment

- Assess patient for previous sensitivity reaction
- Assess patient for signs and symptoms of infection: characteristics of wounds, sputum, urine, stool, WBC >10,000/mm^3, fever; baseline and during treatment
- Obtain C&S before beginning drug therapy to identify if correct treatment has been initiated
- Assess for allergic reactions and anaphylaxis: rash, urticaria, pruritus, chills, fever, joint pain; may occur a few days after therapy begins; epinephrine and resuscitation equipment should be available for anaphylactic reaction
- Monitor blood studies: AST, ALT, CBC, Hct, bilirubin, LDH, alkaline phosphatase, Coombs' test monthly if patient is on long-term therapy
- Assess bowel pattern qd; if severe diarrhea occurs, drug should be discontinued
- Assess for overgrowth of infection: perineal itching, fever, malaise, redness, pain, swelling, drainage, rash, diarrhea, change in cough, sputum
- Assess for CNS symptoms: insomnia,

L

vertigo, headaches, agitation, confusion

Nursing diagnoses

- ✓ Infection, risk for (uses)
- ✓ Diarrhea (adverse reactions)
- ✓ Injury, risk for (adverse reactions)
- ✓ Knowledge deficit (teaching)
- ✓ Noncompliance (teaching)

Implementation

- Give with food for GI symptoms; give with 8 oz of water
- Give 2 hr before or 2 hr after iron, calcium, zinc, magnesium products, or antacids, which decrease absorption

Patient/family education

- Instruct patient to take all medication prescribed for the length of time ordered; drug must be taken around the clock to maintain blood levels; do not give medication to others
- Teach patient to use sunscreen when outdoors to decrease phototoxicity
- Advise patient to increase fluids to 2 L/day to prevent crystalluria
- Caution patient to avoid driving and other hazardous activities until response is known; dizziness, confusion, drowsiness may occur
- Advise patient to rinse mouth frequently, use sugarless candy or gum for dry mouth
- Instruct patient to avoid other medications unless approved by prescriber

Evaluation

Positive therapeutic outcome

- Negative C&S, absence of signs/symptoms of infection (WBC <10,000/mm^3, temp WNL)
- Reported improvement in symptoms of infection

lomustine (℞)

(loe-mus'teen)

CCNU, CeeNU

Func. class.: Antineoplastic alkylating agent

Chem. class.: Nitrosourea

Pregnancy category D

Action: Changes essential cellular ions to covalent bonding with resultant alkylation; this interferes with normal biologic function of DNA; activity is not phase specific; action is due to myelosuppression

➔ **Therapeutic Outcome:** Prevention of rapid growth of malignant cells in chronic myelocytic leukemia

Uses: Hodgkin's disease, lymphomas, multiple myeloma

Investigational uses: Brain, breast, renal, GI tract, bronchogenic carcinoma; melanomas

Dosage and routes

Adult: PO 100, 130 mg/m^2 as a single dose q6 wk; titrate dosage to WBC level; do not give repeat dose unless WBCs are >4000/mm^3, platelet count >100,000/mm^3

Available forms: Caps 10, 40, 100 mg

Adverse effects

GI: *Nausea, vomiting, anorexia, stomatitis,* **hepatotoxicity**

GU: **Azotemia, renal failure**

HEMA: **Thrombocytopenia, leukopenia, myelosuppression, anemia**

INTEG: Burning at inj site

RESP: **Fibrosis, pulmonary infiltrate**

Contraindications: Radiation, chemotherapy, lactation, pregnancy **D** (3rd trimester), "blastic" phase of chronic myelocytic leukemia, hypersensitivity, lactation

Precautions: Childbearing age men and women, leukopenia, thrombocytopenia, anemia, hepatotoxicity, renal toxicity

Pharmacokinetics

Absorption	Rapidly absorbed
Distribution	Widely
Metabolism	Liver
Excretion	Kidneys, breast milk
Half-life	16-48 hr

Pharmacodynamics

Unknown

Interactions

Individual drugs

Radiation: ↑ toxicity, bone marrow suppression

Drug classifications

Antineoplastics: ↑ toxicity, bone marrow suppression

Lab test interferences

False positive: Cytology tests for breast, bladder, cervix, lung

NURSING CONSIDERATIONS

Assessment

- Monitor CBC, differential, platelet count weekly; withhold drug if WBC is <4000/mm^3 or platelet count is <100,000/mm^3; notify prescriber of results if WBC <20,000/mm^3, platelets <150,000/mm^3
- Monitor pulmonary function tests, chest x-ray films before, during therapy; chest film should be obtained q2 wk during treatment; assess for dyspnea, rales, unproductive cough, chest pain, tachypnea
- Monitor renal function studies: BUN, serum uric acid, urine CrCl before, during therapy; I&O ratio; report fall in urine output of 30 ml/hr; check for decreased hyperuricemia
- Monitor for cold, fever, sore throat (may indicate beginning of infection); identify edema in feet, joint and stomach pain, shaking; prescriber should be notified
- Assess for bleeding: hematuria, guaiac, bruising or petechiae, mucosa or orifices q8h, no rec temp

Nursing diagnoses

- ✓ Injury, risk for (adverse reactions)
- ✓ Body image disturbance (adverse reactions)
- ✓ Infection, risk for (adverse reactions)
- ✓ Knowledge deficit (teaching)

Implementation

- Give drug after evening meal, before hs; administer antiemetic 30-60 min before giving drug to prevent vomiting
- Antiinfectives for prophylaxis of infection may be prescribed since infection potential is high
- Store in tight container

Patient/family education

- Teach patient to avoid use of products containing aspirin or ibuprofen, razors, commercial mouthwash, since bleeding may occur; to report symptoms of bleeding (hematuria, tarry stools)
- Advise patient to report signs of anemia (fatigue, headache, irritability, faintness, shortness of breath)
- Caution patient to report any changes in breathing or coughing even several mo after treatment; to avoid crowds and persons with respiratory tract or other infections
- Caution patient not to have any vaccinations without the advice of prescriber; serious reactions can occur
- Tell patient contraception is needed during treatment and for several mo after the completion of therapy

Evaluation

Positive therapeutic outcome

- Decreased tumor sizes
- Decreased spread of malignancy

L

loperamide (OTC, ℞)
(loe-per'a-mide)

loperamide solution, Imodium, Imodium A-D, Imodium A-D Caplet, Loperamide, A-D Kaopectate II Caplets, Maalox Antidiarrheal Caplets, Pepto Diarrhea Control

Func. class.: Antidiarrheal
Chem. class.: Piperidine derivative

Pregnancy category B

Action: Direct action on intestinal muscles to decrease GI peristalsis; reduces volume, increases bulk; electrolytes are not lost

Therapeutic Outcome: Absence of diarrhea

Uses: Diarrhea (cause undetermined), chronic diarrhea, ileostomy discharge

Dosage and routes
Adult: PO 4 mg, then 2 mg after each loose stool, max 16 mg/day

P ***Child 9-11 yr:*** PO 2 mg, then 1 mg after each loose stool, max 6 mg/24 hr

P ***Child 2-5 yr:*** PO 1 mg on day 1, then 0.1 mg/kg after each loose stool, max 4 mg/24 hr

Available forms: Caps 2 mg; liq 1 mg/5 ml; tabs 2 mg

Adverse effects
CNS: Dizziness, drowsiness, fatigue, fever
GI: *Nausea, dry mouth, vomiting, constipation,* abdominal pain, anorexia, **toxic megacolon**
INTEG: Rash

Contraindications: Hypersensitivity, severe ulcerative colitis, pseudomembranous colitis, acute diarrhea associated with *Escherichia coli*

Precautions: Pregnancy **B**, lactation, P children <2 yr, liver disease, dehydration, bacterial disease

Pharmacokinetics

Absorption	Poor
Distribution	Unknown
Metabolism	Liver
Excretion	Feces, unchanged; small amount in urine
Half-life	7-14 hr

Pharmacodynamics

Onset	½-1 hr
Peak	Unknown
Duration	4-5 hr

Interaction
Solutions: Do not mix with other oral sol

NURSING CONSIDERATIONS
Assessment
- Monitor electrolytes (potassium, sodium, chloride) if patient is on long-term therapy; check fluid status, skin turgor
- Assess bowel pattern before, during treatment; check for rebound constipation after termination of medication; check bowel sounds
- Check response after 48 hr; if no response, drug should be discontinued and other treatment initiated
- Assess for abdominal distention, toxic megacolon, which may occur in ulcerative colitis
- Assess for dehydration, CNS symptoms in children P

Nursing diagnoses
- ✓ Diarrhea (uses)
- ✓ Constipation (adverse reactions)
- ✓ Knowledge deficit (teaching)
- ✓ Noncompliance (teaching)

Implementation
- ⊘ Do not chew, crush caps
- Store in airtight containers

Patient/family education
- Caution patient to avoid alcohol and OTC products unless directed by prescriber; may cause increased CNS depression
- Advise patient not to exceed recom-

mended dosage; drug may be habit forming
- Advise patient that drug may cause drowsiness and to avoid hazardous activities until response to drug is determined
- Teach patient that dry mouth can be decreased by frequent sips of water, hard candy, sugarless gum

Evaluation
Positive therapeutic outcome
- Decreased diarrhea

loracarbef
See cephalosporins—2nd generation

loratadine (℞)
(lor-a'ti-deen)
Claritin
Func. class.: Antihistamine (2nd generation)
Chem. class.: Selective histamine (H_1) receptor antagonist
Pregnancy category B

Action: Binds to peripheral histamine receptors, which provides antihistamine action without sedation

Therapeutic Outcome: Decreased nasal stuffiness, itching, swollen eyes

Uses: Seasonal rhinitis

Dosage and routes
P ***Adult and child ≥12 yr:*** PO 10 mg qd, tabs rapid-disintegrating 10 mg; syrup 1 mg/ml

P ***Child 2-12 yr:*** PO 5 mg (10 ml) qd

Available forms: Tabs 10 mg; tab rapid-disintegrating 10 mg; syrup 5 mg/5 ml

Adverse effects
CNS: Sedation (more common with increased dosages), headache

Contraindications: Hypersensitivity, acute asthma attacks, lower respiratory tract disease

Precautions: Pregnancy **B**, increased intraocular pressure, bronchial asthma

Pharmacokinetics

Absorption	Well absorbed
Distribution	Unknown
Metabolism	Liver, extensively, to active metabolites
Excretion	Kidneys
Half-life	8½-28 hr

Pharmacodynamics

Onset	Unknown
Peak	1½ hr
Duration	Unknown

Interactions
Individual drugs
Alcohol: ↑ CNS depression
Drug classifications
CNS depressants: ↑ CNS depression
Opiates: ↑ CNS depression
Sedative/hypnotics: ↑ CNS depression
Food/drug
↑ Absorption
Herb/drug
Henbane: ↑ anticholinergic effect
Lab test interferences
False negative: Skin allergy tests (discontinue antihistamine 3 days before testing)

NURSING CONSIDERATIONS
Assessment
- Assess allergy: hives, rash, rhinitis
- Assess respiratory status: rate, rhythm, increase in bronchial secretions, wheezing, chest tightness; provide fluids to 2 L/day to decrease secretion thickness

Nursing diagnoses
- ✓ Airway clearance, ineffective (uses)
- ✓ Knowledge deficit (teaching)
- ✓ Noncompliance (teaching, overuse)

L

Implementation

- Give on an empty stomach, 1 hr ac or 2 hr pc to facilitate absorption
- Place rapidly disintegrating tabs on tongue, then swallow after disintegrated with or without water
- Store in airtight, light-resistant container

Patient/family education

- Teach all aspects of drug uses; to notify prescriber if confusion, sedation, hypotension occur; to avoid driving and other hazardous activity if drowsiness occurs; to avoid alcohol and other CNS depressants that may potentiate effect
- Teach patient to take 1 hr ac or 2 hr pc to facilitate absorption
- Advise patient to use sunscreen or stay out of the sun to prevent burns
- Caution patient not to exceed recommended dosage; dysrhythmias may occur
- Teach patient hard candy, gum, frequent rinsing of mouth may be used for dryness

Evaluation

Positive therapeutic outcome

- Absence of running or congested nose, other allergy symptoms

lorazepam (℞)

(lor-az′e-pam)

Apo-Lorazepam ♣, Ativan, lorazepam, Novolorazem ♣, Nu-Loraz ♣

Func. class.: Sedative/hypnotic, antianxiety agent

Chem. class.: Benzodiazepine

Pregnancy category D

Controlled substance schedule IV

Action: Potentiates the actions of GABA, an inhibitory neurotransmitter, especially in the limbic system and reticular formation, which depresses the CNS

➔ **Therapeutic Outcome:** Decreased anxiety, relaxation

Uses: Anxiety, irritability in psychiatric or organic disorders, preoperatively, insomnia

Investigational uses: Antiemetic before chemotherapy, status epilepticus, rectal use

Dosage and routes

Anxiety

Adult: PO 2-6 mg/day in divided doses, not to exceed 10 mg/day

G ***Elderly:*** PO 0.5-1 mg/day in divided doses; or 0.5-1 mg hs

P ***Child:*** PO 0.05 mg/kg/dose, q4-8 hr

Insomnia

Adult: PO 2-4 mg hs; only minimally effective after 2 wk continuous therapy

G ***Elderly:*** PO 1-2 mg initially

Preoperatively

Adult: IM 50 μg/kg 2 hr before surgery; **IV** 44 μg/kg 15-20 min before surgery

P ***Child:*** 0.05 mg/kg

Status epilepticus

P ***Neonate:*** 0.05 mg/kg

P ***Child:*** 0.1 mg/kg up to 4 mg/dose; rect (off label) 0.05-0.1 mg × 2; wait 7 min before giving 2nd dose

Available forms: Tabs 0.5, 1, 2 mg; inj 2, 4 mg/ml; conc sol 2 mg/ml

Adverse effects

CNS: *Dizziness, drowsiness,* confusion, headache, anxiety, tremors, stimulation, fatigue, depression, insomnia, hallucinations, weakness, unsteadiness

CV: *Orthostatic hypotension,* **ECG changes, tachycardia,** hypotension; **apnea, cardiac arrest (IV, rapid)**

EENT: *Blurred vision,* tinnitus, mydriasis

GI: Constipation, dry mouth, nausea, vomiting, anorexia, diarrhea

INTEG: Rash, dermatitis, itching

Contraindications: Hypersensitivity to benzodiazepines, narrow-angle glaucoma, psychosis, pregnancy **D**, P child <12 yr, history of drug abuse, COPD

G **Precautions:** Elderly, debilitated patients, hepatic disease, renal disease

Do Not Confuse:
lorazepam/alprazolam

Pharmacokinetics

Absorption	Well absorbed (PO); completely absorbed (IM)
Distribution	Widely distributed; crosses placenta, blood-brain barrier
Metabolism	Liver, extensively
Excretion	Kidneys, breast milk
Half-life	14 hr

Pharmacodynamics

	PO	IM	IV
Onset	½ hr	15-30 min	5-15 min
Peak	1-3 hr	1-1½ hr	Unknown
Duration	3-6 hr	3-6 hr	3-6 hr

Interactions

Individual drugs

Alcohol: ↑ CNS depression
Cimetidine: ↑ action
Disulfiram: ↑ action
Fluoxetine: ↑ action
Levodopa: ↓ action of levodopa

Drug classifications

Antidepressants: ↑ CNS depression
Antihistamines: ↑ CNS depression
Opiates: ↑ CNS depression

Smoking

↑ Metabolism, ↓ effect

Herb/drug

Kava: ↑ action

Lab test interferences

↑ AST, ↑ ALT, ↑ serum bilirubin
False: ↑ 17-OHCS
↓ Radioactive iodine uptake

NURSING CONSIDERATIONS

Assessment

- Assess degree of anxiety; what precipitates anxiety and whether drug controls symptoms; other signs of anxiety: dilated pupils, inability to sleep, restlessness, inability to focus
- Assess for alcohol withdrawal symptoms, including hallucinations (visual, auditory), delirium, irritability, agitation, fine to coarse tremors
- Monitor B/P (with patient lying/standing), pulse, check respiratory rate; if systolic B/P drops 20 mm Hg, hold drug, notify prescriber; respirations q5-15 min if given **IV**
- Monitor CBC during long-term therapy; blood dyscrasias have occurred (rarely)
- Monitor for seizure control; type, duration, and intensity of seizures; what precipitates seizures
- Monitor hepatic studies: AST, ALT, bilirubin, creatinine, LDH, alkaline phosphatase
- Assess mental status: mood, sensorium, affect, sleeping pattern, drowsiness, dizziness, suicidal tendencies, and ability of drug to control these symptoms; check for tolerance, withdrawal symptoms: headache, nausea, vomiting, muscle pain, weakness after longterm use

Nursing diagnoses

- ✓ Sleep pattern disturbance (uses)
- ✓ Coping, ineffective individual (uses)
- ✓ Knowledge deficit (teaching)
- ✓ Noncompliance (teaching)

Implementation

PO route

- Give with food or milk for GI symptoms; crush tab if patient is unable to swallow medication whole; provide sugarless gum, hard candy, frequent sips of water for dry mouth
- Use by SL route for rapid response (investigational use)

IM route

- Give deep in muscle mass; if using for preoperative sedation, give 2 hr or more before surgical procedure

IV **IV route**

- Dilute with sterile water for inj, 0.9% NaCl, or D_5W just before using;

L

give by Y-site or 3-way stopcock at 2 mg/min
- Do not use sol that is discolored or contains a precipitate

Syringe compatibilities: Cimetidine, hydromorphone

Y-site compatibilities: Acyclovir, albumin, allopurinol, amifostine, amikacin, amoxicillin, amoxicillin/clavulanate, amsacrine, atracurium, bumetanide, cefepime, cefmetazole, cefotaxime, ciprofloxacin, cisatracurium, cisplatin, cladribine, clonidine, cyclophosphamide, cytarabine, dexamethasone, diltiazem, dobutamine, dopamine, doxorubicin, epinephrine, erythromycin, etomidate, famotidine, fentanyl, filgrastim, fluconazole, fludarabine, furosemide, gentamicin, granisetron, haloperidol, heparin, hydrocortisone, hydromorphone, ketanserin, labetalol, melphalan, methotrexate, metronidazole, midazolam, milrinone, morphine, nicardipine, nitroglycerin, norepinephrine, paclitaxel, pancuronium, piperacillin, piperacillin/tazobactam, potassium chloride, propofol, ranitidine, tacrolimus, teniposide, thiotepa, trimethoprim-sulfamethoxazole, vancomycin, vecuronium, vinorelbine, zidovudine

Y-site incompatibilities: Idarubicin, ondansetron, sargramostim

Patient/family education
- Advise patient that drug may be taken with food; that drug is not to be used for everyday stress or used longer than 4 mo unless directed by a prescriber; to take no more than prescribed amount; may be habit forming
- Caution patient to avoid OTC preparations unless approved by prescriber; to avoid alcohol, other psychotropic medications unless prescribed by physician; not to discontinue medication abruptly after long-term use
- Inform patient to avoid driving and activities that require alertness; drowsiness may occur; to rise slowly or fainting may occur, especially in [G] elderly
- Inform patient that drowsiness may worsen at beginning of treatment

Evaluation
Positive therapeutic outcome
- Decreased anxiety, restlessness, insomnia

Treatment of overdose:
Lavage, VS, supportive care

losartan (℞)
(low-sar'tan)
Cozaar
Func. class.: Antihypertensive
Chem. class.: Angiotensin II receptor (type AT_1)

Pregnancy category
C (1st trimester);
D (2nd/3rd trimesters)

Action: Blocks the vasoconstrictor and aldosterone-secreting effects of angiotensin II; selectively blocks the binding of angiotensin II to the AT_1 receptor found in tissues

➡ **Therapeutic Outcome:** Decreased B/P

Uses: Hypertension, alone or in combination

Dosage and routes
Adult: PO 50 mg qd alone or 25 mg qd when used in combination

Hepatic dose
Adult: PO 25 mg qd

Available forms: Tabs 25, 50 mg

Adverse effects
CNS: Dizziness, insomnia, anxiety, confusion, abnormal dreams, migraine, tremor, vertigo
CV: Angina pectoris, 2nd- degree AV block, **CVA,** hypotension, **MI, dysrhythmias**

EENT: Blurred vision, burning eyes, conjunctivitis
GI: *Diarrhea, dyspepsia,* anorexia, constipation, dry mouth, flatulence, gastritis, vomiting
GU: Impotence, nocturia, urinary frequency, urinary tract infection
HEMA: Anemia
INTEG: Alopecia, dermatitis, dry skin, flushing, photosensitivity, rash, pruritus, sweating
META: Gout
MS: Cramps, myalgia, pain, stiffness
RESP: *Cough, upper respiratory infection,* congestion, dyspnea, bronchitis

Contraindications: Hypersensitivity, pregnancy **D** (2nd/3rd trimesters)

Precautions: Hypersensitivity to ACE inhibitors; pregnancy **C** (1st trimester); lactation, children, elderly

P G

Do Not Confuse:
Cozaar/Zocor

Pharmacokinetics

Absorption	Well
Distribution	Bound to plasma proteins
Metabolism	Extensive
Excretion	Feces, urine
Half-life	Biphasic, 2 hr, 6-9 hr

Pharmacodynamics

Unknown

Interactions

Individual drugs

Lithium: ↑ toxicity

NURSING CONSIDERATIONS

Assessment

- Assess B/P with position changes, pulse q4h; note rate, rhythm, quality
- Monitor electrolytes: potassium, sodium, chloride
- Obtain baselines for renal, liver function tests before therapy begins
- Monitor for edema in feet, legs daily
- Assess for skin turgor, dryness of mucous membranes for hydration status

Nursing diagnoses

- ✓ Fluid volume deficit (side effects)
- ✓ Noncompliance (teaching)
- ✓ Knowledge deficit (teaching)

Implementation

- Administer without regard to meals

Patient/family education

- Teach patient to avoid sunlight or wear sunscreen if in sunlight; photosensitivity may occur
- Advise patient to comply with dosage schedule, even if feeling better
- Teach patient to notify prescriber of mouth sores, fever, swelling of hands or feet, irregular heartbeat, chest pain
- Advise patient that excessive perspiration, dehydration, vomiting, diarrhea may lead to fall in blood pressure, consult prescriber if these occur
- Inform patient that drug may cause dizziness, fainting; light-headedness may occur
- Caution patient to rise slowly to sitting or standing position to minimize orthostatic hypotension
- Advise patient to use contraception while taking this product

Evaluation

Positive therapeutic outcome

- Decreased B/P

lovastatin (℞)

(loe'va-sta-tin)
Mevacor
Func. class.: Antilipemic
Chem. class.: *Aspergillus terreus* strain derivative

Pregnancy category X

Action: By inhibiting HMG-CoA reductase, inhibits biosynthesis of VLDL and LDL, which are responsible for cholesterol development

L

Therapeutic Outcome: Decreased cholesterol levels and LDLs, increased HDLs

Uses: As an adjunct in primary hypercholesterolemia (types IIa, IIb), mixed hyperlipidemia, other sclerosis

Dosage and routes

(Patient should first be consuming a cholesterol-lowering diet)

Adult: PO 20 mg qd with evening meal; may increase to 20-80 mg/day in single or divided doses; not to exceed 80 mg/day; dosage adjustments should be made monthly; reduce dose in renal disease

Available forms: Tabs 10, 20, 40 mg

Adverse effects

CNS: Dizziness, headache, tremor
EENT: Blurred vision, dysgeusia, lens opacities
GI: Nausea, constipation, diarrhea, dyspepsia, flatus, abdominal pain, heartburn, **liver dysfunction**
HEMA: **Thrombocytopenia, hemolytic anemia, leukopenia**
INTEG: Rash, pruritus, photosensitivity
MS: Muscle cramps, myalgia, **myositis, rhabdomyolysis**

Contraindications: Hypersensitivity, pregnancy **X,** lactation, active liver disease

Precautions: Past liver disease, alcoholism, severe acute infections, trauma, hypotension, uncontrolled seizure disorders, severe metabolic disorders, electrolyte imbalances, visual condition, children

Pharmacokinetics

Absorption	Poorly absorbed, erratic
Distribution	Crosses placenta, blood-brain barrier
Metabolism	Liver, extensively
Excretion	Feces, kidneys
Half-life	3-4 hr

Pharmacodynamics

Onset	Unknown
Peak	2-4 hr
Duration	Unknown

Interactions

Individual drugs

Cholestyramine: ↓ action of lovastatin
Clofibrate: ↑ myopathy risk
Cyclosporine: ↑ risk of myopathy
Erythromycin: ↑ risk of myopathy
Gemfibrozil: ↑ risk of myopathy
Niacin: ↑ risk of myopathy
Propranolol: ↓ antihyperlipidemic effect
Warfarin: ↑ bleeding

Food/drug

↑ Levels of lovastatin with food

Lab test interferences

↑ CPK, ↑ liver function tests

NURSING CONSIDERATIONS

Assessment

- Assess nutrition: fat, protein, carbohydrates; nutritional analysis should be completed by dietitian before treatment
- Monitor bowel pattern daily; diarrhea may be a problem
- Monitor triglycerides, fasting cholesterol LDL, HDL at baseline and throughout treatment; watch LDL and VLDL closely; if increased, drug should be discontinued
- Assess for muscle pain, tenderness, obtain CPK; if these occur, drug may need to be discontinued

Nursing diagnoses

✓ Diarrhea (adverse reactions)
✓ Knowledge deficit (teaching)
✓ Noncompliance (teaching)

Implementation

- Give with evening meal; if dosage is increased, take with breakfast and evening meal
- Store in cool environment in airtight, light-resistant container

Patient/family education

- Inform patient that compliance is needed for positive results to occur; not to double doses
- Inform patient that blood work and eye exam will be necessary during treatment
- Teach patient that risk factors should be decreased: high-fat diet, smoking, alcohol consumption, absence of exercise
- Advise patient to report if pregnancy is suspected
- Advise patient to notify prescriber if the GI symptoms of diarrhea, abdominal or epigastric pain, nausea, vomiting occur; or if chills, fever, sore throat, blurred vision, dizziness, headache, muscle pain, weakness occur
- Advise patient to stay out of the sun or use sunscreen to prevent burns

Evaluation

Positive therapeutic outcome

- Decreased cholesterol, serum triglyceride levels
- Improved ratio of HDLs

loxapine (℞)

(lox'a-peen)

Loxapac ♣, loxapine succinate, Loxitane IM, Loxitane, Loxitane-C

Func. class.: Antipsychotic/neuroleptic

Chem. class.: Dibenzoxazepine

Pregnancy category C

Action: Depresses cerebral cortex, hypothalamus, limbic system, which control activity and aggression; blocks neurotransmission produced by dopamine at synapse; exhibits strong α-adrenergic, anticholinergic blocking action; mechanism for antipsychotic effects is unclear

➔ **Therapeutic Outcome:** Decreased psychotic behavior

Uses: Psychotic disorders, nonpsychotic symptoms associated with dementia

Investigational uses: Depression, anxiety

Dosage and routes

Adult: PO 10 mg bid-qid initially; may be rapidly increased depending on severity of condition; maintenance 60-100 mg/day; IM 12.5-50 mg q4-6h or more until desired response, then start PO form

G ***Elderly:*** PO 5-10 mg qd bid, increase q4-7 days by 5-10 mg, max 125 mg

Available forms: Caps 5, 10, 25, 50 mg; conc 25 mg/ml; inj 50 mg/ml; tabs 5, 10, 25, 50 mg

Adverse effects

CNS: *Extrapyramidal symptoms (EPS): pseudoparkinsonism, akathisia, dystonia, tardive dyskinesia, drowsiness, headache,* **seizures,** confusion, **neuroleptic malignant syndrome**

CV: *Orthostatic hypotension,* **cardiac arrest,** ECG changes, tachycardia

EENT: Blurred vision, glaucoma

GI: *Dry mouth, nausea, vomiting, anorexia, constipation,* diarrhea, jaundice, weight gain

GU: Urinary retention, urinary frequency, enuresis, impotence, amenorrhea, gynecomastia

HEMA: **Anemia, leukopenia, leukocytosis, agranulocytosis**

INTEG: *Rash,* photosensitivity, dermatitis

RESP: **Laryngospasm,** dyspnea, **respiratory depression**

Contraindications: Hypersensitivity, blood dyscrasias, coma, severe CNS depression, brain damage, bone marrow depression, alcohol and barbiturate withdrawal states

Precautions: Pregnancy **C,** lactation, seizure disorders, hepatic disease, cardiac disease, prostatic hyper-

L

P G trophy, cardiac conditions, child <16 yr, glaucoma, GI obstruction, elderly

Pharmacokinetics

Absorption	Well absorbed (PO)
Distribution	Unknown
Metabolism	Liver, extensively
Excretion	Kidneys
Half-life	Biphasic 5 hr, 19 hr

Pharmacodynamics

	PO	IM
Onset	½ hr	15-30 min
Peak	2-4 hr	15-20 min
Duration	12 hr	12 hr

Interactions

Individual drugs

Alcohol: ↑ effects of both drugs, oversedation
Aluminum hydroxide: ↓ absorption
Epinephrine: ↑ toxicity
Guanadrel: ↓ antihypertensive response
Guanethidine: ↓ antihypertensive response
Magnesium hydroxide: ↓ absorption

Drug classifications

Anticholinergics: ↑ anticholinergic effects
Antidepressants: ↑ CNS depression
Antihistamines: ↑ CNS depression
Barbiturate anesthetics: ↑ CNS depression
MAOIs: ↑ CNS depression
Opiates: ↑ CNS depression
Sedative/hypnotics: ↑ CNS depression

Herb/drug

Kava: ↑ action

NURSING CONSIDERATIONS

Assessment

- Assess mental status: orientation, mood, behavior, presence and type of hallucinations before initial administration and monthly; this drug should significantly reduce psychotic behavior
- Check for swallowing of PO medication; check for hoarding or giving of medication to other patients
- Monitor I&O ratio; palpate bladder if low urinary output occurs, G especially in elderly; urinalysis recommended before, during prolonged therapy
- Monitor bilirubin, CBC, liver function studies monthly
- Assess affect, orientation, LOC, reflexes, gait, coordination, sleep pattern disturbances
- Monitor B/P with patient sitting, standing, and lying; take pulse and respirations q4h during initial treatment; establish baseline before starting treatment; report drops of 30 mm Hg
- Check for dizziness, faintness, palpitations, tachycardia on rising; severe orthostatic hypotension is common
- ! Identify for neuroleptic malignant syndrome: hyperpyrexia, muscle rigidity, increased CPK, altered mental status; drug should be discontinued
- Assess for EPS including akathisia (inability to sit still, no pattern to movements), tardive dyskinesia (bizarre movements of the jaw, mouth, tongue, extremities), pseudoparkinsonism (ragged tremors, pill rolling, shuffling gait); an antiparkinsonian drug should be prescribed
- Assess for constipation, urinary retention daily; if these occur, increase bulk, water in diet

Nursing diagnoses

✓ Thought processes, altered (uses)
✓ Coping, ineffective individual (uses)
✓ Knowledge deficit (teaching)
✓ Noncompliance (teaching)

Implementation

PO route

- Administer drug in liq form mixed in glass of juice or cola if hoarding is suspected; do not mix in caffeine drinks, tannics, pectins
- G Administer lowered dose in elderly, since metabolism is slowed

• Administer with full glass of water or milk; or give with food to decrease GI upset
• Store in airtight, light-resistant container, oral sol in amber bottle

IM route
• Inject deep in muscle mass; do not give SC; do not administer sol with a precipitate; amber-colored sol can be used

Patient/family education
• Teach patient to use good oral hygiene; suggest frequent rinsing of mouth, sugarless gum for dry mouth
• Caution patient to avoid hazardous activities until drug response is determined; dizziness, blurred vision may occur
• Inform patient that orthostatic hypotension occurs often and to rise from sitting or lying position gradually; to remain lying down after IM inj for at least 30 min; caution patient to avoid hot tubs, hot showers, tub baths, since hypotension may occur; tell patient that in hot weather heat stroke may occur; take extra precautions to stay cool
• Advise patient to avoid abrupt withdrawal of this drug, or EPS may result; drug should be withdrawn slowly
• Advise patient to avoid use with alcohol, CNS depressants; increased drowsiness may occur
• Advise patient to use a sunscreen and sunglasses to prevent burns
• Teach patient about EPS and necessity of meticulous oral hygiene, since oral candidiasis may occur
• Suggest patient take antacids 2 hr before or after taking this drug
• Instruct patient to report sore throat, malaise, fever, bleeding, mouth sores; if these occur, CBC should be performed and drug discontinued

Evaluation
Positive therapeutic outcome
• Decrease in emotional excitement, hallucinations, delusions, paranoia
• Reorganization of patterns of thought, speech

Treatment of overdose:
Lavage if orally ingested; barbiturates; provide airway, **IV** fluids; do not use epinephrine, which may increase hypotension

lymphocyte immune globulin, (anti-thymocyte) (℞)
Atgam
Func. class.: Immune globulins-immunosuppressant

Pregnancy category C

Action: Produces immunosuppression by inhibiting the function of T-lymphocytes

Therapeutic Outcome: Absence of transplant rejection; hematologic remission (aplastic anemia)

L

Uses: Organ transplants to prevent rejection, aplastic anemia

Investigational uses: Multiple sclerosis, myasthenia gravis, immunosuppressant in liver, bone marrow, heart and other organ transplants, pure red cell aplasia, scleroderma

Dosage and routes
Adult: **IV** 10-30 mg/kg/day

P ***Child:*** **IV** 5-25 mg/kg/day

Available forms: Inj 50 mg horse gamma globulin/ml

Adverse effects
Renal transplant
CNS: Fever, chills, headache, dizziness, weakness, faintness, seizures
CV: Chest pain, hypertension, tachycardia
GI: Diarrhea, nausea, vomiting, epigastric pain
INTEG: Rash, pruritus, urticaria, wheal
SYST: Anaphylaxis

Aplastic anemia

CNS: Fever, chills, headache, seizures, light-headedness, encephalitis, postviral encephalopathy
CV: Bradycardia, myocarditis, irregularity
GI: Nausea, LFT abnormality

Contraindications: Hypersensitivity

Precautions: Severe renal disease, severe hepatic disease, pregnancy **C**, P lactation, children

Pharmacokinetics	
Absorption	Unknown
Distribution	Unknown
Metabolism	Unknown
Excretion	Unknown
Half-life	5.7 days

Pharmacodynamics	
Onset	Rapid
Peak	Unknown
Duration	Unknown

Interactions

None known

NURSING CONSIDERATIONS

Assessment

- Assess for infection, if infection occurs evaluation will be needed to continue treatment
- Monitor renal studies: BUN, creatinine at least monthly during treatment, 3 mo after treatment
- Monitor liver function studies: alkaline phosphatase, AST, ALT, bilirubin

Nursing diagnoses

✓ Mobility, impaired (uses)
✓ Infection, risk for (uses)
✓ Knowledge deficit (teaching)

Implementation

IV **IV route**

- Do not infuse <4 hr

Delay of renal allograft rejection
Adult: **IV** 15 mg/kg/day × 14 days, then qod × 14 days for a total of 21 doses in 28 days

Aplastic anemia
Adult: **IV** 10-20 mg/kg/day × 8-14 days

- Keep emergency equipment nearby for severe allergic reactions
- Skin testing must be completed before treatment; use intradermal inj of 0.1 ml of a 1:1000 dilution (5 μg of horse IgG) in 0.9% NaCl, if a wheal or rash >10 mm or both, use caution during inf
- Dilute in saline sol before inf; invert **IV** bag, so undiluted drug does not contact the air inside, concentration should not be >1 mg/ml

Patient/family education

- Advise patient to report fever, rash, chills, sore throat, fatigue, since serious infections may occur
- Caution patient to use contraceptive measures during treatment and for 12 wk after ending therapy; drug is teratogenic
- Caution patient to avoid crowds and persons with known infections to reduce risk of infection

Evaluation

Positive therapeutic outcome

- Absence of graft rejection
- Hematologic recovery (aplastic anemia)

magaldrate (OTC)

(mag′al-drate)

Antiflux ✤, Losopan ✤, Lowsium, Riopan, Riopan Extra Strength ✤

Func. class.: Antacid
Chem. class.: Aluminum/magnesium hydroxide

Pregnancy category C

Action: Neutralizes gastric acidity; drug is dissolved in gastric contents; this drug is a combination of aluminum and magnesium

Therapeutic Outcome: Decreased pain of ulcers

Uses: Antacid, peptic ulcer disease (adjunct), indigestion/heartburn, duodenal and gastric ulcers, reflex esophagitis, hyperacidity

Dosage and routes

Adult: SUSP 5-10 ml (400-800 mg) with water between meals, hs, not to exceed 100 ml/day

Available forms: Susp 540 mg/5 ml; liq 540 mg/5 ml

Adverse effects

GI: Constipation, diarrhea
META: Hypermagnesemia, hypophosphatemia

Contraindications: Hypersensitivity to this drug or aluminum products

G **Precautions:** Elderly, fluid restriction, decreased GI motility, GI obstruction, dehydration, renal disease, sodium-restricted diets, pregnancy **C**

Pharmacokinetics

Absorption	Not absorbed
Distribution	Not distributed
Metabolism	Not metabolized
Excretion	Kidneys
Half-life	Unknown

Pharmacodynamics

Onset	Unknown
Peak	½ hr
Duration	1 hr

Interactions

Individual drugs

Chlordiazepoxide: ↓ absorption of chlordiazapoxide
Cimetidine: ↓ absorption of cimetidine
Ketoconazole: ↓ effect of ketoconazole
Phenytoin: ↓ absorption of phenytoin
Tetracycline: ↓ effect of tetracycline

Drug classifications

Anticholinergics: ↓ absorption of anticholinergics
Corticosteroids: ↓ absorption of corticosteroids
Iron salts: ↓ absorption of iron salts
Phenothiazines: ↓ absorption of phenothiazines
Salicylates: ↓ absorption of salicylates

NURSING CONSIDERATIONS

Assessment

- Assess GI status: location of pain, intensity, characteristics, what aggravates, ameliorates pain; heartburn/indigestion; hematemesis
- Monitor serum magnesium, calcium, phosphate, potassium if using long term or with impaired renal function
- Assess for constipation: increase bulk in diet if needed or obtain order for stool softener

Nursing diagnoses

✓ Pain (uses)
✓ Knowledge deficit (teaching)

Implementation

- Give laxatives or stool softeners if constipation occurs
- Give susp after shaking; give between meals and hs
- Give when stomach is empty pc and hs

Patient/family education

- Advise patient to separate ingestion of enteric-coated drugs and antacid by 2 hr
- Advise patient to use 2 wk or less; drug should not be used for long periods
- Teach patient to notify prescriber immediately if coffee-ground emesis, emesis with frank blood, or black tarry stools occur

Evaluation

Positive therapeutic outcome

- Absence of abdominal pain
- Decreased acidity

M

magnesium chloride (OTC)

Chloromag, Slo-Mag

magnesium citrate (OTC)

Citrate of Magnesia, Citroma, Citromag ✱, Evac-Q-Mag

magnesium hydroxide (OTC)

Phillips Magnesium Tablets, Phillips Milk of Magnesia, MOM

magnesium oxide (OTC)

Mag-Ox 400, Maox, Uro-Mag

magnesium salts (OTC)

(mag-neez'ee-um)

HIGH ALERT

magnesium sulfate (OTC)

Epsom Salt

Func. class.: Laxative, saline; antacid

Pregnancy category A

Action: Increases osmotic pressure, draws fluid into colon, neutralizes HCl

➔ **Therapeutic Outcome:** Magnesium levels WNL, absence of constipation

Uses: Constipation, bowel preparation before surgery or exam, electrolyte, anticonvulsant

Dosage and routes

Laxative

Adult: PO 30-60 ml hs (Milk of Magnesia), 300 mg

P ***Adult and child >6 yr:*** PO 15 g in 8 oz of H_2O (magnesium sulfate); PO 10-20 ml (Concentrated Milk of Magnesia); PO 5-10 oz hs (magnesium citrate)

P ***Child 2-6 yr:*** 5-15 ml (Milk of Magnesia)

Prevention of magnesium deficiency

P ***Adult and child ≥10 yr:*** PO male: 270-400 mg/day; female: 280-300 mg/day; lactation: 335-350 mg/day; pregnancy 320 mg/day

P ***Child 8-10 yr:*** PO 170 mg/day

P ***Child 4-7 yr:*** PO 120 mg/day

P ***Infant to 4 yr:*** 40-80 mg/day

Deficiency

Adult: PO 200-400 mg in divided doses tid-qid; IM 1 g q6h × 4 doses; **IV** 5 g (severe)

P ***Child 6-12 yr:*** 3-6 mg/kg/day in divided doses tid-qid

Preeclampsia/eclampsia magnesium sulfate

Adult: IM/**IV** 4-5 g **IV** inf; with 5 g IM in each gluteus, then 5 g q4h or 4 g **IV** inf then 1-2 g/hr cont inf

Available forms: *Chloride:* sus rel tabs 535 mg (64 mg Mg); enteric tabs 833 mg (100 mg Mg) *Hydroxide:* liq 400 mg/5 ml (164 mg Mg/5 ml); conc liq 800 mg/5 ml (328 mg Mg/5 ml); chew tabs 300 mg (130 Mg); chew tabs 300, 600 mg
Oxide: tabs 400 mg (241.3 mg Mg); caps 140 mg (84.5 mg Mg)
Sulfate: powder for oral; bulk packages; Epsom salts, bulk packages; inj 10, 12.5, 25, 50%

Adverse effects

CNS: Muscle weakness, flushing, sweating, confusion, sedation, depressed reflexes, **flaccidity, paralysis, hypothermia**

CV: Hypotension, heart block, **circulatory collapse**

GI: *Nausea, vomiting, anorexia, cramps*

META: Electrolyte, fluid imbalances

Contraindications: Hypersensitivity, renal diseases, abdominal pain, nausea/vomiting, obstruction, acute surgical abdomen, rectal bleeding

Precautions: Pregnancy **A**

Pharmacokinetics	
PO	Onset 3-6 hr
IM	Onset 1 hr, duration 4 hr
IV	Duration ½ hr

Interactions
Drug classifications
Antiinfectives, other: ↓ absorption
Neuromuscular blockers: ↑ effect
Tetracyclines: ↓ absorption

NURSING CONSIDERATIONS
Assessment
- Assess I&O ratio; check for decrease in urinary output
- Assess cause of constipation; lack of fluids, bulk, exercise
- Assess cramping, rectal bleeding, nausea, vomiting; drug should be discontinued
- Assess Mg toxicity: thirst, confusion, decrease in reflexes
- Assess visual changes: blurring, halos, corneal and retinal damage
- Assess edema in feet, ankles, legs
- Assess prior drug history; there are many drug interactions

Implementation
PO route
- Administer with 8 oz of H_2O
- Refrigerate magnesium citrate before administration
- Shake susp before using
- Give as antacid at least 2 hr pc
- Administer to patient crushed or whole; chewable tablets may be chewed
- Administer with food or milk to decrease gastric symptoms; give 30 min before or 2 hr after antacids

IV route
- Administer only when calcium gluconate available for magnesium toxicity
- Administer **IV** undiluted 1.5 ml of 10% sol over 1 min; may dilute to 20% sol, infuse over 3 hr
- Administer **IV** at less than 150 mg/min; circulatory collapse may occur

Y-site compatibilities: Acyclovir, aldesleukin, amifostine, amikacin, ampicillin, aztreonam, cefamandole, cefazolin, cefmetazole, cefoperazone, cefotaxime, cefoxitin, cephalothin, cephapirin, chloramphenicol, cisatracurium, clindamycin, dobutamine, doxycycline, doxorubicin liposome, enalaprilat, erythromycin, esmolol, famotidine, fludarabine, gallium, gentamicin, granisetron, heparin, hydrocortisone, hydromorphone, idarubicin, insulin, kanamycin, labetalol, meperidine, metronidazole, minocycline, morphine, moxalactam, nafcillin, ondansetron, oxacillin, paclitaxel, penicillin G potassium, piperacillin, piperacillin/tazobactam, potassium chloride, propofol, remifentanil, sargramostim, thiotepa, ticarcillin, tobramycin, trimethoprim/sulfamethoxazole, vancomycin, vit B complex/C

Additive compatibilities: Calcium gluconate, cephalothin, chloramphenicol, cisplatin, heparin, hydrocortisone, isoproterenol, meropenem, methyldopate, norepinephrine, penicillin G potassium, potassium phosphate, verapamil

Patient/family education
- Inform patient to report any symptoms of hepatotoxicity, renal toxicity, visual changes, ototoxicity, allergic reactions, bleeding (long-term therapy)
- Inform patient not to exceed recommended dosage; acute poisoning may result
- Inform patient to read label on other OTC drugs; many contain aspirin
- Inform patient that therapeutic response takes 2 wk (arthritis)
- Inform patient to avoid alcohol ingestion; GI bleeding may occur
- Inform patient that if anticoagulants are given with this drug, both should be discontinued 2 wk before surgery

M

Evaluation

Positive therapeutic outcomes

- Decreased pain, fever

Treatment of overdose:

Lavage, activated charcoal, monitor electrolytes, VS

mannitol (℞)

(man'i-tole)

mannitol, Osmitrol, Resectisol

Func. class.: Osmotic diuretic

Chem. class.: Hexahydric alcohol

Pregnancy category C

Action: Increases osmolarity of glomerular filtrate, which raises osmotic pressure of fluid in renal tubules; there is a decrease in reabsorption of water, electrolytes; increases in urinary output, sodium, chloride, potassium, calcium, phosphorus, uric acid, urea, magnesium

Uses: Edema; promote systemic diuresis in cerebral edema, decrease intraocular pressure, improve renal function in acute renal failure, chemical poisoning

Dosage and routes

Oliguria, prevention

Adult: **IV** 50-100 g of a 5%-25% sol, may use test dose 0.2 g/kg over 3-5 min

Oliguria, treatment

Adult: **IV** 300-400 mg/kg of a 20%-25% sol up to 100 g of a 15%-20% sol over 30-60 min

P ***Child:*** **IV** 0.25-2 g/kg as a 15%-20% sol, run over 2-6 hr

Intraocular pressure/ICP

Adult: **IV** 1.5-2 g/kg of a 15%-25% sol over 30-60 min

P ***Child:*** **IV** 1-2 g/kg (30-60 g/m^2) as a 15%-20% sol run over 30-60 min

Renal failure

Adult: **IV** 50-200 g/24 hr, adjusting to maintain output of 30-50 mg/hr

Diuresis in drug intoxication

P ***Adult and child >12 yr:*** 5%-10% sol continuously up to 200 g **IV**, while maintaining 100-500 ml urine output/hr

Available forms: Inj 5%, 10%, 15%, 20%, 25%; GU irrigation 5%

Adverse effects

CNS: Dizziness, headache, *seizures,* **rebound increased ICP,** confusion

CV: Edema, hypotension, hypertension, **tachycardia, CHF,** thrombophlebitis

EENT: Loss of hearing, blurred vision, nasal congestion, decreased intraocular pressure

ELECT: Fluid, electrolyte imbalances, **acidosis,** electrolyte loss, dehydration

GI: *Nausea, vomiting,* dry mouth, diarrhea

GU: Marked diuresis, urinary retention, thirst

RESP: Pulmonary congestion

Contraindications: Active intracranial bleeding, hypersensitivity, anuria, severe pulmonary congestion, edema, severe dehydration, progressive heart disease, renal failure

Precautions: Dehydration, pregnancy **C,** severe renal disease, CHF, lactation

Pharmacokinetics	
Absorption	Complete
Distribution	Extracellular spaces
Metabolism	Minimal
Excretion	Renal
Half-life	100 min

Pharmacodynamics	
Onset	½-1 hr
Peak	1 hr
Duration	6-8 hr

Interactions

Individual drugs

EDTA: ↑ effects

Lithium: ↓ action, ↑ excretion

Food/drug
Potassium foods: ↑ hyperkalemia
Lab test interferences
Interference: Inorganic phosphorus, ethylene glycol

NURSING CONSIDERATIONS
Assessment
- Assess neurologic status: LOC, ICP reading, pupil size and reaction when drug is given for increased ICP
- Assess for visual changes or eye discomfort or pain before and during treatment; (increases intraocular pressure); neurologic checks, ICP during treatment (increased ICP)
- Assess patient for tinnitus, hearing loss, ear pain; periodic testing of hearing is needed when high doses of this drug are given by **IV** route
- Monitor manifestations of hypokalemia: acidic urine, reduced urine osmolality, nocturia, polyuria, polydipsia; hypotension, broad T wave, U wave, ectopy, tachycardia, weak pulse; muscle weakness, altered LOC, drowsiness, apathy, lethargy, confusion, depression; anorexia, nausea, cramps, constipation, distention, paralytic ileus; hypoventilation, respiratory muscle weakness
- Monitor for manifestations of hyponatremia: increased B/P, cold, clammy skin, hypovolemia or hypervolemia; anorexia, nausea, vomiting, diarrhea, abdominal cramps; lethargy, increased ICP, confusion, headache, seizures, coma, fatigue, tremors, hyperreflexia
- Assess fluid volume status: check I&O ratios and record hourly urine values, CVP, breath sounds, weight, distended red veins, crackles in lung, color, quality and sp gr of urine, skin turgor, adequacy of pulses, moist mucous membranes, bilateral lung sounds, peripheral pitting edema
- Assess for dehydration; symptoms of decreasing output, thirst, hypotension, dry mouth and mucous membranes should be reported
- Monitor electrolytes: potassium, sodium, calcium, magnesium; also include BUN, ABGs, CVP, PAP, CBC; regularly monitor serum and urine levels of sodium and potassium
- Assess B/P before and during therapy with patient lying, standing, and sitting as appropriate; orthostatic hypotension can occur rapidly
- Monitor for rebound ICP: headache, confusion

Nursing diagnoses
✓ Urinary elimination, altered (adverse reactions)
✓ Fluid volume deficit (adverse reactions)
✓ Fluid volume excess (uses)
✓ Knowledge deficit (teaching)

Implementation
- Administer potassium replacement if potassium level is less than 3 mg/ml
- Use an in-line filter for 15%, 20%, 25% give with infusion pump; check **IV** patency at infusion site before and during administration; do not use sol that is yellow or has a precipitate or crystals; to redissolve, run bottle in hot water and shake vigorously; cool to body temp before giving
- Run at 30-50 ml/hr in oliguria
- Run over 30-60 min in increased ICP
- Run over 30 min for intraocular pressure; 60-90 min after surgery

Irrigation
- Use 100 ml of 25%/900 ml of sterile water for inj (2.5% sol)

Y-*site compatibilities:*
Allopurinol, amifostine, aztreonam, cladribine, fludarabine, fluorouracil, gallium, idarubicin, melphalan, ondansetron, paclitaxel, piperacillin, propofol, sargramostim, teniposide, thiotepa, vinorelbine

Y-*site incompatibilities:*
Amsacrine, bleomycin, doxorubicin, fluconazole, gentamicin, quinidine, vinblastine, vincristine

M

Additive compatibilities: Amikacin, bretylium, cefamandole, cefoxitin, cimetidine, cisplatin, dopamine, fosphenytoin, furosemide, gentamicin, metoclopramide, netilmicin, nizatidine, ofloxacin, ondansetron, sodium bicarbonate, tobramycin, verapamil

Additive incompatibilities: Blood, blood products, imipenem/cilastatin, potassium chloride, sodium chloride

Patient/family education

- Teach patient reason for and method of treatment

Evaluation

Positive therapeutic outcome

- Decreased intraocular pressure
- Prevention of hypokalemia (diuretic use)
- Decreased edema
- Decreased ICP
- Increased diuresis of >30 ml/hr
- Increased excretion of toxic substances

Treatment of overdose: Discontinue inf, correct fluid, electrolyte imbalances, hemodialysis, monitor hydration, CV, renal function

mebendazole (℞)

(me-ben'da-zole)

Vermox

Func. class.: Anthelmintic

Chem. class.: Carbamate

Pregnancy category C

Action: Inhibits glucose uptake, degeneration of cytoplasmic microtubules in the cell; interferes with absorption, secretory function

➡ **Therapeutic Outcome:** Parasite, cyst, egg death

Uses: Infestation with pinworms, roundworms, hookworms, whipworms, threadworms, pork tapeworms, dwarf tapeworms, beef tapeworms; hydatid cyst

Dosage and routes

P ***Adult and child >2 yr:*** PO 100 mg as a single dose (pinworms) or bid × 3 days (whip-, round-, or hookworms); course may be repeated in 3 wk if needed

Available forms: Chew tab 100 mg

Adverse effects

CNS: Dizziness, fever, headache

GI: Transient diarrhea, abdominal pain, nausea, vomiting

Contraindication: Hypersensitivity

P **Precautions:** Child <2 yr, lactation, pregnancy **C** (1st trimester)

Pharmacokinetics	
Absorption	Minimal
Distribution	Highly bound to plasma proteins
Metabolism	Liver
Excretion	Feces in metabolites (>95%); urine, unchanged
Half-life	2½-9 hr; increased in hepatic disease

Pharmacodynamics	
Onset	Unknown
Peak	½-7 hr
Duration	Unknown

Interactions

Individual drugs

Carbamazepine: ↓ effect of mebendazole

Drug classifications

Hydantoins: ↓ effect of hydantoins

Food/drug

High-fat foods: ↑ absorption

NURSING CONSIDERATIONS

Assessment

- Assess stools during entire treatment, also 1-3 wk after treatment is completed; specimens must be sent to lab while still warm; monitor for

diarrhea during expulsion of worms; avoid self-contamination with patient's feces
- Assess for allergic reaction: rash (rare)
- Identify infestation in other family members, since transmission from person to person is common
- If pinworms are suspected, place a piece of cellophane tape over the anal area at night for 1 wk after treatment at night to identify ova; negative perianal swabs taken every AM for 3 days confirm that the patient is no longer infested
- Monitor blood studies: AST, ALT, alkaline phosphatase, BUN, CBC during treatment

Nursing diagnoses
✓ Infection, risk for (uses)
✓ Knowledge deficit (teaching)

Implementation
- Tabs may be chewed or crushed and mixed with food if patient is unable to swallow whole
- Give PO after meals to avoid GI symptoms, since absorption is not decreased by food
- Give second course after 3 wk if needed; usually recommended (pinworms)
- Store in airtight container

Patient/family education
- Teach patient proper hygiene after bowel movements, including hand-washing technique; tell patient to avoid putting fingers in mouth; clean fingernails
- Advise patient that infested person should sleep alone; do not shake bed linen; wash bed linen daily in hot water; change and wash undergarments daily; that all members of the family should be treated (pinworms)
- Advise patient to clean toilet daily with disinfectant (green soap sol)
- Inform patient that compliance is needed with dosage schedule, duration of treatment
- Tell patient to wear shoes, wash all fruits and vegetables well before eating, use commercial fruit and vegetable cleaner solution

Evaluation
Positive therapeutic outcome
- Expulsion of worms
- Three negative stool cultures after completion of treatment

mechlorethamine (℞)
(me-klor-eth'a-meen)
Mustargen, nitrogen mustard
Func. class.: Antineoplastic alkylating agent
Chem. class.: Nitrogen mustard
Pregnancy category D

Action: Alkylates DNA, RNA; inhibits enzymes that allow synthesis of amino acids in proteins; activity is not cell cycle phase specific; a vesicant

➔ **Therapeutic Outcome:** Prevention of rapidly growing malignant cells

Uses: Hodgkin's disease, lymphomas, leukemias, lymphosarcoma; ovarian, breast, lung carcinoma; neoplastic effusions

Dosage and routes
Adult: **IV** 0.4 mg/kg as 1 dose or 2-4 divided doses over 2-4 days; second course after 3 wk depending on blood cell count

Neoplastic effusions
Adult: Intracavity 0.4 mg/kg

Available forms: Inj 10 mg/vial

Adverse effects
CNS: *Headache, dizziness, drowsiness, paresthesia,* peripheral neuropathy, **coma**
EENT: Tinnitus, hearing loss
GI: *Nausea, vomiting, diarrhea, stomatitis, weight loss,* colitis, **hepatotoxicity**
HEMA: **Thrombocytopenia, leukopenia, agranulocytosis,** anemia
INTEG: *Alopecia,* pruritus, herpes zoster, extravasation

M

Contraindications: Lactation, pregnancy **D**, myelosuppression, acute herpes zoster

Precautions: Radiation therapy, chronic lymphocytic leukopenia

Pharmacokinetics

Absorption	Complete (**IV**)
Distribution	Unknown
Metabolism	Tissues/fluids
Excretion	Kidneys
Half-life	Unknown

Pharmacodynamics

	IV
Onset	1 day
Peak	1-2 wk
Duration	1-3 wk

Interactions

Individual drugs

Radiation: ↑ toxicity, bone marrow suppression

Drug classifications

Antineoplastics: ↑ toxicity, bone marrow suppression

Bone marrow–suppressing drugs: ↑ bone marrow suppression

Live virus vaccines: ↑ adverse reactions, ↓ antibody reaction

Lab test interferences

↑ Uric acid

NURSING CONSIDERATIONS

Assessment

- Monitor CBC, differential, platelet count weekly; withhold drug if WBC is <1000/mm³ or platelet count is <75,000/mm³; notify prescriber of results if WBC <20,000/mm³, platelets <150,000/mm³; recovery of WBC platelets within 20 days
- Monitor pulmonary function tests, chest x-ray films before, during therapy; chest film should be obtained q2 wk during treatment; assess for dyspnea, rales, unproductive cough, chest pain, tachypnea
- Assess for increased uric acid levels, swelling, joint pain primarily in extremities; patient should be well hydrated to prevent urate deposits
- Monitor renal function studies: BUN, serum uric acid, urine CrCl before, during therapy; I&O ratio; report fall in urine output of 30 ml/hr; for decreased hyperuricemia
- Monitor for cold, fever, sore throat (may indicate beginning of infection); identify edema in feet, joint and stomach pain, shaking; prescriber should be notified
- Assess for bleeding: hematuria, guaiac, bruising or petechiae, mucosa or orifices q8h; no rec temp

Nursing diagnoses

- ✓ Injury, risk for (adverse reactions)
- ✓ Body image disturbance (adverse reactions)
- ✓ Infection, risk for (adverse reactions)
- ✓ Knowledge deficit (teaching)

Implementation

- Give fluids **IV** or PO before chemotherapy to hydrate patient
- Give antacid before oral agent; give drug after evening meal, before hs; administer antiemetic 30-60 min before giving drug and prn to prevent vomiting; give antibiotics for prophylaxis of infection
- Give top or systemic analgesics for pain
- Give in AM so drug can be eliminated before hs
- Use a liq diet: carbonated beverages; gelatin may be added if patient is not nauseated or vomiting

IV route

- Give **IV** after diluting 10 mg/10 ml sterile water or 0.9% NaCl; leave needle in vial, shake, withdraw dose, give through Y-tube or 3-way stopcock or directly over 3-5 min into running **IV** of 0.9% NaCl

Y-site compatibilities:

Amifostine, aztreonam, filgrastim, fludarabine, granisetron, melphalan, ondansetron, sargramostim, teniposide, vinorelbine

Additive incompatibilities: Methohexital

Solution incompatibilities: D_5W, 0.9% NaCl (**IV** only)

Intracavity route

- Further dilute in 100 ml of 0.9% NaCl; administration is completed by prescriber
- Watch for infiltration; if infiltration occurs, infiltrate area with isotonic sodium thiosulfate or 1% lidocaine; apply ice for 6-12 hr

Patient/family education

- Teach patient to avoid use of products containing aspirin or ibuprofen, razors, commercial mouthwash, since bleeding may occur; to report symptoms of bleeding (hematuria, tarry stools)
- Teach patient to report signs of anemia (fatigue, headache, irritability, faintness, shortness of breath)
- Advise patient to report any changes in breathing or coughing even several mo after treatment; to avoid crowds and persons with respiratory tract or other infections
- Tell patient hair loss is common; discuss the use of wigs or hairpieces
- Caution patient not to have any vaccinations without the advice of the presciber, serious reactions can occur
- Advise patient that contraception is needed during treatment and for several mo after the completion of therapy
- Have patient rinse mouth tid-qid with water, club soda; brush teeth bid-qid with soft brush or cotton-tipped applicators for stomatitis; use unwaxed dental floss

Evaluation

Positive therapeutic outcome

- Decreased size of tumor
- Decreased spread of malignancy
- Improved blood values
- Absence of sweating at night
- Increased appetite, increased weight

medroxyprogesterone (℞)

(me-drox-ee-proe-jess'te-rone)

Amen, Curretab, Cycrin, Depo-Provera, medroxyprogesterone, Provera

Func. class.: Hormone—progestogen; contraceptive; antineoplastic

Chem. class.: Progesterone derivative

Pregnancy category X

Action: Inhibits secretion of pituitary gonadotropins, which prevents follicular maturation and ovulation; stimulates growth of mammary tissue; antineoplastic action against endometrial cancer

➔ Therapeutic Outcome: Decreased abnormal uterine bleeding, absence of amenorrhea

Uses: Uterine bleeding (abnormal), secondary amenorrhea, endometrial cancer, renal cancer, contraceptive, prevention of endometrial changes associated with estrogen replacement therapy (ERT)

Investigational uses: Pickwickian syndrome, sleep apnea, hypersomnolence

Dosage and routes

Secondary amenorrhea

Adult: PO 5-10 mg qd × 5-10 days

Endometrial/renal cancer

Adult: IM 400-1000 mg/wk; may repeat q wk, dose may be decreased after adequate response

Uterine bleeding

Adult: PO 5-10 mg qd × 5-10 days starting on 16th or 21st day of menstrual cycle

Contraceptive

Adult: Inj q3 mo

M

With ERT

Adult: PO monophasic 2.5 mg qd; biphasic 5 mg days 15-28 of cycle

Available forms: Tabs 2.5, 5, 10, 100 mg; inj susp 50, 100, 150, 400 mg/ml; contraceptive injectable

Adverse effects

CNS: Dizziness, headache, migraines, depression, fatigue

CV: Hypotension, thrombophlebitis, edema, **thromboembolism, stroke, pulmonary embolism, MI**

EENT: Diplopia

GI: *Nausea,* vomiting, anorexia, cramps, increased weight, **cholestatic jaundice**

GU: Amenorrhea, cervical erosion, breakthrough bleeding, dysmenorrhea, vaginal candidiasis, breast changes, *gynecomastia, testicular atrophy, impotence,* endometriosis, **spontaneous abortion**

INTEG: Rash, urticaria, acne, hirsutism, alopecia, oily skin, seborrhea, purpura, melasma, photosensitivity

META: Hyperglycemia

SYST: **Angioedema, anaphylaxis**

Contraindications: Breast cancer, hypersensitivity, thromboembolic disorders, reproductive cancer, genital bleeding (abnormal, undiagnosed), pregnancy **X**

Precautions: Lactation, hypertension, asthma, blood dyscrasias, gallbladder disease, CHF, diabetes mellitus, bone disease, depression, migraine headache, seizure disorders, hepatic disease, renal disease, family history of cancer of breast or reproductive tract

Do Not Confuse:
Amen/Ambien, medroxyprogesterone/methylprednisolone, Provera/Premarin

Pharmacokinetics

Absorption	Unknown
Distribution	Unknown
Metabolism	Unknown
Excretion	Unknown
Half-life	Unknown

Pharmacodynamics

	PO	IM
Onset	Unknown	Unknown
Peak	Unknown	Unknown
Duration	2-4 hr	Unknown

Interactions

Individual drugs

Aminoglutethimide: ↓ contraceptive effect

Bromocriptine: ↓ effectiveness

Lab test interferences

↑ Alkaline phosphatase, ↑ pregnanediol, ↑ amino acids

↓ GTT, ↓ HDL

NURSING CONSIDERATIONS

Assessment

- Assess for symptoms indicating severe allergic reaction, angioedema; have epinephrine and resuscitative equipment available
- Monitor B/P at beginning of treatment and periodically; check weight daily; notify prescriber of weekly weight gain >5 lb
- Monitor I&O ratio: be alert for decreasing urinary output, increasing edema, hypertension
- Assess liver function studies: ALT, AST, bilirubin, periodically during long-term therapy
- Assess for edema, hypertension, cardiac symptoms, jaundice
- Assess mental status: affect, mood, behavioral changes, depression

Nursing diagnoses

✓ Sexual dysfunction (uses)
✓ Tissue perfusion, altered (adverse reactions)
✓ Injury, risk for (adverse reactions)
✓ Knowledge deficit (teaching)

Implementation

PO route

- Give with food or milk to decrease GI symptoms

IM route

- Store in dark area
- Give titrated dosage; use lowest effective dosage; give oil sol deep in large muscle mass (IM); rotate sites; use after warming to dissolve crystals

Patient/family education

- Advise patients to avoid sunlight or use sunscreen; photosensitivity and melasma (brown patches on the face) can occur
- Teach patient about cushingoid symptoms
- Teach women patient to report breast lumps, vaginal bleeding, edema, jaundice, dark urine, clay-colored stools, dyspnea, headache, blurred vision, abdominal pain, numbness or stiffness in legs, chest pain; men to report impotence or gynecomastia
- Teach patient to report suspected pregnancy immediately

Evaluation

Positive therapeutic outcome

- Decreased abnormal uterine bleeding
- Absence of amenorrhea
- Prevention of pregnancy
- Arrested spread of malignant cells

megestrol (℞)

(me-jess'trole)

Megace, megestrol

Func. class.: Antineoplastic

Chem. class.: Hormone, progestin, contraceptive

Pregnancy category D (tabs), X (susp)

Action: Affects endometrium by antiluteinizing effect; this is thought to bring about cell death

Therapeutic Outcome: Prevention of rapidly growing malignant cells; weight gain, increased appetite in AIDS

Uses: Breast, endometrial, renal cell cancer; increase weight, decrease cachexia and anorexia associated with AIDS

Investigational uses: Hot flashes

Dosage and routes

Endometrial/ovarian carcinoma

Adult: PO 40-320 mg/day in divided doses

Breast carcinoma

Adult: PO 40 mg qid or 160 mg qd

Anorexia (AIDS)

Adult: PO 800 mg qd (oral susp)

Hot flashes (off-label)

Adult: PO 20 mg qd

Available forms: Tabs 20, 40 mg; oral susp 200 mg/5 ml

Adverse effects

CNS: Mood swings

CV: **Thrombophlebitis, thromboembolism**

GI: Nausea, vomiting, diarrhea, abdominal cramps, weight gain

GU: Gynecomastia, fluid retention, **hypercalcemia,** vaginal bleeding, discharge, impotence, decreased libido

INTEG: Alopecia, rash, pruritus, purpura, itching

Contraindications: Hypersensitivity, pregnancy **X** (susp), **D** (tabs)

Do Not Confuse:
Megace/Reglan

Pharmacokinetics	
Absorption	Well absorbed
Distribution	Unknown
Metabolism	Liver, completely
Excretion	Unknown
Half-life	1 hr

M

Pharmacodynamics

Onset	Several wk-mo
Peak	Unknown
Duration	1-3 days

Interactions: None

Lab test interferences

↑ Alkaline phosphatase, ↑ urinary pregnanediol, ↑ plasma amino acids

↓ HDL, ↓ GTT

False positive: Urine glucose

NURSING CONSIDERATIONS

Assessment

- Monitor effects of alopecia on body image; discuss feelings about body changes
- In AIDS patients monitor calorie counts, weight, appetite
- Assess for thrombophlebitis: pain, redness, swelling in legs; notify prescriber if these occur

Nursing diagnoses

✓ Knowledge deficit (teaching)

Implementation

- Administer with meals for GI symptoms
- Oral susp is usually used for AIDS patients

Patient/family education

- Teach patient to report any complaints or side effects to prescriber
- Advise patient that contraceptive measures must be used during and several mo after treatment; drug is teratogenic
- Explore with patient the need for wig a or hairpiece for hair loss
- Caution patient to report vaginal bleeding to prescriber
- Review with patient the need to comply with dosage schedule, not to miss or double doses; missed doses may be taken up to 1 hr before next dose
- Teach patient how to recognize signs of fluid retention, thromboembolism

Evaluation

Positive therapeutic outcome

- Decreased spread of malignant cells
- Weight gain, increased appetite in AIDS patients

meloxicam (℞)

(mel-ox'i-kam)

Mobic

Func. class.: Nonsteroidal antiinflammatory/nonopioid analgesic

Chem. class.: Oxicam

Pregnancy category C

Action: Inhibits prostaglandin synthesis by decreasing an enzyme needed for biosynthesis; analgesic, antiinflammatory, antipyretic effects

➔ **Therapeutic Outcome:** Decreased pain, swelling of joints; improved mobility

Uses: Osteoarthritis

Dosage and routes

Adult: PO 7.5 mg qd, may increase to 15 mg qd

Available forms: Tabs 7.5 mg

Adverse effects

CV: Hypertension, angina, **cardiac failure, MI,** hypotension, palpitations, **dysrhythmias,** tachycardia

CNS: Dizziness, drowsiness, tremors, headache, nervousness, malaise, fatigue, insomnia, depression, **seizures**

EENT: Tinnitus, hearing loss

GI: Pancreatitis, nausea, colitis, GERD, vomiting, diarrhea, constipation, flatulence, cramps, dry mouth, peptic ulcer, **GI bleeding, perforation**

GU: **Nephrotoxicity: dysuria, hematuria, oliguria, azotemia**

HEMA: **Blood dyscrasias,** anemia, prolonged bleeding

INTEG: Rash, urticaria, photosensitivity

SYST: **Angioedema, anaphylaxis**

Contraindications: Hypersensitivity, asthma, severe renal disease, severe hepatic disease, peptic ulcer disease, labor and delivery, lactation, CV bleeding

Precautions: Pregnancy **C**, P children, bleeding disorders, GI disorders, cardiac disorders, hypersensitivity to other antiinflammatory G agents, elderly, CrCl <25 ml/min

Pharmacokinetics

Absorption	Unknown
Distribution	Unknown
Metabolism	Liver <50%
Excretion	Breast milk, kidneys
Half-life	6 hr

Pharmacodynamics

	PO	IM
Onset	Unknown	Unknown
Peak	4-5 hr	50 min
Duration	Unknown	Unknown

Interactions

Individual drugs

Cholestyramine: ↓ action of meloxicam

Cyclosporine: ↑ nephrotoxicity

Phenytoin: ↑ action of meloxicam

Drug classifications

Aminoglycosides: ↑ action of aminoglycosides

Anticoagulants: ↑ action of anticoagulants

β-Adrenergic blockers: ↓ action of β-blockers

Diuretics: ↑ action of diuretics

Hydantoins: ↑ action of hydantoins

Salicylates: ↑ action of meloxicam

Sulfonamides: ↑ action of meloxicam

NURSING CONSIDERATIONS

Assessment

- Monitor renal, liver, blood studies: BUN, creatinine, AST, ALT, Hgb before treatment, periodically thereafter
- Assess for bleeding times; check for bruising, bleeding; test for occult blood in urine

❗ Assess for anaphylaxis and angioedema; emergency equipment should be nearby

❗ Assess for hepatic dysfunction: jaundice, yellow sclera and skin, clay-colored stools

- Assess for audiometric, ophth exam before, during, after treatment
- Assess for GI condition, hypertension, cardiac conditions

Nursing diagnoses

✓ Impaired mobility (uses)

✓ Pain (uses)

✓ Knowledge deficit (teaching)

Implementation

- May take without regard to meals, take with food for GI upset
- Store at room temp

Patient/family education

- Advise patient to report blurred vision or ringing, roaring in ears (may indicate toxicity)
- Advise patient to avoid driving, other hazardous activities if dizziness or drowsiness occurs
- Teach patient to report change in urine pattern, weight increase, edema, pain increase in joints, fever, blood in urine (indicates nephrotoxicity); to report rash, black stools, or continuing headache
- Teach patient to avoid alcohol, aspirin

Evaluation

Positive therapeutic outcome

- Decreased pain, stiffness, swelling in joints, able to move more easily

M

HIGH ALERT

melphalan (℞)
(mel'fa-lan)

Alkeran, Alkeran IV, L-Pam, phenylalanine mustard

Func. class.: Antineoplastic, alkylating agent

Chem. class.: Nitrogen mustard

Pregnancy category D

Action: Alkylates DNA, RNA; inhibits enzymes that allow synthesis of amino acids in proteins; activity is not cell cycle phase specific

➡ **Therapeutic Outcome:** Prevention of rapidly growing malignant cells

Uses: Multiple myeloma, malignant melanoma, advanced ovarian cancer

Investigational uses: Breast, testicular, prostate carcinoma; osteogenic sarcoma, chronic myelogenous leukemia

Dosage and routes

Multiple myeloma

Adult: 150 μg/kg/day × 1 wk, then 21 days off, then 50 μg/kg/day or 100-150 μg/kg/day or 250 μg/kg/day × 4 days for 2-3 wk, then 2-4 wk off, then 2-4 mg/day or 7 mg/m^2 × 5 days q5-6 wk

Ovarian carcinoma

Adult: **IV** inf 16 mg/m^2; reduce in renal insufficiency; give over 15-20 min; give at 2-wk intervals × 4 doses, then at 4-wk intervals

Available forms: Tabs 2 mg; inj 50 mg

Adverse effects

GI: *Nausea, vomiting,* stomatitis, diarrhea

GU: Amenorrhea, hyperuricemia, gonadal suppression

HEMA: **Thrombocytopenia, neutropenia, leukopenia,** anemia

INTEG: Rash, urticaria, alopecia, pruritus

RESP: **Fibrosis, dysplasia**

SYST: **Anaphylaxis,** allergic reaction

Contraindications: Lactation, pregnancy **D**, hypersensitivity to this drug or other nitrogen mustards

Precautions: Radiation therapy, bone marrow depression, infection, P renal disease, children

Pharmacokinetics

Absorption	Variable; incompletely absorbed
Distribution	Rapidly distributed
Metabolism	Bloodstream
Excretion	Kidneys, unchanged (10%)
Half-life	1½ hr

Pharmacodynamics

Unknown

Interactions

Individual drugs

Radiation: ↑ toxicity, bone marrow suppression

Drug classifications

Antineoplastics: ↑ toxicity, bone marrow suppression

Bone marrow–suppressing drugs: ↑ bone marrow suppression

Live virus vaccines: ↑ adverse reactions, ↓ antibody reaction

Lab test interferences

Increase: Uric acid

NURSING CONSIDERATIONS

Assessment

- Monitor CBC, differential, platelet count weekly; withhold drug if WBC is $<3000/mm^3$ or platelet count is $<100,000/mm^3$; notify prescriber of results if WBC $<20,000/mm^3$, platelets $<100,000/mm^3$
- Monitor pulmonary function tests, chest x-ray films before, during therapy; chest film should be obtained q2 wk during treatment; check for dyspnea, rales, unproductive cough, chest pain, tachypnea

• Assess for increased uric acid levels, swelling, joint pain primarily in extremities; patient should be well hydrated to prevent urate deposits
• Monitor renal function studies: BUN, serum uric acid, urine CrCl before, during therapy; check I&O ratio; report fall in urine output of 30 ml/hr; check for decreased hyperuricemia; monitor AST, ALT
• Monitor for cold, fever, sore throat (may indicate beginning of infection); identify edema in feet, joint and stomach pain, shaking; prescriber should be notified
• Assess for bleeding: hematuria, guaiac, bruising or petechiae, from mucosa or orifices q8h; no rec temp

Nursing diagnoses

✓ Injury, risk for (adverse reactions)
✓ Body image disturbance (adverse reactions)
✓ Infection, risk for (adverse reactions)
✓ Knowledge deficit (teaching)

Implementation

• Give fluids **IV** or PO before chemotherapy to hydrate patient
• Give antacid before oral agent; give drug after evening meal, before hs; provide antiemetic 30-60 min before giving drug and prn to prevent vomiting; give antibiotics for prophylaxis of infection
• Give in AM so drug can be eliminated before hs
• Use a liq diet: carbonated beverages; gelatin may be added if patient is not nauseated or vomiting

PO route

• Give 1 hr ac or 2 hr pc to prevent nausea/vomiting

IV **IV route**

• Give as intermittent inf: reconstitute with provided diluent (10 ml) to 5 mg/ml; shake until clear; further dilute with 0.9% NaCl to <0.45 mg/ml; give over 15 min

Y-site compatibilities:

Acyclovir, amikacin, aminophylline, ampicillin, aztreonam, bleomycin, bumetanide, buprenorphine, butorphanol, calcium gluconate, carboplatin, carmustine, cefazolin, cefepime, cefoperazone, cefotaxime, cefotetan, ceftazidime, ceftizoxime, ceftriaxone, cefuroxime, cimetidine, cisplatin, clindamycin, cyclophosphamide, cytarabine, dacarbazine, dactinomycin, daunorubicin, dexamethasone, diphenhydramine, doxorubicin, doxycycline, droperidol, enalaprilat, etoposide, famotidine, floxuridine, fluconazole, fludarabine, fluorouracil, furosemide, gallium, ganciclovir, gentamicin, granisetron, haloperidol, heparin, hydrocortisone sodium phosphate, hydromorphone, hydroxyzine, idarubicin, ifosfamide, imipenem-cilastatin, lorazepam, mannitol, mechlorethamine, meperidine, mesna, methylprednisolone, metoclopramide, methotrexate, metronidazole, miconazole, minocycline, mitomycin, mitoxantrone, morphine, nalbuphine, netilmicin, ondansetron, pentostatin, piperacillin, plicamycin, potassium chloride, prochlorperazine, promethazine, ranitidine, sodium bicarbonate, streptozocin, teniposide, thiotepa, ticarcillin, ticarcillin/clavulanate, tobramycin, trimethoprim-sulfamethoxazole, vancomycin, vinblastine, vincristine, vinorelbine, zidovudine

Patient/family education

• Teach patient to avoid use of products containing aspirin or ibuprofen, razors, commercial mouthwash, since bleeding may occur; to report symptoms of bleeding (hematuria, tarry stools)
• Instruct patient to report signs of anemia (fatigue, headache, irritability, faintness, shortness of breath)
• Instruct patient to report any changes in breathing or coughing even several mo after treatment; to avoid crowds and persons with respiratory tract or other infections

M

• Tell patient hair loss is common; discuss the use of wigs or hairpieces
• Caution patient not to have any vaccinations without the advice of the prescriber, serious reactions can occur
• Advise patient that contraception is needed during treatment and for several mo after the completion of therapy
• Teach patient to rinse mouth tid-qid with water, club soda; brush teeth bid-qid with soft brush or cotton-tipped applicators for stomatitis; use unwaxed dental floss

Evaluation
Positive therapeutic outcome
• Decreased size of tumor
• Decreased spread of malignancy

menotropins (℞)
(men-oh-troe'pinz)
HMG, Pergonal, Repronex
Func. class.: Gonadotropin
Chem. class.: Exogenous gonadotropin
Pregnancy category X

Action: In women, increases follicular growth, maturation; in men, when given with hCG, stimulates spermatogenesis; contains FSH and LH

Therapeutic Outcome: Pregnancy, ovulation

Uses: Infertility, anovulation in women; stimulates spermatogenesis in men; usually used with hCG

Dosage and routes
Infertility
Adult (men): IM 1 ampule 3 times a wk with hCG 2000 U 2 times a wk × 4 mo
Anovulation
Adult (women): IM 75 IU of FSH, LH qd × 9-12 days, then 10,000 U of hCG 1 day after these drugs; repeat × 2 menstrual cycles, then increase to 150 IU of FSH, LH qd × 9-12 days, then 10,000 U of hCG 1 day after these drugs × 2 menstrual cycles

Available forms: Powder for inj 17 IU/ampule

Adverse effects
CNS: Fever
CV: **Hypovolemia,** thrombophlebitis, **pulmonary embolism, thromboembolism**
GI: Nausea, vomiting, diarrhea, anorexia, abdominal distention/pain
GU: **Ovarian enlargement,** multiple births, ovarian hyperstimulation, sudden ovarian enlargement, ascites with or without pain, pleural effusion, gynecomastia in men
HEMA: **Hemoperitoneum, arterial thromboembolism**
RESP: **ARDS, pulmonary embolism, pulmonary infarction**
OTHER: **Anaphylaxis**

Contraindications: Primary ovarian failure, abnormal bleeding, thyroid/adrenal dysfunction, organic intracranial lesion, ovarian cysts, primary testicular failure, pregnancy **X**

Pharmacokinetics	
Absorption	Well absorbed
Distribution	Unknown
Metabolism	Unknown
Excretion	Kidneys, unchanged (8%)
Half-life	70 hr (FSH); 4 hr (LH)

Pharmacodynamics
Unknown

Interactions: None

NURSING CONSIDERATIONS
Assessment
• Monitor weight qd; notify prescriber if weight gain increases rapidly
• Monitor estrogen excretion level; if >100 μg/24 hr, drug is withheld; hyperstimulation syndrome may occur
• Monitor I&O ratio; be alert for decreasing urinary output
• Assess for ovarian enlargement,

abdominal distention/pain; report symptoms immediately

Nursing diagnoses

✓ Sexual dysfunction (uses)
✓ Knowledge deficit (teaching)

Implementation

- Give after reconstituting with 1-2 ml of sterile saline inj; use immediately

Patient/family education

- Advise patient that multiple births are possible; if pregnancy occurs, it is usually 4-6 wk after start of treatment
- Instruct patient to keep daily appointment for 2 wk during treatment

Evaluation

Positive therapeutic outcome

- Pregnancy

HIGH ALERT

meperidine (Rx)

(me-per'i-deen)

Demerol, meperidine HCl, Pethandol, Pethidine

Func. class.: Opiate analgesic

Chem. class.: Phenylpiperidine derivative

Pregnancy category B

Controlled substance schedule II

Action: Depresses pain impulse transmission at the spinal cord level by interacting with opioid receptors; produces CNS depression

Therapeutic Outcome: Relief of pain

Uses: Moderate to severe pain, preoperatively, during labor

Dosage and routes

Pain

Adult: PO/SC/IM 50-150 mg q3-4h prn; dosage should be decreased if given **IV**

P *Child:* PO/SC/IM 1 mg/kg q3-4h prn, not to exceed 100 mg q4h

Preoperatively

Adult: IM/SC 50-100 mg q30-90 min before surgery; dosage should be reduced if given **IV**

P *Child:* IM/SC 1-2.2 mg/kg 30-90 min before surgery

Renal dose

CrCl 10-50 ml/min 75% of dose; CrCl <10 ml/min 50% of dose

Labor analgesia

Adult: SC/IM 50-100 mg given when contractions are regulary spaced, repeat q1-3h prn

Available forms: Inj 10, 25, 50, 75, 100 mg/ml; tabs 50, 100 mg; syrup 50 mg/5 ml

Adverse effects

CNS: Drowsiness, dizziness, confusion, headache, sedation, euphoria, **increased ICP, seizures**

CV: Palpitations, bradycardia, change in B/P, tachycardia (**IV**)

EENT: Tinnitus, blurred vision, miosis, diplopia, depressed corneal reflex

GI: Nausea, vomiting, anorexia, constipation, cramps

GU: Urinary retention, dysuria

INTEG: Rash, urticaria, bruising, flushing, diaphoresis, pruritus

***RESP:* Respiratory depression**

Contraindications: Hypersensitivity, addiction (opiate)

Precautions: Addictive personality, pregnancy **B,** lactation, increased ICP, MI (acute), severe heart disease, respiratory depression, hepatic disease, renal disease, P child <18 yr, G elderly

Do Not Confuse: Demerol/Dilaudid, meperidine/hydromorphone

M

Pharmacokinetics

Absorption	Well absorbed (IM, SC); 50% (PO)
Distribution	Widely distributed; crosses placenta
Metabolism	Liver, extensively
Excretion	Kidneys; breast milk
Half-life	3-4 hr

Pharmacodynamics

	PO	IM/SC	IV
Onset	15 min	10 min	Rapid
Peak	½-1 hr	½-1 hr	5-7 min
Duration	2-4 hr	2-4 hr	2-4 hr

Interactions

Individual drugs

Alcohol: ↑ respiratory depression, hypotension, sedation
Cimetidine: ↑ recovery
Chlorpromazine: ↑ adverse ractions
Erythromycin: ↑ recovery
Nalbuphine: ↓ analgesia
Pentazocine: ↓ analgesia
Phenytoin: ↓ meperidine effect
Procarbazine: Fatal reaction, do not use together

Drug classifications

Antihistamines: ↑ respiratory depression, hypotension
Barbiturates: ↑ respiratory depression
CNS depressants: ↑ respiratory depression, hypotension
MAOIs: Do not use for 2 wk before taking meperidine
Phenothiazines: ↑ respiratory depression, hypotension
Protease inhibitor antiretrovirals: ↑ adverse reactions
Sedative/hypnotics: ↑ respiratory depression, hypotension

Lab test interferences

↑ Amylase

NURSING CONSIDERATIONS

Assessment

- Assess pain: location, duration, intensity before and 1 hr after administration
- Assess renal function before initiating therapy; poor renal function can lead to accumulation of toxic metabolite and seizures
- Monitor VS after parenteral route; note muscle rigidity, drug history, liver, kidney function tests, respiratory dysfunction: respiratory depression, character, rate, rhythm; notify prescriber if respirations are <10/min
- Monitor CNS changes: dizziness, drowsiness, hallucinations, euphoria, LOC, pupil reaction; these are due to metabolite produced
- Monitor allergic reactions: rash, urticaria

Nursing diagnoses

- ✓ Pain (uses)
- ✓ Sensory perceptual alteration: visual, auditory (adverse reactions)
- ✓ Breathing pattern, ineffective (adverse reactions)
- ✓ Injury, risk for (adverse reactions)
- ✓ Knowledge deficit (teaching)

Implementation

- Give with antiemetic if nausea, vomiting occur
- Administer when pain is beginning to return; determine dosage interval by patient response; continuous dosing of medication is more effective given prn
- Medication should be slowly withdrawn after long-term use to prevent withdrawal symptoms
- Store in light-resistant container at room temp

PO route

- May be given with food or milk to lessen GI upset
- Syrup should be mixed with 4 oz of water

IM/SC route

- Do not give if cloudy or a precipitate has formed
- Patient should remain recumbent for 1 hr after administration

IV IV route

- Give by direct **IV** after diluting to 10 mg/ml with sterile water, 0.9% NaCl for inj; give slowly at 25 mg/1 min; rapid administration may cause respiratory depression, hypotension, circulatory collapse

• Give cont inf after diluting to 1 mg/ml with D_5W, $D_{10}W$, dextrose/saline combinations, dextrose/Ringer's, inj combinations, 0.45% NaCl, 0.9% NaCl, Ringer's, LR; give by infusion pump; titrate according to response

Syringe compatibilities: Atropine, benzquinamide, butorphanol, chlorpromazine, cimetidine, dimenhydrinate, diphenhydramine, droperidol, fentanyl, glycopyrrolate, hydroxyzine, ketamine, metoclopramide, midazolam, pentazocine, perphenazine, prochlorperazine, promazine, promethazine, ranitidine, scopolamine

Syringe incompatibilities: Heparin, morphine, pentobarbital

Y-site compatibilities: Amifostine, amikacin, ampicillin, atenolol, aztreonam, bumetanide, cefamandole, cefazolin, cefmetazole, cefotaxime, cefotetan, cefoxitin, ceftazidime, ceftizoxime, ceftriaxone, cefuroxime, cephalothin, cephapirin, chloramphenicol, cladribine, clindamycin, dexamethasone, diltiazem, diphenhydramine, dobutamine, dopamine, doxycycline, droperidol, erythromycin lactobionate, famotidine, filgrastim, fluconazole, fludarabine, gallium, gentamicin, granisetron, heparin, hydrocortisone, regular insulin, kanamycin, labetalol, lidocaine, magnesium sulfate, melphalan, methyldopate, methylprednisolone, metoclopramide, metoprolol, metronidazole, moxalactam, ondansetron, oxacillin, oxytocin, paclitaxel, penicillin G potassium, piperacillin, potassium chloride, propofol, propranolol, ranitidine, sargramostim, teniposide, thiotepa, ticarcillin, ticarcillin/clavulanate, tobramycin, trimethoprim/sulfamethoxazole, vancomycin, verapamil, vinorelbine

Y-site incompatibilities: Cefoperazone, idarubicin, imipenem/cilastatin, mezlocillin, minocycline

Additive compatibilities: Cefazolin, dobutamine, ondansetron, scopolamine, succinylcholine, triflupromazine, verapamil

Patient/family education

• Advise patients to avoid CNS depressants (alcohol, sedative/hypnotics) for at least 24 hr after taking this drug

• Discuss with patient that dizziness, drowsiness, and confusion are common; to avoid getting up without assistance

• Discuss in detail with patient all aspects of the drug, including its purpose and what to expect

• Caution patient to make position changes carefully to lessen orthostatic hypotension

Evaluation

Positive therapeutic outcome

• Decreased pain

Treatment of overdose: Naloxone 0.2-0.8 mg **IV**, O_2, **IV** fluids, vasopressors

meprobamate (℞)

(me-proe-ba′mate)

Apo-Meprobamate ✦, Equanil, Meditran ✦, meprobamate, Meprospan, Miltown, Miltown 400, Miltown 600, Neuramate, Neo-Tran ✦, Novomepro ✦, Sedabamate, Trancot

Func. class.: Sedative/hypnotic; antianxiety

Chem. class.: Propanediol carbamate derivative

Pregnancy category D

Controlled substance schedule IV

Action: Produces widespread depression of the CNS

M

Therapeutic Outcome: Decreased anxiety, sedation

Uses: Anxiety, sedation

Dosage and routes

Adult: PO 1.2-1.6 g/day in 2-3 divided doses, not to exceed 2.4 g/day or 800-1600 mg/day in 2 divided doses (sus rel); max 2.4 g/day

G ***Elderly:*** PO 200 mg bid-tid, adjust to lowest possible dose

P ***Child 6-12 yr:*** PO 100-200 mg bid-tid or 200 mg (sus rel) bid

Available forms: Tabs 200, 400, 600 mg; sus rel caps 200, 400 mg

Adverse effects

CNS: *Dizziness, drowsiness,* headache, **seizures,** ataxia

CV: Hypotension, tachycardia, palpitations, **hyperthermia**

EENT: Blurred vision, tinnitus, mydriasis, slurred speech

GI: Nausea, vomiting, anorexia, diarrhea, stomatitis

HEMA: **Thrombocytopenia, leukopenia, eosinophilia**

INTEG: Urticaria, pruritus, maculopapular rash

Contraindications: Hypersensitivity, renal failure, porphyria, pregnancy **D,** history of drug abuse or dependence

Precautions: Suicidal patients, severe depression, renal disease, G hepatic disease, elderly

Pharmacokinetics

Absorption	Well absorbed
Distribution	Widely distributed; crosses placenta
Metabolism	Liver
Excretion	Kidneys, feces, breast milk
Half-life	6-16 hr

Pharmacodynamics

	PO	PO–SUS REL
Onset	1 hr	Unknown
Peak	1-3 hr	Unknown
Duration	6-12 hr	Up to 12 hr

Interactions

Individual drugs

Alcohol: ↑ CNS depression

Fluoxetine: ↑ action

Propoxyphene: ↑ action

Drug classifications

Antidepressants: ↑ CNS depression

Antihistamines: ↑ CNS depression

Opiates: ↑ CNS depression

Sedative/hypnotics: ↑ CNS depression

Lab test interferences

False: ↑ 17-OHCS

False positive: Phentolamine test

NURSING CONSIDERATIONS

Assessment

- Assess patient's sleep pattern and note physical (sleep apnea, obstructed airway, pain/discomfort, urinary frequency) and psychologic (fear, anxiety) circumstances that interrupt sleep
- Assess patient's bedtime routine, presleep cues, props
- Assess potential for abuse; this drug may lend to physical and psychologic dependency; amount of drug should be limited
- Monitor blood studies: Hct, Hgb, RBCs, serum folate (if on long-term therapy), pro-time in patients receiving anticoagulants, since action of anticoagulant may be increased
- Monitor mental status: mood, sensorium, affect, memory (long, short)
- Monitor physical dependency: more frequent requests for medication, shakes, anxiety, pinpoint pupils
- Monitor respiratory dysfunction: respiratory depression, character, rate, rhythm; hold drug if respirations are <10/min or if pupils are dilated (rare)

- Assess for blood dyscrasias: fever, sore throat, bruising, rash, jaundice, epistaxis (rare)
- Assess previous history of substance abuse, cardiac disease, or gastritis

Nursing diagnoses

✓ Anxiety (uses)
✓ Knowledge deficit (teaching)
✓ Noncompliance (teaching)

Implementation

- Give with food to minimize GI symptoms
- Do not break, crush, or chew sus rel caps
- Store in airtight container in cool environment

Patient/family education

- Advise patient to avoid driving and other activities requiring alertness; to avoid alcohol and CNS depressants; serious CNS depression may result, as well as tachycardia, flushing, headache, hypotension
- Caution patient not to discontinue medication quickly after long-term use; drug should be tapered over 1-2 wk; effects may take 2 nights for benefits to be noticed; withdrawal symptoms include tremors, anxiety, hallucinations, delirium
- Teach patient alternate measures to improve sleep (reading, exercise several hr before hs, warm bath, warm milk, TV, self-hypnosis, deep breathing)
- Instruct patient that hangover is common in elderly but less common than with barbiturates
- Teach patient symptoms of withdrawal: nausea, vomiting, anxiety, hallucinations, insomnia, tachycardia, fever, cramps, tremors, seizures
- Teach patient to watch for blood dyscrasias: fever, sore throat, bruising, rash, jaundice (rare)
- Teach patient to watch for allergic reaction (rash); discontinue drug if rash occurs

Evaluation

Positive therapeutic outcome

- Decreased anxiety, restlessness, insomnia

Treatment of overdose:

Lavage, VS, supportive care

mercaptopurine (℞)

(mer-kap-toe-pyoor′een)

6-MP, Purinethol

Func. class.: Antineoplastic, antimetabolite

Chem. class.: Purine analog

Pregnancy category D

Action: Inhibits purine metabolism at multiple sites, which inhibits DNA and RNA synthesis S phase of cell cycle

Therapeutic Outcome: Prevention of rapidly growing malignant cells

Uses: Chronic myelocytic leukemia, acute lymphoblastic leukemia in children, acute myelogenous leukemia

Investigational uses: Polycythemia vera, psoriatic arthritis, colitis, lymphoma

Dosage and routes

Adult: PO 80-100 mg/m^2 qd, max 5 mg/kg/day; maintenance 1.5-2.5 mg/kg/day

Child: 75 mg/m^2/day (2.5 mg/kg/day); maintenance 1.5-2.5 mg/kg/day

Available forms: Tabs 50 mg

Adverse effects

CNS: Fever, headache, weakness

GI: *Nausea, vomiting, anorexia, diarrhea, stomatitis,* **hepatotoxicity** (with high doses), jaundice, gastritis

GU: **Renal failure**, hyperuricemia, **oliguria,** crystalluria, **hematuria**

HEMA: **Thrombocytopenia, leukopenia, myelosuppression, anemia**

INTEG: *Rash,* dry skin, urticaria

Contraindications: Patients with prior drug resistance, leukopenia (<2500/mm^3), thrombocytopenia

($<100,000/mm^3$), anemia, pregnancy **D**

Precautions: Renal disease

Pharmacokinetics

Absorption	Variable
Distribution	Widely—body water
Metabolism	Liver—extensively
Excretion	Kidneys unchanged (small amounts)
Half-life	Unknown

Pharmacodynamics

Unknown

Interactions

Individual drugs

Allopurinol: ↑ toxicity
Cotrimoxazole: ↑ bone marrow depression
Cyclophosphamide: ↑ cardiotoxicity, CHF
Radiation: ↑ toxicity, bone marrow suppression
Warfarin: ↑ or ↓ effect of warfarin

Drug classifications

Antineoplastics: ↑ toxicity, bone marrow suppression
Hepatotoxic agents: ↑ hepatotoxicity
Live virus vaccines: ↓ antibodies
Nondepolarizing muscle relaxants: Reversal of neuromuscular blockade

NURSING CONSIDERATIONS

Assessment

- Assess buccal cavity q8h for dryness, sores or ulceration, white patches, oral pain, bleeding, dysphagia; obtain prescription for viscous lidocaine (Xylocaine)
- (Alert) Assess symptoms indicating severe allergic reaction: rash, pruritus, urticaria, purpuric skin lesions, itching, flushing
- Monitor CBC, differential, platelet count weekly; withhold drug if WBC is $<4000/mm^3$ or platelet count is $<100,000/mm^3$; notify prescriber of results if WBC $<20,000/mm^3$, platelets $<150,000/mm^3$
- Assess for increased uric acid levels, swelling, joint pain primarily in extremities; patient should be well hydrated to prevent urate deposits
- Monitor renal function studies: BUN, creatinine, serum uric acid, urine CrCl before and during therapy; check I&O ratio; report fall in urine output to <30 ml/hr
- Monitor temp q4h (may indicate beginning of infection)
- Monitor liver function tests before and during therapy (bilirubin, AST, ALT, LDH) as needed or monthly; check for yellowing of skin or sclera, dark urine, clay-colored stools, itchy skin, abdominal pain, fever, diarrhea
- Assess for bleeding: hematuria, stool guaiac, bruising or petechiae, mucosa or orifices q8h; check for inflammation of mucosa, breaks in skin

Nursing diagnoses

- ✓ Injury, risk for (adverse reactions)
- ✓ Body image disturbance (adverse reactions)
- ✓ Infection, risk for (adverse reactions)
- ✓ Knowledge deficit (teaching)

Implementation

- Give fluids **IV** or PO before chemotherapy to hydrate patient
- Give antiemetic 30-60 min before giving drug and prn to prevent vomiting; give antibiotics for prophylaxis of infection
- Give in AM so drug can be eliminated before hs
- Provide liq diet: carbonated beverages; gelatin may be added if patient is not nauseated or vomiting
- Encourage patient to rinse mouth tid-qid with water, club soda; brush teeth bid-qid with soft brush or cotton-tipped applicators for stomatitis; use unwaxed dental floss
- Tab may be crushed and added to fluids or food to facilitate swallowing

Patient/family education

- Advise patient that contraceptive measures are recommended during therapy; serious teratogenic effects may occur, to avoid breast-feeding
- Teach patient to avoid use of products containing aspirin or NSAIDs, razors, commercial mouthwash, since bleeding may occur; to report symptoms of bleeding (hematuria, tarry stools)
- Instruct patient to report signs of anemia (fatigue, headache, irritability, faintness, shortness of breath)
- Instruct patient to report any changes in breathing or coughing even several mo after treatment; to avoid crowds and persons with respiratory tract or other infections
- Caution patient not to have any vaccinations without the advice of the prescriber; serious reactions can occur

Evaluation

Positive therapeutic outcome

- Prevention of rapid division of malignant cells

meropenem (℞)

(mer-oh-pen′em)

Merrem **IV**

Func. class.: Antiinfective, misc.

Pregnancy category B

Action: Interferes with cell wall replication of susceptible organisms; osmotically unstable cell wall swells and bursts from osmotic pressure

➔ **Therapeutic Outcome:** Bactericidal action against the following: *Streptococcus pneumoniae,* group A β-hemolytic streptococci, *viridans* group streptococci, enterococcus; gram-negative organisms *Klebsiella, Proteus, Escherichia coli, Pseudomonas aeruginosa, Bacteroides fragilis, Bacteroides thetaiotamicron,* bacterial meningitis (>3 mo old) P

Uses: Serious infections caused by gram-positive or gram-negative organisms (appendicitis, peritonitis)

Dosage and routes

Adult: **IV** 1 g q8h, given over 15-30 min or as an **IV** bolus 5-20 ml given over 3-5 min

Renal dose

Adult: **IV** CrCl 26-50 ml/min 1 g q12h; CrCl 10-25 ml/min 500 mg q12h; CrCl <10 ml/min 500 mg q24h

P ***Child ≥ 3 mo:*** **IV** 20-40 mg/kg q8h (max 2 g q8h meningitis)

P ***Child >50 kg:*** **IV** 1 g q8h (intraabdominal infection) or 2 g q8h (meningitis) given over 15-30 min or as an **IV** bolus 5-20 ml over 3-5 min

Available forms: Inj 500 mg

Adverse effects

CNS: Fever, somnolence, *seizures,* dizziness, weakness, *headache*
CV: Hypotension, palpitations
GI: Diarrhea, nausea, vomiting, **pseudomembranous colitis, hepatitis,** glossitis
HEMA: **Eosinophilia, neutropenia,** decreased Hgb, Hct
INTEG: Rash, urticaria, *pruritus,* pain at inj site, phlebitis, erythema at inj site
RESP: Chest discomfort, dyspnea, hyperventilation
SYST: **Anaphylaxis**

Contraindications: Hypersensitivity to meropenem or imipenem

Precautions: Pregnancy **B,** lactation, elderly, renal disease G

Pharmacokinetics

Absorption	Complete bioavailability
Distribution	Widely distributed
Metabolism	Liver
Excretion	Kidneys
Half-life	1 hr; increased in renal disease

M

Pharmacodynamics

Onset	Rapid
Peak	Dose dependent

Interactions
Individual drugs
Probenecid: ↓ renal excretion, ↑ blood level
Lab test interferences
False: ↑ Creatinine (serum urine), ↑ urinary 17-KS
False positive: Urinary protein, direct Coombs' test, urine glucose
Interference: Cross-matching

NURSING CONSIDERATIONS
Assessment
- Assess patient for previous sensitivity reaction to carbapenem antiinfectives, penicillins
- Assess patient for signs and symptoms of infection, including characteristics of wounds, sputum, urine, stool, WBC >10,000/100 mm^3, fever; obtain baseline information before and during treatment
- Complete C&S tests before beginning drug therapy to identify if correct treatment has been initiated
- Assess for allergic reactions, anaphylaxis: rash, urticaria, pruritus, chills, fever, joint pain; angioedema may occur a few days after therapy begins; epinephrine and resuscitation equipment should be available for anaphylactic reaction
- Identify urine output; if decreasing, notify prescriber (may indicate nephrotoxicity); also check for increased BUN, creatinine
- Monitor blood studies: AST, ALT, CBC, Hct, bilirubin, LDH, alkaline phosphatase, Coombs' test monthly if patient is on long-term therapy
- Monitor electrolytes: potassium, sodium, chloride monthly if patient is on long-term therapy
- Assess bowel pattern qd; if severe diarrhea occurs, drug should be discontinued; may indicate pseudomembranous colitis
- Monitor for bleeding: ecchymosis, bleeding gums, hematuria, stool guaiac daily if on long-term therapy
- Assess for overgrowth of infection: perineal itching, fever, malaise, redness, pain, swelling, drainage, rash, diarrhea, change in cough, sputum

Nursing diagnoses
- ✓ Infection, risk for (uses)
- ✓ Diarrhea (adverse reactions)
- ✓ Injury, risk for (adverse reactions)
- ✓ Knowledge deficit (teaching)
- ✓ Noncompliance (teaching)

Implementation
IV IV route
- Reconstitute with 0.9% NaCl, D_5W, LR, dilute in 5-20 ml of compatible sol; give by direct **IV** over 3-5 min
- Give by intermittent inf, dilute in 5-20 ml of compatible sol, give over 15-30 min

Y-site compatibilities: Aminophylline, atenolol, atropine, cimetidine, dexamethasone, digoxin, diphenhydramine, enalaprilat, fluconazole, furosemide, gentamicin, heparin, insulin (regular), metoclopramide, morphine, norepinephrine, phenobarbital, vancomycin

Additive compatibilities: Aminophylline, atropine, cimetidine, dexamethasone, dobutamine, dopamine, enalaprilat, fluconazole, furosemide, gentamicin, heparin, insulin (regular), magnesium sulfate, metoclopramide, morphine, norepinephrine, phenobarbital, ranitidine, vancomycin

Patient/family education
- Teach patient to report sore throat, bruising, bleeding, joint pain; may indicate blood dyscrasias (rare)
- Advise patient to contact prescriber if vaginal itching, loose foul-smelling stools, furry tongue occur; may indicate superinfection
- Advise patient to avoid breast-

feeding, drug is excreted in breast milk
- Advise patient to notify prescriber of diarrhea with blood or pus, may indicate pseudomembranous colitis

Evaluation
Positive therapeutic outcome
- Absence of signs/symptoms of infection (WBC <10,000/mm^3, temp WNL, absence of red draining wounds)
- Reported improvement in symptoms of infection

Treatment of anaphylaxis:
Epinephrine, antihistamines, resuscitate if needed

mesalamine (℞)
(mez-al'a-meen)

Asacol, Mesasal, Pentasa, Rowasa, Salofulk ✦

Func class.: GI antiinflammatory

Chem class.: 5-Aminosalicylic acid

Pregnancy category B

Action: May diminish inflammation by blocking cyclooxygenase, inhibiting prostaglandin production in colon, local action only

Therapeutic Outcome: Decreased cramping, pain in GI conditions

Uses: Mild to moderate active distal ulcerative colitis, proctosigmoiditis, proctitis

Dosage and routes
Adult: REC 60 ml (4 g) hs, retained for 8 hr × 3-6 wk; PO 800 mg tid for 6 wk; supp 500 mg bid for 3-6 wk

Available forms: Rec susp 4 g/60 ml; supp 500 mg; delayed rel tabs 400 mg; caps cont rel 250 mg (Pentasa)

Adverse effects
CNS: *Headache, fever, dizziness,* insomnia, asthenia, weakness, fatigue

CV: Pericarditis, myocarditis

EENT: Sore throat, cough, pharyngitis, rhinitis

GI: *Cramps, gas, nausea, diarrhea,* rectal pain, constipation

INTEG: *Rash, itching,* acne

SYST: *Flu, malaise,* back pain, peripheral edema, leg and joint pain, arthralgia, dysmenorrhea

Contraindications: Hypersensitivity to this drug or salicylates

Precautions: Renal disease, pregnancy **B**, lactation, children, sulfite sensitivity

Do Not Confuse:
Asacol/Ansaid

Pharmacokinetics

Absorption	20%-30% (PO), 10%-25% (rec)
Distribution	Unknown
Metabolism	Unknown
Excretion	Feces
Half-life	1 hr; metabolite 5-10 hr

Pharmacodynamics
Unknown

Interactions
Individual drugs
Omeprazole: ↑ mesalamine absorption

NURSING CONSIDERATIONS
Assessment
- Assess for GI symptoms: cramping, gas, nausea, diarrhea, rectal pain, abdominal pain; if severe, the drug should be discontinued
- Assess renal function before treatment

Nursing diagnoses
- ✓ Pain (uses)
- ✓ Diarrhea (uses)
- ✓ Knowledge deficit (teaching)

Implementation
PO route
- Do not crush, chew tabs
- May give orally

Rectal route (susp)
- Give hs, retained until AM
- Store at room temp
- Usual course of therapy is 3-6 wk
- Give after shaking bottle well

Patient/family education
- Advise patient to notify prescriber if abdominal pain, cramping, diarrhea with blood, headache, fever, rash, chest pain occur; drug should be discontinued
- Teach correct administration for PO, or enema

Evaluation
Positive therapeutic outcome
- Absence of pain, bleeding from GI tract

mesoridazine (℞)
(mez-oh-rid′a-zeen)

Serentil, Serentil Concentrate

Func. class.: Antipsychotic/neuroleptic

Chem. class.: Phenothiazine, piperidine

Pregnancy category C

Action: Depresses cerebral cortex, hypothalamus, limbic system, which control activity, aggression; blocks neurotransmission produced by dopamine at synapse; exhibits strong α-adrenergic, anticholinergic blocking action; mechanism for antipsychotic effects is unclear

Therapeutic Outcome: Decreased signs and symptoms of psychosis, reorganization of thought patterns

Uses: Psychotic disorders, schizophrenia, anxiety, alcoholism, behavioral problems in mental deficiency, chronic brain syndrome

Dosage and routes
Schizophrenia

Adult: PO 50 mg tid; optimum dosage 100-400 mg/day; IM 25 mg; may repeat in 30-60 min; dosage range 25-200 mg/day

Behavior problems

Adult: PO 25 mg tid; optimum dosage 75-300 mg/day

G ***Elderly:*** PO 10 mg qd bid, increase q3-7 days by 10-25 mg to desired dose

Alcoholism

Adult: PO 25 mg bid; optimum dosage 50-200 mg/day

Psychoneurotic disorders

Adult: PO 10 mg tid; optimum dosage 30-150 mg/day

Available forms: Tabs 10, 25, 50, 100 mg; conc 25 mg/ml; inj 25 mg/ml

Adverse effects
CNS: *Extrapyramidal symptoms: pseudoparkinsonism, akathisia, dystonia, tardive dyskinesia, drowsiness, headache,* **neuroleptic malignant syndrome**

CV: *Orthostatic hypotension,* hypertension, **cardiac arrest,** ECG changes, tachycardia

EENT: Blurred vision, glaucoma

GI: *Dry mouth, nausea, vomiting, anorexia, constipation,* diarrhea, jaundice, weight gain

GU: Urinary retention, urinary frequency, enuresis, impotence, amenorrhea, gynecomastia

HEMA: **Anemia, leukopenia, leukocytosis, agranulocytosis**

INTEG: *Rash,* photosensitivity, dermatitis

RESP: **Laryngospasm,** dyspnea, **respiratory depression**

Contraindications: Hypersensitivity, circulatory collapse, liver damage, cerebral arteriosclerosis, coronary disease, severe hypertension/hypotension, blood dyscrasias, coma, severe CNS depression, brain damage, bone marrow depression, narrow-angle glaucoma

Precautions: Pregnancy **C,** lactation, seizure disorders, hypertension, hepatic disease, cardiac disease, prostatic hypertrophy, intestinal obstruction, respiratory conditions

Do Not Confuse:
Serentil/Sinequan

Pharmacokinetics

Absorption	Well absorbed (PO, IM)
Distribution	Widely distributed; crosses placenta, blood-brain barrier
Metabolism	Liver, extensively
Excretion	Kidneys, breast milk
Half-life	Unknown

Pharmacodynamics

	PO	IM
Onset	Erratic	15-30 min
Peak	2 hr	30 min
Duration	4-6 hr	6-8 hr

Interactions
Individual drugs
Alcohol: ↑ effects of both drugs, oversedation
Aluminum hydroxide: ↓ absorption
Bromocriptine: ↓ antiparkinsonian activity
Disopyramide: ↑ anticholinergic effects
Guanethidine: ↓ antihypertensive response
Levodopa: ↓ antiparkinsonian activity
Magnesium hydroxide: ↓ absorption
Norepinephrine: ↓ vasoresponse, ↑ toxicity
Phenobarbital: ↓ effectiveness, ↑ metabolism
Drug classifications
Antacids: ↓ absorption
Anticholinergics: ↑ anticholinergic effects
Antidepressants: ↑ CNS depression
Antidiarrheals, adsorbent: ↓ absorption
Antihistamines: ↑ CNS depression
Antihypertensives: ↑ hypotension
Barbiturate anesthetics: ↑ CNS depression
General anesthetics: ↑ CNS depression
MAOIs: ↑ CNS depression
Opiates: ↑ CNS depression
Sedative/hypnotics: ↑ CNS depression
Herb/drug
Henbane: ↑ anticholinergic effect
Lab test interferences
↑ Liver function tests, ↑ cardiac enzymes, ↑ cholesterol, ↑ blood glucose, ↑ prolactin, ↑ bilirubin, ↑ PBI, ↑ cholinesterase, ↑ ^{131}I, ↑ alkaline phosphatase, ↑ leukocytes, ↑ granulocytes, ↑ platelets
↓ Hormones (blood and urine)
False positive: Pregnancy tests, PKU
False negative: Urinary steroids, 17-OHCS

NURSING CONSIDERATIONS
Assessment
- Assess mental status: orientation, mood, behavior, presence and type of hallucinations before initial administration and monthly; this drug should significantly reduce psychotic behavior
- Check for swallowing of PO medication; check for hoarding or giving of medication to other patients
- Monitor I&O ratio; palpate bladder if low urinary output occurs, especially in elderly; urinalysis recommended before, during prolonged therapy
- Monitor bilirubin, CBC, liver function studies monthly
- Assess affect, orientation, LOC, reflexes, gait, coordination, sleep pattern disturbances
- Monitor B/P with patient sitting, standing, and lying; take pulse and respirations q4h during initial treatment; establish baseline before starting treatment; report drops of 30 mm Hg; obtain baseline ECG, Q-wave and T-wave changes
- Check for dizziness, faintness, palpitations, tachycardia on rising; severe orthostatic hypotension is common
- Identify for neuroleptic malignant

M

syndrome: hyperpyrexia, muscle rigidity, increased CPK, altered mental status; drug should be discontinued
- Assess for EPS including akathisia (inability to sit still, no pattern to movements), tardive dyskinesia (bizarre movements of the jaw, mouth, tongue, extremities), pseudoparkinsonism (ragged tremors, pill rolling, shuffling gait); an antiparkinsonism drug should be prescribed
- Assess for constipation, urinary retention daily; if these occur, increase bulk, water in diet

Nursing diagnoses

- ✓ Thought processes, altered (uses)
- ✓ Coping, ineffective individual (uses)
- ✓ Knowledge deficit (teaching)
- ✓ Noncompliance (teaching)

Implementation

PO route

- Administer drug in liq form mixed in glass of juice or cola if hoarding is suspected; do not mix in caffeine drinks or with tannics, pectins
- Administer lowest possible dose to G elderly to minimize side effects, since metabolism is slowed
- Reduce dose in patients treated for behavior problems
- Administer PO with full glass of water, milk; or give with food to decrease GI upset
- Store in airtight, light-resistant container, oral sol in bottle

IM route

- Inject deeply in large muscle mass; do not give SC; do not administer sol with a precipitate; use gloves when preparing sol, prevent contact with skin/clothes

Patient/family education

- Teach patient to use good oral hygiene; frequent rinsing of mouth, sugarless gum for dry mouth
- Tell patient to avoid hazardous activities until drug response is determined; dizziness, blurred vision may occur
- Inform patient that orthostatic hypotension occurs often and to rise from sitting or lying position gradually; to remain lying down after IM inj for at least 30 min; tell patient to avoid hot tubs, hot showers, tub baths, since hypotension may occur; tell patient that in hot weather heat stroke may occur; take extra precautions to stay cool
- Caution patient to avoid abrupt withdrawal of this drug, or extrapyramidal symptoms (EPS) may result; drug should be withdrawn slowly
- Teach patient to avoid OTC preparations (cough, hay fever, cold) unless approved by prescriber, since serious drug interactions may occur; avoid use with alcohol, CNS depressants; increased drowsiness may occur
- Caution patient to use a sunscreen and sunglasses in case of photosensitivity
- Teach patient about EPS and necessity of meticulous oral hygiene, since oral candidiasis may occur
- Advise patient to take antacids 2 hr before or after taking this drug
- Instruct patient to report sore throat, malaise, fever, bleeding, mouth sores; if these occur, CBC should be performed and drug discontinued
- Teach patient that urine may turn pink or red

Evaluation

Positive therapeutic outcome

- Decrease in emotional excitement, hallucinations, delusions, paranoia
- Reorganization of patterns of thought, speech

Treatment of overdose:

Lavage if orally ingested; provide airway; **do not induce vomiting or use epinephrine**

metaproterenol (℞)

(met-a-proe-ter'e-nole)

Alupent, Arm-A-Med, Dey-Lute, metaproterenol sulfate, Metaprel

Func. class.: Selective β_2-agonist, bronchodilator

Pregnancy category C

Action: Relaxes bronchial smooth muscle by direct action on β_2-adrenergic receptors, with increased levels of cAMP and increased bronchodilatation, diuresis, and cardiac and CNS stimulation

Therapeutic Outcome: Bronchodilatation with ease of breathing

Uses: Bronchial asthma, bronchospasm

Dosage and routes

P ***Adult and child >12 yr:*** INH 2-3 puffs; may repeat q3-4h, not to exceed 12 puffs/day

Asthma/bronchospasm

Adult: PO 20 mg q6-8h

G ***Elderly:*** PO 10 mg tid-qid, initially

P ***Child >9 yr or >27 kg:*** PO 20 mg q6-8h or 0.4-0.9 mg/kg tid

P ***Child 6-9 yr or <27 kg:*** PO 10 mg q6-8h or 0.4-0.9 mg/kg tid

P ***Child 2-6 yr:*** PO 1.3-2.6 mg/kg divided q6-8h

Available forms: Tabs 10, 20 mg; aerosol 0.65 mg/dose; syrup 10 mg/5 ml; sol for inh 0.4%, 0.6%, 5%

Adverse effects

CNS: *Tremors,* anxiety, insomnia, headache, dizziness, stimulation

CV: Palpitations, tachycardia, hypertension, **dysrhythmias, cardiac arrest** (high dose)

GI: Nausea, vomiting

RESP: **Paradoxical bronchospasm**

Contraindications: Hypersensitivity to sympathomimetics, narrow-angle glaucoma

Precautions: Pregnancy **C**, cardiac disorders, hyperthyroidism, diabetes mellitus, prostatic hypertrophy

Do Not Confuse:

Alupent/Atrovent

Pharmacokinetics

Absorption	Well absorbed (PO)
Distribution	Unknown
Metabolism	Liver, tissues
Excretion	Unknown
Half-life	2-4 hr

Pharmacodynamics

	PO	INH
Onset	15 min	5 min
Peak	1 hr	1 hr
Duration	4 hr	4 hr

Interactions

Drug classifications

β-Adrenergic blockers: Block therapeutic effect

Bronchodilators, aerosol: ↑ action of bronchodilator

MAOIs: ↑ chance of hypertensive crisis

Sympathomimetics: ↑ adrenergic side effects

Herb/drug

Ephedra: ↑ effect

NURSING CONSIDERATIONS

Assessment

- Monitor respiratory function: vital capacity, FEV, ABGs, lung sounds, heart rate, rhythm (baseline)
- Determine that patient has not received theophylline therapy before giving dose; identify client's ability to self-medicate
- Monitor for evidence of allergic reactions; paradoxic bronchospasm; withhold dose; notify prescriber

Nursing diagnoses

- ✓ Airway clearance, ineffective (uses)
- ✓ Impaired gas exchange (uses)
- ✓ Knowledge deficit (teaching)

Implementation

Aerosol route

- Give after shaking, exhale, place

M

mouthpiece in mouth, inhale slowly, hold breath, remove, exhale slowly; allow at least 1 min between inhalations

• Store in light-resistant container, do not expose to temp over 86° F (30° C)

G • Provide spacer device for elderly

PO route

• Give PO with meals to decrease gastric irritation; syrup to children (no alcohol, sugar) P

Patient/family education

• Advise patient not to use OTC medications; excess stimulation may occur; to use this medication before other medications and allow at least 5 min between each to prevent overstimulation

• Teach patient use of inhaler; review package insert with patient; teach patient to avoid getting aerosol in eyes, since blurring may result; to wash inhaler in warm water qd and dry; to avoid smoking, smoke-filled rooms, persons with respiratory tract infections

• Advise patient that paradoxic bronchospasm may occur and to stop drug immediately and notify prescriber; to limit caffeine products such as chocolate, coffee, tea, and colas

• Instruct patient on administration of dose; not to use more than prescribed; serious side effects may occur

Evaluation

Positive therapeutic outcome

• Absence of dyspnea, wheezing after 1 hr

• Improved airway exchange

• Improved ABGs

Treatment of overdose:

Administer a β_1-adrenergic blocker

metformin (℞)

(met-for′min)

Glucophage, Glucophage XR

Func. class.: Antidiabetic, oral

Chem. class.: Biguanide

Pregnancy category B

Action: Inhibits hepatic glucose production and increases sensitivity of peripheral tissue to insulin

➔ **Therapeutic Outcome:** Blood glucose at normal levels

Uses: Stable adult-onset diabetes mellitus, type II (NIDDM)

Dosage and routes

Adult: PO 500 mg bid initially, then increase to desired response 1-3 g; dosage adjustment q2-3 wk or 850 mg qd with morning meal with dosage increased every other week, max 2500 mg/day

G ***Elderly:*** PO use lowest effective dose

Available forms: Tabs 500, 850 mg

Adverse effects:

CNS: *Headache, weakness, dizziness, drowsiness,* tinnitus, fatigue, vertigo, *agitation*

ENDO: **Lactic acidosis**

GI: Nausea, vomiting, diarrhea, heartburn, anorexia, metallic taste

HEMA: **Thrombocytopenia,** decreased vit B_{12} concentration

INTEG: Rash

Contraindications: Hypersensitivity, hepatic, renal disease, alcoholism, cardiopulmonary disease, history of lactic acidosis

G **Precautions:** Pregnancy **B,** elderly, thyroid disease, previous hypersensitivity to phenformin or buformin, CHF, renal disease

Pharmacokinetics

Absorption	Unknown
Distribution	Unknown
Metabolism	Unknown
Excretion	Kidneys, unchanged (35-50%)
Half-life	1½-5, Terminal 6-20 hr

Pharmacodynamics

Onset	Unknown
Peak	1-3 hr
Duration	Unknown

Interactions
Individual drugs
Acetazolamide: ↑ blood glucose levels
Cimetidine: ↑ hypoglycemia
Digoxin: ↑ hypoglycemia
Ethanol: ↑ risk of lactic acidosis
Morphine: ↑ hypoglycemia
Procainamide: ↑ hypoglycemia
Ranitidine: ↑ hypoglycemia
Triamterone: ↑ hypoglycemia
Vancomycin: ↑ hypoglycemia
Drug classifications
Calcium channel blockers: ↑ hypoglycemia
Diuretics: ↑ hypoglycemia
Estrogens: ↑ hypoglycemia
Glucocorticoids: ↑ risk of lactic acidosis
Oral contraceptives: ↑ hypoglycemia
Phenothiazines: ↑ hypoglycemia
Thyroid agents: ↑ hypoglycemia
Sympathomimetics: ↑ hypoglycemia
Herb/drug
Quinine: ↑ metformin level

NURSING CONSIDERATIONS
Assessment
- Assess for hypoglycemic reactions (sweating, weakness, dizziness, anxiety, tremors, hunger), hyperglycemic reactions soon after meals
- Monitor CBC (baseline, q3 mo) during treatment; check liver function tests (AST, LDH) and renal studies (BUN, creatinine) periodically during treatment
- Monitor for lactic acidosis: malaise, myalgia, abdominal distress; risk increases with age, poor renal function

Nursing diagnoses
✓ Knowledge deficit (teaching)

Implementation
- Conversion from other oral hypoglycemic agents; change may be made without gradual dosage change; monitor serum or urine glucose and ketones tid during conversion
- Give twice a day with meals to decrease GI upset and provide best absorption, may also be taken as a single dose
- Give tabs crushed and mixed with meal or fluids for patients with difficulty swallowing
- Store in tight container in cool environment

Patient/family education
- Teach patient to use capillary blood glucose test or Chemstrip tid
- Teach patient symptoms of hypo/hyperglycemia, what to do about each
- Advise patient that drug must be continued on daily basis; explain consequence of discontinuing drug abruptly
- Advise patient to take drug in morning to prevent hypoglycemic reactions at night
- Advise patient to avoid OTC medications unless approved by the prescriber
- Teach patient that diabetes is a lifelong illness; that this drug controls symptoms, but does not cure the condition
- Teach patient symptoms of lactic acidosis: fatigue, malaise, myalgia, somnolence
- Teach patient that all food included in diet plan must be eaten to prevent hypoglycemia
- Teach patient to carry ID and

glucagon emergency kit for emergencies

Evaluation

- Therapeutic response: decrease in polyuria, polydipsia, polyphagia; clear sensorium; absence of dizziness; stable gait, blood glucose at normal level

Treatment of overdose: Glucose 25 g **IV** via dextrose 50% sol, 50 ml or 1 mg glucagon

HIGH ALERT

methadone (℞)

(meth'a-done)

Dolophine, methadone HCl, Methadose

Func. class.: Opiate analgesic

Chem. class.: Synthetic diphenylheptane derivative

Pregnancy category C

Controlled substance schedule II

Action: Depresses pain impulse transmission at the spinal cord level by interacting with opioid receptors; produces CNS depression

Therapeutic Outcome: Relief of pain; successful opiate withdrawal

Uses: Severe pain, opiate withdrawal

Dosage and routes

Severe pain

Adult: PO/SC/IM 2.5-10 mg q3-4h prn

Opiate withdrawal

Adult: PO 15-40 mg/day individualized initially, then 20-120 mg/day titrated to patient response

P ***Child:*** 0.05-0.1 mg/kg/dose q6-12h

Renal dose

CrCl 10-50 ml/min dose q8h; CrCl <10 ml/min dose q8-12h

Available forms: Inj 10 mg/ml; tabs 5, 10 mg; oral sol 5, 10 mg/5 ml; dispersible tabs 40 mg; oral conc 10 mg/ml; oral sol 5, 10 mg/5 ml, 10 mg/10 ml

Adverse effects

CNS: ***Drowsiness, dizziness, confusion, headache, sedation,*** euphoria, **seizures**

CV: Palpitations, bradycardia, change in B/P, **cardiac arrest, shock**

EENT: Tinnitus, blurred vision, miosis, diplopia

GI: ***Nausea, vomiting, anorexia, constipation, cramps,*** biliary tract spasm

GU: Increased urinary output, dysuria, urinary retention

INTEG: ***Rash,*** urticaria, bruising, flushing, diaphoresis, pruritus

RESP: **Respiratory depression, respiratory arrest**

Contraindications: Hypersensitivity to this drug, or hypersensitivity to chlorobutanol (inj route), addiction (opiate)

Precautions: Addictive personality, pregnancy **C,** lactation, increased ICP, MI (acute), severe heart disease, respiratory depression, hepatic disease, renal disease, child <18 yr, elderly

Do Not Confuse:
methadone/methylphenidate

Pharmacokinetics	
Absorption	Well absorbed (PO, SC, IM)
Distribution	Widely distributed; crosses placenta
Metabolism	Liver, extensively
Excretion	Kidneys, breast milk
Half-life	15-30 hr; extended interval with continued dosing

Pharmacodynamics	PO	IM/SC
Onset	½-1hr	20 min
Peak	1½-2 hr	1½-2 hr
Duration	4-12 hr	4-6 hr

Interactions

Individual drugs

Alcohol: ↑ respiratory depression, hypotension, sedation
Cimetidine: ↑ recovery
Erythromycin: ↑ recovery
Nalbuphine: ↓ analgesia
Pentazocine: ↓ analgesia

Drug classifications

Antihistamines: ↑ respiratory depression, hypotension
CNS depressants: ↑ respiratory depression, hypotension
MAOIs: Do not use for 2 wk before taking methadone
Phenothiazines: ↑ respiratory depression, hypotension
Sedative/hypnotics: ↑ respiratory depression, hypotension

Lab test interferences

↑ amylase, ↑ lipase

NURSING CONSIDERATIONS

Assessment

- Assess for pain: type, location, intensity, grimacing before and 1½-2 hr after administration; use pain scoring
- Monitor VS after parenteral route; note muscle rigidity, drug history, liver, kidney function tests, respiratory dysfunction: respiratory depression, character, rate, rhythm; notify prescriber if respirations are <10/min
- Monitor CNS changes: dizziness, drowsiness, hallucinations, euphoria, LOC, pupil reaction
- Monitor allergic reactions: rash, urticaria

Nursing diagnoses

✓ Pain (uses)
✓ Sensory-perceptual alteration: visual, auditory (adverse reactions)
✓ Breathing pattern, ineffective (adverse reactions)
✓ Knowledge deficit (teaching)

Implementation

- Medication should be slowly withdrawn after long-term use to prevent withdrawal symptoms

PO route

- May be given with food or milk to lessen GI upset
- Store in light-resistant container at room temp

IM/SC route

- Do not give if cloudy or a precipitate has formed
- Give deeply in large muscle mass; rotate inj sites

Patient/family education

- Instruct patient to report any symptoms of CNS changes, allergic reactions; to avoid CNS depressants: alcohol, sedative/hypnotics for at least 24 hr after taking this drug
- Discuss with patient that dizziness, drowsiness, and confusion are common; to avoid getting up without assistance
- Discuss in detail with patient all aspects of the drug
- Caution patient to make position changes slowly to prevent orthostatic hypotension

Evaluation

Positive therapeutic outcome

- Decreased pain
- Successful narcotic withdrawal

Treatment of overdose:

Naloxone (Narcan) 0.2-0.8 mg **IV**, O_2, **IV** fluids, vasopressors

M

methimazole (℞)

(meth-im'a-zole)

Tapazole

Func. class.: Thyroid hormone antagonist (antithyroid)
Chem. class.: Thioamide

Pregnancy category D

Action: Inhibits synthesis of thyroid hormones by decreasing iodine use in the manufacture of thyroglobin and iodothyronine; does not affect already formed hormones

Therapeutic Outcome: Decreased T_4 levels, hyperthyroid symptoms

Uses: Hyperthyroidism, preparation for thyroidectomy, thyrotoxic crisis, thyroid storm

Dosage and routes

Hyperthyroidism

Adult: PO 5-20 mg tid depending on severity of condition; continue until euthyroid; maintenance dosage 5-10 mg qd-tid; max dosage 150 mg qd

P ***Child:*** PO 0.4 mg/kg/day in divided doses q8h; continue until euthyroid; maintenance dosage 0.2 mg/kg/day in divided doses q8h

Preparation for thyroidectomy

P ***Adult and child:*** PO same as above; iodine may be added for 10 days before surgery

Thyrotoxic crisis

P ***Adult and child:*** PO same as hyperthyroidism with iodine and propranolol

Available forms: Tabs 5, 10 mg

Adverse effects

CNS: *Drowsiness, headache, vertigo, fever,* paresthesias, neuritis
ENDO: *Enlarged thyroid*
GI: *Nausea, diarrhea, vomiting, jaundice,* **hepatitis,** loss of taste
GU: **Nephritis**
HEMA: **Agranulocytosis, leukopenia, thrombocytopenia, hypothrombinemia, lymphadenopathy,** bleeding, vasculitis
INTEG: *Rash, urticaria, pruritus, alopecia, hyperpigmentation,* lupus-like syndrome
MS: Myalgia, arthralgia, nocturnal muscle cramps

Contraindications: Hypersensitivity, pregnancy **D**, lactation

Precautions: Infection, bone marrow depression, hepatic disease, patient >40 yr

Pharmacokinetics	
Absorption	Rapidly absorbed
Distribution	Crosses placenta
Metabolism	Liver, extensively
Excretion	Kidneys, unchanged; breast milk
Half-life	1-2 hr

Pharmacodynamics	
Onset	½ hr
Peak	Unknown
Duration	2-4 hr

Interactions

Individual drugs

Amiodarone: ↓ effectiveness
Digitalis: Altered response
Lithium: ↑ antithyroid effect
Potassium iodide: ↑ antithyroid effect, ↓ effectiveness
Radiation: ↑ bone marrow depression
Warfarin: Altered response

Drug classifications

Antineoplastics: ↑ bone marrow depression
Phenothiazines: ↑ granulocytosis

Lab test interferences

↑ Pro-time, ↑ AST, ↑ ALT, ↑ alkaline phosphatase

NURSING CONSIDERATIONS

Assessment

- Monitor pulse, B/P, temp; check I&O ratio; check for edema (puffy hands, feet, periorbits); indicates hypothyroidism
- Check weight qd; same clothing, scale, time of day
- Monitor T_3, T_4, which are increased; serum TSH, which is decreased; free thyroxine index, which is increased if dosage is too low; discontinue drug 3-4 wk before radioactive iodine uptake
- Monitor blood studies: CBC for blood dyscrasias (leukopenia, thrombocytopenia, agranulocytosis); liver function tests
- (Alert) Assess for overdose (peripheral

edema, heat intolerance, diaphoresis, palpitations, dysrhythmias, severe tachycardia, increased temp, delirium, CNS irritability); drug should be discontinued
- Assess for hypersensitivity (rash, enlarged cervical lymph nodes); drug may have to be discontinued
- Assess for hypoprothrombinemia (bleeding, petechiae, ecchymosis)
- Monitor clinical response: after 3 wk should include increased weight, pulse, decreased T_4
- Assess for bone marrow depression: sore throat, fever, fatigue

Nursing diagnoses

✓ Knowledge deficit (teaching)
✓ Noncompliance (teaching)

Implementation

- Give with meals to decrease GI upset; give at same time each day to maintain drug level
- Give lowest dosage that relieves symptoms
- Store in light-resistant container
- Increase fluids to 3-4 L/day, unless contraindicated

Patient/family education

- Advise patient to abstain from breast-feeding after delivery; drug appears in breast milk
- Instruct patient to take pulse daily; to keep graph of weight, pulse, mood
- Advise patient to report redness, swelling, sore throat, mouth lesions, which indicate blood dyscrasias
- Caution patient to avoid OTC products that contain iodine; that seafood and other iodine-containing products may be restricted by prescriber
- Caution patient not to discontinue this medication abruptly; thyroid crisis may occur; stress patient compliance
- Advise patient that response may take several mo if thyroid is large
- Teach patient symptoms/signs of overdose: periorbital edema, cold intolerance, mental depression; notify prescriber at once
- Teach patient symptoms of inadequate dosage: tachycardia, diarrhea, fever, irritability; prescriber should be notified to adjust
- Teach patient to take medication exactly as prescribed, not to skip or double doses; missed doses should be taken when remembered up to 1 hr before next dose
- Instruct patient to carry ID describing medication taken and condition being treated

Evaluation

Positive therapeutic outcome

- Decreased weight gain
- Decreased pulse
- Decreased T_4
- Decreased B/P

methocarbamol (℞)

(meth-oh-kar'ba-mole)

Carbacot, methocarbamol, Robaxin, Robaxin-750, Skelex

Func. class.: Skeletal muscle relaxant, central acting

Chem. class.: Carbamate derivative

Pregnancy category C

Action: Depresses multisynaptic pathways in the spinal cord, causing skeletal muscle relaxation

Therapeutic Outcome: Decreased pain, spasm

Uses: Adjunct for relief of spasm and pain in musculoskeletal conditions, tetanus management

Dosage and routes

Pain of muscle spasm

Adult: PO 1.5 g × 2-3 days, then 1 g qid; IM 500 mg in each gluteal region; may repeat q8h; **IV** bol 1-3 g/day at 3 ml/min; **IV** inf 1 g/250 ml D_5W or 0.9% NaCl, not to exceed 3 g/day

G ***Elderly:*** PO 500 mg qid, titrate to needed dose

Tetanus

Adult: **IV** inf 1-3 g/L of sol q6h; **IV** bol 1-2 g injected into running **IV**

M

P *Child:* **IV** 15 mg/kg q6h

Available forms: Tabs 500, 750 mg; inj 100 mg/ml

Adverse effects

CNS: Dizziness, weakness, drowsiness, headache, tremor, depression, insomnia; **seizures** (**IV** only)
CV: Postural hypotension, *bradycardia*
EENT: Diplopia, temporary loss of vision, blurred vision, nystagmus
GI: Nausea, vomiting, hiccups, anorexia, metallic taste
GU: Brown, black, green urine
HEMA: Hemolysis, increased hemoglobin (**IV** only)
INTEG: Rash, pruritus, fever, facial flushing, urticaria
MISC: **Anaphylaxis** (IM, **IV**)

Contraindications: Hypersensitivity, P child <12 yr, intermittent porphyria

Precautions: Renal disease, hepatic disease, addictive personalities, pregnancy **C**, myasthenia gravis, epilepsy

Pharmacokinetics

Absorption	Rapidly absorbed (PO)
Distribution	Widely distributed; crosses placenta
Metabolism	Liver, partially
Excretion	Kidney, unchanged
Half-life	1-2 hr

Pharmacodynamics

	PO	IM	IV
Onset	½ hr	Rapid	Rapid
Peak	1-2 hr	Unknown	Inf end
Duration	>8 hr	Unknown	Unknown

Interactions

Individual drugs

Alcohol: CNS depression

Drug classifications

Antidepressants, tricyclic: ↑ CNS depression
Barbiturates: ↑ CNS depression
Narcotics: ↑ CNS depression
Sedative/hypnotics: ↑ CNS depression

Lab test interferences

False: ↑ VMA, ↑ urinary 5-HIAA

NURSING CONSIDERATIONS

Assessment

- Assess for pain and spasm: location, duration, intensity, range of motion
- Monitor during and after inj: CNS effects, rash, conjunctivitis, and nasal congestion may occur
- Monitor ECG in epileptic patients; poor seizure control has occurred in patients taking this drug
- Assess allergic reactions: rash, fever, respiratory distress; check for severe weakness, numbness in extremities
- Assess for tolerance: increased need for medication, more frequent requests for medication, increased pain
- Assess for CNS depression: dizziness, drowsiness, psychiatric symptoms

Nursing diagnoses

✓ Physical mobility, impaired (uses)
✓ Injury, risk for (adverse reactions)
✓ Knowledge deficit (teaching)

Implementation

PO route

- Give with meals if GI symptoms occur
- Store in airtight container at room temp

IV **IV route**

- Give **IV** undiluted over 1 min or more; give 300 mg or less/1 min or longer; may be diluted in 250 ml or less D_5 or isotonic NaCl sol
- Give by slow **IV** to prevent phlebitis; keep recumbent for 15 min to prevent orthostatic hypotension; check for extravasation

IM route

- Give deep in large muscle mass; rotate sites

Patient/family education

- Advise patient not to discontinue medication quickly; insomnia, nausea, headache, spasticity, tachycardia will occur; drug should be tapered off over 1-2 wk

- Inform patient that urine may turn green, black, or brown
- Caution patient not to take with alcohol, other CNS depressants; increased CNS depression can occur
- Advise patient to avoid altering activities while taking this drug
- Caution patient to avoid hazardous activities if drowsiness, dizziness occur; driving should be avoided until drug response is known
- Advise patient to avoid using OTC medications that are CNS depressants (cough preparations, antihistamines) unless directed by prescriber; CNS depression can occur

Evaluation

Positive therapeutic outcome

- Decreased pain, spasticity

Treatment of overdose:

Induce emesis in conscious patient; lavage, dialysis; have epinephrine, antihistamines, and corticosteroids available

---

HIGH ALERT

methotrexate (℞)

(meth-oh-trex′ate)

Amethopterin, Folex, Folex PFS, methotrexate, methotrexate LPF, Rheumatrex, Trexall

Func. class.: Antineoplastic, antimetabolite

Chem. class.: Folic acid antagonist

Pregnancy category X

Action: Inhibits an enzyme that reduces folic acid, which is needed for nucleic acid synthesis in all cells; cell cycle specific (S phase); immunosuppressive

Therapeutic Outcome: Prevention of rapidly growing malignant cells; immunosuppression

Uses: Acute lymphocytic leukemia, in combination for breast, lung, head, neck carcinoma, lymphosarcoma, gestational choriocarcinoma, hydatidiform mole, psoriasis, rheumatoid arthritis, mycosis fungoides

Dosage and routes

Acute lymphocytic leukemia

P ***Adult and child:*** PO 3.3 mg/m^2/day given with prednisone IT 12 mg/m^2; maintenance 30 mg/m^2/day 2 times a wk; **IV** 2.5 mg/kg q2 wk

Burkitt's lymphoma (stages I, II, III)

Adult: PO 10-25 mg qd × 4-8 days with 7-day rest period

Lymphosarcoma (stage III)

Adult: PO/IM/IV, 0.625-2.5 mg/kg/day

Meningeal leukemia

P ***Adult and child:*** 12 mg/m^2 IT q2-5 days until CSF is normal, then one additional dose, max 15 mg

Choriocarcinoma

P ***Adult and child:*** PO 15-30 mg/m^2 qd × 5 days, then off 1 wk; may repeat

Breast cancer

Adult: **IV** 40 mg/m^2 on days 1 and 8 with other antineoplastics

Rheumatoid arthritis

Adult: PO 7.5 mg/wk, max 20 mg/wk

Osteosarcoma

P ***Adult and child:*** **IV** 12 g/m^2 given over 4 hr, then leucovorin rescue is given

Mycosis fungoides

Adult: PO 2.5-10 mg/day until cleared (may be many mo); IM 50 mg qwk or 25 mg 2 ×/wk

Psoriasis

Adult: PO/IM/**IV** 10 mg qwk; may increase to 25 mg qwk

Available forms: Tabs 2.5, 5, 7.5, 10, 15 mg; inj 25 mg/ml; powder

M

for inj 20, 25, 50, 100, 250 mg/g; sodium inj 2.5, 25 mg/ml

Adverse effects

CNS: Dizziness, **seizures,** headache, confusion, hemiparesis, malaise, fatigue, chills, fever
GI: Nausea, vomiting, anorexia, diarrhea, stomatitis, **hepatotoxicity,** cramps, ulcer, gastritis, **GI hemorrhage,** abdominal pain, hematemesis
GU: Urinary retention, **renal failure,** menstrual irregularities, defective spermatogenesis, **hematuria, azotemia, uric acid nephropathy**
HEMA: **Leukopenia, thrombocytopenia, myelosuppression, anemia**
INTEG: Rash, alopecia, dry skin, urticaria, photosensitivity, folliculitis, vasculitis, petechiae, ecchymosis, acne, alopecia

Contraindications: Hypersensitivity, leukopenia (<2500/mm^3), thrombocytopenia (<100,000/mm^3), anemia, psoriatic patients with severe renal/hepatic disease, pregnancy **X**, alcoholism, HIV infection

Precautions: Renal disease, lactation

Do Not Confuse:

methotrexate/metolazone

Pharmacokinetics

Absorption	Well absorbed (GI)
Distribution	Widely distributed; crosses placenta
Metabolism	Not metabolized
Excretion	Kidneys, unchanged; breast milk (minimal)
Half-life	2-4 hr; increased in renal disease

Pharmacodynamics

	PO	IM/IV	IT
Onset	Unknown	Unknown	Unknown
Peak	1-4 hr	½-2 hr	Unknown
Duration	Unknown	Unknown	Unknown

Interactions

Individual drugs

Acyclovir: ↑ neurologic reactions (IT route)
Allopurinol: ↑ toxicity
Asparaginase: ↓ effects of methotrexate
Chloramphenicol: ↑ toxicity
Cyclophosphamide: ↑ cardiotoxicity, CHF
Phenylbutazone: ↑ toxicity
Phenytoin: ↑ toxicity
Probenecid: ↑ toxicity
Radiation: ↑ toxicity, bone marrow suppression
Theophylline: ↑ toxicity
Warfarin: ↑ or ↓ effect of warfarin

Drug classifications

Antineoplastics: ↑ toxicity, bone marrow suppression
Hepatotoxic agents: ↑ hepatotoxicity
Live virus vaccines: ↓ antibodies
Nephrotoxic drugs: ↑ toxicity
Nondepolarizing muscle relaxants: Reversal of neuromuscular blockade
NSAIDs: ↑ toxicity
Penicillins: ↑ toxicity
Salicylates: ↑ toxicity
Sulfonylureas: ↑ toxicity
Tetracylines: ↑ toxicity

NURSING CONSIDERATIONS

Assessment

- Assess buccal cavity q8h for dryness, sores or ulceration, white patches, oral pain, bleeding, dysphagia; obtain prescription for viscous lidocaine (Xylocaine)
- Assess symptoms indicating severe allergic reaction: rash, pruritus, urticaria, purpuric skin lesions, itching, flushing
- Assess tachypnea, ECG changes, dyspnea, edema, fatigue; identify dyspnea, rales, unproductive cough, chest pain, tachypnea
- Monitor CBC, differential, platelet count weekly; withhold drug if WBC is <4000/mm^3 or platelet count is

<100,000/mm^3; notify prescriber of results if WBC <20,000/mm^3, platelets <150,000/mm^3
- Assess for increased uric acid levels, swelling, joint pain primarily in extremities; patient should be well hydrated to prevent urate deposits
- Monitor renal function studies: BUN, creatinine, serum uric acid, urine CrCl before and during therapy; check I&O ratio; report fall in urine output to <30 ml/hr
- Monitor temp q4h (may indicate beginning of infection)
- Monitor liver function tests before and during therapy (bilirubin, AST, ALT, LDH) as needed or monthly; check for jaundice of skin and sclera, dark urine, clay-colored stools, itchy skin, abdominal pain, fever, diarrhea (hepatotoxicity)
- Assess for bleeding: hematuria, stool guaiac, bruising or petechiae, mucosa or orifices q8h; check for inflammation of mucosa, breaks in skin
- Identify effects of alopecia on body image; discuss feelings about body changes
- Identify edema in feet, joint and stomach pain, shaking; prescriber should be notified

Nursing diagnoses

✓ Injury, risk for (adverse reactions)
✓ Body image disturbance (adverse reactions)
✓ Infection, risk for (adverse reactions)
✓ Knowledge deficit (teaching)

Implementation

- Avoid contact with skin, since drug is very irritating; wash completely to remove
- ❗ Administer leucovorin calcium within 12 hr of giving this drug to prevent tissue damage; check agency policy
- Give fluids **IV** or PO before chemotherapy to hydrate patient
- Give antacid before oral agent; give drug after evening meal, before hs; give antiemetic 30-60 min before giving drug and prn to prevent vomiting; administer antibiotics for infection prophylaxis
- Give in AM so drug can be eliminated before hs
- Provide liq diet: carbonated beverages; gelatin may be added if patient is not nauseated or vomiting
- Encourage patient to rinse mouth tid-qid with water, club soda; brush teeth bid-qid with soft brush or cotton-tipped applicators for stomatitis; use unwaxed dental floss

PO route
- Give 1 hr ac or 2 hr pc to prevent vomiting

IM route
- Give deeply in large muscle mass

IV **IV route**
- Give **IV** after diluting 5 mg/2 ml of sterile water for inj; give through Y-tube or 3-way stopcock at 10 mg or less/min
- Give **IV** inf after diluting in 0.9% NaCl, D_5W, D_5/0.9% NaCl and give as prescribed

Syringe compatibilities:
Bleomycin, cisplatin, cyclophosphamide, doxapram, doxorubicin, fluorouracil, furosemide, heparin, leucovorin, mitomycin, vinblastine, vincristine

Syringe incompatibilities:
Droperidol, ranitidine

Y-site compatibilities:
Allopurinol, amifostine, asparaginase, aztreonam, bleomycin, cefepime, ceftriaxone, cimetidine, cisplatin, cyclophosphamide, cytarabine, daunorubicin, dexchlorpheniramine, diphenhydramine, doxorubicin, etoposide, famotidine, filgrastim, fludarabine, fluorouracil, furosemide, gallium, ganciclovir, granisetron, heparin, hydromorphone, imipenem-cilastatin, leucovorin, lorazepam, melphalan, mesna, methylprednisolone, metoclopramide, mitomycin, morphine, ondansetron, oxacillin, paclitaxel, piperacillin/tazobactam,

M

prochlorperazine, ranitidine, sargramostim, teniposide, thiotepa, vinblastine, vincristine, vinorelbine

Y-site incompatibilities: Droperidol, idarubicin

Additive compatibilities: Cephalothin, cyclophosphamide, cytarabine, fluorouracil, hydroxyzine, mercaptopurine, ondansetron, sodium bicarbonate, vincristine

Additive incompatibilities: Bleomycin, prednisolone

Solution compatibilities: Amino acids, 4.25%/D_{25}, D_5W, sodium bicarbonate 0.05 mol/L, sodium chloride 0.9%

Patient/family education

- Advise patient that contraceptive measures are recommended during therapy; drug is teratogenic; contraception should be used for 3 mo (male) and 4-6 wk (female)
- Teach patient to avoid use of products containing aspirin or NSAIDs, razors, commercial mouthwash, since bleeding may occur; to report symptoms of bleeding (hematuria, tarry stools)
- Caution patient to report signs of anemia (fatigue, headache, irritability, faintness, shortness of breath)
- Advise patient to report any changes in breathing or coughing even several mo after treatment; to avoid crowds and persons with respiratory tract or other infections
- Teach patient that hair may be lost during treatment; a wig or hairpiece may make patient feel better; new hair may be different in color, texture
- Caution patient not to have any vaccinations without the advice of the prescriber; serious reactions can occur
- Advise patient to use sunblock or protective clothing to prevent burns

Evaluation

Positive therapeutic outcome

- Prevention of rapid division of malignant cells

methyldopa/ methyldopate (℞)

(meth-ill-doe'pa)

Aldomet, Apo-methyldopa ✦, Dopamet ✦, methyldopa/ methyldopate HCl, Novamedopa, Nu-Medopa ✦

Func. class.: Antihypertensive

Chem. class.: Centrally acting α-adrenergic inhibitor

Pregnancy category C

Action: Stimulates central α_2-adrenergic receptors in the CNS, resulting in decreased sympathetic outflow from the brain with decreased peripheral resistance

➔ **Therapeutic Outcome:** Decreased B/P in hypertension

Uses: Hypertension

Dosage and routes

Adult: PO 250-500 mg bid or tid, then adjusted q2 days prn, 0.5-2 g qd in 2-4 divided doses (maintenance), max 3 g/day; **IV** 250-500 mg in 100 ml D_5W q6h, run over 30-60 min, not to exceed 1 g q6h, switch to PO as soon as possible

G ***Elderly:*** PO 125 mg bid tid, increase q2 days as needed, max 3 g/day

P ***Child:*** PO 10 mg/kg/day in 2-4 divided doses, max 65 mg/kg or 3 g/day, whichever is less; **IV** 20-40 mg/kg/day in 4 divided doses, max 65 mg/kg or 3 g, whichever is less

Available forms: Methyldopa tabs 125, 250, 500 mg; oral susp 50 mg/ml; methydopate inj 50 mg/ml (250 mg/5 ml)

Adverse effects

CNS: *Drowsiness, weakness, dizziness, sedation, headache,* depression, psychosis, paresthesias, parkinsonism, Bell's palsy, nightmares
CV: Bradycardia, **myocarditis,** orthostatic hypotension, angina, edema, weight gain, CHF
EENT: Nasal congestion, eczema
ENDO: Breast enlargement, gynecomastia, lactation, amenorrhea
GI: Nausea, vomiting, diarrhea, constipation, **hepatic dysfunction,** sore or "black" tongue, **pancreatitis**
GU: Impotence, failure to ejaculate
HEMA: **Leukopenia, thrombocytopenia, hemolytic anemia, granulocytopenia,** positive Coombs' test
INTEG: Lupus-like syndrome, rash, toxic epidural necrolysis

Contraindications: Active hepatic disease, hypersensitivity, blood dyscrasias

Precautions: Pregnancy **B** (PO), **C** (**IV**) liver disease, eclampsia, severe cardiac disease

Do Not Confuse:
methyldopa/L-dopa (levodopa)

Pharmacokinetics

Absorption	50% (PO)
Distribution	Crosses placenta, blood-brain barrier
Metabolism	Liver, moderately
Excretion	Kidneys, unchanged (partially)
Half-life	1½ hr

Pharmacodynamics

	PO	IV
Onset	Unknown	Unknown
Peak	2-4 hr	2 hr
Duration	12-24 hr	10-16 hr

Interactions

Individual drugs

Alcohol: ↑ hypotension
Haloperidol: ↑ psychosis
Levodopa: ↑ hypotension, toxicity
Lithium: ↑ lithium toxicity
Tolbutamide: ↑ hypoglycemia

Drug classifications

Amphetamines: ↓ antihypertensive effect
Antidepressants, tricyclic: ↓ effects of methyldopa
Antihypertensives: ↑ hypotension
β-Adrenergic blockers: ↑ B/P
Barbiturates: ↓ effects of methyldopa
MAOIs: ↑ pressor effect
Nitrates: ↑ hypotension
NSAIDs: ↓ antihypertensive effect
Phenothiazines: ↓ antihypertensive effect

Herb/drug

Indian snakeroot: ↓ methyldopa effect
Capsicum: ↓ methyldopa effect

Lab test interferences

Interference: Urinary uric acid, serum creatinine, AST
False: ↑ Urinary catecholamines

NURSING CONSIDERATIONS

Assessment

- Monitor blood studies: neutrophils, decreased platelets
- Monitor renal studies: protein, BUN, creatinine; watch for increased levels that may indicate nephrotic syndrome: polyuria, oliguria, frequency
- Obtain baselines in renal, liver function tests before therapy begins; check potassium levels, although hyperkalemia rarely occurs
- Monitor B/P, pulse if the drug is being used for hypertension; notify prescriber of changes
- Monitor edema in feet, legs daily; monitor I&O; check weight for decreasing output
- Assess for allergic reaction: rash, fever, pruritus, urticaria; drug should be discontinued if antihistamines fail to help
- Monitor CNS symptoms, especially G in the elderly

Nursing diagnoses

✓ Cardiac output, decreased (uses)
✓ Injury, risk for (side effects)

M

✓ Knowledge deficit (teaching)
✓ Noncompliance (teaching)

Implementation

PO route

- Give ac
- Shake susp before using
- Store in airtight container at room temp

IV **IV route**

- Give by intermittent inf after diluting in 100 ml of 0.9% NaCl, D_5W, D_5/0.9% NaCl, 5% sodium bicarbonate, Ringer's; administer over 30-60 min

Y-site compatibilities: Esmolol, heparin, meperidine, morphine, theophylline

Additive compatibilities: Aminophylline, ascorbic acid, chloramphenicol, diphenhydramine, heparin, magnesium sulfate, multivitamins, netilmicin, potassium chloride, promazine, sodium bicarbonate, succinylcholine, verapamil, vit B/C

Additive incompatibilities: Amphotericin B, barbiturates, methohexital, sulfonamides

Solution compatibilities: D_5W, D_5/0.9% NaCl, Ringer's, sodium bicarbonate 5%, 0.9% NaCl, amino acids 4.25%/D_{25}, Dextran$_6$/0.9% NaCl, Normosol R, Normosol M/D_5W

Patient/family education

- Instruct patient not to discontinue drug abruptly, or withdrawal symptoms may occur: anxiety, increased B/P, headache, insomnia, increased pulse, tremors, nausea, sweating
- Caution patient not to use OTC (cough, cold, or allergy) products unless directed by prescriber
- Teach patient to comply with dosage schedule even if feeling better; drug controls symptoms, does not cure
- Caution patient to change position slowly, to rise slowly to sitting or standing position to minimize ortho- G static hypotension, especially elderly
- Teach patient about excessive perspiration, dehydration, vomiting, diarrhea, may lead to fall in B/P; consult prescriber if these occur
- Advise patient that drug may cause dizziness, fainting; lightheadedness may occur during 1st few days of therapy; that drug may cause dry mouth; use hard candy, saliva product, or frequent rinsing of mouth
- Caution patient that compliance is necessary; not to skip or stop drug unless directed by prescriber
- Teach patient that drug may cause skin rash
- Teach patient to avoid hazardous activities, since drug may cause drowsiness, dizziness
- Teach patient to take ac

Evaluation

Positive therapeutic outcome

- Decreased B/P

Treatment of overdose: Gastric evacuation, sympathomimetics, may be indicated if severe; hemodialysis

methylergonovine (℞)

(meth-ill-er-goe-noe′veen)

Methergine, methylergonovine

Func. class.: Oxytocic

Chem. class.: Ergot alkaloid

Pregnancy category C

Action: Stimulates uterine and vascular smooth muscle, causing contractions, decreased bleeding

➡ **Therapeutic Outcome:** Absence of hemorrhage

Uses: Treatment of hemorrhage postpartum or after abortion

Dosage and routes

Adult: IM 0.2 mg q2-5h, not to exceed 5 doses; **IV** 0.2 mg given over 1 min; PO 0.2 mg given over 1 min; PO 0.2-0.4 mg q6-12h × 2-7 days after initial IM or **IV** dose

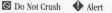

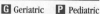

Available forms: Inj 0.2 mg/ml; tabs 0.2 mg

Adverse effects

CNS: *Headache, dizziness,* **seizures**
CV: Chest pain, palpitations, hypertension, *hypotension,* **dysrhythmias; CVA (IV)**
EENT: Tinnitus
GI: *Nausea, vomiting*
GU: Cramping
INTEG: Sweating, rash, allergic reactions
RESP: *Dyspnea*

Contraindications: Hypersensitivity to ergot preparations, indication of labor, before delivery of placenta, hypertension, pelvic inflammatory disease, respiratory disease, cardiac disease, peripheral vascular disease

Precautions: Pregnancy **C**, severe hepatic disease, severe renal disease, jaundice, diabetes mellitus, convulsive disorders

Pharmacokinetics

Absorption	Well absorbed (PO, IM)
Distribution	Unknown
Metabolism	Liver, possibly
Excretion	Unknown
Half-life	½-2 hr

Pharmacodynamics

	PO	IM	IV
Onset	5-15 min	5 min	Immediate
Peak	Unknown	Unknown	Unknown
Duration	3 hr	3 hr	Unknown

Interactions

Individual drugs

Cyclopropane anesthesia: ↑ hypotension

Drug classifications

Vasopressors: ↑ hypertension

Smoking

↑ Vasoconstriction

NURSING CONSIDERATIONS

Assessment

- Monitor B/P, pulse; watch for change that may indicate hemorrhage; check respiratory rate, rhythm, depth; notify prescriber of abnormalities
- Assess fundal tone, nonphasic contractions; check for relaxation or severe cramping
- Assess for ergotism or overdose: nausea, vomiting, weakness, muscular pain, insensitivity to cold, paresthesia of extremities; drug should be decreased or inf discontinued
- Before administering ergonovine, check calcium levels; if hypocalcemia is present, correction should be made to increase effectiveness of this drug
- Monitor prolactin levels and for decreased breast milk production

Nursing diagnoses

- ✓ Tissue perfusion, decreased (uses)
- ✓ Injury, risk for (adverse reactions)
- ✓ Knowledge deficit (teaching)

Implementation

PO route
- PO is the preferred route

IM route
- Give deeply in large muscle mass

IV **IV route**
- Give by this route for severe, life-threatening hemorrhage
- Give directly undiluted or diluted with 5 ml of 0.9% NaCl given through Y-site or 3-way stopcock; give 0.2 mg/min; use clear, colorless sol
- Store up to 2 mo if unused

Y-site compatibilities:

Heparin, hydrocortisone sodium succinate, potassium chloride, vit B/C

Patient/family education

- Advise patient to stop smoking, since increased vasoconstriction will result
- Inform patient that abdominal cramps are a side effect of this medication
- Instruct patient to notify prescriber if chest pain, nausea, vomiting, headache, muscle pain, weakness or cold, numb extremities occur

Evaluation

Positive therapeutic outcome
- Prevention of hemorrhage

M

methylphenidate (℞)

(meth-ill-fen'i-date)

Concerta, Metadate CD, Metadate ER, Methidate, Methylin, Methylin ER, PMS-methylphenidate, Ritalin, Ritalin SR

Func. class.: Cerebral stimulant
Chem. class.: Piperidine derivative

Pregnancy category C

Controlled substance schedule II

Action: Increases release of norepinephrine and dopamine in cerebral cortex to reticular activating system; exact action not known

Therapeutic Outcome: Increased alertness, decreased fatigue, ability to stay awake (narcolepsy), increased attention span, decreased hyperactivity (ADHD)

Uses: Attention deficit disorder with hyperactivity (ADHD), narcolepsy

Investigational uses: Depression in the elderly, cancer, poststroke, HIV, brain injury, anesthesia-related hiccups

Dosage and routes

ADHD

Adult: PO 5-20 bid-tid

Child >6 yr: PO 5 mg before breakfast and lunch, increasing by 5-10 mg/wk, not to exceed 60 mg/day; sus rel 20 mg qd-tid

Narcolepsy

Adult: PO 10 mg bid-tid, 30-45 min ac; may increase up to 40-60 mg/day

Depression

Elderly: PO 2.5 mg q AM, increase q 3rd day by 2.5 mg to desired dose, max 20 mg/day

Available forms: Tabs 5, 10, 20 mg; sus rel tabs 20 mg; ext rel caps 20 mg; ext rel tabs 10, 18, 20, 36, 54 mg

Adverse effects

CNS: *Hyperactivity, insomnia, restlessness, talkativeness,* dizziness, headache, akathisia, dyskinesia, masking or worsening of Gilles de la Tourette's syndrome, **seizures,** drowsiness, toxic psychosis

CV: *Palpitations, tachycardia,* B/P changes, angina, **dysrhythmias**

ENDO: Growth retardation

GI: Nausea, anorexia, dry mouth, weight loss, abdominal pain

HEMA: **Leukopenia,** anemia, **thrombocytopenic purpura**

INTEG: **Exfoliative dermatitis,** urticaria, rash, erythema multiforme

MISC: Fever, arthralgia, scalp hair loss

Contraindications: Hypersensitivity, anxiety, history of Gilles de la Tourette's syndrome; children <6 yr, glaucoma

Precautions: Hypertension, depression, pregnancy **C,** seizures, lactation, drug abuse

Do Not Confuse:
methylphenidate/methadone

Pharmacokinetics

Absorption	Well absorbed (PO); delayed (sus rel)
Distribution	Widely distributed; crosses placenta
Metabolism	Liver
Excretion	Kidneys
Half-life	1-3 hr

Pharmacodynamics

	PO	PO–SUS REL
Onset	½-1 hr	2 hr
Peak	1-3 hr	4 hr
Duration	4-6 hr	6-8 hr

Interactions

Drug classifications

Anticonvulsants: ↑ effects
Antidepressants, tricyclic: ↑ effects
MAOIs: Hypertensive crisis
Oral anticoagulants: ↓ effects

Selective serotonin reuptake inhibitors: ↑ effect
Sympathomimetics: ↑ effects
Vasopressors: Hypertensive crisis
Food/drug
Caffeine: ↑ stimulation

NURSING CONSIDERATIONS
Assessment
- Monitor VS, B/P, since this drug may reverse antihypertensives; check patients with cardiac disease more often for increased B/P
- Perform CBC, urinalysis; for diabetic patients monitor blood glucose, urine glucose; insulin changes may be required, since eating will decrease
- Monitor height and weight q3 mo since growth rate in children may be decreased; appetite is suppressed, weight loss is common during the first few mo of treatment
- Monitor mental status: mood sensorium, affect, stimulation, insomnia; aggressiveness may occur; depression with crying spells may occur after drug has worn off
- Assess for tolerance; should not be used for extended time except in ADHD; dosage should be discontinued gradually to prevent withdrawal symptoms
- Assess for narcoleptic symptoms before medication and after; ability to stay awake should increase significantly
- In children or adults with ADHD, monitor for improved organizational skills, attention span, attending to tasks, impulse control, socialization, and ability to get along better with others
- Assess for withdrawal symptoms: headache, nausea, vomiting, muscle pain, weakness; drug tolerance will develop after long-term use; dosage should not be increased if tolerance develops
- Assess appetite, sleep, speech patterns

Nursing diagnoses
- ✓ Thought processes, altered (uses, adverse reactions)
- ✓ Coping, ineffective individual (uses)
- ✓ Knowledge deficit (teaching)
- ✓ Family coping, impaired (uses)

Implementation
- Give at least 6 hr before hs (regular release); at least 10 hr (sus rel, ext rel) to avoid sleeplessness; titrate to patient's response; lowest dosage should be used to control symptoms
- Do not chew, crush time rel tabs
- Give gum, hard candy, frequent sips of water for dry mouth at beginning of treatment; these symptoms tend to lessen with time

Patient/family education
- Teach patient to decrease caffeine consumption (coffee, tea, cola, chocolate), which may increase irritability and stimulation; to avoid OTC preparations unless approved by prescriber; to avoid alcohol ingestion; these may cause serious drug interactions
- Advise patient to taper off drug over several wk, or depression, increased sleeping, lethargy may occur
- Caution patient to avoid hazardous activities until stabilized on medication
- Instruct patient not to double doses if medication is missed; prescriber may suggest drug holidays (ADHD) during the school year to assess progress and determine continued drug necessity
- Instruct patient/family to notify presciber if significant side effects occur: tremors, insomnia, palpitations, restlessness; drug changes may be needed
- Inform patient that if dry mouth occurs to use frequent sips of water, sugarless gum, hard candy during beginning therapy; dry mouth lessens with continued treatment
- Encourage patient to get needed rest; patient will feel more tired at

M

end of day; to take last dose at least 6 hr before hs to avoid insomnia

Evaluation

Positive therapeutic outcome

- Decreased hyperactivity in ADHD
- Improved attention span in ADHD
- Absence of sleeping during day in narcolepsy

Treatment of overdose: Administer fluids, hemodialysis, peritoneal dialysis, antihypertensives for increased B/P

methylprednisolone (℞)

(meth-ill-pred-niss'oh-lone)

A-Methapred, dep Medalone, Depoject, Depo-Medrol, Depopred, Depo-Predate, Duralone, Medralone, Medrol, Rep-Pred, Solu-Medrol

Func. class.: Corticosteroid

Chem. class.: Glucocorticoid, immediate acting

Pregnancy category C

Action: Decreases inflammation by suppression of migration of polymorphonuclear leukocytes, fibroblasts; reverses increased capillary permeability and lysosomal stabilization; antipruritic, antiinflammatory (top)

Therapeutic Outcome: Decreased inflammation

Uses: Severe inflammation, shock, adrenal insufficiency, collagen disorders, psoriasis, eczema, contact dermatitis, pruritus (top)

Dosage and routes

Adrenal insufficiency/ inflammation

Adult: PO 2-60 mg in 4 divided doses; IM 10-80 mg (acetate); IM/**IV** 10-250 mg (succinate); intraarticular 4-30 mg (acetate)

P ***Child:*** **IV** 117 µg-1.66 mg/kg in 3-4 divided doses (succinate)

Shock

Adult: **IV** 100-250 mg q2-6h or 30 mg/kg, then q4-6h prn × 2-3 days (succinate)

Multiple sclerosis

Adult: PO 160 mg/day × 1 wk, then 64 mg qod × 30 days

Pruritus

P ***Adult and child:*** TOP apply to affected area qd-qid

Available forms: Tabs 2, 4, 6, 8, 16, 24, 32 mg; inj 20, 40, 80 mg/ml acetate; inj 40, 125, 500, 1000 mg/vial succinate, 1%; dosepack 4 mg tabs

Adverse effects

CNS: Depression, flushing, sweating, headache, mood changes

CV: Hypertension, **circulatory collapse, thrombophlebitis, embolism,** tachycardia

EENT: Fungal infections, increased intraocular pressure, blurred vision, cataracts

GI: Diarrhea, nausea, abdominal distention, **GI hemorrhage,** increased appetite, **pancreatitis**

HEMA: **Thrombocytopenia**

INTEG: Burning, dryness, itching, irritation, acne, folliculitis, hypertrichosis, perioral dermatitis, hypopigmentation, atrophy, striae, miliaria, allergic contact dermatitis, secondary infection, poor wound healing, ecchymosis, petechiae

MS: Fractures, osteoporosis, weakness

Contraindications: Hypersensitivity to corticosteroids, fungal infections, psychosis, idiopathic thrombocytopenia, acute glomerulonephritis, amebiasis, nonasthmatic bronchial P disease, child <2 yr, AIDS, TB

Precautions: Pregnancy **C,** lactation, viral or bacterial infections, diabetes mellitus, glaucoma, osteoporosis

Do Not Confuse:
methylprednisolone/ medroxyprogesterone, methylprednisolone/prednisone

Pharmacokinetics

Absorption	Well absorbed (PO); systemic (top)
Distribution	Crosses placenta
Metabolism	Liver, extensively
Excretion	Kidney
Half-life	3-5 hr; adrenal suppression 3-4 days

Pharmacodynamics

	PO	IM	IV	TOP
Onset	Unknown	Unknown	Rapid	Min to hr
Peak	2 hr	4-8 days	Unknown	Hr to days
Duration	1½ days	1-4 wk	Unknown	Hr to days

Interactions

Individual drugs

Amphotericin B: ↑ hypokalemia
Insulin: ↑ need for insulin
Mezlocillin: ↑ hypokalemia
Phenytoin: ↓ action, ↑ metabolism
Rifampin: ↓ action, ↑ metabolism
Ticarcillin: ↑ hypokalemia

Drug classifications

Barbiturates: ↓ action, ↑ metabolism
Diuretics: ↑ hypokalemia
Hypoglycemic agents: ↑ need for hypoglycemic agents

Herb/drug

Aloe: ↑ hypokalemia
Buckthorn: ↑ hypokalemia
Cascara sagrada: ↑ hypokalemia
Rhubarb root: ↑ hypokalemia
Senna: ↑ hypokalemia

Lab test interferences

↑ Cholesterol, ↑ sodium, ↑ blood glucose, ↑ uric acid, ↑ calcium, ↑ urine glucose
↓ calcium, ↓ potassium, ↓ T_4, ↓ T_3, ↓ thyroid radioactive iodine uptake test, ↓ urine 17-OHCS, ↓ 17-KS, ↓ PBI
False negative: Skin allergy tests

NURSING CONSIDERATIONS

Assessment

- Monitor potassium, blood glucose, urine glucose while patient is on long-term therapy; hypokalemia and hyperglycemia
- Monitor weight daily; notify prescriber of weekly gain >5 lb
- Monitor B/P q4h, pulse; notify prescriber if chest pain occurs
- Monitor I&O ratio; be alert for decreasing urinary output and increasing edema
- Monitor plasma cortisol levels during long-term therapy (normal level 138-635 nmol/L when drawn at 8 AM)
- Monitor adrenal function periodically for hypothalamic-pituitary-adrenal axis suppression
- Assess for infection: increased temp, WBC even after withdrawal of medication; drug masks infection symptoms
- Assess for potassium depletion: paresthesias, fatigue, nausea, vomiting, depression, polyuria, dysrhythmias, weakness
- Assess for edema, hypertension, cardiac symptoms
- Assess mental status: affect, mood, behavioral changes, aggression
- Check temp; if fever develops, drug should be discontinued
- Assess for systemic absorption: increased temp, inflammation, irritation (top)

Nursing diagnoses

- ✓ Infection, risk for (adverse reactions)
- ✓ Knowledge deficit (teaching)
- ✓ Noncompliance (teaching)

Implementation

IV route

- Give **IV**, use only sodium phosphate product; give >1 min; may be given by **IV** inf in compatible sol
- Give after shaking susp (parenteral)
- Give titrated dosage; use lowest effective dosage

Syringe compatibilities: Granisetron, metoclopramide

Y-site compatibilities: Acyclovir, amifostine, amrinone,

M

aztreonam, cefepime, cisplatin, cladribine, cyclophosphamide, cytarabine, dopamine, doxorubicin, enalaprilat, famotidine, fludarabine, granisetron, heparin, melphalan, meperidine, methotrexate, metronidazole, midazolam, morphine, piperacillin/tazobactam, sodium bicarbonate, tacrolimus, teniposide, theophylline, thiotepa, vit B with C

Y-site incompatibilities: Ondansetron, paclitaxel, sargramostim, vinorelbine

Additive compatibilities: Chloramphenicol, cimetidine, clindamycin, dopamine, granisetron, heparin, norepinephrine, penicillin G potassium, ranitidine, theophylline, verapamil

IM route

- Give IM inj deep in large muscle mass; rotate sites; avoid deltoid; use 21-G needle
- Give in one dose in AM to prevent adrenal suppression; avoid SC administration; may damage tissue

PO route

- Give with food or milk to decrease GI symptoms

Inhalation route

- Give inh with water to decrease possibility of fungal infections
- Give titrated dosage; use lowest effective dosage
- Clean aerosol top daily with warm water; dry thoroughly
- Store in cool environment; do not puncture or incinerate container

Topical route

- Cleanse area before applying drug
- Apply only to affected areas; do not get in eyes
- Apply medication, then cover with occlusive dressing (only if prescribed); seal to normal skin; change q12h; systemic absorption may occur
- Apply only to dermatoses; do not use on weeping, denuded, or infected area
- Apply treatment for a few days after area has cleared
- Store at room temp

Patient/family education

- Teach patient that ID as steroid user should be carried
- Advise patient to notify prescriber if therapeutic response decreases; dosage adjustment may be needed
- Caution patient not to discontinue abruptly; adrenal crisis can result
- Caution patient to avoid OTC products: salicylates, alcohol in cough products, cold preparations unless directed by prescriber
- Teach patient all aspects of drug usage including cushingoid symptoms
- Teach patient symptoms of adrenal insufficiency: nausea, anorexia, fatigue, dizziness, dyspnea, weakness, joint pain
- Inform patient that long-term therapy may be needed to clear infection (1-2 mo depending on type of infection)

Nasal route

- Advise patient to clear nasal passages if sneezing attack occurs; repeat dose
- Advise patient to continue using product even if mild nasal bleeding occurs; is usually transient
- Teach patient method of instillation after providing written instructions from manufacturer

Topical route

- Advise patient to avoid sunlight on affected area; burns may occur

Evaluation

Positive therapeutic outcome

- Ease of respirations, decreased inflammation
- Absence of severe itching, patches on skin, flaking (top)

methysergide (℞)
(meth-i-ser'jide)
Sansert
Func. class.: Adrenergic blocker, serotonin antagonist
Chem. class.: Ergot derivative
Pregnancy category X

Action: Competitively blocks serotonin (hydroxytryptamine) receptors in CNS and periphery; potent vasoconstrictor

Therapeutic Outcome: Absence of migraines and other vascular headaches

Uses: Prophylaxis for migraine and other vascular headaches; if no improvement is noted in 3 wk, drug is unlikely to be beneficial

Dosage and routes
Adult: PO 2 mg bid with meals; 3-4 wk rest period after each 6-mo treatment

Available forms: Tabs 2 mg

Adverse effects
CNS: *Tremors, anxiety,* insomnia, headache, dizziness, euphoria, confusion, depersonalization, hallucinations, paresthesias, drowsiness
CV: **Retroperitoneal fibrosis,** valvular thickening, palpitations, tachycardia, postural hypertension, angina, thrombophlebitis, ECG changes, **cardiac fibrosis**
GI: Nausea, vomiting, weight gain
HEMA: **Blood dyscrasias**
INTEG: Flushing, rash, alopecia
MS: Arthralgia, myalgia

Contraindications: Hypersensitivity to ergot, tartrazine, peripheral vascular occlusion, CAD, hepatic disease, renal disease, peptic ulcer, hypertension, connective tissue disease, fibrotic pulmonary disease

Precautions: Pregnancy **X,** lactation, children

Pharmacokinetics

Absorption	Rapidly absorbed
Distribution	Widely distributed
Metabolism	Liver
Excretion	Kidneys, breast milk
Half-life	10 hr

Pharmacodynamics
Unknown

Interactions
Drug classifications
β-Adrenergic blockers: ↑ vasoconstriction
Opiates: ↓ effect of opiates
Smoking
↑ Vasoconstriction

NURSING CONSIDERATIONS
Assessment
- Monitor stress level, activity, reaction, coping mechanisms of patient
- Assess neurologic status: LOC, blurring vision, nausea, vomiting, tingling in extremities preceding headache
- Assess for ingestion of tyramine-containing foods (pickled products, beer, wine, aged cheese), food additives, preservatives, colorings, artificial sweeteners, chocolate, caffeine, which may precipitate these types of headaches

Nursing diagnoses
- ✓ Pain, chronic (uses)
- ✓ Injury, risk for (adverse reactions)
- ✓ Knowledge deficit (teaching)

Implementation
- Provide quiet, calm environment with decreased stimulation; no noise, bright lights, or excessive talking
- Give with or pc to avoid GI symptoms
- Store in dark area

Patient/family education
- Caution patient to avoid OTC medications and alcohol; serious drug interactions may occur
- Caution patient to maintain dosage

M

at approved level; not to increase even if drug does not relieve headache
- Advise patient that an increase in headaches may occur when this drug is discontinued after long-term use
- Caution patient to keep drug out of P the reach of children; death may occur
- Caution patient to use drug for less than 6 mo continuously; a 3-4 wk drug-free period must follow each 6 mo period

Evaluation
Positive therapeutic outcome
- Decrease in frequency, severity of headache

metoclopramide (Rx)
(met-oh-kloe-pra'mide)
Apo-Metoclop ♣, Clopra, Emex ♣, Maxeran ♣, Maxolon, metoclopramide, Octamide PFS, Reclomide, Reglan
Func. class.: Cholinergic, antiemetic
Chem. class.: Central dopamine receptor antagonist
Pregnancy category B

Action: Enhances response to acetylcholine of tissue in upper GI tract, which causes contraction of gastric muscle, relaxes pyloric, duodenal segments, increases peristalsis without stimulating secretions, blocks dopamine in chemoreceptor trigger zone of CNS

➔ **Therapeutic Outcome:** Decreased symptoms of delayed gastric emptying, decreased nausea, vomiting

Uses: Prevention of nausea, vomiting induced by chemotherapy, radiation; delayed gastric emptying, gastroesophageal reflux

Investigational uses: Hiccups, migraines

Dosage and routes
Nausea/vomiting
Adult: **IV** 1-2 mg/kg 30 min before administration of chemotherapy, then q2h × 2 doses, then q3h × 3 doses
P ***Child:*** **IV** 0.1-0.2 mg/kg/dose

Facilitation of small bowel intubation in radiologic exams
P ***Adult and child >14 yr:*** **IV** 10 mg over 1-2 min
P ***Child <6 yr:*** **IV** 0.1 mg/kg
P ***Child 6-14 yr:*** **IV** 2.5-5 mg

Delayed gastric emptying
Adult: PO 10 mg 30 min ac, hs × 2-8 wk
G ***Elderly:*** PO 5 mg ½ hr ac hs, increase to 10 mg if needed

Gastroesophageal reflux
Adult: PO 10-15 mg qid 30 min ac
P ***Child:*** 0.4-0.8 mg/kg/day divided in 4 doses

Renal dose: CrCl <40 ml/min 50% of dose

Available forms: Tabs 5, 10 mg; syrup 5 mg/5 ml; inj 5 mg/ml

Adverse effects
CNS: *Sedation, fatigue, restlessness, headache, sleeplessness, dystonia,* dizziness, drowsiness, suicide ideation, **seizures**
CV: Hypotension, **supraventricular tachycardia**
GI: Dry mouth, constipation, nausea, anorexia, vomiting, diarrhea
GU: Decreased libido, prolactin secretion, amenorrhea, galactorrhea
HEMA: **Neutropenia, leukopenia, agranulocytosis**
INTEG: Urticaria, rash

Contraindications: Hypersensitivity to this drug or procaine or procainamide, seizure disorder, pheochromocytoma, breast cancer (prolactin dependent), GI obstruction

Precautions: Pregnancy **B**, lactation, GI hemorrhage, CHF, Parkinson's disease

Do Not Confuse:
metoclopramide/metolazone, Reglan/Megace

Pharmacokinetics

Absorption	Well absorbed (PO)
Distribution	Widely distributed; crosses blood-brain barrier, placenta
Metabolism	Liver, minimally
Excretion	Kidneys, breast milk
Half-life	4 hr

Pharmacodynamics

	PO	IM	IV
Onset	½-1 hr	10-15 min	1-3 min
Peak	Unknown	Unknown	Unknown
Duration	1-2 hr	1-2 hr	1-2 hr

Interactions
Individual drugs
Alcohol: ↓ action of metoclopramide
Digoxin: ↓ action
Haloperidol: ↑ extrapyramidal reaction
Drug classifications
Anticholinergics: ↓ action of metoclopramide
Antidepressants: ↑ CNS depression
Antihistamines: ↑ CNS depression
CNS depressants: ↑ sedation
MAOIs: Avoid use
Opiates: ↑ sedation
Phenothiazines: ↑ extrapyramidal reaction
Sedative/hypnotics: ↑ CNS depression
Lab test interferences
↑ Prolactin, ↑ aldosterone, ↑ thyrotropin

NURSING CONSIDERATIONS
Assessment
- Assess GI complaints: nausea, vomiting, anorexia, constipation, abdominal distention before and after administration
- Assess for extrapyramidal symptoms (EPS) and tardive dyskinesia, more likely to occur in elderly patient: rigidity, grimacing, shuffling gait, tremors, rhythmic involuntary movements of tongue, mouth, jaw, feet, hands; these side effects should be reported to prescriber immediately; some effects may be irreversible
- Assess mental status: depression, anxiety, irritability during treatment

Nursing diagnoses
✓ Injury, risk for (adverse reactions)
✓ Knowledge deficit (teaching)

Implementation
IV route
- Give **IV** undiluted if dose is <10 mg; give over 2 min
- Dilute 10 mg or more in 50 ml or more D_5W, NaCl, Ringer's, LR and give over 15 min or more
- Give diphenhydramine **IV** for EPS
- Discard open ampules

Syringe compatibilities:
Aminophylline, ascorbic acid, atropine, benztropine, bleomycin, butorphanol, chlorpromazine, cisplatin, cyclophosphamide, cytarabine, dexamethasone, dimenhydrinate, diphenhydramine, doxorubicin, droperidol, fentanyl, fluorouracil, heparin, hydrocortisone, hydroxyzine, regular insulin, leucovorin, lidocaine, magnesium sulfate, meperidine, methotrimeprazine, methylprednisolone, midazolam, mitomycin, morphine, pentazocine, perphenazine, prochlorperazine, promazine, promethazine, ranitidine, scopolamine, sufentanil, vinblastine, vincristine, vit B/C

Syringe incompatibilities:
Ampicillin, calcium gluconate, cephalothin, chloramphenicol, furosemide, penicillin G potassium, sodium bicarbonate

Y-site compatibilities:
Acyclovir, aldesleukin, amifostine, aztreonam, bleomycin, ciprofloxacin, cisplatin, cladribine, cyclophosphamide, cytarabine, diltiazem, doxorubicin, droperidol, famotidine, filgrastim, fluconazole, fludarabine, fluorouracil, foscarnet, gallium, granisetron,

M

heparin, idarubicin, leucovorin, melphalan, meperidine, meropenem, methotrexate, mitomycin, morphine, ondansetron, paclitaxel, piperacillin/tazobactam, propofol, sargramostim, sufentanil, tacrolimus, teniposide, thiotepa, vinblastine, vincristine, vinorelbine, zidovudine

Y-site incompatibilities: Furosemide

Additive compatibilities: Clindamycin, meropenem, morphine, multivitamins, potassium acetate/chloride/phosphate, verapamil

Additive incompatibilities: Cisplatin, erythromycin, tetracycline

PO route

- Give 30-60 min ac for better absorption and at hs
- Use gum, hard candy, frequent rinsing of mouth for dryness of oral cavity

Patient/family education

- Instruct patient to avoid driving, other hazardous activities until stabilized on this medication
- Advise patient to avoid alcohol and other CNS depressants that enhance sedating properties of this drug
- Advise patient to notify prescriber if involuntary movements occur

Evaluation

Positive therapeutic outcome

- Absence of nausea, vomiting, anorexia, fullness

metolazone (℞)

(me-tole′a-zone)

MyKrox, Zaroxolyn

Func. class.: Diuretic, antihypertensive

Chem. class.: Thiazide-like quinazoline derivative

Pregnancy category B

Action: Acts on the distal tubule and cortical thick ascending limb of the loop of Henle in the kidney, increasing excretion of sodium, water, chloride, magnesium, potassium, and bicarbonate

➔ **Therapeutic Outcome:** Decreased B/P, decreased edema in lung tissue and peripherally

Uses: Edema in CHF, nephrotic syndrome; may be used alone or as adjunct with antihypertensives for mild to moderate hypertension

Dosage and routes

Edema

Adult: PO 5-20 mg/day

Hypertension

Adult: PO 2.5-5 mg/day (Zaroxolyn)

P ***Child:*** PO 0.2-0.4 mg/kg/day divided q12-24h

Adult: PO 0.5 mg (MyKrox) qd in AM: may increase to 1 mg

Available forms: MyKrox tabs 0.5; Zaroxolyn tabs 2.5, 5, 10 mg

Adverse effects

CNS: Drowsiness, paresthesia, anxiety, depression, headache, *dizziness, fatigue, weakness*

CV: Irregular pulse, orthostatic hypotension, palpitations, volume depletion, chest pain

EENT: Blurred vision

ELECT: *Hypokalemia,* hypercalcemia, hyponatremia, hypochloremia, hypomagnesemia, hypophosphatemia

GI: *Nausea, vomiting, anorexia,* constipation, diarrhea, cramps, **pancreatitis,** GI irritation, **hepatitis**

GU: *Frequency,* polyuria, **uremia,** glucosuria

HEMA: **Aplastic anemia, hemolytic anemia, leukopenia, agranulocytosis, neutropenia**

INTEG: *Rash,* urticaria, purpura, photosensitivity, fever

META: *Hyperglycemia, hypomagnesemia, increased creatinine, BUN*

Contraindications: Hypersensitivity to thiazides or sulfonamides, anuria, renal decompensation

Precautions: Hypokalemia, renal disease, hepatic disease, gout, COPD, lupus erythematosus, diabetes mellitus, elderly, pregnancy **B**, lactation

Do Not Confuse:
metolazone/methotrexate, metolazone/metoclopramide

Pharmacokinetics

Absorption	GI tract (10%-20%)
Distribution	Crosses placenta
Metabolism	Urine, unchanged
Excretion	Breast milk
Half-life	8 hr (extended); 14 hr (prompt)

Pharmacodynamics

Onset	1 hr
Peak	2 hr
Duration	12-24 hr

Interactions
Individual drugs
Amphotericin B: ↑ hypokalemia
Cholestyramine: ↓ absorption of metolazone
Colestipol: ↓ absorption of metolazone
Diazoxide: ↓ hyperglycemia, hyperuricemia, hypotension
Digoxin: ↑ toxicity
Indomethacin: ↓ hypotensive response
Lithium: ↑ toxicity
Mezlocillin: ↑ hypokalemia
Piperacillin: ↑ hypokalemia
Ticarcillin: ↑ hypokalemia
Drug classifications
Antidiabetics: ↓ effect of antidiabetic agent
Antihypertensives: ↑ antihypertensive effect
Barbiturates: ↑ hypotension
Cardiac glycosides: ↑ hypokalemia
Glucocorticoids: ↑ hypokalemia
Nitrates: ↑ hypotension
Nondepolarizing skeletal muscle relaxants: ↑ toxicity
NSAIDs: ↓ action of metolazone
Opioids: ↑ hypotension
Salicylates: ↓ action of metolazone
Sulfonylureas: ↓ effect of sulfonylurea
Food/drug
↑ Absorption
Lab test interferences
Interference: Urine steroid tests
↑ BSP retention, ↑ calcium, ↑ amylase, ↑ parathyroid test
↓ PBI, ↓ PSP

NURSING CONSIDERATIONS
Assessment
- Monitor blood glucose if patient is diabetic
- Check for rashes, temp elevation qd
- Monitor patients receiving cardiac glycosides for increased hypokalemia
- Monitor manifestations of hypokalemia; acidic urine, reduced urine, osmolality, nocturia; hypotension, broad T wave, U wave, ectopy, tachycardia, weak pulse; muscle weakness, altered LOC, drowsiness, apathy, lethargy, confusion, depression; anorexia, nausea, cramps, constipation, distention, paralytic ileus; hypoventilation, respiratory muscle weakness
- Monitor for manifestations of hypomagnesemia: agitation, muscle twitching, paresthesias, hyperactive reflexes, positive Babinski reflex, dysphagia, nystagmus seizures, tetany; nausea, vomiting, diarrhea, anorexia, abdominal distention; ectopy, tachycardia, broad, flat, or inverted T waves, depressed ST segment, prolonged QT interval, decreased cardiac output, hypotension
- Monitor for manifestations of hyponatremia; increased B/P, cold, clammy skin, hypovolemia or hypervolemia; anorexia, nausea, vomiting, diarrhea, abdominal cramps; lethargy, increased ICP, confusion, headache, seizures, coma, fatigue, tremors, hyperreflexia
- Monitor for manifestations of hyperchloremia: weakness, lethargy, coma, deep rapid breathing

M

• Assess and record fluid volume status: I&O ratios; monitor weight, distended red veins, crackles in lung, color, quality and sp gr of urine, skin turgor, adequacy of pulses, moist mucous membranes, bilateral lung sounds, peripheral pitting edema; dehydration symptoms of decreasing output, thirst, hypotension, dry mouth and mucous membranes should be reported
• Monitor electrolytes: potassium, sodium, calcium, magnesium; also include BUN, blood pH, ABGs, uric acid, CBC, blood glucose
• Assess B/P before and during therapy with patient lying, standing, and sitting as appropriate; orthostatic hypotension can occur rapidly

Nursing diagnoses

✓ Altered urinary elimination (adverse reactions)
✓ Fluid volume deficit (adverse reactions)
✓ Fluid volume excess (uses)
✓ Knowledge deficit (teaching)

Implementation

• Give in AM to avoid interference with sleep
• Provide potassium replacement if potassium level is 3.0; drug may be crushed if patient is unable to swallow
• Give with food; if nausea occurs, absorption may be increased; extended release product is Zaroxolyn; prompt action product is MyKrox; the two formulations are not equivalent

Patient/family education

• Teach patient to take the medication early in the day to prevent nocturia
• Instruct patient to take with food or milk if GI symptoms of nausea and anorexia occur
• Teach patient to maintain a weekly record of weight and notify prescriber of weight loss >5 lb
• Caution patient that this drug causes a loss of potassium, so foods rich in potassium should be added to the diet; refer to a dietitian for assistance in planning
• Caution the patient not to exercise in hot weather or stand for prolonged periods, since orthostatic hypotension will be enhanced
• Teach patient not to use alcohol or any OTC medications without prescriber's approval; serious drug reactions may occur
• Emphasize the need to contact prescriber immediately if muscle cramps, weakness, nausea, dizziness, or numbness occurs
• Teach patient to take own B/P and pulse and record
• Advise patient to use sunscreen to prevent burns
• Caution the patient that orthostatic hypotension may occur and to rise slowly from sitting or reclining positions, lie down if dizziness occurs
• Teach patient to continue taking medication even if feeling better; this drug controls symptoms but does not cure the condition
• Advise patient with hypertension to continue other medical regimen (exercise, weight loss, relaxation techniques, cessation of smoking)

Evaluation

Positive therapeutic outcome

• Decreased edema
• Decreased B/P

Treatment of overdose:

Lavage if taken orally, monitor electrolytes; administer dextrose in saline; monitor hydration, CV, renal status

metoprolol (℞)
(met-oh-proe'lole)

Apo-Metoprolol ✤, Betaloc ✤, Betaloc Durules ✤, Lopressor, Lopressor SR ✤, Novometoprol ✤, Toprol XL

Func. class.: Antihypertensive, antianginal

Chem. class.: β_1-Adrenergic blocker

Pregnancy category C

Action: Competitively blocks stimulation of β_1-adrenergic receptor within vascular smooth muscle; produces chronotropic, inotropic activity (decreases rate of SA node discharge, increases recovery time), slows conduction of AV node, decreases heart rate, which decreases O_2 consumption in myocardium; also decreases renin-aldosterone-angiotensin system at high doses

Therapeutic Outcome: Decreased B/P, heart rate, AV conduction

Uses: Mild to moderate hypertension, acute MI to reduce cardiovascular mortality, angina pectoris, New York Heart Association class II, III heart failure

Investigational uses: Dysrhythmias, hypertrophic cardiomyopathy, mitral valve prolapse, pheochromocytoma, tremors, prevention of vascular headaches, aggression

Dosage and routes

Hypertension

Adult: PO 50 mg bid, or 100 mg qd; may give 200-450 mg in divided doses; ext rel tabs give qd

Elderly: PO 25 mg/day initially, increase weekly as needed

MI

Adult: Early treatment, **IV** bol 5 mg q2 min × 3 doses, then 50 mg PO 15 min after last dose and q6h × 48 hr; late treatment, PO maintenance 100 mg bid for 3 mo

Angina

Adult: PO 100 mg qd, increase qwk as needed or 100 mg ext rel tab qd

Available forms: Tabs 50, 100 mg; inj 1 mg/ml; ext rel tabs 25, 50, 100, 200 mg

Adverse effects

CNS: *Insomnia, dizziness,* mental changes, hallucinations, **depression,** anxiety, headaches, nightmares, confusion, fatigue

CV: **CHF,** *palpitations,* dysrhythmias, **cardiac arrest, AV block**, hypotension, **bradycardia**

EENT: Sore throat, dry burning eyes

GI: *Nausea, vomiting,* colitis, cramps, *diarrhea,* constipation, flatulence, dry mouth, *hiccups*

GU: Impotence

HEMA: **Agranulocytosis, eosinophilia, thrombocytopenic purpura**

INTEG: Rash, purpura, alopecia, dry skin, urticaria, pruritus

RESP: **Bronchospasm,** dyspnea, wheezing

Contraindications: Hypersensitivity to β-blockers, cardiogenic shock, heart block (2nd- and 3rd-degree), sinus bradycardia, CHF, bronchial asthma

Precautions: Major surgery, pregnancy **C,** lactation, diabetes mellitus, renal disease, thyroid disease, COPD, heart failure, CAD, nonallergic bronchospasm, hepatic disease

Do Not Confuse:
metoprolol/misoprostol

Pharmacokinetics	
Absorption	Well absorbed (PO); completely absorbed (**IV**)
Distribution	Crosses blood-brain barrier, placenta
Metabolism	Liver, extensively
Excretion	Kidneys, breast milk
Half-life	3-4 hr

M

Pharmacodynamics	PO	IV
Onset	15 min	Immediate
Peak	2-4 hr	20 min
Duration	6-19 hr	5-8 hr

Interactions

Individual drugs

Alcohol: ↑ hypotension (large amounts)
Dobutamine: ↓ effect of dobutamine
Dopamine: ↓ dopamine
Epinephrine: α-Adrenergic stimulation
Hydralazine: ↑ hypotension, bradycardia
Indomethacin: ↓ antihypertensive effect
Insulin: ↑ hypoglycemia
Methyldopa: ↑ hypotension, bradycardia
Prazosin: ↑ hypotension, bradycardia
Reserpine: ↑ hypotension, bradycardia
Thyroid: ↓ effectiveness
Verapamil: ↑ myocardial depression

Drug classifications

Amphetamines: ↑ hypertension, bradycardia **Antidiabetics:** ↑ hypoglycemia
Antihypertensive: ↑ hypotension
β_2-Adrenergic agonists: ↓ bronchodilatation
Cardiac glycosides: ↑ bradycardia
Histamine H_2 antagonists: ↑ hypotension, bradycardia
MAOIs: Do not use together
Nitrates: ↑ hypotension
Sulfonylureas: ↓ hypoglycemic effect
Theophyllines: ↓ bronchodilatation

Food/drug

↑ Absorption with food

Lab test interferences

False: ↑ urinary catecholamines

NURSING CONSIDERATIONS

Assessment

- Monitor B/P during beginning treatment, periodically thereafter; pulse q4h; note rate, rhythm, quality; check apical/radial pulse before administration; notify prescriber of any significant changes (pulse <50 bpm)
- Check for baselines in renal, liver function tests before therapy begins and periodically thereafter
- Assess for edema in feet, legs daily; monitor I&O, daily weight; check for jugular vein distention, rales bilaterally, dyspnea (CHF)
- Monitor skin turgor, dryness of mucous membranes for hydration status, especially elderly [G]

Nursing diagnoses

- ✓ Cardiac output, decreased (uses)
- ✓ Injury, risk for (adverse reactions)
- ✓ Knowledge deficit (teaching)
- ✓ Noncompliance (teaching)

Implementation

PO route

- Given ac, hs; tab may be crushed or swallowed whole; give with food to prevent GI upset; reduced dosage in renal dysfunction
- [Do Not Crush] Do not crush or chew ext rel tabs
- Store protected from light, moisture; place in cool environment

IV route

- Give by direct **IV** 5 mg/2 min or more; keep patient recumbent for 3 hr

Y-site compatibilities:
Alteplase, meperidine, morphine

Patient/family education

- Teach patient not to discontinue drug abruptly; taper over 2 wk; may cause precipitate angina if stopped abruptly
- Teach patient not to use OTC products containing α-adrenergic stimulants (such as nasal decongestants, cold preparations); to avoid alcohol, smoking and to limit sodium intake as prescribed
- Teach patient how to take pulse and B/P at home; advise when to notify prescriber
- Instruct patient to comply with weight control, dietary adjustments, modified exercise program

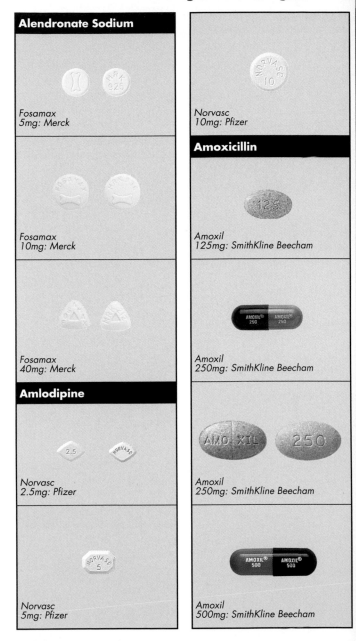

Alendronate Sodium

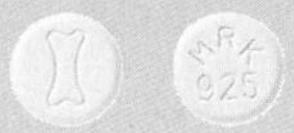

Fosamax
5mg: Merck

Fosamax
10mg: Merck

Fosamax
40mg: Merck

Amlodipine

Norvasc
2.5mg: Pfizer

Norvasc
5mg: Pfizer

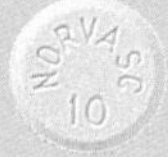

Norvasc
10mg: Pfizer

Amoxicillin

Amoxil
125mg: SmithKline Beecham

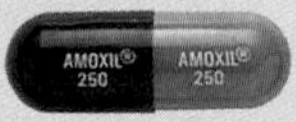

Amoxil
250mg: SmithKline Beecham

Amoxil
250mg: SmithKline Beecham

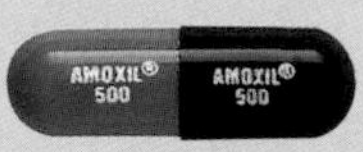

Amoxil
500mg: SmithKline Beecham

Amoxicillin; Clavulanate

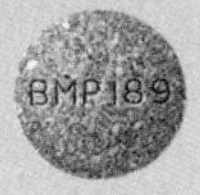

Augmentin
125/31.25mg: SmithKline Beecham

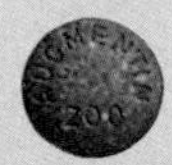

Augmentin
200mg: SmithKline Beecham

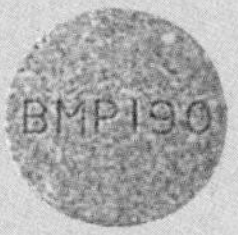

Augmentin
250/62.5mg: SmithKline Beecham

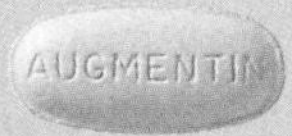

Augmentin
250/125mg: SmithKline Beecham

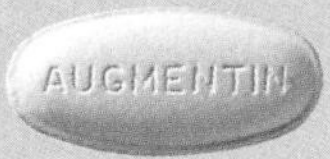

Augmentin
500/125mg: SmithKline Beecham

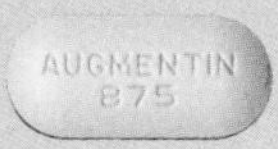

Augmentin
875/125mg: SmithKline Beecham

Atorvastatin Calcium

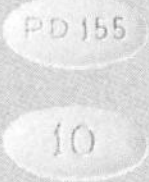

Lipitor
10mg: Parke-Davis

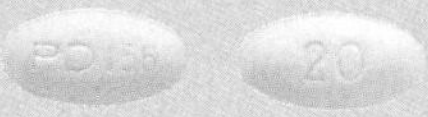

Lipitor
20mg: Parke-Davis

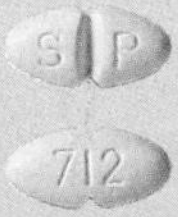

Lipitor
40mg: Parke-Davis

Azithromycin

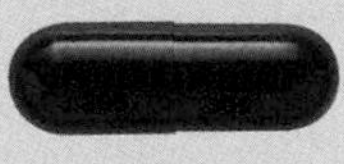

Zithromax
250mg: Pfizer

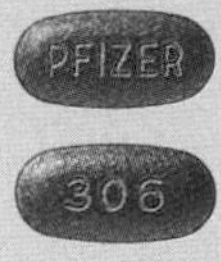

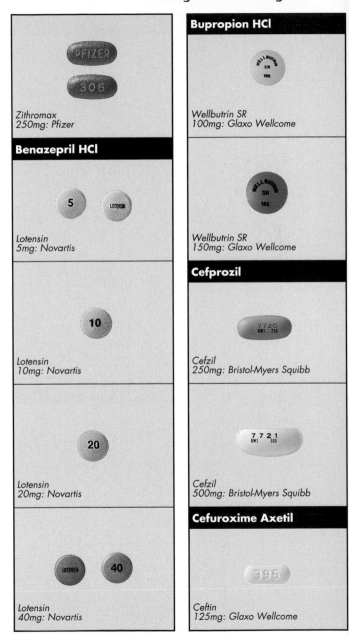

Zithromax
250mg: Pfizer

Benazepril HCl

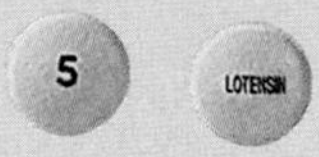

Lotensin
5mg: Novartis

Lotensin
10mg: Novartis

Lotensin
20mg: Novartis

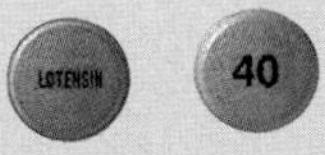

Lotensin
40mg: Novartis

Bupropion HCl

Wellbutrin SR
100mg: Glaxo Wellcome

Wellbutrin SR
150mg: Glaxo Wellcome

Cefprozil

Cefzil
250mg: Bristol-Myers Squibb

Cefzil
500mg: Bristol-Myers Squibb

Cefuroxime Axetil

Ceftin
125mg: Glaxo Wellcome

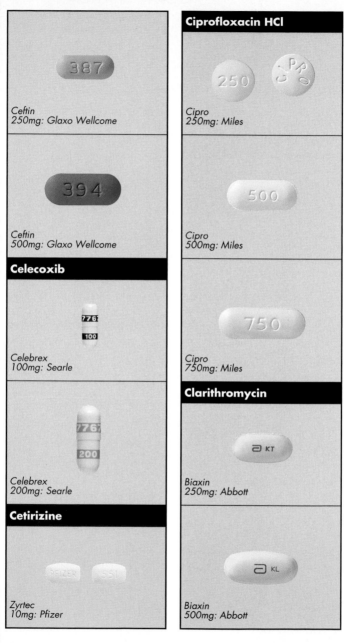

Ceftin
250mg: Glaxo Wellcome

Ceftin
500mg: Glaxo Wellcome

Celecoxib

Celebrex
100mg: Searle

Celebrex
200mg: Searle

Cetirizine

Zyrtec
10mg: Pfizer

Ciprofloxacin HCl

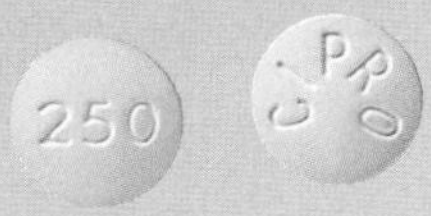

Cipro
250mg: Miles

Cipro
500mg: Miles

Cipro
750mg: Miles

Clarithromycin

Biaxin
250mg: Abbott

Biaxin
500mg: Abbott

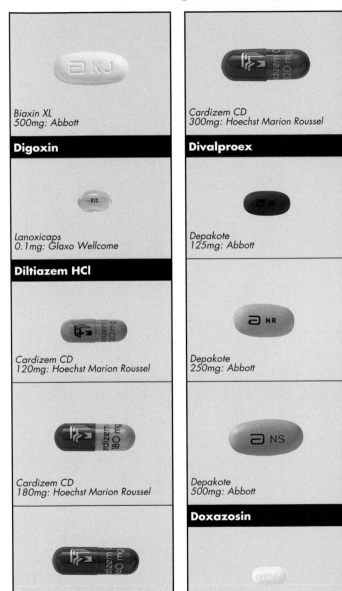

Biaxin XL
500mg: Abbott

Digoxin

Lanoxicaps
0.1mg: Glaxo Wellcome

Diltiazem HCl

Cardizem CD
120mg: Hoechst Marion Roussel

Cardizem CD
180mg: Hoechst Marion Roussel

Cardizem CD
240mg: Hoechst Marion Roussel

Cardizem CD
300mg: Hoechst Marion Roussel

Divalproex

Depakote
125mg: Abbott

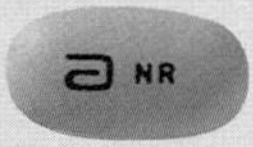

Depakote
250mg: Abbott

Depakote
500mg: Abbott

Doxazosin

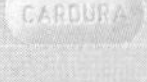

Cardura
1mg: Roerig

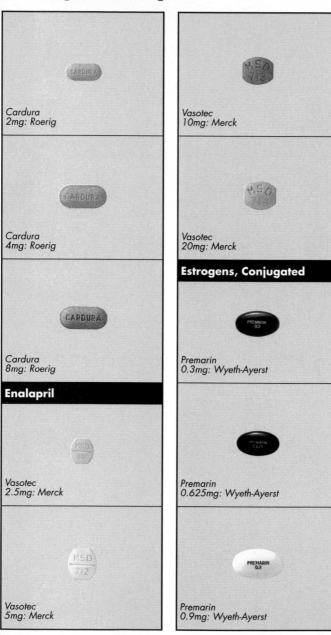

Cardura
2mg: Roerig

Cardura
4mg: Roerig

Cardura
8mg: Roerig

Enalapril

Vasotec
2.5mg: Merck

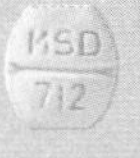

Vasotec
5mg: Merck

Vasotec
10mg: Merck

Vasotec
20mg: Merck

Estrogens, Conjugated

Premarin
0.3mg: Wyeth-Ayerst

Premarin
0.625mg: Wyeth-Ayerst

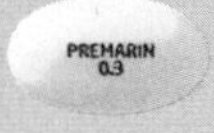

Premarin
0.9mg: Wyeth-Ayerst

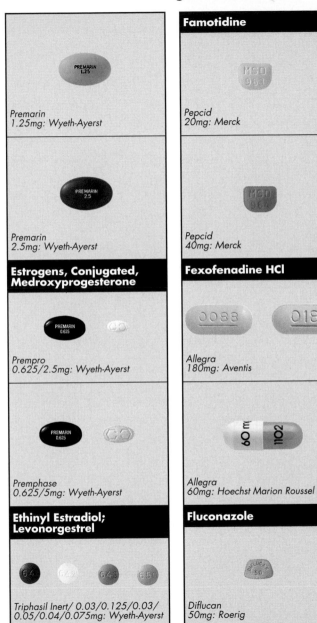

Premarin
1.25mg: Wyeth-Ayerst

Premarin
2.5mg: Wyeth-Ayerst

Estrogens, Conjugated, Medroxyprogesterone

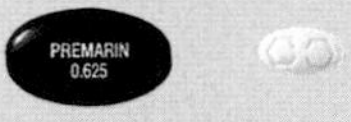

Prempro
0.625/2.5mg: Wyeth-Ayerst

Premphase
0.625/5mg: Wyeth-Ayerst

Ethinyl Estradiol; Levonorgestrel

Triphasil Inert/ 0.03/0.125/0.03/ 0.05/0.04/0.075mg: Wyeth-Ayerst

Famotidine

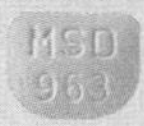

Pepcid
20mg: Merck

Pepcid
40mg: Merck

Fexofenadine HCl

Allegra
180mg: Aventis

Allegra
60mg: Hoechst Marion Roussel

Fluconazole

Diflucan
50mg: Roerig

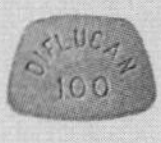

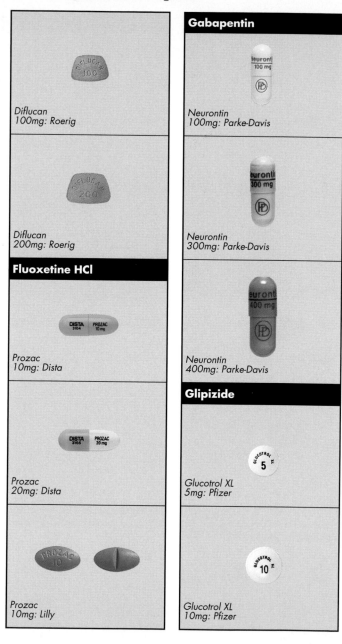

Diflucan
100mg: Roerig

Diflucan
200mg: Roerig

Fluoxetine HCl

Prozac
10mg: Dista

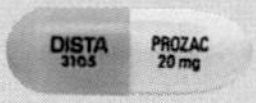

Prozac
20mg: Dista

Prozac
10mg: Lilly

Gabapentin

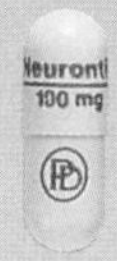

Neurontin
100mg: Parke-Davis

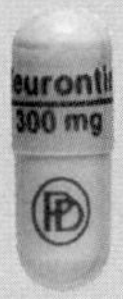

Neurontin
300mg: Parke-Davis

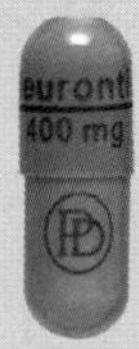

Neurontin
400mg: Parke-Davis

Glipizide

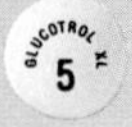

Glucotrol XL
5mg: Pfizer

Glucotrol XL
10mg: Pfizer

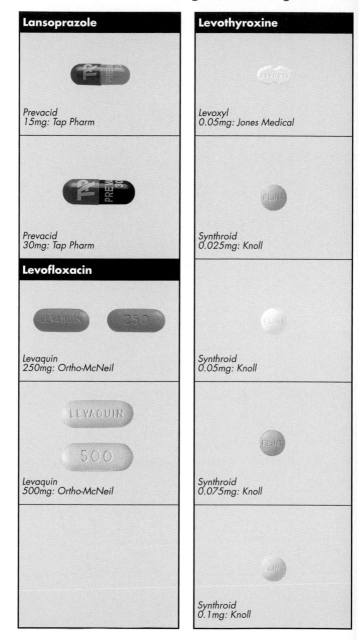

Lansoprazole

Prevacid
15mg: Tap Pharm

Prevacid
30mg: Tap Pharm

Levofloxacin

Levaquin
250mg: Ortho-McNeil

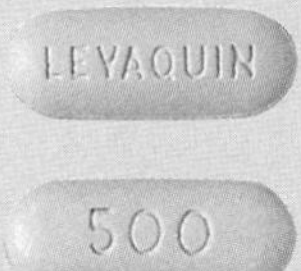

Levaquin
500mg: Ortho-McNeil

Levothyroxine

Levoxyl
0.05mg: Jones Medical

Synthroid
0.025mg: Knoll

Synthroid
0.05mg: Knoll

Synthroid
0.075mg: Knoll

Synthroid
0.1mg: Knoll

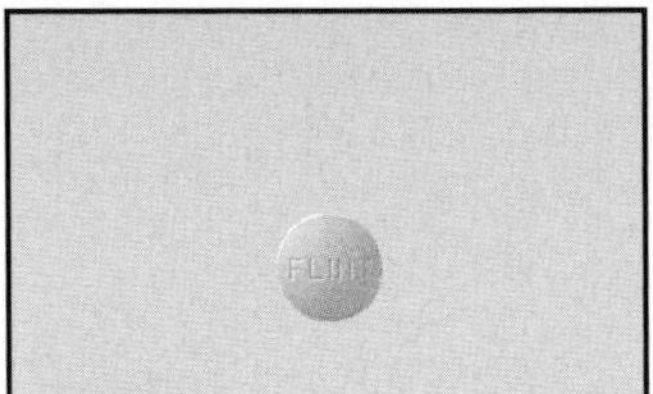

Synthroid
0.125mg: Knoll

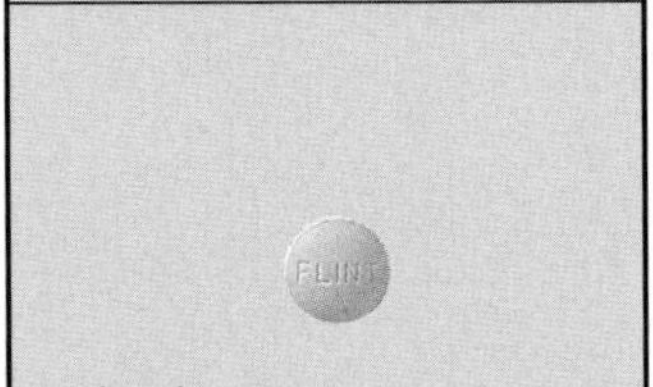

Synthroid
0.15mg: Knoll

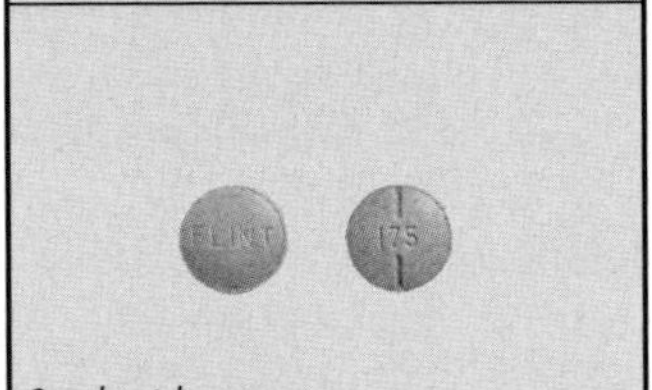

Synthroid
0.175mg: Knoll

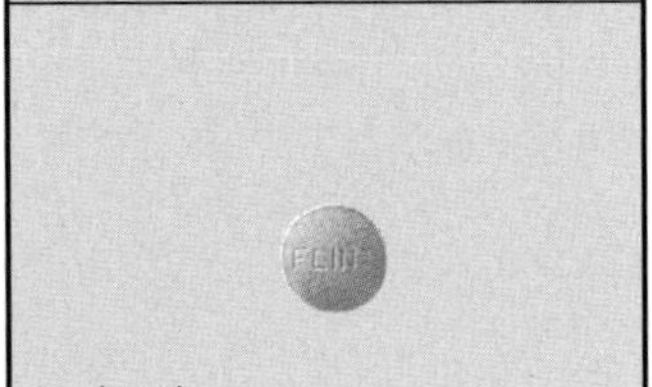

Synthroid
0.2mg: Knoll

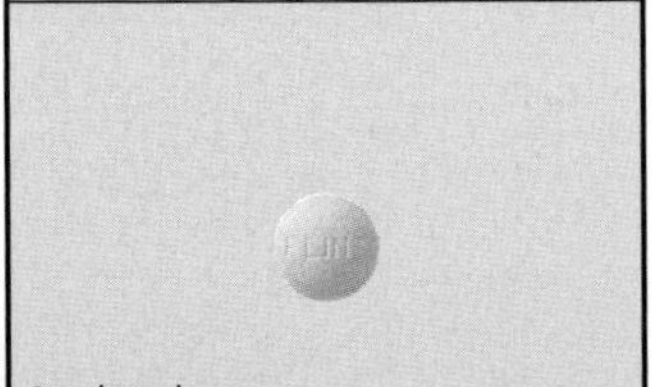

Synthroid
0.3mg: Knoll

Lisinopril

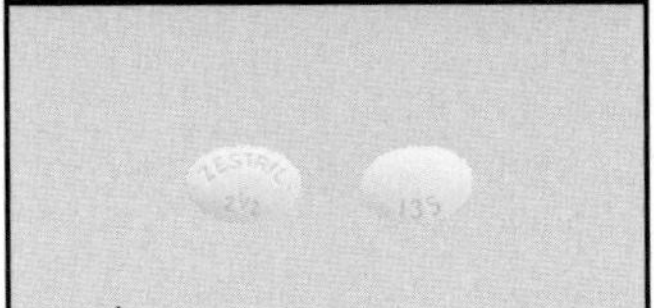

Zestril
2.5mg: Astra Zeneca

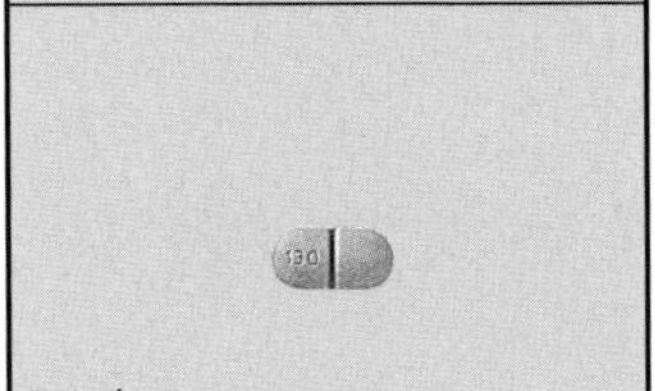

Zestril
5mg: Astra Zeneca

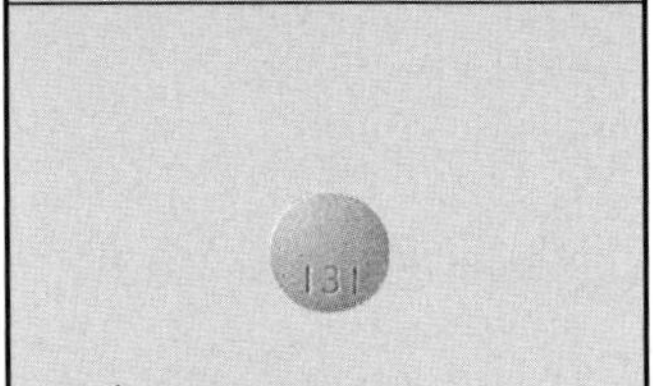

Zestril
10mg: Astra Zeneca

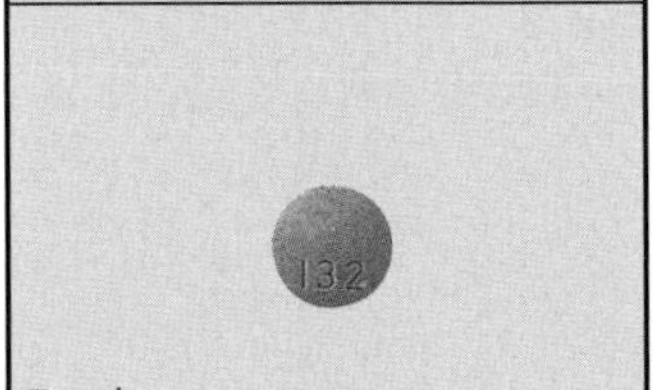

Zestril
20mg: Astra Zeneca

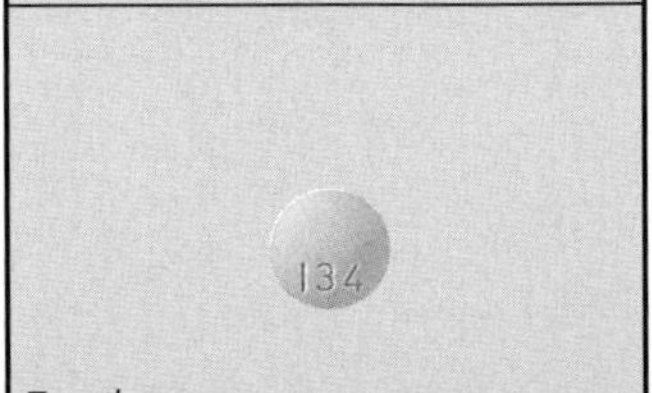

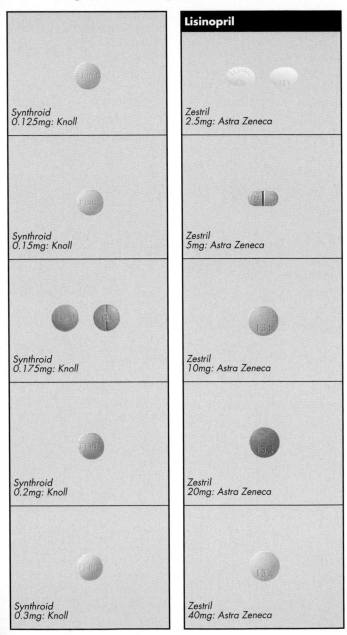

Zestril
40mg: Astra Zeneca

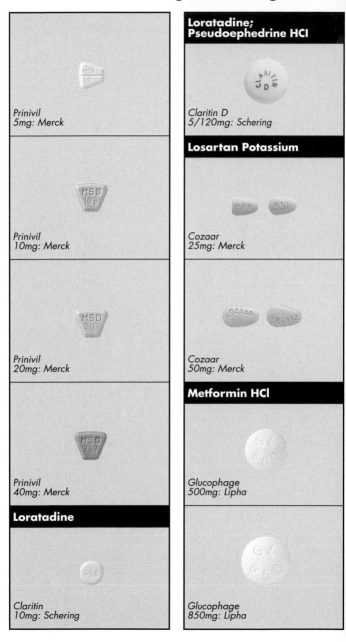

Prinivil
5mg: Merck

Prinivil
10mg: Merck

Prinivil
20mg: Merck

Prinivil
40mg: Merck

Loratadine

Claritin
10mg: Schering

Loratadine; Pseudoephedrine HCl

Claritin D
5/120mg: Schering

Losartan Potassium

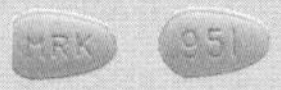

Cozaar
25mg: Merck

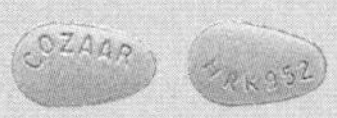

Cozaar
50mg: Merck

Metformin HCl

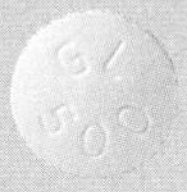

Glucophage
500mg: Lipha

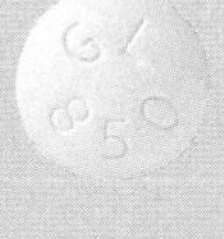

Glucophage
850mg: Lipha

Metoprolol Succinate

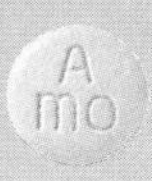

Toprol XL
50mg: Astra Zeneca

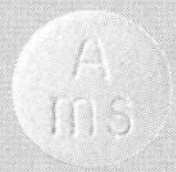

Toprol XL
100mg: Astra Zeneca

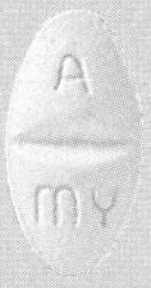

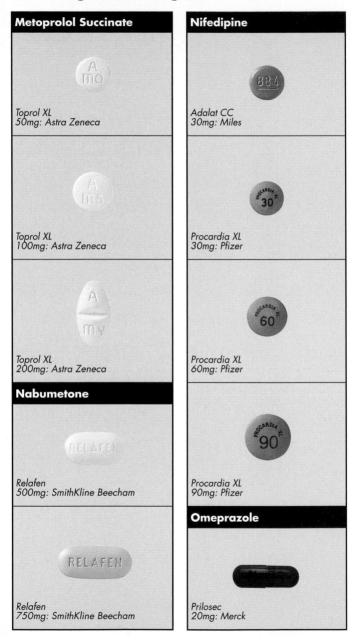

Toprol XL
200mg: Astra Zeneca

Nabumetone

Relafen
500mg: SmithKline Beecham

Relafen
750mg: SmithKline Beecham

Nifedipine

Adalat CC
30mg: Miles

Procardia XL
30mg: Pfizer

Procardia XL
60mg: Pfizer

Procardia XL
90mg: Pfizer

Omeprazole

Prilosec
20mg: Merck

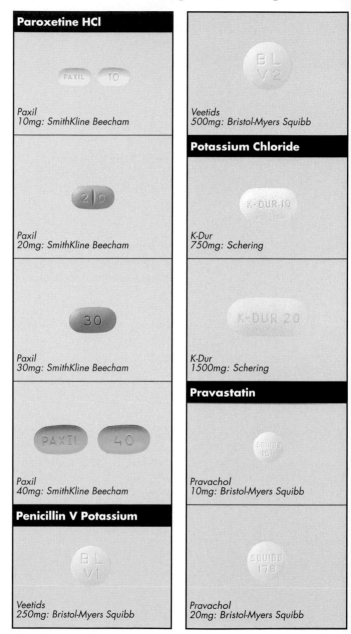

Paroxetine HCl

Paxil
10mg: SmithKline Beecham

Paxil
20mg: SmithKline Beecham

Paxil
30mg: SmithKline Beecham

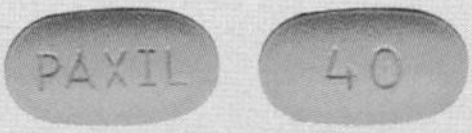

Paxil
40mg: SmithKline Beecham

Penicillin V Potassium

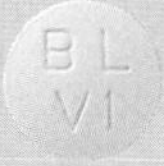

Veetids
250mg: Bristol-Myers Squibb

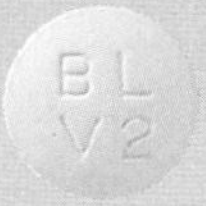

Veetids
500mg: Bristol-Myers Squibb

Potassium Chloride

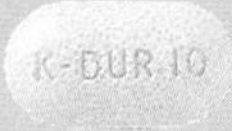

K-Dur
750mg: Schering

K-Dur
1500mg: Schering

Pravastatin

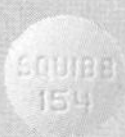

Pravachol
10mg: Bristol-Myers Squibb

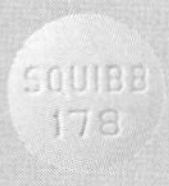

Pravachol
20mg: Bristol-Myers Squibb

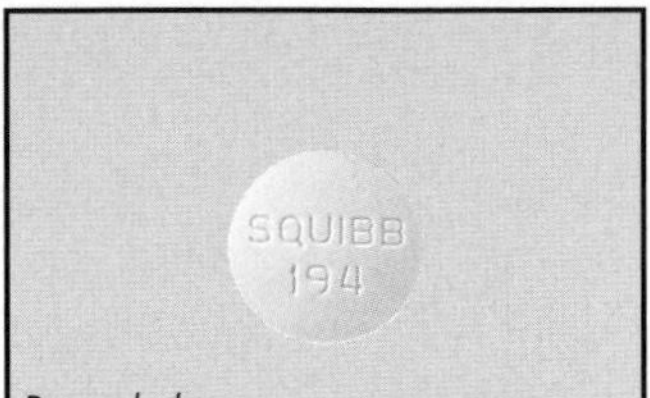

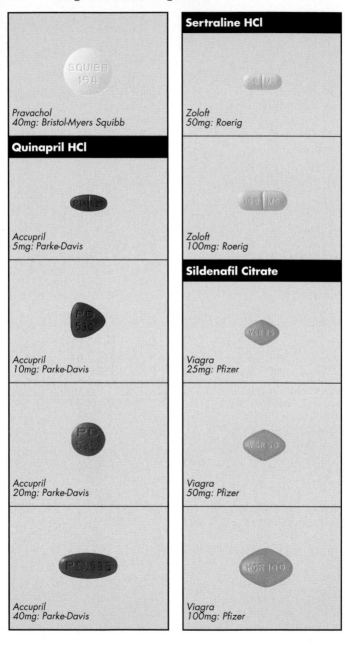

Pravachol
40mg: Bristol-Myers Squibb

Quinapril HCl

Accupril
5mg: Parke-Davis

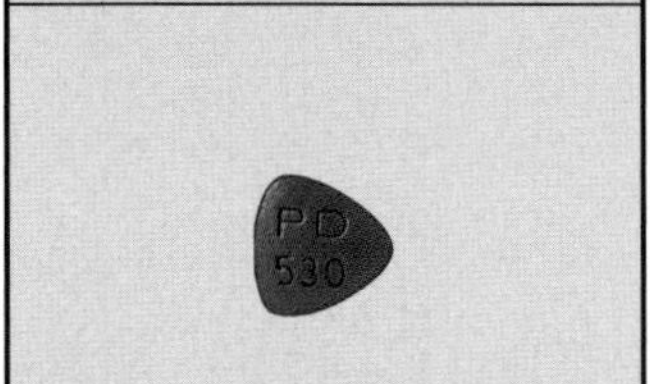

Accupril
10mg: Parke-Davis

Accupril
20mg: Parke-Davis

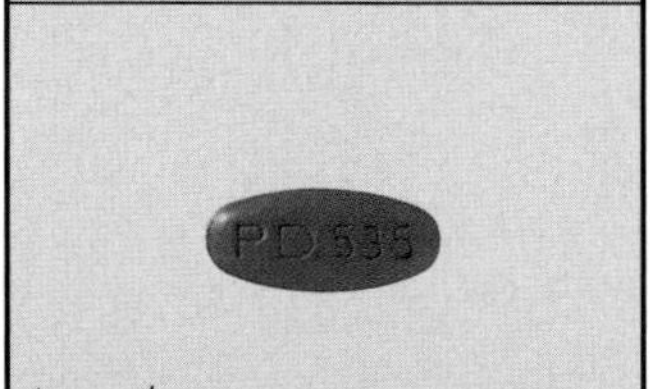

Accupril
40mg: Parke-Davis

Sertraline HCl

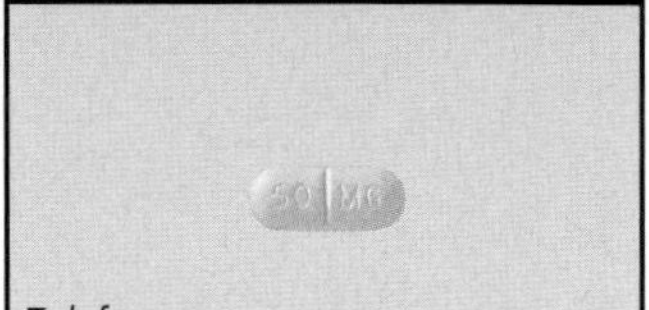

Zoloft
50mg: Roerig

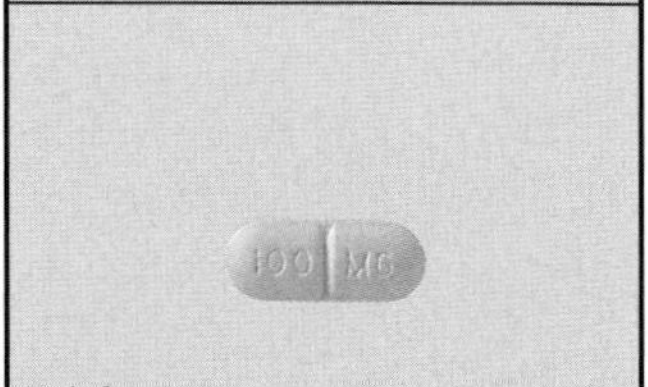

Zoloft
100mg: Roerig

Sildenafil Citrate

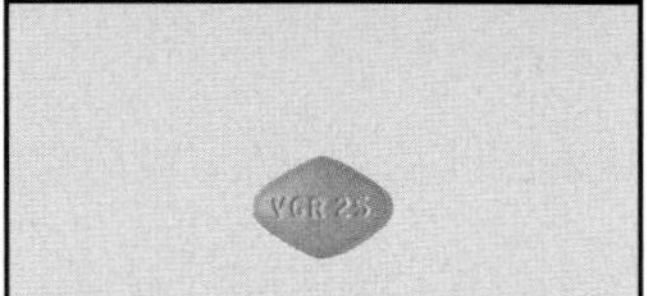

Viagra
25mg: Pfizer

Viagra
50mg: Pfizer

Viagra
100mg: Pfizer

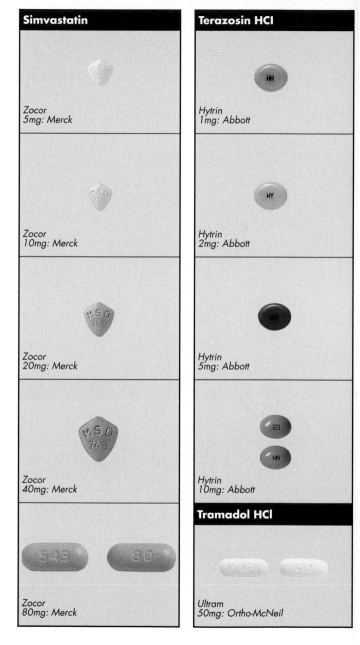

Simvastatin

Zocor
5mg: Merck

Zocor
10mg: Merck

Zocor
20mg: Merck

Zocor
40mg: Merck

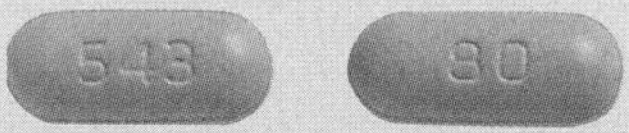

Zocor
80mg: Merck

Terazosin HCl

Hytrin
1mg: Abbott

Hytrin
2mg: Abbott

Hytrin
5mg: Abbott

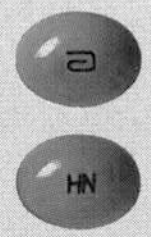

Hytrin
10mg: Abbott

Tramadol HCl

Ultram
50mg: Ortho-McNeil

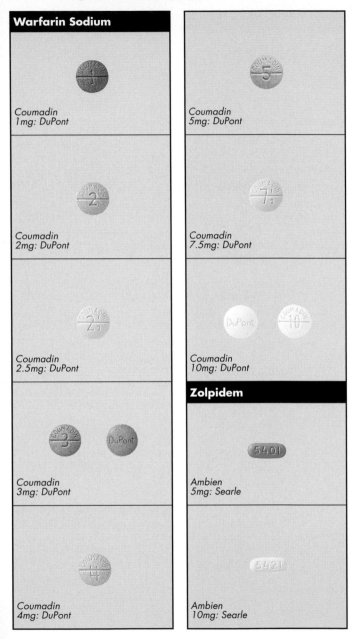

Warfarin Sodium

Coumadin
1mg: DuPont

Coumadin
2mg: DuPont

Coumadin
2.5mg: DuPont

Coumadin
3mg: DuPont

Coumadin
4mg: DuPont

Coumadin
5mg: DuPont

Coumadin
7.5mg: DuPont

Coumadin
10mg: DuPont

Zolpidem

Ambien
5mg: Searle

Ambien
10mg: Searle

PHOTO ATLAS OF DRUG ADMINISTRATION*

*All color plates are from Potter PA and Perry AG: *Fundamentals of Nursing*, ed. 5, St. Louis, 2001, Mosby.

Standard Precautions

The following precautions are used in the care of all patients regardless of their diagnosis or disease. They are also applied when handling or cleaning equipment or supplies that are potentially contaminated.

1. Wear gloves any time that you may contact blood, any moist body fluid (except sweat), secretions, excretions, nonintact skin, or mucous membranes.
2. Remove your gloves, wash your hands, and reapply clean gloves if your gloves become soiled with infective material.
3. Even if you are wearing gloves, remove them, wash your hands, and apply clean gloves *immediately before* contact with mucous membranes or nonintact skin.
4. Wear a protective cover gown of waterproof material if your clothing is likely to have substantial contact with infective material or if splashing of body fluids is likely.
5. Wear a face shield or goggles to protect your eyes if splashing of secretions is likely.
6. Any time a face shield or goggles is worn, wear a surgical mask to protect the mucous membranes of your nose and mouth. A surgical mask may be worn during certain sterile procedures without protective eyewear. However, protective eyewear is *never* worn without a surgical mask.
7. Handle needles, razors, broken glass, and other sharp objects with care. Needles should never be recapped. All sharps should be disposed of in a puncture-resistant sharps container.
8. Wash your hands before and after each patient contact.
9. Wash your hands before you apply and after you remove gloves. Do not assume that handwashing is unnecessary because gloves were worn. Do not wash your hands with gloves on them.
10. Gloves are used for the care of one patient only, then discarded.
11. Follow your facility policy for disposal of gloves and other contaminated items. These items are generally not disposed of in open trash containers. Facilities have designated disposal sites for these biohazardous waste materials.
12. Use resuscitation barrier devices as an alternative to mouth-to-mouth resuscitation.
13. Linen should be handled in a manner that prevents contamination of the outside of the container. Linen from isolation rooms was previously double bagged. Double bagging is no longer recommended, since all linen is handled as potentially infectious. Double bag linen only if the outside of the bag becomes contaminated during the bagging process.

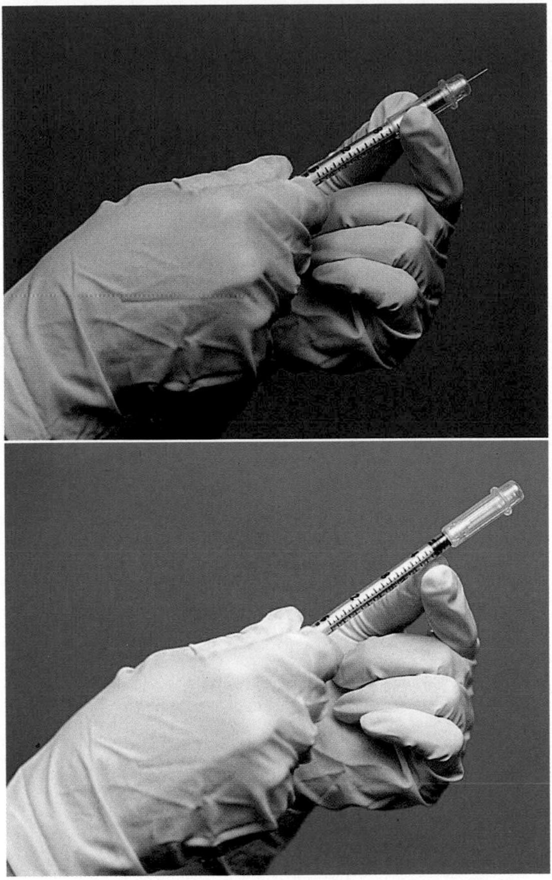

A

B

Plate 1 Needle with plastic guard to prevent needle sticks. **A,** Position of guard before injection. **B,** After injection, the guard locks in place, covering the needle.

A

B

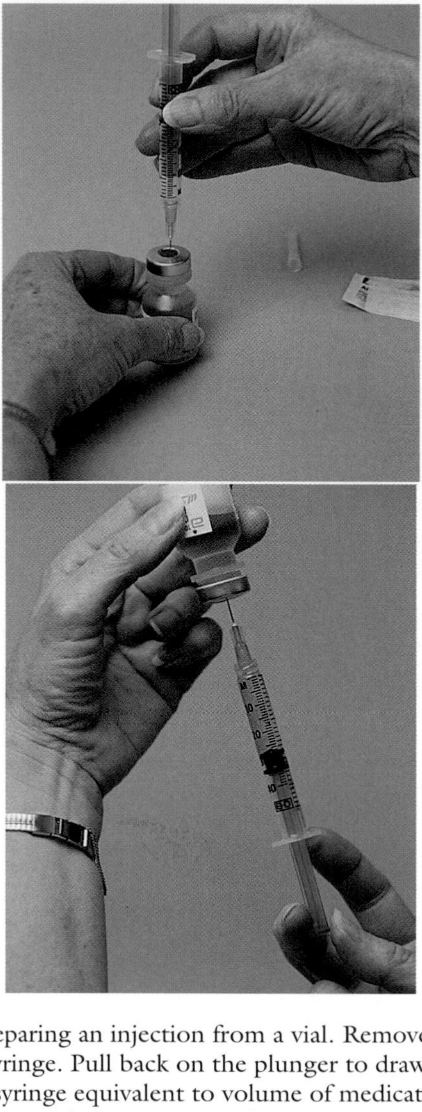

Plate 2 Preparing an injection from a vial. Remove needle cap from syringe. Pull back on the plunger to draw amount of air into syringe equivalent to volume of medication to be aspirated from vial. **A,** Insert tip of needle, with bevel pointing up, through center of rubber seal. Apply pressure on tip of needle during insertion. **B,** Allow air pressure to fill syringe gradually with medication. Pull back slightly on plunger if necessary.

Continued

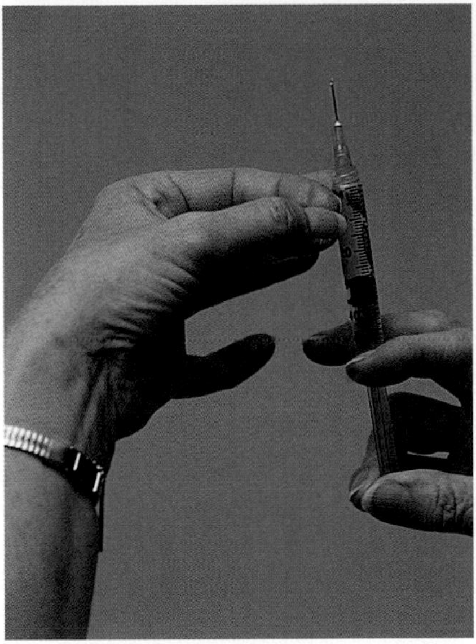

C

Plate 2, cont'd C, Remove remaining air from syringe by holding it and needle upright. Tap barrel to dislodge air bubbles. Draw back slightly on plunger and then push plunger upward to eject air. Do not eject fluid.

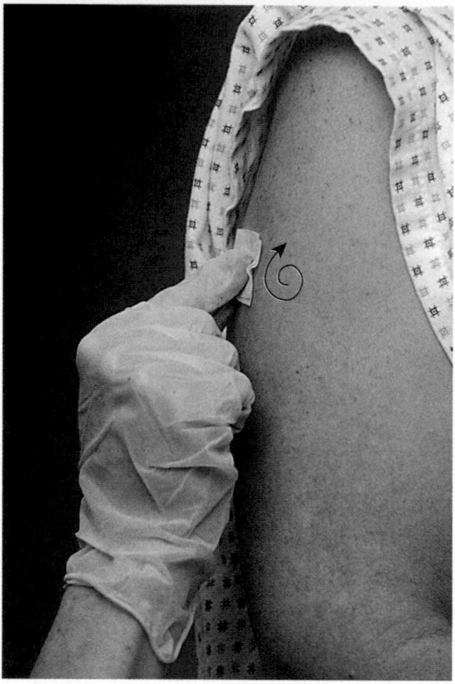

Plate 3 Administering an injection. Cleanse site with antiseptic swab. Apply swab at center of site and rotate outward in circular direction for about 5 cm (2 in).

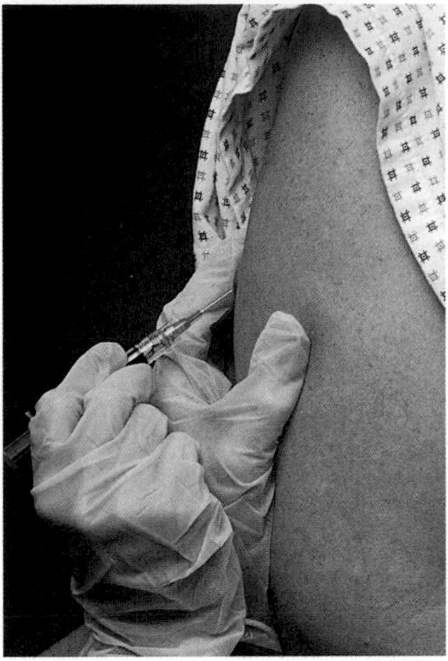

A

Plate 4 **A,** For a subcutaneous injection, hold the syringe between the thumb and forefinger of the dominant hand as a dart, with the palm down.

B

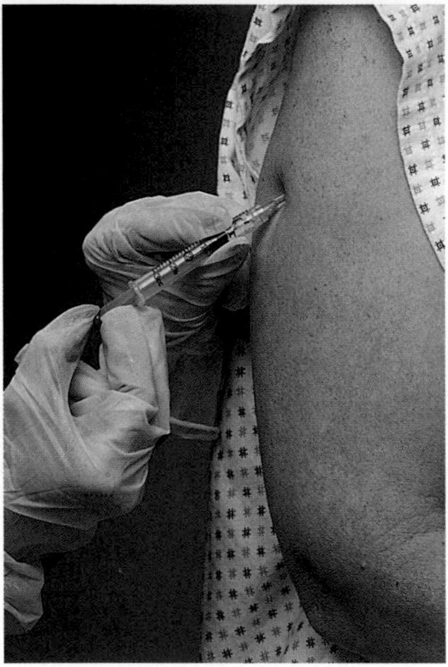

Plate 4, cont'd B, After injecting the needle at a 45- to 90-degree angle, grasp lower end of syringe barrel with nondominant hand to end of plunger. Avoid moving syringe while slowly pulling back on plunger to aspirate drug. If blood appears in syringe, remove needle, discard medication and syringe, and repeat procedure. *Exception:* do not aspirate when giving heparin.

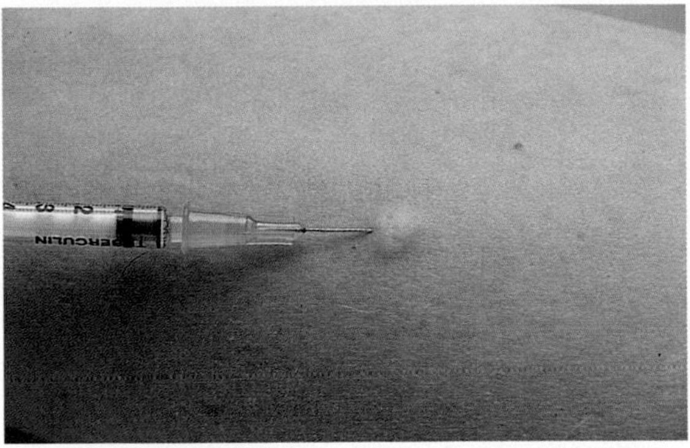

Plate 5 For an intradermal injection, note formation of small bleb approximately 6 mm (½ in) in diameter at injection site.

A

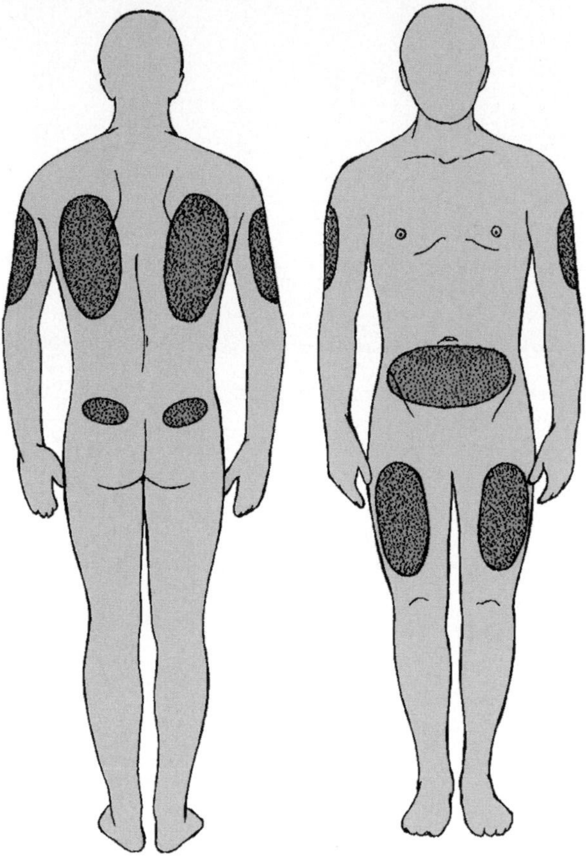

Plate 6 **A,** Sites recommended for subcutaneous injections.

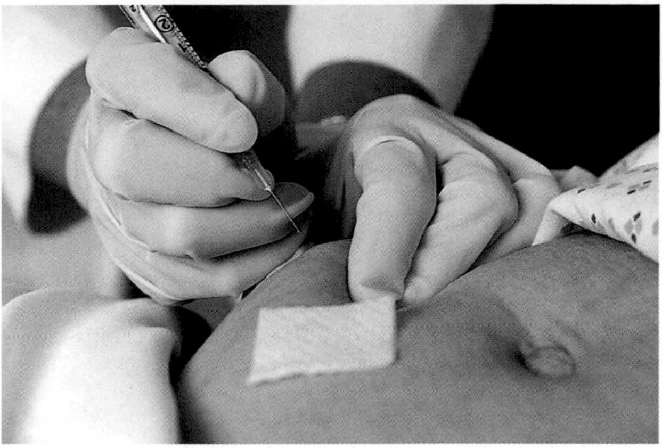

B

Plate 6 B, Giving SQ injection in the abdomen.

A

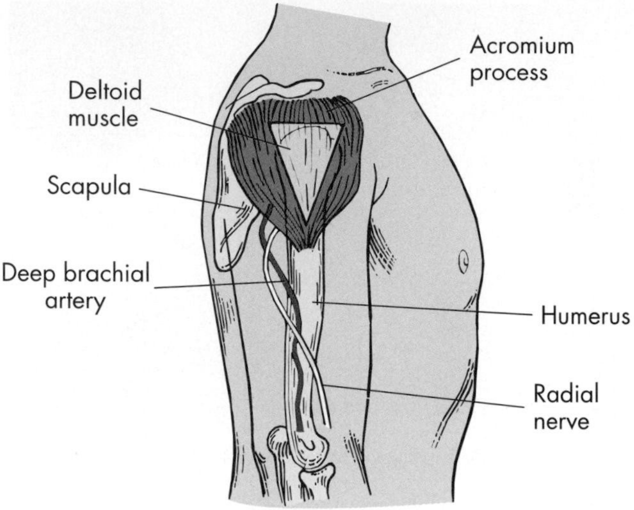

Plate 7 A, Landmarks for IM injection into the deltoid muscle.

Continued

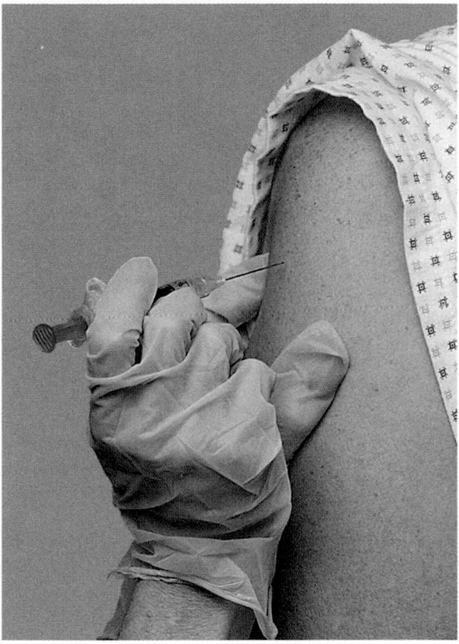

B

Plate 7, cont'd B, Giving IM injection in deltoid muscle.

A

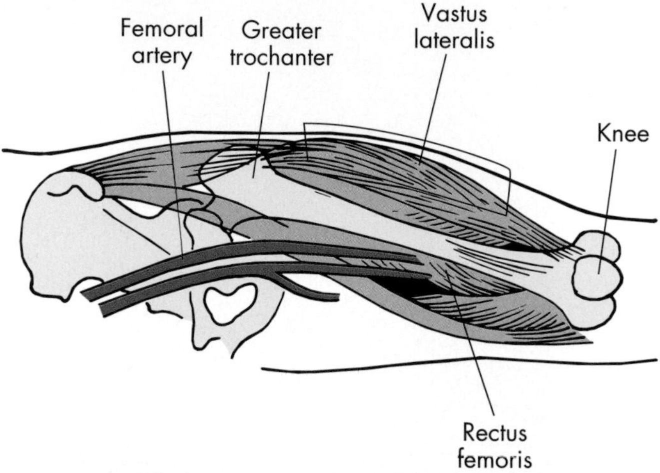

B

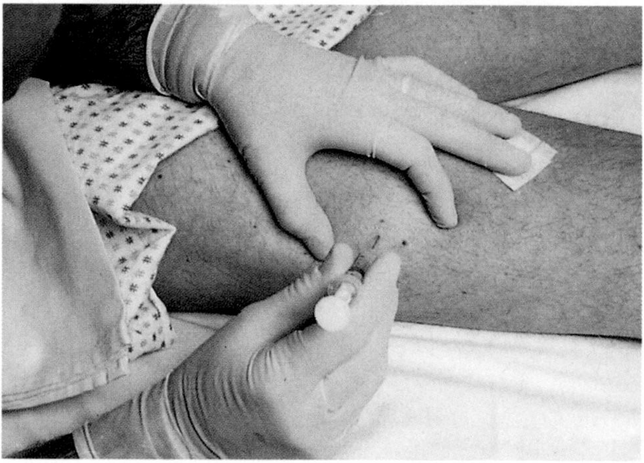

Plate 8 **A,** Landmarks for IM injection in vastus lateralis. **B,** Giving IM injection in vastus lateralis site.

A

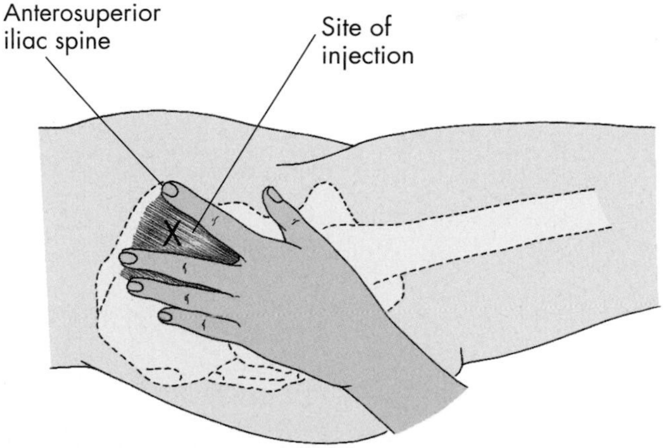

B

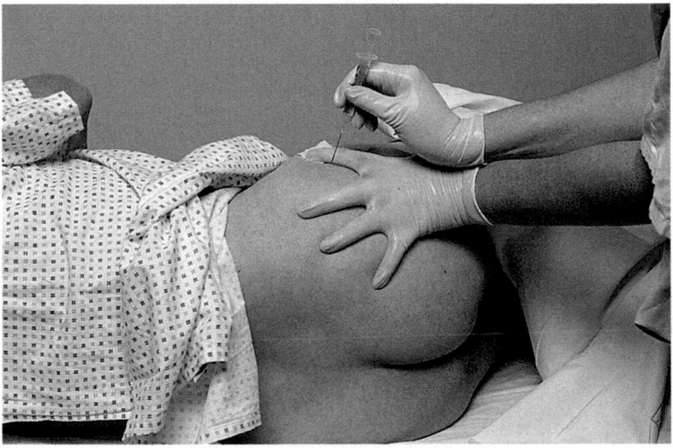

Plate 9 **A,** Anatomical view of ventrogluteal site. **B,** Giving IM injection into ventrogluteal muscle to avoid major nerves and blood vessels.

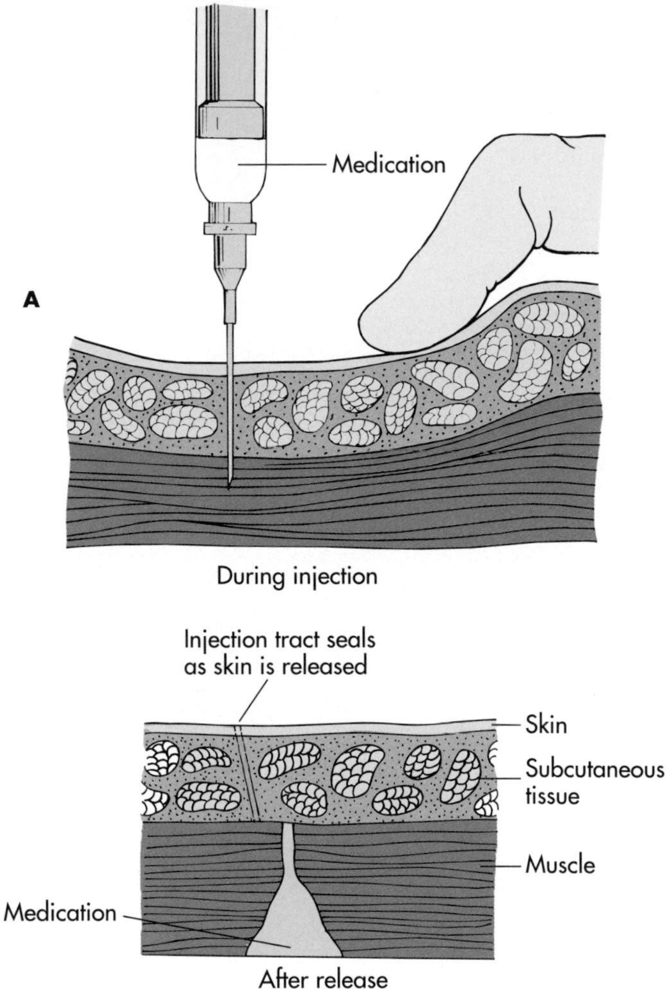

Plate 10 Z-track method of injection. **A,** Pulling on overlying skin during IM injection moves tissues to prevent later tracking. **B,** The Z-track left after injection prevents the deposit of medication through sensitive tissue.

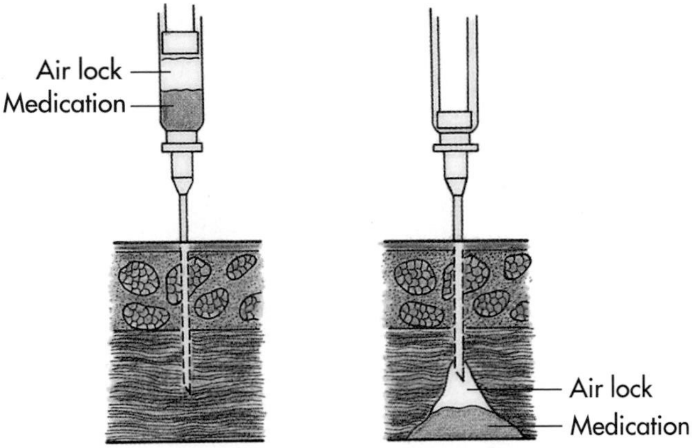

Plate 11 Administering IM injection by the air-lock technique prevents tracing of medication through SQ tissue.

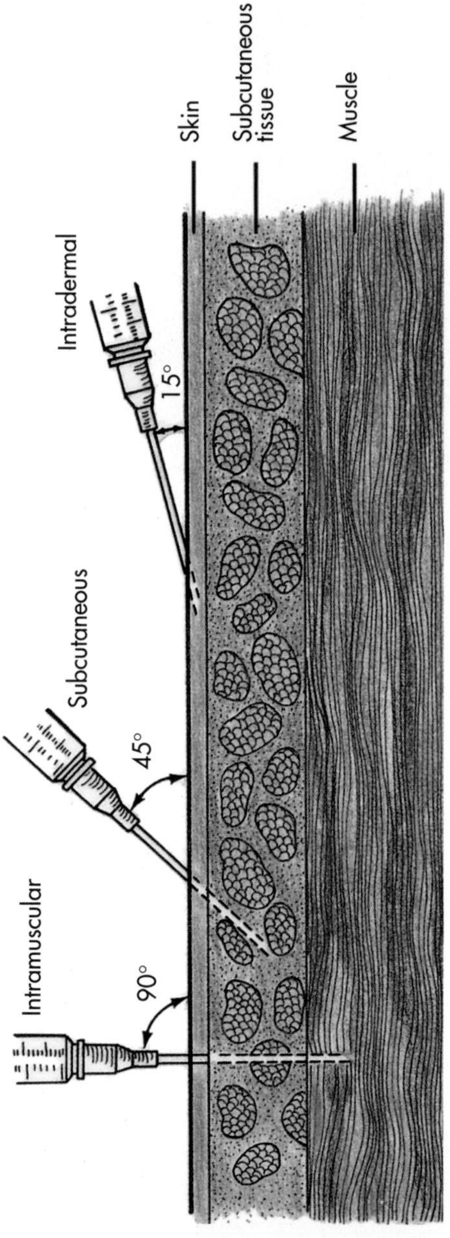

Plate 12 Comparison of angles of insertion for IM (90 degrees), SQ (45 degrees), and ID (15 degrees) injections.

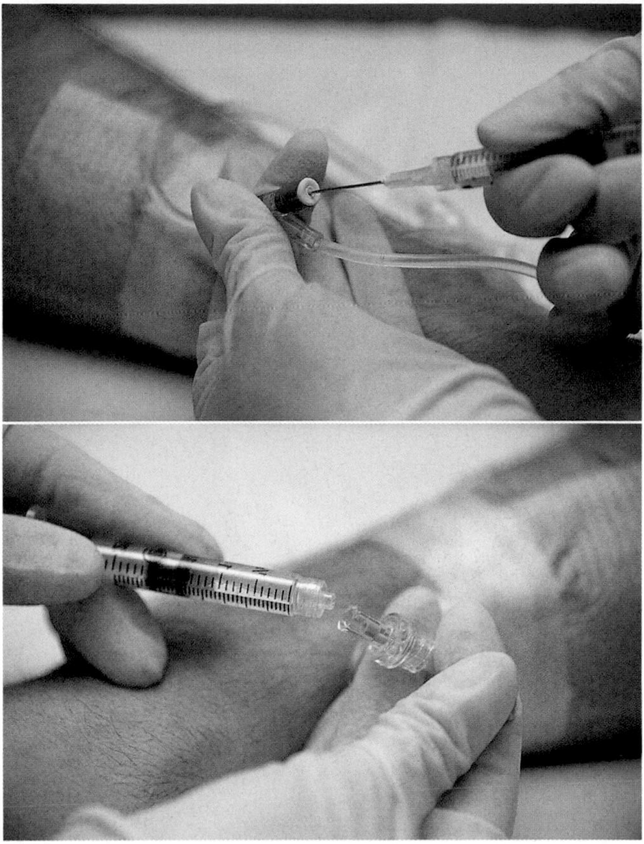

A

B

Plate 13 Administering medication by IV bolus (push). **A,** Needle system: insert small-gauge needle of syringe containing prepared drug through center of injection port. **B,** Needleless system: Remove cap of needleless injection port. Connect tip of syringe directly.

Continued

C

D

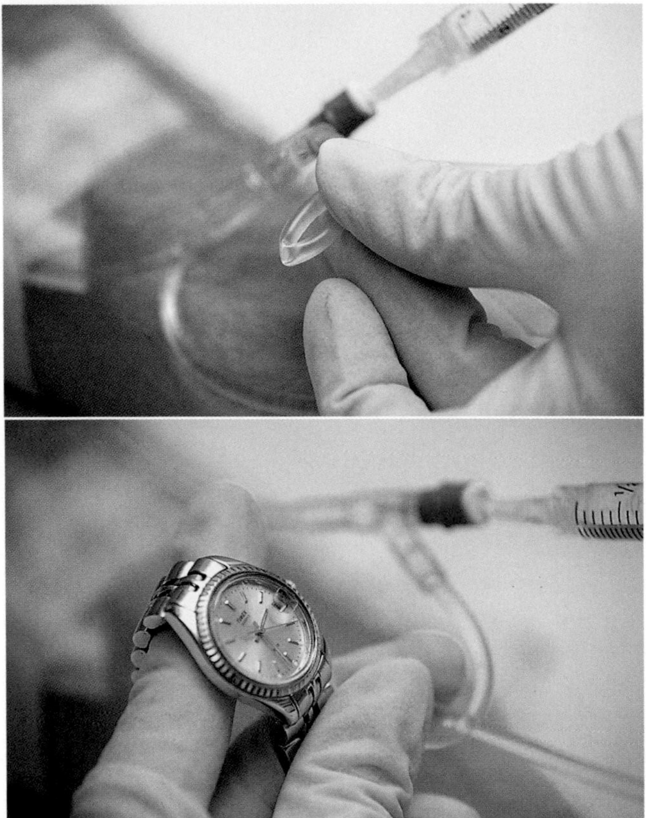

Plate 13, cont'd **C,** Occlude IV line by pinching tubing just above injection port. Pull back gently on syringe's plunger to aspirate blood return. **D,** After noting blood return, continue to occlude tubing and inject medication slowly over several minutes (read directions on drug package). Use watch to time administration.

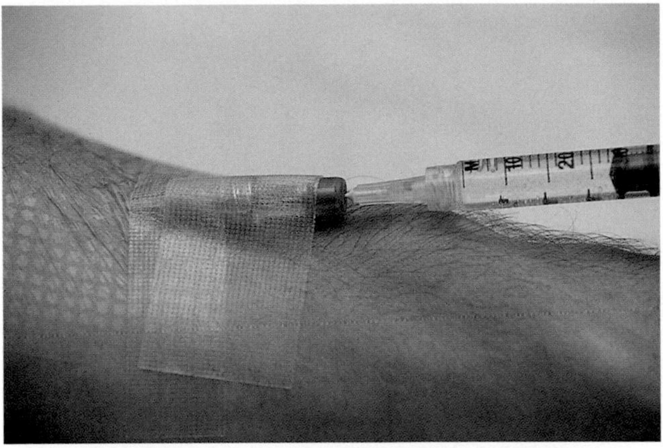

E

Plate 13, cont'd **E,** IV lock: Insert needle of syringe containing prepared drug through center of diaphragm.

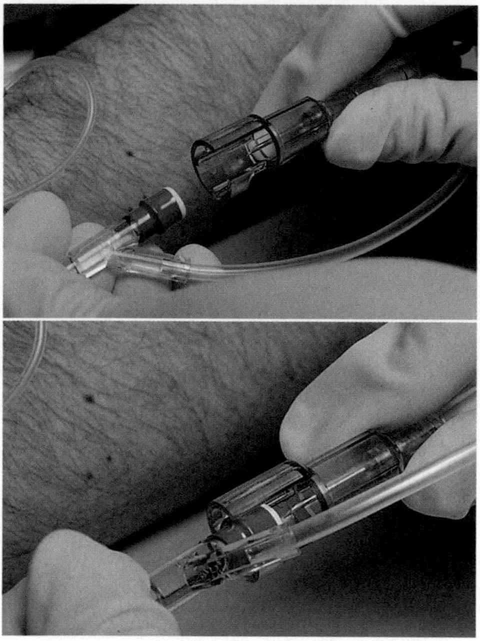

Plate 14 Administering IV medication by piggyback, volume administration sets or miniinfusors (syringe pump). Use needle-lock device to secure needle of secondary piggyback line through injection port of main line.

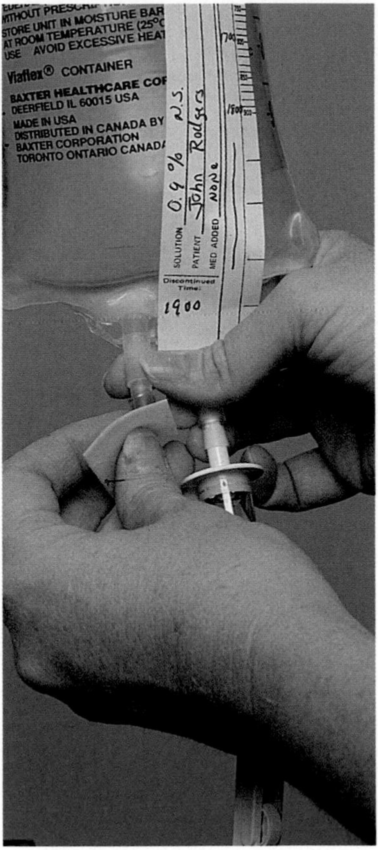

A

Plate 15 Adding medications to IV fluid containers. **A,** Wipe off port or injection site with alcohol or antiseptic swab.

Continued

B

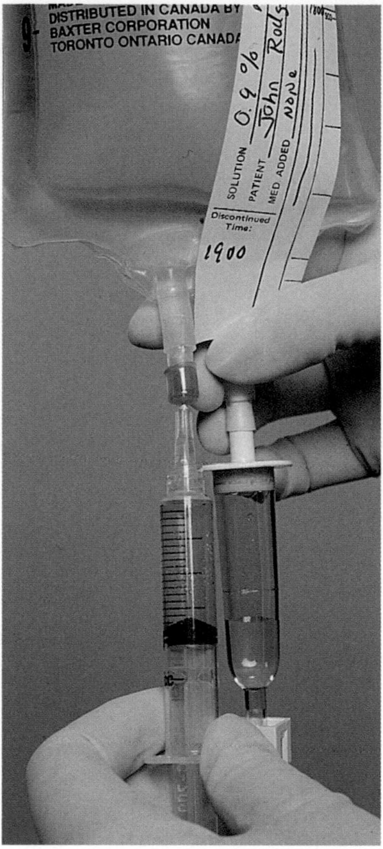

Plate 15, cont'd B, Remove needle cap from syringe and insert needle of syringe through center of injection port or site, and inject medication.

- Tell patient to carry/wear ID to identify drug being taken, allergies; tell patient drug controls symptoms but does not cure
- Caution patient to avoid hazardous activities if dizziness, drowsiness is present, to avoid driving until drug response is known
- Teach patient to report symptoms of CHF; difficult breathing, especially with exertion or when lying down, night cough, swelling of extremities or bradycardia, dizziness, confusion, depression, fever
- Teach patient to take drug as prescribed, not to double doses or skip doses; take any missed doses as soon as remembered if at least 4 hr until next dose

Evaluation

Positive therapeutic outcome

- Decreased B/P in hypertension (after 1-2 wk)
- Absence of dysrhythmias

Treatment of overdose: Lavage, **IV** atropine for bradycardia, **IV** theophylline for bronchospasm, digitalis, O_2, diuretic for cardiac failure, hemodialysis, **IV** glucose for hyperglycemia, **IV** diazepam (or phenytoin) for seizures

metronidazole (℞)

(me-troe-ni′da-zole)

Apo-Metronidazole ♣, Flagyl, Flagyl ER, Flagyl IV, Flagyl IV RTU, Metronidazole, Novonidazole ♣, Protostat, Trikacide ♣

Func. class.: Trichomonacide, amebicide, antiinfective

Chem. class.: Nitroimidazole derivative

Pregnancy category C (2nd, 3rd trimesters)

Action: Direct-acting amebicide/trichomonacide; binds, degrades DNA in organism

→ **Therapeutic Outcome:** Trichomonacidal, amebicidal, bactericidal for the following susceptible organisms: *Bacteroides, Clostridium, Trichomonas vaginalis, Giardia lamblia, Entamoeba histolytica*

Uses: Intestinal amebiasis, amebic abscess, trichomoniasis, refractory trichomoniasis, bacterial anaerobic infections, giardiasis; septicemia, endocarditis, bone, joint, and lower respiratory tract infections

Dosage and routes

Trichomoniasis

Adult: PO 250 mg tid × 7 days or 2 g in single dose; do not repeat treatment for 4-6 wk

P ***Child:*** PO 5 mg/kg/day in divided doses × 7-10 days

Refractory trichomoniasis

Adult: PO 250 mg bid × 10 days

Amebic hepatic abscess

Adult: PO 500-750 mg tid × 5-10 days

P ***Child:*** PO 35-50 mg/kg/day in 3 divided doses × 10 days

Intestinal amebiasis

Adult: PO 750 mg tid × 5-10 days

P ***Child:*** PO 35-50 mg/kg/day in 3 divided doses × 10 days; then oral iodoquinol

Anaerobic bacterial infections

Adult: **IV** inf 15 mg/kg/over 1 hr, then 7.5 mg/kg **IV** or PO q6h, max 4 g/day; first maintenance dose should be administered 6 hr after loading dose

Giardiasis

Adult: PO 250 mg tid × 5 days

P ***Child:*** PO 5 mg/kg tid × 5 days

Antibiotic-associated pseudomembranous colitis

Adult: PO 250-500 mg 3-4 ×/day × 10-14 days

M

P *Child:* PO 20 mg/kg/day (max 2 g) divided q6h

Available forms: Tabs 250, 500 mg; caps 375 mg; ext rel tabs 750 mg; inj 500 mg/100 ml; powder for inj 500 mg single dose

Adverse effects

CNS: *Headache, dizziness,* confusion, irritability, restlessness, ataxia, depression, fatigue, drowsiness, insomnia, paresthesia, peripheral neuropathy, **seizures,** incoordination, depression

CV: Flat T waves

EENT: Blurred vision, sore throat, retinal edema, dry mouth, metallic taste, furry tongue, glossitis, stomatitis

GI: *Nausea, vomiting, diarrhea,* epigastric distress, *anorexia,* constipation, *abdominal cramps,* metallic taste, **pseudomembranous colitis**

GU: Darkened urine, vaginal dryness, polyuria, **albuminuria,** dysuria, cystitis, decreased libido, **nephrotoxicity,** incontinence, dyspareunia

HEMA: **Leukopenia, bone marrow depression, aplasia**

INTEG: Rash, pruritus, urticaria, flushing

SYST: Superinfection

Contraindications: Hypersensitivity to this drug, renal disease, hepatic disease, contracted visual or color fields, blood dyscrasias, lactation, CNS disorders

Precautions: Candidal infections, pregnancy **C** (2nd, 3rd trimesters)

Pharmacokinetics

Absorption	80% (PO)
Distribution	Widely distributed, crosses placenta
Metabolism	Liver
Excretion	Urine, unchanged; feces
Half-life	6-11 hr

Pharmacodynamics

	PO	IV
Onset	Rapid	Immediate
Peak	1-2 hr	Infusion's end

Interactions

Individual drugs

Alcohol: ↑ disulfiram-like reaction
Azathioprine: ↑ leukopenia
Cimetidine: ↑ toxicity
Disulfiram: ↑ risk of psychosis
Fluorouracil: ↑ leukopenia
Lithium: ↑ toxicity
Phenobarbital: ↓ effect of metronidazole
Phenytoin: ↓ action of metronidazole

Drug classifications

Anticoagulants, oral: ↑ risk of bleeding

Lab test interferences

↓ AST, ↓ ALT

NURSING CONSIDERATIONS

Assessment

- Assess patient for signs and symptoms of infection including characteristics of wounds, WBC >10,000/mm^3, vaginal secretions, fever; obtain baseline information and during treatment
- Obtain C&S before beginning drug therapy to identify if correct treatment has been initiated
- Assess for allergic reactions: rash, urticaria, pruritus
- Identify urine output; if decreasing, notify prescriber (may indicate nephrotoxicity); also check for increased BUN, creatinine
- Assess bowel pattern qd; if severe diarrhea occurs, drug should be discontinued
- Assess for overgrowth of infection: perineal itching, fever, malaise, redness, pain, swelling, drainage, rash, diarrhea, change in cough, sputum

Nursing diagnoses

✓ Infection, risk for (uses)
✓ Diarrhea (adverse reactions)
✓ Injury, risk for (adverse reactions)

✓ Knowledge deficit (teaching)
✓ Noncompliance (teaching)

Implementation

IV route

- Give intermittent **IV** prediluted; for Flagyl **IV** dilute with 4.4 ml of sterile water or 0.9% NaCl; must be diluted further with 8 mg/ml or more 0.9% NaCl, D_5W, or LR; must neutralize with 5 mEq of $NaHCO_3$/500 mg; CO_2 gas will be generated and may require venting; run over 1 hr or more; primary **IV** must be discontinued; may be given as cont inf; do not use aluminum products; **IV** may require venting

Y-site compatibilities:
Acyclovir, allopurinol, amifostine, amiodarone, cefepime, cyclophosphamide, diltiazem, dopamine, enalaprilat, esmolol, fluconazole, foscarnet, granisetron, heparin, hydromorphone, labetalol, lorazepam, magnesium sulfate, melphalan, meperidine, methylprednisolone, midazolam, morphine, perphenazine, piperacillin/tazobactam, sargramostim, tacrolimus, teniposide, theophylline, thiotepa, vinorelbine

Additive compatibilities:
Amikacin, aminophylline, cefazolin, cefotaxime, cefotiam, ceftazidime, ceftizoxime, ceftriaxone, cefuroxime, chloramphenicol, ciprofloxacin, clindamycin, disopyramide, floxacillin, fluconazole, gentamicin, heparin, moxalactam, multielectrolyte concentrate, multivitamins, netilmicin, penicillin G potassium, tobramycin

Topical route

- A thin coating should be applied to affected area after cleaning with soap and water and patting dry

PO route

- Give with or after a meal to avoid GI symptoms, metallic taste; crush tab if needed
- Store in light-resistant container; do not refrigerate

Patient/family education

- Teach patient to report sore throat, bruising, bleeding, joint pain; may indicate blood dyscrasias (rare)
- Advise patient to contact prescriber if vaginal itching, loose, foul-smelling stools, furry tongue occur; may indicate superinfection
- Advise patient to notify physician of numbness or tingling of extremities
- Teach trichomoniasis patient that both partners need to be treated; condoms should be used during intercourse to prevent reinfection
- Advise patient of disulfiram-like reaction to alcohol ingestion; alcohol should not be used when taking this antiinfective
- Inform patient drug has a metallic taste and urine may turn dark
- Advise patient to contact prescriber if pregnancy is suspected

Evaluation

Positive therapeutic outcome

- Decreased symptoms of infection

M

mexiletine (℞)

(mex-il'e-teen)
Mexitil
Func. class.: Antidysrhythmic (class IB)
Chem. class.: Lidocaine analog
Pregnancy category C

Action: Increases electrical stimulation threshold of ventricle and His-Purkinje system, which stabilizes cardiac membrane and decreases automaticity

➔ Therapeutic Outcome: Decreased ventricular dysrhythmia

Uses: Ventricular tachycardia, ventricular dysrhythmias during cardiac surgery, MI

Investigational uses: Diabetic neuropathy

Dosage and routes

Adult: PO 200-400 mg (loading dose), then 200 mg q8h, then 200-400 mg q8h

Diabetic neuropathy (off-label)

Adult: PO 75 mg tid with gradual titration to 450-675 mg/day; maintenance 150-675 mg/day in 3 divided doses

Available forms: Caps 100 ✤, 150, 200, 250 mg

Adverse effects

CNS: Headache, dizziness, confusion, **seizures,** tremors, psychosis, nervousness, paresthesias, weakness, fatigue, coordination difficulties, change in sleep habits

CV: Hypotension, bradycardia, angina, PVCs, **heart block, cardiovascular collapse, arrest,** sinus node slowing, **left ventricular failure,** syncope, **cardiogenic shock**

EENT: Blurred vision, hearing loss, tinnitus

GI: Nausea, vomiting, anorexia, diarrhea, abdominal pain, **hepatitis,** dry mouth, peptic ulcer, altered taste, GI bleeding

GU: Urinary hesitancy, decreased libido

HEMA: **Thrombocytopenia, leukopenia, agranulocytosis, hypoplastic anemia,** systemic lupus erythematosus syndrome

INTEG: Rash, alopecia, dry skin

MISC: Edema, arthralgia, fever

RESP: Dyspnea, **fibrosis, embolism,** pneumonia

Contraindications: Hypersensitivity to amides, cardiogenic shock, blood dyscrasias, severe heart block

Precautions: Pregnancy **C,** lactation, **P** children, renal disease, liver disease, CHF, respiratory depression, myasthenia gravis

Pharmacokinetics

Absorption	Well absorbed
Distribution	Body tissues
Metabolism	Liver, extensively
Excretion	Kidneys, unchanged (10%)
Half-life	12 hr

Pharmacodynamics

Onset	½-2 hr
Peak	2-3 hr
Duration	8-12 hr

Interactions

Individual drugs

Cimetidine: ↑ toxicity
Digoxin: ↑ blood levels, toxicity
Disopyramide: ↑ levels, toxicity
Flecainide: ↑ levels, toxicity
Lidocaine: ↑ or ↓ effects of mexiletine
Metoclopramide: ↑ effects of mexiletine
Phenobarbital: ↓ effectiveness
Phenytoin: ↑ effectiveness
Procainamide: ↑ levels, toxicity
Quinidine: ↑ levels, toxicity
Rifampin: ↓ effectiveness
Warfarin: ↑ level, bleeding

Drug classifications

Analgesics, opioid: ↓ absorption
Antacids: ↓ absorption
Theophyllines: ↑ theophylline levels

Smoking

↓ Effectiveness

Herb/drug

Aloe: ↑ hypokalemia, ↑ antidysrhythmic action
Buckthorn: ↑ hypokalemia, ↑ antidysrhythmic action
Cascara sagrada: ↑ hypokalemia, ↑ antidysrhythmic action
Rhubarb: ↑ hypokalemia, ↑ antidysrhythmic action
Senna: ↑ hypokalemia, ↑ antidysrhythmic action

Lab test interferences

↑ CPK

NURSING CONSIDERATIONS

Assessment

- Assess for oxygenation or perfusion deficit: decreased B/P, chest pain, dizziness, loss of consciousness
- Assess respiratory status: auscultate lung fields for bibasilar crackles in patients with advanced CHF
- Assess for urinary retention: check for pain, abdominal absorption, palpate bladder; check males with benign prostatic hypertrophy; anticholinergic reaction may cause retention
- Monitor I&O ratio; electrolytes potassium, sodium, chloride; watch for decreasing urinary output, possible retention
- Monitor liver function studies: AST, ALT, bilirubin, alkaline phosphatase
- Monitor ECG periodically to determine drug effectiveness; measure PR, QRS, QT intervals; check for PVCs, other dysrhythmias; assess B/P for hypotension, hypertension, for rebound hypertension after 1-2 hr; for prolonged PR/QT intervals, QRS complex, if QT or QRS increase by 50% or more, withhold next dose, notify prescriber
- Monitor for dehydration and hypovolemia
- Monitor blood levels (therapeutic level 0.5-2 μg/ml), notify prescriber of abnormal results
- Assess pulmonary toxicity: dyspnea, fatigue, cough, fever, chest pain; drug should be discontinued
- Assess cardiac rate, respiration: rate, rhythm, character, chest pain, ventricular tachycardia, supraventricular tachycardia, fibrillation

Nursing diagnoses

✓ Cardiac output, decreased (uses)
✓ Impaired gas exchange (adverse reactions)
✓ Knowledge deficit (teaching)

Implementation

- Give with meals for GI upset

Patient/family education

- Teach patient to report side effects immediately to prescriber; to take exactly as prescribed; if dose is missed, take when remembered if within 3-4 hr of next dose; do not double doses
- Caution patient to avoid temp extremes; impairment of heat-regulating mechanism can occur
- Encourage patient to complete follow-up appointment with health care provider, including pulmonary function studies, chest x-ray
- Instruct patient that dry mouth may be relieved by frequent sips of water, hard candy, sugarless gum
- Caution patient to make position changes from lying to standing slowly to prevent orthostatic hypotension

Evaluation

Positive therapeutic outcome

- Decreased B/P, dysrhythmias
- Decreased heart rate
- Normal sinus rhythm

Treatment of overdose:

O_2, artificial ventilation, ECG monitoring, administer dopamine for circulatory depression, administer diazepam or thiopental for convulsions, isoproterenol

mezlocillin (℞)

(mez-loe-sill'in)

Mezlin

Func. class.: Antiinfective, broad-spectrum

Chem. class.: Extended-spectrum penicillin

Pregnancy category B

Action: Interferes with cell wall replication of susceptible organisms; osmotically unstable cell wall swells, bursts from osmotic pressure

Uses: Infection due to penicillinase-producing staphylococci, streptococci; respiratory tract, skin, skin structure, urinary tract, bone, joint infections; sinusitis, endocarditis, septicemia, meningitis; may be combined with an aminoglycoside for *Pseudomonas* infection

Therapeutic Outcome: Bactericidal effects on the following: gram-positive cocci *Staphylococcus aureus, Streptococcus viridans, Streptococcus faecalis, Streptococcus pneumoniae;* gram-negative coccus *Neisseria gonorrhoeae;* gram-positive bacilli *Clostridium perfringens, Clostridium tetani;* gram-negative bacilli *Bacteroides, Escherichia coli, Haemophilus influenzae, Klebsiella, Peptococcus, Peptostreptococcus, Morganella morganii, Enterobacter, Serratia, Pseudomonas, Proteus mirabilis, Proteus vulgaris, Proteus rettgeri, Shigella, Citrobacter, Veillonella*

Dosage and routes

Adult: IM/**IV** 200-300 mg/kg/day (serious infections) q4-6h or **IV** 500 mg q8h; may give up to 24 g/day for severe infections

P ***Child:*** IM/**IV** 50 mg/kg q4-6h

P ***Infants >8 days:*** (>2000 g) 75 mg/kg q6h; <2000 g, 75 mg/kg q8h

P ***Infants <8 days:*** 75 mg/kg q12h

Renal dose

Adult: Dose reduction indicated if CrCl <30 ml/min

Hepatic dose

Adult: Give 50% of dose

Available forms: Powder for inj 1, 2, 3, 4 g; **IV** inf 2, 3, 4 g

Adverse effects

CNS: Lethargy, hallucinations, anxiety, depression, twitching, **coma, seizures**

GI: Nausea, vomiting, diarrhea, increased AST, ALT, abdominal pain, glossitis, colitis, abnormal taste

GU: Oliguria, proteinuria, hematuria vaginitis, moniliasis, **glomerulonephritis,** increased BUN, creatinine

HEMA: Anemia, increased bleeding time, **bone marrow depression, granulocytopenia**

META: Hyperkalemia, hypokalemia, alkalosis, hypernatremia

Contraindications: Hypersensitivity to penicillins

Precautions: Pregnancy **B,** hypersensitivity to cephalosporins, P neonates, renal disease

Pharmacokinetics

Absorption	Well absorbed
Distribution	Widely distributed; crosses placenta
Metabolism	Liver, small amounts
Excretion	Kidneys, unchanged (40%-70%); breast milk, bile (15%-30%)
Half-life	50-55 min; increased in renal disease

Pharmacodynamics

	IM	IV
Onset	Rapid	Rapid
Peak	5 min	Inf end

Interactions

Individual drugs

Aspirin: ↑ mezlocillin levels, ↓ renal excretion

Chloramphenicol: ↑ half-life of chloramphenicol, ↓ effectiveness of mezlocillin

Cholestyramine: ↓ effectiveness of mezlocillin

Colestipol: ↓ effectiveness of mezlocillin

Digoxin: ↑ hypokalemia

Heparin: ↑ effect

Lithium: ↓ excretion, ↑ toxicity

Probenecid: ↑ mezlocillin levels, ↓ renal excretion

Vecuronium: ↑ effect

Drug classifications

Aminoglycosides: ↓ effectiveness of aminoglycosides if mixed together

Diuretics: ↑ hypokalemia

Erythromycins: ↓ antimicrobial effectiveness

Oral anticoagulants: ↑ anticoagulant effects
Oral contraceptives: ↓ contraceptive effectiveness
Tetracyclines: ↓ antimicrobial effectiveness

Food

Food, carbonated drinks, citrus fruit juices: ↓ absorption

Herb/drug

Khat: ↓ absorption

Lab test interferences

False positive: Urine glucose, urine protein

NURSING CONSIDERATIONS

Assessment

- Assess patient for previous sensitivity reaction to penicillins or other cephalosporins; cross-sensitivity between penicillins and cephalosporins is common
- Assess patient for signs and symptoms of infection including characteristics of wounds, sputum, urine, stool, WBC >10,000/mm^3, fever; obtain baseline information and during treatment
- Obtain C&S before beginning drug therapy to identify if correct treatment has been initiated
- Assess for allergic reactions: rash, urticaria, pruritus, chills, fever, joint pain; angioedema may occur a few days after therapy begins; epinephrine, resuscitation equipment should be available for anaphylactic reaction
- Identify urine output; if decreasing, notify prescriber (may indicate nephrotoxicity); also check for increased BUN, creatinine
- Monitor blood studies: AST, ALT, CBC, Hct, bilirubin, LDH, alkaline phosphatase, Coombs' test monthly if patient is on long-term therapy
- Monitor electrolytes: potassium, sodium, chloride monthly if patient is on long-term therapy
- Assess bowel pattern qd; if severe diarrhea occurs, drug should be discontinued; may indicate pseudomembranous colitis
- Monitor for bleeding: ecchymosis, bleeding gums, hematuria, stool guaiac daily if on long-term therapy
- Assess for overgrowth of infection: perineal itching, fever, malaise, redness, pain, swelling, drainage, rash, diarrhea, change in cough, sputum
- Assess for possible seizures; use seizure precautions in those receiving high doses

Nursing diagnoses

- ✓ Infection, risk for (uses)
- ✓ Diarrhea (adverse reactions)
- ✓ Injury, risk for (adverse reactions)
- ✓ Knowledge deficit (teaching)
- ✓ Noncompliance (teaching)

Implementation

IV route

- Dilute 1 g or less/10 ml of sterile water, for inj; D_5, 0.9% NaCl, for inj; shake, dilute further with D_5W or 0.45 NaCl, give over 3-5 min, change site q48h

Syringe compatibilities:
Heparin

Y-site compatibilities:
Amifostine, aztreonam, cyclophosphamide, famotidine, fludarabine, granisetron, hydromorphone, morphine, perphenazine, sargramostim, tacrolimus, teniposide, thiotepa

Patient/family education

- Teach patient to report sore throat, bruising, bleeding, joint pain; may indicate blood dyscrasias (rare)
- Advise patient to contact prescriber if vaginal itching, loose, foul-smelling stools, furry tongue occur; may indicate superinfection
- Advise patient to notify prescriber of diarrhea with blood or pus, which may indicate pseudomembranous colitis

Evaluation

Positive therapeutic outcome

- Absence of signs/symptoms of infection (WBC <10,000/mm^3, temp

M

WNL, absence of red, draining wounds)
• Reported improvement in symptoms of infection

Treatment of anaphylaxis: Withdraw drug, maintain airway, administer epinephrine, aminophylline, O_2, **IV** corticosteroids

mibefradil (℞)

(mi-be-fray'dill)

Posicor

Func. class.: Calcium channel blocker; antihypertensive; antianginal

Chem. class.: Benzimidazole-substituted tetraline derivative

Pregnancy category C

Action: Inhibits calcium ion influx across cell membrane during cardiac depolarization; produces relaxation of coronary vascular smooth muscle; peripheral vascular smooth muscle; dilates coronary vascular arteries; increases myocardial oxygen delivery in patients with vasospastic angina; only calcium channel blocker that blocks both T-type and L-type channels

Therapeutic Outcome: Decreased angina pectoris

Uses: Chronic stable angina pectoris

Dosage and routes

Adult: PO 50-100 mg qd

Available forms: Tabs 50, 100 mg

Adverse effects

CNS: *Headache,* dizziness

CV: Bradycardia, hypotension, palpitation, AV block, Wenckebach episodes

GI: Gastric upset, heartburn

HEMA: **Intravascular hemolysis**

Contraindications: Sick sinus syndrome, 2nd- or 3rd-degree heart block, hypotension less than 90 mm Hg systolic, cardiogenic shock, severe CHF

Precautions: CHF, hypotension, hepatic injury, pregnancy **C**, lactation, P children, renal disease, concomitant β-blocker therapy, G elderly

Pharmacokinetics	
Absorption	Unknown
Distribution	Unknown
Metabolism	Liver
Excretion	Kidneys
Half-life	27 hr

Pharmacodynamics	
Onset	Unknown
Peak	2 hr
Duration	24 hr

Interactions

Drug classifications

β-Adrenergic blockers: ↑ depressant effects on myocardial contractility

NURSING CONSIDERATIONS

Assessment

• Assess fluid volume status: I&O ratio and record; weight; distended red veins; crackles in lung; color, quality, and sp gr of urine; skin turgor; adequacy of pulses; moist mucous membranes; bilateral lung sounds; peripheral pitting edema; dehydration symptoms of decreasing output, thirst, hypotension, dry mouth, and mucous membranes should be reported
• Monitor if platelets are $<150,000/mm^3$; if so, drug is usually discontinued and another drug started
• Assess for extravasation: change site q48h
• Monitor cardiac status: B/P, pulse, respiration, ECG

Nursing diagnoses

✓ Cardiac output, decreased (uses)
✓ Knowledge deficit (teaching)

Implementation

• Give once a day, with food for GI symptoms

Patient/family education

• Caution patient to avoid hazardous

activities until stabilized on drug, dizziness is no longer a problem

- Instruct patient to limit caffeine consumption; to avoid alcohol and OTC drugs unless directed by prescriber
- Advise patient to comply with medical regimen: diet, exercise, stress reduction, drug therapy; to notify prescriber of irregular heart beat, shortness of breath, swelling of feet and hands, pronounced dizziness, constipation, nausea, hypotension
- Teach patient to use as directed even if feeling better; may be taken with other cardiovascular drugs (nitrates, β-blockers)

Evaluation

Positive therapeutic outcome

- Decreased anginal pain

Treatment of overdose:

Defibrillation, atropine for AV block, vasopressor for hypotension

miconazole (OTC)

(mi-kon′a-zole)

Monistat, Monistat I.V.; topical: Micatin, Micatin Liquid, miconazole nitrate, Monistat-Derm, Monistat 3, Monistat 7, Monistat Dual-Pak

Func. class.: Antifungal

Chem. class.: Imidazole

Pregnancy category C

Action: Alters cell membranes, inhibits fungal enzymes, inhibits sterols so intracellular contents are lost, prevents biosynthesis of phospholipids/triglycerides

Therapeutic Outcome: Fungistatic/fungicidal against *Aspergillus, Coccidioides, Cryptococcus, Candida, Dermatophytes, Histoplasma*

Uses: Coccidioidomycosis, candidiasis, cryptococcosis, paracoccidioidomycosis, chronic mucocutaneous candidiasis, fungal meningitis; **IV** used for severe infections only; (top) tinea pedis, tinea cruris, tinea corporis, tinea versicolor, vaginal or vulva candidal infections

Dosage and routes

Adult: **IV** inf 200-3600 mg/day; may be divided in 3 inf at 200-1200 mg/inf; may have to repeat course; IT 20 mg given simultaneously with **IV** for fungal meningitis q1-2 days

P ***Child:*** **IV** 20-40 mg/kg/day, max 15 mg/kg/day

P ***Adult and child:*** TOP apply to affected area bid × 2-4 wk

Adult: Intravaginal give 1 applicator or supp × 7 days hs

Available forms: Inj 10 mg/ml; aerosol 2%; cream 2%; lotion 2%; powder 2%; spray 2%; vag cream 2%; vag supp 100, 200 mg

Adverse effects

CNS: Drowsiness, headache, lethargy
CV: Tachycardia, **dysrhythmias** (rapid **IV**)
GI: Nausea, vomiting, anorexia, diarrhea, cramps
GU: Vulvovaginal burning, itching, hyponatremia, pelvic cramps (topical forms)
HEMA: **Decreased Hct, thrombocytopenia, hyperlipidemia**
INTEG: Pruritus, rash, fever, flushing, hives
SYST: **Anaphylaxis**

Contraindications: Hypersensitivity

Precautions: Renal disease, hepatic disease, pregnancy **C**

Pharmacokinetics	
Absorption	Poorly absorbed (PO)
Distribution	Widely distributed (**IV**); bound to serum proteins (90%)
Metabolism	Liver, extensively
Excretion	Unknown
Half-life	Triphasic: 0.4, 2.1, 24 hr

M

Pharmacodynamics

	IV	TOP	VAG
Onset	Rapid	Unknown	Unknown
Peak	Infusion's end	Unknown	Unknown

Interactions

Individual drugs

Amphotericin B: ↓ effect of miconazole and amphotericin B
Isoniazid: ↓ effect of miconazole
Phenytoin: ↑ effect
Rifampin: ↓ effect of miconazole
Warfarin: ↑ anticoagulant effect

Drug classifications

Sulfonylureas: ↑ effect

Lab test interferences

False positive: Urine glucose, urine protein

NURSING CONSIDERATIONS

Assessment

- Assess for signs and symptoms of infection: drainage, sore throat, urinary pain, hematuria, fever
- Obtain C&S before beginning treatment; therapy may be started after culture is taken; monitor signs of infection before and throughout treatment
- Monitor bowel pattern before and during treatment; diarrhea may occur
- Monitor cardiac system: B/P, pulse; watch for increasing pulse, cardiac dysrhythmias; drug should be discontinued
- Monitor blood studies: WBC, RBC, Hgb, Hct, bleeding time; patients taking anticoagulants may need a decreased dosage; monitor liver and renal studies periodically for patients on long-term therapy
- Monitor I&O ratio; watch for decreasing urinary output, change in sp gr; discontinue drug to prevent renal damage; patients with renal disease may require lowered dose
- Monitor **IV** site for thrombophlebitis; site should be changed q48-72h
- Monitor for allergies before initiation of treatment and reaction to each medication; highlight allergies on chart; check for allergic reaction: burning, stinging, swelling, redness (top); observe for skin eruptions after administration of drug to 1 wk after discontinuing drug

Nursing diagnoses

- ✓ Skin integrity, impaired (uses)
- ✓ Infection, risk (uses)
- ✓ Injury, risk for (adverse reactions)
- ✓ Knowledge deficit (teaching)

Implementation

- Have adrenalin, suction, tracheostomy set, endotracheal intubation equipment available

IV IV route

- Give 200 mg initially to prevent severe hypersensitive reaction
- Give **IV** after diluting ≤1 g/10 ml of sterile water, D_5W, or 0.45% NaCl over 3-5 min
- Give by intermittent **IV** after diluting in 200 ml or more, D_5W or 0.9% NaCl; give over 30-60 min
- Store at room temp; reconstituted sol is stable for 24 hr refrigerated

Y-site compatibilities:

Allopurinol, filgrastim, foscarnet, granisetron, melphalan, ondansetron, propofol, sargramostim, teniposide, thiotepa, vinorelbine

Y-site incompatibilities:

Fludarabine

Topical route

- Apply after cleansing area with soap and water before each application; use enough medication to cover lesions completely; dry well
- Store at room temp in dry place

Vaginal route

- Administer 1 applicatorfull every night high into the vagina
- Store at room temp in dry place

Patient/family education

- Inform patient that culture may be performed after completed course of medication
- Advise patient to notify nurse of

diarrhea, symptoms of candidal vaginitis

Topical route

- Teach patient to use medical asepsis (hand washing) before, after each application; to apply with glove to prevent further infection; to avoid contact with eyes; not to use occlusive dressings
- Caution patient to avoid use of OTC creams, ointments, lotions unless directed by prescriber
- Instruct patient to notify prescriber if no improvement in condition in 4 wk or if symptoms return in 2 mo; pregnancy or a serious medical condition may be the cause
- Teach patient to use for full prescribed treatment time, or reinfection may occur

Vaginal route

- Instruct patient in asepsis (hand washing) before, after each application
- Teach patient to apply with applicator only; to avoid use of any other vaginal product unless directed by prescriber; sanitary napkin may prevent soiling of undergarments; to abstain from sexual intercourse until treatment is completed; reinfection and irritation may occur
- Instruct patient to notify prescriber if symptoms persist

Evaluation

Positive therapeutic outcome

- Decreasing oral candidiasis, fever, malaise, rash
- Negative C&S for infectious organism
- Decrease in size, number of lesions
- Decrease in itching or white discharge (vaginal)

Treatment of overdose: Withdraw drug; maintain airway; administer epinephrine, aminophylline, O_2, **IV** corticosteroids for anaphylaxis

midazolam (℞)

(mid'ay-zoe-lam)

Versed

Func. class.: Sedative/hypnotic, antianxiety

Chem. class.: Benzodiazepine, short-acting

Pregnancy category D

Controlled substance schedule IV

Action: Depresses subcortical levels in CNS; may act on limbic system, reticular formation; may potentiate GABA by binding to specific benzodiazepine receptors

➔ **Therapeutic Outcome:** Sedation for anesthesia induction and procedures

Uses: Preoperative sedation, general anesthesia induction, sedation for diagnostic endoscopic procedures, intubation

Investigational uses: Epileptic seizures, refractory status epilepticus

Dosage and routes

Preoperative sedation

Adult: IM 0.07-0.08 mg/kg 30-60 min before general anesthesia

P ***Child:*** IM 0.1-0.15 mg/kg, may give up to 0.5 mg/kg if needed

Induction of general anesthesia

P ***Adult and child 12-16 yr:*** Unpremedicated patients, **IV** 0.3-0.35 mg/kg over 30 sec, wait 2 min, follow with 25% of initial dose if needed; premedicated patients, 0.15-0.35 mg/kg over 20-30 sec, allow 2 min for effect

P ***Child 6-12 yr:*** **IV** 0.025-0.05 mg/kg, total dose up to 0.4 mg/kg if needed

P ***Child 6 mo-5 yr:*** **IV** 0.05-0.1 mg/kg, total dose up to 0.6 mg/kg may be needed

M

P ***Child <6 mo:*** Titrate with small increments

Available forms: Inj 1, 5 mg/ml; syrup 2 mg/ml

Adverse effects

CNS: Retrograde amnesia, euphoria, confusion, headache, anxiety, insomnia, slurred speech, paresthesia, tremors, weakness, chills

CV: Hypotension, PVCs, tachycardia, bigeminy, nodal rhythm, **cardiac arrest**

EENT: Blurred vision, nystagmus, diplopia, blocked ears, loss of balance

GI: *Nausea, vomiting,* increased salivation, hiccups

INTEG: Urticaria, pain, swelling at inj site, rash, pruritus

RESP: Coughing, **apnea, bronchospasm, laryngospasm,** dyspnea, **respiratory depression**

Contraindications: Pregnancy **D**, hypersensitivity to benzodiazepines, shock, coma, alcohol intoxication, acute narrowangle glaucoma

Precautions: COPD, CHF, chronic renal failure, chills, debilitated, G elderly, P children, lactation

Do Not Confuse:
Versed/Vepesid, Versed/Vistaril

Pharmacokinetics

Absorption	Well absorbed
Distribution	Crosses placenta, blood-brain barrier
Metabolism	Liver
Excretion	Kidneys, breast milk
Half-life	1-12 hr

Pharmacodynamics

	IM	IV
Onset	15 min	3-5 min
Peak	½-1 hr	Unknown
Duration	2-6 hr	2-6 hr

Interactions

Individual drugs

Alcohol: ↑ CNS depression
Cimetidine: ↑ levels of midazolam
Erythromycin: May alter midazolam metabolism
Fluvoxamine: ↑ respiratory depression
Indinavir: ↑ respiratory depression
Ritonavir: ↑ respiratory depression
Theophylline: May alter midazolam metabolism
Verapamil: ↑ respiratory depression

Drug classifications

Antifungals, azole: ↑ levels of midalozam
Antihistamines: ↑ CNS depression
Antihypertensives: ↑ hypotension
Nitrates: ↑ hypotension
Opiates: ↑ CNS depression
Oral contraceptives: ↑ half-life of midazolam
Sedative/hypnotics: ↑ CNS depression
Theophyllines: ↓ effect of midazolam

NURSING CONSIDERATIONS

Assessment

- Monitor B/P, pulse, respiration during **IV**; O_2 and emergency equipment should be nearby
- Monitor inj site for redness, pain, swelling
- Assess degree of amnesia in G elderly; may be increased
- Assess anterograde amnesia
- Assess vital signs for recovery period in obese patient, since half-life may be extended
- Assess for apnea, respiratory depression, which may be increased in G the elderly

Nursing diagnoses

✓ Knowledge deficit (teaching)

Implementation

IV **IV route**

- Give **IV** undiluted or after diluting with D_5W or 0.9% NaCl to a conc of 0.25 mg/ml; give over 2 min (conscious sedation) or over 30 sec (anesthesia induction)
- Ensure immediate availability of

resuscitation equipment, O_2 to support airway; do not give by rapid bol

Syringe compatibilities: Atracurium, atropine, benzquinamide, buprenorphine, butorphanol, chlorpromazine, cimetadine, diphenhydramine, droperidol, fentanyl, glycopyrrolate, hydromorphine, hydroxyzine, meperidine, metoclopramide, morphine, nalbuphine, promazine, promethazine, scopolamine, sufentanil, thiethylperazine, trimethobenzamide

Syringe incompatibilities: Dimenhydrinate, pentobarbital, perphenazine, prochlorperazine, ranitidine

Y-site compatibilities: Amikacin, amiodarone, atracurium, calcium gluconate, cefazolin, cefmetazole, cefotaxime, cimetidine, ciprofloxacin, clindamycin, digoxin, diltiazem, dopamine, epinephrine, erythromycin, esmolol, etomidate, famotidine, fentanyl, fluconazole, gentamicin, haloperidol, heparin, hydromorphone, insulin (regular), labetalol, lorazepam, methylprednisolone, metronidazole, milrinone, morphine, nicardipine, nitroglycerin, norepinephrine, pancuronium, piperacillin, potassium chloride, ranitidine, sodium nitroprusside, sufentanil, theophylline, tobramycin, vancomycin, vecuronium

Y-site incompatibilities: Foscarnet

IM route

- Give IM deep in large muscle mass
- Store at room temp

Patient/family education

- Inform patient that amnesia occurs; events may not be remembered
- Caution patient to avoid CNS depressants including alcohol for 24 hr after taking this drug

Evaluation

Positive therapeutic outcome

- Induction of sedation, amnesia

Treatment of overdose: O_2, vasopressors, physostigmine, resuscitation; flumazenil will reverse effects

midodrine (℞)

(mye'doh-dreen)

ProAmatine

Func. class.: Prodrug

Pregnancy category C

Action: Activates α-adrenergic receptors of arteriolar venous vasculature; increases vascular tone

➔ Therapeutic Outcome: Decreased feeling of faintness upon rising, absence of significant change in B/P

Uses: Orthostatic hypotension

Dosage and routes

Adult: PO 10 mg

Renal dose

Adult: PO 2.5 mg tid

Available forms: Tabs 2.5, 5 mg

Adverse effects

CNS: Drowsiness, restlessness, headache, paresthesia, pain, chills

CV: **Supine hypertension**

EENT: Dry mouth, blurred vision

GI: Nausea, anorexia

GU: Urinary urgency

INTEG: Pruritus, piloerection, rash

Contraindications: Hypersensitivity, severe organic heart disease, acute renal disease, urinary retention, pheochromocytoma, thyrotoxicosis, persistent/excessive supine hypertension

P Precautions: Children, urinary retention, lactation, prostatic hypertrophy, pregnancy **C**

M

Pharmacokinetics

Absorption	Unknown
Distribution	Unknown
Metabolism	Unknown
Excretion	Unknown
Half-life	3-4 hr

Pharmacodynamics

Onset	Unknown
Peak	1-2 hr
Duration	Unknown

Interactions
Individual drugs:
Fludrocortisone: ↑ supine hypertension
Drug classifications
α-Adrenergic agonists: ↑ pressor effects
β-Adrenergic blockers: ↑ bradycardia
Cardiac glycosides: ↑ bradycardia
Psychotropics: ↑ bradycardia
Steroids: ↑ intraocular pressure

NURSING CONSIDERATIONS
Assessment
- Monitor VS, B/P (standing, supine); notify prescriber if B/P supine is increased
- Observe for drowsiness, dizziness, LOC

Implementation
- Tablets may be swallowed whole, chewed, or allowed to dissolve
- Administer upon arising, at midday, and in late afternoon (no later than 6 PM)
- Avoid administering if patient is to be supine during day

Nursing diagnoses
✓ Knowledge deficit (teaching)

Patient/family education
- Advise to avoid hazardous activities; activities requiring alertness; dizziness may occur; instruct patient to request assistance with ambulation
- Advise to avoid alcohol, other depressants

Evaluation
Positive therapeutic outcome
- Decreased orthostatic hypotension

mifepristone (℞)
(mif-ee-press′tone)
Mifeprex
Func. class.: Abortifacient

Pregnancy category C

Action: Stimulates uterine contractions, causing complete abortion

➔ **Therapeutic Outcome:** Termination of pregnancy

Uses: Abortion through 49 days gestation

Investigational uses: Postcoital contraception/contragestation, intrauterine fetal death, endometriosis, Cushing's syndrome, unresectable meningioma

Dosage and routes
Coadministration of mifepristone/misoprostol
- Day 1: PO single dose 600 mg mifepristone
- Day 3: If abortion has not taken place, as evidenced by clinical exam or ultrasound, give PO single dose 400 µg misoprostol
- Day 14: Patient returns for post-treatment exam to determine complete termination of pregnancy

Available forms: Tabs 200 mg

Adverse effects
CNS: Dizziness, insomnia, anxiety, syncope, fainting, headache
GI: *Nausea, vomiting, diarrhea,* dyspepsia
GU: Uterine cramping, uterine hemorrhage, vaginitis, pelvic pain
MISC: Fatigue, back pain, fever, viral infections, chills, sinusitis

Contraindications: Hypersensitivity, severe hepatic disease, severe renal disease, PID, respiratory disease, cardiac disease

Precautions: Asthma, anemia, jaundice, diabetes mellitus, convulsive disorders, past uterine surgery, pregnancy **C**

Pharmacokinetics

Absorption	Rapidly
Distribution	98% protein binding, albumin, glycoprotein
Metabolism	Unknown
Excretion	Feces, urine
Half-life	Unknown

Pharmacodynamics

Onset	Unknown
Peak	90 min
Duration	Unknown

Interactions
Individual drugs
Erythromycin: ↓ metabolism of erythromycin
Itraconazole: ↓ metabolism of itraconazole
Ketoconazole: ↓ metabolism of ketoconazole

NURSING CONSIDERATIONS
Assessment
- Monitor B/P, pulse; watch for change that may indicate hemorrhage
- Monitor respiratory rate, rhythm, depth; notify prescriber of abnormalities
- Assess for length, duration of contraction; notify prescriber of contractions lasting over 1 min or absence of contractions
- Assess for incomplete abortion, pregnancy must be terminated by another method; drug is teratogenic

Nursing diagnoses
✓ Pain (adverse reactions)
✓ Knowledge deficit (teaching)

Implementation
- Provide emotional support before and after abortion

Patient/family education
- Advise patient to report increased blood loss, abdominal cramps, increased temperature, foul-smelling lochia
- Teach patient some methods of comfort control and pain control
- Advise patient to continue with follow-up
- Advise patient that cramping and vaginal bleeding will occur

Evaluation
Positive therapeutic outcome
- Expulsion of fetus

miglitol (℞)
(mig'le-tol)
Glyset
Func. class.: Oral hypoglycemic
Chem. class.: α-Glucosidase inhibitor

Pregnancy category B

Action: Delays the digestion of ingested carbohydrates, results in a smaller rise in blood glucose after meals; does not increase insulin production

➔ **Therapeutic Outcome:** Decreased blood glucose levels in diabetes mellitus

Uses: Stable adult-onset diabetes mellitus, (type 2) NIDDM

Dosage and routes
Initial dose
Adult: PO 25 mg tid with first bite of meal

Maintenance dose
Adult: PO may be increased to 50 mg tid; may increase to 100 mg tid if needed only in patients >60 kg; dosage adjustment at 4-8 wk intervals

Available forms: Tabs 25, 50, 100 mg

Adverse effects
GI: *Abdominal pain, diarrhea, flatulence,* **hepatotoxicity**
HEMA: Low iron
INTEG: Rash

M

Contraindications: Hypersensitivity, diabetic ketoacidosis, cirrhosis, inflammatory bowel disease, colonic ulceration, partial intestinal obstruction, chronic intestinal disease

Precautions: Pregnancy **B**, renal disease, lactation, children, hepatic disease

P

Pharmacokinetics	
Absorption	Unknown
Distribution	Unknown
Metabolism	Not metabolized
Excretion	Kidneys, unchanged drug
Half-life	2 hr

Pharmacodynamics	
Onset	Unknown
Peak	2-3 hr
Duration	Unknown

Interactions

Individual drugs

Digoxin: ↓ levels of digoxin
Propranolol: ↓ levels of propranolol
Ranitidine: ↓ levels of ranitidine

Drug classifications

Adsorbents, intestinal: ↓ miglitol levels; do not use together
Enzymes, digestive: ↓ miglitol levels; do not use together

Herb/drug

Broom: ↓ hypoglycemia
Buchu: ↓ hypoglycemia
Chromium: ↑ or ↓ hypoglycemic effect
Dandelion: ↓ hypoglycemia
Fenugreek: ↑ or ↓ hypoglycemic effect
Ginseng: ↑ or ↓ hypoglycemic effect
Juniper: ↓ hypoglycemia
Karela: Improved glucose tolerance

NURSING CONSIDERATIONS

Assessment

- Assess for hypoglycemia, hyperglycemia; even though this drug does not cause hypoglycemia, if taking a sulfonylurea or insulin, hypoglycemia may be additive
- Monitor blood glucose levels, glycosylated hemoglobin, LFTs

Nursing diagnoses

- ✓ Nutrition altered, more than body requirements (uses)
- ✓ Nutrition altered, less than body requirements (adverse reactions)
- ✓ Knowledge deficit (teaching)
- ✓ Noncompliance (teaching)

Implementation

- Give tid with first bite of each meal
- Provide storage in airtight container in cool environment

Patient/family education

- Teach patient the symptoms of hypoglycemia, hyperglycemia and what to do about each
- Instruct that medication must be taken as prescribed; explain consequences of discontinuing the medication abruptly; that during periods of stress, infection, surgery, insulin may be required
- Tell patient to avoid OTC medications unless approved by prescriber
- Teach patient that diabetes is a life-long illness; drug will not cure condition
- Instruct patient to carry/wear ID as diabetic
- Teach patient that diet and exercise regimen must be followed

Evaluation

Positive therapeutic outcome

- Decreased signs, symptoms of diabetes mellitus (polyuria, polydipsia, polyphagia, clear sensorium, absence of dizziness, stable gait)

HIGH ALERT

milrinone (℞)

(mill-re′none)

Primacor

Func. class.: Inotropic/vasodilator agent with phosphodiesterase activity

Chem. class.: Bipyridine derivative

Pregnancy category C

Action: Positive inotropic agent with vasodilator properties; increases contractility of cardiac muscle; reduces preload and afterload by direct relaxation of vascular smooth muscle; increases myocardial contractility

➔ **Therapeutic Outcome:** Increased inotropic effect resulting in increased cardiac output

Uses: Short-term management of advanced CHF that has not responded to other medication; can be used with digitalis products

Dosage and routes

***Adult:* IV** bol 50 μg/kg given over 10 min; start inf of 0.375-0.75 μg/kg/min; reduce dosage in renal impairment

Available forms: Inj 1 mg/ml; premixed inj 200 μg/ml in D^5W

Adverse effects

CV: Dysrhythmias, hypotension, chest pain

GI: Nausea, vomiting, anorexia, abdominal pain, **hepatotoxicity**, jaundice

***HEMA:* Thrombocytopenia**

MISC: Headache, hypokalemia, tremor

Contraindications: Hypersensitivity to this drug, severe aortic disease, severe pulmonic valvular disease, acute MI

Precautions: Lactation, pregnancy **P** C, children, renal disease, hepatic disease, atrial flutter/fibrillation, **G** elderly

Pharmacokinetics	
Absorption	Completely absorbed
Distribution	Unknown
Metabolism	Liver (50%)
Excretion	Kidney, unchanged and metabolites (60%-90%)
Half-life	3½-6 hr; increased in CHF

Pharmacodynamics	
Onset	2-5 min
Peak	10 min
Duration	Variable

Interactions: None

NURSING CONSIDERATIONS

Assessment

- Monitor manifestations of hypokalemia: acidic urine, reduced urine, osmolality, nocturia; hypotension, broad T wave, U wave, ectopy, tachycardia, weak pulse; muscle weakness, altered LOC, drowsiness, apathy, lethargy, confusion, depression; anorexia, nausea, cramps, constipation, distention, paralytic ileus; hypoventilation, respiratory muscle weakness
- Assess fluid volume status: complete I&O ratio and record; note weight, distended red veins, crackles in lung, color, quality, and sp gr of urine, skin turgor, adequacy of pulses, moist mucous membranes, bilateral lung sounds, peripheral pitting edema; dehydration symptoms of decreasing output, thirst, hypotension, dry mouth and mucous membranes should be reported
- Monitor electrolytes: potassium, sodium, calcium, magnesium; also include BUN, blood pH, ABGs
- Monitor B/P and pulse, PCWP, CVP, index often during inf; if B/P drops 30 mm Hg, stop inf and call prescriber
- Monitor ALT, AST, bilirubin daily; if these are elevated, hepatoxicity is suspected
- Monitor platelets; if <150,000/

M

mm^3, drug is usually discontinued and another drug started

- Assess for extravasation: change site q48h

Nursing diagnoses

✓ Cardiac output, decreased (uses)
✓ Fluid volume excess (uses)
✓ Knowledge deficit (teaching)

IV **IV route**

Implementation

- Do not mix directly with glucose sol; chemical reaction occurs over 24 hr; precipitate forms if milrinone and furosemide come in contact
- Administer by direct **IV** into inf through Y-connector or directly into tubing; may give undiluted over 2-3 min
- Give by cont inf diluted with 0.9% NaCl to conc of 1-3 mg/ml, run at prescribed rate; give by infusion pump for doses other than bol
- Administer potassium supplements if ordered for potassium levels <3.0 mg/dl

Syringe compatibilities: Atropine, calcium chloride, digoxin, epinephrine, lidocaine, morphine, propranolol, sodium bicarbonate, verapamil

Y-site compatibilities: Digoxin, diltiazem, dobutamine, dopamine, epinephrine, fentanyl, heparin, hydromorphone, labetalol, lorazepam, midazolam, morphine, nicardipine, nitroglycerin, norepinephrine, propranolol, quinidine, ranitidine, thiopental, vecuronium

Additive compatibilities: Quinidine

Patient/family education

- Teach patient reason for medication and expected results
- Instruct patient to make position changes slowly; orthostatic hypotension may occur
- Teach patient signs and symptoms of hypersensitivity reactions and hypokalemia

Evaluation

Positive therapeutic outcome

- Increased cardiac output
- Decreased PCWP, adequate CVP
- Decreased dyspnea, fatigue, edema, ECG

Treatment of overdose:
Discontinue drug, support circulation

minocycline (℞)

(min-oh-sye'kleen)

Apo-Minocycline ✱, Arestin, Dynacin, Minocin, Minocin IV, Vectrin

Func. class.: Antiinfective
Chem. class.: Tetracycline

Pregnancy category D

Action: Inhibits protein synthesis and phosphorylation in microorganisms by binding to 30S ribosomal subunits and reversibly binding to 50S ribosomal subunits; bacteriostatic

➡ **Therapeutic Outcome:** Bactericidal action against susceptible organisms, including *Neisseria meningitidis, Neisseria gonorrhoeae, Treponema pallidum, Chlamydia trachomatis, Ureaplasma urealyticum, Mycoplasma pneumoniae, Nocardia, Rickettsia*

Uses: Syphilis, chlamydial infection, gonorrhea, lymphogranuloma venereum, rickettsial infections, inflammatory acne, meningitis carriers, periodontitis

Investigational uses: Rheumatoid arthritis

Dosage and routes

Adult: PO/**IV** 200 mg, then 100 mg q12h or 50 mg q6h, max 400 mg/24 hr **IV**

P ***Child >8 yr:*** PO/**IV** 4 mg/kg then 4 mg/kg/day PO in divided doses q12h

Gonorrhea

Adult: PO 200 mg, then 100 mg q12h × 4 days

C. trachomatis infection
Adult: PO 100 mg bid × 7 days
Syphilis
Adult: PO 200 mg, then 100 mg q12h × 10-15 days
Uncomplicated gonococcal urethritis in men
Adult: PO 100 mg bid × 5 days
Rheumatoid arthritis (off-label)
Adult: PO 100 mg bid for ≤48 wk

Available forms: Tabs 50, 100 mg; caps 50, 100 mg; oral susp 50 mg/5 ml; inj 100 mg; microspheres

Adverse effects

CNS: *Dizziness,* fever, lightheadedness, vertigo
CV: Pericarditis
EENT: Dysphagia, glossitis, decreased calcification, permanent discoloration of deciduous teeth, oral candidiasis
GI: *Nausea,* abdominal pain, *vomiting, diarrhea,* anorexia, enterocolitis, **hepatotoxicity,** flatulence, abdominal cramps, epigastric burning, stomatitis
GU: Increased BUN, polyuria, polydipsia, **renal failure, nephrotoxicity**
HEMA: **Eosinophilia, neutropenia, thrombocytopenia, hemolytic anemia**
INTEG: *Rash, urticaria, photosensitivity, increased pigmentation,* **exfoliative dermatitis,** pruritus, angioedema, blue-gray color of skin and mucous membranes

Contraindications: Hypersensitivity to tetracyclines, children <8 yr, P pregnancy **D**

Precautions: Hepatic disease, lactation

Pharmacokinetics

Absorption	Well absorbed (PO)
Distribution	Widely distributed (70%-75% protein bound); some distribution in CSF, crosses placenta
Metabolism	Liver, some
Excretion	Kidneys, unchanged (20%), bile, feces
Half-life	11-17 hr

Pharmacodynamics

	PO	IV
Onset	Rapid	Rapid
Peak	2-3 hr	Infusion's end

Interactions

Individual drugs
Calcium: Forms chelates, ↓ absorption
Carbamazepine: ↓ effect
Iron: Forms chelates, ↓ absorption
Magnesium: Forms chelates, ↓ absorption
Phenytoin: ↓ effect
Sodium bicarbonate: ↓ minocycline effect
Warfarin: ↑ effect
Drug classifications
Antidiarrheals, adsorbent: ↓ absorption
Barbiturates: ↓ effect
Oral contraceptives: ↓ effect of oral contraception **Penicillins:** ↓ effect
Lab test interferences
False negative: Urine glucose with Clinistix, Tes-Tape

NURSING CONSIDERATIONS

Assessment

- Assess patient for previous sensitivity reaction
- Assess patient for signs and symptoms of infection including characteristics of wounds, sputum, urine, stool, WBC >10,000/mm^3, fever; obtain baseline information, before and during treatment
- Obtain C&S before beginning drug therapy to identify if correct treatment has been initiated

M

- Assess for allergic reactions: rash, urticaria, pruritus
- Monitor blood studies: AST, ALT, CBC, Hct, bilirubin, alkaline phosphatase, amylase monthly if patient is on long-term therapy
- Assess bowel pattern qd; if severe diarrhea occurs, drug should be discontinued
- Monitor for bleeding: ecchymosis, bleeding gums, hematuria, stool guaiac daily if on long-term therapy; blood dyscrasias may occur
- Assess for overgrowth of infection: perineal itching, fever, malaise, redness, pain, swelling, drainage, rash, diarrhea, change in cough, sputum; black, furry tongue

Nursing diagnoses

- ✓ Infection, risk for (uses)
- ✓ Diarrhea (adverse reactions)
- ✓ Knowledge deficit (teaching)
- ✓ Noncompliance (teaching)

Implementation

PO route

- Give around the clock to maintain proper blood levels; give with food to increase absorption of drug; do not give within 3 hr of other agents; drug interactions may occur
- Give with 8 oz of water 1 hr before hs to prevent ulceration
- Shake liq preparation well before giving; use calibrated device for proper dosing
- Do not give with iron, calcium, magnesium products, or antacids, which decrease absorption and form insoluble chelate

IV **IV route**

- Check for irritation, extravasation, phlebitis daily; change site q72h
- For intermittent inf, dilute each 100 mg/10 ml of 0.9% NaCl, sterile water for inj; further dilute in 500-1000 ml of 0.9% NaCl, D_5W, Ringer's, LR, D_5/LR; give over 6 hr

Y-site compatibilities:
Cyclophosphamide, fludarabine, granisetron, heparin, hydrocortisone, magnesium sulfate, melphalan, perphenazine, potassium chloride, sargramostim, sodium succinate, vinorelbine, vit B/C

Y-site incompatibilities:
Aztreonam, filgrastim, hydromorphone, meperidine, morphine, teniposide

Patient/family education

- Teach patient to use sunscreen when outdoors to decrease photosensitivity reaction
- Teach patient to report sore throat, bruising, bleeding, joint pain; may indicate blood dyscrasias (rare)
- Advise patient to contact prescriber if vaginal itching, loose, foul-smelling stools, furry tongue occur; may indicate superinfection; report itching, rash, pruritus, urticaria
- Instruct patient to take all medication prescribed for the length of time ordered; drug must be taken around the clock to maintain blood levels; do not give medication to others; take with a full glass of water; may take with food; not to use outdated product, Fanconi's syndrome may occur
- Advise patient to use a form of contraception other than hormonal

Evaluation

Positive therapeutic outcome

- Absence of signs/symptoms of infection (WBC <10,000/mm^3, temp WNL, absence of red, draining wounds)
- Reported improvement in symptoms of infection

minoxidil (℞, OTC)

(mi-nox'i-dill)

Loniten, minoxidil, Rogaine (top)

Func. class.: Antihypertensive, hair growth stimulant

Chem. class.: Vasodilator, peripheral

Pregnancy category C

Action: Directly relaxes arteriolar smooth muscle, causing vasodilatation; increased cutaneous blood flow; stimulation of hair follicles

Therapeutic Outcome: Decreased B/P in hypertension; hair growth

Uses: Severe hypertension unresponsive to other therapy (use with diuretic); topically to treat alopecia

Dosage and routes

Severe hypertension

Adult: PO 2.5-5 mg/day max 100 mg daily; usual range 10-40 mg/day in single doses

G ***Elderly:*** PO 2.5 mg qd, may be increased gradually

P ***Child <12 yr:*** Initial, 0.2 mg/kg/day; effective range, 0.25-1 mg/kg/day; max, 50 mg/day

Alopecia

Adult: TOP rub into scalp daily

Available forms: Tabs 2.5, 10 mg; top 20, 50 mg/ml

Adverse effects

CNS: Drowsiness, dizziness, sedation, headache, depression, fatigue

CV: Severe rebound hypertension, tachycardia, angina, increased T wave, **CHF, pulmonary edema, pericardial effusion,** edema, sodium retention, water retention

GI: Nausea, vomiting

GU: Gynecomastia, breast tenderness

HEMA: Hct, Hgb, erythrocyte count may decrease initially

INTEG: Pruritus, **Stevens-Johnson syndrome,** rash, hirsutism

Contraindications: Acute MI, dissecting aortic aneurysm, hypersensitivity, pheochromocytoma

Precautions: Pregnancy **C,** lactation, P children, renal disease, CAD, CHF

Do Not Confuse:

Loniten/Lotensin, minoxidil/Monopril

Pharmacokinetics

Absorption	Well absorbed (PO); minimally absorbed (top)
Distribution	Widely distributed
Metabolism	Liver
Excretion	Kidneys, breast milk
Half-life	4.2 hr

Pharmacodynamics

	PO	TOP
Onset	½ hr	4 mo
Peak	2-3 hr	Unknown
Duration	75 hr	4 mo

Interactions

Individual drugs

Alcohol: ↑ hypotension

Drug classifications

Antihypertensives: ↑ hypotension

Glucocorticoids (top route): ↑ absorption

Nitrates: ↑ nitrates

NSAIDs: ↓ antihypertensive effect

Retinoids (top route): ↑ absorption

NURSING CONSIDERATIONS

Assessment

- Monitor B/P, pulse, jugular venous distention periodically throughout treatment
- Monitor electrolytes, blood studies: potassium, sodium, chloride, carbon dioxide, CBC, serum glucose
- Monitor weight daily, I&O; assess edema in feet, legs daily; check skin turgor, dryness of mucous membranes for hydration status
- Assess for rales, dyspnea, orthopnea, peripheral edema, fatigue, weight gain, jugular vein distention (CHF)
- Assess for signs of hyperglycemia: acetone breath, increased urinary output, severe thirst, lethargy, dizziness

M

Nursing diagnoses
✓ Cardiac output, decreased (adverse reactions)
✓ Injury, risk for (side effects)
✓ Knowledge deficit (teaching)

Implementation
PO route
- Give with meals to decrease GI symptoms
- Give with β-blockers and/or diuretic for hypertension
- Store protected from light and heat

Topical route
- Administer 1 ml dose no matter how much balding has occurred; increasing dose does not speed hair growth
- Treatment must continue long term or new hair will be lost again

Patient/family education
Topical route
- Teach patient that new hair will be soft and hardly visible
- Caution patient not to use on other parts of the body; drug is to be used on the scalp only
- Instruct patient that hair should be clean before applying medication; do not get on clothing
- Caution patient not to get medication near mucous membranes (mouth, nose, eyes) and to contact prescriber if burning, stinging, or rash occurs

Evaluation
Positive therapeutic outcome
- Decreased B/P in hypertension
- Hair growth (TOP)

mirtazapine (℞)
(mer-ta'za-peen)
Remeron, Remeron SolTab
Func. class.: Antidepressant
Chem. class.: Tetracyclic
Pregnancy category C

Action: Blocks reuptake of norepinephrine, serotonin into nerve endings, increasing action of norepinephrine, serotonin in nerve cells; has anticholinergic action

➔ **Therapeutic Outcome:** Decreased symptoms of depression after 2-3 wk

Uses: Depression, dysthymic disorder, bipolar disorder: depression, agitated depression

Dosage and routes
Adult: PO 15 mg/day at hs, maintenance to continue for 6 mo; orally disintegrating tabs, open blister pack, place tab on tongue, allow to disintegrate, swallow

G ***Elderly:*** PO 7.5 mg qhs, increase by 7.5 mg q1-2 wk to desired dose, max 45 mg/day

Available forms: Tabs 15, 30 mg; orally disintegrating tabs 15, 30, 45 mg

Adverse effects
CNS: Dizziness, drowsiness, confusion, headache, anxiety, tremors, stimulation, weakness, insomnia, nightmares, extrapyramidal symptoms G (elderly), increased psychiatric symptoms, *seizures*
CV: Orthostatic hypotension, ECG changes, tachycardia, hypertension, palpitations
EENT: Blurred vision, tinnitus, mydriasis
GI: Diarrhea, dry mouth, nausea, vomiting, **paralytic ileus,** increased appetite; cramps, epigastric distress, jaundice, *hepatitis,* stomatitis
GU: Retention, **acute renal failure**
HEMA: **Agranulocytosis, thrombocytopenia, eosinophilia, leukopenia**
INTEG: Rash, urticaria, sweating, pruritus, photosensitivity

Contraindications: Hypersensitivity to tricyclic antidepressants, recovery phase of MI, seizure disorders, prostatic hypertrophy

Precautions: Suicidal patients, severe depression, increased intraocular pressure, narrow-angle glaucoma, urinary retention, cardiac disease, hepatic disease, hypothyroidism, hyperthyroidism, electroshock therapy, G elective surgery, elderly, pregnancy **C**

Pharmacokinetics

Absorption	Slow, complete
Distribution	Widely distributed; crosses placenta
Metabolism	Liver, extensively
Excretion	Feces; breast milk
Half-life	20-40 hr

Pharmacodynamics

Onset	Unknown
Peak	2 hr
Duration	Unknown

Interactions

Individual drugs

Alcohol: ↑ CNS depression
Cimetidine: ↑ levels, ↑ toxicity
Clonidine: Severe hypotension; avoid use
Disulfiram: Organic brain syndrome
Fluoxetine: ↑ levels, toxicity

Drug classifications

Analgesics: ↑ CNS depression
Anticholinergics: ↑ side effects
Antihistamines: ↑ CNS depression
Antihypertensives: May block antihypertensive effect
Barbiturates: ↑ effects
CNS depressants: ↑ effects
MAOIs: Hypertensive crisis, seizures
Oral contraceptives: ↑ effects, toxicity
Phenothiazines: ↑ toxicity
Sedative/hypnotics: ↑ CNS depression

Smoking

↑ Metabolism, ↓ effects

Herb/drug

Belladonna: ↑ anticholinergic effect
Henbane: ↑ anticholinergic effect
Scopolia: ↑ antidepressant effect

Lab test interferences

↑ Serum bilirubin, ↑ blood glucose, ↑ alkaline phosphatase
↓ VMA, ↓ 5-HIAA
False: ↑ Urinary catecholamines

NURSING CONSIDERATIONS

Assessment

- Monitor B/P (with patient lying, standing), pulse q4h during beginning treatment; if systolic B/P drops 20 mm Hg, hold drug, notify prescriber; take VS q4h in patients with CV disease
- Monitor blood studies: CBC, leukocytes, differential, cardiac enzymes if patient is receiving long-term therapy
- Monitor hepatic studies: AST, ALT, bilirubin
- Check weight weekly, drug may increase appetite
- Assess ECG for flattening of T wave, bundle branch block, AV block, dysrhythmias in cardiac patients
- G Assess for EPS primarily in elderly: rigidity, dystonia, akathisia
- Assess mental status: mood, sensorium, affect, suicidal tendencies; assess increase in psychiatric symptoms: depression, panic
- Identify alcohol consumption; if alcohol is consumed, hold dose until AM

Nursing diagnoses

✓ Coping, ineffective individual (uses)
✓ Injury, risk for (side effects)
✓ Knowledge deficit (teaching)
✓ Noncompliance (teaching)

Implementation

- Give with food or milk for GI symptoms; crush if patient is unable to swallow medication whole
- Give dose hs if oversedation occurs during day; may take entire dose hs; G elderly may not tolerate once/day dosing
- Store at room temp; do not freeze

Orally disintegrating tablets

- No water needed, allow to dissolve on tongue

Patient/family education

- Inform patient that therapeutic effects may take 2-3 wk

M

• Advise patient to use caution in driving and other activities requiring alertness because of drowsiness, dizziness, blurred vision; to avoid rising quickly from sitting to standing, G especially elderly
• Caution patient to avoid alcohol ingestion, other CNS depressants
• Teach patient to increase fluids, bulk in diet if constipation, urinary G retention occur, especially elderly
• Teach patient to use gum, hard sugarless candy, or frequent sips of water for dry mouth

Evaluation

Positive therapeutic outcome

• Decrease in depression
• Absence of suicidal thoughts

Treatment of overdose: ECG monitoring, induce emesis, lavage, activated charcoal, administer anticonvulsant

misoprostol (℞)

(mye-soe-prost'ole)

Cytotec

Func. class.: Gastric mucosa protectant; antiulcer

Chem. class.: Prostaglandin E_1 analog

Pregnancy category X

Action: Inhibits gastric acid secretion; may protect gastric mucosa; can increase bicarbonate, mucus production

➔ **Therapeutic Outcome:** Prevention of gastric ulcers

Uses: Prevention of NSAID-induced gastric ulcers

Dosage and routes

Adult: PO 200 µg qid with food for duration of NSAID therapy; if 200 µg is not tolerated, 100 µg may be given

Available forms: Tabs 100, 200 µg

Adverse effects

GI: Diarrhea, nausea, vomiting, flatulence, constipation, dyspepsia, abdominal pain

GU: Spotting, cramps, hypermenorrhea, menstrual disorders

Contraindications: Hypersensitivity, pregnancy **X**

P **Precautions:** Lactation, children, G elderly, renal disease

Do Not Confuse: Cytotec/Cytoxan, misoprostol/metoprolol

Pharmacokinetics	
Absorption	Well absorbed
Distribution	Unknown
Metabolism	Liver
Excretion	Kidneys
Half-life	½-1 hr

Pharmacodynamics	
Onset	½ hr
Peak	Unknown
Duration	3 hr

Interactions

Drug classifications

Antacids, magnesium: ↑ diarrhea

Food/drug

↓ Absorption with food

NURSING CONSIDERATIONS

Assessment

• Assess patient for GI symptoms: hematemesis, occult or frank blood in stools, also severe abdominal pain, cramping, severe diarrhea
• Obtain a negative pregnancy test in women of childbearing age before starting medication; miscarriages are common

Nursing diagnoses

✓ Pain (uses)
✓ Knowledge deficit (teaching)

Implementation

• Give with meals for prolonged drug effect; avoid use of magnesium antacids

Patient/family education

- Advise patient to avoid black pepper, caffeine, alcohol, harsh spices, extremes in temp of food, which may aggravate condition
- Caution patient to avoid OTC preparations: aspirin, cough, cold preparations; condition may worsen
- Teach patient that drug must be continued for prescribed time to be effective and taken exactly as prescribed; doses are not to be doubled
- Instruct patient to report to prescriber diarrhea, black tarry stools, abdominal pain, cramping, menstrual disorders
- Caution patient to prevent pregnancy while taking this drug; spontaneous abortion may occur

Evaluation

Positive therapeutic outcome

- Prevention of ulcers

HIGH ALERT

mitomycin (℞)

(mye-toe-mye'sin)

mitomycin, Mutamycin

Func. class.: Antineoplastic, antibiotic

Pregnancy category D

Action: Inhibits DNA synthesis, primarily; derived from *Streptomyces caespitosus;* appears to cause cross-linking of DNA, a vesicant

➔ **Therapeutic Outcome:** Prevention of rapidly growing malignant cells

Uses: Pancreas, stomach, head and neck, breast cancer

Investigational uses: Palliative treatment of head, neck, colon, breast, biliary, cervical, lung malignancies

Dosage and routes

Adult: **IV** 20 mg/m²/day × 5 days, stop drug for 2 days, then repeat cycle; or 10-20 mg/m² as a single dose; repeat cycle in 6-8 wk; stop drug if platelets are <75,000/mm³ or WBC is <3000/mm³

Available forms: Inj 5, 20, 40 mg/vial

Adverse effects

CNS: Fever, headache, confusion, drowsiness, syncope, fatigue

EENT: Blurred vision, drowsiness, syncope

GI: *Nausea, vomiting, anorexia, stomatitis,* **hepatotoxicity,** diarrhea

GU: Urinary retention, **renal failure,** edema

HEMA: **Thrombocytopenia, leukopenia, anemia**

INTEG: *Rash,* alopecia, ***extravasation***

RESP: **Fibrosis, pulmonary infiltrate,** dyspnea

Contraindications: Hypersensitivity, pregnancy **D** (1st trimester), as a single agent, thrombocytopenia, coagulation disorders, lactation

Precautions: Renal disease, bone marrow depression

Pharmacokinetics	
Absorption	Complete bioavailability
Distribution	Widely distributed; concentrates in tumor
Metabolism	Liver, extensively
Excretion	Kidneys, unchanged
Half-life	1 hr

Pharmacodynamics

Unknown

Interactions

Individual drugs

Radiation: ↑ toxicity, bone marrow suppression

Drug classifications

Antineoplastics: ↑ toxicity, bone marrow suppression

M

NURSING CONSIDERATIONS

Assessment

- Assess buccal cavity q8h for dryness, sores or ulceration, white patches, oral pain, bleeding, dysphagia; obtain prescription for viscous lidocaine (Xylocaine)
- Assess symptoms indicating severe allergic reaction: rash, pruritus, urticaria, purpuric skin lesions, itching, flushing
- Monitor CBC, differential, platelet count weekly; withhold drug if WBC is <2000/mm^3 or platelet count is <100,000/mm^3 or granulocyte count is <1000/mm^3, notify prescriber of results if WBC <20,000/mm^3, platelets <150,000/mm^3
- Monitor renal function studies: BUN, creatinine, serum uric acid, urine CrCl before and during therapy; check I&O ratio; report fall in urine output to <30 ml/hr
- Monitor temp q4h (may indicate beginning of infection)
- Monitor liver function tests before and during therapy (bilirubin, AST, ALT, LDH) as needed or monthly; check for jaundiced skin and sclera, dark urine, clay-colored stools, itchy skin, abdominal pain, fever, diarrhea
- Assess for bleeding: hematuria, stool guaiac, bruising or petechiae, mucosa or orifices q8h; inflammation of mucosa, breaks in skin
- Identify effects of alopecia on body image; discuss feelings about body changes
- Identify edema in feet, joint pain, stomach pain, shaking; check for inflammation of mucosa, breaks in skin

Nursing diagnoses

✓ Injury, risk for (adverse reactions)
✓ Body image disturbance (adverse reactions)
✓ Infection, risk for (adverse reactions)
✓ Knowledge deficit (teaching)

Implementation

- Avoid contact with skin, since medication is very irritating; wash completely to remove
- Give fluids **IV** or PO before chemotherapy to hydrate patient
- Provide antacid before oral agent; give drug after evening meal, before hs; administer antiemetic 30-60 min before giving drug and prn to prevent vomiting; use antibiotics for prophylaxis of infection
- Give top or syst analgesics for pain
- Give in AM so drug can be eliminated before hs
- Provide a liq diet: carbonated beverages; gelatin may be added if patient is not nauseated or vomiting
- Encourage patient to rinse mouth tid-qid with water, club soda, brush teeth bid-qid with soft brush or cotton-tipped applicators for stomatitis, use unwaxed dental floss
- Drug should be prepared by experienced personnel using proper precautions in a biologic cabinet using gown, gloves, mask
- Give by direct **IV** after diluting 5 mg/10 sterile water for inj; shake, allow to stand, give through Y-tube or 3 way stopcock; give over 5-10 min through running D_5W, 0.9% NaCl **IV**
- Apply ice compress for extravasation

Syringe compatibilities:

Bleomycin, cisplatin, cyclophosphamide, doxorubicin, droperidol, fluorouracil, furosemide, heparin, leucovorin, methotrexate, metoclopramide, vinblastine, vincristine

Y-site compatibilities:

Allopurinol, amifostine, bleomycin, cisplatin, cyclophosphamide, doxorubicin, droperidol, fluorouracil, furosemide, granisetron, heparin, leucovorin, melphalan, methotrexate, metoclopramide, ondansetron, teniposide, thiotepa, vinblastine, vincristine

Y-site incompatibilities:

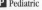

Sargramostim, vinorelbine

Additive compatibilities:
Dexamethasone, hydrocortisone

Additive incompatibilities:
Bleomycin

Solution compatibilities:
LR, 0.3% NaCl, 0.5% NaCl

Patient/family education

- Teach patient to avoid use of products containing aspirin or ibuprofen, razors, commercial mouthwash, since bleeding may occur; to report symptoms of bleeding (hematuria, tarry stools)
- Caution patient to report signs of anemia (fatigue, headache, irritability, faintness, shortness of breath)
- Advise patient to report any changes in breathing or coughing even several mo after treatment; to avoid crowds and persons with respiratory tract or other infections
- Inform patient that hair may be lost during treatment; a wig or hairpiece may make patient feel better; new hair may be different in color, texture
- Advise patient not to have any vaccinations without the advice of the prescriber, serious reactions can occur
- Teach patient that contraception is needed during treatment and for several mo after completion of therapy

Evaluation

Positive therapeutic outcome

- Prevention of rapid division of malignant cells

HIGH ALERT

mitoxantrone (℞)

(mye-toe-zan'trone)

Novantrone

Func. class.: Antineoplastic-antibiotic, immunomodulator

Chem. class.: Synthetic anthraquinone

Pregnancy category D

Action: DNA reactive agent; cytocidal effect on both proliferating and nonproliferating cells, suggesting lack of cell cycle phase specificity; a vesicant

Therapeutic Outcome: Prevention of rapidly growing malignant cells

Uses: Acute nonlymphocytic leukemia (adult), relapsed leukemia, breast cancer, multiple sclerosis

Investigational uses: Breast and liver malignancies, non-Hodgkin's lymphoma

Dosage and routes

Induction

***Adult:* IV** inf 12 mg/m^2/day on days 1-3, and 100 mg/m^2 cytosine arabinoside × 7 days as a cont 24-hr inf; if complete remission occurs, 2nd inductor may be used

Consolidation

***Adult:* IV** inf 12 mg/m^2/day × 2 days, given with cytosine arabinoside 100 mg/m^2/day × 5 days as cont inf usually 6 wk after induction

Available forms: Inj 2 mg/ml

Adverse effects

CNS: Headache, seizures

CV: **CHF, cardiomyopathy, dysrhythmias,** ECG changes

EENT: Conjunctivitis, blue-green sclera

GI: *Nausea, vomiting, diarrhea, anorexia, mucositis,* **hepatoxicity**

HEMA: **Thrombocytopenia, leukopenia, myelosuppression, anemia**

M

INTEG: ***Rash, necrosis at inj site,*** alopecia, dermatitis, thrombophlebitis at inj site
MISC: Fever, hypersensitivity, hyperuricemia
RESP: Cough, dyspnea

Contraindications: Hypersensitivity, pregnancy **D**

Precautions: Myelosuppression, P lactation, cardiac disease, children, renal, hepatic disease, gout

Pharmacokinetics

Absorption	Completely absorbed
Distribution	Widely distributed
Metabolism	Liver
Excretion	Bile; kidneys, unchanged (<10%)
Half-life	24-72 hr

Pharmacodynamics

Unknown

Interactions

Individual drugs

Radiation: ↑ toxicity, bone marrow suppression

Drug classifications

Antineoplastics: ↑ toxicity, bone marrow suppression
Live virus vaccines: ↑ adverse reactions

NURSING CONSIDERATIONS

Assessment

- Multiple sclerosis: obtain baseline multigated angiogram, left ventricular ejection fraction (LVEF) if symptoms of CHF occur, repeat LVEF or if cumulative dose is >100 mg/m^2; do not administer to patients who have received a lifetime dose of ≥140 mg/m^2 or if LVEF <50% or significant decrease in LVEF
- Do not administer in multiple sclerosis if neutrophils <1500/mm^3
- Obtain pregnancy test in all women of childbearing age
- Monitor ECG; watch for ST-T wave changes, low QRS and T, possible dysrhythmias (sinus tachycardia, heart block, PVCs)
- Assess buccal cavity q8h for dryness, sores or ulceration, white patches, oral pain, bleeding, dysphagia; obtain prescription for viscous lidocaine (Xylocaine)
- Assess symptoms indicating severe allergic reaction: rash, pruritus, urticaria, purpuric skin lesions, itching, flushing
- Assess tachypnea, ECG changes, dyspnea, edema, fatigue
- Monitor CBC, differential, platelet count weekly; withhold drug if WBC is <4000/mm^3 or platelet count is <100,000/mm^3, notify prescriber of results if WBC <20,000/mm^3, platelets <150,000/mm^3
- Assess for increased uric acid levels, swelling, joint pain primarily in extremities; patient should be well hydrated to prevent urate deposits
- Monitor renal function studies: BUN, creatinine, urine CrCl before and during therapy; determine I&O ratio
- Monitor temp q4h (may indicate beginning of infection)
- Monitor liver function tests before and during therapy (bilirubin, AST, ALT, LDH) as needed or monthly; check for jaundiced skin and sclera, dark urine, clay-colored stools, itchy skin, abdominal pain, fever, diarrhea
- Assess for bleeding: hematuria, stool guaiac, bruising or petechiae, mucosa or orifices q8h; check for inflammation of mucosa, breaks in skin
- Identify effects of alopecia on body image; discuss feelings about body changes

Nursing diagnoses

- ✓ Injury, risk for (adverse reactions)
- ✓ Body image disturbance (adverse reactions)
- ✓ Infection, risk for (adverse reactions)
- ✓ Knowledge deficit (teaching)

Implementation

- Avoid contact with skin, since

medication is very irritating; wash completely to remove

- Give fluids **IV** or PO before chemotherapy to hydrate patient
- Give antacid before oral agent; give drug after evening meal, before hs; provide antiemetic 30-60 min before giving drug and prn to prevent vomiting; administer antibiotics for prophylaxis of infection
- Give top or systemic analgesics for pain
- Liq diet: carbonated beverages; gelatin may be added if patient is not nauseated or vomiting
- Encourage patient to rinse mouth tid-qid with water, club soda, brush teeth bid-qid with soft brush or cotton-tipped applicators for stomatitis, use unwaxed dental floss
- Sol should be prepared by qualified personnel only under controlled conditions in a biologic cabinet using mask, gloves, gown
- Use Luer-Lok tubing to prevent leakage; do not let sol come in contact with skin; if contact occurs wash well with soap and water
- Give by direct **IV** after diluting with 50 ml or more of 0.9% NaCl or D_5W; give over 3-5 min, running **IV** of D_5W or 0.9% NaCl
- Intermittent inf may be diluted further in D_5W, 0.9% NaCl and run over 15-30 min; check for extravasation

Y-site compatibilities: Allopurinol, amifostine, cladribine, filgrastim, fludarabine, granisetron, melphalan, ondansetron, sargramostim, teniposide, thiotepa, vinorelbine

Y-site incompatibilities: Paclitaxel

Additive compatibilities: Cyclophosphamide, cytarabine, fluorouracil, hydrocortisone, potassium chloride

Additive incompatibilities: Heparin

Solution compatibilities: D_5/0.9 NaCl, D_5W, 0.9% NaCl

Patient/family education

- Teach patient to avoid use of products containing aspirin or NSAIDs, razors, commercial mouthwash, since bleeding may occur; to report symptoms of bleeding (hematuria, tarry stools)
- Caution patient to report signs of anemia (fatigue, headache, irritability, faintness, shortness of breath)
- Inform patient that hair may be lost during treatment; a wig or hairpiece may make patient feel better; new hair may be different in color, texture
- Caution patient not to have any vaccinations without the advice of the prescriber; serious reactions can occur
- Advise patient that contraception is needed during treatment and for several mo after completion of therapy
- Advise patient that sclera, urine may turn blue or green

M

Evaluation

Positive therapeutic outcome

- Prevention of rapid division of malignant cells

HIGH ALERT

mivacurium (℞)

(mi-va-kure′ee-um)

Mivacron

Func. class.: Nondepolarizing neuromuscular blocker

Pregnancy category C

Action: Inhibits transmission of nerve impulses by binding with cholinergic receptor sites, antagonizing action of acetylcholine; no analgesic response

➔ **Therapeutic Outcome:** Paralysis of all skeletal muscles

Uses: Facilitation of endotracheal intubation; skeletal muscle relaxation during mechanical ventilation, surgery, or general anesthesia; reduction of fractures/dislocations

Dosage and routes

Adult: **IV** 0.15 mg/kg; maintenance q15 min

P ***Child 2-12:*** **IV** 0.2 mg/kg for a 10-min block

Available forms: 5, 10 ml single-use vial (2 mg/ml); premixed inf in D_5W 50 ml flexible container

Adverse effects

CV: Decreased B/P, bradycardia, tachycardia
EENT: Diplopia
INTEG: Rash, urticaria
MS: Weakness, prolonged skeletal muscle relaxation, **paralysis**
RESP: **Prolonged apnea, bronchospasm, wheezing, respiratory depression**

Contraindications: Hypersensitivity

Precautions: Pregnancy **C**, renal or hepatic disease, lactation, P children <3 mo, fluid and electrolyte imbalances, neuromuscular disease, respiratory disease, obesity, G elderly

Do Not Confuse:
Mivacron/Mazicon

Pharmacokinetics	
Absorption	Completely absorbed
Distribution	Extracellular spaces; crosses placenta
Metabolism	Plasma
Excretion	Kidneys
Half-life	2 hr

Pharmacodynamics	
Onset	2-2½ min
Peak	2-3 min
Duration	20-30 min

Interactions

Individual drugs

Clindamycin: ↑ paralysis length and intensity
Colistin: ↑ paralysis length and intensity
Lidocaine: ↑ paralysis length and intensity
Lithium: ↑ paralysis length and intensity
Magnesium: ↑ paralysis length and intensity
Polymyxin B: ↑ paralysis length and intensity
Procainamide: ↑ paralysis length and intensity
Quinidine: ↑ paralysis length and intensity
Succinylcholine: ↑ paralysis length and intensity

Drug classifications

Aminoglycosides: ↑ paralysis length and intensity
β-Adrenergic blockers: ↑ paralysis length and intensity
Diuretics, potassium-losing: ↑ paralysis length and intensity
General anesthesia: ↑ paralysis length and intensity

NURSING CONSIDERATIONS

Assessment

- Monitor VS (B/P, pulse, respirations, airway) until fully recovered; rate, depth, pattern of respirations, strength of hand grip; patient should be intubated before use
- Monitor for electrolyte imbalances (potassium, magnesium) before drug is used; electrolyte imbalances may lead to increased action of this drug
- Monitor for recovery: decreased paralysis of face, diaphragm, leg, arm, rest of body; residual weakness and respiratory problems may occur during recovery period
- Assess for hypersensitive reactions: rash, fever, respiratory distress, pruritus; drug should be discontinued

Nursing diagnoses

✓ Breathing pattern, ineffective (uses)

✓ Communication, impaired verbal (adverse reactions)
✓ Fear (adverse reactions)
✓ Knowledge deficit (teaching)

Implementation

- Use peripheral nerve stimulator (anesthesiologist) to determine neuromuscular blockade; deep tendon reflexes should be monitored during extended periods
- Give direct **IV** undiluted over 5-15 min
- Give cont **IV** diluted to 0.5 mg ml in D_5W, 0.9% NaCl, D_5/0.9% NaCl, LR, D_5/LR and give as an inf at prescribed rate (only by qualified person, usually an anesthesiologist); do not administer IM
- Store in light-resistant container
- Give anticholinesterase to reverse neuromuscular blockade

Y-site compatibilities: Etomidate, thiopental

Y-site incompatibilities: Barbiturates

Patient/family education

- Provide reassurance if communication is difficult during recovery from neuromuscular blockade
- Provide explanation to patients regarding all procedures or treatments; patient will remain conscious if anesthesia is not given also

Evaluation

Positive therapeutic outcome

- Paralysis of jaw, eyelid, head, neck, rest of body as evaluated by peripheral nerve stimulator

Treatment of overdose: Edrophonium or neostigmine, atropine; monitor VS; may require mechanical ventilation

modafinil (Ɍ)

(mod-aa-fen'ill)

Provigil

Func. class.: Cerebral stimulant

Pregnancy category C (1st trimester)

Controlled substance schedule IV

Action: Promotes wakefullness, exact mechanism is unknown

➔ **Therapeutic Outcome:** Increased alertness, decreased fatigue, ability to stay awake (narcolepsy)

Uses: Narcolepsy

Dosage and routes

Adult: PO 200 mg qd in the AM, may increase to 400 mg qd if needed

Hepatic dose
Reduce dose by 50%

Available forms: Tabs 100, 200 mg

Adverse effects

CNS: *Hyperactivity, insomnia, restlessness,* dizziness, headache, chills, stimulation
CV: *Palpitations, tachycardia,* hypertension, dysrhythmias
EENT: Abnormal vision, amblyopia
GI: Anorexia, dry mouth, diarrhea, nausea, vomiting, mouth ulcer, gingivitis, thirst
GU: Urinary retention, abnormal ejaculation
INTEG: Herpes simplex, dry skin
META: Hyperglycemia, albuminuria
RESP: Rhinitis, pharyngitis, lung disorder, dyspnea, asthma, epistaxis

Contraindications: Hypersensitivity, hyperthyroidism, hypertension, glaucoma, severe arteriosclerosis, drug abuse, CV disease, anxiety

Precautions: Gilles de la Tourette's disorder, G elderly, pregnancy **C,** lactation, P children <16 yr

Pharmacokinetics

Absorption	Rapid
Distribution	Well distributed; protein binding 60%; crosses placenta
Metabolism	Liver extensively
Excretion	10%
Half-life	15 hr with multiple dosing

Pharmacodynamics

Onset	Unknown
Peak	2-4 hr
Duration	Unknown

Interactions
Individual drugs
Carbamazepine: ↑ levels
Clomipramine: ↑ levels of clomipramine
Cyclosporine: ↓ level of cyclosporine
Diazepam: ↑ level of diazepam
Itraconazole: ↑ altered levels
Ketoconazole: ↑ altered levels
Methylphenidate: ↓ modafinil absorption
Phenobarbital: ↑ altered levels
Phenytoin: ↑ phenytoin toxicity
Propranolol: ↑ propranolol level
Rifampin: ↑ altered levels
Theophylline: ↓ level of theophylline
Warfarin: ↑ warfarin level
Drug classifications
Antidepressants, tricyclic: ↑ levels, reduce dose
MAOIs: Use caution when giving together
Oral contraceptives: ↓ oral contraceptive effect

NURSING CONSIDERATIONS
Assessment
- Assess for improvement in narcolepsy

Nursing diagnoses
✓ Sleep pattern disturbance (uses)
✓ Knowledge deficit (teaching)

Implementation
- Titrate to patient's response; lowest dosage should be used to control symptoms
- Give gum, hard candy, frequent sips of water for dry mouth at beginning of treatment; these symptoms tend to lessen with time

Patient/family education
- Advise patient to decrease caffeine consumption (coffee, tea, cola, chocolate), which may increase irritability and stimulation; to avoid OTC preparations unless approved by prescriber; to avoid alcohol ingestion; these may cause serious drug interactions
- Inform patient to notify prescriber if rash or other symptoms of allergy occur
- Advise patient to notify prescriber if pregnancy is suspected, or if breastfeeding; another form of contraception is needed if using hormonal contraception while on this drug and for a month afterward
- Caution patient to avoid hazardous activities until patient is stabilized on medication
- Instruct patient/family to notify prescriber if significant side effects occur: tremors, insomnia, palpitations, restlessness; drug changes may be needed

Evaluation
Positive therapeutic outcome
- Absence of sleeping during day in narcolepsy

moexipril (℞)
(moe-ex'i-pril)
Univasc
Func. class.: Antihypertensive
Chem. class.: Angiotensin-converting enzyme (ACE) inhibitor

Pregnancy category
C (1st trimester),
D (2nd/3rd trimesters)

Action: Selectively suppresses renin-angiotensin-aldosterone system; inhibits ACE; prevents conversion of angiotensin I to angiotensin II; results in dilation of arterial, venous vessels

→ **Therapeutic Outcome:** Decreased B/P in hypertension

Uses: Hypertension, alone or in combination with thiazide diuretics

Dosage and routes

Initial treatment

Adult: PO 7.5 mg 1 hr ac, may be increased or divided depending on B/P response

Maintenance

Adult: PO 7.5-30 mg qd in 1-2 divided doses 1 hr ac

Renal dose

CrCl <40 ml/min 3.75 mg/day titrate to desired dose

Available forms: Tabs 7.5, 15 mg

Adverse effects

CNS: Fever, chills
CV: Hypotension, postural hypotension
GI: Loss of taste
GU: Impotence, dysuria, nocturia, proteinura, nephrotic syndrome, acute reversible renal failure, polyuria, oliguria, frequency
HEMA: **Neutropenia**
INTEG: Rash
META: Hypokalemia
RESP: **Bronchospasm**, dyspnea, dry cough
SYST: **Angioedema**, anaphylaxis

Contraindications: Hypersensitivity, children, lactation, heart block, bilateral renal stenosis, K-sparing diuretics, pregnancy **D** (2nd/3rd trimesters)

P

Precautions: Dialysis patients, hypovolemia, leukemia, scleroderma, lupus erythematosus, blood dyscrasias, CHF, diabetes mellitus, renal disease, thyroid disease, COPD, asthma, pregnancy **C** (1st trimester)

Pharmacokinetics

Absorption	Unknown
Distribution	Unknown
Metabolism	Liver to metabolites
Excretion	Via kidneys, crosses placenta, excreted in breast milk
Half-life	Unknown

Pharmacodynamics

Unknown

Interactions

Drug classification

Adrenergic blockers: ↑ hypotension
Antihypertensives: ↑ hypotension
Diuretics: ↑ hypotension
Diuretics, potassium-sparing: Do not use together
Ganglionic blockers: ↑ hypotension
Potassium supplements: Do not use together
Sympathomimetics: Do not use together

Lab test interferences

False positive: Urine acetone

NURSING CONSIDERATIONS

Assessment

- Monitor blood studies: neutrophils, decreased platelets
- Monitor B/P
- Monitor renal studies: protein, BUN, creatinine; watch for increased levels that may indicate nephrotic syndrome
- Monitor baselines in renal, liver function tests before therapy begins
- Monitor potassium levels, although hyperkalemia rarely occurs
- Assess edema in feet, legs daily
- Assess allergic reaction: rash, fever, pruritus, urticaria; drug should be discontinued if antihistamines fail to help
- Assess for symptoms of CHF: edema, dyspnea, wet rales, B/P
- Monitor for renal symptoms: polyuria, oliguria, frequency

Implementation

- Give PO 1 hr ac

M

- Store in airtight container at 86° F or less

Nursing diagnoses

✓ Knowledge deficit (teaching)

Patient/family education

- Teach patient to take 1 hr ac
- Instruct patient not to discontinue drug abruptly
- Tell patient not to use OTC (cough, cold, allergy) products unless directed by prescriber
- Teach patient to comply with dosage schedule, even if feeling better
- Encourage patient to rise slowly to sitting or standing position to minimize orthostatic hypotension
- Teach patient to notify prescriber of mouth sores, sore throat, fever, swelling of hands or feet, irregular heartbeat, chest pain, signs of angioedema
- Tell patient that excessive perspiration, dehydration, vomiting, diarrhea may lead to fall in B/P; consult prescriber if this occurs
- Teach patient that dizziness, fainting, light-headedness may occur during first few days of therapy
- Tell patient that skin rash or impaired perspiration may occur
- Teach patient how to take B/P

Evaluation

Positive therapeutic outcome

- Decreased B/P in hypertension

Treatment of overdose: 0.9% NaCl **IV** inf, hemodialysis

montelukast (℞)

(mon-teh-loo'kast)

Singulair

Func. class.: Bronchodilator

Chem. class.: Leukotriene receptor

Pregnancy category B

Action: Inhibits leukotriene (LTD_4) formation; leukotrienes exert their effects by increasing neutrophil, eosinophil migration; aggregation of neutrophils, monocytes; smooth muscle contraction, capillary permeability; these actions further lead to bronchoconstriction, inflammation, edema

➔ **Therapeutic Outcome:** Ability to breathe with ease

Uses: Chronic asthma

Dosage and routes

Asthma

P ***Adult and child ≥15 yr:*** PO 10 mg qd PM

P ***Child 6-14 yr:*** PO 5 mg chew tabs qd PM

P ***Child 2-5 yr:*** PO chew tabs 4 mg qd

Available forms: Tabs 10 mg; chewable tabs 4, 5 mg

Adverse effects

CNS: Dizziness, fatigue, headache

GI: Abdominal pain, dyspepsia

INTEG: Rash

MS: Asthenia

RESP: Influenza, cough, nasal congestion

Contraindications: Hypersensitivity

Precautions: Acute attacks of asthma, alcohol consumption, pregnancy **B**, lactation, child <6 yr, aspirin sensitivity (P)

Pharmacokinetics	
Absorption	Rapidly
Distribution	Protein binding 99%
Metabolism	Liver
Excretion	Bile
Half-life	2.7-5.5 hr

Pharmacodynamics	
Onset	Unknown
Peak	3-4 hr
Duration	Unknown

Interactions

Individual drugs

Phenobarbitol: ↑ montelukast levels
Rifampin: ↑ montelukast levels

NURSING CONSIDERATIONS

Assessment

- Assess adult patients carefully for symptoms of Churg-Strauss syndrome (rare), including eosinophilia, vasculitic rash, worsening pulmonary symptoms, cardiac complications and/or neuropathy
- Monitor CBC, blood chemistry during treatment
- Assess respiratory rate, rhythm, depth; auscultate lung fields bilaterally; notify prescriber of abnormalities
- Assess allergic reactions: rash, urticaria; drug should be discontinued

Nursing diagnoses

- ✓ Airway clearance, ineffective (uses)
- ✓ Activity intolerance (uses)
- ✓ Knowledge deficit (teaching)

Implementation

PO route

- Give PO in PM qd

Patient/family education

- Instruct patient to check OTC and current prescription medications for ephedrine, which will increase stimulation; to avoid alcohol
- Advise patient to avoid hazardous activities; dizziness may occur
- Teach patient that drug is not to be used for acute asthma attacks

Evaluation

Positive therapeutic outcome

- Increased ease of breathing
- Decreased bronchospasm

moricizine (℞)

(more-i'siz-een)

Ethmozine

Func. class.: Antidysrhythmic, group I

Chem. class.: Phenothiazine

Pregnancy category B

Action: Decreased rate of rise of action potential, prolonging refractory period and shortening the action potential duration; depression of inward influx if sodium mediates the effects; may slow atrial and AV nodal conduction

Therapeutic Outcome: Resolution of life-threatening dysrhythmias

Uses: Life-threatening ventricular dysrhythmias

Dosage and routes

Adult: PO 10-15 mg/kg/day in 2-3 divided doses or 600-900 mg/day given in 2-3 divided doses

Hepatic dose

Adult: PO 600 mg or less qd

Available forms: Film-coated tabs 200, 250, 300 mg

Adverse effects

CNS: *Dizziness, headache, fatigue, perioral numbness, euphoria,* nervousness, sleep disorders, depression, tinnitus, fatigue

CV: Palpitations, chest pain, CHF, hypertension, syncope, **dysrythmias,** bradycardia, **MI,** thrombophlebitis

GI: Nausea, abdominal pain, vomiting, diarrhea

GU: Sexual dysfunction, difficult urination, dysuria, incontinence

MISC: Sweating, musculoskeletal pain

RESP: Dyspnea, hyperventilation, **apnea,** asthma, pharyngitis, cough

Contraindications: 2nd- to 3rd-degree AV block, right bundle branch block, cardiogenic shock, hypersensitivity

Precautions: CHF, hypokalemia,

M

hyperkalemia, sick sinus syndrome, P pregnancy **B**, lactation, children, impaired hepatic and renal function, cardiac dysfunction

Pharmacokinetics

Absorption	Well absorbed
Distribution	Plasma protein binding (95%)
Metabolism	Liver, extensively
Excretion	Kidneys, breast milk
Half-life	1½-3½ hr

Pharmacodynamics

Onset	Unknown
Peak	½-2 hr
Duration	8-12 hr

Interactions

Individual drugs

Cimetidine: ↑ effect of moricizine
Theophylline: ↓ effect of theophylline

Herb/drug

Aloe: ↑ hypokalemia, ↑ antidysrhythmic effect
Buckthorn: ↑ hypokalemia, ↑ antidysrhythmic effect
Cascara sagrada: ↑ hypokalemia, ↑ antidysrhythmic effect
Henbane: ↑ anticholinergic effect
Rhubarb: ↑ hypokalemia, ↑ antidysrhythmic effect
Senna: ↑ hypokalemia, ↑ antidysrhythmic effect

NURSING CONSIDERATIONS

Assessment

- Monitor ECG at baseline and periodically to determine drug effectiveness; measure PR, QRS, QT intervals, check for PVCs, other dysrhythmias; check B/P for hypotension, hypertension and for rebound hypertension after 1-2 hr; check for dehydration or hypovolemia
- Monitor I&O ratio and electrolytes: potassium, sodium, chloride; check weight daily and for signs of CHF or pulmonary toxicity: dyspnea, fatigue, cough, fever, chest pain; drug should be discontinued
- Monitor liver function studies: AST, ALT, bilirubin, alkaline phosphatase
- Monitor cardiac rate; monitor respiration rate, rhythm, character, and chest pain; watch for ventricular tachycardia, supraventricular tachycardia, or fibrillation

Nursing diagnoses

- ✓ Cardiac output, decreased (uses)
- ✓ Impaired gas exchange (adverse reactions)
- ✓ Knowledge deficit (teaching)

Implementation

- Give with meals for GI upset; may be given in 2 divided doses if adverse reactions are minimal
- Make dosage adjustment q3 days or more

Patient/family education

- Instruct patient to report side effects to prescriber immediately
- Instruct patient to complete follow-up appointment with health care provider including pulmonary function studies, chest x-ray, ophth and otoscopic examinations
- Advise patient to carry ID indicating condition and treatment
- Caution patient to avoid driving and other hazardous activities until drug response is determined
- Instruct patient to take medication as prescribed, not to double doses; missed doses may be taken up to 6 hr after previous dose

Treatment of overdose:

O_2, artificial ventilation, ECG, administer dopamine for circulatory depression, administer diazepam or thiopental for convulsions, isoproterenol

HIGH ALERT

morphine 🔑 (℞)

(mor'feen)

Astramorph PF, Duramorph, Epimorph ✤, Infumorph 200, Infumorph 500, Morphine H.P. ✤, morphine sulfate, Morphitec ✤, M.O.S. ✤, M.O.S.-S.R. ✤, MS Contin, MSIR, MSIR, OMS Concentrate, Oramorph SR, RMS, Roxanol, Roxanol 100, Roxanol Rescudose, Roxanol SR

Func. class.: Opioid analgesic

Pregnancy category C

Controlled substance schedule II

Action: Depresses pain impulse transmission at the spinal cord level by interacting with opioid receptors, produces CNS depression

Therapeutic Outcome: Decreased pain

Uses: Severe pain; often given after or during an MI

Dosage and routes

Adult: SC/IM 4-15 mg q4h prn; PO 10-30 mg q4h prn; ext rel q8-12h; rec 10-20 mg q4h prn; **IV** 4-10 mg diluted in 4-5 ml of water for inj, over 5 min; epidural 2-10 mg/day

P ***Child:*** SC/**IV** 0.1-0.2 mg/kg, max 15 mg; IM/**IV** 50-100 μg/kg, max 10 mg/dose initially; PO 0.2-0.5 mg/ kg q4-6h (regular rel), q12h (sus rel)

Available forms: Inj 0.5, 1, 2, 3, 4, 5, 8, 10, 15, 25, 50 mg/ml; sol tabs 10, 15, 30 mg; oral sol 10, 20 mg/5 ml, 20 mg/10 ml, 20 mg/ml; oral tabs 15, 30 mg; rec supp 5, 10, 20, 30 mg; ext rel tabs 15, 30, 60, 100, 200 mg; caps 15, 30 mg; syrup 1, 5 mg/ml

Adverse effects

CNS: Drowsiness, dizziness, *confusion*, headache, *sedation*, euphoria, hallucinations, dysphoria

CV: Palpitations, **bradycardia,** *hypotension,* **shock, cardiac arrest**

EENT: Tinnitus, blurred vision, miosis, diplopia

GI: Nausea, vomiting, anorexia, *constipation,* cramps, biliary tract pressure

GU: Urinary retention

HEMA: **Thrombocytopenia**

INTEG: Rash, urticaria, bruising, flushing, diaphoresis, pruritus

RESP: **Respiratory depression, respiratory arrest, apnea**

Contraindications: Hypersensitivity, addiction (narcotic), hemorrhage, bronchial asthma, increased intracranial pressure

Precautions: Addictive personality, pregnancy **C,** lactation, acute MI, G severe heart disease, elderly, respiratory depression, hepatic disease, renal P disease, child <18 yr

Do Not Confuse: morphine/hydromorphone, Roxanol/Roxicet

Pharmacokinetics

Absorption	Variably absorbed (PO); well absorbed (IM, SC, rec); completely absorbed (**IV**)
Distribution	Widely distributed; crosses placenta
Metabolism	Liver, extensively
Excretion	Kidneys
Half-life	1½-2 hr

Pharmacodynamics

	PO	PO–EXT REL	IM	SC	REC	IV	IT
Onset	Variable	Unknown	10-30 min	20 min	Unknown	Rapid	Rapid
Peak	1 hr	Unknown	½-1 hr	1-1½ hr	½-1 hr	20 min	Unknown
Duration	4-5 hr	8-12 hr	3-7 hr	4-5 hr	4-5 hr	4-5 hr	Ext

M

Interactions

Individual drugs

Alcohol: ↑ respiratory depression, hypotension, sedation
Nalbuphine: ↓ analgesia
Pentazocine: ↓ analgesia
Rifampin: ↓ analgesic action

Drug classifications

Antihistamines: ↑ respiratory depression, hypotension
CNS depressants: ↑ respiratory depression, hypotension
MAOIs: Reduce dosage; unpredictable reaction may occur
Sedative/hypnotics: ↑ respiratory depression, hypotension

Lab test interferences

↑ Amylase

NURSING CONSIDERATIONS

Assessment

- Assess pain: location, type, character, intensity; give dose before pain becomes extreme
- Monitor I&O ratio; check for decreasing output; may indicate urinary retention; check for constipation; increase fluids, bulk in diet if needed or stool softeners may be prescribed
- Monitor CNS changes: dizziness, drowsiness, hallucinations, euphoria, LOC, pupil reactions
- Monitor allergic reactions: rash, urticaria
- Assess respiratory dysfunction: depression, character, rate, rhythm; notify prescriber if respirations are <10/min

Nursing diagnoses

✓ Pain (uses)
✓ Sensory-perceptual alteration: visual, auditory (adverse reactions)
✓ Breathing pattern, ineffective (adverse reactions)
✓ Knowledge deficit (teaching)

Implementation

- Give with antiemetic if nausea, vomiting occur
- Administer when pain is beginning to return; determine dosage interval by patient response; continuous dosing of medication is more effective than giving prn
- Withdraw medication slowly after long-term use to prevent withdrawal symptoms
- Store in light-resistant container at room temp

PO route

- May be given with food or milk to lessen GI upset; may be crushed and mixed with food or fluids; ext rel tabs should be swallowed whole

IM/SC route

- Do not give if cloudy or a precipitate has formed

IV **IV route**

- Give direct **IV** by diluting with ≥5 ml of sterile water or 0.9% NaCl for inj; give 2.5-15 mg/4-5 min; rapid administration may lead to increased respiratory depression, death
- Give cont inf by adding to D_5W, $D_{10}W$, 0.9% NaCl, 0.45% NaCl, Ringer's, LR, any dextrose/saline sol, or any dextrose/Ringer's, 0.1-1 mg/ml
- Give by infusion pump to deliver correct dosage; titrate to provide adequate pain relief without serious sedation, respiratory depression, hypotension
- May be given by patient-controlled analgesia (PCA) pump in terminal illnesses; patient is able to control amount of morphine
- Administer epidurally with caution G in the elderly

Syringe compatibilities:

Atropine, benzquinamide, bupivacaine, butorphanol, cimetidine, dimenhydrinate, diphenhydramine, droperidol, fentanyl, glycopyrrolate, hydroxyzine, ketamine, metoclopramide, midazolam, milrinone, pentazocine, perphenazine, promazine, ranitidine, scopolamine

Syringe incompatibilities:

Meperidine, thiopental

Y-site compatibilities:
Allopurinol, amifostine, amikacin, aminophylline, amiodarone, ampicillin, ampicillin/sulbactam, amsacrine, atenolol, atracurium, aztreonam, bumetanide, calcium chloride, cefamandole, cefazolin, cefmetazole, cefoperazone, cefotaxime, cefotetan, cefoxitin, ceftazidime, ceftizoxime, ceftriaxone, cefuroxime, cephalothin, cephapirin, chloramphenicol, cisplatin, cladribine, clindamycin, cyclophosphamide, cytarabine, dexamethasone, digoxin, diltiazem, dobutamine, dopamine, doxycycline, enalaprilat, epinephrine, erythromycin, esmolol, etomidate, famotidine, fentanyl, filgrastim, fluconazole, fludarabine, foscarnet, gentamicin, granisetron, heparin, hydrocortisone, hydromorphone, IL-2, insulin (regular), kanamycin, labetalol, lidocaine, lorazepam, magnesium sulfate, melphalan, meropenem, methotrexate, methyldopate, methylprednisolone, metoclopramide, metoprolol, metronidazole, mezlocillin, midazolam, milrinone, moxalactam, nafcillin, nicardipine, nitroglycerin, norepinephrine, ondansetron, oxacillin, oxytocin, paclitaxel, pancuronium, penicillin G potassium, piperacillin, piperacillin/tazobactam, potassium chloride, propofol, propranolol, ranitidine, sodium bicarbonate, sodium nitroprusside, teniposide, thiotepa, ticarcillin, ticarcillin/clavulanate, tobramycin, trimethoprim-sulfamethoxazole, vancomycin, vecuronium, vinorelbine, vit B/C, warfarin, zidovudine

Y-site incompatibilities:
Furosemide, minocycline, tetracycline

Additive compatibilities:
Alteplase, atracurium, baclofen, bupivacaine, dobutamine, fluconazole, furosemide, meropenem, metoclopramide, ondansetron, succinylcholine, verapamil

Additive incompatibilities:
Aminophylline

Patient/family education
- Advise patient to report any symptoms of CNS changes, allergic reactions
- Caution patients to avoid CNS depressants (alcohol, sedative/hypnotics) for at least 24 hr after taking this drug
- Discuss with patient that dizziness, drowsiness, and confusion are common; to avoid getting up without assistance
- Discuss in detail all aspects of the drug and expected response

Evaluation
Positive therapeutic outcome
- Decreased pain

Treatment of overdose:
Naloxone (Narcan) 0.2-0.8 **IV**, O_2, **IV** fluids, vasopressors

M

moxifloxacin (℞)
(mox-i-floks′a-sin)
Avelox, cephalosporins—3rd generation
Func. class.: Antiinfective
Chem. class.: Fluoroquinolone
Pregnancy category C

Action: Interferes with conversion of intermediate DNA fragments into high-molecular-weight DNA in bacteria; DNA gyrase inhibitor

➔ **Therapeutic Outcome:** Bactericidal action against the following: *Staphylococcus aureus, Streptococcus pneumoniae, Haemophilus influenza, Haemophilus parainfluenzae, Moraxella catarrhalis, Klebsiella pneumoniae, Mycoplasma pneumoniae, Chlamydia pneumoniae;* uncomplicated skin/skin structure infections: *Staphylococcus aureus, Streptococcus pyogenes*

Uses: Acute bacterial sinusitis, acute bacterial exacerbation of chronic bronchitis, community-acquired pneumoniae (mild to moderate)

Dosage and routes

Urinary tract infections

Adult: 400 mg qd × 5-10 days depending on condition

Available forms: Tabs 400 mg

Adverse effects

CNS: Headache, dizziness, fatigue, insomnia, depression, restlessness
CV: Prolonged QT interval, ***dysrhythmias***
GI: Nausea, constipation, increased ALT, AST, flatulence, insomnia, heartburn, vomiting, diarrhea, oral candidiasis, dysphagia
INTEG: Rash, pruritus, urticaria, photosensitivity, flushing, fever, chills
MS: Blurred vision, tinnitus
SYST: **Anaphylaxis, Stevens-Johnson syndrome**

Contraindications: Hypersensitivity to quinolones

Precautions: Pregnancy **C,** lactation, P children, renal disease, uncorrected hypokalemia, prolonged QT interval, patients receiving class IA, III antidysrhythmics

Pharmacokinetics

Absorption	Well absorbed (75%) (PO)
Distribution	Widely distributed
Metabolism	Liver
Excretion	Kidneys
Half-life	Increased in renal disease

Pharmacodynamics

	PO
Onset	Rapid
Peak	1 hr

Interactions

Individual drugs

Caffeine: ↓ effect of moxifloxacin
Cyclosporine: ↑ nephrotoxicity
Nitrofurantoin: ↓ effectiveness
Probenecid: ↑ blood levels
Sucralfate: ↓ absorption of moxifloxacin
Theophylline: ↑ toxicity
Warfarin: ↑ warfarin effect
Zinc sulfate: ↓ absorption of moxifloxacin

Drug classifications

Antacids: ↓ absorption of moxifloxacin
Antidysrhythmics IA, III: Prolonged QT interval
Antineoplastics: ↓ moxifloxacin
Iron salts: ↓ absorption of moxifloxacin
Oral anticoagulants: ↑ effect of anticoagulants

Lab test interferences

↑ AST, ↑ ALT, ↑ BUN, ↑ creatinine, ↑ alkaline phosphatase

NURSING CONSIDERATIONS

Assessment

- Assess patient for previous sensitivity reaction
- Assess patient for signs and symptoms of infection including characteristics of wounds, sputum, urine, stool, WBC >10,000/mm^3, fever; baseline and during treatment
- Obtain C&S before beginning drug therapy to identify if correct treatment has been initiated
- Assess for allergic reactions and anaphylaxis: rash, urticaria, pruritus, chills, fever, joint pain; may occur a few days after therapy begins; epinephrine and resuscitation equipment should be available for anaphylactic reaction
- Identify urine output; if decreasing, notify prescriber (may indicate nephrotoxicity); also check for increased BUN, creatinine
- Monitor blood studies: AST, ALT, CBC, Hct, bilirubin, LDH, alkaline phosphatase, Coombs' test monthly if patient is on long-term therapy
- Monitor electrolytes: potassium, sodium chloride monthly if patient is on long-term therapy
- Assess bowel pattern qd; if severe

diarrhea occurs, drug should be discontinued
- Monitor for bleeding: ecchymosis, bleeding gums, hematuria, stool guaiac daily if on long-term therapy
- Assess for overgrowth of infection: perineal itching, fever, malaise, redness, pain, swelling, drainage, rash, diarrhea, change in cough, sputum

Nursing diagnoses
- ✓ Infection, risk for (uses)
- ✓ Diarrhea (side effects)
- ✓ Injury, risk for (side effects)
- ✓ Knowledge deficit (teaching)
- ✓ Noncompliance (teaching)

Implementation
PO route
- Give once a day for 5-10 days depending on condition

Patient/family education
- Teach patient to report sore throat, bruising, bleeding, joint pain; may indicate blood dyscrasias (rare)
- Advise patient to contact prescriber if vaginal itching, loose, foul-smelling stools, furry tongue occur; may indicate superinfection; report itching, rash, pruritus, urticaria
- Instruct patient to take all medication prescribed for the length of time ordered; do not give medication to others
- Advise patient to notify prescriber of diarrhea with blood or pus
- Advise patient to rinse mouth frequently, use sugarless candy or gum for dry mouth
- Advise patient to take as prescribed, not to double or miss doses
- Instruct patient not to use theophylline with this product, may cause toxicity; contact prescriber if taking theophylline

Evaluation
Positive therapeutic outcome
- Absence of signs/symptoms of infection (WBC <10,000/mm^3, temp WNL)
- Reported improvement in symptoms of infection

multivitamins
(PO, OTC, IV, ℞)
Adavite, Dayalets, LKV Drops, Multi-75, Multi-Day, One-A-Day, Optilets, Poly-Vi-Sol, Quintabs, Rulets, Sesame Street Vitamins, Tab-A-Vite, Therabid, Theragran, Unicaps, Vita-Bob, Vita-Kid, many other brands; Berocca Parenteral, M.V.C. 9+3, M.V.I. Pediatric

Func. class.: Vitamins, multiple

Pregnancy category A

Action: Needed for adequate metabolism

➔ **Therapeutic Outcome:** Prevention and treatment of vitamin deficiencies

Uses: Prevention and treatment of vitamin deficiencies

Dosage and routes
P ***Adult and child:*** PO depends on brand

Available forms: Many forms available

Adverse effects
Rare at recommended dosage

Precautions: Pregnancy **A**

Do Not Confuse:
Theragran/Phenergan

Pharmacokinetics

Absorption	Well absorbed (PO)
Distribution	Widely distributed; crosses placenta
Metabolism	Widely metabolized
Excretion	Kidney, unchanged (water soluble)
Half-life	Unknown

Pharmacodynamics
Unknown

M

Interactions

Individual drugs

Levodopa: ↓ effect of levodopa (large amounts of vit B_6)

NURSING CONSIDERATIONS

Assessment

- Assess patient for vitamin deficiency; usually more than one vitamin deficiency is present

Nursing diagnoses

✓ Nutrition, less than body requirements (uses)

✓ Knowledge deficit (teaching)

Implementation

PO route

- Liq multivitamins can be diluted or dropped into patients' mouth using dropper provided with some brands
- Chew tabs should be chewed and not swallowed whole

IV **IV route**

- Give by cont inf only after diluting 5-10 ml (multivitamins)/500-1000 ml of D_5W, $D_{10}W$, $D_{20}W$, LR, D_5/LR, D_5/0.9% NaCl, 0.9% NaCl, 3% NaCl
- Do not use sol with crystals, precipitate, or color other than bright yellow

Y-site compatibilities:
Acyclovir, ampicillin, cefazolin, cephalothin, cephapirin, diltiazem, erythromycin, fludarabine, gentamicin, tacrolimus, tetracycline

Additive compatibilities:
Cefoxitin, isoproterenol, methyldopate, metoclopramide, metronidazole, netilmicin, norepinephrine, sodium bicarbonate, verapamil

Additive incompatibilities:
Penicillin G, erythromycin, tetracycline, kanamycin, streptomycin, doxycycline, lincomycin should not be admixed

Patient/family education

- Advise patient that adequate nutrition must be maintained to prevent further deficiencies; to comply with treatment regimen
- Advise patient to avoid treating P flavored multivitamins as candy; child may overdose
- Caution patient to store vitamins out P of children's reach

Evaluation

Positive therapeutic outcome

- Check each individual vitamin for guidelines
- Absence of vitamin deficiencies

muromonab-CD3 (℞)

(mur-oe-mone'ab)

Orthoclone OKT3

Func. class.: Immunosuppressive

Chem. class.: Murine monoclonal antibody

Pregnancy category C

Action: Reverses graft rejection by blocking T-cell function

➔ **Therapeutic Outcome:** Prevention of graft rejection

Uses: Acute allograft rejection in renal, cardiac, hepatic transplant patients

Dosage and routes

***Adult:* IV** bol 5 mg/day × 10-14 days; usually methylprednisolone sodium succinate, 1 mg/kg **IV**, is given before muromonab-CD3, 100 mg **IV** hydrocortisone sodium succinate is given 30 min after muromonab-CD3

P ***Child:* IV** 100 μg/kg/day × 10-14 day

Cardiac/hepatic allograft rejection, steroid resistant

***Adult:* IV** bol 5 mg/day × 10-14 days; begin when it is known that rejection has not been reversed by steroids

Available forms: Inj 5 mg/5 ml

Adverse effects

CNS: *Pyrexia, chills, tremors,* **aseptic meningitis**

CV: *Chest pain*

GI: *Vomiting, nausea, diarrhea*
MISC: Infection, cytokine release syndrome, **anaphylaxis**
RESP: *Dyspnea, wheezing,* **pulmonary edema**

Contraindications:
Hypersensitivity to murine origin, fluid overload

P Precautions:
Pregnancy **C**, child <2 yr, fever

Pharmacokinetics

Absorption	Completely absorbed
Distribution	Unknown
Metabolism	Unknown
Excretion	Unknown
Half-life	Unknown

Pharmacodynamics

Unknown

Interactions
Individual drugs
Allopurinol: ↑ toxicity
Azathioprine: ↑ risk of infection
Cyclosporine: ↑ myelosuppression
Drug classifications
Antineoplastics: ↑ myelosuppression
Corticosteroids: ↑ risk of infection
Immunosuppressants: ↑ immunosuppressant
Live virus vaccines: ↓ antibody response

NURSING CONSIDERATIONS
Assessment
- ! Assess for cytosine release syndrome (CRS): nausea, vomiting, chills, fever, joint pain, weakness, dizziness, diarrhea, tremors, abdominal pain; occurs 30-60 min after first dose; methylprednisolone sodium succinate may be prescribed to lessen this reaction
- Assess for hypersensitivity reaction, anaphylaxis: dyspnea, bronchospasm, urticaria, tachycardia, hypotension, angioedema; discontinue drug; emergency equipment must be nearby
- Assess for headache, photophobia, fever, rigidity; indicate aseptic meningitis has developed
- Assess for sore throat, fever, chills, rash, dysuria, which may indicate infection; therapy may be discontinued
- Assess for fluid overload: edema, pulmonary edema, increasing weight
- Monitor blood studies: CBC with differential, platelets, BUN, creatinine, alkaline phosphatase, bilirubin during treatment monthly
- Monitor AST, ALT, BUN, creatinine, alkaline phosphatase, bilirubin
- Obtain human-mouse antibody; if titer is >1:1000, this drug should not be used
- Monitor T cell with CD3, CD4, CD8 antigen qd; report should be CD3 positive and T cells <25/mm^3

Nursing diagnoses
- ✓ Infection, risk for (uses)
- ✓ Knowledge deficit (teaching)

Implementation
- Give by direct **IV** undiluted; withdraw with a 0.2-0.22 low–protein binding μm filter; discard and use new needle for administration; give over 1 min
- Give for several days before transplant surgery

Patient/family education
- Instruct patient to report fever, chills, sore throat, fatigue, since serious infections may occur; rash, rapid heart beat
- Advise patient to use contraceptive measures during treatment and for 12 wk after ending therapy; drug is mutagenic
- Advise patient to avoid crowds and persons with known infections to reduce risk of infection
- Advise patient to report symptoms of cytokine release syndrome, aseptic meningitis, give list of symptoms
- Instruct patient to avoid vaccinations during treatment

Evaluation

Positive therapeutic outcome

- Absence of graft rejection

mycophenolate mofetil (℞)

(mie-koe-feen'oh-late moe-feh-til)

CellCept

Func. class.: Immunosuppressant

Pregnancy category C

Action: Inhibits inflammatory responses that are mediated by the immune system; prolongs survival of allogenic transplants

Therapeutic Outcome: Absence of graft rejection

Uses: Organ transplants to prevent rejection (renal); prophylaxis of rejection in allogenic cardiac, hepatic, renal transplants

Investigational uses: Refractory uveitis, 2nd-line therapy for Churg-Strauss syndrome, diffuse proliferative lupus nephritis (in combination)

Dosage and routes

Renal transplant

Adult: PO/**IV** give initial dose 72 hr before transplantation; 1 g bid given to renal transplant patients in combination with corticosteroids and cyclosporine

Renal dose

Adult: PO/**IV** GFR <25 ml/min, max 2 g/day

Cardiac transplant

Adult: PO/**IV** 1.5 g bid, **IV** can be started ≤24 hr after transplant, switch to PO when able

Hepatic transplant

Adult: PO/**IV** 1.5 g bid, give **IV** over ≥2 hr

Available forms: Caps 250 mg; tabs 500 mg; inj (powder) 500 mg/20 ml vial; powder for oral susp 200 mg/ml

Adverse effects

CNS: *Tremor, dizziness, insomnia, headache, fever*

CV: *Hypertension, chest pain*

GI: *Nausea, vomiting,* stomatitis, *diarrhea, constipation,* GI bleeding

GU: *UTI, hematuria,* **renal tubular necrosis**

HEMA: **Leukopenia, thrombocytopenia, anemia, pancytopenia**

INTEG: *Rash*

META: *Peripheral edema, hypercholesteremia, hypophosphatemia, edema, hyperkalemia, hypokalemia, hyperglycemia*

MS: Arthralgia, muscle wasting

RESP: *Dyspnea, respiratory infection, increased cough, pharyngitis, bronchitis, pneumonia*

SYST: **Lymphoma, nonmelanoma skin carcinoma**

Contraindications: Hypersensitivity to this drug or mycophenolic acid

Precautions: Lymphomas, malignancies, neutropenia, renal disease, pregnancy **C,** lactation

Pharmacokinetics

Absorption	Rapidly and completely absorbed
Distribution	Unknown
Metabolism	To active metabolite (MPA)
Excretion	Urine, feces
Half-life	Unknown

Pharmacodynamics

Unknown

Interactions

Individual drugs

Acyclovir: ↑ concentration of both drugs

Azathioprine: Avoid use

Cholestyramine: ↓ levels of mycophenolate

Ganciclovir: ↑ concentration of both drugs
Phenytoin: ↓ protein binding of phenytoin
Probenecid: ↑ levels of mycophenolate
Theophylline: ↓ protein binding of theophylline

Drug classifications

Antacids: ↓ levels of mycophenolate
Salicylates: ↑ levels of mycophenolate

Food/drug

Decreased absorption if taken with food

NURSING CONSIDERATIONS

Assessment

- Monitor blood studies: CBC monthly during treatment
- Monitor liver function studies: alkaline phosphatase, AST, ALT, bilirubin

Nursing diagnoses

✓ Infection, risk for (uses)
✓ Knowledge deficit (teaching)

Implementation

- Give 72 hr before transplantation; may be given in combination with corticosteroids and cyclosporine

PO route

- Give alone for better absorption
- ⊘ Do not crush, chew tabs, do not open caps

IV route

- Do not give by rapid or bolus inj: reconstitute and dilute to 6 mg/ml with D_5, give over ≥2 hr
- Do not admix with mycophenolate **IV** in infusion catheter or with other **IV** drug or infusion admixtures

Patient/family education

- Teach patient to report fever, rash, severe diarrhea, chills, sore throat, fatigue, since serious infections may occur
- Instruct patient to avoid crowds to reduce risk of infection
- Advise patient that repeated lab tests are necessary
- Advise patient to limit exposure to sunlight/UV light
- Instruct patient to use contraception before, during, and 6 wk after therapy

Evaluation

Positive therapeutic outcome

- Absence of graft rejection

nabumetone (℞)

(na-byoo'me-tone)

Relafen

Func. class.: Nonsteroidal antiinflammatory

Chem. class.: Acetic acid derivative

Pregnancy category C (1st trimester), B (2nd trimester)

Action: Inhibits prostaglandin synthesis by decreasing an enzyme needed for biosynthesis; analgesic, antiinflammatory

➔ **Therapeutic Outcome:** Decreased pain, swelling of joints

Uses: Osteoarthritis, rheumatoid arthritis, acute or chronic treatment

Dosage and routes

Adult: PO 1 g as a single dose; may increase to 1.5-2 g/day if needed; may give qd or bid (as a divided dose)

Available forms: Tabs 500, 750 mg

Adverse effects

CNS: Dizziness, headache, drowsiness, fatigue, tremors, confusion, insomnia, anxiety, depression, nervousness

CV: Tachycardia, peripheral edema, palpitations, **dysrhythmias, CHF**

EENT: Tinnitus, hearing loss, blurred vision

GI: Nausea, anorexia, vomiting, diarrhea, jaundice, cholestatic hepatitis, constipation, flatulence, cramps, dry mouth, peptic ulcer, gastritis, **ulceration, perforation**

GU: **Nephrotoxicity, dysuria,**

M

hematuria, oliguria, azotemia, cystitis
HEMA: **Blood dyscrasias**
INTEG: Purpura, rash, pruritus, sweating, photosensitivity
RESP: Dyspnea, pharyngitis, **bronchospasm**
SYST: **Anaphylaxis, angioneurotic edema**

Contraindications: Hypersensitivity to this drug or aspirin, iodides, NSAIDs, asthma, severe renal disease

Precautions: **C** (1st trimester), **B** (2nd trimester), lactation, children, bleeding disorders, GI disorders, cardiac disorders, renal disorders, hepatic dysfunction, elderly

P G

Pharmacokinetics

Absorption	Well absorbed
Distribution	Unknown
Metabolism	Liver, extensively, to inactive metabolite
Excretion	Unknown
Half-life	22-30 hr

Pharmacodynamics

Onset	Unknown
Peak	2½-4 hr
Duration	Unknown

Interactions
Individual drugs
Acetaminophen (long-term use): ↑ renal reactions
Alcohol: ↑ adverse reactions
Aspirin: ↓ effectiveness, ↑ adverse reactions
Cefamandole: ↑ risk of bleeding
Cefoperazone: ↑ risk of bleeding
Cefotetan: ↑ risk of bleeding
Clopidogrel: ↑ risk of bleeding
Digoxin: ↑ toxicity, levels
Eptifibatide: ↑ risk of bleeding
Insulin: ↓ insulin effect
Lithium: ↑ toxicity
Methotrexate: ↑ toxicity
Phenytoin: ↑ toxicity
Plicamycin: ↑ risk of bleeding
Probenecid: ↑ toxicity
Radiation: ↑ risk of hematologic toxicity
Sulfonylurea: ↑ toxicity
Ticlopidine: ↑ risk of bleeding
Valproic acid: ↑ risk of bleeding

Drug classifications
Anticoagulants: ↑ risk of bleeding
Antihypertensives: ↓ effect of antihypertensives
Antineoplastics: ↑ risk of hematologic toxicity
Cephalosporins: ↑ risk of bleeding
Diuretics: ↓ effectiveness of diuretics
Glucocorticoids: ↑ adverse reactions
Hypoglycemics, oral: ↓ hypoglycemic effect
NSAIDs: ↑ adverse reactions
Potassium supplements: ↑ adverse reactions
Salicylates: possible ↑ action or toxicity
Sulfonamides: ↑ toxicity
Thrombolytics: ↑ bleeding

NURSING CONSIDERATIONS
Assessment
- Assess for pain: frequency, characteristics, location, duration, intensity, relief of pain after medication; and for inflammation of joints, ROM
- Monitor blood counts during therapy; watch for decreasing platelets; if low, therapy may need to be discontinued, restarted after hematologic recovery; check for blood dyscrasias (thrombocytopenia): brusing, fatigue, bleeding, poor healing; monitor liver function tests: AST, ALT, alkaline phosphatase; LDH, blood glucose, WBC, CrCl
- Assess for asthma, aspirin sensitivity, nasal polyps; increased hypersensitivity reactions

Nursing diagnoses
- ✓ Pain (uses)
- ✓ Mobility, impaired (uses)
- ✓ Injury, risk for (adverse reactions)
- ✓ Knowledge deficit (teaching)

Implementation

- Administer tab to patient crushed or whole
- Give with food or milk to decrease gastric symptoms

Patient/family education

- Tell patient that drug must be continued for prescribed time to be effective; to avoid aspirin, alcoholic beverages, NSAIDs, and OTC medications unless approved by prescriber
- Caution patient to report bleeding, bruising, fatigue, malaise, since blood dyscrasias do occur
- Instruct patient to use caution when driving; drowsiness, dizziness may occur
- Advise patient to use sunscreen, hat, and other protective clothing to prevent burns
- Instruct patient to take with a full glass of water and sit upright
- Advise patient to report dark stools, a change in urine pattern, increased weight, edema, increased pain in joints, fever, blood in urine, blurred vision, ringing or roaring in ears

Evaluation

Positive therapeutic outcome

- Decreased pain
- Decreased inflammation
- Increased mobility

nadolol (℞)

(nay-doe'lole)

Corgard

Func. class.: Antihypertensive, antianginal

Chem. class.: β-Adrenergic receptor blocker

Pregnancy category C

Action: Competitively blocks stimulation of β-adrenergic receptor within vascular smooth muscle; produces chronotropic, inotropic activity (decreases rate of SA node discharge, increases recovery time), slows conduction of AV node, decreases heart rate, which decreases O_2 consumption in myocardium; also decreases renin-aldosterone-angiotensin system at high doses, inhibits β_2-receptors in bronchial system

➔ **Therapeutic Outcome:** Decreased B/P, heart rate

Uses: Chronic stable angina pectoris, mild to moderate hypertension

Investigational uses: Tachydysrhythmias, aggression, anxiety, tremors, esophageal varices (rebleeding only), prophylaxis of migraine headaches, hyperthyroidism adjunctive therapy

Dosage and routes

Adult: PO 40 mg qd; increase by 40-80 mg q3-7 days; maintenance 40-240 mg/day for angina, 40-320 mg/day for hypertension

G ***Elderly:*** PO 20 mg/day, may increase by 20 mg until desired dose

Renal dose

CrCl 31-50 ml/min give q24-36h; CrCl 10-30 ml/min give q24-48h

Available forms: Tabs 20, 40, 80, 120, 160 mg

Adverse effects

CNS: Depression, hallucinations, dizziness, fatigue, lethargy, paresthesia, headache

CV: **Bradycardia,** *hypotension,* **CHF,** palpitations, AV block, chest pain, peripheral ischemia, flushing, edema, vasodilatation, conduction disturbances, **pulmonary edema**

EENT: Sore throat

GI: Nausea, vomiting, diarrhea, colitis, constipation, cramps, dry mouth, flatulence, hepatomegaly, **pancreatitis,** taste distortion

GU: *Impotence*

HEMA: **Agranulocytosis, thrombocytopenia**

INTEG: Rash, pruritus, fever

RESP: Dyspnea, respiratory dysfunction, **bronchospasm,** cough, wheez-

N

ing, nasal stuffiness, pharyngitis, **laryngospasm**

Contraindications: Hypersensitivity to this drug, cardiac failure, cardiogenic shock, 2nd- or 3rd-degree heart block, bronchospastic disease, sinus bradycardia, CHF, COPD

Precautions: Diabetes mellitus, pregnancy **C**, renal disease, lactation, hyperthyroidism, peripheral vascular disease, myasthenia gravis

Do Not Confuse:
Corgard/Cognex

Pharmacokinetics

Absorption	Variably absorbed
Distribution	Crosses placenta; minimal concentration in CNS, protein binding 30%
Excretion	Kidneys, unchanged
Half-life	10-24 hr; increased in renal disease

Pharmacodynamics

Onset	Variable
Peak	3-4 hr
Duration	20-24 hr

Interactions

Individual drugs

Alcohol: ↑ hypotension (large amounts)
Epinephrine: α-Adrenergic stimulation
Hydralazine: ↑ hypotension, bradycardia
Insulin: ↑ hypoglycemia
Methyldopa: ↑ hypotension, bradycardia
Norepinephrine: ↑ hypotension, bradycardia
Phenylephrine: ↑ hypotension, bradycardia
Prazosin: ↑ hypotension, bradycardia
Pseudoephedrine: ↑ hypotension, bradycardia
Reserpine: ↑ hypotension, bradycardia
Thyroid: ↓ effect of nadolol
Verapamil: ↑ myocardial depression

Drug classifications

Amphetamines: ↑ hypotension, bradycardia
Antihypertensives: ↑ hypertension
β_2-Agonists: ↓ bronchodilatation
Cardiac glycosides: ↑ bradycardia
MAOIs: ↑ hypertension, do not use together
Nitrates: ↑ hypotension
NSAIDs: ↓ antihypertensive effect
Theophyllines: ↓ bronchodilatation

Lab test interferences

False: ↑ urinary catecholamines

NURSING CONSIDERATIONS

Assessment

- Monitor B/P at beginning of treatment, periodically thereafter; note rate, rhythm, quality of apical/radial pulse before administration; notify prescriber of any significant changes (pulse <55 bpm), orthostatic hypotension
- Check for baselines in renal, liver function tests before therapy begins
- Assess for edema in feet, legs daily; monitor I&O, daily weight; check for jugular vein distention and rales bilaterally, dyspnea (CHF)
- Monitor skin turgor, dryness of mucous membranes for hydration status, especially elderly

Nursing diagnoses

- ✓ Cardiac output, decreased (uses)
- ✓ Injury, potential for (adverse reactions)
- ✓ Knowledge deficit (teaching)
- ✓ Noncompliance (teaching)

Implementation

- Given ac, hs, tab may be crushed or swallowed whole; give with food to prevent GI upset; give reduced dosage in renal dysfunction
- Store protected from light, moisture; place in cool environment

Patient/family education

- Teach patient not to discontinue drug abruptly; taper over 2 wk; may cause precipitate angina, serious dysrhythmias if stopped abruptly

- Teach patient not to use OTC products containing α-adrenergic stimulants (such as nasal decongestants, cold preparations); to avoid alcohol, smoking and to limit sodium intake as prescribed
- Teach patient how to take pulse and B/P at home; advise when to notify prescriber
- Instruct patient to comply with weight control, dietary adjustments, modified exercise program
- Advise patient to carry/wear ID to identify drug being taken, allergies; teach patient drug controls symptoms but does not cure condition
- Caution patient to avoid hazardous activities if dizziness, drowsiness present; to rise slowly to prevent orthostatic hypotension
- Teach patient to report symptoms of CHF: difficult breathing, especially on exertion or when lying down, night cough, swelling of extremities or bradycardia, dizziness, confusion, depression, fever
- Teach patient to take drug as prescribed, not to double doses, skip doses; take any missed doses as soon as remembered if at least 4 hr until next dose

Evaluation

Positive therapeutic outcome

- Decreased B/P in hypertension

nafcillin (℞)

(naf-sill'in)

Nafcil, nafcillin sodium, Nallpen, Unipen

Func. class.: Antiinfective, broad-spectrum

Chem. class.: Penicillinase-resistant penicillin

Pregnancy category B

Action: Interferes with cell wall replication of susceptible organisms; osmotically unstable cell wall swells, bursts from osmotic pressure

➔ **Therapeutic Outcome:** Bactericidal effects for gram-positive cocci *Staphylococcus aureus, Streptococcus viridans, Streptococcus pneumoniae* and infections caused by penicillinase-producing *Staphylococcus*

Uses: Infections caused by penicillinase-producing staphylococci, streptococci; respiratory tract, skin, skin structure, urinary tract, bone, joint infections, sinusitis, endocarditis, septicemia, meningitis

Dosage and routes

Adult: PO 250-1000 mg q4-6h; IM 500 mg q4-6h; **IV** 500-1500 mg q4-6h

P ***Child and infants, most infections:*** PO 6.25-12.5 mg/kg q6h; pharyngitis PO 250 mg q8h; IM 25 mg/kg q12h; **IV** most infections 10-20 mg/kg q4h or 20-40 mg/kg q8h, max 200 mg/kg/day

P ***Neonates:*** PO 10 mg/kg q6-8h; IM 10 mg/kg q12h; **IV**: most infections 10-20 mg/kg q4h or 20-40 mg/kg q8h, max 200 mg/kg/day

Meningitis

P ***Neonates ≥2 kg:*** 50 mg/kg q8h × 1 wk of life, then 50 mg/kg q6h

P ***Neonates <2 kg:*** 25-50 mg/kg q12h × 1 wk of life, then 50 mg/kg q8h

Available forms: Caps 250 mg; tabs 500 mg; powder for inj 1, 2, 10 g, 500 mg, 4 mg; sol 250 mg/5 ml

Adverse effects

CNS: Lethargy, hallucinations, anxiety, depression, muscle twitching, **coma, seizures**

GI: Nausea, vomiting, diarrhea, increased AST, ALT, abdominal pain, glossitis, **pseudomembranous colitis**

GU: Oliguria, **proteinuria, hematu-**

N

ria, vaginitis, moniliasis, glomerulonephritis, interstitial nephritis
HEMA: Anemia, increased bleeding time, **bone marrow depression, granulocytopenia**

Contraindications: Hypersensitivity to penicillins

Precautions: Pregnancy **B**, hypersensitivity to cephalosporins, P neonates

Pharmacokinetics

Absorption	Well absorbed (IM); erratic (PO)
Distribution	Widely distributed; crosses placenta
Metabolism	Not metabolized
Excretion	Kidneys, unchanged; breast milk
Half-life	1 hr; increased in renal disease

Pharmacodynamics

	PO	IM	IV
Onset	½ hr	½ hr	Immediate
Peak	1-2 hr	1-2 hr	Inf end

Interactions

Individual drugs

Aspirin: ↑ nafcillin levels, ↓ renal excretion
Dilsulfiram: ↑ nafcillin concentrations
Probenecid: ↑ nafcillin levels, ↓ renal excretion

Drug classifications

Oral anticoagulants: ↑ anticoagulant effects
Oral contraceptives: ↓ contraceptive effectiveness

Food/drug

Food, carbonated drinks, citrus fruit juices: ↓ absorption

Herb/drug

Khat: ↓ absorption

Lab test interferences

False positive: Urine glucose, urine protein

NURSING CONSIDERATIONS

Assessment

- Assess patient for previous sensitivity reaction to penicillins or other cephalosporins; cross-sensitivity between penicillins and cephalosporins is common
- Assess patient for signs and symptoms of infection including characteristics of wounds, sputum, urine, stool, WBC >10,000/mm^3, earache, fever; obtain baseline information and during treatment
- Obtain C&S before beginning drug therapy to identify if correct treatment has been initiated
- Assess for allergic reactions, anaphylaxis: rash, urticaria, pruritus, chills, fever, dyspnea, laryngeal edema, joint pain; angioedema may occur a few days after therapy begins; epinephrine, resuscitation equipment should be available for anaphylactic reaction
- Assess renal studies: urinalysis, protein, blood, BUN, creatinine
- (Alert) Identify urine output; if decreasing, notify prescriber (may indicate nephrotoxicity)
- Monitor blood studies: AST, ALT, CBC, Hct, bilirubin, LDH, alkaline phosphatase, Coombs' test monthly if patient is on long-term therapy
- Monitor electrolytes: potassium, sodium, chloride monthly if patient is on long-term therapy
- Assess bowel pattern qd; if severe diarrhea occurs, drug should be discontinued; may indicate pseudomembranous colitis
- Monitor for bleeding: ecchymosis, bleeding gums, hematuria, stool guaiac daily if on long-term therapy
- Assess for overgrowth of infection: perineal itching, fever, malaise, redness, pain, swelling, drainage, rash, diarrhea, change in cough, sputum

Nursing diagnoses

- ✓ Infection, risk for (uses)
- ✓ Diarrhea (adverse reactions)
- ✓ Injury, risk for (adverse reactions)
- ✓ Knowledge deficit (teaching)
- ✓ Noncompliance (teaching)

Implementation

PO route

- Give in even doses around the clock; if GI upset occurs, give with food; drug must be given for 10-14 days to ensure organism death and prevent superinfection; store in tight container.
- Do not crush, chew caps
- Shake susp; store in refrigerator for 2 wk, 1 wk at room temp

IM route

- Reconstitute 500 mg/1.7-1.8 ml; 1 g/3.4 ml; 2 g/6.6-6.8 ml with sterile water or bacteriostatic water for a conc of 250 mg/ml; store unused portion in refrigerator for up to 7 days
- Give deep in large muscle mass

IV route

- Reconstitute 1 g/3.4 ml, 2 g/6.6-6.8 ml with sterile water or bacteriostatic water for a conc of 250 mg/ml; store unused portion in refrigerator for up to 7 days
- Give by direct **IV** by diluting reconstituted sol with 15-30 ml of sterile water or 0.9% NaCl; give over 5-10 min
- Give by intermittent inf by diluting to a conc of 2-40 mg/ml with 0.9% NaCl, D_5W, $D_{10}W$, D_5/0.9% NaCl, D_5/LR, LR, Ringer's; store in refrigerator for up to 96 hr or 24 hr room temp; run over 30-60 min

Syringe compatibilities:
Cimetidine, heparin

Y-site compatibilities:
Acyclovir, atropine, cyclophosphamide, diazepam, enalaprilat, esmolol, famotidine, fentanyl, fluconazole, foscarnet, hydromorphone, magnesium sulfate, morphine, perphenazine, propofol, theophylline, zidovudine

Y-site incompatibilities:
Droperidol, fentanyl/droperidol, labetalol, nalbuphine, pentazocine, regular insulin, verapamil

Additive compatibilities:
Chloramphenicol, chlorothiazide, dexamethasone, diphenhydramine, ephedrine, heparin, hydroxyzine, lidocaine, potassium chloride, prochlorperazine, sodium bicarbonate, sodium lactate

Additive incompatibilities:
Ascorbic acid, aztreonam, bleomycin, cytarabine, gentamicin, hydrocortisone sodium succinate, methylprednisolone sodium succinate, promazine

Patient/family education

- Teach patient to report sore throat, bruising, bleeding, joint pain; may indicate blood dyscrasias (rare)
- Advise patient to contact prescriber if vaginal itching, loose, foul-smelling stools, furry tongue occur; may indicate superinfection
- Instruct patient to take all medication prescribed for the length of time ordered
- Advise patient to notify prescriber of diarrhea with blood or pus, which may indicate pseudomembranous colitis

Evaluation

Positive therapeutic outcome

- Absence of signs/symptoms of infection (WBC <10,000/mm^3, temp WNL, absence of red, draining wounds, earache)
- Reported improvement in symptoms of infection

Treatment of anaphylaxis:
Withdraw drug, maintain airway, administer epinephrine, aminophylline, O_2, **IV** corticosteroids

N

HIGH ALERT

nalbuphine (℞)

(nal'byoo-feen)

Nubain, nalbuphine HCl

Func. class.: Opioid analgesic

Chem. class.: Synthetic opioid agonist/antagonist

Pregnancy category C

Action: Inhibits ascending pain pathways in limbic system, thalamus, midbrain, hypothalamus by binding to opiate receptor sites, thus altering pain perception and response

Therapeutic Outcome: Relief of pain

Uses: Moderate to severe pain, labor analgesia, balanced anesthesia (adjunct)

Dosage and routes

Analgesic

Adult: SC/IM/**IV** 10-20 mg q3-6h prn, not to exceed 160 mg/day

Balanced anesthesia supplement

Adult: **IV** 0.3-3 mg/kg given over 10-15 min; may give 0.25-0.5 mg/kg as needed (maintenance)

Available forms: Inj 10, 20 mg/ml

Adverse effects

CNS: *Drowsiness, dizziness, confusion, headache, sedation, euphoria,* dysphoria (high doses), hallucinations, dreaming, tolerance, physical and psychologic dependency

CV: Palpitations, bradycardia, change in B/P, orthostatic hypotension

EENT: Tinnitus, blurred vision, miosis (high doses), diplopia

GI: *Nausea, vomiting, anorexia, constipation, cramps*

GU: Increased urinary output, dysuria, urinary retention, urgency

INTEG: *Rash,* urticaria, bruising, flushing, *diaphoresis,* pruritus

RESP: **Respiratory depression**

Contraindications: Hypersensitivity, addiction (narcotic)

Precautions: Addictive personality, pregnancy **C**, lactation, increased intracranial pressure, MI (acute), severe heart disease, respiratory depression, hepatic disease, renal disease

Pharmacokinetics

Absorption	Well absorbed (SC, IM); completely absorbed (**IV**)
Distribution	Crosses placenta
Metabolism	Liver, extensively
Excretion	Feces, kidneys, unchanged (small amounts); breast milk
Half-life	5 hr

Pharmacodynamics

	IM	SC	IV
Onset	Up to 15 min	Up to 15 min	Rapid
Peak	1 hr	Unknown	½ hr
Duration	3-6 hr	3-6 hr	3-6 hr

Interactions

Individual drugs

Alcohol: ↑ respiratory depression, hypotension, sedation

Drug classifications

Antihistamines: ↑ respiratory depression, hypotension

CNS depressants: ↑ respiratory depression, hypotension

MAOIs: Use cautiously, results are unpredictable

Opiates: ↑ opioid withdrawals (dependency)

Phenothiazines: ↑ respiratory depression, hypotension

Sedative/hypnotics: ↑ respiratory depression, hypotension

Lab test interferences

↑ amylase, ↑ lipase

NURSING CONSIDERATIONS

Assessment

- Assess pain characteristics (location, intensity, type) before medication administration and after treatment
- Monitor VS after parenteral route; note muscle rigidity, drug history, liver, kidney function tests; respiratory dysfunction: respiratory depression, character, rate, rhythm; notify prescriber if respirations are <10/min
- Monitor CNS changes: dizziness, drowsiness, hallucinations, euphoria, LOC, pupil reaction
- Monitor allergic reactions: rash, urticaria

Nursing diagnoses

✓ Pain (uses)
✓ Sensory-perceptual alteration: visual, auditory (adverse reactions)
✓ Breathing pattern, ineffective (adverse reactions)
✓ Knowledge deficit (teaching)

Implementation

- Give by inj (IM, **IV**), only with resuscitative equipment available; give slowly to prevent rigidity
- Store in light-resistant area at room temp

IM route

- Give deeply in large muscle mass; rotate inj sites

IV **IV route**

- Give direct **IV** undiluted 10 mg or less over 3-5 min or more

Syringe compatibilities: Atropine, cimetidine, diphenhydramine, droperidol, glycopyrrolate, hydroxyzine, lidocaine, midazolam, prochlorperazine, promethazine, ranitidine, scopolamine, trimethobenzamide

Syringe incompatibilities: Diazepam, pentobarbital

Y-site compatibilities: Amifostine, aztreonam, cefmetazole, cladribine, filgrastim, fludarabine, granisetron, melphalan, paclitaxel, propofol, teniposide, thiotepa, vinorelbine

Y-site incompatibilities: Nafcillin, sargramostim

Patient/family education

- Instruct patient to report any symptoms of CNS changes, allergic reactions
- Caution patients to avoid CNS depressants: alcohol, sedative/hypnotics for at least 24 hr after taking this drug
- Discuss with patient that dizziness, drowsiness, confusion are common; to avoid getting up without assistance
- Discuss in detail all aspects of the drug: reason for taking drug and expected results
- Instruct patient to change position slowly to prevent orthostatic hypotension
- Teach patient to turn, cough, deep breathe after surgery to prevent atelectasis

Evaluation

Positive therapeutic outcome

- Relief of pain

Treatment of overdose:

Naloxone (Narcan) 0.2-0.8 **IV**, O_2, **IV** fluids, vasopressors

naloxone (℞)

(nal-oks'one)

naloxone HCl, Narcan

Func. class.: Opioid antagonist, antidote

Chem. class.: Thebaine derivative

Pregnancy category B

Action: Competes with opioids at opioid receptor sites

➔ **Therapeutic Outcome:** Absence of opioid overdose

Uses: Respiratory depression induced by narcotics, pentazocine, propoxyphene; refractory circulatory shock

N

Dosage and routes

Opioid-induced respiratory depression, CNS depression

Adult: **IV**/SC/IM 0.4-2 mg; repeat q2-3 min if needed

P ***Child:*** **IV**/SC/IM 0.5-2 μg/kg as small, frequent qmin bolus or as an inf titrated to response

Postoperative respiratory depression

Adult: **IV** 0.1-0.2 mg q2-3 min prn

P ***Child:*** **IV**/IM/SC 0.01 mg/kg q2-3 min prn

Asphyxia neonatorum

P ***Neonates:*** **IV** 0.01 mg/kg given into umbilical vein after delivery; may repeat in q2-3 min × 3 doses

Available forms: Inj 0.4, 1 P mg/ml; neonatal inj 0.02 mg/ml

Adverse effects

CNS: Drowsiness, nervousness

CV: **Ventricular tachycardia, fibrillation,** increased systolic B/P (high doses)

GI: Nausea, vomiting

RESP: Hyperpnea

Contraindications: Hypersensitivity, respiratory depression

Precautions: Pregnancy **B,** chil-P dren, CV disease, opioid dependency, lactation

Do Not Confuse:

Narcan/Norcuron

Pharmacokinetics

Absorption	Well absorbed (SC, IM); completely absorbed (**IV**)
Distribution	Rapidly distributed; crosses placenta
Metabolism	Liver
Excretion	Kidneys
P **Half-life**	1 hr; up to 3 hr (neonates)

Pharmacodynamics

	IV	IM/SC
Onset	1 min	2-5 min
Peak	Unknown	Unknown
Duration	45 min	45-60 min

Interactions

Drug classifications

Analgesics, opioids: ↑ withdrawal in those addicted to opioids

Lab test interferences

Interference: Urine VMA, 5-HIAA, urine glucose

NURSING CONSIDERATIONS

Assessment

- Assess for signs of opioid withdrawal in drug-dependent individuals: cramping, hypertension, anxiety, vomiting; may occur up to 2 hr after administration
- Monitor VS q3-5 min; ABGs including Po_2, Pco_2
- Assess cardiac status: tachycardia, hypertension; monitor ECG
- Assess for pain: duration, intensity, location before and after administration; may be used for respiratory depression
- Assess for respiratory dysfunction: respiratory depression, character, rate, rhythm; if respirations are <10/min, probably due to opioid overdose, administer naloxone; monitor LOC

Nursing diagnoses

- ✓ Breathing pattern, ineffective (uses)
- ✓ Coping, ineffective individual (uses)
- ✓ Pain (adverse reactions)
- ✓ Knowledge deficit (teaching)

Implementation

IV route

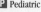

- Give by direct **IV** undiluted; give 0.4 mg or less over 15 sec or titrate inf to response
- Give cont inf **IV** further diluted with 0.9% NaCl and D_5 and give as an inf
- Give only with resuscitative equipment, O_2 nearby
- Use only sol prepared within 24 hr
- Store at room temp in darkness

Syringe compatibilities:
Benzquinamide, heparin

Y-site compatibilities:
Propofol

Additive compatibilities:
Verapamil

Patient/family education
- Explain reason for and expected results of medication when patient alert

Evaluation
Positive therapeutic outcome
- Reversal of respiratory depression
- LOC: alert

naproxen (℞)
(na-prox'en)

Apo-Naproxen ✤, EC-Naprosyn, Naprelan, Napron X, Naprosyn, Naprosyn-E ✤, Naprosyn-SR ✤, Naxen ✤, Novo-Naprox ✤, Nu-Naprox ✤

naproxen sodium

Aleve, Anaprox, Anaprox DS, Apo-Napro-Na ✤, Apo-Napro-Na DS, Naprelan, Novo-Naprox Sodium ✤, Novo-Naprox Sodium DS ✤, Synflex ✤, Synflex DS ✤

Func. class.: Nonsteroidal antiinflammatory, nonopioid analgesic

Chem. class.: Propionic acid derivative

Pregnancy category B

Action: Inhibits prostaglandin synthesis by decreasing enzyme needed for biosynthesis; analgesic, antiinflammatory

➔ **Therapeutic Outcome:** Decreased pain, inflammation

Uses: Mild to moderate pain, osteoarthritis, rheumatoid arthritis, gouty arthritis, juvenile arthritis, primary dysmenorrhea

Dosage and routes

Adult: PO 250-500 mg bid, not to exceed 1 g/day (base); 525 mg, then 275 mg q6-8h prn, not to exceed 1475 mg (sodium)

P ***Child:*** PO 10 mg/kg in 2 divided doses

Available forms: Naproxen, tabs 250, 375, 500 mg; del rel tabs 375, 500 mg; ext rel tabs 750, 1000 mg; oral susp 125 mg/5 ml; naproxen sodium, cont rel tabs 421.5, 550 mg; tabs 220, 275, 550 mg

Adverse effects

CNS: Dizziness, drowsiness, fatigue, tremors, confusion, insomnia, anxiety, depression

CV: Tachycardia, peripheral edema, palpitations, **dysrhythmias**

EENT: Tinnitus, hearing loss, blurred vision

GI: Nausea, anorexia, vomiting, diarrhea, jaundice, **cholestatic hepatitis**, constipation, flatulence, cramps, dry mouth, peptic ulcer, **GI ulceration, bleeding, perforation**

GU: **Nephrotoxicity: dysuria, hematuria, oliguria, azotemia**

HEMA: **Blood dyscrasias**

INTEG: Purpura, rash, pruritus, sweating

Contraindications: Hypersensitivity, asthma, severe renal disease, severe hepatic disease, ulcer disease

Precautions: Pregnancy **B** (1st trimester), P lactation, children <2 yr, bleeding disorders, GI disorders, cardiac disorders, hypersensitivity to G other antiinflammatory agents, elderly, CrCl <25 ml/min

Pharmacokinetics

Absorption	Completely absorbed
Distribution	Crosses placenta, 99% protein binding
Metabolism	Liver, extensively
Excretion	Breast milk
Half-life	10-20 hr

N

Pharmacodynamics	
Onset	1 hr
Peak	2-4 hr
Duration	<7 hr

Interactions
Individual drugs
Acetaminophen (long-term use): ↑ renal reactions
Alcohol: ↑ adverse reactions
Aspirin: ↓ effectiveness, ↑ adverse reactions
Cefamandole: ↑ bleeding
Cefoperazone: ↑ bleeding
Cefotetan: ↑ bleeding
Digoxin: ↑ toxicity, levels
Insulin: ↓ insulin effect
Lithium: ↑ toxicity
Methotrexate: ↑ toxicity
Phenytoin: ↑ toxicity
Probenecid: ↑ toxicity
Radiation: ↑ risk of hematologic toxicity
Sulfonylurea: ↑ toxicity
Valproic acid: ↑ bleeding
Drug classifications
Anticoagulants: ↑ risk of bleeding
Antihypertensives: ↓ effect of antihypertensives
Antineoplastics: ↑ risk of hematologic toxicity
β-Adrenergic blockers: ↑ antihypertension
Cephalosporins: ↑ risk of bleeding
Diuretics: ↓ effectiveness of diuretics
Glucocorticoids: ↑ adverse reactions
Hypoglycemics, oral: ↓ hypoglycemic effect
NSAIDs: ↑ adverse reactions
Potassium supplements: ↑ adverse reactions
Sulfonamides: ↑ toxicity
Lab test interferences
↑ BUN, ↑ alkaline phosphatase
False: ↑ 5-HIAA, ↑ 17KS

NURSING CONSIDERATIONS
Assessment
- Monitor liver function, renal function, other blood studies: AST, ALT, bilirubin, creatinine, BUN, CBC, Hct, Hgb, pro-time, LDH, blood glucose, WBC, platelets; if patient is on long-term therapy
- Check I&O ratio; decreasing output may indicate renal failure (long-term therapy)
- Assess hepatotoxicity: dark urine, clay-colored stools, yellowing of the skin and sclera, itching, abdominal pain, fever, diarrhea if patient is on long-term therapy
- Assess for allergic reactions: rash, urticaria; if these occur, drug may have to be discontinued
- Assess for ototoxicity: tinnitus, ringing, roaring in ears; audiometric testing needed before, after long-term therapy
- Assess for visual changes: blurring, halos; may indicate corneal, retinal damage
- Check for edema in feet, ankles, legs
- Identify prior drug history; there are many drug interactions
- Monitor pain: location, frequency, duration, characteristics, type, intensity before dose and 1 hour after; assess ROM before dose and after
- Assess for asthma, aspirin hypersensitivity, or nasal polyps, increased risk of hypersensitivity

Nursing diagnoses
✓ Pain (uses)
✓ Mobility, impaired (uses)
✓ Injury, risk for (adverse reactions)
✓ Knowledge deficit (teaching)

Implementation
- Administer to patient crushed or whole
- Give with food or milk to decrease gastric symptoms; give ½ hr ac or 2 hr pc for better absorption

Patient/family education
- Teach patient to report any symptoms of hepatotoxicity, renal toxicity, visual changes, ototoxicity, allergic reactions, bleeding (long-term therapy)

• Advise patient to take with 8 oz of water and sit upright for 30 min after dose to prevent ulceration
• Caution patient not to exceed recommended dosage; acute poisoning may result; to take as prescribed, do not double dose
• Advise patient to use sunscreen to prevent photosensitivity reactions
• Teach patient to read label on other OTC drugs; many contain other antiinflammatories; caution patient to avoid alcohol ingestion; GI bleeding may occur
• Inform patient that the therapeutic response takes 2 wk (arthritis)
• Teach patient to report tinnitus, confusion, diarrhea, sweating, hyperventilation, blurred vision, fever, joint aches, black stools, flu-like symptoms

Evaluation

Positive therapeutic outcome

• Decreased pain
• Decreased inflammation
• Increased mobility

naratriptan (℞)

(nair'ah-trip-tan)

Amerge

Func. class.: Migraine agent

Chem. class.: $5\text{-}HT_1$-like receptor agonist

Pregnancy category C

Action: Binds selectively to the vascular $5\text{-}HT_1$ receptor subtype, exerts antimigraine effect; causes vasoconstriction in cranial arteries

Therapeutic Outcome: Decreased intensity and incidence of migraines

Uses: Acute treatment of migraine with or without aura

Dosage and routes

Adult: PO 1 or 2.5 mg with fluids, if headache returns, repeat once after 4 hr, max 5 mg/24 hr

Hepatic/renal dose

Max 2.5 mg/24 hr

Available forms: Tab 1, 2.5 mg

Adverse effects

CV: Increased B/P, palpitations, **tachydysrhythmias, PR, QT_C prolongation, ST/T wave changes, PVCs, atrial flutter, fibrillation, coronary vasospasm**

EENT: EENT infections, photophobia

GI: Nausea, vomiting

MISC: Temperature change sensations, tightness, pressure sensations

MS: Weakness, neck stiffness, myalgia

NEURO: Dizziness, sedation, fatigue

Contraindications: Angina pectoris, history of MI, documented silent ischemia, ischemic heart disease, concurrent ergotamine-containing preparations, uncontrolled hypertension, hypersensitivity, severe renal disease (CrCl <15 ml/min); severe hepatic disease(Child-Pugh grade C), CV syndromes, hemiplegic or basilar migraines

Precautions: Postmenopausal women, men >40 yr, risk factors for CAD, hypercholesterolemia, obesity, diabetes, impaired hepatic or renal function, pregnancy **C**, lactation, P children, elderly, peripheral vascular G disease

Pharmacokinetics	
Absorption	Unknown
Distribution	28%-31% protein binding
Metabolism	Liver (metabolite)
Excretion	Urine/feces
Half-life	6 hr

Pharmacodynamics	
Onset	Unknown
Peak	2-3 hr
Duration	Unknown

Interactions

Drug classifications

5-HT agonists: ↑ vasospastic effect

N

Ergot derivatives: ↑ vasospastics effects
Selective serotonin release inhibitors: ↑ weakness, hyperreflexia, incoordination

NURSING CONSIDERATIONS

Assessment

- Assess for stress level, activity, recreation, coping mechanisms
- Assess neurologic status: LOC, blurred vision, nausea, ties preceding headache

Nursing diagnoses

- ✓ Pain (uses)
- ✓ Knowledge deficit (teaching)
- ✓ Noncompliance (teaching)

Implementation

- Give with fluids as soon as symptoms appear, may take another dose after 4 hr; do not take >5 mg in any 24 hr period
- Provide a quiet, calm environment with decreased stimulation for noise, bright light, excessive talking

Patient/family education

- Teach patient to report pain, tightness in chest, neck, throat, or jaw; notify prescriber immediately if sudden, severe abdominal pain occurs
- Teach patient to use contraception while taking drug, to notify prescriber if pregnancy is planned or suspected
- Advise patient not to use if another 5-HT agonist or an ergot preparation has been used in the past 24 hr

Evaluation

Positive therapeutic outcome

- Absence of migraine headaches

nedocromil (℞)

(ned-o-kroe'mil)
Tilade
Func. class.: Antiasthmatic
Chem. class.: Mast cell stabilizer
Pregnancy category B

Action: Stabilizes the membrane of the sensitized mast cell, preventing release of chemical mediators after an antigen-IgE interaction

➔ **Therapeutic Outcome:** Reduced symptoms of asthma

Uses: Allergic rhinitis, severe perennial bronchial asthma, exercise-induced bronchospasm (prevention), prevention of acute bronchospasm induced by environmental pollutants, mastocytosis

Dosage and routes

P ***Adult and child >12 yr:*** 2 inh 2-4 ×/day at regular intervals to provide 14 g/day

Available forms: 1.75 mg of nedocromil per activation in 16.2-g canisters providing at least 112 metered inhalations

Adverse effects

CNS: Headache, dizziness, neuritis, dysphonia
EENT: Throat irritation, cough, nasal congestion, burning eyes, rhinitis
GI: Nausea, vomiting, anorexia, dry mouth, bitter taste

Contraindications: Hypersensitivity to this drug or lactose, status asthmaticus

Precautions: Pregnancy **B,** lactation, children P

Pharmacokinetics	
Absorption	Poorly, 3%
Distribution	Unknown
Metabolism	Not usually metabolized
Excretion	Small amounts in bile, urine unchanged
Half-life	80 min

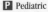

Pharmacodynamics

Onset	Unknown
Peak	15 min
Duration	4-6 hr

Interactions: None

NURSING CONSIDERATIONS
Assessment
- Assess pulmonary function testing baseline (asthma)
- Assess respiratory status: respiratory rate, rhythm, characteristics, cough, wheezing, dyspnea

Nursing diagnoses
✓ Airway clearance, ineffective (uses)
✓ Knowledge deficit (teaching)

Implementation
- Give by inh only with spacer device if needed
- Encourage patient to gargle, sip water to decrease irritation in throat

Patient/family education
- Instruct patient to clear mucus before using
- Teach patient proper inhalation technique: exhale; using inhaler, inhale deeply with head tipped back to open airway; remove, hold breath, exhale; use Halermatic or Spinhaler with Intal caps
- Inform patient that therapeutic effect may take up to 4 wk
- Teach patient that drug is preventive only, not restorative

Evaluation
Positive therapeutic outcome
- Decrease in asthmatic symptoms

nefazodone (℞)
(nef-az'oe-done)
Serzone
Func. class.: Antidepressant—misc
Chem. class.: Phenylpiperazine

Pregnancy category C

Action: Selectively inhibits serotonin uptake by brain, potentiates behavioral changes, occupies central HT_2 receptors

→ **Therapeutic Outcome:** Decreased symptoms of depression after 2-3 wk

Uses: Major depression

Dosage and routes
Adult: PO 200 mg/day (100 mg bid); dosage may be increased to 300 mg/day (150 bid); max 600 mg/day

G ***Elderly:*** PO 100 mg/day (50 mg bid); increase to 100 mg bid after 2 wk to desired dose

Available forms: Tabs 50, 100, 150, 200, 250 mg

Adverse effects
CNS: Dizziness, headache, insomnia
CV: *Postural hypotension*
EENT: *Blurred vision*
GI: *Nausea, constipation, dry mouth*
GU: *Urinary frequency,* retention, UTI
RESP: Pharyngitis, cough

Contraindications: Hypersensitivity to this drug or phenylpiperazines

P G **Precautions:** Pregnancy **C**, lactation, children, elderly, CV disease, seizure disorder

Pharmacokinetics

Absorption	Well absorbed
Distribution	Widely distributed; crosses placenta
Metabolism	Liver, extensively, to metabolites
Excretion	Kidneys, breast milk
Half-life	2-4 hr

N

Pharmacodynamics

Onset	Unknown
Peak	1-3 hr
Duration	Unknown

Interactions
Individual drugs
Alcohol: ↑ CNS depression
Alprazolam: ↑ toxicity
Midazolam: ↑ toxicity
Phenytoin: ↑ toxicity
Triazolam: ↑ toxicity
Drug classifications
Benzodiazepines: ↑ plasma concentrations
Barbiturates: ↑ effects
CNS depressants: ↑ effects
MAOIs: ↑ toxicity

NURSING CONSIDERATIONS
Assessment
- Monitor B/P (with patient lying, standing), pulse q4h; if systolic B/P drops 20 mm Hg hold drug, notify prescriber; take VS q4h in patients with CV disease
- Monitor blood studies: CBC, leukocytes, differential, cardiac enzymes if patient is receiving long-term therapy
- Monitor hepatic studies: AST, ALT, bilirubin
- Assess mental status: mood, sensorium, affect, suicidal tendencies; increase in psychiatric symptoms: depression, panic
- Monitor urinary retention, constipation; constipation is more G likely to occur in the elderly
- Identify alcohol consumption; if alcohol is consumed, hold dose until AM

Nursing diagnoses
✓ Coping, ineffective individual (uses)
✓ Knowledge deficit (teaching)
✓ Noncompliance (teaching)

Implementation
- Give with food or milk to decrease GI symptoms
- Give crushed if patient is unable to swallow medication whole
- Store at room temp; do not freeze

Patient/family education
- Teach patient that therapeutic effects may take 3-4 wk
- Teach patient to use caution in driving and other activities requiring alertness because of drowsiness, dizziness; to avoid rising quickly from G sitting to standing, especially elderly
- Teach patient to avoid alcohol ingestion, other CNS depressants, benzodiazepines
- Teach patient to increase bulk in diet if constipation occurs, especially G elderly
- Teach patient to take gum, hard sugarless candy, or frequent sips of water for dry mouth

Evaluation
Positive therapeutic outcome
- Decrease in depression
- Absence of suicidal thoughts

Treatment of overdose: ECG monitoring, induce emesis, lavage, activated charcoal, administer anticonvulsant

nelfinavir (℞)
(nell-fin′a-ver)
Viracept
Func. class.: Antiretroviral
Chem. class.: HIV protease inhibitor
Pregnancy category B

Action: Inhibits HIV protease

➔ **Therapeutic Outcome:** Prevents maturation of the infectious virus

Uses: HIV alone or in combination

Dosage and routes
Adult: PO 750 mg tid
P ***Child 2-13 yr:*** PO 20-30 mg/kg tid

Available forms: Tabs 250 mg; oral powder 50 mg/g

Adverse effects

CNS: Headache, poor concentration, fatigue, anxiety, depression, **seizures**
CV: Bleeding
ENDO: Hypoglycemia, hyperlipidemia
GI: Diarrhea, nausea, anorexia, dyspepsia
HEMA: **Anemia, leukopenia, thrombocytopenia, Hgb abnormalities**
INTEG: Rash, dermatitis
MISC: Asthenia
MS: Arthralgia, myalgia, myopathy

Contraindications: Hypersensitivity to protease inhibitors

Precautions: Liver disease, pregnancy **B**, lactation, hemophilia, PKU, renal disease

Pharmacokinetics	
Absorption	Unknown
Distribution	98% protein binding
Metabolism	Liver, (minimal)
Excretion	Feces
Half-life	3½-5 hr

Pharmacodynamics	
Onset	Unknown
Peak	2-4 hr
Duration	Unknown

Interactions

Individual drugs

Amiodarone: ↑ serious dysrhythmias
Carbamazepine: ↓ nelfinavir levels
Dexamethasone: ↓ nelfinavir levels
Indinavir: ↑ nelfinavir effect
Lamivudine: ↓ effect of lamivudine
Midazolam: ↑ serious dysrhythmias
Nevirapine: ↓ nelfinavir effect
Phenobarbital: ↓ nelfinavir level
Phenytoin: ↓ nelfinavir level
Quinidine: ↑ serious dysrhythmias
Rifamycin: ↓ nelfinavir levels
Ritonavir: ↑ nelfinavir effect
Triazolam: ↑ serious dysrhythmias
Zidovudine: ↓ effect of zidovudine

Drug classifications

Ergots: ↑ serious dysrhythmias
Oral contraceptives: ↓ effect of contraceptive

Food/drug

↑ Absorption with food

NURSING CONSIDERATIONS

Assessment

- Assess signs of infection, anemia
- Monitor liver studies: ALT, AST
- Monitor C&S before drug therapy; drug may be taken as soon as culture is performed; repeat C&S after treatment; determine the presence of other sexually transmitted diseases
- Assess bowel pattern before, during treatment; if severe abdominal pain with bleeding occurs, drug should be discontinued; monitor hydration
- Assess skin eruptions, rash, urticaria, itching
- Assess allergies before treatment, reaction of each medication; place allergies on chart
- Monitor viral load, CD_4 cell counts baseline and throughout treatment

Nursing diagnoses

✓ Infection, risk for (uses)
✓ Knowledge deficit (teaching)

Implementation

- Administer with food
- Oral powder can be mixed with fluids, do not mix with juice or acidic fluids, stable mixed for 6 hr

Patient/family education

- Advise patient to take with meal or snack; if dose is missed, take as soon as remembered up to 1 hr before next dose; do not double dose
- Advise patient to avoid taking with other medications, unless directed by prescriber
- Teach patient that drug does not cure, but manages symptoms, does not prevent transmission of HIV to others
- Teach patient to use nonhormonal form of contraception while taking this drug

N

neomycin (℞)

(nee-oh-mye'sin)

Mycifradin, Myciguent

Func. class.: Antiinfective

Chem. class.: Aminoglycoside

Pregnancy category C

Action: Interferes with protein synthesis in bacterial cell by binding to 30S ribosomal subunit causing inaccurate peptide sequence to form in protein chain, resulting in bacterial death

➔ **Therapeutic Outcome:** Bactericidal effects for *Pseudomonas aeruginosa, Escherichia coli, Enterobacter,* enteropathogenic *Escherichia coli, Klebsiella pneumoniae, Proteus vulgaris*

Uses: Severe systemic infections of CNS, respiratory tract, GI tract, urinary tract, eye, bone, skin, soft tissues, also used for hepatic coma, preoperatively to sterilize bowel, infectious diarrhea; minor skin infections (top)

Dosage and routes

Hepatic encephalopathy

Adult: PO 4-12 g/day in divided doses times 5-6 days

P ***Child:*** PO 50-100 mg/kg/day in divided doses

Preoperative intestinal antisepsis

Adult: PO on 3rd day of a 3-day regimen; give 1 g early PM; repeat in 1 hr; repeat at hs (given with erythromycin); give saline cathartic before giving this drug

P ***Child:*** PO 14.7 mg/kg or 4.7 mg/m^2 q4h × 3 days

Skin infection

P ***Adult and child:*** TOP 0.5% cream or ointment qd-tid

Available forms: Tabs 500 mg; top 500 mg; oral sol 125 mg/5 ml

Adverse effects

CNS: Confusion, depression, numbness, tremors, **seizures,** muscle twitching, **neurotoxicity,** dizziness, vertigo

CV: Hypotension, hypertension, palpitations

EENT: *Ototoxicity,* deafness, visual disturbances, tinnitus

GI: *Nausea, vomiting, anorexia,* increased ALT, AST, bilirubin, hepatomegaly, **hepatic necrosis,** splenomegaly

GU: **Oliguria, hematuria, renal damage, azotemia, renal failure, nephrotoxicity**

HEMA: **Agranulocytosis, thrombocytopenia,** leukopenia, eosinophilia, anemia

INTEG: *Rash,* burning, urticaria, photosensitivity, dermatitis, alopecia

Contraindications: Bowel obstruction (PO use), severe renal P disease, hypersensitivity, infants, children

Precautions: Mild renal disease, pregnancy **C,** hearing deficits, lactation, myasthenia gravis, Parkinson's disease

Pharmacokinetics

Absorption	Well absorbed (IM); minimally absorbed (top)
Distribution	Unknown
Metabolism	Liver, minimal
Excretion	Feces, unchanged
Half-life	2-3 hr

Pharmacodynamics

	IM
Onset	Rapid
Peak	1-2 hr
Duration	6-8 hr

Interactions

Individual drugs

Amphotericin B: ↑ ototoxicity, neurotoxicity, nephrotoxicity

Cisplatin: ↑ ototoxicity, neurotoxicity, nephrotoxicity

Ethacrynic acid: ↑ ototoxicity, neurotoxicity, nephrotoxicity

Furosemide: ↑ ototoxicity, neurotoxicity, nephrotoxicity
Mannitol: ↑ ototoxicity, neurotoxicity, nephrotoxicity
Methoxyflurane: ↑ ototoxicity, neurotoxicity, nephrotoxicity
Polymyxin: ↑ ototoxicity, neurotoxicity, nephrotoxicity
Succinylcholine: ↑ neuromuscular blockade, respiratory depression
Vancomycin: ↑ ototoxicity, neurotoxicity, nephrotoxicity

Drug classifications

Aminoglycosides: ↑ otoxicity, neurotoxicity, nephrotoxicity
Anesthetics, inhalation: ↑ neuromuscular blockade, respiratory depression
Nondepolarizing neuromuscular blockers: ↑ neuromuscular blockade, respiratory depression

NURSING CONSIDERATIONS

Assessment

- Assess patient for previous sensitivity reaction
- Assess patient for signs and symptoms of infection: characteristics of skin; obtain baseline information and during treatment
- Obtain C&S before beginning drug therapy to identify if correct treatment has been initiated
- Assess for allergic reactions: rash, urticaria, pruritus, chills, fever, joint pain

Nursing diagnoses

✓ Infection, risk for (uses)
✓ Knowledge deficit (teaching)
✓ Noncompliance (teaching)

Implementation

PO route

- Give as a preoperative medication before bowel surgery

Patient/family education

- Instruct patient to take all medication prescribed for the length of time ordered
- Advise patient to report headache, dizziness, symptoms of overgrowth of infection and loss of hearing, ringing or roaring in ears

Evaluation

Positive therapeutic outcome

- Reported improvement in symptoms of infection (top)

Treatment of overdose:

Withdraw drug; hemodialysis; monitor serum levels of drug

neostigmine (℞)

(nee-oh-stig'meen)

neostigmine, Prostigmin

Func. class.: Cholinergic stimulant; anticholinesterase

Chem. class.: Quaternary compound

Pregnancy category C

Action: Inhibits destruction of acetylcholine, which increases concentration at sites where acetylcholine is released; this facilitates transmission of impulses across the myoneural junction

➔ **Therapeutic Outcome:** Increased strength in myasthenia gravis, reversal of nondepolarizing muscular blockers

Uses: Myasthenia gravis, nondepolarizing neuromuscular blocker, antagonist, bladder distention, postoperative ileus

Dosage and routes

Myasthenia gravis

Adult: PO 15 mg q3-4h, may increase to 375 mg/day; IM/**IV** 0.5-2 mg q1-3h

P ***Child:*** PO 2 mg/kg/day q3-4h

Nondepolarizing neuromuscular blocker antagonist

Adult: **IV** 0.5-2 mg slowly; may repeat if needed (give 0.6-1.2 mg atropine before this drug)

P ***Infant/child:*** **IV** 0.025-0.1 mg/kg/dose

Abdominal distention/ postoperative ileus

Adult: IM/SC 0.25-1 mg (1 : 4000) q4-6h depending on condition × 2-3 days

Renal dose

CrCl 10-50 ml/min 50% of dose; CrCl <10 ml/min 25% of dose

Available forms: Tabs 15 mg; inj 1 : 1000, 1 : 2000, 1 : 4000

Adverse effects

CNS: Dizziness, headache, sweating, weakness, **seizures,** incoordination, **paralysis,** drowsiness, LOC
CV: Tachycardia, **dysrhythmias,** bradycardia, hypotension, AV block, ECG changes, **cardiac arrest,** syncope
EENT: Miosis, blurred vision, lacrimation, visual changes
GI: *Nausea, diarrhea, vomiting, cramps,* increased peristalsis, salivary and gastric secretions
GU: Frequency, incontinence, urgency
INTEG: Rash, urticaria, flushing
RESP: **Respiratory depression, bronchospasm, constriction, laryngospasm, respiratory arrest, dyspnea**

Contraindications: Obstruction of intestine, renal system, bromide sensitivity, peritonitis

Precautions: Bradycardia, hypotension, seizure disorders, bronchial asthma, coronary occlusion, hyperthyroidism, dysrhythmias, peptic ulcer, pregnancy **C**, megacolon, poor GI motility, lactation, children [P]

Pharmacokinetics

Absorption	Poorly absorbed (PO), completely absorbed (**IV**)
Distribution	Unknown
Metabolism	Liver
Excretion	Kidneys
Half-life	40-90 min

Pharmacodynamics

	PO	IM	IV
Onset	45-75 min	10-30 min	4-8 min
Peak	Unknown	30 min	30 min
Duration	2½-4 hr	2½-4 hr	2-4 hr

Interactions

Individual drugs

Atropine: ↓ action of atropine
Mecamylamine: ↓ action of neostigmine
Polymyxin: ↓ action of neostigmine
Procainamide: ↓ action of neostigmine
Quinidine: ↓ action of neostigmine

Drug classifications

Antidepressants: ↑ antagonism
Antihistamines: ↑ antagonism
Cholinesterase inhibitors: ↑ toxicity
Muscle relaxants, depolarizing: ↑ action of muscle relaxants
Phenothiazines: ↑ antagonism

NURSING CONSIDERATIONS

Assessment

- Monitor VS, respiration during rest
- [Alert] Monitor for bradycardia, hypotension, bronchospasm, headache, dizziness, seizures, respiratory depression; drug should be discontinued if toxicity occurs

Nursing diagnoses

✓ Breathing pattern, ineffective (uses)
✓ Knowledge deficit (teaching)

Implementation

PO route

- Give only after all other cholinergics have been discontinued
- Increased dosage as ordered may be needed if tolerance develops
- Give larger doses as ordered after exercise or fatigue
- Administer on empty stomach for better absorption
- Store at room temp

[IV] **IV route**

- Give direct **IV** undiluted, through Y-tube or 3-way stopcock; give 0.5 mg or less over 1 min

- Give only with atropine sulfate available for cholinergic crisis

Syringe compatibilities: Glycopyrrolate, heparin, pentobarbital, thiopental

Y-site compatibilities: Heparin, hydrocortisone sodium succinate, potassium chloride, vit B/C

Additive compatibilities: Netilmicin

Patient/family education

- Teach patient to wear ID specifying myasthenia gravis, drugs taken, prescriber's phone number

Evaluation

Positive therapeutic outcome

- Increased muscle strength, hand grasp
- Improved gait
- Absence of labored breathing (if severe)

Treatment of overdose: Respiratory support, **IV** atropine 1-4 mg

nesiritide

See Appendix A, Selected New Drugs

nevirapine (℞)

(ne-veer'a-peen)

Viramune

Func. class.: Antiretroviral

Chem. class.: Non-nucleoside reverse transcriptase inhibitor (NNRTI)

Pregnancy category C

Action: Binds directly to reverse transcriptase and blocks RNA, DNA causing a disruption of the enzyme's site

➔ **Therapeutic Outcome:** Improvement of HIV-1 infection

Uses: HIV-1 in combination with nucleoside analogs in those experiencing deterioration

Dosage and routes

Adult: PO 200 mg qd × 2 wk, then 200 mg bid in combination with nucleoside analogs

P ***Child ≥8 yr:*** PO 4 mg/kg qd × 2 wk, then 4 mg/kg bid

P ***Child 2 mo-8 yr:*** PO 4 mg/kg qd × 2 wk, then 7 mg/kg bid

Available forms: Tabs 200 mg; oral susp 50 mg/5 ml

Adverse effects

CNS: *Paresthesia, headache, fever, peripheral neuropathy*

GI: *Diarrhea,* abdominal pain, *nausea, stomatitis,* hepatitis, **hepatotoxicity**

HEMA: **Neutropenia, anemia, thrombocytopenia**

INTEG: *Rash,* **toxic epidermal necrolysis**

MISC: **Stevens-Johnson syndrome**

MS: Pain, myalgia

Contraindications: Hypersensitivity

Precautions: Liver disease, pregnancy **C**, lactation, P children, renal disease

Pharmacokinetics

Absorption	Rapid
Distribution	60% bound to plasma proteins
Metabolism	Liver
Excretion	Unknown
Half-life	Unknown

Pharmacodynamics

Unknown

Interactions

Drug classifications

Oral contraceptives: ↓ action

Protease inhibitors: ↓ action

Rifamycins: ↓ nevirapine levels

NURSING CONSIDERATIONS

Assessment

- Assess signs of infection, anemia
- Assess liver, renal, blood studies: ALT, AST; viral load, CD_4
- Assess C&S before drug therapy; drug may be taken as soon as culture is performed; repeat C&S after treatment; determine the presence of other sexually transmitted disease
- Assess bowel pattern before, during treatment; if severe abdominal pain with bleeding occurs, drug should be discontinued; monitor hydration
- Assess skin eruptions; rash, urticaria, itching
- Assess allergies before treatment, reaction to each medication; place allergies on chart

Nursing diagnoses

- ✓ Infection, risk for (uses)
- ✓ Diarrhea (side effects)
- ✓ Knowledge deficit (teaching)

Implementation

- Give without regard to meals

Patient/family education

- Instruct patient to report any right quadrant pain, jaundice, rash immediately
- Inform patient that drug may be taken with food, antacids, didanosine
- Advise patient to take as prescribed; if dose is missed, take as soon as remembered up to 1 hr before next dose; do not double dose
- Advise patient that drug must be taken in equal intervals around the clock to maintain blood levels for duration of therapy
- Advise patient that drug is not a cure, controls symptoms of HIV
- Instruct patient to avoid OTC agents unless approved by prescriber
- Advise patient to use a nonhormonal form of contraception during treatment

niacin

(nye'a-sin)

Edur-Acin, Nia-Bid, Niac, Niacels, Niacor, Niaspan, Nico-400, Nicobid, Nicolar, Nicotinex

nicotinic acid

(nick-oh-tin'ick)

Novo-Niacin ✤, Slo-Niacin, vitamin B

niacinamide

(nye-a-sin'a-mide)

nicotinamide

(nick-oh-tin'ah-mide)

Func. class.: Vitamin B_3
Chem. class.: Water-soluble vitamin, lipid-lowering drug

Pregnancy category C

Action: Needed for conversion of fats, protein, carbohydrates by oxidation-reduction; acts directly on vascular smooth muscle, causing vasodilatation; high dosages decrease serum lipids

➔ **Therapeutic Outcome:** Decreasing cholesterol and LDL levels, vitamin B_3 supplementation

Uses: Pellagra, hyperlipidemias, peripheral vascular disease

Dosage and routes

Niacin deficiency

Adult: PO 100-500 mg/day in divided doses; IM/SC 5-100 mg 5 or more times a day; **IV** 25-100 mg bid or tid

P ***Child:*** PO up to 300 mg/day in divided doses

Adjunct in hyperlipidemia

Adult: PO 500 mg qd in 3 divided doses pc; may be increased to 4 g/day

Pellagra

Adult: PO 300-500 mg qd in divided doses

P ***Child:*** PO 100-300 mg qd in divided doses

Peripheral vascular disease

Adult: PO 250-800 mg qd in divided doses

Available forms: Niacin, tabs 25, 50, 100, 125, 500 mg; time rel caps 125, 250, 300, 400, 500 mg; time ext tabs 125, 250, 375, 500, 750, 1000 mg; elixir 50 mg/5 ml; ext rel caps 125, 250, 300, 400, 500 mg; nicotinamide, tabs 50, 100, 125, 250, 500 mg

Adverse effects

CNS: Paresthesias, headache, dizziness, anxiety
CV: Postural hypotension, vasovagal attacks, dysrhythmias, vasodilatation
EENT: Blurred vision, ptosis
GI: Nausea, vomiting, anorexia, flatulence, xerostomia, *jaundice,* diarrhea, peptic ulcer
GU: Hyperuricemia, **glycosuria, hypoalbuminemia**
INTEG: Flushing, dry skin, rash, pruritus
RESP: Wheezing

Contraindications: Hypersensitivity, peptic ulcer, hepatic disease, lactation, hemorrhage, severe hypotension

Precautions: Glaucoma, CV disease, CAD, diabetes mellitus, gout, schizophrenia, pregnancy **C**

Do Not Confuse:
Nicobid/Nitro-Bid

Pharmacokinetics

Absorption	Well absorbed (PO)
Distribution	Widely distributed
Metabolism	Converted to niacinamide
Excretion	Urine, unchanged (30%); breast milk
Half-life	45 min

Pharmacodynamics

	PO	IV
Onset	Unknown	Unknown
Peak	30-70 min	Unknown
Duration	Unknown	Unknown

Interactions

Individual drugs

Guanadrel: ↑ hypotension
Guanethidine: ↑ hypotension
Lovastatin: ↑ myopathy
Probenecid: ↑ uricosuric effects
Sulfinpyrazone: ↑ uricosuric effects

Lab test interferences

↑ Bilirubin, ↑ alkaline phosphatase, ↑ liver enzymes, ↑ LDH, ↑ uric acid
↓ Cholesterol
False: ↑ Urinary catecholamines
False positive: Urine glucose

NURSING CONSIDERATIONS

Assessment

- Assess for niacin deficiency (pellagra): nausea, vomiting, stomatitis, confusion, hallucinations before and throughout treatment
- Assess for symptoms of niacin deficiency: nausea, vomiting, anemia, poor memory, confusion, dermatitis
- Assess for lipid, triglyceride, cholesterol level, if using for hyperlipidemia
- Assess nutrition: fat, protein, carbohydrates, nutritional analysis should be completed by dietitian
- Monitor liver function studies: AST, ALT, bilirubin, uric acid, alkaline phosphatase; blood glucose before and during treatment; liver dysfunction: clay-colored stools, itching, dark urine, jaundice
- Monitor niacin levels during administration of this drug
- Monitor cardiac status: rate, rhythm, quality; postural hypotension, dysrhythmias
- Monitor nutritional status: liver, yeast, legumes, organ meat, lean poultry; high-level niacin products should be included in the diet
- Assess for CNS symptoms: headache, paresthesias, blurred vision

Nursing diagnoses

✓ Nutrition, less than body requirements (uses)
✓ Knowledge deficit (teaching)
✓ Noncompliance (teaching)

N

Implementation

PO route

- Give with meals or milk for GI symptoms, and 325 mg of aspirin ½ hr before dose to decrease flushing
- Do not crush, break, or chew ext rel products

IV route

- Give by direct **IV** after diluting to 2 mg/ml at a rate of ≤2 mg/min
- Give by inf by adding 500 ml of 0.9% NaCl at a rate of ≤2 mg/min

Additive incompatibilities: Acids (strong), alkalis, erythromycin, kanamycin, streptomycin

Additive compatibilities: TPN sol

Patient/family education

- Advise patient that flushing and increase in feelings of warmth will occur several hr after taking drug (PO); after 2 wk of therapy these side effects diminish
- Instruct patient to remain recumbent if postural hypotension occurs; to rise slowly from sitting or recumbent
- Caution patient to abstain from alcohol if drug is prescribed for hyperlipidemia
- Caution patient to avoid sunlight if skin lesions are present

Evaluation

Positive therapeutic outcome

- Decreased lipid levels
- Warm extremities
- Absence of numbness in extremities

nicardipine (℞)

(nye-card'i-peen)

Cardene, Cardene IV, Cardene SR

Func. class.: Calcium channel blocker, antianginal, antihypertensive

Chem. class.: Dihydropyridine

Pregnancy category C

Action: Inhibits calcium ion influx across cell membrane during cardiac depolarization, produces relaxation of coronary vascular smooth muscle and peripheral vascular smooth muscle, dilates coronary arteries, increases myocardial oxygen delivery in patients with vasospastic angina

Therapeutic Outcome: Decreased angina pectoris, decreased B/P in hypertension

Uses: Chronic stable angina pectoris, hypertension

Dosage and routes

Adult: PO 20 mg tid initially; may increase after 3 days (range 20-40 mg tid) or 30 mg bid sus rel, may increase to 60 mg bid

Available forms: Caps 20, 30 mg; sus rel caps 30, 45, 60 mg; inj 2.5 mg/ml

Adverse effects

CNS: Headache, fatigue, drowsiness, dizziness, anxiety, depression, weakness, insomnia, confusion, paresthesia, somnolence

CV: **Dysrhythmia,** edema, **CHF,** bradycardia, hypotension, palpitations, **MI, pulmonary edema**

GI: Nausea, vomiting, diarrhea, gastric upset, constipation, **hepatitis,** abdominal cramps

GU: Nocturia, polyuria, **acute renal failure**

INTEG: Rash, pruritus, urticaria, photosensitivity, hair loss

MISC: Blurred vision, flushing, nasal congestion, sweating, shortness of breath, gynecomastia, hyperglycemia, sexual difficulties, **Stevens-Johnson syndrome**

Contraindications: Sick sinus syndrome, 2nd- or 3rd-degree heart block, hypotension <90 mm Hg systolic, hypersensitivity

Precautions: CHF, hypotension, hepatic injury, pregnancy **C,** lactation, children, renal disease, elderly

Do Not Confuse:
Cardene/Cardizem, Cardene SR/ Cardizem SR

Pharmacokinetics

Absorption	Well absorbed (PO); bioavailability poor
Distribution	Unknown
Metabolism	Liver, extensively
Excretion	Kidneys, minimal
Half-life	2-5 hr

Pharmacodynamics

	PO	PO–SUS REL
Onset	½ hr	Unknown
Peak	1-2 hr	2-6 hr
Duration	8 hr	10-12 hr

Interactions
Individual drugs
Alcohol: ↑ hypotension
Carbamazepine: ↑ risk of toxicity
Cimetidine: ↑ risk of toxicity
Cyclosporine: ↑ risk of toxicity
Digoxin: ↑ digoxin levels, bradycardia, CHF
Phenobarbital: ↓ effectiveness
Phenytoin: ↓ effectiveness
Prazosin: ↑ risk of toxicity
Propranolol: ↑ toxicity
Quinidine: ↑ risk of toxicity
Drug classifications
Antihypertensives: ↑ hypotension
β-Adrenergic blockers: ↑ bradycardia, CHF
Nitrates: ↑ hypotension
NSAIDs: ↓ antihypertensive effect
Food/drug
Grapefruit juice: ↑ hypotensive effect

NURSING CONSIDERATIONS
Assessment
- Assess fluid volume status (I&O ratio) and record weight, color, quality and sp gr of urine, skin turgor, adequacy of pulses, moist mucous membranes, bilateral lung sounds, peripheral pitting edema; dehydration symptoms of decreasing output, thirst, hypotension, dry mouth, and mucous membranes should be reported
- Monitor for CHF: weight gain, rales, jugular venous distention, dyspnea
- Monitor B/P and pulse
- Assess anginal pain: intensity, location, duration, alleviating factors
- Monitor potassium, LFTs, renal studies periodically

Nursing diagnoses
✓ Cardiac output, decreased (uses)
✓ Knowledge deficit (teaching)

Implementation
- Give with or without regard to meals
- Store in airtight container at room temp

IV route
- Dilute each 25 mg/240 ml of compatible sol (0.1 mg/ml), give slowly, stable for 24 hr at room temp

Y-site compatibilities:
Diltiazem, dobutamine, dopamine, epinephrine, fentanyl, hydromorphone, labetalol, lorazepam, midazolam, milrinone, morphine, nitroglycerin, norepinephrine, ranitidine, vecuronium

Patient/family education
- Advise patient to avoid hazardous activities until stabilized on drug and dizziness is no longer a problem
- Instruct patient to limit caffeine consumption; to avoid alcohol and OTC drugs unless directed by a prescriber
- Instruct patient to comply in all areas of medical regimen: diet, exercise, stress reduction, drug therapy; to notify prescriber of irregular heart beat, shortness of breath, swelling of feet and hands, pronounced dizziness, constipation, nausea, hypotension
- Teach patient to use medication as directed even if feeling better; may be taken with other cardiovascular drugs (nitrates, β-blockers)
- Teach patient to take medication exactly as prescribed
- Advise patient to contact prescriber if anginal attacks continue or become worse

N

Evaluation

Positive therapeutic outcome

- Decreased angina attacks
- Decreased B/P

Treatment of overdose: Defibrillation, atropine for AV block, vasopressor for hypotension

nicotinamide

See niacin

nicotine (OTC)

(nik'o-teen)

nicotine chewing gum (OTC)

Nicorette, Nicotine Gum

nicotine inhaler (℞)

Nicotrol Inhaler

nicotine nasal spray (℞)

Nicotrol NS

nicotine transdermal (OTC)

Habitrol, NicoDerm CQ, Nicotine Transdermal System, Nicotrol

Func. class.: Smoking deterrent

Chem. class.: Ganglionic cholinergic agonist

Pregnancy category D

Action: Agonist at nicotinic receptors in the peripheral and central nervous systems; acts at sympathetic ganglia, on chemoreceptors of the aorta and carotid bodies; also affects adrenalin-releasing catecholamines

➔ **Therapeutic Outcome:** Decreased withdrawal effects when smoking cessation is attempted

Uses: Deter cigarette smoking

Investigational uses: Gilles de la Tourette's syndrome

Dosage and routes

Habitrol, NicoDerm

Adult: 21 mg/day × 4-8 wk; 14 mg/day × 2-4 wk; 7 mg/day × 2-4 wk

Nicotine chewing gum

Adult: Gum 1 piece chewed × 30 min as needed to abstain from smoking; not to exceed 30/day

Nicotine inhaler

Adult: Inhale 6 cartridges/day for first 3-6 wk, max 16/day × 12 wk

Nicotine nasal spray

Adult: 1 spray in each nostril 1-2 ×/hr, max 5 ×/hr or 40 ×/day, max 3 mo

Nicotrol

Adult: 15 mg/day × 12 wk; 10 mg/day × 2 wk; 5 mg/day × 2 wk

Nicotrol Inhaler

Adult: Delivers 30% of what a smoker receives from an actual cigarette

Prostep

Adult: 22 mg/day × 4-8 wk; 11 mg/day × 2-4 wk

Available forms: Gum 2, 4 mg/piece; nicotine transdermal system 7, 14, 21 mg/day delivered (Habitrol, NicoDerm, Nicotine Transdermal System); NicoDerm 5, 10, 15 mg/day; nicotine inhaler 4 mg delivered; nasal spray 0.5 mg of nicotine/actuation

Adverse effects

CNS: Dizziness, vertigo, insomnia, headache, confusion, convulsions, depression, euphoria, numbness, tinnitus, strange dreams

CV: **Dysrhythmias,** tachycardia, palpitations, edema, flushing, hypertension

EENT: Jaw ache, irritation in buccal cavity

GI: Nausea, vomiting, anorexia, indigestion, diarrhea, abdominal pain, constipation, eructation

RESP: Breathing difficulty, cough, hoarseness, sneezing, wheezing

Contraindications: Hypersensitivity, immediate post-MI recovery period, severe angina pectoris, pregnancy **D**

Precautions: Vasospastic disease, dysrhythmias, diabetes mellitus, hyperthyroidism, pheochromocytoma, coronary disease, esophagitis, peptic ulcer, lactation, hepatic/renal disease

Pharmacokinetics

Absorption	Slowly absorbed, buccal cavity
Distribution	Unknown
Metabolism	Liver; some by lungs, kidneys
Excretion	Kidneys, unchanged (20%); breast milk
Half-life	1-2 hr

Pharmacodynamics

Onset	Rapid
Peak	½ hr
Duration	Unknown

Interactions
Individual drugs
Acetaminophen: ↑ effects of acetaminophen
Caffeine: ↑ effects of caffeine
Furosemide: ↑ effects of furosemide
Imipramine: ↑ effects of imipramine
Oxazepam: ↑ effects of oxazepam
Pentazocine: ↑ effects of pentazocine
Propranolol: ↑ effects of propranolol

NURSING CONSIDERATIONS
Assessment
- Assess for adverse reaction to gum: irritation of buccal cavity, dislike of taste, jaw ache
- Assess for withdrawal symptoms: headache, fatigue, drowsiness, restlessness, irritability, severe cravings for nicotine products before, during, and after treatment
- Obtain a nicotine assessment: brand of cigarettes, chewing tobacco, cigars, number of each used per day; what increases need or activities performed when each is used
- Gum should not be used if temporomandibular condition exists
- Assess for nicotine toxicity: GI symptoms (nausea, vomiting, diarrhea), cardiopulmonary symptoms (decreased B/P, dyspnea, change in pulse), weakness, abdominal cramping, headache, blurred vision, tinnitus; drug should be discontinued

Nursing diagnoses
- ✓ Coping, ineffective individual (uses)
- ✓ Knowledge deficit (teaching)
- ✓ Noncompliance (teaching)

Implementation
- Give only prescribed amount, or toxicity may occur
- Protect gum from light and heat

Patient/family education
Transdermal patch
- Caution patient that patch is as toxic as cigarettes; to be used only to deter smoking
- Caution patient not to use during pregnancy; birth defects may occur
- Instruct patient to keep used and unused system out of reach of children and pets
- Instruct patient to apply once a day to a nonhairy, clean, dry area of skin on upper body or upper outer arm; to rotate sites to prevent skin irritation
- Instruct patient to stop smoking immediately when beginning patch treatment
- Teach patient to apply promptly after removing from protective pouch; system may lose strength

Inhaler
- Advise patient that puffing on mouthpiece delivers nicotine through the mouth lining
- Instruct patient to chew gum slowly for 30 min to promote buccal absorption of the drug; do not chew over 45 min
- Advise patient to begin drug withdrawal after 3 mo use; do not exceed 6 mo

N

- Teach patient all aspects of drug; give package insert to patient and explain; caution patient not to exceed prescribed dose
- Inform patient that gum will not stick to dentures, dental appliances
- Caution patient that gum is as toxic as cigarettes; it is to be used only to deter smoking
- Caution patient not to use during pregnancy; birth defects may occur

Evaluation

Positive therapeutic outcome

- Decrease in urge to smoke
- Decreased need for gum after 3-6 mo

nifedipine (℞)

(nye-fed'i-peen)

Adalat, Adalat CC, Apo-Nifed ♣, Novo-Nifedin ♣, Nu-Nifed ♣, nifedipine, Procardia, Procardia XL

Func. class.: Calcium channel blocker, antianginal, antihypertensive

Chem. class.: Dihydropyridine

Pregnancy category C

Action: Inhibits calcium ion influx across cell membrane during cardiac depolarization, produces relaxation of coronary vascular smooth muscle and peripheral vascular smooth muscle, dilates coronary vascular arteries, increases myocardial oxygen delivery in patients with vasospastic angina

➔ **Therapeutic Outcome:** Decreased angina pectoris, decreased B/P in hypertension

Uses: Chronic stable angina pectoris, vasospastic angina, hypertension

Investigational uses: Migraines, CHF, Raynaud's disease, anal fissures

Dosage and routes

Adult: PO immediate release, 10 mg tid; increase in 10-mg increments q4-6h, not to exceed 180 mg/24 hr or single dose of 30 mg; sus rel, 30-60 mg/day; may increase q7-14 days; doses >120 mg not recommended

P ***Child:*** PO 0.25-0.5 mg/kg/dose q4-6h, max 1-2 mg/kg/day

Anal fissures (off-label)

Adult: TOP 0.2% gel q12h × 21 days

Available forms: Caps 5, 10, 20 mg; ext rel tabs 10, 20, 30, 60, 90 mg; tabs 10 mg

Adverse effects

CNS: *Headache,* fatigue, drowsiness, *dizziness,* anxiety, depression, weakness, insomnia, ***lightheadedness,*** paresthesia, tinnitus, blurred vision, nervousness

CV: **Dysrhythmias,** edema, **CHF,** hypotension, palpitations, **MI, pulmonary edema,** tachycardia

GI: *Nausea,* vomiting, diarrhea, gastric upset, constipation, increased liver function studies, dry mouth

GU: Nocturia, polyuria

INTEG: Rash, pruritus, *flushing,* photosensitivity, hair loss

MISC: Sexual difficulties, cough, fever, chills

Contraindications: Hypersensitivity

Precautions: CHF, hypotension, sick sinus syndrome, 2nd- or 3rd-degree heart block, hypotension less than 90 mm Hg systolic, hepatic injury, P pregnancy **C,** lactation, children, renal disease

Pharmacokinetics	
Absorption	Well absorbed (PO)
Distribution	Unknown
Metabolism	Liver, extensively
Excretion	Unknown
Half-life	2-5 hr

Pharmacodynamics

	PO	PO-EXT REL
Onset	½ hr	Unknown
Peak	Unknown	Unknown
Duration	6-8 hr	24 hr

Interactions

Individual drugs

Alcohol: ↑ hypotension
Carbamazepine: ↑ risk of toxicity
Cimetidine: ↑ risk of toxicity
Cyclosporine: ↑ risk of toxicity
Digoxin: ↑ digoxin levels, bradycardia, CHF
Prazosin: ↑ risk of toxicity
Propranolol: ↑ toxicity
Quinidine: ↑ risk of toxicity

Drug classifications

Antihypertensives: ↑ hypotension
β-Adrenergic blockers: ↑ bradycardia, CHF
Nitrates: ↑ nitrates
NSAIDs: ↓ antihypertensive effect

Food/drug

Grapefruit juice: ↑ nifedipine level

Lab test interferences

Positive: ANA titer, direct Coombs' test

NURSING CONSIDERATIONS

Assessment

- Assess anginal pain: location, intensity, duration, character, alleviating, aggravating factors
- Monitor potassium, LFTs, renal studies periodically during treatment
- Assess fluid volume status (I&O ratio) and record weight, distended red veins, crackles in lung, color, quality and sp gr of urine, skin turgor, adequacy of pulses, moist mucous membranes, bilateral lung sounds, peripheral pitting edema; dehydration symptoms of decreasing output, thirst, hypotension, dry mouth, and mucous membranes should be reported
- Monitor ALT, AST, bilirubin daily; if these are elevated, hepatotoxicity is suspected
- Monitor cardiac status: B/P, pulse, respirations, ECG

Nursing diagnoses

- ✓ Cardiac output, decreased (uses)
- ✓ Pain (uses)
- ✓ Knowledge deficit (teaching)

Implementation

PO route

- Give without regard to meals
- Store in airtight container at room temp

Sublingual route

- Using a sterile needle puncture the cap and squeeze medication in buccal area (not an FDA-approved use)

Patient/family education

- Advise patient to avoid hazardous activities until stabilized on drug and dizziness is no longer a problem
- Instruct patient to limit caffeine consumption; to avoid alcohol and OTC drugs unless directed by prescriber
- Tell patient that ext rel tab has nonabsorbable shell, may appear in stools
- Instruct patient to comply in all areas of medical regimen: diet, exercise, stress reduction, drug therapy; to notify prescriber of irregular heart beat, shortness of breath, swelling of feet and hands, pronounced dizziness, constipation, nausea, hypotension
- Teach patient to use as directed even if feeling better; may be taken with other cardiovascular drugs (nitrates, β-blockers)

Evaluation

Positive therapeutic outcome

- Decreased angina attacks
- Decreased B/P

Treatment of overdose:

Defibrillation, atropine for AV block, vasopressor for hypotension

N

nilutamide (℞)
(nil-u'ta-mide)
Anandron ♣, Nilandron
Func. class.: Antineoplastic, hormone
Chem. class.: Antiandrogen

Pregnancy category C

Action: Interferes with testosterone uptake in the nucleus or testosterone activity in target tissues; arrests tumor growth in androgen-sensitive tissue, i.e., prostate gland, prostatic carcinoma is androgen-sensitive, so tumor growth is arrested

➡ **Therapeutic Outcome:** Decreased tumor size

Uses: Metastatic prostatic carcinoma, stage D2 in combination with surgical castration

Dosage and routes
Adult: PO 300 mg qd × 30 days, then 150 mg qd

Available forms: Tabs 50, 100 ♣, 150 mg

Adverse effects
CNS: Hot flashes, drowsiness, insomnia, dizziness, hyperthesia, depression
EENT: Delay in adaptation to dark
GI: Diarrhea, nausea, vomiting, elevated liver function studies, constipation, dyspepsia, **hepatotoxicity**
GU: Decreased libido, impotence, testicular atrophy, UTI, hematuria, nocturia, gynecomastia
HEMA: Anemia
INTEG: Rash, sweating, alopecia, dry skin
MISC: Edema
RESP: Dyspnea, URI, pneumonia, **interstitial pneumonitis**

Contraindications: Hypersensitivity, severe hepatic impairment, severe respiratory disease, women

Precautions: Pregnancy **C**

Pharmacokinetics

Absorption	Rapidly, completely
Distribution	Unknown
Metabolism	Unknown
Excretion	Urine, feces
Half-life	Unknown

Pharmacodynamics
Unknown

Interactions
Individual drugs
Phenytoin: ↑ toxicity
Theophylline: ↑ toxicity
Vitamin K: ↑ toxicity

NURSING CONSIDERATIONS
Assessment
- Monitor liver function studies: AST, ALT, alkaline phosphatase, which may be elevated
- Monitor for CNS symptoms: drowsiness, insomnia, dizziness
- Monitor chest x-rays routinely, baseline pulmonary function studies, dyspnea, cough, may indicate interstitial pneumonitis, discontinue treatment if this condition is suspected

Nursing diagnoses
☑ Infection, risk of (side effects)
☑ Knowledge deficit (teaching)

Implementation
- Administer without regard to meals
- Store at room temp

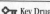

Patient/family education
- Advise patient to report side effects: decreased libido, impotence, breast enlargement, hot flashes, diarrhea, dyspnea, cough; symptoms of hepatotoxicity; notify prescriber immediately if shortness of breath occurs
- Advise patient to wear tinted lens to alleviate delay in adapting to the dark
- Advise patient that drug is started on day of or day after surgical castration
- Advise patient to avoid alcohol consumption

Evaluation

Positive therapeutic outcome

- Decrease in prostatic tumor size, decrease in spread of cancer

Treatment of overdose:

Induce vomiting, provide supportive care

nimodipine (℞)

(ni-moe'dip-een)

Nimotop

Func. class.: Calcium channel blocker

Chem. class.: Dihydropyridine

Pregnancy category C

Action: Unknown, may have greater effect on cerebral arteries

➔ **Therapeutic Outcome:** Prevention of vascular spasm (subarachnoid hemorrhage)

Uses: Prevention of cerebral vascular spasm in subarachnoid hemorrhage

Dosage and routes

Adult: PO Begin therapy within 96 hr, 60 mg q4h × 21 days

Available forms: Caps 30 mg

Adverse effects

CNS: Headache, fatigue, drowsiness, dizziness, anxiety, depression, weakness, insomnia, confusion, paresthesia, somnolence

CV: Dysrhythmia, edema, CHF, bradycardia, hypotension, palpitations, **MI, pulmonary edema**

GI: Nausea, vomiting, diarrhea, gastric upset, constipation, ***hepatitis,*** abdominal cramps

GU: Nocturia, polyuria, **acute renal failure**

INTEG: Rash, pruritus, urticaria, photosensitivity, hair loss

MISC: Blurred vision, flushing, nasal congestion, sweating, shortness of breath, gynecomastia, hyperglycemia, sexual difficulties

Contraindications: Sick sinus syndrome, 2nd- or 3rd-degree heart block, hypotension less than 90 mm Hg systolic, hypersensitivity

Precautions: CHF, hypotension, hepatic injury, pregnancy **C,** lactation, children, renal disease, elderly

Pharmacokinetics

Absorption	Well absorbed, bioavailability poor
Distribution	Crosses blood-brain barrier
Metabolism	Liver, extensively
Excretion	Kidneys
Half-life	1-2 hr

Pharmacodynamics

Onset	Unknown
Peak	1 hr
Duration	Unknown

Interactions

Individual drugs

Alcohol: ↑ hypotension

Digoxin: ↑ digoxin levels, bradycardia

Phenobarbital: ↓ effectiveness

Phenytoin: ↓ effectiveness

Propranolol: ↑ toxicity

Drug classifications

Antihypertensives: ↑ hypotension

β-Adrenergic blockers: ↑ bradycardia

Nitrates: ↑ nitrates

NURSING CONSIDERATIONS

Assessment

- Assess fluid volume status (I&O ratio) and record weight, distended red veins, crackles in lung, color, quality and sp gr of urine, skin turgor, adequacy of pulses, moist mucous membranes, bilateral lung sounds, peripheral pitting edema; dehydration symptoms of decreasing output, thirst, hypotension, dry mouth and mucous membranes should be reported
- Monitor B/P and pulse; if B/P drops 30 mm Hg, call prescriber

- Monitor ALT, AST, bilirubin daily; if these are elevated, hepatotoxicity is suspected

Nursing diagnoses

✓ Injury, risk for (uses)
✓ Knowledge deficit (teaching)

Implementation

- May puncture cap and dilute in water and give through nasogastric tube; flush tube with 0.9% NaCl
- Store in airtight container at room temp

Evaluation

Positive therapeutic outcome

- Prevention of neurologic damage from subarachnoid hemorrhage

nisoldipine (℞)

(nye'sol-dye-peen)

Sular

Func. class.: Antihypertensive, calcium channel blocker

Chem. class.: Dihydropyridine

Pregnancy category C

Action: Inhibits calcium ion influx across cell membrane, resulting in dilation of peripheral arteries

➔ **Therapeutic Outcome:** Decreased B/P in hypertension

Uses: Essential hypertension, alone or with other antihypertensives

Dosage and routes

Adult: PO 20 mg qd initially, may increase by 10 mg/wk, usual dose 20-40 mg qd

G ***Elderly:*** PO 10 mg/day, increase by 10 mg/wk

Available forms: Tabs, ext rel 10, 20, 30, 40 mg

Adverse effects

CNS: Headache, fatigue, drowsiness, dizziness, anxiety, depression, nervousness, insomnia, light-headedness, paresthesia, tinnitus, psychosis, somnolence

CV: **Dysrhythmias,** edema, **CHF,** hypotension, palpitations, **MI, pulmonary edema,** tachycardia, syncope, AV block, angina

GI: Nausea, vomiting, diarrhea, gastric upset, constipation, elevated liver function studies, dry mouth

HEMA: Anemia

INTEG: Rash, pruritus

MISC: Flushing, sexual difficulties, cough, nasal congestion, shortness of breath, wheezing, epistaxis, respiratory infection, chest pain

Contraindications: Hypersensitivity, sick sinus syndrome, 2nd- or 3rd-degree heart block

Precautions: CHF, hypotension <90 mm Hg systolic, hepatic injury, P pregnancy **C,** lactation, children, renal G disease, elderly

Pharmacokinetics

Absorption	Well absorbed
Distribution	Unknown
Metabolism	Liver
Excretion	Kidneys
Half-life	Unknown

Pharmacodynamics

Unknown

Interactions

Individual drugs

Alcohol: ↑ hypotension
Carbamazepine: ↑ toxicity
Digoxin: ↑ digoxin levels, ↑ bradycardia, CHF
Phenobarbital: ↓ effectiveness
Phenytoin: ↓ effectiveness
Propranolol: ↑ toxicity

Drug classifications

Antihypertensives: ↑ hypotension
β-Adrenergic blockers: ↑ bradycardia, CHF
Nitrates: ↑ nitrates

Herb/drug

Angelica: ↑ antidysrhythmic effect
Cat's claw: ↑ antidysrhythmic effect
Chicory: ↑ antidysrhythmic effect

Food/drug
High-fat: ↑ nisoldipine level
Grapefruit juice: ↑ hypotension

NURSING CONSIDERATIONS
Assessment
- Assess fluid volume status: I&O ratio and record; weight; skin turgor; adequacy of pulses; moist mucous membranes; bilateral lung sounds; peripheral pitting edema; dehydration symptoms of decreasing output, thirst, hypotension, dry mouth, and mucous membranes should be reported
- Monitor ALT, AST, bilirubin daily, if these are elevated and hepatotoxicity is suspected
- Monitor cardiac status: B/P, pulse, respiration, ECG

Nursing diagnoses
✓ Cardiac output, decreased (uses)
✓ Knowledge deficit (teaching)

Implementation
- Give once a day, with food to decrease GI symptoms, avoid high-fat foods, grapefruit

Patient/family education
- Caution patient to avoid hazardous activities until stabilized on drug, and dizziness is no longer a problem
- Instruct patient to limit caffeine consumption; to avoid alcohol and OTC drugs unless directed by prescriber
- Urge patient to comply in all areas of medical regimen: diet, exercise, stress reduction, drug therapy; to notify prescriber of irregular heart beat, shortness of breath, swelling of feet and hands, pronounced dizziness, constipation, nausea, hypotension
- Teach patient to use as directed even if feeling better; may be taken with other cardiovascular drugs (nitrates, beta blockers)
- Advise patient to rise slowly to prevent orthostatic hypotension
- Teach patient to report nausea, dizziness, edema, shortness of breath, palpitations

Evaluation
Positive therapeutic outcome
- Decreased B/P

nitric oxide (℞)
INOmax
Func. class.: Respiratory inhalant
Pregnancy category C

Action: Increases partial pressure of arterial oxygen (PaO_2) by dilating pulmonary vessels, and redistributing pulmonary blood flow

➔ **Therapeutic Outcome:** Ability
P of neonate to breathe without assistance

Uses: Treatment of term and near term (>34 wk) neonates with hypoxic respiratory failure associated with pulmonary hypertension; used with other agents and ventilatory support

Dosage and routes
P ***Neonate:*** INH 20 ppm × up to 2 wk until O_2 desaturation has been resolved and neonate is ready to be weaned from therapy

Available forms: Cylinders side D, size 88

Adverse effects
CV: *Hypotension*
GU: *Hematuria*
MISC: *Hyperglycemia,* **sepsis,** *infection, cellulitis,* **stridor,** *withdrawal syndrome,* **methemoglobinemia, intracranial hemorrhage, cerebral infarction, seizures, pulmonary/GI hemorrhage**
RESP: *Atelectasis*

Contraindications: Dependence on right to left shunting of blood, hypersensitivity

Precautions: Bradycardia, rales, infections, pregnancy **C**

N

Pharmacokinetics

Absorption	Unknown
Distribution	Lung
Metabolism	Unknown
Excretion	Unknown
Half-life	Unknown

Pharmacodynamics

Unknown

Interactions

Individual drugs

Nitroglycerin: ↑ effect possible
Nitroprusside: ↑ effect possible

NURSING CONSIDERATIONS

Assessment

- Assess respiratory rate, rhythm, character, chest expansion, color, transcutaneous saturation, ABGs; monitor ECG, for methemoglobinemia

Nursing diagnoses

✓ Gas exchange, impaired (uses)
✓ Knowledge deficit (teaching)

Implementation

P • Use only in neonates, not indicated for other populations
P • Neonate must be weaned off therapy; do not discontinue abruptly

Patient/family education

- Explain disease process and purpose of medication to parents; communicate neonate's progress P

Evaluation

Positive therapeutic outcome

- Significant improvement of hypoxia, pulmonary hypertension

nitroglycerin 🔑 (℞)

(nye-troe-gli'ser-in)

extended-release buccal tablets (℞)
Nitrogard, Nitrogard SR ✱

extended-release capsules (℞)
Nitrocap TD, Nitroglyn, Nitrolin, Nitrospan, Nitro-Time

extended-release tablets (℞)
Nitrong

intravenous (℞)
Nitro-Bid IV, Tridil

spray (℞)
Nitrolingual

sublingual (℞)
Nitrostat, NitroQuick

topical ointment (℞)
Nitro-Bid, Nitrol

transdermal (℞)
Deponit, Minitran, Nitrek, Nitrocine, Nitrodisc, Nitro-Dur, Transderm-Nitro

Func. class.: Coronary vasodilator, antianginal
Chem. class.: Nitrate

Pregnancy category C

Action: Decreases preload and afterload, which thus decreases left ventricular end-diastolic pressure and systemic vascular resistance; dilates coronary arteries and improves blood flow through coronary vasculature

➡ **Therapeutic Outcome:** Prevention of anginal attack

Uses: Chronic stable angina pectoris, prophylaxis of angina pain, CHF associated with acute MI, controlled hypotension in surgical procedures

Dosage and routes

Adult: SL dissolve tab under tongue when pain begins; may repeat q5 min until relief occurs; take no more than 3 tab/15 min; use 1 tab prophylactically 5-10 min before activities; sus rel cap q6-12h on empty stomach; top 1-2 in q8h; increase to 4 in q4h as needed; **IV** 5 µg/min, then increase by 5 µg/min q3-5 min; if no response after 20 µg/min, increase by 10-20 µg/min until desired response; TD apply a pad qd to a site free from hair; remove patch hs to provide 10-12 hr nitrate-free interval to avoid tolerance; translingual spray 1-2 metered doses onto or under the tongue, max 3 sprays; transmucosal insert between lip and gums above incisors or between gum and cheek 1 mg q3-5 hr during waking hr

P ***Child:*** **IV** initial 0.25-0.5 mg/kg/min, titrate to patient response, usual dose 1-3 mg/kg/min

Available forms: Buccal tabs 1, 2, 3 mg; aerosol 0.4 mg/m spray; sus rel caps 2.5, 6.5, 9, 13 mg; sus rel tabs 2.6, 6.5, 9 mg; inj 0.5, 5 mg/ml; SL tabs 0.15, 0.3, 0.4, 0.6 mg; trans oint 2%; trans syst 0.1, 0.2, 0.3, 0.4, 0.6 mg/24 hr; inj 25, 50, 100 mg/250 ml, 50, 200 mg/500 ml; patches 22.4, 44.8, 67.2 mg

Adverse effects

CNS: *Headache, flushing, dizziness*
CV: *Postural hypotension,* tachycardia, **collapse,** syncope
GI: Nausea, vomiting
INTEG: Pallor, sweating, rash

Pharmacokinetics

Absorption	Well absorbed (PO, buccal, SL)
Distribution	Unknown
Metabolism	Liver, extensively
Excretion	Kidney
Half-life	1-4 min

Contraindications: Hypersensitivity to this drug or nitrites, severe anemia, increased ICP, cerebral hemorrhage

Precautions: Postural hypotension, pregnancy **C**, lactation

Interactions

Individual drugs
Alcohol: ↑ hypotension
Haloperidol: ↑ hypotension

Do Not Confuse:
Nitro-Bid/Nicobid

Drug classifications
Antidepressants, tricyclic: ↓ absorption of SL, transmucosal
Antihistamines: ↓ absorption of SL, transmucosal
Antihypertensives: ↑ hypotension
β-Adrenergic blockers: ↑ hypotension
Calcium channel blockers: ↑ hypotension
Phenothiazines: ↓ absorption of SL, transmucosal

NURSING CONSIDERATIONS

Assessment

- Monitor orthostatic B/P, pulse
- Assess pain: duration, time started, activity being performed, character; check for tolerance if taken over long period
- Monitor for headache, lightheadedness, decreased B/P; may indicate a need for decreased dosage

Nursing diagnoses

- ✓ Cardiac output, decreased (uses)
- ✓ Poisoning (uses)
- ✓ Tissue perfusion, decreased (uses)
- ✓ Knowledge deficit (teaching)
- ✓ Noncompliance (teaching)

Pharmacodynamics

	SUS REL	SL	TD	IV	TRANSMUCOSAL	AEROSOL	TOP OINT
Onset	20-45 min	1-3 min	½-1 hr	1-2 min	3 min	2 min	½-1 hr
Peak	Unknown	Unknown	Unknown	Unknown	Unknown	Unknown	Unknown
Duration	3-8 hr	½ hr	12-24 hr	3-5 min	3-5 hr	½-1 hr	2-12 hr

N

Implementation

IV route

- Give **IV** diluted in amount specified D_5W, or 0.9% NaCl for inf; use glass inf bottles, non–polyvinyl chloride inf tubing; titrate to patient response; do not use filters

Syringe compatibilities:
Heparin

Y-site compatibilities:
Amiodarone, amphotericin B cholesteryl, amrinone, atracurium, cefmetazole, cisatracurium, diltiazem, dobutamine, dopamine, epinephrine, esmolol, famotidine, fentanyl, fluconazole, furosemide, haloperidol, heparin, hydromorphone, regular insulin, labetalol, lidocaine, lorazepam, midazolam, milrinone, morphine, nicardipine, nitroprusside, norepinephrine, pancuronium, ranitidine, remifentanil, streptokinase, tacrolimus, theophylline, vecuronium

Y-site incompatibilities:
Alteplase

Additive compatibilities:
Alteplase, aminophylline, dobutamine, dopamine, enalaprilat, furosemide, lidocaine, verapamil

Additive incompatibilities:
Manufacturer recommends that nitroglycerin not be admixed with other medications

SL route

- Keep tab in original container
- If 3 SL tab in 15 min do not relieve pain, consider diagnosis of MI
- SL tab should be held under tongue until dissolved (a few min); do not take anything by mouth when SL tab is in place

PO route

- Give 1 hr ac or 2 hr pc with 8 oz of water
- Sus rel tab should not be chewed or crushed

Transmucosal route

- Tab should be placed between cheek and gum line
- Do not take anything PO when tab is in place

Topical route

- Apply ointment using dose-measuring papers supplied; apply to an area without hair; ointment should cover 2-3 in area; may apply an occlusive dressing as directed
- Apply TD patches to area without hair; press hard to adhere; if patch becomes dislodged, apply a new one

Patient/family education

- Teach patient to place buccal tab between lip and gum above incisors or between cheek and gum; sus rel tab must be swallowed whole, do not chew; SL should be dissolved under tongue, do not swallow; aerosol should be sprayed under tongue, do not inhale; use inhaler only when lying down; do not inhale spray
- Instruct patient to avoid alcohol
- Advise patient that drug may cause headache; tolerance usually develops; use nonnarcotic analgesic
- Teach patient that drug may be taken before stressful activity, exercise, sexual activity
- Inform patient that SL tab may sting when drug comes in contact with mucous membranes
- Caution patient to avoid hazardous activities if dizziness occurs
- Instruct patient to comply with complete medical regimen
- Advise patient to make position changes slowly to prevent fainting

Evaluation

Positive therapeutic outcome

- Decreased, prevention of anginal pain

HIGH ALERT

nitroprusside (℞)

(nye-troe-pruss'ide)

Nitropress, Sodium nitroprusside

Func. class.: Antihypertensive, vasodilator

Pregnancy category C

Action: Directly relaxes arteriolar, venous smooth muscle, resulting in reduction in cardiac preload, afterload

Therapeutic Outcome: Decreased B/P in hypertensive crisis, decreased preload, afterload

Uses: Hypertensive crisis, to decrease bleeding by creating hypotension during surgery, acute CHF, cardiogenic shock

Dosage and routes

Adult: **IV** inf dissolve 50 mg in 2-3 ml of D_5W, then dilute in 250-1000 ml of D_5W; run at 0.5-8 μg/kg/min

P ***Child:*** **IV** 0.3-0.5 mg/kg/min, titrate to response

Available forms: Inj 50 mg

Adverse effects

CNS: ***Dizziness, headache,*** agitation, twitching, decreased reflexes, **coma,** restlessness

CV: Palpitations, severe hypotension, dyspnea

EENT: Tinnitus, blurred vision

GI: Nausea, vomiting, abdominal pain

GU: Impotence

INTEG: Pain, irritation at inj site, sweating

MISC: **Cyanide, thiocyanate toxicity**

Contraindications: Hypersensitivity, hypertension (compensatory)

Precautions: Pregnancy **C,** lactation, P children, fluid, electrolyte imbalances, hepatic disease, renal disease, G hypothyroidism, elderly

Pharmacokinetics

Absorption	Complete bioavailability
Distribution	Not known
Metabolism	RBCs, tissues
Excretion	Kidneys
Half-life	Unknown

Pharmacodynamics

Onset	1-2 min
Peak	Rapid
Duration	1-10 min

Interactions

Drug classifications

Antihypertensives: ↑ hypotension

Ganglionic blockers: ↑ hypotension

Herb/drug

Angelica: ↑ nitroprusside effect

NURSING CONSIDERATIONS

Assessment

- Monitor B/P q5 min × 2 hr, then q1h × 2 hr; monitor pulse q4h; monitor jugular venous distention q4h; ECG should be monitored continuously; monitor PCWP
- Monitor electrolytes, blood studies: potassium, sodium, chloride, CO_2, CBC, serum glucose, serum methemoglobin if pulmonary oxygen levels are decreased
- Check weight, I&O, edema in feet and legs daily; assess skin turgor, dryness of mucous membranes for hydration status
- Assess for signs of CHF: dyspnea, edema, wet rales
- Monitor for increased lactate, cyanide, thiocyanate levels
- Monitor for decrease in bicarbonate, Pco_2 and blood pH; acidosis may occur with this drug

Nursing diagnoses

- ✓ Tissue perfusion, altered (uses)
- ✓ Injury, risk for (adverse reactions)
- ✓ Knowledge deficit (teaching)

Implementation

- Give by cont inf after diluting 50 mg/2-3 ml of D_5W; further dilute in 250 ml of D_5W; use an infusion pump only; wrap bottle with aluminum foil to protect from light; observe for color change in inf; discard if highly discolored (blue, green, red); titrate to patient response; avoid extravasation

Syringe compatibilities: Heparin

Y-site compatibilities: Amrinone, atracurium, diltiazem, dobutamine, dopamine, enalaprilat, famotidine, lidocaine, nitroglycerin, pancuronium, tacrolimus, theophylline, vecuronium

Additive incompatibilities: Do not give with any other drugs

Patient/family education

- Teach patient to report headache, dizziness, loss of hearing, blurred vision, dyspnea, faintness; may indicate adverse reactions

Evaluation

Positive therapeutic outcome

- Decreased B/P in hypertension
- Absence of bleeding in surgery

Treatment of overdose: Administer amyl nitrite inh until 3% sodium nitrate sol can be prepared for **IV** administration, then inject sodium thiosulfate **IV**; correct drop in B/P with vasopressor

nizatidine (℞, OTC)

(ni-za'ti-deen)

Axid, Axid AR

Func. class.: H_2-Receptor antagonist

Chem. class.: Substituted thiazole

Pregnancy category C

Action: Blocks H_2 receptors thereby reducing gastric acid output

Therapeutic Outcome: Healing of duodenal ulcers or gastric ulcers; prevention of duodenal ulcers; decreases symptoms of gastroesophageal reflex disease (GERD)

Uses: Benign gastric and duodenal ulceration, prevention of duodenal ulcer recurrence, symptomatic relief of gastroesophageal reflux, heartburn prevention

Dosage and routes

Prophylaxis of duodenal ulcer

Adult: PO 150 mg qd hs

Gastric and duodenal ulcer disease

Adult: PO 300 mg at night or 150 mg bid for 4-8 wk; maintenance 150 mg at night

Gastroesophageal reflux

Adult: PO 150 mg bid

Heartburn prevention

Adult: PO 75 mg ac

Renal dose

CrCl 20-50 ml/min give 150 mg/day; CrCl <20 ml/min give 150 mg qod

Available forms: Caps 150, 300 mg; tabs 75 mg

Adverse effects

CNS: Headache, somnolence, confusion, abnormal dreams

ENDO: Gynecomastia

GI: Elevated liver enzymes, hepatitis, jaundice, nausea

HEMA: **Thrombocytopenia**

INTEG: Pruritus, sweating, urticaria, exfoliative dermatitis

METAB: Hyperuricemia

MS: Myalgia

RESP: **Bronchospasm, laryngeal edema**

Contraindications: Hypersensitivity

Precautions: Renal or hepatic impairment (reduce dose in renal impairment), pregnancy **C**, lactation

Pharmacokinetics

Absorption	PO 70%
Distribution	Breast milk, crosses placenta
Metabolism	Liver, partially
Excretion	Kidney
Half-life	1½ hr

Pharmacodynamics

Onset	Variable
Peak	½-3 hr
Duration	Unknown

NURSING CONSIDERATIONS

Assessment

- Assess patient with ulcers or suspected ulcers: epigastric or abdominal pain, hematemesis, occult blood in stools, blood or gastric aspirate before and throughout treatment, monitor gastric pH (5 should be maintained)
- Monitor I&O ratio, BUN, creatinine, CBC with differential monthly

Nursing diagnoses

✓ Pain (uses)
✓ Knowledge deficit (teaching)

Implementation

- May be given with or without meals
- Give antacids 1 hr before or 1 hr after this drug

Patient/family education

- Caution patient that gynecomastia, impotence may occur and are reversible after treatment is discontinued
- Advise patient to avoid driving, other hazardous activities until stabilized on this medication; drowsiness or dizziness may occur
- Caution patient to avoid black pepper, caffeine, alcohol, harsh spices, extremes in temp of food; tell patient to avoid OTC preparations: aspirin, cough, cold preparations because condition may worsen
- Caution patient not to take OTC and ℞ forms concurrently
- Inform patient that smoking decreases the effectiveness of the drug; that smoking cessation should be considered
- Instruct patient that drug must be continued for prescribed time to be effective and taken exactly as prescribed; doses should not be doubled; a missed dose should be taken as soon as remembered up to 1 hr before next dose
- Advise patient to report bruising, fatigue, malaise; blood dyscrasias may occur
- Advise patient to report diarrhea, black tarry stools, sore throat, rash, dizziness, confusion, or delirium to prescriber immediately

Evaluation

Positive therapeutic outcome

- Decreased pain in abdomen
- Healing of ulcers
- Absence of gastroesophageal reflux

norfloxacin (℞)

(nor-flox'a-sin)

Noroxin

Func. class.: Urinary antiinfective

Chem. class.: Fluoroquinolone antibacterial

Pregnancy category C

Action: Interferes with conversion of intermediate DNA fragments into high-molecular-weight DNA in bacteria

➔ **Therapeutic Outcome:** Bactericidal action against gram-positive *Staphylococcus epidermidis,* methicillin-resistant strains of *Staphylococcus aureus,* group D streptococci; gram-negative *Escherichia coli, Klebsiella pneumoniae, Enterobacter cloacae, Proteus mirabilis, Proteus vulgaris, Providencia rettgeri, Morganella morganii, Pseudomonas aeruginosa, Citrobacter freundii*

Uses: Adult UTIs (including complicated), uncomplicated gonorrhea, ocular infections

Dosage and routes

Uncomplicated infections

Adult: PO 400 mg bid × 3-10 days 1 hr ac or 2 hr pc

Complicated infections

Adult: PO 400 mg bid × 10-21 days; 400 mg qd × 7-10 days in impaired renal function

N

Uncomplicated gonorrhea
Adult: PO 800 mg as a single dose
Prostatitis
Adult: PO 400 mg bid × 4 wk
Occular infection
P ***Adult and child:*** Ophth i gtt qid; may increase to i gtt q2h for severe infections
Renal dose
CrCl ≤30 ml/min 400 mg PO qd

Available forms: Tabs 400 mg

Adverse effects

CNS: ***Headache, dizziness,*** fatigue, somnolence, depression, insomnia
EENT: Visual disturbances
GI: ***Nausea,*** constipation, increased ALT, AST, flatulence, heartburn, vomiting, diarrhea, dry mouth
INTEG: Rash

Contraindications: Hypersensitivity to quinolones

Precautions: Pregnancy **C**, lactation, P children, renal disease, seizure disorders

Pharmacokinetics	
Absorption	30% (PO)
Distribution	Concentration in urinary system
Metabolism	Liver (minimal)
Excretion	Kidneys, unchanged (30%)
Half-life	3-4 hr; increased in renal disease

Pharmacodynamics	PO
Onset	Unknown
Peak	1 hr

Interactions

Individual drugs
Cyclosporine: ↑ concentrations
Nitrofurantoin: ↓ effectiveness
Probenecid: ↑ blood levels
Sucralfate: ↓ absorption of norfloxacin
Theophylline: ↑ toxicity
Zinc sulfate: ↓ absorption of norfloxacin

Drug classifications
Antacids: ↓ absorption of norfloxacin
Anticoagulants, oral: ↑ effect of anticoagulants
Antineoplastics: ↓ norfloxacin levels
Iron salts: ↓ absorption of norfloxacin

Lab test interferences
↑ AST, ↑ ALT, ↑ BUN, ↑ creatinine, ↑ alkaline phosphatase

NURSING CONSIDERATIONS

Assessment

- Assess patient for previous sensitivity reaction
- Assess patient for signs and symptoms of infection including characteristics of urine, WBC >10,000/mm^3, temp; obtain baseline information before and during treatment
- Obtain C&S before beginning drug therapy to identify if correct treatment has been initiated
- Assess for allergic reactions: rash, urticaria, pruritus
- Monitor blood studies: AST, ALT, BUN, creatinine, alkaline phosphatase monthly if patient is on long-term therapy
- Assess bowel pattern qd; if severe diarrhea occurs, drug should be discontinued
- Assess for overgrowth of infection: perineal itching, fever, malaise, redness, pain, swelling, drainage, rash, diarrhea, change in cough, sputum

Nursing diagnoses

✓ Infection, risk for (uses)
✓ Diarrhea (adverse reactions)
✓ Injury, risk for (adverse reactions)
✓ Knowledge deficit (teaching)
✓ Noncompliance (teaching)

Implementation

PO route

- Give in equal intervals q12h around the clock to maintain proper blood levels; give with food to increase absorption of drug; do not give within

3 hr of other agents; drug interactions may occur; give with 8 oz of water
- Do not give with iron, zinc products, or antacids, which decrease absorption

Patient/family education
- Instruct patient to take all medication prescribed for the length of time ordered; drug must be taken around the clock to maintain blood levels; do not give medication to others; do not double doses; take any missed dose when remembered
- Advise patient to increase fluids to 2 L/day to prevent crystalluria
- Caution patient to avoid driving and other hazardous activities until response is known; dizziness may occur
- Instruct patient to use sunglasses to prevent photophobia
- Have patient use hard candy, frequent sips of water for dry mouth
- Teach patient correct instillation procedure (ophth)

Evaluation
Positive therapeutic outcome
- Reported improvement in symptoms of infection
- Absence of red or itching eyes (ophth)

nortriptyline (℞)
(nor-trip'ti-leen)

Aventyl, Pamelor

Func. class.: Antidepressant, tricyclic

Chem. class.: Dibenzocycloheptene, secondary amine

Pregnancy category C

Action: Blocks reuptake of norepinephrine, serotonin into nerve endings, increasing action of norepinephrine, serotonin in nerve cells; has anticholinergic effects

➡ **Therapeutic Outcome:** Decreased symptoms of depression after 2-3 wk

Uses: Major depression

Investigational uses: Chronic pain management

Dosage and routes
Adult: PO 25 mg tid or qid; may increase to 150 mg/day; may give daily dose hs

P G ***Adolescents and elderly:*** PO 10-25 mg qhs, increase by 10-25 mg at weekly intervals to desired dose; usual maintenance 30-50 mg qd

Available forms: Caps 10, 25, 50, 75 mg; sol 10 mg/5 ml

Adverse effects
CNS: *Dizziness, drowsiness,* confusion, headache, anxiety, tremors, stimulation, weakness, insomnia, G nightmares, EPS (elderly), increased psychiatric symptoms

CV: *Orthostatic hypotension, ECG changes, tachycardia,* **hypertension,** palpitations

EENT: Blurred vision, tinnitus, mydriasis

GI: *Constipation, dry mouth,* nausea, vomiting, **paralytic ileus,** increased appetite, cramps, epigastric distress, jaundice, **hepatitis,** stomatitis

GU: *Retention,* **acute renal failure**

HEMA: **Agranulocytosis, thrombocytopenia, eosinophilia, leukopenia**

INTEG: Rash, urticaria, sweating, pruritus, photosensitivity

Contraindications: Hypersensitivity to tricyclic antidepressants, recovery phase of MI, seizure disorders, prostatic hypertrophy

Precautions: Suicidal patients, severe depression, increased intraocular pressure, narrowangle glaucoma, urinary retention, cardiac disease, hepatic disease, hyperthyroidism, electroshock therapy, elective surgery, pregnancy **C**

Do Not Confuse:
nortriptyline/amitriptyline

N

Pharmacokinetics

Absorption	Well absorbed
Distribution	Widely distributed; crosses placenta
Metabolism	Liver, extensively
Excretion	Kidneys, breast milk
Half-life	18-28 hr; steady state 4-19 days

Pharmacodynamics

Unknown

Interactions

Individual drugs

Alcohol: ↑ CNS depression
Cimetidine: ↑ levels, toxicity
Clonidine: Severe hypotension; avoid use
Disulfiram: Organic brain syndrome
Fluoxetine: ↑ levels, toxicity
Guanethidine: ↓ effects

Drug classifications

Analgesics: ↑ CNS depression
Anticholinergics: ↑ side effects
Antihistamines: ↑ CNS depression
Antihypertensives: May block antihypertensive effect
Barbiturates: ↑ effects
Benzodiazepines: ↑ effects
CNS depressants: ↑ effects
MAOIs: Hypertensive crisis, convulsions
Oral contraceptives: ↑ effects, toxicity
Phenothiazines: ↑ toxicity
Sedative/hypnotics: ↑ CNS depression
Sympathomimetics, indirect-acting: ↓ effects

Smoking

↑ Metabolism, ↓ effects

▨ *Herb/drug*

Belladonna: ↑ anticholinergic effect
Henbane: ↑ anticholinergic effect
Scopolia: ↑ antidepressant effect

Lab test interferences

↑ Serum bilirubin, ↑ blood glucose, ↑ alkaline phosphatase
↓ VMA, ↓ 5-HIAA, ↓ blood glucose
False: ↑ Urinary catecholamines

NURSING CONSIDERATIONS

Assessment

- Monitor B/P (with patient lying, standing), pulse q4h; if systolic B/P drops 20 mm Hg, hold drug, notify prescriber; take VS q4h of patients with CV disease
- Monitor blood studies: CBC, leukocytes, differential, cardiac enzymes if patient is receiving long-term therapy
- Monitor hepatic studies: AST, ALT, bilirubin
- Check weight weekly; appetite may increase with drug
- Assess ECG for flattening of T wave, bundle branch block, AV block, dysrhythmias in cardiac patients
- G • Assess for EPS primarily in elderly: rigidity, dystonia, akathisia
- Assess mental status: mood, sensorium, affect, suicidal tendencies; increase in psychiatric symptoms: depression, panic
- Monitor urinary retention, P constipation; constipation is more G likely to occur in children or elderly
- ◆ • Assess for withdrawal symptoms: headache, nausea, vomiting, muscle pain, weakness; do not usually occur unless drug was discontinued abruptly
- Identify alcohol consumption; if alcohol is consumed, hold dose until AM

Nursing diagnoses

✓ Coping, ineffective individual (uses)
✓ Injury, risk for (adverse reactions)
✓ Knowledge deficit (teaching)
✓ Noncompliance (teaching)

Implementation

- Give with food or milk to decrease GI symptoms; mix conc with water, milk, fruit juice to disguise taste
- Give dose hs if oversedation occurs during day; may take entire dose hs; G elderly may not tolerate once/day dosing
- Store at room temp; do not freeze

Patient/family education

- Teach patient that therapeutic effects may take 2-3 wk

• Teach patient to use caution in driving and other activities requiring alertness because of drowsiness, dizziness, blurred vision; to avoid rising quickly from sitting to standing, G especially elderly
• Teach patient to avoid alcohol ingestion, other CNS depressants; teach patient not to discontinue medication quickly after long-term use; may cause nausea, headache, malaise
• Teach patient to wear sunscreen or large hat, since photosensitivity occurs
• Teach patient to increase fluids, bulk in diet if constipation, urinary G retention occur, especially elderly
• Teach patient to take gum, hard sugarless candy, or frequent sips of water for dry mouth

Evaluation

Positive therapeutic outcome

• Decrease in depression
• Absence of suicidal thoughts

Treatment of overdose: ECG monitoring, induce emesis, lavage, activated charcoal, administer anticonvulsant

nystatin (℞, OTC)

(nis′ta-tin)

Mycostatin, Mycostatin Pastilles, Nadostine ✤, Nyaderm ✤, nystatin, Nystex; topical: Mycostatin, Nilstat, Nodostine ✤, Nyoderm ✤, Nystatin, Nystex; vaginal: Mycostatin, Nilstat, Nadostine ✤, Nyoderm ✤, O-V Statin

Func. class.: Antiinfective
Chem. class.: Antifungal

Pregnancy category B; A (vaginal)

Action: Interferes with fungal DNA replication; binds sterols in fungal cell membrane, which increases permeability, resulting in leaking of cell nutrients

→ Therapeutic Outcome: Fungistatic/fungicidal against *Candida* organisms

Uses: *Candida* species causing oral, vaginal, intestinal infections; vag: cutaneous vulvovaginal candidiasis; top: mucocutaneous fungal infections, P infant eczema, pruritus ani and vulvae

Dosage and routes

Oral infection

Adult: Susp 400,000-600,000 U qid, use ½ dose in each side of mouth, swish and swallow

P ***Infants:*** 200,000 U qid (100,000 U in each side of mouth)

P ***Newborn and premature infants:*** Susp 100,000 U qid

P ***Adult and child:*** Troches 200,000-400,000 U qid × up to 2 wk

GI infection

Adult: PO 500,000-1,000,000 U tid

Topical

P ***Adult and child:*** Apply to affected area bid-tid × 14 days

Vaginal: 1-2 tabs (100,000 U each) inserted into vagina

Available forms: Tabs 500,000 U; powder 50, 150, 500 million, 1, 2, 5 billion U; troches 200,000 U; susp 100,000 U; cream, oint, powder, spray, vag tab 100,000 U; vag cream, lotion 2%

Adverse effects

GI: Nausea, vomiting, anorexia, diarrhea, cramps
INTEG: Rash, urticaria, stinging, burning

Contraindication: Hypersensitivity

Precautions: Pregnancy **B,** lactation

N

Pharmacokinetics

Absorption	Poorly absorbed
Distribution	Unknown
Metabolism	Not metabolized
Excretion	Feces, unchanged
Half-life	Unknown

Pharmacodynamics

Onset	Rapid
Peak	Unknown
Duration	6-12 hr

Interactions: None

NURSING CONSIDERATIONS
Assessment
- Assess for allergic reaction: rash, urticaria; drug may have to be discontinued
- Assess for predisposing factors for candidal infection: antibiotic therapy, pregnancy, diabetes mellitus, sexual partner infection (vag infections), AIDS

Nursing diagnoses
☑ Skin integrity, impaired (uses)
☑ Infection, risk for (uses)
☑ Knowledge deficit (teaching)

Implementation
PO route
- Give oral susp dose by placing ½ in each cheek, swish for several min, then swallow; shake susp before use
- Store oral susp in refrigerator, tab in airtight, light-resistant containers at room temp

Topical route
- Administer by moistening lesions with a swab coated with cream or ointment; use enough medication to cover lesions completely; give after cleansing with soap, water before each application; dry well

Vaginal route
- Insert vag tab high into vagina with applicator provided; administer in gravid client 3-6 wk before term to P decrease candidiasis in the newborn
- Store at room temp in dry place; protect from light, air, heat

Patient/family education
- Instruct patient that long-term therapy may be needed to clear infection; to complete entire course of medication
- Teach patient proper hygiene: use no commercial mouthwashes for mouth infection
- Advise patient to avoid getting preparation on hands
- Instruct patient to wear light-day pad for vag preparations to avoid soiling clothing; to avoid sexual contact during treatment to minimize reinfection
- Instruct patient to notify prescriber if irritation occurs; drug may have to be discontinued
- Inform patient that relief from itching may occur after 24-72 hr

Topical
- Advise patient to discontinue use and notify prescriber if irritation occurs
- Teach patient to apply with glove to prevent further infection; drug may stain
- Caution patient not to use occlusive dressings; to avoid use of OTC creams, ointments, lotions unless directed by prescriber

Evaluation
Positive therapeutic outcome
- Culture negative for *Candida*
- Decrease in size, number of lesions
- Decreased itching, white patches on vulva (vag)

octreotide (℞)
(ok-tree'-o-tide)
Sandostatin, Sandostatin LAR Depot
Func. class.: Hormone, antidiarrheal
Chem. class.: Octapeptide
Pregnancy category B

Action: Action similar to somatostatin

Therapeutic Outcome: Decreased diarrhea; decreased symptoms of acromegaly, carcinoid tumors, vasoactive intestinal peptide tumors (VIPomas)

Uses: Sandostatin: acromegaly, carcinoid tumors, VIPomas; LAR Depot: long-term maintenance of acromegaly, carcinoid tumors, VIPomas

Investigational uses: GI fistula, variceal bleeding, diarrheal conditions, pancreatic fistula, irritable bowel syndrome, dumping syndrome, acromegaly

Dosage and routes

Initial dose

Adult: **IV**/SC 50 μg bid-tid; cont SC inf has been used but is not approved

Acromegaly

Adult: SC 50 μg tid, adjust q2 wk based on Somatomedin C

VIPomas

Adult: SC 0.2-0.3 mg qd in 2-4 doses for 2 wk, not to exceed 0.45 mg qd

Carcinoid tumors

Adult: SC 0.1-0.6 mg qd in 2-4 doses for 2 wk, titrated to patient response

GI fistula

Adult: SC 50-200 μg q8h

Irritable bowel syndrome

Adult: SC 100 μg single dose to 125 μg bid

Dumping syndrome

Adult: SC 50-150 μg/day

Variceal bleeding

Adult: **IV** 25-50 μg/hr cont IV inf for 18 hr-5 days

Available forms: Sandostatin: inj 0.05, 0.1, 0.2, 0.5, 1 mg/ml; LAR Depot: inj 10 mg, 20, 30 mg/5 ml

Adverse effects

CNS: *Headache, dizziness, fatigue, weakness,* depression, anxiety, tremors, **seizures,** paranoia

CV: *Sinus bradycardia, conduction abnormalities,* **dysrhythmias,** chest pain, shortness of breath, thrombophlebitis, ischemia, **CHF,** hypertension, palpitations, edema

ENDO: *Hyperglycemia, ketosis, hypothyroidism, hypoglycemia,* galactorrhea, diabetes insipidus

GI: *Diarrhea, nausea, abdominal pain, vomiting, flatulence, distension, constipation,* **hepatitis,** elevated LFTs, **GI bleeding, pancreatitis,** fat malabsorption

GU: UTI, pollakiuria

HEMA: Hematoma of inj site, bruise

INTEG: Rash, urticaria, pain, inflammation at inj site

MS: Joint and muscle pain

Contraindications: Hypersensitivity

Precautions: Diabetes mellitus, G hypothyroidism, pregnancy **B,** elderly, P lactation, children, renal disease

Pharmacokinetics	
Absorption	Rapidly, completely
Distribution	Unknown
Metabolism	Little
Excretion	Urine, unchanged
Half-life	1.7 hr

Pharmacodynamics	
Onset	Unknown
Peak	½ hr
Duration	12 hr

Interactions

Individual drugs

Cyclosporine: Possible ↑ rejection

Food/drug

↓ Absorption of dietary fat, ↓ vit B_{12} levels

NURSING CONSIDERATIONS

Assessment

- Identify growth hormone antibodies, IGF-1, 1-4 hr intervals for 8-12 hr after dose in acromegaly; 5-HIAA, plasma serotonin, plasma substance P in carcinoid; VIP in VIPomas

O

- Fecal fat, serum carotene
- Monitor thyroid function tests: T_3, T_4, T_7, TSH to identify hypothyroidism
- Assess for allergic reaction: rash, itching, fever, nausea, wheezing
- Assess for cardiac status: bradycardia, conduction abnormalities, dysrhythmias; monitor ECG for QT prolongation, low voltage, axis shifts, early repolarization, R/S transition, early wave progression

Nursing diagnoses

✓ Body image disturbance (uses)
✓ Knowledge deficit (teaching)

Implementation

- Store unopened amps, vials in refrigerator; or room temp for 2 wk, protect from light; do not use discolored or cloudy sol

SC route

- Rotate inj sites

Patient/family education

- Explain reason for medication and expected results
- Advise patient that routine follow-up is needed
- Instruct parents on procedure for medication preparation and inj use; request demonstration, return demonstration; provide written instructions

Evaluation

Positive therapeutic outcome

- Decreased symptoms of acromegaly, carcinoid, VIPoma
- Decreased diarrhea

ofloxacin (Rx)

(o-flox'a-sin)

Floxin, Ocuflox

Func. class.: Antiinfective

Chem. class.: Fluoroquinolone

Pregnancy category C

Action: Interferes with conversion of intermediate DNA fragments into high-molecular-weight DNA in bacteria

Therapeutic Outcome: Bactericidal action against gram-positive pathogens *Staphylococcus epidermidis,* methicillin-resistant strains of *Staphylococcus aureus, Streptococcus pyogenes, Streptococcus pneumoniae;* gram-negative pathogens *Escherichia coli, Klebsiella* species, *Enterobacter, Salmonella, Shigella, Proteus vulgaris, Proteus rettgeri, Providencia stuartii, Morganella morganii, Pseudomonas aeruginosa, Serratia, Haemophilus* species, *Acinetobacter, Neisseria gonorrhoeae, Neisseria meningitidis, Yersinia, Vibrio, Brucella, Campylobacter,* and *Aeromonas* species; anaerobic pathogens *Bacteroides fragilis intermedius, Clostridium perfrigens, Gardnerella vaginalis, Peptococcus niger, Peptostreptococcus* species; *Chlamydia pneumoniae, Chlamydia trachomatis, Legionella pneumoniae, Mycobacterium tuberculosis, Mycoplasma pneumoniae*

Uses: Treatment of lower respiratory tract infections (pneumonia, bronchitis), genitourinary infections (prostatitis, UTIs), skin and skin structure infections, conjunctivitis (ophth)

Dosage and routes

Lower respiratory tract infection/skin and skin structure infections

Adult: PO/**IV** 200-400 mg q12h × 10 days

Cervicitis, urethritis

Adult: PO/**IV** 300 mg q12h × 7 days

Prostatitis

Adult: PO 300 mg q12h × 6 wk

Acute, uncomplicated gonorrhea

Adult: PO/**IV** 400 mg as a single dose

Urinary tract infection

Adult: PO/**IV** 200-400 mg q12h × 3-10 days

Conjunctivitis

P ***Adult and child:*** Ophth 1-2 gtt q2-4h × 2 days, then qid × 5 days

Renal dose

CrCl 10-50 ml/min give q24h; CrCl <10 ml/min give ½ of dose q24h

Available forms: Tabs 200, 300, 400 mg; inj 200, 400 mg; ophth sol 0.3%

Adverse effects

CNS: Dizziness, headache, fatigue, somnolence, depression, insomnia, lethargy, malaise
EENT: Visual disturbances
GI: Diarrhea, nausea, vomiting, anorexia, flatulence, heartburn, dry mouth, increased AST, ALT, abdominal pain, constipation
INTEG: Rash, pruritus

Contraindication: Hypersensitivity to quinolones

Precautions: Pregnancy **C**, lactation, P children, G elderly, renal disease, seizure disorders, excessive sunlight

Do Not Confuse:
Ocuflox/Ocufen

Pharmacokinetics

Absorption	Well absorbed (PO)
Distribution	Widely distributed
Excretion	Kidneys, unchanged; breast milk
Half-life	5-9 hr; increased in renal disease

Pharmacodynamics

	PO	IV	OPHTH
Onset	Rapid	Rapid	Unknown
Peak	1-2 hr	Inf end	Unknown

Interactions

Individual drugs

Calcium: ↓ ofloxacin effect
Cimetidine: ↑ ofloxacin effect
Nitrofurantoin: ↓ effectiveness
Probenecid: ↑ blood levels
Procainamide: ↑ procainamide level
Sucralfate: ↓ absorption of ofloxacin
Theophylline: ↑ toxicity
Zinc sulfate: ↓ absorption of ofloxacin

Drug classifications

Antacids: ↓ absorption of ofloxacin
Anticoagulants, oral: ↑ effect of anticoagulants
Antidiabetics: Altered blood glucose levels
Antineoplastics: ↓ ofloxacin levels
Iron salts: ↓ absorption of ofloxacin
NSAIDs: ↑ CNS stimulation, seizures
Theophyllines: ↑ theophylline effect

Food/drug

↓ absorption

Lab test interferences

Increase: ↑ AST, ↑ ALT, BUN, creatinine, alkaline phosphatase

NURSING CONSIDERATIONS

Assessment

- Assess patient for previous sensitivity reaction
- Assess patient for signs and symptoms of infection including characteristics of wounds, sputum, urine, stool, WBC >10,000/mm³, fever; obtain baselines and monitor during treatment
- Obtain C&S before beginning drug therapy to identify if correct treatment has been initiated
- Assess for allergic reactions: rash, urticaria, pruritus
- Monitor blood studies: AST, ALT, CBC, serum glucose monthly if patient is on long-term therapy
- Assess bowel pattern qd; if severe diarrhea occurs, drug should be discontinued
- Assess for overgrowth of infection: perineal itching, fever, malaise, redness, pain, swelling, drainage, rash, diarrhea, change in cough, sputum
- Assess for CNS symptoms: seizures, vertigo, drowsiness, agitation, confusion, tremors

Nursing diagnoses

- ✓ Infection, risk for (uses)
- ✓ Diarrhea (adverse reactions)
- ✓ Injury, risk for (adverse reactions)

O

☑ Knowledge deficit (teaching)
☑ Noncompliance (teaching)

Implementation

PO route

- Give in equal intervals q12h around the clock to maintain proper blood levels; do not give within 2 hr of other agents, since drug interactions are possible: give with 8 oz of water
- Do not give with iron, aluminum, zinc products or antacids, which decrease absorption and form insoluble chelate

IV route

- For intermittent inf, dilute to 4 mg/ml with D_5W, D_5/0.9% NaCl, 0.9% NaCl, D_5/LR, sodium bicarbonate, sodium lactate, D_5/Plasmalyte 56; give over 1 hr or more

Syringe compatibilities: cefotaxime

Y-site compatibilities: Ampicillin, cisatracurium, granisetron, propofol, remifentanil, thiotepa

Additive compatibilities: Amoxicillin, ceftazidime, clindamycin, gentamicin, piperacillin, tobramycin, vancomycin

Patient/family education

- Store for 2 wk refrigerated or 6 mo frozen, after reconstitution
- Instruct patient to take all medication prescribed for the length of time ordered; drug must be taken around the clock to maintain blood levels; do not give medication to others
- Teach patient to use sunscreen when outdoors to decrease phototoxicity
- Advise patient to increase fluids to 2 L/day to prevent crystalluria
- Caution patient to avoid driving and other hazardous activities until response is known; dizziness, confusion, drowsiness may occur

Evaluation

Positive therapeutic outcome

- Absence of signs/symptoms of infection (WBC <10,000/mm^3, temp WNL)
- Reported improvement in symptoms of infection
- Absence of red or itching eyes (ophth)

olanzapine (℞)

(oh-lanz'a-peen)

Zyprexa, Zyprexa Zydis

Func. class.: Antipsychotic/neuroleptic

Chem. class.: Thienbenzodiazepine

Pregnancy category C

Action: Unknown; may mediate antipsychotic activity by both dopamine and serotonin type 2 (5-HT_2) antagonism; also, may antagonize muscarinic receptors, histaminic (H_1)- and α-adrenergic receptors

Therapeutic Outcome: Decreased psychotic symptoms

Uses: Schizophrenia, acute manic episodes in bipolar disorder

Dosage and routes

Schizophrenia

Adult: PO 5-10 mg initially qd, may increase dosage by 5 mg at 1 wk or more intervals; orally disintegrating tabs: open blister pack, place tab on tongue, let disintegrate, swallow

Elderly: PO 5 mg, may increase cautiously at 1 wk intervals

Bipolar mania

Adult: PO 10-15 mg qd, may increase dose after 24 hr, by 5 mg

Available forms: Tabs 2.5, 5, 7.5, 10, 15, 20 mg

Adverse effects

CNS: EPS (pseudoparkinsonism, akathisia, dystonia, tardive dyskinesia), **seizures,** headache, **neuroleptic malignant syndrome (rare),**

fever, insomnia, somnolence, agitation, nervousness, hostility, dizziness, hypertonia, tremor, euphoria
CV: Orthostatic hypotension, tachycardia, chest pain
EENT: Blurred vision
GI: Dry mouth, nausea, vomiting, anorexia, constipation, abdominal pain, weight gain
GU: Urinary retention, urinary frequency, enuresis, impotence, amenorrhea, gynecomastia, breast engorgement, premenstrual syndrome
INTEG: Rash
MS: Joint pain, twitching
RESP: Dyspnea, rhinitis, cough, pharyngitis

Contraindications: Hypersensitivity

Precautions: Pregnancy **C**, lactation, hypertension, hepatic disease, G cardiac disease, elderly

Pharmacokinetics

Absorption	Well
Distribution	93% plasma protein binding
Metabolism	Liver
Excretion	Kidneys
Half-life	Unknown

Pharmacodynamics

Onset	Unknown
Peak	6 hr
Duration	Unknown

Interactions
Individual drugs
Alcohol: ↑ sedation
Bromocriptine: ↓ antiparkinson activity
Carbamazepine: ↓ levels of olanzapine
Diazepam: ↑ hypotension
Levodopa: ↓ antiparkinson activity
Omeprazole: ↓ olanzapine level
Rifampin: ↓ olanzapine level
Drug classifications
Anesthetics, barbiturates: ↑ sedation
Anticholinergics: ↑ anticholinergic effects
Antidepressants: ↑ sedation
Antihistamines: ↑ sedation
Antihypertensives: ↑ hypotension
Lab test interferences
↑ Liver function tests, ↑ prolactin, ↑ CPK

NURSING CONSIDERATIONS
Assessment
- Assess mental status, orientation, mood, behavior, presence of hallucinations and type before initial administration and monthly
- Monitor swallowing of PO medication: check for hoarding or giving of medication to other patients
- Monitor I&O ratio; palpate bladder if low urinary output occurs, especially G in elderly
- Monitor bilirubin, CBC
- Monitor urinalysis; recommended before, during prolonged therapy
- Assess affect, orientation, LOC, reflexes, gait, coordination, sleep pattern disturbances
- Monitor B/P sitting, standing, lying; take pulse and respirations q4h during initial treatment; establish baseline before starting treatment; report drops of 30 mm Hg; obtain baseline ECG
- Assess dizziness, faintness, palpitations, tachycardia on rising
- Assess for neuroleptic malignant syndrome: hyperpyrexia, muscle rigidity, increased CPK, altered mental status, for acute dystonia (check chewing, swallowing, eyes, pin rolling)
- EPS, including akathisia (inability to sit still, no pattern to movements), tardive dyskinesia (bizarre movements of the jaw, mouth, tongue, extremities), pseudoparkinsonism (rigidity, tremors, pill rolling, shuffling gait)
- Monitor skin turgor daily
- Monitor constipation, urinary retention daily; increase bulk, H_2O in diet

O

Nursing diagnoses
☑ Thought processes, altered (uses)
☑ Knowledge deficit (teaching)
☑ Noncompliance (teaching)

Implementation
- Give antiparkinsonian agent for EPS
- G Give decreased dose in elderly
- Give PO with full glass of water, milk; or with food to decrease GI upset
- Provide decreased stimuli by dimming light, avoiding loud noises
- Provide supervised ambulation until stabilized on medication; do not involve in strenuous exercise program because fainting is possible; patients should not stand still for long periods
- Give increased fluids to prevent constipation
- Give sips of water, candy, gum for dry mouth
- Store in airtight, light-resistant container
- Give orally disintegrating tabs: open blister pack, place tab on tongue until dissolved, swallow; no water needed

Patient/family education
- Teach patient to use good oral hygiene; frequent rinsing of mouth, sugarless gum for dry mouth
- Advise patient to avoid hazardous activities until drug response is determined
- Advise patient that orthostatic hypotension occurs often and to rise from sitting or lying position gradually
- Advise patient to avoid hot tubs, hot showers, tub baths, since hypotension may occur
- Advise patient to avoid abrupt withdrawal of this drug, or EPS may result; drug should be withdrawn slowly
- Advise patient to avoid OTC preparations (cough, hay fever, cold) unless approved by prescriber, since serious drug interactions may occur; avoid use with alcohol, CNS depresssants, increased drowsiness may occur
- Advise patient that in hot weather, heat stroke may occur; take extra precautions to stay cool

Evaluation
Positive therapeutic outcome
- Decrease in emotional excitement, hallucinations, delusion, paranoia, reorganization of patterns of thought, speech

Treatment of overdose:
Lavage if orally ingested; provide airway; do not induce vomiting or use epinephrine

omeprazole (℞)
(oh-mep'ra-zole)
Losec 🍁, Prilosec
Func. class.: Antiulcer, proton pump inhibitor
Chem. class.: Benzimidazole
Pregnancy category C

Action: Suppresses gastric secretion by inhibiting hydrogen/potassium ATPase enzyme system in the gastric parietal cell; characterized as a gastric acid pump inhibitor, since it blocks the final step of acid production

➔ **Therapeutic Outcome:** Absence of duodenal ulcers; decreased gastroesophageal reflux

Uses: Gastroesophageal reflux disease (GERD), severe erosive esophagitis, poorly responsive systemic GERD, pathologic hypersecretory conditions (Zollinger-Ellison syndrome, systemic mastocytosis, multiple endocrine adenomas); possibly effective for treatment of duodenal ulcers with or without antiinfectives for *Helicobacter pylori*

Investigational uses: Posterior laryngitis, enhancing pancreatin

Dosage and routes
Active duodenal ulcers
Adult: PO 20 mg qd × 4-8 wk; associated with *H. pylori* 40 mg QAM

and clarithromycin 500 mg tid on days 1-14, then 20 mg qd days 15-28

Severe erosive esophagitis/ poorly responsive GERD

Adult: PO 20 mg qd × 4-8 wk

Pathologic hypersecretory conditions

Adult: PO 60 mg/day; may increase to 120 mg tid; daily doses >80 mg should be divided

Gastric ulcer

Adult: PO 40 mg qd × 4-8 wk

G ***Elderly:*** Max 20 mg/day

Laryngitis (off-label)

Adult: PO 20-40 mg qhs × 6-24 wk or 20 mg bid × 4-12 wk

Available forms: Sus rel caps 20, 40 mg

Adverse effects

CNS: *Headache, dizziness, asthenia*
CV: Chest pain, angina, tachycardia, bradycardia, palpitations, peripheral edema
EENT: Tinnitus, taste perversion
GI: *Diarrhea, abdominal pain, vomiting, nausea, constipation, flatulence, acid regurgitation,* abdominal swelling, anorexia, irritable colon, esophageal candidiasis, dry mouth
GU: UTI, frequency, increased creatinine, **proteinuria, hematuria,** testicular pain, glycosuria
HEMA: **Pancytopenia, thrombocytopenia, neutropenia, leukocytosis,** anemia
INTEG: Rash, dry skin, urticaria, pruritus, alopecia
META: Hypoglycemia, increased hepatic enzymes, weight gain
MISC: *Back pain,* fever, fatigue, malaise
RESP: *Upper respiratory tract infections, cough,* epistaxis

Contraindications: Hypersensitivity

Precautions: Pregnancy **C**, lactation, children
P

Do Not Confuse:
Prilosec/Prinivil, Prilosec/prednisone, Prilosec/Prozac

Pharmacokinetics

Absorption	Rapidly absorbed
Distribution	Protein binding (95%); gastric parietal cells
Metabolism	Liver, extensively
Excretion	Kidneys, feces
Half-life	½-1 hr; increased in the G elderly, hepatic disease

Pharmacodynamics

Onset	1 hr
Peak	½-3½ hr
Duration	3-4 days

Interactions

Individual drugs

Ampicillin: ↓ absorption of omeprazole
Clarithromycin: ↑ omeprazole level
Diazepam: ↑ serum levels of diazepam
Flurazepam: ↑ omeprazole level
Ketoconazole: ↓ absorption of ketoconazole
Phenytoin: ↑ serum levels of phenytoin
Sucralfate: ↓ absorption
Triazolam: ↑ omeprazole level
Warfarin: ↑ bleeding tendencies

Drug classifications

Iron products: ↓ absorption of iron

Herb/drug

Angelica: ↓ omeprazole effect

NURSING CONSIDERATIONS

Assessment

- Assess GI system: bowel sounds q8h, abdomen for pain and swelling, anorexia
- Monitor hepatic enzymes: AST, ALT, increased alkaline phosphatase during treatment

Nursing diagnoses

✓ Pain (uses)
✓ Knowledge deficit (teaching)

O

Implementation

- Give before patient eats; patient should swallow cap whole
- Do not open, chew, or crush; may give with antacids

Patient/family education

- Advise patient to report severe diarrhea; drug may have to be discontinued
- Caution patient to avoid driving and other hazardous activities until response to drug is known
- Caution patient to avoid alcohol, salicylates, ibuprofen; may cause GI irritation

Evaluation

Positive therapeutic outcome

- Absence of epigastric pain, swelling, fullness

ondansetron (℞)

(on-dan'sa-tron)

Zofran

Func. class.: Antiemetic

Chem. class.: 5-HT receptor antagonist

Pregnancy category B

Action: Prevents nausea, vomiting by blocking serotonin (5-HT) peripherally, centrally, and in the small intestine

Therapeutic Outcome: Control of nausea, vomiting

Uses: Prevention of nausea, vomiting associated with cancer chemotherapy and prevention of postopertive nausea, vomiting

Investigational uses: Bulimia, pruritus, rectal use

Dosage and routes

Prevention of nausea/vomiting associated with cancer chemotherapy

Adult/child 4-18 yr: **IV** 0.15 mg/kg infused over 15 min, 30 min before start of cancer chemotherapy; 0.15 mg/kg is given 4 and 8 hr after first dose or 32 mg as a single dose; dilute in 50 ml of D_5 or 0.9% NaCl before giving; rectal (off-label) 16 mg qd 2 hr before chemotherapy

Prevention of nausea/vomiting of radiotherapy

Adult: PO 8 mg tid

Prevention of postoperative nausea/vomiting

Adult: **IV** 4 mg undiluted over >30 sec

Child 2-12 yr: **IV** 0.1 mg/kg (≤40 kg); 4 mg (≥40 kg) give ≥30 sec

Hepatic dose

Max dose 8 mg qd

Bulimia (off-label)

Adult: PO 4 mg tid (base dose) prn during bingeing/purging

Pruritus (off-label)

Adult: PO 4 mg bid

Available forms: Inj 2 mg/ml, 32 mg/50 ml (premixed); tabs 4, 8 mg; oral sol 4 mg/5 ml; oral disintegrating tabs 4, 8 mg

Adverse effects

CNS: *Headache,* dizziness, drowsiness, fatigue, extrapyramidal syndrome

GI: *Diarrhea, constipation, abdominal pain*

MISC: Rash, **bronchospasm** (rare), *MS pain, wound problems, shivering, fever, hypoxia, urinary retention*

Contraindications: Hypersensitivity

Precautions: Pregnancy **B,** lactation, children, elderly

Do Not Confuse:

Zofran/Zantac

Pharmacokinetics

Absorption	Completely absorbed (**IV**)
Distribution	Unknown
Metabolism	Liver, extensively
Excretion	Kidneys
Half-life	3.5-4.7 hr

Pharmacodynamics

Unknown

Interactions: Unknown

NURSING CONSIDERATIONS

Assessment

- Assess for absence of nausea, vomiting during chemotherapy
- Assess for hypersensitivity reaction: rash, bronchospasm
- Assess for EPS: shuffling gait, tremors, grimacing, rigidity

Nursing diagnoses

✓ Knowledge deficit (teaching)
✓ Noncompliance (teaching)

Implementation

IV route

- Give **IV** after diluting a single dose in 50 ml of 0.9% NaCl or D_5W, 0.45% NaCl; give over 15 min
- Store at room temp for 48 hr after dilution

Y-site compatibilities: Aldesleukin, amifostine, amikacin, aztreonam, bleomycin, carboplatin, carmustine, cefazolin, ceforanide, cefotazime, cefoxitin, ceftazidime, ceftizoxime, cefuroxime, chlorpromazine, cimetidine, cisatracurium, cisplatin, cladribine, clindamycin, cyclophosphamide, cytarabine, dacarbazine, dactinomycin, daunorubicin, dexamethasone, diphenhydramine, doxorubicin, doxorubicin liposome, doxycycline, droperidol, etoposide, famotidine, filgrastim, floxuridine, fluconazole, fludarabine, gentamicin, haloperidol, heparin, hydrocortisone, hydromorphone, hydroxyzine, ifosfamide, imipenem/cilastatin, magnesium sulfate, mannitol, mechlorethamine, melphalan, meperidine, mesna, methotrexate, metoclopramide, miconazole, mitomycin, mitoxantrone, morphine, paclitaxel, pentostatin, potassium chloride, prochlorperazine, ranitidine, remifentanil, streptozocin, teniposide, thiotepa, ticarcillin, ticarcillin/clavulanate, vancomycin, vinblastine, vincristine, vinorelbine, zidovudine

Y-site incompatibilities: Acyclovir, aminophylline, amphotericin B, ampicillin, ampicillin/sulbactam, cefoperazone, furosemide, ganciclovir, lorazepam, methylprednisolone, mezlocillin, piperacillin, sargramostim, sodium bicarbonate

Additive compatibilities: Cisplatin, cyclophosphamide, cytarabine, dacarbazine, dexamethasone, doxorubicin, etoposide, meperidine, methotrexate

Solution compatibilities: May also be diluted with D_5W, LR, D_5/0.9% NaCl, D_5/0.45% NaCl

Patient/family education

- Instruct patient to report diarrhea, constipation, rash, changes in respirations, or discomfort at insertion site
- Teach patient reason for medication and expected results

Evaluation

Positive therapeutic outcome

- Absence of nausea, vomiting during cancer chemotherapy

O

oral contraceptives (℞)

Func. class.: Hormone
Chem. class.: Estrogen/progestin combinations

Pregnancy category X

Action: Prevents ovulation by suppressing FSH, LH; **monophasic:** estrogen/progestin (fixed dose) used during a 21-day cycle; ovulation is inhibited by suppression of FSH and LH; thickness of cervical mucus and endometrial lining prevents pregnancy; **biphasic:** ovulation is inhibited by suppression of FSH and LH; alteration of cervical mucus, endometrial lining prevents pregnancy; **triphasic:** ovulation is inhibited by suppression of FSH and LH; change of cervical mucus, endometrial lining prevents pregnancy; variable doses of estrogen/progestin combinations may be similar to natural hormonal fluctuations; **progestin-only pill and implant:** change of cervical mucus and endometrial lining prevents pregnancy; ovulation may be suppressed

➔ Therapeutic Outcome: Prevention of pregnancy, decreased severity of endometriosis, hypermenorrhea

Uses: To prevent pregnancy, endometriosis, hypermenorrhea

Dosage and routes

Adult: PO 1 qd starting on day 5 of menstrual cycle; day 1 is 1st day of period

21-tablet packs

Adult: PO 1 qd starting on day 7 of menstrual cycle; day 1 is 1st day of period; then on 20 or 21 days, off 7 days

28-tablet packs

Adult: PO 1 qd continuously

Biphasic

Adult: 1 qd × 10 days, then next color 1 qd × 11 days

Triphasic

Adult: 1 qd; check package insert for each brand

Implant

Adult: Subdermal 6 cap implanted during the first wk of menses

Endometriosis

Adult: PO 1 qd × 20 days from day 5 to day 24 of cycle

Adult: PO 1 qd; check package insert for specific instructions

Available forms: Check specific brand

Adverse effects

CNS: Depression, fatigue, dizziness, nervousness, anxiety, headache

CV: Increased B/P, **cerebral hemorrhage, thrombosis, pulmonary embolism,** fluid retention, edema

EENT: Optic neuritis, retinal thrombosis, cataracts

ENDO: Decreased glucose tolerance, increased TBG, PBI, T_4, T_3

GI: *Nausea,* vomiting, cramps, diarrhea, bloating, constipation, change in appetite, **cholestatic jaundice**

GU: Breakthrough bleeding, amenorrhea, spotting, dysmenorrhea, galactorrhea, endocervical hyperplasia, vaginitis, cystitis-like syndrome, breast change

HEMA: Increased fibrinogen, clotting factor

INTEG: *Chloasma, melasma,* acne, rash, urticaria, erythema, pruritus, hirsutism, alopecia, photosensitivity

Contraindications: Pregnancy **X,** lactation, reproductive cancer, thrombophlebitis, MI, hepatic tumors, hepatic disease, CAD, women 40 yr and over, CVA

Precautions: Depression, hypertension, renal disease, seizure disorders, lupus erythematosus, rheumatic disease, migraine headache, amenorrhea, irregular menses, breast cancer (fibrocystic), gallbladder disease, diabetes mellitus, heavy smoking, acute mononucleosis, sickle cell disease

Pharmacokinetics	
Absorption	Well absorbed
Distribution	Unknown
Metabolism	Liver, extensively
Excretion	Kidneys
Half-life	Unknown

Pharmacodynamics

	PO	IM	IMPLANT
Onset	1 mo	1 mo	1 mo
Peak	1 mo	1 mo	1 mo
Duration	1 mo	3 mo	5 yr

Interactions

Individual drugs

Aminocaproic acid: ↑ clotting
Bromocriptine: ↓ effectiveness of bromocriptine
Carbamazepine: ↓ effectiveness of oral contraceptive
Chenodiol: ↓ effectiveness of oral contraceptive
Chloramphenicol: ↓ effectiveness of oral contraceptive
Dantrolene: ↑ hepatic toxicity (estrogen only)
Dihydroergotamine: ↓ effectiveness of oral contraceptive
Griseofulvin: ↓ effectiveness of oral contraceptive
Mineral oil: ↓ effectiveness of oral contraceptive
Phenylbutazone: ↓ effectiveness of oral contraceptive
Phenytoin: ↓ effectiveness of oral contraceptive
Primidone: ↓ effectiveness of oral contraceptive
Rifampin: ↓ effectiveness of oral contraceptive
Warfarin: ↑ or ↓ effect of warfarin

Drug classifications

Analgesics: ↓ action of oral contraceptives
Antibiotics: ↓ action of oral contraceptives
Anticonvulsants: ↓ action of oral contraceptives
Antidepressants, tricyclic: ↑ toxicity
Antihistamines: ↓ action of oral contraceptives
Glucocorticoids: ↓ action of oral contraceptives
Oral anticoagulants: ↓ action of oral anticoagulants

Food/drug

Grapefruit juice: ↑ peak level

Lab test interferences

↑ Pro-time; ↑ clotting factors VII, VIII, IX, X; ↑ TBG, ↑ PBI, ↑ T_4, ↑ platelet aggregation, ↑ BSP, ↑ triglycerides, ↑ bilirubin, ↑ AST, ↑ ALT
↓ T_3, ↓ antithrombin III, ↓ folate, ↓ metyrapone test, ↓ GTT, ↓ 17-OHCS

Herb/drug

St. John's wort: ↓ oral contraceptive effect

NURSING CONSIDERATIONS

Assessment

- Assess for reproductive changes: change in breasts, tumors, positive Pap smear; drug should be discontinued if changes occur
- Monitor glucose, thyroid function, liver function tests, B/P

Nursing diagnoses

- ✓ Injury, risk for (adverse reactions)
- ✓ Body image disturbance (adverse reactions)
- ✓ Knowledge deficit (teaching)
- ✓ Noncompliance (teaching)

Implementation

PO route

- If GI symptoms occur, medication may be taken with food; take at same time each day

Implant route

- Inject 6 cap subdermally
- Implant is effective for 5 yr, should be removed after that

IM route

- Administer deep in large muscle mass after shaking susp well; ensure pregnancy has not occurred if inj are 2 wk or more apart

Patient/family education

- Teach patient about detection of clots using Homans' sign; teach monitoring technique for heat, redness, pain, swelling
- Teach patient to use sunscreen or to avoid sunlight; photosensitivity can occur

O

• Teach patient to take at same time each day to ensure equal drug level; to take another tab as soon as possible if one is missed
• Teach patient that after drug is discontinued, pregnancy may not occur for several mo
• Instruct patient to report GI symptoms that occur after 4 mo
• Advise patient to use another birth control method during first 3 wk of oral contraceptive use
• Teach patient to report abdominal pain, change in vision, shortness of breath, change in menstrual flow, spotting, breakthrough bleeding, breast lumps, swelling, headache, severe leg pain, mental changes; that continuing medical care is needed: Pap smear and gynecologic exam q6 mo
• Teach patient to notify physicians and dentist of oral contraceptive use

Evaluation

Positive therapeutic outcome
• Absence of pregnancy
• Decreased severity of endometriosis
• Decreased severity of hypermenorrhea

orlistat (℞)

(or-li′-stat)
Xenical
Func. class.: Lipase inhibitor
Pregnancy category B

Action: Inhibits the absorption of dietary fat

➔ Therapeutic Outcome: Decrease in weight

Uses: Obesity management

Dosage and routes

Adult: PO 120 mg tid with each main meal containing fat

Available forms: Caps 120 mg

Adverse effects

CNS: *Insomnia,* dizziness, headache, depression, anxiety, fatigue
GI: *Oily spotting, flatus with discharge, fecal urgency, fatty/oily stool, oily evacuation, fecal incontinence,* nausea, vomiting, abdominal pain, infectious diarrhea, rectal pain, tooth disorder
GU: UTI, vaginitis, menstrual irregularity
INTEG: Dry skin, rash
MS: Back pain, arthritis, myalgia, tendinitis
RESP: Influenza, upper, lower respiratory tract infection
EENT: Symptoms

Contraindications: Hypersensitivity, malabsorption syndrome, cholestasis

Precautions: Hypothyroidism, other organic causes of obesity, [P] lactation, children, pregnancy **B**

Pharmacokinetics	
Absorption	Minimal
Distribution	99% protein binding
Metabolism	Unknown
Excretion	Feces
Half-life	1-2 hr

Pharmacodynamics	
Onset	Unknown
Peak	8 hr
Duration	Unknown

Interactions

Individual drugs
Cyclosporine: ↓ absorption
Pravastatin: ↑ lipid-lowering effect
Drug classifications
Fat-soluble vitamins: ↓ absorption

NURSING CONSIDERATIONS

Assessment

• Monitor weight weekly, diabetic patients may need reduction in oral hypoglycemics
• Assess for misuse in certain populations (anorexia nervosa, bulimia)

Nursing diagnoses
✓ Knowledge deficit (teaching)
✓ Noncompliance (teaching)

Implementation
- Patient should be on a diet with 30% of calories from fat, omit dose of orlistat if a meal contains no fat

Patient/family education
- Warn patient that safety and effectiveness beyond 2 yr have not been determined
- Instruct patient to read patient's information sheet
- Advise patient to avoid hazardous activities until stabilized on medication
- Instruct patient to take a multivitamin containing fat-soluble vitamins, take 2 hr before or after orlistat
- Instruct patient/family to notify prescriber if significant side effects occur

Evaluation
Positive therapeutic outcome
- Decreased weight

oseltamivir (℞)
(oh-sell-tam'ih-ver)
Tamiflu
Func. class.: Antiviral
Chem. class.: Ethyl ester prodrug
Pregnancy category C

Action: Inhibits influenza virus neuraminidase with possible alteration of virus particle aggregation and release

➔ **Therapeutic Outcome:** Decreased symptoms of influenza type A

Uses: Prevention/treatment of influenza type A

Dosage and routes
Treatment
Adult: PO 75 bid mg × 5 days, begin treatment within 2 days of onset of symptoms

Prevention
Adult: PO 75 mg qd × ≥7 days

Available forms: Caps 75 mg; powder for oral susp 12 mg/ml after reconstitution

Adverse effects
CNS: Headache, fatigue, insomnia, vertigo
GI: *Nausea, vomiting,* diarrhea, abdominal pain
RESP: Cough

Contraindications: Hypersensitivity

Precautions: Hepatic disease, renal disease, lactation, children <18 yr, pregnancy **C**

Pharmacokinetics

Absorption	Rapidly absorbed
Distribution	Protein binding is low
Metabolism	Converted to oseltamivir carboxylate
Excretion	Eliminated by conversion
Half-life	1-3 hr

Pharmacodynamics
Unknown

NURSING CONSIDERATIONS
Assessment
- Assess for symptoms of influenza A: increased temperature, malaise, aches and pains

Nursing diagnoses
✓ Infection, risk for (uses)
✓ Knowledge deficit (teaching)

Implementation
- Give within 2 days of symptoms of influenza; continue for 5 days
- Give at least 4 hr before hs to prevent insomnia
- Administer after meals for better absorption, to decrease GI symptoms: caps may be opened and mixed with food for easy swallowing
- Store in airtight, dry container

Patient/family education
- Teach patient about aspects of drug therapy: the need to report dyspnea,

O

weight gain, dizziness, poor concentration, dysuria, behavioral changes
- Teach patient to avoid hazardous activities if dizziness occurs
- Advise patient to take missed dose as soon as remembered if within 2 hr of next dose

Evaluation

Positive therapeutic outcome
- Absence of fever, malaise, cough, dyspnea in influenza A

oxacillin (℞)

(ox-a-sill'in)

Bactocill, oxacillin sodium

Func. class.: Broad-spectrum antiinfective

Chem. class.: Penicillinase-resistant penicillin

Pregnancy category B

Action: Interferes with cell wall replication of susceptible organisms; osmotically unstable cell wall swells, bursts from osmotic pressure

➡ **Therapeutic Outcome:** Bactericidal effects for gram-positive cocci *Staphylococcus aureus, Streptococcus pneumoniae,* infections caused by penicillinase-producing staphylococci

Uses: Infections caused by penicillinase-producing staphylococci, streptococci; respiratory tract, skin, skin structure, urinary tract, bone, joint infections, sinusitis, endocarditis, septicemia, meningitis

Dosage and routes

Adult: PO 2-6 g/day in divided doses q4-6h; IM/**IV** 2-12 g/day in divided doses q4-6h

P ***Child:*** PO 50-100 mg/kg/day in divided doses q6h; IM/**IV** 50-100 mg/kg/day in divided doses q4-6h

Available forms: Caps 250, 500 mg; powder for oral susp 250 mg/5 ml; powder for inj 250, 500 mg, 1, 2, 4, 10 g

Adverse effects

CNS: Lethargy, hallucinations, anxiety, depression, twitching, **coma, convulsions**

GI: Nausea, vomiting, diarrhea, increased AST, ALT, abdominal pain, glossitis, colitis

GU: **Oliguria, proteinuria, hematuria, vaginitis, moniliasis, glomerulonephritis**

HEMA: Anemia, increased bleeding time, **bone marrow depression, granulocytopenia**

Contraindications: Hypersensitivity to penicillins

Precautions: Pregnancy **B**, hypersensitivity to cephalosporins, P neonates

Do Not Confuse:
Bactocill/Pathocil

Pharmacokinetics

Absorption	Rapid, incomplete (PO); well absorbed (IM); completely (**IV**)
Distribution	Widely distributed; crosses placenta
Metabolism	Liver
Excretion	Kidneys, unchanged (51%); breast milk
Half-life	20-50 min; increased in severe hepatic disease

Pharmacodynamics

	PO	IM	IV
Onset	Rapid	Rapid	Rapid
Peak	½-1 hr	½ hr	Inf end

Interactions

Individual drugs

Aspirin: ↑ oxacillin levels, ↓ renal excretion

Chloramphenicol: ↑ half-life of chloramphenicol, ↓ effectiveness of oxacillin

Cholestyramine: ↓ effectiveness of oxacillin

Colestipol: ↓ effectiveness of oxacillin

Disulfiram: ↑ oxacillin effect
Probenecid: ↑ oxacillin levels, ↓ renal excretion

Drug classifications
Erythromycins: ↓ antimicrobial effectiveness
Oral anticoagulants: ↑ anticoagulant effects
Oral contraceptives: ↓ contraceptive effectiveness
Tetracyclines: ↓ antimicrobial effectiveness

Food/drug
Food, carbonated drinks, citrus fruit juices: ↓ absorption

Herb/drug
Khat: ↓ absorption

Lab test interferences
False positive: Urine glucose, urine protein

NURSING CONSIDERATIONS
Assessment
- Assess patient for previous sensitivity reaction to penicillins or other cephalosporins; cross-sensitivity between penicillins and cephalosporins is common
- Assess patient for signs and symptoms of infection including characteristics of wounds, sputum, urine, stool, WBC >10,000/mm^3, fever; obtain baseline information and during treatment
- Obtain C&S before beginning drug therapy to identify if correct treatment has been initiated
- Assess for allergic reactions: rash, urticaria, pruritus, chills, fever, joint pain; angioedema may occur a few days after therapy begins; epinephrine, resuscitation equipment should be available for anaphylactic reaction
- Assess urine output; if decreasing, notify prescriber (may indicate nephrotoxicity); also check for increased BUN, creatinine
- Monitor blood studies: AST, ALT, CBC, Hct, bilirubin, LDH, alkaline phosphatase, Coombs' test monthly if patient is on long-term therapy
- Monitor electrolytes: potassium, sodium, chloride monthly if patient is on long-term therapy
- Assess bowel pattern qd; if severe diarrhea occurs, drug should be discontinued; may indicate pseudomembranous colitis
- Monitor for bleeding: ecchymosis, bleeding gums, hematuria, stool guaiac daily if on long-term therapy
- Assess for overgrowth of infection: perineal itching, fever, malaise, redness, pain, swelling, drainage, rash, diarrhea, change in cough, sputum

Nursing diagnoses
- ✓ Infection, risk for (uses)
- ✓ Diarrhea (adverse reactions)
- ✓ Injury, risk for (adverse reactions)
- ✓ Knowledge deficit (teaching)
- ✓ Noncompliance (teaching)

Implementation
PO route
- Give in even doses around the clock; if GI upset occurs, give with food; drug must be given for 10-14 days to ensure organism death and prevent superinfection; store in airtight container
- Shake susp; store in refrigerator for 2 wk, 1 wk at room temp

IM route
- Reconstitute 250 mg/1.4 ml, 500 mg/2.7-2.8 ml, 1 g/5.7 ml, 2 g/11.4-11.5 ml, 4 g/21.8-23 ml of sterile water for a conc of 250 mg/1.5 ml; store unused portion in refrigerator for 1 wk or 3 days at room temp
- Inject deeply in large muscle mass

IV route
- Reconstitute 250 mg/1.4 ml, 500 mg/2.7-2.8 ml, 1 g/5.7 ml, 2 g/11.4-11.5 ml, 4 g/21.8-23 ml of sterile water for a conc of 250 mg/1.5 ml; store unused portion in refrigerator for 1 week or 3 days at room temp
- Give direct **IV** by diluting reconstituted sol with 250-500 mg/5 ml, 1 g/10 ml, 2 g/20 ml, 4 g/40 ml of sterile water or 0.9% NaCl, give over 10 min

O

- Give intermittent inf by diluting to a conc of 0.5-40 mg/ml with D_5W, 0.9% NaCl, D_5/0.9% NaCl, LR; give over 6 hr or less

Y-site compatibilities: Acyclovir, cyclophosphamide, diltiazem, famotidine, fluconazole, foscarnet, heparin, hydrocortisone, hydromorphone, labetalol, magnesium sulfate, meperidine, methotrexate, morphine, perphenazine, potassium chloride, tacrolimus, vit B with C, zidovudine

Y-site incompatibilities: Verapamil

Additive compatibilities: Cephapirin, chloramphenicol, dopamine, potassium chloride, sodium bicarbonate

Additive incompatibilities: Cytarabine, tetracycline

Patient/family education

- Teach patient to report sore throat, bruising, bleeding, joint pain; may indicate blood dyscrasias (rare)
- Advise patient to contact prescriber if vaginal itching, loose, foul-smelling stools, furry tongue occur; may indicate superinfection
- Instruct patient to take all medication prescribed for the length of time ordered
- Advise patient to notify prescriber of diarrhea with blood or pus, which may indicate pseudomembranous colitis

Evaluation

Positive therapeutic outcome

- Absence of signs/symptoms of infection (WBC <10,000/mm^3, temp WNL, absence of red, draining wounds)
- Reported improvement in symptoms of infection

Treatment of anaphylaxis: Withdraw drug, maintain airway, administer epinephrine, aminophylline, O_2, **IV** corticosteroids

oxaprozin (℞)

(ox-a-proe'zin)

Daypro

Func. class.: Nonsteroidal antiinflammatory

Chem. class.: Propionic acid derivative

Pregnancy category C

Action: Inhibits prostaglandin synthesis by decreasing an enzyme needed for biosynthesis; analgesic, antiinflammatory

➔ Therapeutic Outcome: Decreased pain, inflammation

Uses: Acute and long-term management of osteoarthritis, rheumatoid arthritis

Dosage and routes

Adult: PO 600-1200 mg qd; maximum dose 1800 mg/day or 26 mg/kg, whichever is lower in divided doses

Available forms: Tabs 600 mg

Adverse effects

CNS: Dizziness, headache, drowsiness, fatigue, tremors, confusion, insomnia, anxiety, malaise, depression

CV: Tachycardia, peripheral edema, palpitations, dysrhythmias

EENT: Tinnitus, hearing loss, blurred vision

GI: Nausea, *anorexia,* vomiting, *diarrhea,* jaundice, **cholestatic hepatitis,** constipation, flatulence, *cramps,* dry mouth, peptic ulcer, **bleeding,** melena, gastroenteritis

GU: **Nephrotoxicity: dysuria, hematuria, oliguria, azotemia**

HEMA: Increased bleeding time

INTEG: Purpura, rash, pruritus, sweating, photosensitivity

SYST: **Anaphylaxis, angioneurotic edema**

Contraindications: Hypersensitivity, asthma, patients in whom aspirin and iodides have induced symptoms of allergic reactions or asthma

Precautions: Pregnancy **C**, lacta-

P tion, children, bleeding disorders, GI disorders, cardiac disorders, CHF, hypersensitivity to other antiinflammatory agents, severe renal and hepatic G disease, elderly

Do Not Confuse:
Daypro/Diupres

Pharmacokinetics	
Absorption	Well absorbed
Distribution	Unknown
Metabolism	Liver, extensively
Excretion	Breast milk
Half-life	40-50 hr

Pharmacodynamics	
Onset	Unknown
Peak	2 hr
Duration	Unknown

Interactions
Individual drugs
Acetaminophen (long-term use): ↑ renal reactions
Alcohol: ↑ adverse reactions
Aspirin: ↓ effectiveness, ↑ adverse reactions
Cyclosporine: ↑ toxicity
Digoxin: ↑ toxicity, levels
Insulin: ↑ insulin effect
Lithium: ↑ toxicity
Methotrexate: ↑ toxicity
Phenytoin: ↑ phenytoin level
Radiation: ↑ risk of hematologic toxicity
Sulfonylurea: ↑ toxicity

Drug classifications
Anticoagulants: ↑ risk of bleeding
Antihypertensives: ↓ effect of antihypertensives
Antineoplastics: ↑ risk of hematologic toxicity
β-Adrenergic blockers: ↑ antihypertension
Diuretics: ↓ effectiveness of diuretics
Glucocorticoids: ↑ adverse reactions
NSAIDs: ↑ adverse reactions
Potassium supplements: ↑ adverse reactions
Sulfonamides: ↑ toxicity

Lab test interferences
↑ BUN, ↑ alkaline phosphatase
False: ↑ 5-HIAA, false ↑ 17KS

NURSING CONSIDERATIONS
Assessment
- Assess for pain and ROM: intensity, location, duration
- Monitor blood studies: alkaline phosphatase, LDH, AST, ALT, and bleeding time (may be increased)
- Assess for asthma, aspirin hypersensitivity, nasal polyps; increased hypersensitivity reactions

Nursing diagnoses
- ✓ Pain (uses)
- ✓ Mobility, impaired (uses)
- ✓ Injury, risk for (adverse reactions)
- ✓ Knowledge deficit (teaching)

Implementation
- Give with food or milk to decrease gastric symptoms

Patient/family education
- Teach patient that drug must be continued for prescribed time to be effective; to avoid aspirin, alcoholic beverages
- Instruct patient to use caution when driving; drowsiness, dizziness may occur
- Teach patient to take with a full glass of water to enhance absorption; patient should sit upright for 30 min to prevent stomach irritation and ulceration
- Do not crush, break, or chew
- Instruct patient to use sunscreen and protective clothing to prevent burns
- Advise patient to report to prescriber severe abdominal pain, rash, itching, yellowing of skin or eyes, depression

Evaluation
Positive therapeutic outcome
- Decreased pain
- Decreased inflammation
- Increased mobility

O

oxazepam (℞)

(ox-az'e-pam)

Apo-Oxazepam ✦, Novoxapam ✦, oxazepam, Serax

Func. class.: Sedative/hypnotic; antianxiety

Chem. class.: Benzodiazepine

Pregnancy category D

Controlled substance schedule IV

Action: Depresses subcortical levels of CNS, including limbic system, reticular formation; potentiates GABA

➔ **Therapeutic Outcome:** Decreased anxiety, successful alcohol withdrawal, relaxation

Uses: Anxiety, alcohol withdrawal

Dosage and routes

Anxiety

Adult: PO 10-30 mg tid-qid

Alcohol withdrawal

Adult: PO 15-30 mg tid-qid

Available forms: Caps 10, 15, 30 mg; tabs 10, 15, 30 mg

Adverse effects

CNS: ***Dizziness, drowsiness,*** confusion, headache, anxiety, tremors, fatigue, depression, insomnia, hallucinations, paradoxic excitement, transient amnesia

CV: ***Orthostatic hypotension,*** **ECG changes, tachycardia,** hypotension

EENT: ***Blurred vision,*** tinnitus, mydriasis

GI: Nausea, vomiting, anorexia

INTEG: Rash, dermatitis, itching

Contraindications: Hypersensitivity to benzodiazepines, narrow-angle glaucoma, psychosis, pregnancy **D**, [P] child <12 yr

[G] **Precautions:** Elderly, debilitated, hepatic disease, renal disease

Pharmacokinetics

Absorption	Well absorbed
Distribution	Widely distributed; crosses placenta, blood-brain barrier
Metabolism	Liver
Excretion	Kidneys, breast milk
Half-life	5-15 hr

Pharmacodynamics

Onset	½-1½ hr
Peak	Unknown
Duration	6-12 hr

Interactions

Individual drugs

Alcohol: ↑ CNS depression

Cimetidine: ↑ action

Fluoxetine: ↑ action

Levodopa: ↓ action of levodopa

Metoprolol: ↑ action

Phenytoin: ↓ effect

Propoxyphene: ↑ action

Theophylline: ↓ sedative effects

Drug classifications

Antidepressants: ↑ CNS depression

Antihistamines: ↑ CNS depression

Opiates: ↑ CNS depression

Oral contraceptives: ↑ effect

Lab test interferences

↑ AST, ↑ ALT, ↑ serum bilirubin

False: ↑ 17-OHCS

↓ radioactive iodine uptake

NURSING CONSIDERATIONS

Assessment

- Assess mental status: mood, sensorium, anxiety, affect, sleeping pattern, drowsiness, dizziness, especially [G] elderly; physical dependency, withdrawal symptoms: anxiety, panic attacks, agitation, convulsions, headache, nausea, vomiting, muscle pain, weakness; suicidal tendencies; indications of increasing tolerance and abuse
- Monitor B/P with patient lying, standing, pulse; if systolic B/P drops 20 mm Hg, hold drug, notify prescriber
- Monitor blood studies: CBC during long-term therapy; blood dyscrasias

have occurred rarely; decreased hematocrit, neutropenia may occur
- Monitor hepatic studies: AST, ALT, bilirubin, creatinine LDH, alkaline phosphatase if taking long term
- Monitor I&O; indicate renal dysfunction

Nursing diagnoses
- ✓ Anxiety (uses)
- ✓ Depression (uses)
- ✓ Injury, risk for (adverse reactions)
- ✓ Knowledge deficit (teaching)

Implementation
- Give with food or milk for GI symptoms; tab may be crushed if patient is unable to swallow medication whole; give sugarless gum, hard candy, frequent sips of water for dry mouth

Patient/family education
- Teach patient that drug may be taken with food or fluids; tab may be crushed or swallowed whole
- Caution patient not to use for everyday stress or longer than 3 mo unless directed by prescriber; not to take more than prescribed amount; not to double doses or skip doses
- Advise patient to avoid OTC preparations unless approved by prescriber; alcohol and CNS depressants will increase CNS depression
- Caution patient to avoid driving and activities that require alertness, since drowsiness may occur; to avoid alcohol and other psychotropic medications; to rise slowly or fainting may occur, especially elderly; that drowsiness may worsen at beginning of treatment
- Caution patient not to discontinue medication abruptly after long-term use; withdrawal symptoms include vomiting, cramping, tremors, seizures

Evaluation
Positive therapeutic outcome
- Decreased anxiety, restlessness, sleeplessness (short-term treatment only)

Treatment of overdose:
Lavage, VS, supportive care

oxcarbazepine (℞)
ox'kar-baz'uh-peen)

Trileptal

Func. class.: Anticonvulsant

Pregnancy category C

Action: May inhibit nerve impulses by limiting influx of sodium ions across cell membrane in motor cortex

→ Therapeutic Outcome: Absence of seizures

Uses: Partial seizures

Dosage and routes
Seizures

Adult: PO 300 mg bid, may be increased to 600 mg/day in divided doses bid; maintenance 1200 mg/day

P ***Child:*** PO 8-10 mg/kg/day divided bid, max 600 mg/day; dose is determined by weight

Conversion to monotherapy in partial seizures

Adult: PO 300 mg bid with reduction in other anticonvulsants, increase oxcarbazepine to max 600 mg/day q1 wk over 2-4 wk; withdraw other anticonvulsants over 3-6 wk

Initiation of monotherapy in partial seizures

Adult: PO 300 mg bid, increase by 300 mg/day q3 days to 1200 mg divided bid

Renal dose

CrCl <30 ml/min 150 mg bid and increase slowly

Available forms: Tabs, film-coated, 150, 300, 600 mg

Adverse effects
CNS: *Dizziness, confusion, fatigue,* feeling abnormal, ataxia, abnormal gait, tremors, anxiety, agitation, headache, **worsening of seizures**

CV: *Hypotension,* chest pain, edema

O

EENT: *Blurred vision, diplopia, nystagmus,* rhinitis, sinusitis
GI: *Nausea, constipation, diarrhea,* anorexia, vomiting, abdominal pain, gastritis, dry mouth, thirst, **rectal hemorrhage**
GU: *Frequency,* UTI, vaginitis
INTEG: Purpura, rash, acne, bruising, sweating

Contraindications: Hypersensitivity

Precautions: Hypersensitivity to carbamazepine, pregnancy **C**, lactation, P child <4 yr

Pharmacokinetics	
Absorption	Unknown
Distribution	Unknown
Metabolism	Liver
Excretion	Unknown
Half-life	Unknown

Pharmacodynamics	
Onset	Unknown
Peak	Unknown
Duration	Unknown

Interactions
Individual drugs
Alcohol: ↑ CNS depression
Felodipine: ↓ effects of felodipine
Phenobarbital: ↓ oxcarbazepine level
Phenytoin: ↓ oxcarbazepine level

NURSING CONSIDERATIONS
Assessment
- Assess seizure activity including frequency, duration, and aura; provide seizure precautions
- Assess mental status including mood, sensorium, affect, behavioral changes; if mental status changes, notify prescriber
- Assess eye problems: ophthalmic examinations (slit lamp, funduscopy, tonometry) are needed before, during, after treatment
- Assess for allergic reaction including purpura or red, raised rash; if these occur, drug should be discontinued

Nursing diagnoses
- ✓ Injury, risk for (side effects)
- ✓ Knowledge deficit (teaching)

Implementation
- Store drug at room temp
- Provide assistance with ambulation during early part of treatment; dizziness may occur

PO route
- Give drug with food, milk to decrease GI symptoms

Patient/family education
- Caution patient to avoid driving, other activities that require alertness
- Advise patient not to discontinue medication quickly after long-term use
- Caution patient to inform prescriber if hypersensitive to carbamazepine
- Instruct patient to avoid use of alcohol while taking this medication
- Instruct patient to use alternate contraception if using hormonal method
- Advise patient to use hard candy or gum for dry mouth, rinse mouth frequently
- Advise patient to carry ID stating name, drugs taken, condition, prescriber's name and phone number

Evaluation
Positive therapeutic outcome
- Decreased seizure activity

oxtriphylline (℞)
(ox-trye′fi-lin)
Choledyl, Choledyl SA
Func. class.: Bronchodilator, spasmolytic
Chem. class.: Choline salt of theophylline

Pregnancy category C

Action: Relaxes smooth muscle of respiratory system by blocking phosphodiesterase, which increases cAMP; 64% theophylline

Therapeutic Outcome: Bronchodilatation with ease of breathing

Uses: Acute bronchial asthma, reversible bronchospasm in chronic bronchitis and COPD

Dosage and routes

P ***Adult and child >12 yr:*** PO 4.7 mg/kg q8h or sus action q12h

P ***Child 9-16 yr and smokers (adult):*** 4.7 mg/kg q6h

P ***Child 1-9 yr:*** 6.2 mg/kg q6h

Available forms: Elixir 100 mg/5 ml ✤; syrup 50 mg/5 ml; tabs 100, 200 mg; sus rel tabs 400, 600 mg

Adverse effects

CNS: *Anxiety, restlessness, insomnia, dizziness,* **seizures,** headache, lightheadedness

CV: **Palpitations, sinus tachycardia,** hypotension

GI: Nausea, vomiting, anorexia, diarrhea, bitter taste, dyspepsia

INTEG: Flushing, urticaria, alopecia

RESP: Increased rate, **respiratory arrest**

Contraindications: Hypersensitivity to xanthines, tachydysrhythmias

G **Precautions:** Elderly, CHF, cor pulmonale, hepatic disease, active peptic ulcer disease, diabetes mellitus, P hyperthyroidism, hypertension, children, pregnancy **C,** glaucoma, prostatic hypertrophy

Pharmacokinetics

Absorption	Well absorbed (PO); slow (PO-SUS REL)
Distribution	Widely distributed; crosses placenta
Metabolism	Liver to caffeine
Excretion	Kidneys, breast milk
Half-life	3-13 hr; increased in renal disease, CHF

Pharmacodynamics

	PO	PO-SUS REL
Onset	15-60 min	Unknown
Peak	1-5 hr	4-8 hr
Duration	6-8 hr	8-12 hr

Interactions

Individual drugs

Allopurinol: ↓ metabolism, ↑ toxicity
Carbamazepine: ↑ or ↓ oxtriphylline levels
Cimetidine: ↓ metabolism, ↑ toxicity
Disulfiram: ↓ metabolism, ↑ toxicity
Erythromycin: ↓ metabolism, ↑ toxicity
Fluvoxamine: ↑ toxicity
Halothane: ↑ risk of dysrhythmias
Interferon: ↓ metabolism, ↑ toxicity
Isoniazid: ↑ or ↓ oxtriphylline level
Ketoconazole: ↑ metabolism, ↓ effect
Lithium: ↓ effect of lithium
Mexiletine: ↓ metabolism, ↑ toxicity
Nicotine: ↓ oxtriphylline level
Phenytoin: ↑ metabolism, ↓ effect
Rifampin: ↑ metabolism, ↓ effect
Thiabendazole: ↓ metabolism, ↑ toxicity

Drug classifications

Barbiturates: ↓ effect of oxtriphylline
β-Adrenergic blockers: ↓ metabolism, ↑ toxicity
Diuretics, loop: ↑ or ↓ oxtriphylline levels
Fluoroquinolones: ↓ metabolism, ↑ toxicity
Glucocorticoids: ↓ metabolism, ↑ toxicity
Oral contraceptives: ↑ toxicity
Sympathomimetics: ↑ CNS, CV adverse reactions

Food/drug

Caffeinated foods (cola, coffee, tea, chocolate): ↑ CNS, CV adverse reactions
Charbroiled foods: ↓ effect

Smoking

↑ metabolism, ↓ effect

O

Herb/drug
Cola tree: ↑ action of both
Ephedra: ↑ action of both
Lab test interferences
↑ Plasma free fatty acids

NURSING CONSIDERATIONS
Assessment
- Monitor blood levels (therapeutic level is 10-20 μg/ml); toxicity may occur with small increase above 20 μg/ml, especially elderly; check whether theophylline was given recently (24 hr); watch for toxicity: nausea, vomiting, diarrhea, restlessness, tachycardia
- Monitor I&O; diuresis can occur; dehydration may result in elderly or children
- Monitor respiratory rate, rhythm, depth; auscultate lung fields bilaterally; notify prescriber of abnormalities
- Monitor allergic reactions: rash, urticaria; if these occur, drug should be discontinued
- Monitor pulmonary function studies baseline and during treatment

Nursing diagnoses
- Airway clearance, ineffective (uses)
- Activity intolerance (uses)
- Injury, risk for (uses, adverse reactions)
- Knowledge deficit (teaching)

Implementation
- Give PO pc to decrease GI symptoms; absorption may be affected with a full glass of water; do not crush or chew enteric coated or sus rel tab

Patient/family education
- Teach patient to take doses as prescribed, not to skip dose; to check OTC medications, current prescription medications for ephedrine, which will increase CNS stimulation; not to drink alcohol or caffeine products (tea, coffee, chocolate, colas)
- Caution patient to avoid hazardous activities; dizziness may occur
- Instruct patient if GI upset occurs, to take drug with 8 oz of water or food
- Teach patient to notify prescriber of change in smoking habit; a change in dosage may be required
- Teach patient to increase fluids to 2 L/day to decrease viscosity of secretions

Evaluation
Positive therapeutic outcome
- Decreased dyspnea
- Clear lung fields bilaterally

oxybutynin (℞)
(ox-i-byoo′ti-nin)
Ditropan, Ditropan XL, oxybutynin
Func. class.: Anticholinergic
Chem. class.: Synthetic tertiary amine
Pregnancy category B

Action: Relaxes smooth muscles in urinary tract by inhibiting acetylcholine at postganglionic sites

Therapeutic Outcome: Decreased symptoms of urgency, nocturia, incontinence

Uses: Antispasmodic for neurogenic bladder

Dosage and routes
Adult: PO 5 mg bid-tid, not to exceed 5 mg qid; ext rel tabs 5 mg qd, may increase by 5 mg, max 30 mg/day

Elderly: PO 2.5-5 mg tid, increase by 2.5 mg q several days

Child >5 yr: PO 5 mg bid, not to exceed 5 mg tid

Child 1-5 yrs: PO 0.2 mg/kg/dose 2-4 × /day

Available forms: Syrup 5 mg/5 ml; tabs 5 mg; ext rel tabs 5, 10, 15 mg

Adverse effects
CNS: *Anxiety, restlessness, dizziness,* **seizures,** headache, drowsiness, confusion

CV: *Palpitations, sinus tachycardia,* hypotension
EENT: Blurred vision, increased intraocular tension, dry mouth, throat
GI: *Nausea, vomiting, anorexia,* abdominal pain, constipation
GU: Dysuria, retention, hesitancy

Contraindications: Hypersensitivity, GI obstruction, GI hemorrhage, GU obstruction, glaucoma, severe colitis, myasthenia gravis, unstable CV status in acute hemorrhage

Precautions: Pregnancy **B,** lactation, suspected glaucoma, children <12 yr, elderly

Do Not Confuse:
Ditropan/diazepam

Pharmacokinetics

Absorption	Rapidly absorbed
Distribution	Unknown
Metabolism	Liver
Excretion	Unknown
Half-life	Unknown

Pharmacodynamics

Onset	½-1 hr
Peak	3-4 hr
Duration	6-10 hr

Interactions

Individual drugs

Acetaminophen: ↓ levels of acetaminophen
Alcohol: ↑ CNS depression
Atenolol: ↑ levels of atenolol
Digoxin: ↑ levels of digoxin
Disopyramide: ↑ anticholinergic effects
Haloperidol: ↑ anticholinergic effects
Levodopa: ↓ levels of levodopa
Nitrofurantoin: ↑ levels of nitrofurantoin

Drug classifications

Antidepressants: ↑ anticholinergic effects
Antihistamines: ↑ CNS depression
Opiates: ↑ CNS depressants
Phenothiazines: ↑ anticholinergic effects
Sedative/hypnotics: ↑ CNS depression

NURSING CONSIDERATIONS

Assessment

- Assess for allergic reactions: rash, urticaria; if these occur, drug should be discontinued
- Assess urinary patterns: distention, nocturia, frequency, urgency, incontinence; catheterization may be required to remove residual urine

Nursing diagnoses

✓ Urinary elimination, altered patterns (uses)
✓ Pain (uses)
✓ Knowledge deficit (teaching)

Implementation

- May be given with meals or fluids or given on an empty stomach

Patient/family education

- Advise patient to avoid hazardous activities until response to drug is known; dizziness, blurred vision may occur
- Caution patient to avoid OTC medication with alcohol or other CNS depressants
- Advise patient to prevent photophobia by wearing sunglasses
- Caution patient to stay cool, since overheating may occur
- Teach patient to use frequent rinsing of mouth, sips of water for dry mouth
- Teach patient to avoid hot weather, strenuous activity; drug decreases perspiration
- Advise patient to report CNS effects: confusion, anxiety, anticholinergic effect in the elderly
- Do not crush, break, or chew ext rel product

Evaluation

Positive therapeutic outcome

- Absence of dysuria, frequency, nocturia, incontinence

HIGH ALERT

oxycodone (℞)

(ox-i-koe'done)

Endocodone, M-oxy, Oxycontin, OxyFast, Oxyl R, Percolone, Roxicodone, Roxicodone Supeudol ♣

oxycodone/acetaminophen

Endocet ♣, Oxycocet ♣, Percocet, Roxicet, Roxilox, Tylox

oxycodone/aspirin

Endodan ♣, Oxycodan ♣, Percodan, Percodan-Demi, Roxiprin

Func. class.: Opiate analgesic
Chem. class.: Semisynthetic derivative

Pregnancy category B

Controlled substance schedule II

Action: Inhibits ascending pain pathways in CNS, increases pain threshold, alters pain perception

Therapeutic Outcome: Decreased pain

Uses: Moderate to severe pain

Investigational uses: Postherpetic neuralgia (cont rel)

Dosage and routes

Adult: PO 10-30 mg q4h (5 mg q6h for Oxyl R, OxyFast) OxyFast conc sol is extremely concentrated, do not use interchangeably

P ***Child:*** PO 0.05-0.15 mg/kg/dose up to 5 mg/dose q4-6h; not recommended in children

Available forms: *Oxycodone:* Cont rel tabs 10, 20, 40, 80, 160 mg; immediate rel tabs 15, 30 mg; tabs 5 mg; caps, oral sol 5 mg/5 ml, 20 mg/ml; *oxycodone with acetaminophen:* tabs 5 mg/325 mg; caps 5 mg/500 mg; oral sol 5 mg/325 mg/5 ml; *oxycodone with aspirin:* 2.44, 4.88 mg/325 mg

Adverse effects

CNS: *Drowsiness, dizziness, confusion, headache, sedation, euphoria*
CV: Palpitations, bradycardia, change in B/P
EENT: Tinnitus, blurred vision, miosis, diplopia
GI: *Nausea, vomiting, anorexia, constipation, cramps*
GU: Increased urinary output, dysuria, urinary retention
INTEG: *Rash,* urticaria, bruising, flushing, diaphoresis, pruritus
RESP: **Respiratory depression**

Contraindications: Hypersensitivity, addiction (opiate)

Precautions: Addictive personality, pregnancy **B,** lactation, increased ICP, MI (acute), severe heart disease, respiratory depression, hepatic disease, renal disease, P child <18 yr

Do Not Confuse:

Percodan/Decadron, Roxicet/Roxanol, Tylox/Trimox, Tylox/Wymox, Tylox/Xanax

Pharmacokinetics

Absorption	Well absorbed
Distribution	Widely distributed; crosses placenta
Metabolism	Liver, extensively
Excretion	Kidneys, breast milk
Half-life	2-3 hr

Pharmacodynamics

	PO	REC
Onset	15-30 min	Unknown
Peak	½-1 hr	Unknown
Duration	4-6 hr	4-6 hr

Interactions

Individual drugs

Alcohol: ↑ respiratory depression, hypotension, sedation
Nalbuphine: ↓ analgesia
Pentazocine: ↓ analgesia

Drug classifications

Antihistamines: ↑ respiratory depression, hypotension

CNS depressants: ↑ respiratory depression, hypotension
MAOIs: Do not use 2 wk before oxycodone
Phenothiazines: ↑ respiratory depression, hypotension
Sedative/hypnotics: ↑ respiratory depression, hypotension

Lab test interferences
↑ Amylase

NURSING CONSIDERATIONS

Assessment

- Monitor VS after parenteral route; note muscle rigidity, drug history, liver, kidney function tests, respiratory dysfunction: respiratory depression, character, rate, rhythm; notify prescriber if respirations are <10/min
- Monitor CNS changes: dizziness, drowsiness, hallucinations, euphoria, LOC, pupil reaction
- Monitor allergic reactions: rash, urticaria

Nursing diagnoses

- ✓ Pain (uses)
- ✓ Sensory-perceptual alteration: visual, auditory (adverse reactions)
- ✓ Breathing pattern, ineffective (adverse reactions)
- ✓ Injury, risk for (adverse reactions)
- ✓ Knowledge deficit (teaching)

Implementation

- Give with antiemetic if nausea, vomiting occur
- Give when pain is beginning to return; determine dosage interval by patient response; continuous dosing of medication is more effective than when given prn
- Medication should be slowly withdrawn after long-term use to prevent withdrawal symptoms
- Store in light-resistant container at room temp

PO route

- May be given with food or milk to lessen GI upset
- Use 80, 160 mg cont rel tabs only in opioid-tolerant patients
- Do not break, crush, or chew cont rel tabs

Rectal route

- Store supp in the refrigerator; run under warm water before insertion

Patient/family education

- Advise patients to avoid CNS depressants: alcohol, sedative/hypnotics
- Discuss with patient that dizziness, drowsiness, and confusion are common; to avoid getting up without assistance
- Discuss in detail all aspects of the drug, including purpose and what to expect
- Advise patient to make position changes slowly to lessen orthostatic hypotension

Evaluation

Positive therapeutic outcome

- Decreased pain

Treatment of overdose:

Naloxone 0.2-0.8 **IV**, O_2, **IV** fluids, vasopressors

HIGH ALERT

oxymorphone (℞)

(ox-i-mor'fone)

Num orphan

Func. class.: Opiate analgesic

Chem. class.: Semisynthetic phenanthrene derivative

Pregnancy category B

Controlled substance schedule II

Action: Depresses pain impulse transmission at the spinal cord level by interacting with opioid receptors

Therapeutic Outcome: Decreased pain

Uses: Moderate to severe pain

Dosage and routes

Adult: IM/SC 1-1.5 mg q4-6h prn; **IV** 0.5 mg q4-6h prn; rec 5 mg q4-6h prn

Labor analgesia

Adult: IM 0.5-1 mg

Available forms: Inj 1, 1.5 mg/ml; supp 5 mg

Adverse effects

CNS: *Drowsiness, dizziness, confusion, headache, sedation, euphoria,* **seizures**

CV: Palpitations, **bradycardia,** change in B/P

EENT: Tinnitus, blurred vision, miosis, diplopia

GI: *Nausea, vomiting, anorexia, constipation, cramps*

GU: Increased urinary output, dysuria, urinary retention

INTEG: *Rash,* urticaria, bruising, flushing, diaphoresis, pruritus

RESP: **Respiratory depression**

Contraindications: Hypersensitivity, addiction (narcotic)

Precautions: Addictive personality, pregnancy **B** (short- term), lactation, increased ICP, MI (acute), severe heart disease, respiratory depression, hepatic disease, renal disease, [P] child <18 yr

Pharmacokinetics

Absorption	Well absorbed (rec, IM, SC); completely absorbed (**IV**)
Distribution	Widely distributed; crosses placenta
Metabolism	Liver, extensively
Excretion	Kidneys
Half-life	2½-4 hr

Pharmacodynamics

	IM/SC	IV	REC
Onset	15 min	10 min	30 min
Peak	1-1½ hr	15-30 min	Unknown
Duration	3-6 hr	3-4 hr	3-6 hr

Interactions

Individual drugs

Alcohol: ↑ respiratory depression, hypotension, sedation

Nalbuphine: ↓ analgesia

Pentazocine: ↓ analgesia

Drug classifications

Antihistamines: ↑ respiratory depression, hypotension

CNS depressants: ↑ respiratory depression, hypotension

MAOIs: Do not use 2 wk before oxymorphone

Sedative/hypnotics: ↑ respiratory depression, hypotension

Lab test interferences

↑ Amylase, ↑ lipase

NURSING CONSIDERATIONS

Assessment

- Monitor VS after parenteral route; note muscle rigidity, drug history, liver, kidney function tests, respiratory dysfunction: respiratory depression, character, rate, rhythm; notify prescriber if respirations are <10/min
- Monitor CNS changes: dizziness, drowsiness, hallucinations, euphoria, LOC, pupil reaction
- Monitor allergic reactions: rash, urticaria

Nursing diagnoses

- ✓ Pain (uses)
- ✓ Sensory-perceptual alteration: visual, auditory (adverse reactions)
- ✓ Breathing pattern, ineffective (adverse reactions)
- ✓ Injury, risk for (adverse reactions)
- ✓ Knowledge deficit (teaching)

Implementation

- Give with antiemetic if nausea, vomiting occur
- Give when pain is beginning to return; determine dosage interval by patient response; continuous dosing of medication is more effective than when given prn
- Medication should be slowly withdrawn after long-term use to prevent withdrawal symptoms

- Store in light-resistant container at room temp

Rectal route

- Store in refrigerator

IV route

- Give by direct **IV** undiluted over 2-3 min

Y-site compatibilities: Glycopyrrolate, hydroxyzine, ranitidine

Patient/family education

- Advise patients to avoid CNS depressants: alcohol, sedative/hypnotics
- Discuss with patient that dizziness, drowsiness, and confusion are common; to avoid getting up without assistance
- Discuss in detail all aspects of the drug, including purpose and what to expect
- Advise patient to make position changes slowly to lessen orthostatic hypotension

Evaluation

Positive therapeutic outcome

- Decreased pain

Treatment of overdose: Naloxone (Narcan) 0.2-0.8 mg **IV**, O_2, **IV** fluids, vasopressors

HIGH ALERT

oxytocin (℞)

(ox-i-toe′sin)

Pitocin, Syntocinon

Func. class.: Oxytocic hormone

Pregnancy category N/A

Action: Acts directly on myofibrils, producing uterine contraction; stimulates breast milk letdown

Therapeutic Outcome: Stimulation of labor, control of bleeding; stimulation of milk letdown

Uses: Stimulation, induction of labor; missed or incomplete abortion, postpartum bleeding, postpartum breast engorgement

Dosage and routes

Labor induction

Adult: **IV** 1-2 mU/min, increase by 1-2 mU q15-60 min until regular contractions occur, then decrease dosage

Postpartum hemorrhage

Adult: **IV** 10 U infused at 20-40 mU/min

Adult: IM 10 U after placenta delivery

Incomplete abortion

Adult: **IV** 10 U at a rate of 20-40 mU/min

Fetal stress test

Adult: **IV** 0.5 mU/min; increase q20 min until 3 contractions occur at 10 min; not to exceed 20 mU only with fetal monitoring

Available forms: Inj 10 U/ml

Adverse effects

CNS: Hypertension, **seizures, tetanic contractions**

CV: Hypotension, dysrhythmias, increased pulse, bradycardia, tachycardia, premature ventricular contractions

FETUS: Dysrhythmias, jaundice, hypoxia, **intracranial hemorrhage**

GI: Anorexia, nausea, vomiting, constipation

GU: **Abruptio placentae, decreased uterine blood flow**

HEMA: Increased hyperbilirubinemia

INTEG: Rash

RESP: **Asphyxia**

Contraindications: Hypersensitivity, pregnancy-induced hypertension, cephalopelvic disproportion, fetal distress, hypertonic uterus

Precautions: Cervical/uterine surgery, uterine sepsis, primipara >35 yr, 1st, 2nd stage of labor

Pharmacokinetics

Absorption	Well absorbed (nasal); completely absorbed (**IV**)
Distribution	Widely distributed (extracellular fluid)
Metabolism	Liver, rapidly
Excretion	Kidneys
Half-life	3-12 min

Pharmacodynamics

	NASAL	IV	IM
Onset	5 min	Rapid	3-7 min
Peak	Unknown	Unknown	Unknown
Duration	20 min	1 hr	1 hr

Interactions

Individual drugs

Cyclopropane anesthesia: ↑ hypotension

Drug classifications

Vasopressors: ↑ hypertension

Herb/drug

Ephedra: ↑ hypertension

NURSING CONSIDERATIONS

Assessment

- Assess labor contractions: fetal heart tones, frequency, duration, intensity of contractions; if fetal heart tones increase or decrease significantly or if contractions are longer than 1 min, notify prescriber; turn patient on left side to increase oxygen to fetus
- Assess for water intoxication: confusion, anuria, drowsiness, headache; notify prescriber
- Watch for fetal distress, acceleration, deceleration, fetal presentation, pelvic dimensions
- Monitor B/P, pulse, respiratory rate, rhythm, depth
- Monitor I&O ratio
- Provide an environment conducive to letdown reflex

Nursing diagnoses

- ✓ Breast-feeding (uses)
- ✓ Injury, risk for (uses)
- ✓ Knowledge deficit (teaching)

Implementation

IV route

- Use an infusion pump; rotate sol for mixing; have magnesium sulfate available
- For labor induction administer after diluting 10 U/L of D_5W, 0.9% NaCl, 0.45% NaCl, LR, Ringer's for a conc of 10 U/ml; start at 1-2 U/min (0.1-0.2 ml); may increase by 1-2 U/min q15-30 min until labor begins
- For threatened abortion administer after diluting 10 U/500 ml of D_5W, $D_{10}W$, 0.9% NaCl, 0.45% NaCl, LR, Ringer's for a conc of 20 U/ml; give at 10-40 U/min
- For postpartum bleeding administer after diluting 10-40 U/L of D_5W, $D_{10}W$, 0.9% NaCl, 0.45% NaCl, LR, Ringer's for a conc of 10-40 U/ml; may titrate to response

Y-site compatibilities:

Heparin, regular insulin, hydrocortisone, meperidine, morphine, potassium chloride, vit B/C, warfarin

Additive compatibilities:

Chloramphenicol, metaraminol, netilmicin, sodium bicarbonate, thiopental, verapamil

Additive incompatibilities:

Fibrinolysin, warfarin

Patient/family education

- Teach patient to report increased blood loss, abdominal cramps, increased temp or foul-smelling lochia
- Advise patient that contractions will be similar to menstrual cramps, gradually increasing in intensity

Evaluation

Positive therapeutic outcome

- Stimulation of milk letdown (nasal)
- Induction of labor
- Decreased postpartum bleeding

paclitaxel (℞)
(pa-kli-tax'el)
Onxol, Taxol
Func. class.: Miscellaneous antineoplastic
Chem. class.: Natural diterpene, antimicrotubule
Pregnancy category D

Action: Inhibits the reorganization of the microtubule network needed for interphase and mitotic cellular functions; also causes abnormal bundles of microtubules during cell cycle and multiple esters of microtubules during mitosis

Therapeutic Outcome: Prevention of rapidly growing malignant cells

Uses: Taxol: metastatic carcinoma of the ovary unresponsive to other treatment, breast carcinoma; AIDS-related Kaposi's sarcoma (2nd-line), non–small-cell lung cancer, adjuvant treatment for node-positive breast cancer; Onxol: failure of other treatment in breast cancer, advanced ovarian cancer

Investigational uses: Advanced head, neck, small-cell lung cancer; non-Hodgkin's lymphoma, adenocarcinoma of the upper GI tract, hormone-refractory prostate cancer

Dosage and routes

Ovarian cancer

Adults: **IV** inf 135 mg/m^2 given over 24 hr q3 wk, then cisplatin 75 mg/m^2 or 175 mg/m^2 over 3 hr q3 wk

Advanced ovarian carcinoma

Adult: **IV** inf 175 mg/m^2 with cisplatin 75 mg/m^2 over 3 hr q3 wk

Breast carcinoma

Adult: **IV** inf 175 mg/m^2 over 3 hr q3 wk × 4 courses

AIDS-related Kaposi's sarcoma

Adult: **IV** inf 135 mg/m^2 over 3 hr q3 wk or 100 mg/m^2 over 3 hr q2 wk

1st line non–small-cell lung cancer

Adult: Inf 135 mg/m^2/24 hr with cisplatin 75 mg/m^2 × 3 wk

Available forms: Inj 30 mg/5 ml vial (6 mg/ml)

Adverse effects

CV: *Bradycardia, hypotension, abnormal ECG*
GI: *Nausea, vomiting, diarrhea, mucositis; increased bilirubin, alkaline phosphatase, AST*
HEMA: **Neutropenia, leukopenia, thrombocytopenia, anemia,** bleeding, infections
INTEG: Alopecia
MS: **Arthralgia, myalgia**
NEURO: *Peripheral neuropathy*
SYST: *Hypersensitivity reactions,* **anaphylaxis**

Contraindications: Hypersensitivity to paclitaxel or other drugs with polyoxyethylated castor oil, neutropenia (neutrophils <1500/mm^3), pregnancy **D**

Precautions: Children, lactation, hepatic disease, CV disease, CNS disorder

Do Not Confuse:
paclitaxel/paroxetine, paclitaxel/Paxil, Taxol/Paxil

Pharmacokinetics

Absorption	Completely absorbed
Distribution	89%-98% protein binding
Metabolism	Liver, extensively
Excretion	Unknown
Half-life	5-17 hr

Pharmacodynamics

Onset	Unknown
Peak	1-2 wk
Duration	3 wk

Interactions

Individual drugs

Cisplatin: ↑ myelosuppression
Cyclosporine: ↓ metabolism of paclitaxel

Dexamethasone: ↓ metabolism of paclitaxel
Diazepam: ↓ metabolism of paclitaxel
Doxorubicin: ↑ levels of doxorubicin
Etoposide: ↓ metabolism of paclitaxel
Ketoconazole: ↑ toxicity
Quinidine: ↓ metabolism of paclitaxel
Radiation: ↑ myelosuppression
Teniposide: ↓ metabolism of paclitaxel
Testosterone: ↓ metabolism of paclitaxel

Drug classifications

Antineoplastics: ↑ myelosuppression
Live virus vaccines: ↓ immune response

NURSING CONSIDERATIONS

Assessment

- Assess CNS changes: confusion, paresthesias, psychosis, tremors, seizures, neuropathies; drug should be discontinued
- Check buccal cavity q8h for dryness, sores or ulceration, white patches, oral pain, bleeding, dysphagia; obtain prescription for viscous lidocaine (Xylocaine) to use in mouth
- Assess symptoms indicating severe allergic reaction, anaphylaxis: rash, pruritus, urticaria, purpuric skin lesions, itching, flushing
- Monitor CBC, differential, platelet count weekly; withhold drug if WBC is <1500/mm^3 or platelet count is <100,000/mm^3, notify prescriber of results
- Monitor renal function studies: BUN, creatinine, serum uric acid, urine CrCl before and during therapy; check I&O ratio; report fall in urine output to <30 ml/hr
- Monitor temp q4h (may indicate beginning of infection)
- Monitor liver function tests before and during therapy (bilirubin, AST, ALT, LDH) as needed or monthly; check for jaundice of skin and sclera, dark urine, clay-colored stools, itchy skin, abdominal pain, fever, diarrhea
- Assess for bleeding: hematuria, stool guaiac, bruising or petechiae, mucosa or orifices q8h; check for inflammation of mucosa, breaks in skin
- Assess effects of alopecia on body image; discuss feelings about body changes

Nursing diagnoses

- ✓ Injury, risk for (adverse reactions)
- ✓ Body image disturbance (adverse reactions)
- ✓ Infection, risk for (adverse reactions)
- ✓ Knowledge deficit (teaching)

Implementation

IV route

- Give after diluting in 0.9% NaCl, D_5, D_5 and 0.9% NaCl, D_5LR to a concentration of 0.3-1.2 mg/ml
- Use an in-line filter ≤0.22 μm
- Give after premedicating with dexamethasone 20 mg PO 12 and 6 hr before paclitaxel, diphenhydramine 50 mg **IV** ½-1 hr before paclitaxel and cimetidine 300 mg or ranitidine 50 mg **IV** ½-1 hr before paclitaxel
- Use only glass bottles, polypropylene, polyolefin bags and administration sets; do not use PVC infusion bags or sets
- Use gloves and cytotoxic handling precautions
- Give fluids PO before chemotherapy to hydrate patient
- Give antacid before oral agent; give drug after evening meal, before hs; provide antiemetic 30-60 min before giving drug and prn to prevent vomiting; administer antibiotics for prophylaxis of infection
- Give top or systemic analgesics for pain to lessen effects of stomatitis
- Give liq diet: carbonated beverages; gelatin may be added if patient is not nauseated or vomiting
- Encourage patient to rinse mouth

tid-qid with water, club soda; brush teeth bid-qid with soft brush or cotton-tipped applicators for stomatitis; use unwaxed dental floss

Y-site compatiblilities: Acyclovir, amikacin, aminophylline, bleomycin, butorphanol, calcium chloride, carboplatin, cefepime, cefotetan, ceftazidime, ceftriaxone, cimetidine, cisplatin, cyclophosphamide, cytarabine, dacarbazine, dexamethasone, diphenhydramine, doxorubicin, droperidol, etoposide, famotidine, floxuridine, fluconazole, fluorouracil, furosemide, ganciclovir, gentamicin, haloperidol, heparin, mannitol, meperidine, mesna, methotrexate, metoclopramide, morphine, nalbuphine, ondansetron, pentostatin, potassium chloride, prochlorperazine, propofol, ranitidine, sodium bicarbonate, vancomycin, vinblastine, vincristine, zidovudine

Patient/family education

- Inform patient that nonhormonal contraceptive measures are recommended during therapy and >4 mo after; teratogenic effects are possible
- Teach patient to avoid use of products containing aspirin or ibuprofen, razors, commercial mouthwash, since bleeding may occur; to report symptoms of bleeding (hematuria, tarry stools)
- Instruct patient to report signs of anemia (fatigue, headache, irritability, faintness, shortness of breath) and CNS reactions (confusion, psychosis, nightmares, seizures, severe headaches)
- Inform patient that hair may be lost during treatment; a wig or hairpiece may make patient feel better; new hair may be different in color, texture
- Inform patient that receiving vaccinations during therapy may cause serious reactions

Evaluation

Positive therapeutic outcome

- Prevention of rapid division of malignant cells

palivizumab (℞)

(pal-ih-viz′uh-mab)

Synagis

Func. class.: Monoclonal antibody

Pregnancy category C

Action: A humanized monoclonal antibody that exhibits neutralizing and fusion-inhibitory activity against respiratory syncytial virus (RSV)

➔ **Therapeutic Outcome:** Absence of RSV

Uses: Prevention of serious lower respiratory tract disease caused by P RSV in pediatric patients

Dosage and routes

P ***Child:*** IM 15 mg/kg, those patients who develop RSV should receive monthly doses during RSV season

Available forms: Lyophilized inj 100 mg

Adverse effects

EENT: Otitis media, rhinitis, pharyngitis

GI: Nausea, vomiting, diarrhea, increased AST

INTEG: Rash, inj site reaction

RESP: Upper respiratory tract infection, **apnea**

Contraindications: Hypersensitivity, adults, cyanotic congenital heart disease

Precautions: Thrombocytopenia, coagulation disorders, established RSV, congenital heart disease, chronic lung disease, systemic allergic reactions, pregnancy **C**

P

Pharmacokinetics	
Absorption	Unknown
Distribution	Unknown
Metabolism	Unknown
Excretion	Unknown
Half-life	20 days

Pharmacodynamics	
Onset	Unknown
Peak	Unknown
Duration	Unknown

Interactions
Unknown

NURSING CONSIDERATIONS
Assessment
- Assess for presence of RSV infection, drug is given to prevent infection
- Assess for side effects and report if allergic reaction is evident

Nursing diagnoses
- ✓ Infection, risk for (uses)
- ✓ Knowledge deficit (teaching)

Implementation
- Give IM only
- Give after adding 1 ml of sterile water for inj per 100 mg vial, gently swirl, let stand at room temperature for 20 min until sol clarifies; given within 6 hr of reconstitution

Patient/family education
- Teach patient to report upper respiratory infections, earaches, rash, sore throat

Evaluation
Positive therapeutic outcome
- Absence of RSV

pamidronate (℞)
(pam-i-drone'ate)
Aredia
Func. class.: Bone resorption inhibitor, electrolyte modifier
Chem. class.: Bisphosphonate

Pregnancy category C

Action: Absorbs calcium phosphate crystals in bone and may directly block dissolution of hydroxyapatite crystals of bone; inhibits bone resorption, apparently without inhibiting bone formation and mineralization

Therapeutic Outcome: Serum calcium at normal level

Uses: Moderate to severe hypercalcemia associated with malignancy with or without bone metastases; osteolytic lesions in breast cancer patients

Dosage and routes
Adult: **IV** inf 60-90 mg in moderate hypercalcemia, 90 mg in severe hypercalcemia given over 24 hr

Paget's disease
Adult: **IV** 90-180 mg/treatment, may use 30 mg qd × 3 days up to 30 mg/wk × 6 wk

Available forms: Inj 30, 60, 90 mg/vial pamidronate disodium and 470 mg of mannitol

Adverse effects
CNS: *Fatigue*
CV: *Hypertension, fluid overload,* dysrhythmias, tachycardia
GI: *Abdominal pain, anorexia, constipation, nausea, vomiting*
GU: UTI, fluid overload
INTEG: Redness, swelling, induration, pain on palpation at site of catheter insertion
META: Anemia, hypokalemia, hypomagnesemia, hypophosphatemia
MS: *Bone pain*

Contraindications: Hypersensitivity to bisphosphonates

P **Precautions:** Children, nursing

mothers, pregnancy **C**, renal dysfunction

Do Not Confuse:

Aredia/Adriamycin

Pharmacokinetics

Absorption	Rapidly cleared from circulation
Distribution	Mainly to bones
Metabolism	Unknown
Excretion	Kidneys, unchanged (50%)
Half-life	Biphasic 1½ hr; 27 hr; from bone to 300 days

Pharmacodynamics

Onset	1 day
Peak	1 wk
Duration	Unknown

Interactions:
Individual drugs

Calcium: ↓ pamidronate effect
Digoxin: ↑ hypomagnesemia, hypokalemia
Vitamin D: ↓ pamidronate effect

NURSING CONSIDERATIONS
Assessment

• Assess for hypocalcemia: Chvostek's, Trousseau's sign, paresthesia, twitching, laryngospasm
• Monitor manifestations of hypocalcemia: personality changes, anxiety, disturbances, depression, psychosis; nausea, vomiting, constipation, abdominal pain from muscle spasm; decreased contractility, decreased cardiac output, hypotension, lengthened ST segment, prolonged QT interval; scaling eczema, alopecia, hyperpigmentation; tetany, muscle twitching, cramping, grimacing, seizure, altered deep tendon reflexes, spasm
• Monitor manifestations of hypomagnesemia: agitation; muscle twitching, paresthesia, hyperactive reflexes, positive Babinski reflex, dysphagia, nystagmus, seizures, tetany; nausea, vomiting, diarrhea, anorexia, abdominal distention; ectopy, tachycardia, broad, flat, or inverted T waves, depressed ST segment, prolonged QT interval, decreased cardiac output, hypotension
• Monitor manifestations of hypokalemia: acidic urine, reduced urine osmolality, nocturia, polyuria, polydipsia; hypotension, broad T wave, U wave, ectopy, tachycardia, weak pulse; muscle weakness, altered LOC, drowsiness, apathy, lethargy, confusion, depression; anorexia, nausea, cramps, constipation, distention, paralytic ileus; hypoventilation, respiratory muscle weakness
• Assess fluid volume status: check I&O ratio and record, assess for distended red veins, crackles in lung, color, quality, and sp gr of urine, skin turgor, adequacy of pulses, moist mucous membranes, bilateral lung sounds, peripheral pitting edema
• Monitor electrolytes: phosphorus, potassium, sodium, calcium, magnesium; also include BUN, creatinine, CBC, platelets, hemoglobin
• Assess B/P before and during therapy
• Assess for pain: in joints or on exertion, duration and characteristics; analgesics may be ordered
• Assess for phlebitis at **IV** site: swelling, redness, pain, warmth

Nursing diagnoses

✓ Injury, risk for (uses, adverse reactions)
✓ Fluid excess (side effects)
✓ Knowledge deficit (teaching)

Implementation

• Give by **IV** inf after reconstituting by adding 10 ml of sterile water for inj to each vial, then adding to 1000 ml of sterile 0.45%, 0.9% NaCl, D_5W, run over 24 hr for hypercalcemia or 60 mg ≥4 hr, 90 mg/24 hr; dilute reconstituted sol in 500 ml of 0.9% NaCl, 0.45% NaCl, or D_5W, give over 4 hr (multiple myeloma, Paget's disease)

P

- Store inf sol for up to 24 hr at room temp
- Reconstituted sol with sterile water may be stored under refrigeration for up to 24 hr

Additive incompatibilities: Calcium products, sol

Patient/family education

- Advise patient to report hypercalcemic relapse: nausea, vomiting, bone pain, thirst
- Advise patient to continue with dietary recommendations, including calcium and vit D

Evaluation

Positive therapeutic outcome

- Decreased calcium levels to normal

pancrelipase (℞)

(pan-kre-li'pase)

Cotazym, Cotazym Capsules, Cotazym-S Capsules, Creon Capsules, Ilozyme, Ku-Zyme HP Capsules, Pancrease Capsules, Pancrease MT 4, Pancrease MT 10, Pancrease MT 16, Ultrase MT 12, Ultrase MT 20, Ultrase MT 24, Viokase Powder, Viokase Tablets, Zymase

Func. class.: Digestant

Chem. class.: Pancreatic enzyme (bovine/porcine)

Pregnancy category C

Action: Pancreatic enzyme needed for breakdown of substances released from the pancreas

➔ **Therapeutic Outcome:** Increases protein, fat, carbohydrate digestion

Uses: Exocrine pancreatic secretion insufficiency, cystic fibrosis (digestive aid), steatorrhea, pancreatic enzyme deficiency

Dosage and routes

P ***Adult and child:*** PO 1-3 cap/tab ac or with meals, or 1 cap/tab with snack or 1-2 powder packets ac

Available forms: Powder 16,800 U lipase/70,000 U protease and amylase; caps 8,000 U lipase/30,000 U protease and amylase; delayed rel caps, 4,000 U lipase/12,000 U protease and amylase, 4,000 U lipase/25,000 U protease/20,000 U amylase, 5,000 U lipase/20,000 U protease and amylase, 10,000 U lipase/30,000 U protease and amylase, 12,000 U lipase/24,000 U protease and amylase, 12,000 U lipase/39,000 U protease and amylase, 16,000 U lipase/48,000 U protease and amylase 20,000 U lipase/65,000 U protease and amylase, 24,000 U lipase/78,000 U protease and amylase

Adverse effects

GI: Anorexia, nausea, vomiting, diarrhea

GU: Hyperuricuria, hyperuricemia

Contraindications: Allergy to pork

Precautions: Pregnancy **C**

Pharmacokinetics	
Absorption	Unknown
Distribution	Unknown
Metabolism	Unknown
Excretion	Unknown
Half-life	Unknown

Pharmacodynamics

Unknown

Interactions

Individual drugs

Cimetidine: ↓ absorption of pancrelipase

Oral iron: ↓ absorption of pancrelipase

Drug classifications

Antacids: ↓ absorption of pancrelipase

Food/drug

Alkaline foods: ↓ enteric coating

Lab test interferences
↑ Uric acid (serum, urine)

NURSING CONSIDERATIONS
Assessment
- Monitor I&O ratio; watch for increasing urinary output
- Monitor fecal fat, nitrogen, protime, during treatment
- Monitor for polyuria, polydipsia, polyphagia (may indicate diabetes mellitus)
- Assess for allergy to pork; patient may also be sensitive to this drug
- Assess for appropriate weight, height, development; there may be a developmental lag
- Check stools for steatorrhea, which signifies undigested fat content

Nursing diagnoses
✓ Nutrition, altered: less than body requirements (uses)
✓ Knowledge deficit (teaching)

Implementation
- Give after antacid or cimetidine; decreased pH inactivates drug
- Give powder mixed in prepared fruit for infants, children (P)
- Administer low-fat diet to decrease GI symptoms
- Store in airtight container at room temp

Patient/family education
- Teach patient to take tab with 8 oz or more water, not to let tab sit in mouth; have patient take tab sitting up only
- Advise patient to notify prescriber of allergic reactions, abdominal pain, cramping, or hematuria
- Teach patient not to inhale powder, very irritating to mucous membranes, some powder may irritate skin

Evaluation
Positive therapeutic outcome
- Absence of steatorrhea
- Improved digestion of carbohydrates, proteins, fat

HIGH ALERT

pancuronium (℞)
(pan-cure-oh'nee-yum)
pancuronium bromide, Pavulon
Func. class.: Neuromuscular blocker (nondepolarizing)
Chem. class.: Synthetic curariform
Pregnancy category C

Action: Inhibits transmission of nerve impulses by binding with cholinergic receptor sites, antagonizing action of acetylcholine; no analgesic response

→ **Therapeutic Outcome:** Paralysis of all skeletal muscles

Uses: Facilitation of endotracheal intubation, skeletal muscle relaxation during mechanical ventilation, surgery, or general anesthesia

Dosage and routes
Adult: **IV** 0.04-0.1 mg/kg, then 0.01 mg/kg q30-60 min

(P) ***Child >10 yr:*** **IV** 0.04-0.1 mg/kg, then 1/5 initial dose q30-60 min

Available forms: Inj 1, 2 mg/ml

Adverse effects
CV: Bradycardia, tachycardia, increased, decreased B/P, ventricular extrasystoles
EENT: Increased secretions
INTEG: Rash, flushing, pruritus, urticaria, sweating, salivation
MS: Weakness to prolonged skeletal muscle relaxation
RESP: **Prolonged apnea, bronchospasm, cyanosis, respiratory depression**

Contraindications: Hypersensitivity to bromide ion

Precautions: Pregnancy **C,** renal disease, cardiac disease, lactation, (P) children <2 yr, electrolyte imbalances, dehydration, neuromuscular disease, respiratory disease

P

Pharmacokinetics

Absorption	Complete bioavailability
Distribution	Extracellular space; crosses placenta
Metabolism	Plasma
Excretion	Kidneys, unchanged
Half-life	2 hr

Pharmacodynamics

Onset	30-45 sec
Peak	3-5 min
Duration	35-40 min

Interactions

Individual drugs

Clindamycin: ↑ paralysis length and intensity
Colistin: ↑ paralysis length and intensity
Lidocaine: ↑ paralysis length and intensity
Lithium: ↑ paralysis length and intensity
Magnesium: ↑ paralysis length and intensity
Polymyxin B: ↑ paralysis length and intensity
Procainamide: ↑ paralysis length and intensity
Quinidine: ↑ paralysis length and intensity
Succinylcholine: ↑ paralysis length and intensity

Drug classifications

Aminoglycosides: ↑ paralysis length and intensity
β-Adrenergic blockers: ↑ paralysis length and intensity
Diuretics, potassium-losing: ↑ paralysis length and intensity
General anesthesia: ↑ paralysis length and intensity

NURSING CONSIDERATIONS

Assessment

- Monitor vital signs (B/P, pulse, respirations, airway) until fully recovered; note rate, depth, pattern of respirations, strength of hand grip; patient should be intubated before use
- Monitor for electrolyte imbalances (potassium, magnesium) before drug is used; electrolyte imbalances may lead to increased action of this drug
- Monitor for recovery: decreased paralysis of face, diaphragm, leg, arm, rest of body; residual weakness and respiratory problems may occur during recovery period
- Assess for hypersensitive reactions: rash, fever, respiratory distress, pruritus; drug should be discontinued

Nursing diagnoses

- ✓ Breathing pattern, ineffective (uses)
- ✓ Communication, impaired verbal (adverse reactions)
- ✓ Fear (adverse reactions)
- ✓ Knowledge deficit (teaching)

Implementation

- Use peripheral nerve stimulator (anesthesiologist) to determine neuromuscular blockade; deep tendon reflexes should be monitored during extended periods
- Give direct **IV** undiluted over 1-2 min, or diluted in D_5W or 0.9% NaCl and give as an inf at prescribed rate; titrate to patient response; should be administered only by qualified person, usually an anesthesiologist; do not administer IM
- Store in light-resistant area
- Give anticholinesterase to reverse neuromuscular blockade

Syringe compatibilities:

Heparin

Y-site compatibilities:

Aminophylline, cefazolin, cefuroxime, cimetidine, dobutamine, dopamine, epinephrine, esmolol, fentanyl, fluconazole, gentamicin, heparin, hydrocortisone, isoproterenol, lorazepam, midazolam, morphine, nitroglycerin, nitroprusside, ranitidine, sulfamethoxazole/trimethoprim, vancomycin

Y-site incompatibilities:

Diazepam

Additive compatibilities:

Verapamil

Additive incompatibilities: Barbiturates

Patient/family education

- Provide reassurance if communication is difficult during recovery from neuromuscular blockade
- Provide explanation to patients regarding all procedures or treatments; patient will remain conscious if anesthesia is not given also

Evaluation

Positive therapeutic outcome

- Paralysis of jaw, eyelid, head, neck, rest of body as evaluated by peripheral nerve stimulator

Treatment of overdose: Edrophonium or neostigmine, atropine; monitor VS; may require mechanical ventilation

pantoprazole (℞)

(pan-toe-pray′zole)

Protonix, Protonix IV

Func. class.: Proton pump inhibitor

Chem. class.: Benzimidazole

Pregnancy category C

Action: Suppresses gastric secretion by inhibiting hydrogen/potassium ATPase enzyme system in gastric parietal cell; characterized as gastric acid pump inhibitor, since it blocks final step of acid production

Therapeutic Outcome: Absence of epigastric fullness, pain, swelling

Uses: Gastroesophageal reflux disease (GERD), severe erosive esophagitis, maintenance

Dosage and routes

Adult: PO 40 mg qd × 8 wk, may repeat course; **IV**

Available forms: Tabs, delayed rel 20, 40 mg; powder for inj, freeze dried 40 mg/vial

Adverse effects

CNS: *Headache,* insomnia

GI: *Diarrhea, abdominal pain,* flatulence

INTEG: *Rash*

META: Hyperglycemia

Contraindications: Hypersensitivity

Precautions: Pregnancy **C,** lactation, children

Pharmacokinetics	
Absorption	Unknown
Distribution	Protein binding 97%
Metabolism	Unknown
Excretion	Urine-metabolites, feces, ↓ rate in elderly
Half-life	1½ hr

Pharmacodynamics	
Onset	Unknown
Peak	2.4 hr
Duration	>24 hr

Interactions

Individual drugs

Clarithromycin: ↑ levels of pantoprazole

Diazepam: ↑ level of pantoprazole

Flurazepam: ↑ level of pantoprazole

Phenytoin: ↑ level of pantoprazole

Sucralfate: ↓ absorption of pantoprazole

Triazolam: ↑ level of pantoprazole

Warfarin: ↑ risk of bleeding

NURSING CONSIDERATIONS

Assessment

- Assess GI system: bowel sounds q8h, abdomen for pain, swelling, anorexia
- Monitor hepatic enzymes: AST, ALT, alkaline phosphatase during treatment

Nursing diagnoses

✓ Knowledge deficit (teaching)

Implementation

- May take with or without food
- Do not crush del rel tabs, swallow whole

P

IV route
- Reconstitute with 10 ml of 0.9% NaCl, further dilute with 100 ml of Ringer's, D_5 (0.4 mg/ml), given over 15 min (≤3 mg/ml) using in-line filter provided

Patient/family education
- Advise patient to report severe diarrhea; drug may have to be discontinued
- Advise patient with diabetes that hypoglycemia may occur
- Advise patient to avoid hazardous activities; dizziness may occur
- Advise patient to avoid alcohol, salicylates, ibuprofen; may cause GI irritation

Evaluation
Positive therapeutic outcome
- Absence of epigastric pain, swelling, fullness

paricalcitol (℞)
(par-ih-cal'sih-tol)
Zemplar
Func. class.: Vitamin D analog
Chem. class.: Fat-soluble vitamin

Pregnancy category C

Action: Reduces parathyroid hormone (PTH) levels; suppresses PTH levels in patients with chronic renal failure with absence of hypercalcemia/hyperphosphatemia; serum PO_4, Ca, calcium-phosphate product (Ca × P) may increase

Therapeutic Outcome: Decreased symptoms of hypoparathyroidism

Uses: Hypoparathyroidism

Dosage and routes
Adult: **IV** bol 0.04-0.1 µg/kg (2.8-7 µg) no more than qod during dialysis; may increase by 2-4 µg q2-4 wk

Available forms: Inj 5 µg/ml

Adverse effects
CNS: Light-headedness
CV: Palpitations
GI: Nausea, vomiting, anorexia, dry mouth
MISC: Pneumonia, edema, chills, fever, flu, sepsis

Contraindications: Hypersensitivity, hypercalcemia

Precautions: CV disease, renal calculi, pregnancy **C**, elderly, lactation, children

Pharmacokinetics	
Absorption	Unknown
Distribution	Unknown
Metabolism	Unknown
Excretion	Unknown
Half-life	Unknown

Pharmacodynamics	
Onset	Unknown
Peak	Unknown
Duration	Unknown

Interactions
Individual drugs
Digitalis: ↑ toxicity

NURSING CONSIDERATIONS
Assessment
- Monitor Ca, PO_4, 2 ×/wk qwk during initial therapy; after dose is established measure calcium and phosphorus q mo

Nursing diagnoses
- Knowledge deficit (teaching)

Implementation
IV route
- Give by **IV** bol only

Patient/family education
- Advise patient to report weakness, lethargy, headache, anorexia, loss of weight
- Teach patient to report nausea, vomiting, palpitations

Evaluation
Positive therapeutic outcome
- Decreased hypoparathyroidism in chronic renal disease

paroxetine (℞)

(par-ox'e-teen)

Paxil

Func. class.: Antidepressant, selective serotonin reuptake inhibitor (SSRI)

Chem. class.: Phenylpiperidine derivative

Pregnancy category B

Action: Inhibits CNS neuron reuptake of serotonin but not of norepinephrine or dopamine

Therapeutic Outcome: Relief of depression

Uses: Major depressive disorder, obsessive-compulsive disorder, panic disorder, generalized anxiety disorder

Investigational uses: Diabetic neuropathy, headache, premature ejaculation, premenstrual disorders, bipolar depression with lithium, fibromyalgia, posttraumatic stress disorder

Dosage and routes

Depression

Adult: PO 20 mg qd in AM; after 4 wk if no clinical improvement is noted, dosage may be increased by 10 mg/day weekly to desired response; not to exceed 50 mg/day; cont rel 25 mg/day

G ***Elderly:*** PO 10 mg qd, increase by 10 mg to desired dose, max 40 mg/day; cont rel 12.5 mg/day

Obsessive-compulsive disorder

Adults: PO 40 mg/day in AM; start with 20 mg/day, increase 10 mg/day increments, max 60 mg/day

Panic disorder

Adults: PO 40 mg/day; start with 10 mg/day and increase in 10 mg/day increments, max 60 mg/day

Renal dose

10 mg qd in AM, may increase by 10 mg/day q wk, max 40 mg qd

Premenstrual disorders (off-label)

Adult: PO 10-30 mg qd

Available forms: Tabs 10, 20, 30, 40 mg; susp 10 mg/5 ml; oral susp 10 mg/5 ml

Adverse effects

CNS: *Headache, nervousness, insomnia, drowsiness, anxiety, tremor, dizziness, fatigue, sedation,* abnormal dreams, agitation, apathy, euphoria, hallucinations, delusions, psychosis

CV: Vasodilatation, postural hypotension, palpitations

EENT: Visual changes, rhinitis, oropharyngeal disorder

GI: *Nausea, diarrhea, constipation, dry mouth, anorexia,* dyspepsia, vomiting, taste changes, flatulence, decreased appetite

GU: Dysmenorrhea, decreased libido, urinary frequency, UTI, amenorrhea, cystitis, impotence, *abnormal ejaculation, male genital disorders*

INTEG: *Sweating,* rash

MS: Pain, arthritis, myalgia, myopathy, myasthenia gravis

RESP: Infection, pharyngitis, nasal congestion, sinus headache, sinusitis, cough, dyspnea

SYST: Asthenia, fever, chills

Contraindications: Hypersensitivity, patients taking MAOIs, alcohol use

Precautions: Pregnancy **B,** lactation, children, elderly, seizure history, patients with history of mania, renal and hepatic disease

Do Not Confuse:
paroxetine/paclitaxel, Paxil/paclitaxel, Paxil/Taxol

P

Pharmacokinetics

Absorption	Well absorbed
Distribution	Widely distributed; crosses blood-brain barrier, protein-binding 95%
Metabolism	Liver, mostly
Excretion	Kidneys, unchanged (2%); breast milk
Half-life	21 hrs

Pharmacodynamics

Onset	Unknown
Peak	5.2 hr
Duration	Unknown

Interactions

Individual drugs

Alcohol: ↑ CNS depression
Digoxin: ↓ effect of digoxin
Phenytoin: ↓ effect of paroxetine
Procycline: ↓ metabolism
Quinidine: ↓ metabolism
Theophylline: ↑ theophylline levels
Warfarin: ↑ warfarin levels

Drug classifications

Antidepressants: ↓ metabolism
Antidysrhythmics, class 1C: ↓ metabolism
Barbiturates: ↑ effects
Benzodiazepines: ↑ effects
CNS depressants: ↑ effects
MAOIs: Hypertensive crisis, seizures; do not use together
Phenothiazines: ↓ metabolism

Lab test interferences

↑ Serum bilirubin, ↑ blood glucose, ↑ alkaline phosphatase
↓ VMA, ↓ 5-HIAA, ↓ blood glucose
False: ↑ Urinary catecholamines

NURSING CONSIDERATIONS

Assessment

- Assess mental status: mood, sensorium, affect, suicidal tendencies; increase in psychiatric symptoms: depression, panic
- Assess for withdrawal symptoms: headache, nausea, vomiting, muscle pain, weakness; do not usually occur unless drug was discontinued abruptly
- Monitor B/P (with patient lying, standing), pulse q4h; if systolic B/P drops 20 mm Hg, hold drug, notify prescriber; take VS q4h in patients with CV disease
- Monitor blood studies: CBC, leukocytes, differential, cardiac enzymes if patient is receiving long-term therapy
- Monitor hepatic studies: AST, ALT, bilirubin
- Check weight weekly; appetite may increase with drug
- Assess ECG for flattening of T wave, bundle branch block, AV block, dysrhythmias in cardiac patients
- G Assess for EPS primarily in elderly: rigidity, dystonia, akathisia
- Monitor urinary retention, P constipation; constipation is more G likely to occur in children or elderly
- Identify alcohol consumption; if alcohol is consumed, hold dose until AM

Nursing diagnoses

- ✓ Coping, ineffective individual (uses)
- ✓ Injury, risk for (adverse reactions)
- ✓ Knowledge deficit (teaching)
- ✓ Noncompliance (teaching)

Implementation

- Give with food or milk for GI symptoms; store at room temp; do not freeze
- Give crushed if patient is unable to swallow whole

Patient/family education

- Advise patient that therapeutic effects may take 1-4 wk
- Teach patient to use caution in driving and other activities requiring alertness because of drowsiness, dizziness, blurred vision; to avoid rising quickly from sitting to standing, G especially elderly
- Caution patient to avoid alcohol ingestion, other CNS depressants, and OTC medication unless prescribed
- Caution patient not to discontinue medication quickly after long-term use; may cause nausea, anxiety, headache, malaise; do not double doses if one is missed

- Advise patient to use gum, hard sugarless candy, or frequent sips of water for dry mouth; if dry mouth continues an artificial saliva product may be used

Evaluation

Positive therapeutic outcome

- Decrease in depression
- Absence of suicidal thoughts

Treatment of overdose: Maintain airway, for seizures give diazepam, symptomatic treatment

HIGH ALERT

pegaspargase (℞)

(peg-as'per-gase)

Oncaspar, PEG-L-asparaginase

Func. class.: Antineoplastic

Chem. class.: Escherichia coli enzyme

Pregnancy category D

Action: Indirectly inhibits protein synthesis in tumor cells; without amino acid, DNA, RNA synthesis is halted; asparagine, protein synthesis is halted; G_1 phase of cell cycle specific; a nonvesicant

Therapeutic Outcome: Prevention of rapidly growing malignant cells

Uses: Acute lymphocytic leukemia unresponsive to other agents in combination with other antineoplastics

Dosage and routes

In combination

P *Adult and child with BSA ≥0.6 m²:* **IV** 1000 IU/kg/day × 10 days given over 30 min; IM 6000 IU/m²/day

P *Child with BSA <0.6 m²:* **IV**/IM 82.5 IU/kg q14 days

Sole induction

Adult: **IV** 200 IU/kg/day × 28 days

Available forms: Inj 10,000 IU

Adverse effects

CNS: Neuritis, dizziness, headache, **coma,** depression, fatigue, confusion, hallucinations, **seizures**

CV: Chest pain

ENDO: Hyperglycemia

GI: *Nausea, vomiting, anorexia, cramps, stomatitis,* **hepatotoxicity, pancreatitis**

GU: Urinary retention, **renal failure,** glycosuria, polyuria, azotemia, uric acid neuropathy

HEMA: **Thrombocytopenia, leukopenia, myelosuppression, anemia, decreased clotting factors**

INTEG: *Rash,* urticaria, chills, fever

RESP: **Fibrosis, pulmonary infiltrate**

SYST: **Anaphylaxis, hypersensitivity**

Contraindications: Hypersensitivity, infants, pregnancy **D,** lactation, pancreatitis

Precautions: Renal disease, hepatic disease

Pharmacokinetics	
Absorption	Complete bioavailability
Distribution	Intravascular spaces
Metabolism	Unknown
Excretion	Reticuloendothelial system
Half-life	5½ days

Pharmacodynamics	
Onset	Rapid
Peak	Unknown
Duration	2 wks

Interactions

Individual drugs

Methotrexate: Blocking action of methotrexate

Vincristine: ↑ neurotoxicity

Drug classifications

Glucocorticosteroids: ↑ hyperglycemia

Hepatotoxic agents: ↑ hepatotoxic agents

P

Lab test interferences

↓ Thyroid function tests
↑ BUN

NURSING CONSIDERATIONS

Assessment

- Assess for signs and symptoms of pancreatitis (nausea, vomiting, severe abdominal pain), anaphylaxis (bronchospasm, dyspnea), cyanosis; monitor amylase, glucose
- Assess symptoms indicating severe allergic reaction: rash, pruritus, urticaria, purpuric skin lesions, itching, flushing; monitor for joint pain, bronchospasm, hypotension; epinephrine and crash carts should be nearby
- Monitor for frequency of stools, characteristics: cramping, acidosis; signs of dehydration: rapid respirations, poor skin turgor, decreased urine output, dry skin, restlessness, weakness
- Monitor CBC, differential, platelet count weekly; withhold drug if WBC is <4000/mm^3 or platelet count is <100,000/mm^3; notify physician of results; also assess pro-time, PTT, and thrombin time, which may be increased
- Monitor renal function studies: BUN, creatinine, serum uric acid, urine CrCl before and during therapy; check I&O ratio; report fall in urine output to <30 ml/hr; patient should be well hydrated with 2-3 L/day to prevent urate deposits
- Monitor temp q4h (may indicate beginning of infection)
- Monitor liver function tests before and during therapy (bilirubin, AST, ALT, LDH) as needed or monthly; check for jaundice of skin and sclera, dark urine, clay-colored stools, itchy skin, abdominal pain, fever, diarrhea; also monitor cholesterol, alkaline phosphatase
- Assess for bleeding: hematuria, stool guaiac, bruising or petechiae, mucosa or orifices q8h; check for inflammation of mucosa, breaks in skin
- Identify edema in feet, joint pain, stomach pain, shaking

Nursing diagnoses

✓ Injury, risk for (adverse reactions)
✓ Infection, risk for (adverse reactions)
✓ Knowledge deficit (teaching)

Implementation

- Preparation by trained personnel is required in controlled environment
- Give fluids **IV** or PO before chemotherapy to hydrate patient
- Provide antiemetic 30-60 min before giving drug and prn to prevent vomiting; administer antibiotics for prophylaxis of infection
- Provide a liq diet: carbonated beverages; gelatin may be added if patient is not nauseated or vomiting

Intradermal route

- After intradermal skin testing and desensitization, give 0.1 ml (2 IU) intradermally after reconstituting with 5 ml of sterile water or 0.9% NaCl for inj; then add 0.1 ml of reconstituted drug to 9.9 ml of diluent (20 IU/ml); observe for 1 hr, check for wheal; desensitization may be required
- For direct **IV** dilute 10,000 IU/5 ml of sterile water for inj or 0.9% NaCl without preservatives; give through 5-μm filter if fibers are present; do not use if sol cloudy or discolored, give over 30 min through Y-site of full-flowing **IV** of 0.9% NaCl or D_5W; run **IV** sol for at least 2 hr after direct administration
- Give **IV** inf using 21-, 23-, 25-G needle; administer by slow **IV** inf via Y-tube or 3-way stopcock of flowing D_5W or 0.9% NaCl inf over 30 min after diluting 10,000 IU/5 ml of sterile water or 0.9% NaCl (no preservatives) to 2000 IU/ml; filter may be necessary if fibers are present
- Provide allopurinol or sodium bicarbonate to reduce uric acid levels, alkalinization of urine

IM route

- Dilute 10,000 IU/2 ml of 0.9% NaCl with preservatives; give 2 ml or less per site

Patient/family education

- Advise patient that contraceptive measures are recommended during therapy; drug is teratogenic
- Teach patient to avoid use of products containing aspirin or NSAIDs, razors, commercial mouthwash, since bleeding may occur; to report symptoms of bleeding (hematuria, tarry stools)
- Teach patient to report signs of anemia (fatigue, headache, irritability, faintness, shortness of breath)
- Tell patient to avoid crowds and persons with respiratory tract infections to prevent patient infection
- Advise patient to avoid vaccinations, since serious reactions can occur
- Teach patient to report nausea, vomiting, bruising, bleeding, stomatitis, severe diarrhea, jaundice, chest pain, abdominal pain, trouble breathing, rash

Evaluation

Positive therapeutic outcome

- Prevention of rapid division of malignant cells

pemoline (℞)

(pem'oh-leen)

Cylert, PemADD, pemoline

Func. class.: Cerebral stimulant

Chem. class.: Oxazolidinone derivative

Pregnancy category B

Controlled substance schedule IV

Action: Exact mechanism unknown; may act through dopaminergic mechanisms; produces CNS stimulation and a paradoxic effect in attention deficit hyperactivity disorder (ADHD)

➔ **Therapeutic Outcome:** Increased alertness, increased attention span, decreased hyperactivity (ADHD)

P **Uses:** ADHD for children >6 yr when other treatments have failed

Investigational uses: Narcolepsy, fatigue, excessive daytime sleepiness

Dosage and routes

P ***Child >6 yr:*** PO 37.5 mg in AM, increasing by 18.75 mg/wk, max 112.5 mg/day

Available forms: Tabs 18.75, 37.5, 75 mg; chewable tabs 37.5 mg

Adverse effects

CNS: Hyperactivity, insomnia, restlessness, dizziness, depression, headache, stimulation, irritability, aggressiveness, hallucinations, **seizures, masking or worsening of Gilles de la Tourette's syndrome,** drowsiness, dyskinetic movements

CV: Tachycardia

GI: Nausea, *anorexia,* diarrhea, abdominal pain, increased liver enzymes, **hepatitis,** jaundice, weight loss, **life-threatening hepatic failure**

MISC: Rashes, growth suppression in P children

Contraindications: Hypersensitivity, hepatic insufficiency

Precautions: Renal disease, pregnancy **B,** lactation, drug abuse, P child <6 yr, psychosis, tics, seizure disorders

Pharmacokinetics

Absorption	Well absorbed
Distribution	Widely distributed; crosses placenta
Metabolism	Liver
Excretion	Kidneys, pH dependent; increased pH, increased reabsorption
Half-life	12 hr; increased when urine is alkaline

P

Pharmacodynamics	
Onset	Unknown
Peak	2-4 hr
Duration	8 hr

Interactions
Drug classifications
Adrenergic blockers: ↑ stimulation
Anticonvulsants: ↓ seizure threshold
Antihypertensive: ↓ effect of pemoline
Decongestants: ↑ stimulation
CNS stimulants: ↑ stimulation
Food/drug
Caffeine (coffee, teas, chocolate): ↑ stimulation

NURSING CONSIDERATIONS
Assessment
- Monitor VS, B/P, since this drug may reverse effects of antihypertensives; check patients with cardiac disease more often for increased B/P
- Monitor height and weight q3 mo, since growth rate in children may be decreased; appetite is suppressed; weight loss is common during the first few mo of treatment
- Monitor mental status: mood, sensorium, affect, stimulation, insomnia; aggressiveness may occur; depression with crying spells may occur after drug has worn off
- Assess for tolerance; should not be used for extended time except in ADHD; dosage should be diminished gradually to prevent withdrawal symptoms
- In children or adults with ADHD, monitor for improved organizational skills, attention span, attending to tasks, impulse control, socialization, and ability to get along better with others
- Assess for withdrawal symptoms: headache, nausea, vomiting, muscle pain, weakness; drug tolerance will develop after long-term use; dosage should not be increased if tolerance develops
- Monitor hepatic and renal function studies: ALT, AST, bilirubin, creatinine, before treatment and periodically thereafter; life-threatening hepatic failure has occurred; discontinue drug if symptoms of hepatic failure occur

Nursing diagnoses
- ✓ Thought processes, altered (uses, adverse reactions)
- ✓ Coping, impaired individual (uses)
- ✓ Knowledge deficit (teaching)
- ✓ Family coping, impaired individual (uses)

Implementation
- Give in AM; titrate to patient's response; lowest dosage should be used to control symptoms
- Provide gum, hard candy, frequent sips of water for dry mouth at beginning of treatment; these symptoms tend to lessen with time

Patient/family education
- Teach patient to decrease caffeine consumption (coffee, tea, cola, chocolate), which may increase irritability and stimulation; to avoid OTC preparations unless approved by prescriber; to avoid alcohol ingestion; these may cause serious drug interactions
- Instruct patient to taper off drug over several wk, or depression, increased sleeping, lethargy may occur
- Caution patient to avoid hazardous activities until stabilized on medication
- Instruct patient not to double doses if medication is missed; prescriber may suggest drug holidays (ADHD) during the school year to assess progress and determine continued drug necessity
- Teach patient/family to notify prescriber if significant side effects occur: tremors, insomnia, palpitations, restlessness, jaundice, bleeding, dark urine; drug changes may be needed
- Inform patient that if dry mouth occurs to use frequent sips of water, sugarless gum, hard candy during beginning therapy; dry mouth lessens with continued treatment

• Advise patient to get needed rest; patients will feel more tired at end of day; to take last dose at least 6 hr before hs to avoid insomnia
• Teach patient about the possibility of hepatotoxicity

Evaluation

Positive therapeutic outcome

• Decreased activity in ADHD

Treatment of overdose: Administer fluids, hemodialysis, peritoneal dialysis, antihypertensives for increased B/P; ammonium chloride for increased excretion

PENICILLINS

penicillin G benzathine (℞)

(pen-i-sill'in)

Bicillin, Bicillin L-A, Megacillin ✤, Permapen

penicillin G potassium (℞)

Pfizerpen

penicillin G procaine (℞)

Crysticillin A.S., Duracillin A.S., Pfizerpen-AS, Wycillin

penicillin G sodium (℞)

Crystapen ✤, Pfizerpen ✤

penicillin V potassium (℞)

Apo-Pen-VK ✤, Betapen-VK, Deltapen-VK, Ledercillin-VK, Nadopen-V ✤, Novopen-VK ✤, Pen-Vee K ✤, PVFK ✤, Veetids

Func. class.: Broad-spectrum antiinfective

Chem. class.: Natural penicillin

Pregnancy category B

Action: Interferes with cell wall replication of susceptible organisms; osmotically unstable cell wall swells and bursts from osmotic pressure, resulting in cell death

➔ **Therapeutic Outcome:** Bactericidal effects on the gram-positive cocci *Staphylococcus, Streptococcus pyogenes, Streptococcus viridans, Streptococcus faecalis, Streptococcus bovis, Streptococcus pneumoniae;* gram-negative cocci *Neisseria gonorrhoeae;* gram-positive bacilli *Bacillus anthracis, Clostridium perfringens, Clostridium tetani, Corynebacterium diphtheriae, Listeria monocytogenes;* gram-negative bacilli *Escherichia coli, Proteus mirabilis, Salmonella, Shigella, Enterobacter, Streptobacillus moniliformis,* spirochete *Treponema pallidum; Actinomyces*

Uses: Respiratory tract infections, scarlet fever, erysipelas, otitis media, pneumonia, skin and soft tissue infections, gonorrhea; prevention of rheumatic fever, glomerulonephritis

Dosage and routes

Penicillin G benzathine

Early syphilis

Adult: IM 2.4 million U in single dose

Congenital syphilis

P ***Child <2 yr:*** IM 50,000 U/kg in single dose

Prophylaxis of rheumatic fever, glomerulonephritis

P ***Adult and child >27 kg:*** IM 1.2 million U in single dose qmo or 600,000 U q2 wk

P ***Child <27 kg:*** IM 25-50,000 U/kg as single dose qmo

Upper respiratory tract infections (group A streptococcal)

Adult: IM 1.2 million U in single dose; PO 400,000-600,000 U q4-6h

P ***Child >27 kg:*** IM 900,000 U in single dose

P ***Child <27 kg:*** IM 300,000-600,000 U in single dose

P

Available forms: Inj 300,000 U/ml; 600,000; 1,200,000; 2,400,000 U/dose

Penicillin G potassium
Pneumococcal/streptococcal infections (mild to moderate)

Adult: IM/**IV** 2-24 million U in divided doses q4h

P ***Child <12 yr:*** 100,000-400,000 U/kg/day in 4-6 divided doses

Renal dose

CrCl <50 ml/min dosage reduction indicated

Available forms: Inj 1, 2, 3 million U/50 ml; powder for inj 1, 5, 10, 20 million U/vial

Penicillin G procaine
Moderate to severe infections

P ***Adult and child:*** IM 600,000-1.2 million U in 1 or 2 doses/day for 10 days to 2 wk

P ***Newborn:*** 50,000 U/kg IM once daily (avoid use in newborns)

Gonorrhea

P ***Adult and child >12 yr:*** IM 4.8 million U in two injections given 30 min after probenecid 1 g

Renal dose

CrCl 10-30 ml/min q8-12h; CrCl <10 ml/min q12-18h

Available forms: Inj 600,000; 1,200,000; 2,400,000 U/dose; 300,000, 500,000, 600,000 U/ml

Penicillin G sodium
Moderate to severe infections

Adult: IM/**IV** 2 million-24 million U/day in divided doses q4h

P ***Child:*** IM/**IV** 50,000-400,000 U/kg/day in divided doses q4-12h

Dental surgery prophylaxis for endocarditis

Adult: IM/**IV** 2 million U ½-1 hr before procedure, then 1 million U 6 hr after procedure

Renal dose

CrCl <50 ml/min dosage reduction indicated

Available forms: Inj 5 million U/vial

Penicillin V potassium
Pneumococcal/staphylococcal infections

Adult: PO 250-500 mg q6h

P ***Child <12 yr:*** PO 25-50 mg/kg/day in divided doses q6-8h

Streptococcal infections

Adult: PO 125-250 mg q6-8h × 10 days

Prevention of recurrence of rheumatic fever/chorea

Adult: PO 125-250 mg bid continuously

P ***Child <5 yr:*** PO 125 mg bid

P ***Child >5 yr:*** PO 250 mg bid

Vincent's gingivitis/pharyngitis

Adult: PO 500 mg q6h

Renal dose

CrCl <50 ml/min dosage reduction indicated

Available forms: Tabs 125, 250, 500 mg; powder for oral sol 125, 250 mg/5 ml

Adverse effects

CNS: Lethargy, hallucinations, anxiety, depression, twitching, **coma, seizures**

GI: *Nausea, vomiting, diarrhea,* increased AST, ALT, abdominal pain, glossitis, colitis

GU: **Oliguria, proteinuria, hematuria, vaginitis, moniliasis, glomerulonephritis**

HEMA: Anemia, increased bleeding time, **bone marrow depression, granulocytopenia**

META: Hyperkalemia, hypokalemia, alkalosis, hypernatremia

MISC: Local pain, tenderness and fever with IM inj

Contraindications: Hypersensitivity to penicillins; neonates

Precautions: Hypersensitivity to cephalosporins, pregnancy **B**, severe renal disease

Penicillin G benzathine

Pharmacokinetics

Absorption	Delayed; prolonged drug levels
Distribution	Widely distributed; crosses placenta
Metabolism	Liver, minimally
Excretion	Kidneys, unchanged; breast milk
Half-life	½-1 hr

Pharmacodynamics

Onset	Slow
Peak	12-24 hr
Duration	1-4 wk

Penicillin G potassium

Pharmacokinetics

Absorption	Variably absorbed (PO); well absorbed (IM)
Distribution	Widely distributed; crosses placenta
Metabolism	Liver, minimally
Excretion	Kidneys, unchanged; breast milk
Half-life	½-1 hr

Pharmacodynamics

	PO	IM	IV
Onset	Rapid	Rapid	Rapid
Peak	1 hr	¼-½ hr	Immediate

Penicillin G procaine

Pharmacokinetics

Absorption	Delayed; prolonged drug levels
Distribution	Widely distributed; crosses placenta
Metabolism	Liver, minimally
Excretion	Kidneys, unchanged; breast milk
Half-life	½-1 hr

Pharmacodynamics

Onset	Slow
Peak	1-4 hr
Duration	15 hr

Penicillin G sodium

Pharmacokinetics

Absorption	Well absorbed
Distribution	Widely distributed; crosses placenta
Metabolism	Liver, minimally
Excretion	Kidneys, unchanged; breast milk
Half-life	½-1 hr

Pharmacodynamics

	IM	IV
Onset	Rapid	Rapid
Peak	1-3 hr	Rapid

Penicillin V potassium

Pharmacokinetics

Absorption	Widely absorbed
Distribution	Widely distributed; crosses placenta
Metabolism	Liver, minimally
Excretion	Kidneys, unchanged; breast milk
Half-life	½-1 hr

Pharmacodynamics

Onset	Rapid
Peak	½ hr

Interactions

Individual drugs

Aspirin: ↑ penicillin levels, ↓ renal excretion

Chloramphenicol: ↑ half-life of chloramphenicol, ↓ effectiveness of penicillin

Cholestyramine: ↓ effectiveness of penicillin

Colestipol: ↓ effectiveness of penicillin

Probenecid: ↑ penicillin levels, ↓ renal excretion

Drug classifications

Erythromycins: ↓ antimicrobial effectiveness

Oral anticoagulants: ↑ anticoagulant effects

Oral contraceptives: ↓ contraceptive effectiveness

Tetracyclines: ↓ antimicrobial effectiveness

Herb/drug

Khat: ↓ absorption of penicillin; separate doses by 2 hr or more

Food/drug

Food, carbonated drinks, citrus fruit juice: ↓ absorption

Lab test interferences

False positive: Urine glucose, urine protein

NURSING CONSIDERATIONS

Assessment

- Assess patient for previous sensitivity reaction to penicillins or cephalosporins; cross-sensitivity between penicillins and cephalosporins is common
- Assess patient for signs and symptoms of infection including characteristics of wounds, sputum, urine, stool, WBC >10,000/mm^3, earache, fever; obtain baseline information and during treatment
- Obtain C&S before beginning drug therapy to identify if correct treatment has been initiated
- Assess for allergic reactions: rash, urticaria, pruritus, chills, fever, joint pain; angioedema may occur a few days after therapy begins; epinephrine, resuscitation equipment should be available for anaphylactic reaction
- Identify urine output; if decreasing, notify prescriber (may indicate nephrotoxicity); also check for increased BUN, creatinine
- Monitor blood studies: AST, ALT, CBC, Hct, bilirubin, LDH, alkaline phosphatase, Coombs' test monthly if patient is on long-term therapy
- Monitor electrolytes: potassium, sodium, chloride monthly if patient is on long-term therapy
- Assess bowel pattern daily; if severe diarrhea occurs, drug should be discontinued; may indicate pseudomembranous colitis
- Monitor for bleeding: ecchymosis, bleeding gums, hematuria, stool guaiac daily if on long-term therapy
- Assess for overgrowth of infection: perineal itching, fever, malaise, redness, pain, swelling, drainage, rash, diarrhea, change in cough, sputum

Nursing diagnoses

- ✓ Infection, risk for (uses)
- ✓ Diarrhea (adverse reactions)
- ✓ Injury, risk for (adverse reactions)
- ✓ Knowledge deficit (teaching)
- ✓ Noncompliance (teaching)

Implementation

Penicillin G benzathine

PO route

- Give in even doses around the clock; if GI upset occurs, give with food, avoid acidic juices; carbonated beverages may decrease PO absorption; drug must be given for 10-14 days to ensure organism death and prevent superinfection
- Shake susp

IM route

- Do not give **IV**
- Give deep in large muscle mass
- Reconstitute with 0.9% NaCl, sterile water for inj, D_5W; refrigerate unused portion

Penicillin G potassium

PO route

- Give in even doses around the clock; if GI upset occurs, give with food; drug must be given for 10-14 days to ensure organism death and prevent superinfection
- Shake susp

IM route

- Reconstitute with D_5W, 0.9% NaCl, sterile water for inj; shake well
- Give deep in large muscle mass; massage

• Do not give SC; may cause severe pain
• If injected near a nerve, loss of function and severe pain may occur

IV **IV route**
• Change **IV** sites q48h to prevent pain and phlebitis
• Give by intermittent inf by diluting 3 million U or less/50 ml or more; dilute 3 million U or more/100 ml of D_5W, $D_{10}W$, 0.45% NaCl, 0.9% NaCl, LR, Ringer's, or any combination run over
P 1-2 hr (adult), 15-30 min (child)
• Give by cont inf by diluting and infusing over 24 hr

Syringe compatibilities: Heparin

Syringe incompatibilities: Metoclopramide

Y-site compatibilities: Acyclovir, amiodarone, cyclophosphamide, diltiazem, enalaprilat, esmolol, fluconazole, foscarnet, heparin, hydromorphone, labetalol, magnesium sulfate, meperidine, morphine, perphenazine, potassium chloride, tacrolimus, theophylline, verapamil, vit B/C

Additive compatibilities: Ascorbic acid, calcium chloride, calcium gluconate, cephapirin, chloramphenicol, cimetidine, clindamycin, colistimethate, corticotropin, dimenhydrinate, diphenhydramine, ephedrine, erythromycin, furosemide, hydrocortisone, kanamycin, lidocaine, magnesium sulfate, methicillin, methylprednisolone, metronidazole, polymyxin B, prednisolone, potassium chloride, procaine, prochlorperazine, verapamil

Additive incompatibilities: Aminoglycosides, aminophylline, amphotericin B, chlorpromazine, dopamine, floxacillin, hydroxyzine, metaraminol, oxytetracycline, pentobarbital, prochlorperazine mesylate, promazine, tetracycline, thiopental

Penicillin G procaine
• Do not give **IV**
• Give deeply in large muscle mass
• Reconstitute with 0.9% NaCl, sterile water for inj, D_5W; refrigerate unused portion
• Shake medication before administering
• IM route may include procaine reactions: fear of death, depression, seizures, anxiety, confusion, hallucinations

Penicillin G sodium

IM route
• Reconstitute with 0.9% NaCl, D_5W, sterile water
• May be diluted with lidocaine (1%, 2%) to prevent pain from inj (IM only); use lidocaine without epinephrine only
• Shake after reconstitution; give deep in large muscle mass; massage
• Do not give SC; severe pain may occur
• Inj near nerves can result in severe pain and loss of function of nerve that was injected

IV **IV route**
• Change **IV** sites q48h to prevent phlebitis and pain at site
• Give by intermittent inf by diluting 3 million U or less/50 ml or more; or doses of 73 million U/100 ml of D_5W, 0.9% NaCl; give over 1-2 hr (adult) or
P 30 min (child)
• Give by cont inf by diluting in compatible sol and run over 24 hr

Syringe compatibilities: Aminoglycosides, chloramphenicol, cimetidine, colistimethate, gentamicin, heparin, kanamycin, lincomycin, polymyxin B, streptomycin

Syringe incompatibilities: Oxytetracycline, tetracycline

Additive compatibilities: Calcium chloride, calcium gluconate, chloramphenicol, clindamycin, colistimethate, diphenhydramine, erythromycin, furosemide, gentamicin,

P

hydrocortisone, kanamycin, methicillin, polymyxin B, prednisolone, procaine, ranitidine, verapamil, vit B/C

Additive incompatibilities: Amphotericin B, bleomycin, cephalothin, chlorpromazine, cytarabine, floxacillin, hydroxyzine, methylprednisolone, oxytetracycline, prochlorperazine, promethazine

Penicillin V potassium

- Give in even doses around the clock; if GI upset occurs, give with food; drug must be given for 10-14 days to ensure organism death and prevent superinfection; store in tight container
- Shake susp; store in refrigerator for 2 wk or for 1 wk at room temp

Patient/family education

- Teach patient to report sore throat, bruising, bleeding, joint pain; may indicate blood dyscrasias (rare)
- Advise patient to contact prescriber if vaginal itching, loose, foul-smelling stools, furry tongue occur; may indicate superinfection
- Instruct patient to take all medication prescribed for the length of time ordered
- Advise patient to notify prescriber of diarrhea with blood or pus, which may indicate pseudomembranous colitis

Evaluation

Positive therapeutic outcome

- Absence of signs/symptoms of infection (WBC <10,000/mm^3, temp WNL, absence of red, draining wounds, earache)
- Reported improvement in symptoms of infection

Treatment of anaphylaxis: Withdraw drug, maintain airway, administer epinephrine, aminophylline, O_2, **IV** corticosteroids

pentamidine (℞)

(pen-tam′i-deen)

Nebupent, Pentam 300, Pentacarinat ✤, Pneumopent ✤

Func. class.: Antiprotozoal

Chem. class.: Aromatic diamide derivative

Pregnancy category C

Action: Interferes with DNA/RNA synthesis in protozoa; has direct effect on islet cells in the pancreas

➔ **Therapeutic Outcome:** Protozoa death

Uses: Treatment/prevention of *Pneumocystis carinii* infections

Investigational uses: Babesiosis, leishmaniasis, African trypanosomiasis

Dosage and routes

P ***Adult and child:*** **IV**/IM 4 mg/kg/day × 2-3 wk; neb 300 mg via specific nebulizer given q4 wk for prevention

Available forms: Inj; aerosol 300 mg/vial; sol for aerosol 60 mg/vial ✤

Adverse effects

CNS: Disorientation, hallucinations, dizziness, confusion

CV: Hypotension, ventricular tachycardia, ECG abnormalities; **dysrhythmias**

GI: Nausea, vomiting, anorexia, increased AST, ALT, **acute pancreatitis,** metallic taste

GU: **Acute renal failure, increased serum creatinine, renal toxicity**

HEMA: Anemia, **leukopenia, thrombocytopenia**

INTEG: Sterile abscess, pain at inj site, pruritus, urticaria, rash

META: Hyperkalemia, hypocalcemia, *hypoglycemia, hyperglycemia*

MISC: Fatigue, chills, night sweats, **anaphylaxis, Stevens-Johnson syndrome**

RESP: Cough, shortness of breath, **bronchospasm** (with aerosol)

Precautions: Blood dyscrasias,

hepatic disease, renal disease, diabetes mellitus, cardiac disease, hypocalcemia, pregnancy **C**, hypertension, hypotension, lactation, children

P

Pharmacokinetics

Absorption	Well absorbed (IM); minimally absorbed (inh); completely absorbed (**IV**)
Distribution	Widely distributed; does not appear in CSF
Metabolism	Not known
Excretion	Kidneys, unchanged (up to 30%)
Half-life	6½-9½ hr; increased in renal disease

Pharmacodynamics

	IM	IV	INH
Onset	Unknown	Unknown	Unknown
Peak	½-1 hr	Inf end	Unknown

Interactions

Individual drugs

Amphotericin B: ↑ nephrotoxicity
Cisplatin: ↑ bone marrow depression
Colistin: ↑ nephrotoxicity
Erythromycin IV: fatal dysrhythmias
Foscarnet: ↑ nephrotoxicity
Methoxyflurane: ↑ bone marrow depression
Polymyxin B: ↑ bone marrow depression
Radiation: ↑ nephrotoxicity, bone marrow depression
Vancomycin: ↑ bone marrow depression

Drug classifications

Aminoglycosides: ↑ nephrotoxicity
Antineoplastics: ↑ nephrotoxicity, bone marrow depression

NURSING CONSIDERATIONS

Assessment

- Assess any patient with compromised renal system: drug is excreted slowly in poor renal system function; toxicity may occur rapidly
- Assess patient for infection including increased temp, thick sputum, WBC >10,000/mm^3; monitor these signs of infection throughout treatment; obtain C&S before beginning therapy; treatment may begin after culture is obtained
- Assess respiratory system including rate, rhythm, bilateral lung sounds, shortness of breath, wheezing, dyspnea
- Monitor ECG for cardiac dysrhythmias; ECG and pulse should be checked frequently during treatment, since cardiotoxicity can occur
- Assess for hypoglycemia including nausea, tremors, anxiety, chills, diaphoresis, headache, hunger, cold, pale skin; this side effect can last for several mo after treatment is completed
- Monitor for hyperglycemia including flushed, dry skin, acetone breath, thirst, anorexia, drowsiness, polyuria; this side effect can last for several mo after treatment is completed
- Monitor renal function studies including BUN, urinalysis, creatinine; obtain at baseline and frequently during treatment; nephrotoxicity may occur; check I&O, report hematuria, oliguria
- Monitor blood studies including blood glucose, CBC, platelets; blood glucose fluctuations are common; anemia, leukopenia, thrombocytopenia can occur
- Monitor liver function studies including AST, ALT, alkaline phosphatase, bilirubin before beginning treatment and every 3 days during therapy
- Monitor calcium and magnesium before beginning treatment and every 3 days during therapy; hypocalcemia may occur

Nursing diagnoses

✓ Infection, risk for (uses)
✓ Knowledge deficit (teaching)

Implementation

IM route

- Reconstitute 300 mg/3 ml of sterile water for inj; give deep in large muscle

P

mass by Z-track; IM is a painful route
• Do not mix in normal saline

IV route
• For intermittent inf reconstitute 300 mg/3-5 ml of sterile water for inj, D_5W; withdraw dose and further dilute in 50-250 ml of D_5W; diluted sol is stable for 48 hr; discard unused sol; give over 1 hr or more

Y-site compatibilities: Zidovudine

Y-site incompatibilities: Foscarnet, fluconazole

Inhalation route
• Dilute 300 mg/600 ml sterile water for inj; put reconstituted sol into nebulizer; do not use with other drugs or sol precipitate may occur; sol stable for 48 hr at room temp; protect from light; administer over 30-45 min

Patient/family education
• Teach patient to report sore throat, fever, fatigue; could indicate superinfection
• Advise patient not to drink alcohol or take aspirin, since gastric bleeding may occur
• Teach patient to make position changes slowly to prevent orthostatic hypotension
• Advise patient to maintain adequate fluid intake

Evaluation

Positive therapeutic outcome
• Decreased signs and symptoms of protozoan infections
• Decreased signs and symptoms of *Pneumocystis carinii* pneumonia in HIV infections

HIGH ALERT

pentazocine (℞)
(pen-taz'oh-seen)
Talwin, Talwin NX
Func. class.: Opiate analgesic
Chem. class.: Synthetic benzomorphan (agonist/antagonist)

Pregnancy category C

Controlled substance schedule IV

Action: Inhibits ascending pain pathways in limbic system, thalamus, midbrain, hypothalamus by binding to opiate receptor sites, altering pain perception and response

Therapeutic Outcome: Relief of pain

Uses: Moderate to severe pain

Dosage and routes

Adult: PO 50-100 mg q3-4h prn, not to exceed 600 mg/day; **IV**/IM/SC 30 mg q3-4h prn, not to exceed 360 mg/day

Labor

Adult: IM 60 mg; **IV** 30 mg q2-3h when contractions are regular

Renal dose

CrCl 10-50 ml/min q24-36h; CrCl <10 ml/min q48h

Available forms: SC, IM, **IV** 30 mg/ml; tabs 50 mg

Adverse effects

CNS: *Drowsiness, dizziness, confusion, headache, sedation, euphoria, hallucinations,* dreaming

CV: Palpitations, bradycardia, change in B/P, tachycardia, increased B/P (high doses)

EENT: Tinnitus, blurred vision, miosis (high doses), diplopia

GI: *Nausea,* vomiting, anorexia, constipation, cramps, dry mouth

GU: Urinary retention

INTEG: *Rash,* urticaria, bruising,

flushing, diaphoresis, pruritus, severe irritation at inj sites
RESP: **Respiratory depression**

Contraindications: Hypersensitivity, addiction (narcotic)

Precautions: Addictive personality, pregnancy **C**, lactation, increased ICP, MI (acute), severe heart disease, respiratory depression, hepatic disease, renal disease, seizure disorder, P child <18 yr, head trauma

Pharmacokinetics

Absorption	Well absorbed (PO, SC, IM); completely absorbed (**IV**)
Distribution	Widely distributed; crosses placenta
Metabolism	Liver, extensively
Excretion	Kidneys, small amounts (unchanged)
Half-life	2-3 hr

Pharmacodynamics

	PO	SC/IM	IV
Onset	15-30 min	15-30 min	Rapid
Peak	1-3 hr	1-2 hr	15 min
Duration	3 hr	2-4 hr	1 hr

Interactions
Individual drugs
Alcohol: ↑ respiratory depression, hypotension, sedation
Drug classifications
Antihistamines: ↑ respiratory depression, hypotension
CNS depressants: ↑ respiratory depression, hypotension
MAOIs: Use cautiously; results are unpredictable
Opiates: ↑ opioid withdrawals (dependency)
Phenothiazines: ↑ respiratory depression, hypotension
Sedative/hypnotics: ↑ respiratory depression, hypotension
Lab test interferences
↑ Amylase, ↑ lipase

NURSING CONSIDERATIONS
Assessment
- Assess pain characteristics: location, intensity, type of pain before medication administration and after treatment
- Monitor VS after parenteral route; note muscle rigidity, drug history, liver, kidney function tests, respiratory dysfunction: respiratory depression, character, rate, rhythm; notify prescriber if respirations are <10/min
- Monitor CNS changes: dizziness, drowsiness, hallucinations, euphoria, LOC, pupil reaction
- Monitor allergic reactions: rash, urticaria
- Assess for withdrawal symptoms in opiate-dependent patients

Nursing diagnoses
✓ Pain (uses)
✓ Sensory-perceptual alteration: visual, auditory (adverse reactions)
✓ Breathing pattern, ineffective (adverse reactions)
✓ Knowledge deficit (teaching)

Implementation
- Give by inj (IM, **IV**), only when resuscitative equipment available; give slowly to prevent rigidity
- Store in light-resistant area at room temp

PO route
- Tabs made in the United States contain naloxone 0.5 mg to prevent abuse if the PO preparation is used **IV**

SC/IM route
- Give IM deeply in large muscle mass; rotate inj sites; repeated SC inj may cause necrosis

IV **IV route**
- Give by direct **IV** after diluting 5 mg/ml of sterile water for inj; give 5 mg or less over 1 min

Syringe compatibilities:
Atropine, benzquinamide, butorphanol, chlorpromazine, cimetidine, dimenhydrinate, diphenhydramine, droperidol, fentanyl, hydromorphone, hydroxyzine, meperidine, metoclopra-

P

mide, morphine, perphenazine, prochlorperazine, promazine, promethazine, propiomazine, ranitidine, scopolamine

Syringe incompatibilities: Glycopyrrolate, heparin, pentobarbital, other barbiturates

Y-site compatibilities: Heparin, hydrocortisone, potassium chloride, vit B/C

Y-site incompatibilities: Nafcillin

Additive incompatibilities: Aminophylline, amobarbital, pentobarbital, phenobarbital, secobarbital, sodium bicarbonate

Patient/family education

- Teach patient to report any symptoms of CNS changes, allergic reactions
- Advise patients to avoid CNS depressants: alcohol, sedative/hypnotics for at least 24 hr after taking this drug
- Discuss with patient that dizziness, drowsiness, and confusion are common; to avoid getting up without assistance
- Discuss in detail all aspects of the drug
- Instruct patient to change position slowly to prevent orthostatic hypotension
- Teach patient to turn, cough, deep breathe after surgery to prevent atelectasis

Evaluation

Positive therapeutic outcome

- Relief of pain

Treatment of overdose: Naloxone (Narcan) 0.2-0.8 mg **IV**, O_2, **IV** fluids, vasopressors

HIGH ALERT

pentobarbital (℞)

(pen-toe-bar′bi-tal)

Nembutal, Novopentobarb ✱, Nova-Rectal ✱, pentobarbital sodium

Func. class.: Sedative/hypnotic barbiturate; anticonvulsant

Chem. class.: Barbitone, short acting

Pregnancy category D

Controlled substance schedule II (USA), schedule G (Canada)

Action: Depresses activity in brain cells, primarily in reticular activating system in brainstem; also selectively depresses neurons in posterior hypothalamus, limbic structures; may decrease cerebral blood flow, intracranial pressure (**IV**) and cerebral edema; may potentiate GABA, an inhibitory neurotransmitter

Therapeutic Outcome: Sedation, sleep

Uses: Insomnia, sedation, preoperative medication, increased intracranial pressure, dental anesthetic

Dosage and routes

Adult: PO 100-200 mg hs; IM 150-200 mg hs; **IV** 100 mg initially, then up to 500 mg; rec 120-200 mg hs

P ***Child:*** IM 2-6 mg/kg, not to exceed 100 mg; PO 2-6 mg/kg/day in divided doses; PO preoperatively 2-6 mg/kg, max 100 mg/dose; **IV** 50 mg (hypnotic/anticonvulsant)

Available forms: Caps 50, 100 mg; elixir 20 mg/5 ml; rec supp 25, 30, 50, 60, 120, 200 mg; inj 50 mg/ml

Adverse effects

CNS: *Lethargy, drowsiness, hangover,* dizziness, paradoxic stimulation in elderly and children, lightheadedness, dependence, **CNS de-**

pression, mental depression, slurred speech
CV: Hypotension, bradycardia
GI: Nausea, vomiting, diarrhea, constipation
HEMA: **Agranulocytosis, thrombocytopenia, megaloblastic anemia** (long-term treatment)
INTEG: Rash, urticaria, pain, abscesses at inj site, angioedema, thrombophlebitis, **Stevens-Johnson syndrome**
RESP: **Depression, apnea, laryngospasm, bronchospasm**

Contraindications: Hypersensitivity to barbiturates, respiratory depression, addiction to barbiturates, severe liver, renal impairment, porphyria, uncontrolled pain, pregnancy **D**

Precautions: Anemia, lactation, hepatic disease, renal disease, hypertension, elderly, acute/chronic pain

Do Not Confuse:
pentobarbital/phenobarbital

Pharmacokinetics

Absorption	Well absorbed
Distribution	Widely distributed; crosses placenta, enters breast milk
Metabolism	Liver
Excretion	Kidneys, unchanged (minimally)
Half-life	15-48 hr

Pharmacodynamics

	PO	IM	IV	REC
Onset	15-30 min	10-25 min	Immediate	Slow
Peak	3-4 hr	Unknown	1 min	Unknown
Duration	4-6 hr	1-4 hr	15 min	4-6 hr

Interactions:
Individual drugs
Alcohol: ↑ CNS depression
Chloramphenicol: ↓ effectiveness
Cyclophosphamide: ↑ hematologic toxicity
Cyclosporine: ↓ effectiveness
Dacarbazine: ↓ effectiveness
Quinidine: ↓ effectiveness
Valproic acid: ↑ sedation
Drug classifications
Anticoagulants: ↓ effectiveness
Antidepressants: ↑ CNS depression
Antidepressants, tricyclic: ↓ effectiveness
Antihistamines: ↑ CNS depression
Glucocorticoids: ↓ effectiveness
MAOIs: ↑ CNS depression
Opiates: ↑ CNS depression
Oral contraceptives: ↓ effectiveness
Sedative/hypnotics: ↑ CNS depression
Herb/drug
Quinine: ↑ pentobarbital level

NURSING CONSIDERATIONS
Assessment
- Assess mental status: mood, sensorium, affect, memory (long, short), especially elderly; if using as a hypnotic, assess sleep patterns during therapy; drug suppresses REM sleep with dreaming; withdrawal insomnia may occur after short-term use; do not start using drug again; insomnia will improve in 1-3 nights; may experience increased dreaming
- Monitor for respiratory dysfunction: respiratory depression, character, rate, rhythm (when using **IV**); hold drug if respirations are <10/min or if pupils are dilated; also check VS q30 min after parenteral route for 2 hr
- Assess for blood dyscrasias: fever, sore throat, bruising, rash, jaundice, epistaxis (long-term treatment only)
- Assess seizure activity including type, location, duration, and character; provide seizure precaution
- Assess for pain in postoperative patients; pain threshold is lowered when patients are taking this medication

Nursing diagnoses
✓ Injury, risk for (side effects)
✓ Knowledge deficit (teaching)

P

Implementation

- Administer only after removal of cigarettes, to prevent fires
- Reserve use until after trying conservative measures for insomnia

PO route

- Give 30 min before bedtime for expected sleeplessness
- May dilute elixir in juice, milk, or water if needed
- Give on empty stomach for best absorption

IM route

- Give deeply in muscle mass (gluteal) to minimize irritation to tissues; split inj >5 ml into 2 inj since irritation to tissues may occur; do not administer SC

IV **IV route**

- Use large vein to prevent extravasation; if extravasation occurs, use moist heat to the area and 5% procaine sol injected into area; give at 50 mg/1 min or more
- Give **IV** only with resuscitative equipment available (and only by qualified personnel)

Syringe compatibilities: Aminophylline, ephedrine, hydromorphone, neostigmine, scopolamine, sodium bicarbonate, thiopental

Syringe incompatibilities: Benzquinamide, butorphanol, chlorpromazine, cimetidine, dimenhydrinate, diphenhydramine, droperidol, fentanyl, glycopyrrolate, hydroxyzine, meperidine, midazolam, nalbuphine, pentazocine, perphenazine, prochlorperazine, promazine, promethazine, ranitidine

Y-site compatibilities: Acyclovir, propofol, regular insulin

Additive compatibilities: Amikacin, aminophylline, calcium chloride, cephapirin, chloramphenicol, dimenhydrinate, erythromycin, lidocaine, thiopental, verapamil

Additive incompatibilities: Chlorpheniramine, codeine, ephedrine, erythromycin gluceptate, hydrocortisone, hydroxyzine, levorphanol, methadone, norepinephrine, pentazocine, penicillin G potassium, phenytoin, promazine, promethazine, regular insulin, sodium succinate, streptomycin, triflupromazine, vancomycin

Patient/family education

- Teach patient to carry ID card or bracelet stating name, drugs taken, condition, prescriber's name, phone number
- Caution patient to avoid driving and other activities that require alertness
- Caution patient to avoid alcohol ingestion and CNS depressants; increased sedation may occur
- Teach patient not to discontinue medication quickly after long-term use; taper off over several wk

Evaluation

Positive therapeutic outcome

- Improved sleeping patterns
- Decreased seizure activity
- Improved energy

Treatment of overdose: Lavage, activated charcoal, warming blanket, vital signs, hemodialysis

---

HIGH ALERT

pentostatin (℞)

(pen'toe-sta-tin)

Nipent

Func. class.: Antineoplastic, enzyme inhibitor

Chem. class.: Streptomyces antibioticus derivative

Pregnancy category D

Action: Inhibits the enzyme adenosine deaminase (ADA), which is able to block DNA synthesis and some RNA synthesis

Therapeutic Outcome: Prevention of rapidly growing malignant cells

Uses: α-Interferon–refractory hairy

cell leukemia, chronic lymphocytic leukemia

Dosage and routes

Adult: **IV** 4 mg/m^2 every other wk; may be given **IV** bol or diluted in a larger volume and given over 20-30 min

Available forms: Inj 10 mg/vial

Adverse effects

CNS: Headache, anxiety, confusion, depression, dizziness, insomnia, nervousness, paresthesia
GI: Nausea, vomiting, anorexia, diarrhea, constipation, flatulence, stomatitis, elevated liver function tests
GU: **Hematuria,** dysuria, increased BUN/creatinine
HEMA: **Leukopenia, anemia, thrombocytopenia, ecchymosis, lymphadenopathy,** petechiae
INTEG: Rash, eczema, dry skin, pruritus, sweating, herpes simplex/zoster
RESP: Cough, upper respiratory tract infection, bronchitis, dyspnea, epistaxis, pneumonia, pharyngitis, rhinitis, sinusitis
SYST: Fever, infection, fatigue, pain, allergic reaction, chills, **death, sepsis,** chest pain, flu syndrome

Contraindications: Hypersensitivity to this drug or mannitol, pregnancy **D**

Precautions: Renal disease, P lactation, children, bone marrow depression

Pharmacokinetics

Absorption	Completely absorbed
Distribution	Unknown; low protein binding
Metabolism	Unknown
Excretion	Kidneys
Half-life	5-7 hr; increased in renal disease

Pharmacodynamics

Onset	4-5 mo
Peak	Unknown
Duration	1½-34 mo

Interactions

Individual drugs

Fludarabine: Fatal pulmonary reaction
Vidarabine: ↑ adverse reactions

NURSING CONSIDERATIONS

Assessment

- Assess CNS changes: confusion, paresthesias, psychosis, tremors, seizures, neuropathies; drug should be discontinued
- Assess for toxicity: facial flushing, epistaxis, increased pro-time, thrombocytopenia; drug should be discontinued
- Assess acidosis, signs of dehydration: rapid respirations, poor skin turgor, decreased urine output, dry skin, restlessness, weakness
- Check buccal cavity q8h for dryness, sores or ulceration, white patches, oral pain, bleeding, dysphagia; obtain prescription for viscous lidocaine (Xylocaine) to use in mouth
- Assess symptoms indicating severe allergic reaction: rash, pruritus, urticaria, purpuric skin lesions, itching, flushing
- Assess tachypnea, ECG changes, dyspnea, edema, fatigue; respiratory and cardiovascular reaction can be severe
- Monitor CBC, differential, platelet count weekly; withhold drug if WBC is <2000/mm^3 or platelet count is <100,000/mm^3, notify prescriber of results
- Monitor renal function studies: BUN, creatinine, serum uric acid, urine CrCl before and during therapy; I&O ratio; report fall in urine output to <30 ml/hr

P

- Monitor temp q4h (may indicate beginning of infection)
- Monitor liver function tests before and during therapy (bilirubin, AST, ALT, LDH) as needed or monthly; check for jaundice of skin and sclera, dark urine, clay-colored stools, itchy skin, abdominal pain, fever, diarrhea
- Assess for bleeding: hematuria, stool guaiac, bruising or petechiae, mucosa or orifices q8h; check for inflammation of mucosa, breaks in skin
- Assess effects of alopecia on body image; discuss feelings about body changes

Nursing diagnoses

- ✓ Injury, risk for (adverse reactions)
- ✓ Body image disturbance (adverse reactions)
- ✓ Infection, risk for (adverse reactions)
- ✓ Knowledge deficit (teaching)

Implementation

- Give fluids **IV** or PO before chemotherapy to hydrate patient
- Give antacid before oral agent, antiemetic 30-60 min before giving drug and prn to prevent vomiting; administer antibiotics for prophylaxis of infection
- Give top or systemic analgesics for pain to lessen effects from stomatitis
- Give liq diet: carbonated beverages; gelatin may be added if patient is not nauseated or vomiting
- Encourage patient to rinse mouth tid-qid with water, club soda; brush teeth bid-qid with soft brush or cotton-tipped applicators for stomatitis; use unwaxed dental floss
- Preparation should be done by personnel knowledgeable in preparing antineoplastics wearing gloves, gown, mask in biologic cabinet
- Give by direct **IV** by reconstituting 10 mg/5 ml of sterile water for inj (2 mg/ml); shake well
- Give over 5 min
- Give by intermittent inf after diluting 10 mg/25-50 ml of 0.9% NaCl, D_5W; give over 30 min
- Diluted sol should be used within 8 hr at room temp

Y-site compatibilities: Fludarabine, melphalan, ondansetron, paclitaxel, sargramostim

Solution compatibilities: D_5W, 0.9% NaCl, LR

Patient/family education

- Teach patient to avoid use of products containing aspirin or NSAIDs, razors, commercial mouthwash, since bleeding may occur; to report symptoms of bleeding (hematuria, tarry stools)
- Advise patient to report signs of anemia (fatigue, headache, irritability, faintness, shortness of breath); CNS reactions including confusion, psychosis, nightmares, seizures, severe headaches
- Inform patient that hair may be lost during treatment; a wig or hairpiece may make patient feel better; new hair may be different in color, texture
- Advise patient to use sunscreen and protective clothing to prevent photosensitive reactions

Evaluation

Positive therapeutic outcome

- Prevention of rapid division of malignant cells
- Decreased bone marrow hairy cells

pentoxifylline (℞)

(pen-tox-if′i-lin)

Trental

Func. class.: Hemorheologic agent

Chem. class.: Dimethylxanthine derivative

Pregnancy category C

Action: Decreases blood viscosity, stimulates prostacyclin formation, increases blood flow by increasing flexibility of RBCs; decreases RBC hyperaggregation; reduces platelet aggregation, decreases fibrinogen concentration

Therapeutic Outcome: Decreased claudication and improved blood flow

Uses: Intermittent claudication related to chronic occlusive vascular disease

Investigational uses: Cerebrovascular insufficiency, diabetic neuropathies, TIAs, leg ulcers, CVA, aphthous stomatitis

Dosage and routes

Adult: PO 400 mg tid with meals

Stomatitis (off-label)

Adult: PO 400 mg tid × 1-6 mo

Available forms: Cont rel tabs 400 mg

Adverse effects

CNS: *Headache,* anxiety, *tremors,* confusion, *dizziness*

CV: Angina, dysrhythmias, palpitations, hypotension, chest pain, dyspnea, edema

EENT: Blurred vision, earache, increased salivation, sore throat, conjunctivitis

GI: *Dyspepsia, nausea, vomiting,* anorexia, bloating, belching, constipation, cholecystitis, dry mouth, thirst, bad taste

INTEG: Rash, pruritus, urticaria, brittle fingernails

MISC: Epistaxis, flulike symptoms, laryngitis, nasal congestion, **leukopenia,** malaise, weight changes

Contraindications: Hypersensitivity to this drug or xanthines, retinal/cerebral hemorrhage

Precautions: Pregnancy **C,** angina pectoris, cardiac disease, lactation, P children, impaired renal function, recent surgery, peptic ulcer

Pharmacokinetics

Absorption	Well absorbed
Distribution	Unknown
Metabolism	Liver, degradation
Excretion	Kidneys
Half-life	½-1 hr

Pharmacodynamics

Onset	Unknown
Peak	1 hr
Duration	Unknown

Interactions

Individual drugs

Plicamycin: ↑ risk of bleeding
Theophylline: ↑ theophylline level
Valproic acid: ↑ risk of bleeding

Drug classifications

Antihypertensives: ↑ hypotension
Nitrates: ↑ hypotension
NSAIDs: ↑ risk of bleeding
Salicylates: ↑ risk of bleeding
Thrombolytics: ↑ risk of bleeding

NURSING CONSIDERATIONS

Assessment

- Monitor B/P, respirations in patient taking antihypertensives
- Assess for intermittent claudication baseline and during treatment

Nursing diagnoses

- ✓ Pain (uses)
- ✓ Activity intolerance (uses)
- ✓ Knowledge deficit (teaching)
- ✓ Noncompliance (teaching)

Implementation

- Give with meals to prevent GI upset
- ⊘ Tab should not be crushed or chewed

Patient/family education

- Teach patient that therapeutic response may take 2-4 wk
- Advise patient that decreased fats, cholesterol, increased exercise, decreased smoking are necessary to correct condition
- Instruct patient to observe feet for arterial insufficiency

P

- Instruct patient to use cotton socks, well-fitted shoes; not to go barefoot
- Advise patient to watch for bleeding, bruises, petechiae, epistaxis

Evaluation

Positive therapeutic outcome

- Decreased pain, cramping
- Increased ambulation

perflutren lipid microsphere

See Appendix A, Selected New Drugs

perindopril (℞) 🗝

(per-in-doe-pril)

Aceon

Func. class.: Antihypertensive

Chem. class.: Angiotensin-converting enzyme (ACE) inhibitor

Pregnancy category
C (1st trimester),
D (2nd/3rd trimesters)

Action: Selectively suppresses renin-angiotensin-aldosterone system; inhibits ACE; prevents conversion of angiotensin I to angiotensin II, resulting in dilatation of arterial and venous vessels

Therapeutic Outcome: Decreased B/P in hypertension

Uses: Hypertension alone or in combination

Dosage and routes

Adult: PO 4 mg/day, may increase or decrease to desired response; range 4-8 mg/day may give in 2 divided doses or as a single dose

Patients taking diuretics
Discontinue diuretic 2-3 days before perindopril, then resume diuretic if needed

Renal dose
CrCl >30 ml/min 2 mg/day, max 8 mg/day

Available forms: Tabs 2, 4, 8 mg scored

Adverse effects

CNS: *Insomnia, dizziness,* paresthesias, headache, fatigue, anxiety
CV: *Hypotension,* chest pain, tachycardia, dysrhythmias
EENT: *Tinnitus,* visual changes, sore throat, double vision, dry burning eyes
GI: Nausea, vomiting, colitis, cramps, diarrhea, constipation, flatulence, dry mouth, loss of taste
GU: **Proteinuria, renal failure,** increased frequency of polyuria or oliguria
HEMA: **Agranulocytosis, neutropenia**
INTEG: Rash, purpura, alopecia, hyperhidrosis
META: Hyperkalemia
RESP: Dyspnea, cough, rales, angioedema

Contraindications: Pregnancy **D** (2nd/3rd trimesters), lactation

Precautions: Renal disease, hyperkalemia, pregnancy **C** (1st trimester)

Pharmacokinetics	
Absorption	Well absorbed
Distribution	Unknown
Metabolism	Liver
Excretion	Kidneys
Half-life	Unknown

Pharmacodynamics
Unknown

Interactions

Individual drugs
Alcohol: ↑ hypotension (large amounts)
Allopurinol: ↑ hypersensitivity
Digoxin: ↑ serum levels
Hydralazine: ↑ toxicity
Indomethacin: ↓ antihypertensive effect
Lithium: ↑ serum levels
Prazosin: ↑ toxicity

Drug classifications

Adrenergic blockers: ↑ hypotension
Antacids: ↓ absorption
Antihypertensives: ↑ hypotension
Diuretics: ↑ hypotension
Diuretics, potassium-sparing: ↑ toxicity
Ganglionic blockers: ↑ hypotension
Potassium supplements: ↑ toxicity
Sympathomimetics: ↑ toxicity

Lab test interferences

Interference: Glucose/insulin tolerance tests

NURSING CONSIDERATIONS

Assessment

- Monitor blood studies: neutrophils, decreased platelets
- Monitor B/P, orthostatic hypotension, syncope; if changes occur dosage change may be required
- Monitor renal studies: protein, BUN, creatinine; increased levels may indicate nephrotic syndrome and renal failure
- Monitor renal symptoms: polyuria, oliguria, frequency, dysuria
- Establish baselines in renal, liver function tests before therapy begins
- Check potassium levels throughout treatment, although hyperkalemia rarely occurs
- Check for edema in feet, legs daily
- Assess for allergic reactions: rash, fever, pruritus, urticaria; drug should be discontinued if antihistamines fail to help

Nursing diagnoses

✓ Cardiac output, decreased (uses)
✓ Injury, potential for (adverse reactions)
✓ Knowledge deficit (teaching)
✓ Noncompliance (teaching)

Implementation

PO route

- Store in airtight container at 86° F (30° C) or less
- Severe hypotension may occur after 1st dose of this medication; decreased hypotension may be prevented by reducing or discontinuing diuretic therapy 3 days before beginning perindopril therapy
- Give by **IV** inf of 0.9% NaCl (as ordered) to expand fluid volume if severe hypotension occurs

Patient/family education

- Advise patient not to discontinue drug abruptly; advise patient to tell all persons associated with health care
- Teach patient not to use OTC products (cough, cold, allergy medications) unless directed by physician; serious side effects can occur; xanthines, such as coffee, tea, chocolate, cola can prevent action of drug
- Instruct patient on the importance of complying with dosage schedule, even if feeling better; to continue with medical regimen to decrease B/P: exercise, cessation of smoking, decreasing stress, diet modifications
- Emphasize the need to rise slowly to sitting or standing position to minimize orthostatic hypotension; not to exercise in hot weather, which can cause increased hypotension
- Advise patient to notify prescriber of mouth sores, sore throat, fever, swelling of hands or feet, irregular heartbeat, chest pain, coughing, shortness of breath
- Caution patient to report excessive perspiration, dehydration, vomiting, diarrhea; may lead to fall in B/P
- Caution patient that drug may cause dizziness, fainting, light-headedness; may occur during 1st few days of therapy; to avoid activities that may be hazardous
- Teach patient how to take B/P, and normal readings for age group

Evaluation

Positive therapeutic outcome

- Decreased B/P in hypertension

Treatment of overdose:

Lavage, **IV** atropine for bradycardia, **IV** theophylline for bronchospasm, digitalis, O_2; diuretic for cardiac failure, hemodialysis

P

perphenazine (℞)

(per-fen'a-zeen)

Apo-Perphenazine ✤, Trilafon, Trilafon concentrate, perphenazine, Phenazine ✤, PMS Perphenazine ✤

Func. class.: Antipsychotic/neuroleptic

Chem. class.: Phenothiazine piperidine

Pregnancy category C

Action: Depresses cerebral cortex, hypothalamus, limbic system, which control activity, aggression; blocks neurotransmission produced by dopamine at synapse; exhibits strong α-adrenergic, anticholinergic blocking action; as antiemetic inhibits medullary chemoreceptor trigger zone; mechanism for antipsychotic effects is unclear

Therapeutic Outcome: Decreased signs and symptoms of psychosis; decreased nausea and vomiting

Uses: Psychotic disorders, schizophrenia, nausea, vomiting

Dosage and routes

G ***Elderly:*** PO 2-4 mg qd-bid, increase by 2-4 mg/wk to desired dose

Nausea/vomiting/alcoholism

P ***Adult and child >12 yr:*** IM 5-10 mg prn, max 15 mg in ambulatory patients, 30 mg in hospitalized patients; PO 8-16 mg/day in divided doses, up to 24 mg; **IV** max 5 mg; give diluted or slow **IV** drip

Psychiatric use in hospitalized patients

Adults: PO 8-16 mg bid-qid, gradually increased to desired dose, max 64 mg/day; IM 5 mg q6h, max 30 mg/day

P ***Child >12 yr:*** PO 6-12 mg in divided doses

Nonhospitalized patients

Adult: PO 4-8 mg tid

Available forms: Tabs 2, 4, 8, 16 mg; oral sol 16 mg/5 ml; inj 5 mg/ml; syrup 2 mg/5 ml ✤

Adverse effects

CNS: EPS (pseudoparkinsonism, akathisia, dystonia, tardive dyskinesia), **neuroleptic malignant syndrome, seizures,** *headache*

CV: Orthostatic hypotension, **cardiac arrest**, ECG changes, **tachycardia**

EENT: Blurred vision, glaucoma

GI: Dry mouth, nausea, vomiting, anorexia, constipation, diarrhea, jaundice, weight gain

GU: Urinary retention, urinary frequency, enuresis, impotence, amenorrhea, gynecomastia

HEMA: Anemia, **leukopenia, leukocytosis, agranulocytosis**

INTEG: Rash, photosensitivity, dermatitis

RESP: **Laryngospasm,** dyspnea, **respiratory depression**

Contraindications: Hypersensitivity, blood dyscrasias, coma, child P <12 yr, brain damage, bone marrow depression

Precautions: Pregnancy **C**, lactation, seizure disorders, hypertension, hepatic disease, cardiac disease, G elderly

Pharmacokinetics

Absorption	Variably absorbed (PO); well absorbed (IM)
Distribution	Widely distributed; high concentrations in CNS; crosses placenta
Metabolism	Liver, extensively; GI mucosa
Excretion	Kidneys

Pharmacodynamics

	PO	IM	IV
Onset	Erratic	10 min	Rapid
Peak	2-4 hr	1-2 hr	Unknown
Duration	6-12 hr	6-12 hr	Unknown

Interactions

Individual drugs

Alcohol: ↑ effects of both drugs, oversedation
Aluminum hydroxide: ↓ absorption
Bromocriptine: ↓ antiparkinson activity
Disopyramide: ↑ anticholinergic effects
Epinephrine: ↑ toxicity
Guanethidine: ↓ antihypertensive response
Levodopa: ↓ antiparkinson activity
Lithium: ↓ perphenazine levels, ↑ EPS, masking of lithium toxicity
Magnesium hydroxide: ↓ absorption
Norepinephrine: ↓ vasoresponse, ↑ toxicity
Phenobarbital: ↓ effectiveness, ↑ metabolism

Drug classifications

Antacids: ↓ absorption
Anticholinergics: ↑ anticholinergic effects
Antidepressants: ↑ CNS depression
Antidiarrheals, adsorbent: ↓ absorption
Antihistamines: ↑ CNS depression
Antihypertensives: ↑ hypotension
Antithyroid agents: ↑ agranulocytosis
Barbiturate anesthetics: ↑ CNS depression
β-Adrenergic blockers: ↑ effects of both drugs
General anesthetics: ↑ CNS depression
MAOIs: ↑ CNS depression
Opiates: ↑ CNS depression
Sedative/hypnotics: ↑ CNS depression

Herb/drug

Henbane: ↑ anticholinergic effect

Lab test interferences

↑ Liver function tests, ↑ cardiac enzymes, ↑ cholesterol, ↑ blood glucose, ↑ prolactin, ↑ bilirubin, ↑ PBI, ↑ cholinesterase, ↑ iodine, ↑ alkaline phosphatase, ↑ leukocytes, ↑ granulocytes, ↑ platelets
↓ Hormones (blood and urine)
False positive: Pregnancy tests, PKU
False negative: Urinary steroids, 17-OHCS

NURSING CONSIDERATIONS

Assessment

- Assess mental status: orientation, mood, behavior, presence and type of hallucinations before initial administration and monthly; this drug should significantly reduce psychotic behavior
- Check for swallowing of PO medication; check for hoarding or giving medication to other patients
- Monitor I&O ratio; palpate bladder if low urinary output occurs, G especially in elderly; urinalysis recommended before, during prolonged therapy
- Monitor bilirubin, CBC, liver function studies monthly
- Assess affect, orientation, LOC, reflexes, gait, coordination, sleep pattern disturbances
- Monitor B/P with patient sitting, standing, and lying; take pulse and respirations q4h during initial treatment; establish baseline before starting treatment; report drops of 30 mm Hg; obtain baseline ECG, with Q- and T-wave changes
- Check for dizziness, faintness, palpitations, tachycardia on rising; severe orthostatic hypotension is common
- ! Identify for neuroleptic malignant syndrome: hyperpyrexia, muscle rigidity, increased CPK, altered mental status; drug should be discontinued
- Assess for EPS including akathisia (inability to sit still, no pattern to movements), tardive dyskinesia (bizarre movements of the jaw, mouth, tongue, extremities), pseudoparkinsonism (ragged tremors, pill rolling, shuffling gait); an antiparkinsonian drug should be prescribed
- Assess for constipation, urinary

P

retention daily; if these occur, increase bulk, water in diet

Nursing diagnoses

- ✓ Thought processes, altered (uses)
- ✓ Coping, ineffective individual (uses)
- ✓ Knowledge deficit (teaching)
- ✓ Noncompliance (teaching)

Implementation

PO route

- Administer drug in liq form mixed in glass of juice or cola if hoarding is suspected; do not mix in caffeine drinks, tannics, pectins
- Administer decreased dose in G elderly, in whom metabolism is slowed
- Administer PO with full glass of water, milk; or give with food to decrease GI upset
- Store in airtight, light-resistant container; oral sol in amber bottle

IM route

- Inject in deep muscle mass; do not give SC; do not administer sol with a precipitate

IV **IV route**

- Give by direct **IV** after diluting with 0.9% NaCl to a conc of 0.5 mg/1 ml; administer at 1 mg/min; may be further diluted and given as an inf

Syringe compatibilities: Atropine, benztropine, butorphanol, chlorpromazine, cimetidine, dimenhydrinate, diphenhydramine, droperidol, fentanyl, hydroxyzine, meperidine, methotrimeprazine, metoclopramide, morphine, pentazocine, prochlorperazine, promethazine, ranitidine, scopolamine

Syringe incompatibilities: Midazolam, opium alkaloids, pentobarbital, thiethylperazine

Y-site compatibilities: Acyclovir, amikacin, ampicillin, azlocillin, cefamandole, cefazolin, cefotaxime, cefoxitin, cefuroxime, cephalothin, cephapirin, chloramphenicol, clindamycin, cotrimoxazole, doxycycline, erythromycin, famotidine, gentamicin, kanamycin, metronidazole, mezlocillin, minocycline, moxalactam, nafcillin, oxacillin, penicillin G potassium, piperacillin, sulfamethoxazole, tacrolimus, ticarcillin, ticarcillin/clavulanate, tobramycin, trimethoprim, vancomycin

Additive compatibilities: Ascorbic acid, ethacrynate, netilmicin

Additive incompatibilities: Cefoperazone

Patient/family education

- Teach patient to use good oral hygiene; frequent rinsing of mouth, sugarless gum for dry mouth
- Advise patient to avoid hazardous activities until drug response is determined, dizziness, blurred vision may occur
- Inform patient that orthostatic hypotension occurs often and to rise from sitting or lying position gradually; to remain lying down after IM inj for at least 30 min; tell patient to avoid hot tubs, hot showers, tub baths, since hypotension may occur; teach patient that in hot weather heat stroke may occur; take extra precautions to stay cool
- Teach patient to avoid abrupt withdrawal of this drug, or EPS may result; drug should be withdrawn slowly
- Teach patient to avoid OTC preparations (cough, hay fever, cold) unless approved by prescriber, since serious drug interactions may occur; avoid use with alcohol, CNS depressants; increased drowsiness may result
- Caution patient to use a sunscreen and sunglasses to prevent burns
- Teach patient about EPS and necessity of meticulous oral hygiene, since oral candidiasis may occur
- Instruct patient to take antacids 2 hr before or after taking this drug
- Teach patient to report sore throat, malaise, fever, bleeding, mouth sores; if these occur, CBC should be performed and drug discontinued

- Teach patient that urine may turn pink or red

Evaluation

Positive therapeutic outcome

- Decrease in emotional excitement, hallucinations, delusions, paranoia
- Reorganization of patterns of thought, speech

Treatment of overdose:

Lavage if orally ingested; provide airway; *do not induce vomiting or use epinephrine*

phenazopyridine

(℞/OTC)

(fen-az-o-peer'i-deen)

AZO-Standard, Baridium, Eridium, Geridium, Phenazo ✦, Phenazodine, phenazopyridine HCl, Prodium, Pyridate, Pyridiate, Pyridium, Urodine, Urogesic, Viridium

Func. class.: Nonopioid analgesic, urinary

Chem. class.: Azodye

Pregnancy category B

Action: Exerts analgesic, anesthetic action on the urinary tract mucosa

Uses: Urinary tract irritation, infection (for symptoms only of pain, burning, itching) used with urinary antiinfectives

Dosage and routes

Adult: PO 200 mg tid × 2 days or less when used with antibacterial for UTI

P ***Child 6-12 yr:*** PO 4 mg/kg tid × 2 days

Renal dose

CrCl <50 ml/min do not use

Available forms: Tabs 95, 100, 200 mg

Adverse effects

CNS: Headache

GI: Nausea, vomiting, diarrhea, heartburn, anorexia, **hepatic toxicity**

GU: **Renal toxicity,** *orange-red urine*

HEMA: **Thrombocytopenia, agranulocytosis, leukopenia, neutropenia, hemolytic anemia, methemoglobinemia**

INTEG: Rash, pruritus, skin pigmentation

Contraindications: Hypersensitivity, renal insufficiency

Precautions: Pregnancy **B,** renal P disease, lactation, children <12 yr

Pharmacokinetics	
Absorption	Well absorbed
Distribution	Unknown; crosses placenta
Metabolism	Unknown
Excretion	Kidneys, unchanged
Half-life	Unknown

Pharmacodynamics	
Onset	Unknown
Peak	5-6 hr
Duration	8 hr

Interactions: None

Lab test interferences

Interference: Urinalysis

NURSING CONSIDERATIONS

Assessment

- Assess urinary status: burning, pain, itching, urgency, frequency, hematuria before, during, and after completion of drug therapy
- Monitor liver function studies: AST, ALT, bilirubin if patient is on long-term therapy
- ❗ Assess for hepatotoxicity: dark urine, clay-colored stools, yellowing of skin and sclera, itching, abdominal pain, fever, diarrhea if patient is on long-term therapy
- Assess for allergic reactions: rash, urticaria; if these occur, drug may have to be discontinued

Nursing diagnoses

✓ Pain (uses)

✓ Urinary elimination, altered patterns (uses)
✓ Knowledge deficit (teaching)

Implementation

- Give to patient crushed or whole; chew tab may be chewed
- Give with food or milk to decrease gastric symptoms

Patient/family education

- Advise patient to report any symptoms of hepatotoxicity
- Caution patient not to exceed recommended dosage and to take with meals; to read label on other OTC drugs
- Teach patient not to discontinue after pain is relieved but continue to take concurrent prescribed antiinfective until finished
- Inform patient urine may turn red-orange, may stain clothing or contact lens

Evaluation

Positive therapeutic outcome

- Decrease in pain, burning, itching when urinating

Treatment of overdose:
Methylene blue 1-2 mg/kg **IV** or vit C 100-200 mg PO

phenelzine (℞)
(fen'el-zeen)
Nardil
Func. class.: Antidepressant, MAOI
Chem. class.: Hydrazine
Pregnancy category C

Action: Increases concentrations of endogenous epinephrine, norepinephrine, serotonin, dopamine in storage sites in CNS by inhibition of MAO; increased concentration reduces depression

➔ **Therapeutic Outcome:** Decreased symptoms of depression after 2-3 wk

Uses: Depression, when uncontrolled by other means

Dosage and routes

Adult: PO 45 mg/day in divided doses; may increase to 60 mg/day

G ***Elderly:*** PO 7.5 mg qd, increase by 7.5-15 mg q3-4 days

Available forms: Tabs 15 mg

Adverse effects

CNS: *Dizziness, drowsiness,* confusion, headache, anxiety, tremors, stimulation, weakness, hyperreflexia, mania, insomnia, fatigue, weight gain
CV: *Orthostatic hypotension, hypertension,* **dysrhythmias, hypertensive crisis**
EENT: Blurred vision
ENDO: **Syndrome of inappropriate antidiuretic hormone–like syndrome**
GI: Constipation, dry mouth, nausea, vomiting, *anorexia,* diarrhea, weight gain
GU: Change in libido, frequency of urination
HEMA: Anemia
INTEG: Rash, flushing, increased perspiration

Contraindications: Hypersensitivity to MAOIs, G elderly, hypertension, CHF, severe hepatic disease, pheochromocytoma, severe renal disease, severe cardiac disease

Precautions: Suicidal patients, seizure disorders, severe depression, schizophrenia, hyperactivity, diabetes mellitus, pregnancy **C**

Pharmacokinetics	
Absorption	Well absorbed
Distribution	Crosses placenta
Metabolism	Liver, extensively
Excretion	Kidneys, breast milk
Half-life	Unknown

Pharmacodynamics
Unknown

Interactions

Individual drugs

Alcohol: ↑ CNS depression
Clonidine: Severe hypotension; avoid use
Guanethidine: ↓ effects
L-Tryptophan: ↑ confusion, shivering, hyperreflexia
Methylphenidate: Hypertensive crisis, seizures, do not use together
Sumatriptan: ↑ toxicity

Drug classifications

Analgesics: ↑ CNS depression
Anticholinergics: ↑ side effects
Antidiabetics: ↑ hypoglycemia
Antihistamines: ↑ CNS depression
Antihypertensives: May block antihypertensive effect
Barbiturates: ↑ effects of barbiturates
Benzodiazepines: ↑ effects of benzodiazepines
CNS depressants: ↑ effects of CNS depressants
Diuretics, thiazide: ↑ hypotension
Oral contraceptives: ↑ effects, toxicity
Phenothiazines: ↑ toxicity
Rauwolfia alkaloids: ↓ serotonin, norepinephrine
Sedative/hypnotics: ↑ CNS depression
Selective serotonin reuptake inhibitors: ↑ Hyperpyretic crisis, seizures, hypertensive episode
Sulfonamides: ↑ toxicity
Sympathomimetics, indirect-acting or mixed: ↑ pressor effect

Food/drug

Caffeine: ↑ hypertension
Tyramine-containing foods: Hypertensive crisis

Herb/drug

Brewer's yeast: ↑ hypertension
Ephedra: ↑ sympathomimetic effect
Ginseng: ↑ tension headache, irritability, visual hallucinations

NURSING CONSIDERATIONS

Assessment

- Monitor B/P (with patient lying, standing), pulse q4h; if systolic B/P drops 20 mm Hg, hold drug, notify prescriber; take VS q4h in patients with CV disease
- Monitor hepatic studies: AST, ALT, bilirubin if patient is on long-term therapy
- Check weight weekly; appetite may increase with drug
- Assess ECG for flattening of T wave, bundle branch block, AV block, dysrhythmias in cardiac patients
- Assess mental status: mood, sensorium, affect, suicidal tendencies; increase in psychiatric symptoms: depression, panic
- Monitor urinary retention, constipation; constipation is more G likely to occur in elderly
- Assess for withdrawal symptoms: headache, nausea, vomiting, muscle pain, weakness; do not usually occur unless drug was discontinued abruptly
- Identify alcohol consumption; if alcohol is consumed, hold dose until AM

Nursing diagnoses

✓ Coping, ineffective individual (uses)
✓ Injury, risk for (adverse reactions)
✓ Knowledge deficit (teaching)
✓ Noncompliance (teaching)

Implementation

- Give with food or milk for GI symptoms; crush if patient is unable to swallow medication whole and mix with food or fluids
- Store at room temp; do not freeze

Patient/family education

- Teach patient that therapeutic effects may take 2-3 wk
- Advise patient to use caution in driving and other activities requiring alertness because of drowsiness, dizziness, blurred vision; to avoid rising quickly from sitting to standing, G especially elderly
- Caution patient to avoid alcohol

P

ingestion, other CNS depressants; serious reaction can occur
- Advise patient not to discontinue medication quickly after long-term use: may cause nausea, headache, malaise, sweating, hallucinations
- Instruct patient to increase fluids, bulk in diet if constipation, urinary G retention occur, especially elderly; a stool softener may be ordered
- Teach patient to take gum, hard sugarless candy, or frequent sips of water for dry mouth
- Teach patient that therapeutic effects may take 1-4 wk
- Teach patient to avoid alcohol ingestion, CNS depressants, OTC medications: cold, weight loss, hay fever, cough syrup
- Teach patient not to discontinue medication quickly after long-term use
- Teach patient to avoid high-tyramine foods: cheese (aged), sour cream, beer, wine, pickled products, liver, raisins, bananas, figs, avocados, meat tenderizers, chocolate, yogurt; increased caffeine
- Teach patient to report headache, palpitations, neck stiffness, dizziness, constriction in chest, throat

Evaluation

Positive therapeutic outcome
- Decrease in depression
- Absence of suicidal thoughts

Treatment of overdose:

Lavage, activated charcoal, monitor electrolytes, VS, diazepam **IV**, sodium bicarbonate

HIGH ALERT

phenobarbital Key Drug (℞)

(fee-noe-bar'bit-tal)

Ancalixir (Canada), Barbita, Luminal, phenobarbital sodium, Solfoton

Func. class.: Anticonvulsant, sedative/hypnotic

Chem. class.: Barbiturate

Pregnancy category D

Controlled substance schedule IV

Action: Depresses activity in brain cells primarily in reticular activating system in brainstem; also selectively depresses neurons in posterior hypothalamus, limbic structures; able to decrease seizure activity by inhibition of impulses in CNS; decreases motor activity

Therapeutic Outcome: Sedation, anticonvulsant, improved energy

Uses: All forms of epilepsy, status P epilepticus, febrile seizures in children, sedation, insomnia

Investigational uses: Hyperbilirubinemia, chronic cholestasis

Dosage and routes

Seizures

Adult: PO 60-200 mg/day in divided doses tid or total dose hs

P ***Child:*** PO 4-6 mg/kg/day in divided doses q12h; may be given as single dose

Status epilepticus

Adult: **IV** inf 10 mg/kg; run no faster than 50 mg/min; may give up to 20 mg/kg

P ***Child:*** **IV** inf 5-10 mg/kg; may repeat q10-15 min up to 20 mg/kg; run no faster than 50 mg/min

Insomnia

Adult: PO/IM 100-320 mg

P ***Child:*** PO/IM 3-5 mg/kg

Sedation
Adult: PO 30-120 mg/day in 2-3 divided doses

P ***Child:*** PO 3-5 mg/kg/day in 3 divided doses

Preoperative sedation
Adult: IM 100-200 mg 1-1½ hr before surgery

P ***Child:*** IM 16-100 mg or PO/IM/**IV** 1-3 mg/kg 1-1½ hr before surgery

Available forms: Caps 15 mg; elixir 15 ✦, 20 mg/5 ml; tabs 8, 15, 30, 60, 100 mg; inj 30, 60, 130 mg/ml

Adverse effects

G *CNS:* Paradoxic excitement (elderly), drowsiness, lethargy, *hangover headache,* flushing, hallucinations, **coma**

GI: Nausea, vomiting, diarrhea, constipation

INTEG: Rash, urticaria, **Stevens-Johnson syndrome, angioedema,** local pain, swelling, necrosis, **thrombophlebitis**

Contraindications: Hypersensitivity to barbiturates, porphyria, hepatic disease, respiratory disease, nephritis, hyperthyroidism, diabetes G mellitus, elderly, lactation, pregnancy **D**

Precautions: Anemia

Do Not Confuse:
phenobarbital/pentobarbital

Pharmacokinetics

Absorption	Slow (70%-90%) (PO/IM/**IV**)
Distribution	Not known; crosses placenta
Metabolism	Liver (75%)
Excretion	Kidneys (25% unchanged)
Half-life	2-6 days

Pharmacodynamics

	PO	IM	IV
Onset	30-60 min	10-30 min	5 min
Peak	Unknown	Unknown	30 min
Duration	6-8 hr	4-6 hr	4-6 hr

Interactions

Individual drugs

Alcohol: ↑ CNS depression
Chloramphenicol: ↓ effectiveness
Cyclophosphamide: ↑ hematologic toxicity
Cyclosporine: ↓ effectiveness
Dacarbazine: ↓ effectiveness
Quinidine: ↓ effectiveness
Valproic acid: ↑ sedation

Drug classifications

Anticoagulants: ↓ effectiveness
Antidepressants: ↑ CNS depression
Antidepressants, tricyclic: ↓ effectiveness
Antihistamines: ↑ CNS depression
Glucocorticoids: ↓ effectiveness
MAOIs: ↑ CNS depression
Opiates: ↑ CNS depression
Oral contraceptives: ↓ effectiveness
Sedative/hypnotics: ↑ CNS depression

Herb/drug

Quinine: ↑ phenobarbital level

NURSING CONSIDERATIONS
Assessment

- Assess mental status: mood, sensorium, affect, memory (long, short), G especially elderly; if using as a hypnotic, assess sleep patterns during therapy; drug suppresses REM sleep with dreaming
- Withdrawal insomnia may occur after short-term use; do not start using drug again; insomnia improves in 1-3 nights; may experience increased dreaming
- Assess respiratory dysfunction: respiratory depression, character, rate, rhythm when using **IV**; hold drug if respirations are <10/min or if pupils are dilated; also check VS q30 min after parenteral route for 2 hr
- Assess for barbiturate toxicity: hypotension, pulmonary constriction, cold, clammy skin, cyanosis of lips, CNS depression, nausea, vomiting, hallucinations, delirium, weakness, coma, pupillary constriction; mild

P

symptoms occur in 8-12 hr without drug

- Assess for pain in postoperative patients; pain threshold is lowered when patients are taking this medication
- Assess for blood dyscrasias: fever, sore throat, bruising, rash, jaundice, epistaxis (long-term treatment only)
- Assess seizure activity including type, location, duration, and character; provide seizure precaution

Nursing diagnoses

✓ Sleep pattern disturbance (uses)
✓ Injury, risk for (adverse reactions)
✓ Knowledge deficit (teaching)

Implementation

- Give medication after removal of cigarettes to prevent fires
- Give medication after trying conservative measures for insomnia

PO route

- Tab may be crushed and mixed with food if swallowing is difficult; also may be mixed with other fluids 30-60 min before bedtime for expected sleeplessness; on empty stomach for best absorption

IM route

- Give in deep muscle mass (gluteal) to minimize irritation to tissues
- Split inj of >5 ml into two, since irritation to tissues may occur

IV Direct IV route

- Use large vein to prevent extravasation; if extravasation occurs, use moist heat to the area and 5% procaine sol injected into area; give at 65 mg or less/min; titrate to patient response

Syringe compatibilities:
Heparin

Syringe incompatibilities:
Benzquinamide, ranitidine

Y-site compatibilities:
Enalaprilat, meropenem, propofol, sufentanil

Y-site incompatibilities:
Hydromorphone

Additive compatibilities:
Amikacin, aminophylline, calcium chloride, calcium gluceptate, cephapirin, colistimethate, dimenhydrinate, meropenem, polymyxin B, sodium bicarbonate, thiopental, verapamil

Additive incompatibilities:
Cephalothin, chlorpromazine, codeine, ephedrine, hydralazine, hydrocortisone sodium succinate, hydroxyzine, insulin, levorphanol, meperidine, methadone, morphine, norepinephrine, pentazocine, procaine, prochlorazine mesylate, promazine, promethazine, streptomycin, vancomycin

Solution compatibilities:
D_5W, $D_{10}W$, 0.45% NaCl, 0.9% NaCl, Ringer's, dextrose/saline combinations, dextrose/Ringer's, dextrose/LR combinations, sodium lactate

Patient/family education

- Teach patient that hangover is common
- Instruct patient that drug is indicated only for short-term treatment of insomnia and is probably ineffective after 2 wk
- Inform patient that physical dependency may result when used for extended time (45-90 days depending on dosage)
- Teach patient to avoid driving and other activities requiring alertness
- Caution patient to avoid alcohol ingestion and CNS depressants; serious CNS depression may result
- Instruct patient not to discontinue medication quickly after long-term use; may cause seizures; drug should be tapered over 1 wk; take exactly as prescribed
- Emphasize the need to tell all prescribers that a barbiturate is being taken
- Teach the patient to make position changes slowly; orthostatic hypotension may occur
- Teach patient that response may take 4 days to 2 wk

• Instruct patient to notify prescriber immediately if bruising, bleeding occur, which may indicate blood dyscrasias

Evaluation

Positive therapeutic outcome

- Improved sleeping patterns
- Decreased seizure activity
- Sedative preoperatively

Treatment of overdose: Lavage, activated charcoal, warming blanket, VS, hemodialysis, alkalinize urine, give **IV** volume expanders, **IV** fluids

phenolphthalein (OTC)

(fee-nol-thay'leen)

Alophen, Correctol, Espotabs, Evac-U-Gen, Evac-U-Lax, Ex-Lax, Feen-A-Mint, Lax-Pills, Modane, Medilax, Phenolax, Prulet

Func. class.: Laxative, stimulant/irritant

Chem. class.: Diphenylmethane

Pregnancy category C

Action: Directly acts on intestinal smooth muscle by increasing motor activity; thought to irritate colonic intramural plexus; increases fluid in small intestine; alters fluid and electrolytes; action requires presence of bile

→ **Therapeutic Outcome:** Decreased constipation

Uses: Constipation, preparation for bowel surgery or examination

Dosage and routes

Adult: PO 30-270 mg hs

P ***Child >6 yr:*** 30-60 mg/day

P ***Child 2-5 yr:*** 15-20 mg/day

Available forms: Tabs 60, 90, 97.2, 130 mg; chew tabs 65, 90, 97.2 mg; chew gum 97.2 mg; wafers 64.8 mg; chew wafers 80 mg

Adverse effects

GI: *Nausea, vomiting, anorexia, diarrhea,* abdominal cramps, rectal burning

INTEG: Rash, urticaria, **Stevens-Johnson syndrome**

META: Hypokalemia, electrolyte and fluid imbalances

Contraindications: Hypersensitivity, GI obstructions, abdominal pain, nausea/vomiting, fecal impaction, rectal fissures, hemorrhoids (ulcerated)

Precautions: Pregnancy **C**, lactation

Pharmacokinetics	
Absorption	Minimally absorbed (15%)
Distribution	Unknown
Metabolism	Not metabolized
Excretion	Kidneys, feces
Half-life	Unknown

Pharmacodynamics	
Onset	6-8 hr
Peak	Unknown
Duration	3-4 days

Interactions

Drug classifications

Oral drugs (any): ↓ absorption

Lab test interferences

Interference: BSP test

NURSING CONSIDERATIONS

Assessment

- Monitor blood, urine electrolytes if drug used often by patient; check I&O ratio to identify fluid loss
- Assess for cramping, rectal bleeding, nausea, vomiting; if these symptoms occur, drug should be discontinued; identify cause of constipation; identify whether fluids, bulk, or exercise is missing from lifestyle
- Assess stool for color, consistency, amount, presence of flatulence

Nursing diagnoses

✓ Constipation (uses)

P

✓ Diarrhea (adverse reaction)
✓ Knowledge deficit (teaching)
✓ Noncompliance (teaching)

Implementation

- Chew well before swallowing; follow with 4 oz of water to prevent undissolved tab entering small intestine
- Give with 8 oz of water (tab); administer on empty stomach for more rapid results; do not give hs

Patient/family education

- Discuss with patient that adequate fluid consumption is necessary
- Teach patient that normal bowel movements do not always occur daily
- Caution patient not to use in presence of abdominal pain, nausea, vomiting; tell patient to notify prescriber if constipation is unrelieved or if symptoms of electrolyte imbalance occur (muscle cramps, pain, weakness, dizziness, excessive thirst)
- Teach patient not to use laxatives for long-term therapy; bowel tone will be lost
- Shake susp well as needed
- Teach patient not to take hs as a laxative; may interfere with sleep; also can cause problems with lipid pneumonia
- Teach patient not to use with food or vitamin preparations; delays digestion and absorption of fat-soluble vitamins

Evaluation

Positive therapeutic outcome

- Decreased constipation in 8-10 hr

phentolamine (℞)

(fen-tole'a-meen)

Regitine, Rogitine ♣

Func. class.: Antihypertensive

Chem. class.: α-Adrenergic blocker

Pregnancy category C

Action: α-Adrenergic blocker, binds to α-adrenergic receptors, dilating peripheral blood vessels, lowering peripheral resistances, lowering blood pressure

→ **Therapeutic Outcome:** Decreased B/P, reversal of vasoconstriction (dermal necrosis)

Uses: Hypertension, pheochromocytoma, prevention, treatment of dermal necrosis after extravasation of norepinephrine or dopamine, impotence

Dosage and routes

Treatment of hypertensive episodes in pheochromocytoma

Adult: **IV**/IM 5 mg; repeat if necessary

P ***Child:*** **IV**/IM 1 mg; repeat if necessary

Diagnosis of pheochromocytoma

Adult: **IV** 2.5 mg; if negative, repeat with 5 mg **IV**

P ***Child:*** **IV** 0.5 mg; if negative, repeat with 1 mg **IV**

Prevention of dermal necrosis

Adult: **IV** 10 mg/100 ml of **IV** fluids with norepinephrine

P ***Child:*** **IV** 0.1-0.2 mg/kg, max 10 mg

Available forms: Inj 5 mg/ml

Adverse effects

CNS: *Dizziness,* flushing, weakness, **cerebrovascular spasm**

CV: *Hypotension,* **tachycardia,** *angina,* **dysrhythmias, MI**

EENT: Nasal congestion

GI: *Dry mouth, nausea, vomiting, diarrhea, abdominal pain*

Contraindications: Hypersensitivity, MI, coronary insufficiency, angina

Precautions: Pregnancy **C**, lactation

Pharmacokinetics

Absorption	Well absorbed (IM); completely absorbed (**IV**)
Distribution	Unknown
Metabolism	Unknown
Excretion	Kidneys, unchanged (10%)
Half-life	Unknown

Pharmacodynamics

	IM	IV
Onset	Unknown	Rapid
Peak	20 min	2 min
Duration	½-1 hr	½ hr

Interactions

Individual drugs

Dopamine: ↓ peripheral vasoconstriction
Ephedrine: ↓ pressor effect
Epinephrine: ↑ effects of epinephrine, hypotension
Guanadrel: ↑ hypotension, bradycardia
Guanethidine: ↑ hypotension, bradycardia
Metaraminol: ↓ pressor effect
Methoxamine: ↑ effects of methoxamine, hypotension
Phenylephrine: ↓ pressor effect

Drug classifications

α-Adrenergic blockers: Antagonistic effect
Antihypertensives: ↑ effects of antihypertensives

NURSING CONSIDERATIONS

Assessment

- Monitor B/P, orthostatic hypotension, syncope, pulse and ECG until stable

Nursing diagnoses

✓ Cardiac output, decreased (uses)
✓ Injury, potential for (adverse reactions)
✓ Knowledge deficit (teaching)
✓ Noncompliance (teaching)

Implementation

- Give with vasopressor nearby

IV IV route

- Give by direct **IV** after diluting 5 mg/1 ml of sterile water for inj or 0.9% NaCl; give 5 mg or less/min
- Give by cont inf by further diluting 5-10 mg/500 ml of D_5W, titrate to patient response

Syringe compatibilities:
Papaverine

Y-site compatibilities:
Amiodarone

Additive compatibilities:
Dobutamine, verapamil

Prevention of dermal necrosis

- Add 10 mg/L to norepinephrine in **IV** sol

Patient/family education

- Caution patient not to discontinue drug abruptly
- Teach patient not to use OTC products (cough, cold, allergy) unless directed by prescriber
- Teach patient the importance of complying with dosage schedule, even if feeling better
- Emphasize the need to rise slowly to sitting or standing position to minimize orthostatic hypotension
- Teach patient to notify prescriber of mouth sores, sore throat, fever, swelling of hands or feet, irregular heartbeat, chest pain
- Caution patient to report excessive perspiration, dehydration, vomiting, diarrhea; may lead to fall in B/P
- Caution patient that drug may cause dizziness, fainting, light-headedness; may occur during 1st few days of therapy
- Teach patient how to take B/P, and normal readings for age group

Evaluation

Positive therapeutic outcome

- Decreased B/P in hypertension
- Resolution of impotence
- Prevention of dermal necrosis

Treatment of overdose:

Administer norepinephrine; discontinue drug

P

phenylephrine (℞)
(fen-ill-ef'rin)

Neo-Synephrine

Func. class.: Adrenergic, direct acting

Chem. class.: Direct sympathomimetic amine (α-agonist)

Pregnancy category C

Action: Powerful and selective receptor agonist causing contraction of blood vessels, vasoconstriction of eye arterioles; decreases eye engorgement by stimulation of α-adrenergic receptors

→ Therapeutic Outcome: Increased B/P, decreased nasal congestion, decreased eye irritation

Uses: Hypotension, paroxysmal supraventricular tachycardia, shock, B/P maintenance during spinal anesthesia, topical ocular vasoconstrictor in uveitis, open-angle glaucoma, preoperatively, diagnostic procedures, refraction without cycloplegia, nasal congestion

Dosage and routes
Hypotension

Adult: SC/IM 2-5 mg; may repeat q10-15 min if needed, do not exceed initial dose; **IV** 0.1-0.5 mg; may repeat q10-15 min if needed, do not exceed initial dose

P ***Child:*** IM/SC 0.1 mg/kg/dose q1-2h prn

Premature ventricular contractions

Adult: **IV** bol 0.5 mg given rapidly, not to exceed prior dose by >0.1 mg; total dose >1 mg

Shock

Adult: **IV** inf 10 mg/500 ml of D_5W given 100-180 μg/min (if 20 gtt/ml device is used), then maintenance of 40-60 μg/min (if 20 gtt/ml device is used)

P ***Child:*** **IV** bol 5-20 μg/kg/dose q10-15 min; **IV** inf 0.1-0.5 mg/kg/min

Available forms: Inj 1% (10 mg/ml)

Adverse effects

CNS: *Headache, dizziness, weakness, anxiety, tremor, insomnia*

CV: Reflex bradycardia, **dysrhythmias**, *hypertension,* **tachycardia,** CV collapse, palpitations, ectopic beats, angina

EENT: Stinging, lacrimation, blurred vision, conjunctival allergy

GI: *Nausea, vomiting*

INTEG: Necrosis, tissue sloughing with extravasation, **gangrene**

MISC: **Anaphylaxis**

Contraindications: Hypersensitivity, narrow-angle glaucoma, ventricular fibrillation, tachydysrhythmias, pheochromocytoma

Precautions: Severe hypertension, diabetes, hyperthyroidism, G elderly, severe arteriosclerosis, cardiac disease, P infants, pregnancy **C**, lactation, arterial embolism, peripheral vascular disease, bradycardia, myocardial disease

Pharmacokinetics

Absorption	Well absorbed (IM); completely absorbed (**IV**); minimally absorbed (nasal, ophth)
Distribution	Unknown
Metabolism	Liver
Excretion	Unknown
Half-life	Unknown

Pharmacodynamics

	IV	SC/IM
Onset	Rapid	15 min
Peak	Unknown	Unknown
Duration	20-30 min	45-60 min

Interactions

Individual drugs

Bretylium: ↑ dysrhythmias
Guanethidine: ↑ pressor effect
Mecamylamine: ↑ hypotension
Methyldopa: ↑ hypotension
Reserpine: ↑ hypotension

Drug classifications
Antidepressants, tricyclic: ↑ pressor effect
β-Adrenergic blockers: ↑ pressor effect
General anesthetics: ↑ dysrhythmias
H_1 antihistamines: ↑ pressor effect
MAOIs: ↑ pressor effect
Oxytocics: ↑ B/P

NURSING CONSIDERATIONS
Assessment
- Monitor I&O ratio; notify prescriber if output <30 ml/hr
- Monitor ECG during administration continuously; if B/P increases, drug is decreased
- Monitor B/P and pulse q5 min after parenteral route; CVP or PWP during inf if possible
- Assess for paresthesias and coldness of extremities; peripheral blood flow may decrease

Nursing diagnoses
✓ Tissue perfusion, altered (uses)
✓ Cardiac output, decreased (uses)
✓ Knowledge deficit (teaching)

Implementation
IV **IV route**
- Give plasma expanders for hypovolemia
- Give **IV** after diluting 1 mg/9 ml of sterile water for inj; give dose over 30-60 sec; may be diluted 10 mg/500 ml of D_5W or 0.9% NaCl; titrate to patient response; low normal B/P; check for extravasation; check site for infiltration; use infusion pump
- Store reconstituted sol in refrigerator for no longer than 24 hr
- Do not use discolored sol

Y-site compatibilities:
Amrinone, famotidine, haloperidol, zidovudine

Additive compatibilities:
Chloramphenicol, dobutamine, lidocaine, potassium chloride, sodium bicarbonate

Patient/family education
- Inform patient of reason for drug administration and expected result
- Advise patient to report pain at inf site immediately
- Instruct patient to report change in vision, blurring, loss of sight; breathing trouble, sweating, flushing

Evaluation
Positive therapeutic outcome
- Increased B/P with stabilization

phenytoin (Rx)
(fen′i-toyn)
Diphenylhydantoin, Dilantin, Dilantin Capsules, Diphenylan, Phenytoin Oral Suspension
Func. class.: Anticonvulsant/ antidysrhythmic (class IB)
Chem. class.: Hydantoin

Pregnancy category D

Action: Inhibits spread of seizure activity in motor cortex by altering ion transport; increases AV conduction to decrease dysrhythmias

➔ **Therapeutic Outcome:** Decreased seizures, absence of dysrhythmias

Uses: Generalized tonic-clonic seizures, status epilepticus, nonepileptic seizures associated with Reye's syndrome or after head trauma, migraines, trigeminal neuralgia, Bell's palsy, ventricular dysrhythmias uncontrolled by antidysrhythmics

Dosage and routes
Seizures
Adult: PO 1 g or 20 mg/kg (ext rel) in 3-4 divided doses given q2h or 400 mg, then 300 mg q2h × 2 doses, maintenance 300-400 mg/day; max 600 mg/day; **IV** 15-20 mg/kg, max 25-50 mg/min then 100 mg q6-8h

P ***Child:*** PO 5 mg/kg/day in 2-3 divided doses, maintenance 4-8 mg/kg/day in

P

2-3 divided doses, max 300 mg/day; **IV** 15-20 mg/kg at 1-3 mg/kg/min

Status epilepticus
Adult: **IV** 15-20 mg/kg, max 25-50 mg/min; may give 100 mg q6-8h thereafter

P ***Child:*** **IV** 15-20 mg/kg given 1-3 mg/kg/min

Neuritic pain
Adult: PO 200-400 mg/day in divided doses

Ventricular dysrhythmias
Adult: PO loading dose 1 g divided over 24 hr, then 500 mg/day × 2 days; **IV** 250 mg given over 5 min until dysrhythmias subside or 1 g is given, or 100 mg q15 min until dysrhythmias subside or 1 g is given

P ***Child:*** PO 3-8 mg/kg or 250 mg/m^2/day as single dose or divided in 2 doses; **IV** 3-8 mg/kg given over several min, or 250 mg/m^2/day as single dose or divided in 2 doses

Renal dose
CrCl <10 ml/min do not use loading dose

Available forms: Susp 30, 125 mg/5 ml; chew tabs 50 mg; inj 50 mg/ml; ext rel caps 100 mg; prompt rel caps 30 🍁, 100 mg

Adverse effects
CNS: Drowsiness, dizziness, insomnia, paresthesias, depression, suicidal tendencies, aggression, headache, confusion, slurred speech
CV: Hypotension, **ventricular fibrillation**
EENT: Nystagmus, diplopia, blurred vision
GI: Nausea, vomiting, constipation, anorexia, weight loss, **hepatitis,** jaundice, gingival hyperplasia
GU: **Nephritis,** urine discoloration
HEMA: **Agranulocytosis, leukopenia, aplastic anemia, thrombocytopenia, megaloblastic anemia**
INTEG: Rash, **lupus erythematosus, Stevens-Johnson syndrome,** hirsutism
SYST: Hypocalcemia

Contraindications: Hypersensitivity, psychiatric condition, pregnancy **D**, bradycardia, SA and AV block, Stokes-Adams syndrome, hepatic failure

Precautions: Allergies, hepatic **G** disease, renal disease, elderly, petit mal seizures

Pharmacokinetics

Absorption	Slowly absorbed from GI tract; erratic (IM)
Distribution	Crosses placenta, highly protein bound
Metabolism	Liver, extensively
Excretion	Kidneys, minimally; enters breast milk
Half-life	22 hr

Pharmacodynamics

	PO	PO–EXT REL	IM	IV
Onset	2-24 hr	2-24 hr	Erratic	1-2 hr
Peak	1.5-3 hr	4-12 hr	Erratic	Unknown
Duration	6-12 hr	12-36 hr	12-24 hr	12-24 hr

Interactions
Individual drugs
Alcohol: ↑ CNS depression
Carbamazepine: ↓ effectiveness
Chloramphenicol: ↑ blood level
Cimetidine: ↓ metabolism, ↑ action, blood level
Disulfiram: ↓ metabolism, ↑ action
Felbamate: ↑ blood level
Fluconazole: ↑ blood level
Isoniazid: ↓ metabolism, ↑ action
Ketoconazole: ↓ metabolism, ↑ action
Metronidazole: ↑ blood level
Miconazole: ↑ blood level
Omeprazole: ↑ blood level
Phenylbutazone: ↑ blood level
Valproic acid: ↑ seizures
Warfarin: ↓ blood level of phenytoin

Drug classifications

Anticonvulsants: ↑ CNS depression
Antidepressants: ↑ CNS depression
Antihistamines: ↑ CNS depression
Barbiturates: ↑ CNS depression, ↓ effect of phenytoin
Benzodiazepines: ↑ blood levels
General anesthetics: ↑ CNS depression
Sedative/hypnotics: ↑ CNS depression
Opiates: ↑ CNS depression
Oral contraceptives: ↓ metabolism, ↑ action
Sulfonamides: ↑ blood levels

Herb/drug

Aloe: ↑ hypokalemia
Buckthorn: ↑ hypokalemia
Cascara sagrada: ↑ hypokalemia
Senna: ↑ hypokalemia

Lab test interferences

↓ Dexamethasone, ↓ metyrapone test serum, ↓ PBI, ↓ urinary steroids
↑ Glucose, ↑ alkaline phosphatase, ↑ BSP

NURSING CONSIDERATIONS

Assessment

- Assess drug level: toxic level 30-50 μg/ml; therapeutic level 7.5-20 μg/ml, wait ≥1 wk to determine level
- Assess mental status: mood, sensorium, affect, memory (long, short), G especially elderly
- Assess for beginning rash that may lead to Stevens-Johnson syndrome or toxic epidermal necrolysis; phenytoin should not be used again
- Assess for blood dyscrasias: fever, sore throat, bruising, rash, jaundice, epistaxis (long-term treatment only)
- Assess seizure activity including type, location, duration, and character; provide seizure precaution
- Assess renal studies: urinalysis, BUN, urine creatinine
- Monitor blood studies: RBC, Hct, Hgb, reticulocyte counts weekly for 4 wk then monthly; also check thyroid function tests, serum calcium
- Monitor hepatic studies: ALT, AST, bilirubin, creatinine; for renal failure
- Assess for signs of physical withdrawal if medication suddenly discontinued
- Assess eye problems: need for ophth exam before, during, after treatment (slit lamp, funduscopy, tonometry)
- Assess allergic reaction: red raised rash, increased temp, lymphadenopathy; if this occurs, drug should be discontinued, usually occurs 3-12 wk after start of treatment; may also cause hepatotoxicity, rhabdomyolysis
- Monitor for toxicity: bone marrow depression, nausea, vomiting, ataxia, diplopia, CV collapse, slurred speech, confusion

Nursing diagnoses

- ✓ Injury, risk for (uses, adverse reactions)
- ✓ Knowledge deficit (teaching)
- ✓ Noncompliance (teaching)

Implementation

PO route

- Give with meals to decrease GI upset
- Chew tab can be crushed or chewed; cap can be opened and mixed with foods or fluids; cap and tab are not interchangeable
- Give by gastric/NG tube: dilute susp before administration, flush tube with 20 ml of H_2O after dose
- Shake oral susp well; use measuring device for correct dose

IV route

- Administer by direct **IV** after diluting with special diluent provided (1 ml/50 mg, 2.2 ml/100 mg, 5.2 ml/250 mg); shake; place vial in warm water to dissolve powder; give through Y-tube or 3-way stopcock; inject slowly <50 mg/min
- Give intermittent **IV** after diluting to a conc of 1-10 mg/ml
- Clear **IV** tubing first with 0.9% NaCl sol; use in-line filter; discard sol 4 hr

P

after preparation; inject into large veins to prevent purple glove syndrome

Additive compatibilities: Bleomycin, verapamil

Y-site compatibilities: Esmolol, famotidine, fluconazole, foscarnet, tacrolimus

Y-site incompatibilities: Enalaprilat, potassium chloride, vit B/C

Patient/family education

- Teach patient to carry ID card or bracelet stating name, drugs taken, condition, prescriber's name and phone number
- Advise patient to avoid driving and other activities that require alertness until drug response is known; dizziness, drowsiness can occur
- Advise patient to avoid alcohol ingestion and CNS depressants unless approved by prescriber; increased sedation may occur
- Teach patient not to discontinue medication quickly after long-term use; taper off over several wk
- Advise patient that urine may turn pink, red, or brown
- Caution patient to avoid antacids or antidiarrheals within 2-3 hr of taking phenytoin
- Instruct patient in proper oral hygiene to prevent gingival hyperplasia; to visit dentist routinely

Evaluation

Positive therapeutic outcome

- Decreased seizure activity
- Decreased dysrhythmias
- Relief of pain

phytonadione (℞)

(fye-toe-na-dye'one)

AquaMEPHYTON, Konakion, Mephyton, vitamin K_1

Func. class.: Vitamin K_1, fat-soluble vitamin

Pregnancy category C

Action: Needed for adequate blood clotting (factors II, VII, IX, X)

➔ **Therapeutic Outcome:** Prevention of bleeding

Uses: Vitamin K malabsorption, hypoprothrombinemia, prevention of hypoprothrombinemia caused by oral anticoagulants, prevention of hemorrhagic disease of the newborn [P]

Dosage and routes

Hypoprothrombinemia caused by vitamin K malabsorption

Adult: PO/IM 2.5-25 mg; may repeat or increase to 50 mg

[P] ***Child:*** PO/IM 5-10 mg

[P] ***Infants:*** PO/IM 2 mg

Prevention of hemorrhagic disease of the newborn

[P] ***Neonate:*** IM 0.5-1 mg within 1 hr after birth; repeat in 2-3 wk if required

Hypoprothrombinemia caused by oral anticoagulants

[P] ***Adult and child:*** PO/SC/IM 2.5-10 mg, may repeat 12-48 hr after PO dose or 6-8 hr after SC/IM dose, based on prothrombin time

Available forms: Tabs 5 mg; inj 2 mg/ml; aqueous colloidal (IM, **IV**); inj aqueous dispersion 10 mg/ml (IM)

Adverse effects

CNS: Headache, **brain damage** (large doses)

GI: Nausea, decreased liver function tests

***HEMA:* Hemolytic anemia, hemoglobinuria, hyperbilirubinemia**
INTEG: Rash, urticaria

Contraindications: Hypersensitivity, severe hepatic disease, last few wk of pregnancy

Precautions: Pregnancy **C**, P neonates

Pharmacokinetics

Absorption	Well absorbed (PO, IM, SC)
Distribution	Crosses placenta
Metabolism	Liver, rapidly
Excretion	Breast milk
Half-life	Unknown

Pharmacodynamics

	PO	SC/IM
Onset	6-12 hr	1-2 hr
Peak	Unknown	6 hr
Duration	Unknown	14 hr

Interactions

Individual drugs

Cholestyramine: ↓ action of phytonadione
Mineral oil: ↓ action of phytonadione
Sucralfate: ↓ phytonadione absorption

Drug classifications

Antiinfectives: ↑ phytonadione need
Oral anticoagulants: ↓ action of phytonadione
Salicylates: ↑ phytonadione need

NURSING CONSIDERATIONS

Assessment

- Monitor pro-time during treatment (2-sec deviation from control time, bleeding time, and clotting time); monitor for bleeding, pulse, and B/P
- Assess nutritional status: liver (beef), spinach, tomatoes, coffee, asparagus, broccoli, cabbage, lettuce, greens
- Assess for bleeding or bruising: hematuria, black tarry stools, hematemesis

Nursing diagnoses

✓ Nutrition, altered: less than body requirements (uses)
✓ Tissue perfusion, altered (uses)
✓ Knowledge deficit (teaching)

Implementation

IV **IV route**

- Give **IV** after diluting with D_5 NS 10 ml or more; give 1 mg/min or more
- Give **IV** only when other routes not possible (deaths have occurred)
- Store in airtight, light-resistant container

Syringe compatibilities:
Doxapram

Y-site compatibilities:
Ampicillin, epinephrine, famotidine, heparin, hydrocortisone, potassium chloride, tolazoline, vit B/C

Additive compatibilities:
Amikacin, calcium gluceptate, cephapirin, chloramphenicol, cimetidine, netilmicin, sodium bicarbonate

Patient/family education

- Teach patient not to take other supplements, unless directed by prescriber; to take this medication as directed
- Teach patient necessary foods high in vit K to be included in diet
- Advise patient to avoid IM inj, hard toothbrush, flossing; use electric razor until treatment is terminated
- Instruct patient to report symptoms of bleeding: bruising, nosebleeds, blood in urine, heavy menstruation, black tarry stools
- Caution patient not to use OTC medications unless approved by prescriber
- Stress the need for periodic lab tests to monitor coagulation levels
- Stress the need for patient to wear ID with condition, treatment, and medications taken

P

Evaluation

Positive therapeutic outcome

- Decreased bleeding tendencies
- Decreased pro-time
- Decreased clotting time

pindolol (℞)

(pin'doe-lole)

Novo-Pindol ✤, Syn-Pindol ✤, Visken

Func. class.: Antihypertensive

Chem. class.: Nonselective β-blocker

Pregnancy category B

Action: Competitively blocks stimulation of β-adrenergic receptor within vascular smooth muscle; produces chronotropic, inotropic activity (decreases rate of SA node discharge, increases recovery time), slows conduction of AV node, decreases heart rate, which decreases O_2 consumption in myocardium; also decreases renin-aldosterone-angiotensin system and at high doses inhibits β_2 receptors in bronchial system

Therapeutic Outcome: Decreased B/P in hypertension, heart rate

Uses: Mild to moderate hypertension

Investigational uses: Angina pectoris

Dosage and routes

Adult: PO 5 mg bid; usual dose 15 mg/day (5 mg tid); may increase by 10 mg/day q3-4 wk to a max of 60 mg/day

Elderly: PO 5 mg qd increase by 5 mg q3-4 wk

Available forms: Tabs 5, 10 mg

Adverse effects

CNS: *Insomnia, dizziness,* hallucinations, anxiety, fatigue

CV: Hypotension, bradycardia, **CHF,** edema, chest pain, palpitations, claudication, tachycardia, **AV block**

EENT: *Visual changes,* sore throat, *double vision,* dry burning eyes

GI: *Nausea,* vomiting, **ischemic colitis,** diarrhea, *abdominal pain,* **mesenteric arterial thrombosis**

GU: Impotence, frequency

HEMA: **Agranulocytosis, thrombocytopenia, purpura**

INTEG: Rash, alopecia, pruritus, fever

MISC: *Joint pain, muscle pain*

RESP: **Bronchospasm,** *dyspnea,* cough, rales

Contraindications: Hypersensitivity to β-blockers, cardiogenic shock, 2nd- or 3rd-degree heart block, sinus bradycardia, CHF, cardiac failure, bronchial asthma

Precautions: Major surgery, pregnancy **B**, lactation, diabetes mellitus, renal disease, thyroid disease, COPD, well-compensated heart failure, CAD, nonallergic bronchospasm

Do Not Confuse: pindolol/Parlodel, pindolol/Plendil

Pharmacokinetics	
Absorption	Well absorbed
Distribution	Crosses placenta; some penetration in CNS, protein binding 40%
Metabolism	Liver, moderately (60%-65%)
Excretion	Kidneys, unchanged (30%-45%)
Half-life	3-4 hr

Pharmacodynamics	
Onset	Unknown
Peak	2-4 hr
Duration	8-24 hr

Interactions

Individual drugs

Alcohol: ↑ hypotension (large amounts)

Epinephrine: α-Adrenergic stimulation

Hydralazine: ↑ hypotension, bradycardia

Insulin: ↑ hypoglycemia

Methyldopa: ↑ hypotension, bradycardia
Prazosin: ↑ hypotension, bradycardia
Reserpine: ↑ hypotension, bradycardia
Thyroid: ↓ effect of β-blockers
Verapamil: ↑ cardiac depression

Drug classifications

Antihypertensives: ↑ hypertension
β_2-Adrenergic agonists: ↓ bronchodilatation
Cardiac glycosides: ↑ bradycardia
Nitrates: ↑ hypotension
NSAIDs: ↓ antihypertensive effect
Oral hypoglycemics: ↑ hypoglycemia
Theophyllines: ↓ bronchodilatation

Lab test interferences

False: ↑ Urinary catecholamines

NURSING CONSIDERATIONS

Assessment

- Monitor B/P during beginning treatment, periodically thereafter; pulse q4h; note rate, rhythm, quality: apical/radial pulse before administration; notify prescriber of any significant changes (pulse <50 bpm)
- Obtain baselines in renal, liver function tests before therapy begins
- Assess for edema in feet, legs daily; monitor I&O, daily weight; check for jugular vein distention, rales bilaterally, dyspnea (CHF)
- Monitor skin turgor, dryness of mucous membranes for hydration G status, especially elderly

Nursing diagnoses

✓ Cardiac output, decreased (uses)
✓ Injury, potential for (adverse reactions)
✓ Knowledge deficit (teaching)
✓ Noncompliance (teaching)

Implementation

- Given ac, hs, tab may be crushed or swallowed whole; give with food to prevent GI upset; reduced dosage in renal impairment
- Store protected from light, moisture; place in cool environment

Patient/family education

- Teach patient not to discontinue drug abruptly; taper over 2 wk; may cause precipitate angina if stopped abruptly
- Teach patient not to use OTC products containing α-adrenergic stimulants (such as nasal decongestants, cold preparations); to avoid alcohol, smoking, and to limit sodium intake as prescribed
- Teach patient how to take pulse and B/P at home; advise when to notify prescriber
- Instruct patient to comply with weight control, dietary adjustments, modified exercise program
- Tell patient to carry/wear ID to identify drug being taken, allergies; tell patient drug controls symptoms but does not cure
- Caution patient to avoid hazardous activities if dizziness, drowsiness present
- Teach patient to report symptoms of CHF: difficult breathing, especially on exertion or when lying down, night cough, swelling of extremities or bradycardia, dizziness, confusion, depression, fever
- Teach patient to take drug as prescribed, not to double doses, skip doses; take any missed doses as soon as remembered if at least 4 hr until next dose

Evaluation

Positive therapeutic outcome

- Decreased B/P in hypertension (after 1-2 wk)

Treatment of overdose:

Lavage, **IV** atropine for bradycardia, **IV** theophylline for bronchospasm, digitalis, O_2, diuretic for cardiac failure, hemodialysis, **IV** glucose for hyperglycemia, **IV** diazepam (or phenytoin) for seizures

P

pioglitazone (℞)
(pie-oh-glye'ta-zone)
Actos
Func. class.: Antidiabetic, oral
Chem. class.: Thiazolidinedione
Pregnancy category C

Action: Improves insulin resistance by hepatic glucose metabolism, insulin receptor kinase activity, insulin receptor phosphorylation

Therapeutic Outcome: Decreased symptoms of diabetes mellitus

Uses: Stable adult-onset diabetes mellitus, type II (NIDDM)

Dosage and routes
Monotherapy
Adult: PO 15-30 mg qd, may increase to 45 mg/day
Combination therapy
Adult: PO 15-30 mg qd with a sulfonylurea, metformin, or insulin; decrease sulfonylurea dose if hypoglycemia occurs; decrease insulin dose by 10-25% if hypoglycemia occurs or if plasma glucose is <100 mg/dl, max 45 mg/day
Hepatic dose
Do not use in active liver disease or if ALT >2.5 × ULN

Available forms: Tabs 15, 30, 45 mg

Adverse effects
CNS: *Headache*
ENDO: *Aggravated diabetes mellitus*
MISC: *Myalgia, sinusitis, upper respiratory tract infection, pharyngitis*

Contraindications: Hypersensitivity to thiazolidinediones, diabetic ketoacidosis, lactation, children

Precautions: Pregnancy **C**, elderly, thyroid disease, hepatic, renal disease, edema, CHF

Pharmacokinetics	
Absorption	Unknown
Distribution	Unknown
Metabolism	Unknown
Excretion	Kidneys
Half-life	3-7 hr, terminal 16-24 hr

Pharmacodynamics	
Onset	Unknown
Peak	6-12 wk
Duration	Unknown

Interactions
Individual drugs
Ketoconazole: ↓ pioglitazone effect
Drug classifications
Oral contraceptives: ↓ effect, use an alternate contraceptive method

NURSING CONSIDERATIONS
Assessment
- Assess for hypoglycemic reactions (sweating, weakness, dizziness, anxiety, tremors, hunger), hyperglycemic reactions soon after meals
- Assess CBC (baseline, q3 mo) during treatment; check liver function tests periodically; AST, LDH, FBS, glycosylated Hgb, fasting plasma insulin, plasma lipids, lipoproteins, B/P, body weight during treatment

Nursing diagnoses
- ✓ Nutrition, altered: more than body requirements (uses)
- ✓ Knowledge deficit (teaching)

Implementation
- Convert from other oral hypoglycemic agents; change may be made without gradual dosage change; monitor serum or urine glucose and ketones tid during conversion
- Give once a day; give with meals to decrease GI upset and provide best absorption
- Give tabs crushed and mixed with meal or fluids for patients with difficulty swallowing
- Store in airtight container in cool environment

Patient/family education

- Teach patient to use capillary blood glucose test or Chemstrip tid
- Teach patient symptoms of hypo/hyperglycemia, what to do about each
- Advise patient that drug must be continued on daily basis; explain consequence of discontinuing drug abruptly
- Advise patient to avoid OTC medications or herbal preparations unless approved by prescriber
- Advise patient that diabetes is life-long illness; that this drug is not a cure, only controls symptoms
- Advise patient that all food included in diet plan must be eaten to prevent hypoglycemia
- Advise patient to carry ID and glucagon emergency kit for emergencies
- Instruct patient to notify prescriber if oral contraceptives are used
- Teach patient not to use if breast-feeding

Evaluation

Positive therapeutic outcome

- Decrease in polyuria, polydipsia, polyphagia; clear sensorium; absence of dizziness; stable gait; blood glucose at normal level

---

HIGH ALERT

pipecuronium (℞)

(pip-e-kyoor'oh'nee-um)

Arduran

Func. class.: Neuromuscular blocker (nondepolarizing)

Chem. class.: Synthetic curariform

Pregnancy category C

Action: Inhibits transmission of nerve impulses by binding with cholinergic receptor sites, antagonizing action of acetylcholine; no analgesic response

➔ **Therapeutic Outcome:** Paralysis of all skeletal muscles

Uses: Facilitation of endotracheal intubation, skeletal muscle relaxation during mechanical ventilation, surgery, or general anesthesia

Dosage and routes

Adult: **IV** dosage is individualized; in patients with normal renal function who are not obese, initial dose 70-85 μg/kg; maintenance dose 10-15 μg/kg

P ***Child 1-14 yr:*** **IV** 57 μg/kg

P ***Child 3 mo-1 yr:*** **IV** 40 μg/kg

Available forms: Inj 10-mg vials

Adverse effects

CNS: Hypesthesia, CNS depression

CV: Bradycardia, tachycardia, increased or decreased B/P, ventricular extrasystole, **myocardial ischemia, CVA, thrombosis, atrial fibrillation**

EENT: Increased secretions

GU: **Anuria**

INTEG: Rash, urticaria

META: Hypoglycemia, hyperkalemia, increased creatinine

MS: Weakness to prolonged skeletal muscle relaxation

RESP: **Prolonged apnea, bronchospasm, cyanosis, respiratory depression**

Contraindications: Hypersensitivity to bromide ion

Precautions: Pregnancy **C**, renal disease, cardiac disease, lactation, P children <3 mo, fluid and electrolyte imbalances, neuromuscular diseases, respiratory disease, obesity

Pharmacokinetics

Absorption	Complete bioavailability
Distribution	Unknown
Metabolism	Unknown
Excretion	Kidneys, unchanged (>75%)
Half-life	1½ hr; increased in renal disease

Pharmacodynamics	
Onset	30-45 sec
Peak	3-5 min
Duration	1-2 hr

Interactions
Individual drugs
Clindamycin: ↑ paralysis length and intensity
Colistin: ↑ paralysis length and intensity
Lidocaine: ↑ paralysis length and intensity
Lithium: ↑ paralysis length and intensity
Magnesium: ↑ paralysis length and intensity
Polymyxin B: ↑ paralysis length and intensity
Procainamide: ↑ paralysis length and intensity
Quinidine: ↑ paralysis length and intensity
Succinylcholine: ↑ paralysis length and intensity
Drug classifications
Aminoglycosides: ↑ paralysis length and intensity
β-Adrenergic blockers: ↑ paralysis length and intensity
Diuretics, potassium-losing: ↑ paralysis length and intensity
General anesthetics: ↑ paralysis length and intensity

NURSING CONSIDERATIONS
Assessment
- Monitor vital signs (B/P, pulse, respirations, airway) until fully recovered; rate, depth, pattern of respirations, strength of hand grip; patient should be intubated before use
- Monitor for electrolyte imbalances (potassium, magnesium) before drug is used; electrolyte imbalances may lead to increased action of this drug
- Monitor for recovery: decreased paralysis of face, diaphragm, leg, arm, rest of body; residual weakness and respiratory problems may occur during recovery period
- Assess for hypersensitive reactions: rash, fever, respiratory distress, pruritus; drug should be discontinued

Nursing diagnoses
✓ Breathing pattern, ineffective (uses)
✓ Communication, impaired verbal (adverse reactions)
✓ Fear (adverse reactions)
✓ Knowledge deficit (teaching)

Implementation
- Use peripheral nerve stimulator (anesthesiologist) to determine neuromuscular blockade; deep tendon reflexes should be monitored during extended periods
- Give **IV** after reconstituting with 0.9% NaCl, D_5W, D_5/0.9% NaCl, LR, sterile water for inj; sol with benzyl alcohol should not be used for **P** newborns; should be administered only by qualified person, usually an anesthesiologist; do not administer IM
- Store in light-resistant area (powder); refrigerate unused portions (sterile water); use within 24 hr

Patient/family education
- Provide reassurance to patient if communication is difficult during recovery from neuromuscular blockade
- Provide patient with explanation of all procedures or treatments; patient will remain conscious if anesthesia is not given also

Evaluation
Positive therapeutic outcome
- Paralysis of jaw, eyelid, head, neck, rest of body as evaluated by peripheral nerve stimulator

Treatment of overdose:
Edrophonium or neostigmine, atropine, monitor VS; may require mechanical ventilation

piperacillin (℞)
(pi-per'a-sill-in)
Pipracil
Func. class.: Broad-spectrum antiinfective
Chem. class.: Extended-spectrum penicillin
Pregnancy category B

Action: Interferes with cell wall replication of susceptible organisms; osmotically unstable cell wall swells and bursts from osmotic pressure

➔ **Therapeutic Outcome:** Bactericidal effects for gram-positive cocci *Staphylococcus aureus, Streptococcus pyogenes, Streptococcus viridans, Streptococcus faecalis, Streptococcus bovis, Streptococcus pneumoniae;* gram-negative cocci *Neisseria gonorrhoeae, Neisseria meningitidis;* gram-positive bacilli *Clostridium perfringens, Clostridium tetani;* gram-negative bacilli *Bacteroides, Fusobacterium nucleatum, Escherichia coli, Klebsiella, Proteus mirabilis, Proteus vulgaris, Proteus rettgeri, Morganella morganii, Enterobacter, Citrobacter, Pseudomonas aeruginosa, Serratia, Acinetobacter, Peptococcus, Peptostreptococcus, Eubacterium*

Uses: Respiratory tract, skin, skin structure, urinary tract, bone, and joint infections; gonorrhea, pneumonia, endocarditis, septicemia, meningitis, sinusitis; infections caused by penicillinase-producing staphylococci, streptococci; may be combined with an aminoglycoside for *Pseudomonas* infection

Dosage and routes
Urinary tract infections
Adult: **IV** 8-16 g/day (125-200 mg/kg/day) in divided doses q6-8h
Serious systemic infections
P ***Adult and child >12 yr:*** IM/**IV** 100-300 mg/kg/day in divided doses q4-6h
P ***Child <12 yr:*** IM/**IV** 200-300 mg/kg/day in divided doses q4-6h
P ***Neonates <36 wk:*** **IV** 75 mg/kg q12h in the 1st wk of life, then q8h in 2nd wk
P ***Full term infants:*** **IV** 75 mg/kg q8h in 1st wk of life, then q6h thereafter
Prophylaxis of surgical infections
Adult: **IV** 2 g 30-60 min before procedure; may be repeated during or after surgery
Renal dose
CrCl 10-50 ml/min give q6-8h; CrCl <10 ml/min give q8h

Available forms: Powder for inj 2, 3, 4, 40 g

Adverse effects
CNS: Lethargy, hallucinations, anxiety, depression, twitching, **coma, seizures**
GI: Nausea, vomiting, diarrhea, increased AST, ALT, abdominal pain, glossitis, colitis, **pseudomembranous colitis**
GU: **Oliguria, proteinuria, hematuria, vaginitis, moniliasis, glomerulonephritis**
HEMA: Anemia, increased bleeding time, **bone marrow depression, thrombocytopenia**
META: Hypokalemia, hypernatremia
SYST: **Serum sickness, anaphylaxis**

Contraindications: Hypersensitivity to penicillins; P neonates

Precautions: Pregnancy **B,** hypersensitivity to cephalosporins, CHF, renal disease, seizures

Pharmacokinetics

Absorption	Well absorbed (80%)
Distribution	Widely distributed; crosses placenta
Metabolism	Not metabolized
Excretion	Kidneys, unchanged (90%); bile (10%); breast milk
Half-life	0.7-1.3 hr

Pharmacodynamics

	IM	IV
Onset	Rapid	Rapid
Peak	30-50 min	Inf end

Interactions

Individual drugs

Aminoglycosides: ↓ half-life in renal disease
Amphotericin B: ↑ hypokalemia
Aspirin: ↑ piperacillin levels, ↓ renal excretion
Chloramphenicol: ↑ half-life of chloramphenicol, ↓ effectiveness of piperacillin
Cholestyramine: ↓ effectiveness of piperacillin
Colestipol: ↓ effectiveness of piperacillin
Erythromycin: ↓ antimicrobial effectiveness
Lithium: ↓ excretion, ↑ toxicity
Probenecid: ↑ piperacillin levels, ↓ renal excretion

Drug classifications

Diuretics: ↑ hypokalemia
Glucocorticoids: ↑ hypokalemia
Hepatotoxic agents: ↑ hepatotoxicity
Oral anticoagulants: ↑ anticoagulant effects
Oral contraceptives: ↓ contraceptive effectiveness
Tetracyclines: ↓ antimicrobial effectiveness

Food/drug

Food, carbonated drinks, citrus fruit juices: ↓ absorption

Herb/drug

Khat: ↓ absorption

Lab test interferences

False positive: Urine glucose, urine protein

NURSING CONSIDERATIONS

Assessment

- Assess patient for previous sensitivity reaction to penicillins or other cephalosporins; cross-sensitivity between penicillins and cephalosporins is common
- Assess patient for signs and symptoms of infection including characteristics of wounds, sputum, urine, stool, WBC >10,000/mm^3, fever; obtain baseline information and during treatment
- Obtain C&S before beginning drug therapy to identify if correct treatment has been initiated
- Assess for allergic reactions: rash, urticaria, pruritus, chills, fever, joint pain; angioedema may occur a few days after therapy begins; epinephrine, resuscitation equipment should be available for anaphylactic reaction
- (Alert) Identify urine output; if decreasing, notify prescriber (may indicate nephrotoxicity); also check for increased BUN, creatinine
- Monitor blood studies: AST, ALT, CBC, Hct, bilirubin, LDH, alkaline phosphatase, Coombs' test monthly if patient is on long-term therapy
- Monitor electrolytes: potassium, sodium, chloride monthly if patient is on long-term therapy
- Assess bowel pattern daily; if severe diarrhea occurs, drug should be discontinued; may indicate pseudomembranous colitis
- Monitor for bleeding: ecchymosis, bleeding gums, hematuria, stool guaiac daily if on long-term therapy
- Assess for overgrowth of infection: perineal itching, fever, malaise, redness, pain, swelling, drainage, rash, diarrhea, change in cough, sputum

Nursing diagnoses

- ✓ Infection, risk for (uses)
- ✓ Diarrhea (adverse reactions)

✓ Injury, risk for (adverse reactions)
✓ Knowledge deficit (teaching)
✓ Noncompliance (teaching)

Implementation

IM route

- Reconstitute 2 g/4 ml, 3 g/6 ml, 4 g/7.8 ml with sterile water, 0.9% NaCl, bacteriostatic water, 0.5% or 1% lidocaine without epinephrine
- Inject deep in large muscle mass, massage; split inj >2 g into 2 inj

IV **IV route**

- Reconstitute with 5 ml or more 0.9% NaCl, bacteriostatic water; shake sol to dissolve
- Change **IV** sites q48h to prevent phlebitis and pain
- Give direct **IV** over 3-5 min
- Give by intermittent inf by diluting in 50 ml or more D_5W, 0.9% NaCl, D_5/0.9% NaCl, LR, give over 20-30 min by Y-site; discontinue primary inf during intermittent inf

Syringe compatibilities:
Heparin

Y-site compatibilities:
Acyclovir, aldesleukin, allopurinol, amifostine, aztreonam, ciprofloxacin, cyclophosphamide, diltiazem, enalaprilat, esmolol, famotidine, fludarabine, foscarnet, heparin, hydromorphone, IL-2, labetalol, lorazepam, magnesium sulfate, melphalan, meperidine, midazolam, morphine, perphenazine, propofol, ranitidine, tacrolimus, teniposide, theophylline, thiotepa, verapamil, zidovudine

Y-site incompatibilities:
Ondansetron, fluconazole, sargramostim, vinorelbine

Additive compatibilities:
Ciprofloxacin, clindamycin, flucloxacillin, fluconazole, hydrocortisone sodium succinate, ofloxacin, potassium chloride, verapamil

Additive incompatibilities:
Aminoglycosides

Patient/family education

- Teach patient to report sore throat, bruising, bleeding, joint pain; may indicate blood dyscrasias (rare)
- Advise patient to contact prescriber if vaginal itching, loose, foul-smelling stools, furry tongue occur; may indicate superinfection
- Advise patient to notify prescriber of diarrhea with blood or pus, which may indicate pseudomembranous colitis

Evaluation

Positive therapeutic outcome

- Absence of signs/symptoms of infection (WBC <10,000/mm^3, temp WNL, absence of red, draining wounds)
- Reported improvement in symptoms of infection

Treatment of anaphylaxis: Withdraw drug, maintain airway, administer epinephrine, aminophylline, O_2, **IV** corticosteroids

piperacillin/tazobactam (℞)

Pipracil

Func. class.: Broad-spectrum antiinfective

Chem. class.: Extended-spectrum penicillin

Pregnancy category B

Action: Interferes with cell wall replication of susceptible organisms; osmotically unstable cell wall swells and bursts from osmotic pressure

➔ **Therapeutic Outcome:** Bactericidal effects for piperacillin-resistant β-lactamase, *Escherichia coli, Staphylococcus aureus, Bacteroides fragilis, Haemophilus influenzae*

Uses: Respiratory tract, skin, skin structure, urinary tract, bone, and joint infections; gonorrhea, pneumonia, infections from penicillinase-producing staphylococci, streptococci

P

Dosage and routes

Nosocomial pneumonia

Adult: **IV** 3.375 g q6-8h with an aminoglycoside × 1-2 wk; continue aminoglycoside only if *Pseudomonas aeruginosa* is isolated

Other infections

Adult: **IV** 6-12 g/day, given 3.375 g q6h × 7-10 days

Renal dose

CrCl 20-40 ml/min 2.25 g q6h; CrCl <20 ml/min 2.25 g q8h

Available forms: Powder for inj 2 g piperacillin/0.25 g tazobactam; 3 g piperacillin/0.375 g tazobactam, 4 g piperacillin/0.5 g tazobactam, 36 g piperacillin/4.5 g tazobactam

Adverse effects

CNS: Headache, insomnia, agitation, dizziness, fever, lethargy, hallucinations, **coma, seizures**
CV: Chest pain, edema, hypertension
EENT: Rhinitis
GI: *Nausea, vomiting, diarrhea,* increased AST, ALT, abdominal pain, glossitis, colitis, constipation, **pseudomembranous colitis**
INTEG: Rash, pruritus
MISC: Fever, superinfection
RESP: Dyspnea
SYST: **Serum sickness, anaphylaxis**

Contraindications: Hypersensitivity to penicillins, cephalosporins, P tazobactam; neonates

Precautions: Pregnancy **B**, CHF, renal disease, lactation, sodium restriction, children, seizures

Pharmacokinetics

Absorption	Well absorbed (80%)
Distribution	Widely distributed; crosses placenta
Metabolism	Not metabolized
Excretion	Kidneys, unchanged (90%); bile (10%); breast milk
Half-life	0.7-1.3 hr

Pharmacodynamics

Onset	Rapid
Peak	Inf end

Interactions

Individual drugs

Aminoglycosides: ↓ half-life in renal disease
Amphotericin B: ↑ hypokalemia
Aspirin: ↑ piperacillin levels, ↑ renal excretion
Chloramphenicol: ↑ half-life of chloramphenicol, ↓ effectiveness of piperacillin
Cholestyramine: ↓ effectiveness of piperacillin
Colestipol: ↓ effectiveness of piperacillin
Diuretics: ↑ hypokalemia
Glucocorticoids: ↑ hypokalemia
Hepatotoxic agents: ↑ hepatotoxicity
Probenecid: ↑ piperacillin levels, ↓ renal excretion

Drug classifications

Erythromycins: ↓ antimicrobial effectiveness
Lithium: ↓ excretion, ↑ toxicity
Oral anticoagulants: ↑ anticoagulant effects
Oral contraceptives: ↓ contraceptive effectiveness
Tetracyclines: ↓ antimicrobial effectiveness

Food/drug

Food, carbonated drinks, citrus fruit juices: ↓ absorption

Herb/drug

Khat: ↓ absorption

Lab test interferences

False positive: Urine glucose, urine protein

NURSING CONSIDERATIONS

Assessment

- Assess patient for previous sensitivity reaction to penicillins or other cephalosporins, cross-sensitivity between penicillins and cephalosporins is common

• Assess patient for signs and symptoms of infection including characteristics of wounds, sptum, urine, stool, WBC >10,000/mm^3, fever; obtain baseline information and during treatment
• Obtain C&S before beginning drug therapy to identify if correct treatment has been initiated
• Assess for allergic reactions: rash, urticaria, pruritus, chills, fever, joint pain; angioedema may occur a few days after therapy begins; epinephrine, resuscitation equipment should be available for anaphylactic reaction
• Identify urine output; if decreasing, notify prescriber (may indicate nephrotoxicity); also check for increased BUN, creatinine
• Monitor blood studies: AST, ALT, CBC, Hct, bilirubin, LDH, alkaline phosphatase, Coombs' test monthly if patient is on long-term therapy
• Monitor electrolytes: potassium, sodium, chloride monthly if patient is on long-term therapy
• Assess bowel pattern daily; if severe diarrhea occurs, drug should be discontinued; may indicate pseudomembranous colitis
• Monitor for bleeding: ecchymosis, bleeding gums, hematuria, stool guaiac daily if on long-term therapy
• Assess for overgrowth of infection: perineal itching, fever, malaise, redness, pain, swelling, drainage, rash, diarrhea, change in cough, sputum

Nursing diagnoses

✓ Infection, risk for (uses)
✓ Diarrhea (adverse reactions)
✓ Injury, risk for (adverse reactions)
✓ Knowledge deficit (teaching)
✓ Noncompliance (teaching)

Implementation

• Reconstitute with 5 ml or more 0.9% NaCl, bacteriostatic water; shake sol to dissolve
• Give by intermittent inf by diluting in 50 ml or more D_5W, 0.9% NaCl, D_5/0.9% NaCl, LR; give over 20-30 min by Y-site; discontinue primary inf during intermittent inf
• Change **IV** sites q48h to prevent phlebitis and pain
• Give direct **IV** over 3-5 min

Y-site compatibilities:

Aminophylline, aztreonam, bleomycin, bumetanide, buprenorphine, butorphanol, calcium gluconate, carboplatin, carmustine, cefepime, cimetidine, clindamycin, cyclophosphamide, cytarabine, dexamethasone, diphenhydramine, dopamine, enalaprilat, etoposide, floxuridine, fluconazole, fludarabine, fluorouracil, furosemide, gallium, granisetron, heparin, hydrocortisone, hydromorphone, ifosfamide, leucovorin, lorazepam, magnesium sulfate, mannitol, meperidine, mesna, methotrexate, methylprednisolone, metoclopramide, metronidazole, morphine, ondansetron, plicomycin, potassium chloride, ranitidine, sargramostim, sodium bicarbonate, thiotepa, trimethoprim/sulfamethoxazole, vinblastine, vincristine, zidovudine

Y-site incompatibilities:

Fluconazole, ondansetron, sargramostim, vinorelbine

Patient/family education

• Teach patient to report sore throat, bruising, bleeding, joint pain; may indicate blood dyscrasias (rare)
• Advise patient to contact prescriber if vaginal itching, loose, foul-smelling stools, furry tongue occur; may indicate superinfection
• Advise patient to notify prescriber of diarrhea with blood or pus, which may indicate pseudomembranous colitis

Evaluation

Positive therapeutic outcome
• Absence of signs/symptoms of infection (WBC <10,000/mm^3, temp WNL, absence of red, draining wounds)
• Reported improvement in symptoms of infection

P

Treatment of anaphylaxis: Withdraw drug, maintain airway, administer epinephrine, aminophylline, O_2, **IV** corticosteroids

pirbuterol (℞)

(peer-byoo'ter-ole)

Maxair

Func. class.: Bronchodilator

Chem. class.: β-Adrenergic agonist

Pregnancy category C

Action: Relaxes bronchial smooth muscle by direct action on β_2-adrenergic receptors, with increased levels of cAMP and increased bronchodilatation, diuresis, and cardiac and CNS stimulation

Therapeutic Outcome: Bronchodilatation with ease of breathing

Uses: Reversible bronchospasm (prevention, treatment), including asthma, may be given with theophylline or steroids

Dosage and routes

P ***Adult and child >12 yr:*** INH 1-2 (0.4 mg) q4-6h; max 12 inh/day

Available forms: Aerosol delivers 0.2 mg pirbuterol/actuation

Adverse effects

CNS: Tremors, anxiety, insomnia, headache, dizziness, stimulation, restlessness, hallucinations, drowsiness, irritability

CV: Palpitations, tachycardia, hypertension, angina, hypotension, **dysrhythmias**

EENT: Dry nose and mouth, irritation of nose, throat

GI: Gastritis, nausea, vomiting, anorexia

MS: Muscle cramps

RESP: **Paradoxical bronchospasm,** dyspnea, coughing

Contraindications: Hypersensitivity to sympathomimetics, tachycardia

Precautions: Lactation, pregnancy **C,** cardiac disorders, hyperthyroidism, diabetes mellitus, prostatic hypertrophy

Pharmacokinetics	
Absorption	Minimally absorbed
Distribution	Unknown
Metabolism	Liver
Excretion	Unknown
Half-life	2 hr

Pharmacodynamics	
Onset	5-15 min
Peak	1-1½ hr
Duration	5 hr

Interactions

Drug classifications

β-Adrenergic blockers: Block therapeutic effect

Bronchodilators, aerosol: ↑ action of bronchodilator

MAOIs: ↑ chance of hypertensive crisis

Sympathomimetics: ↑ adrenergic side effects

Herb/drug

Ephedra: ↑ action of both

NURSING CONSIDERATIONS

Assessment

- Monitor respiratory function: vital capacity, FEV, ABGs, lung sounds, heart rate, rhythm (baseline)
- Monitor for evidence of allergic reactions, paradoxic bronchospasm (can occur rapidly); withhold dose and notify prescriber

Nursing diagnoses

- ✓ Airway clearance, ineffective (uses)
- ✓ Gas exchange, impaired (uses)
- ✓ Knowledge deficit (teaching)

Implementation

- Give after shaking; have patient exhale, place mouthpiece in mouth, inhale slowly, hold breath, remove, exhale slowly; allow at least 1 min between inhalations

- Store in light-resistant container; do not expose to temp over 86° F (30° C)

Patient/family education

- Advise patient not to use OTC medications; extra stimulation may occur; to use this medication before other medications and allow at least 1 min between each to prevent overstimulation
- Teach patient use of inhaler; to avoid getting aerosol in eyes; blurring may result; to wash inhaler in warm water and dry daily; to avoid smoking, smoke-filled rooms, persons with respiratory tract infections; review package insert with patient
- Teach patient that paradoxic bronchospasm may occur and to stop drug immediately and notify prescriber; to limit caffeine products such as chocolate, coffee, tea, and colas
- Instruct patient on administration of dose; not to use more than prescribed; serious side effects may occur

Evaluation

Positive therapeutic outcome

- Absence of dyspnea, wheezing after 1 hr
- Improved airway exchange
- Improved ABGs

Treatment of overdose: Administer a β_2-adrenergic blocker

piroxicam (℞)

(peer-ox'i-kam)

Apo-Piroxicam ✤, Feldene, Novopirocam ✤, Nu-Pirox, PMS-Piroxicam

Func. class.: Nonsteroidal antiinflammatory

Chem. class.: Oxicam derivative

Pregnancy category B

Action: Inhibits prostaglandin synthesis by decreasing an enzyme needed for biosynthesis; analgesic, antiinflammatory

Therapeutic Outcome: Decreased pain, inflammation

Uses: Mild to moderate pain, osteoarthritis, rheumatoid arthritis

Dosage and routes

Adult: PO 20 mg qd or 10 mg bid

Available forms: Caps 10, 20 mg

Adverse effects

CNS: Dizziness, *drowsiness,* fatigue, tremors, confusion, insomnia, anxiety, depression, *headache*

CV: Tachycardia, peripheral edema, palpitations, **dysrhythmias**

EENT: Tinnitus, hearing loss, blurred vision

GI: *Nausea, anorexia, vomiting, diarrhea,* jaundice, **cholestatic hepatitis,** constipation, flatulence, cramps, dry mouth, peptic ulcer, **bleeding, ulceration, perforation**

GU: **Nephrotoxicity: dysuria, hematuria, oliguria, azotemia**

HEMA: **Blood dyscrasias**

INTEG: Purpura, rash, pruritus, sweating, photosensitivity

Contraindications: Hypersensitivity, asthma, severe renal disease, severe hepatic disease, ulcer disease, cardiac disease

Precautions: Pregnancy **B,** lactation, children, bleeding disorders, GI disorders, cardiac disorders, hypersensitivity to other antiinflammatory agents, CHF

Pharmacokinetics	
Absorption	Well absorbed
Distribution	Unknown
Metabolism	Liver, extensively
Excretion	Kidneys, minimal; breast milk
Half-life	30-80 hr

Pharmacodynamics	
Onset	1 hr
Peak	Unknown
Duration	48-72 hr

Interactions

Individual drugs

Acetaminophen (long-term use): ↑ renal reactions
Alcohol: ↑ adverse reactions
Aspirin: ↓ effectiveness, ↑ adverse reactions
Digoxin: ↑ toxicity, levels
Insulin: ↓ insulin effect
Lithium: ↑ toxicity
Methotrexate: ↑ toxicity
Phenytoin: ↑ toxicity
Probenecid: ↑ toxicity
Radiation: ↑ risk of hematologic toxicity
Sulfonylurea: ↑ toxicity
Warfarin: ↑ anticoagulant effects

Drug classifications

Anticoagulants: ↑ risk of bleeding
Antihypertensives: ↓ effect of antihypertensives
Antineoplastics: ↑ risk of hematologic toxicity
β-Adrenergic blockers: ↑ antihypertension
Cephalosporins: ↑ risk of bleeding
Diuretics: ↓ effectiveness of diuretics
Glucocorticoids: ↑ adverse reactions
Hypoglycemic agents: ↓ hypoglycemic effect
NSAIDs: ↑ adverse reactions
Potassium supplements: ↑ adverse reactions
Sulfonamides: ↑ toxicity

Lab test interferences

↑ Serum potassium, ↑ liver function studies
↓ Hct, ↓ Hgb, ↓ blood glucose

NURSING CONSIDERATIONS

Assessment

- Monitor blood counts during therapy; watch for decreasing platelets; if low, therapy may need to be discontinued, restarted after hematologic recovery; check for blood dyscrasia (thrombocytopenia): bruising, fatigue, bleeding, poor healing
- Assess for pain: location, duration, ROM, before and 1-2 hr after administration
- Assess for aspirin sensitivity, asthma, nasal polyps; these may develop into allergic reactions

Nursing diagnoses

- ✓ Pain (uses)
- ✓ Mobility, impaired (uses)
- ✓ Knowledge deficit (teaching)
- ✓ Injury, risk for (adverse reactions)

Implementation

- Administer to patient whole; give with food or milk to decrease gastric symptoms
- ⊘ Do not crush, chew caps

Patient/family education

- Teach patient that drug must be continued for prescribed time to be effective; to avoid aspirin, alcoholic beverages and other OTC medications unless approved by prescriber
- Caution patient to report bleeding, bruising, fatigue, malaise, since blood dyscrasias do occur
- Instruct patient to use caution when driving; drowsiness, dizziness may occur
- Teach patient to take with a full glass of water to enhance absorption; do not crush, break, or chew

Evaluation

Positive therapeutic outcome

- Decreased pain
- Decreased inflammation
- Increased mobility

plasma protein fraction (℞)

Plasmanate, Plasma Plex, Plasmatein, Protenate
Func. class.: Blood derivative
Chem. class.: Human plasma in sodium chloride

Pregnancy category C

Action: Exerts similar oncotic pressure as human plasma, expands blood volume, shifts water from extravascular space to intravascular space

Therapeutic Outcome: Shift of fluid from extravascular into intravascular space

Uses: Hypovolemic shock, hypoproteinemia, ARDS, preoperative cardiopulmonary bypass, acute liver failure, nephrotic syndrome

Dosage and routes

Hypovolemia

Adult: **IV** inf 250-500 ml (12.5-25 g of protein), max 10 ml/min

P ***Child:*** **IV** inf 22-33 ml/kg at 5-10 ml/min

Hypoproteinemia

Adult: **IV** inf 1000-1500 ml qd, max 8 ml/min

Available forms: Inj 5%

Adverse effects

CNS: Fever, chills, headache, paresthesias, flushing

CV: Fluid overload, hypotension, erratic pulse

GI: Nausea, vomiting, increased salivation

INTEG: Rash, urticaria, cyanosis

RESP: Altered respirations, dyspnea, pulmonary edema

Contraindications: Hypersensitivity, CHF, severe anemia, renal insufficiency

Precautions: Decreased salt intake, decreased cardiac reserve, lack of albumin deficiency, hepatic disease, renal disease, pregnancy **C**

Pharmacokinetics	
Absorption	Completely absorbed
Distribution	Intravascular space
Metabolism	Unknown
Excretion	Unknown
Half-life	Unknown

Pharmacodynamics	
Onset	15-30 min
Peak	Unknown
Duration	Unknown

Interactions: None

Lab test interferences

False: ↑ Alkaline phosphatase

NURSING CONSIDERATIONS

Assessment

- Monitor blood studies: Hct, Hgb; electrolytes, serum protein, if serum protein declines, dyspnea, hypoxemia can result
- Monitor B/P (decreased), pulse (erratic), respiration during inf; CVP, jugular vein distention, PWP (increases if overload occurs); shortness of breath, anxiety, insomnia, expiratory rales, frothy blood-tinged cough, cyanosis indicate pulmonary overload
- Monitor I&O ratio; urinary output may decrease
- Assess for allergy: fever, rash, itching, chills, flushing, urticaria, nausea, vomiting, or hypotension requires discontinuation of inf; use new lot if therapy reinstituted, premedicate with diphenhydramine

Nursing diagnoses

✓ Fluid volume deficit (uses)
✓ Cardiac output, decreased (uses)
✓ Fluid volume excess (adverse reactions)

Implementation

- Give by **IV**; no dilution required; use infusion pump, large-gauge needle (≥20 G); discard unused portion; infuse slowly within 4 hr of opening
- Provide adequate hydration before administration
- When storing, check type of albumin, date; may have to refrigerate

Additive compatibilities: Carbohydrate and electrolyte sol, whole blood, packed RBCs, chloramphenicol, tetracycline

Additive incompatibilities: Protein hydrolysate sol, amino acids sol, alcohol, norepinephrine

Patient/family education

- Explain reason for and expected result of medication

P

Evaluation

Positive therapeutic outcome

- Increased B/P
- Decreased edema
- Increased serum albumin

HIGH ALERT

plicamycin (℞)

(plik-a-mi'cin)

Mithramycin, Mithracin

Func. class.: Antineoplastic, antibiotic; hypocalcemic

Chem. class.: Crystalline aglycone

Pregnancy category X

Action: Inhibits DNA, RNA, protein synthesis; derived from *Streptomyces plicatus;* replication is decreased by binding to DNA; demonstrates calcium-lowering effect not related to its tumoricidal activity; also acts on osteoclasts and blocks action of parathyroid hormone; a vesicant

Therapeutic Outcome: Prevention of rapidly growing malignant cells, decreased calcium levels

Uses: Testicular cancer, hypercalcemia, hypercalciuria, symptomatic treatment of advanced neoplasms

Dosage and routes

Testicular tumors

Adult: **IV** 25-30 μg/kg/day × 8-10 days, max 30 μg/kg/day

Hypercalcemia/ hypercalciuria

Adult: **IV** 25 μg/kg/day × 3-4 days; repeat at intervals of 1 wk

Available forms: Inj 2500 μg/vial powder

Adverse effects

CNS: *Drowsiness, weakness, lethargy, headache, flushing,* fever, depression

GI: *Nausea, vomiting, anorexia, diarrhea, stomatitis,* increased liver enzymes

GU: Increased BUN, creatinine, **proteinuria**

HEMA: **Hemorrhage, thrombocytopenia,** decreased pro-time, WBC count

INTEG: *Rash,* cellulitis, **extravasation**, facial flushing

META: Decreased serum calcium, potassium, phosphorus

Contraindications: Hypersensitivity, thrombocytopenia, bone marrow depression, bleeding disorders, P pregnancy **X**, child <15 yr

Precautions: Renal disease, hepatic disease, electrolyte imbalances

Pharmacokinetics

Absorption	Completely absorbed
Distribution	Crosses blood-brain barrier; concentration in bone, liver, renal system
Metabolism	Unknown
Excretion	Kidneys
Half-life	Unknown

Pharmacodynamics

Unknown

Interactions

Individual drugs

Aspirin: ↑ risk of bleeding
Dextran: ↑ risk of bleeding
Heparin: ↑ risk of bleeding
Radiation: ↑ toxicity, bone marrow suppression
Sulfinpyrazone: ↑ risk of bleeding
Valproic acid: ↑ risk of bleeding

Drug classifications

Antineoplastics: ↑ toxicity, bone marrow suppression
Cephalosporins: ↑ risk of bleeding
Hepatotoxic agents: ↑ hepatotoxicity
Neurotoxic agents: ↑ neurotoxicity
NSAIDs: ↑ risk of bleeding
Oral anticoagulants: ↑ risk of bleeding
Thrombolytics: ↑ risk of bleeding

NURSING CONSIDERATIONS

Assessment

- Assess buccal cavity q8h for dryness, sores or ulceration, white patches, oral pain, bleeding, dysphagia; obtain prescription for viscous lidocaine (Xylocaine)
- Assess symptoms indicating severe allergic reaction: rash, pruritus, urticaria, purpuric skin lesions, itching, flushing
- Monitor CBC, differential, platelet count weekly; withhold drug if WBC is $<4000/mm^3$ or platelet count is $<100,000/mm^3$; notify prescriber of results if WBC $<20,000/mm^3$, platelets $<150,000/mm^3$
- Monitor renal function studies: BUN, creatinine, serum uric acid, urine CrCl before and during therapy; I&O ratio; report fall in urine output to <30 ml/hr
- Monitor temp q4h (may indicate beginning of infection)
- Monitor liver function tests before and during therapy (bilirubin, AST, ALT, LDH) as needed or monthly; check for jaundice of skin and sclera, dark urine, clay-colored stools, itchy skin, abdominal pain, fever, diarrhea
- Assess for bleeding: hematuria, stool guaiac, bruising or petechiae, mucosa or orifices q8h, may progress to severe bleeding; check for inflammation of mucosa, breaks in skin

Nursing diagnoses

- ✓ Injury, risk for (adverse reactions)
- ✓ Body image disturbance (adverse reactions)
- ✓ Infection, risk for (adverse reactions)
- ✓ Knowledge deficit (teaching)

Implementation

- Avoid contact with skin; very irritating; wash completely to remove
- Give fluids **IV** or PO before chemotherapy to hydrate patient
- Give antacid before oral agent; give drug after evening meal, before bedtime; provide antiemetic 30-60 min before giving drug and prn to prevent vomiting; administer antibiotics for prophylaxis of infection
- Give top or systemic analgesics for pain
- Give in AM so drug can be eliminated before bedtime
- Provide liq diet: carbonated beverages; gelatin may be added if patient is not nauseated or vomiting
- Encourage patient to rinse mouth tid-qid with water, club soda; brush teeth bid-qid with soft brush or cotton-tipped applicators for stomatitis; use unwaxed dental floss
- Make sure drug is prepared by experienced personnel using proper precautions
- Give **IV** intermittent inf by diluting 2.5 mg/4.9 ml of sterile water; (1 ml = 500 μg); dilute single dose in 1000 ml of D_5W run over 4-6 hr; give slow **IV** inf using 20- or 21-G needle
- Administer EDTA for extravasation; apply ice compress

Y-site compatibilities: Allopurinol, amifostine, aztreonam, filgrastim, melphalan, piperacillin/tazobactam, teniposide, thiotepa, vinorelbine

Patient/family education

- Teach patient to avoid use of products containing aspirin or NSAIDs, razors, commercial mouthwash, since bleeding may occur; to report symptoms of bleeding (hematuria, tarry stools)
- Caution patient to report signs of anemia (fatigue, headache, irritability, faintness, shortness of breath)
- Advise patient to report any changes in breathing or coughing even several mo after treatment; to avoid crowds or persons with respiratory tract and other infections
- Advise patient that hair may be lost during treatment; a wig or hairpiece may make patient feel better; new hair may be different in color, texture
- Caution patient not to have any vaccinations without the advice of the

P

prescriber; serious reactions can occur

- Advise patient that contraception is needed during treatment and for several mo after completion of therapy

Evaluation

Positive therapeutic outcome

- Prevention of rapid division of malignant cells

HIGH ALERT

poractant alfa (℞)

(poor-ak'tant al'fah)

Curosurf

Func. class.: Lung surfactant

Pregnancy category UK

Action: Replenishes surfactant and restores surface activity to lungs in P premature infants

→ **Therapeutic Outcome:** Ability P of neonate to breathe without assistance

Uses: Treatment (rescue) of respiratory distress syndrome (RDS) in P premature infants

Investigational uses: Prophylaxis of RDS, adult RDS due to viral pneumonia, HIV-infected infants with *Pneumocystis carinii* pneumonia, treatment of adult RDS in near drowning

Dosage and routes

Intratracheal instill: Premature infant 2.5 ml/kg birth weight, up to 2 subsequent doses of 1.25 ml/kg birth weight can be administered at 12-hr intervals, max 5 ml/kg

Available forms: Susp 120 mg (1.5 ml); 240 mg (3 ml)

Adverse effects

RESP: **Pulmonary air leaks, pulmonary interstitial emphysema, apnea, pulmonary hemorrhage**

SYST: **Patent ductus arteriosus, intracranial hemorrhage, severe intracranial hemorrhage, necrotizing entercolitis, posttreatment sepsis, posttreatment infection,** bradycardia, oxygen desaturation, pallor, vasoconstriction, hypotension, hypertension

Precautions: Bradycardia, rales, infections

Pharmacokinetics

Absorption	Unknown
Distribution	Lung
Metabolism	Recycled
Excretion	Unknown
Half-life	Unknown

Pharmacodynamics

Onset	Few min
Peak	Unknown
Duration	Becomes lung associated within hours of administration

Interactions: None

NURSING CONSIDERATIONS

Assessment

- Assess respiratory rate, rhythm, character, chest expansion, color, transcutaneous saturation, ABGs; monitor ECG
- Check endotracheal tube placement before dosing; monitor for apnea after endotracheal administration
- Check for reflux of drug into endotracheal tube during administration; stop drug administration if this occurs, and if needed increase peak inspiratory pressure on the ventilator by 4-5 cm H_2O until tube is cleared
- P Assess infant for repeat dosing using radiographic confirmation of RDS; repeat doses should be given as noted above; ventilator settings for repeat doses FIO_2 are decreased by 0.2 or amount to prevent cyanosis; ventilator rate of 30/min; inspiratory time <1 sec; if infant's pretreatment rate was >30, leave unchanged during dosing;

resume usual ventilator management aft er dosing

Nursing diagnoses

✓ Gas exchange, impaired (uses)
✓ Knowledge deficit (teaching)

Implementation

- Administer after suctioning; give endotracheally only by persons trained in neonatal intubation and ventilation
- Use a no. 5 Fr end-hole catheter inserted into the endotracheal tube with the tip at distal end of endotracheal tube; shorten the catheter before insertion; insert the drug into the main bronchi by positioning infant with either right or left side dependent
- Determine dosage by weight of infant; slowly withdraw the contents into the plastic syringe through a 20-G needle; do not filter or shake; attach the premeasured no. 5 Fr catheter to syringe; fill with drug and discard excess through catheter so only dose to be given remains in syringe
- For prevention dosing, stabilize, weigh, and intubate infant; give drug within 15 min of birth if possible; position infant and inject first ¼ of dose through catheter over 2-3 sec; remove catheter and manually ventilate with O_2 to prevent cyanosis (60 bpm) and sufficient positive pressure to promote adequate air exchange and chest wall excursion
- For rescue dosing, give drug as soon as ventilator support is started after birth; immediately before administering dose, change ventilator settings to 60/min, inspiratory time 0.5 sec, FIO_2 1; position infant and inject first ¼ through catheter over 2-3 sec; remove catheter; return to mechanical ventilator
- Ventilate infant for >30 sec or until stable after prevention or rescue strategy; reposition for next dose; same procedure for subsequent dosing; do not suction for at least 1 hr after dosing unless airway obstruction is evident; resume ventilator therapy after dosing
- Reduce peak ventilator inspiratory pressure immediately if chest expansion improves substantially after dose
- Reduce FIO_2 in small, repeated steps when infant becomes pink and transcutaneous oxygen saturation is >95%; oxygen saturation should remain between 90% and 95%
- Suction all infants before administration to prevent mucus plugging; if endotrachcal tube obstruction is suspected, remove the obstruction and replace tube immediately
- Store in refrigerator; protect from light; warm to room temp for ≥20 min or warm in hand 8 min before giving; do not use artificial warming methods; enter a vial only once; unopened, unused vials that have been warmed to room temp may be rerefrigerated within 8 hr of warming; do not warm and return to refrigerator more than once

Patient/family education

- Explain disease process and purpose of medication to parents; communicate neonate's progress

Evaluation

Positive therapeutic outcome

- Significant improvement in respiratory status (oxygenation, ABGs, WNL)

porfirmer (℞)

(pour'fur-meer)

Photofrin

Func. class.: Antineoplastic—misc.
Chem. class.: Photosensitizing agent

Pregnancy category C

Action: Used in photodynamic treatment (PDT) of tumors; antitumor and cytotoxic actions are light and O_2 dependent; used with 630 nm laser light

Therapeutic Outcome: Prevention of growth of tumor

Uses: Esophageal cancer (completely obstructing), endobronchial non–small-cell lung cancer

Dosage and routes

Refer to guide for complete instructions

Adult: **IV** 2 mg/kg, then illumination with laser light 40-50 hr after inj; a second laser light application may be given 96-120 hr after inj; may repeat q30 days × 3

Endobronchial cancer

Adult: 200 joules/cm of tumor length

Available forms: Cake/powder for inj 75 mg

Adverse effects

CNS: *Anxiety, confusion, insomnia*

CV: *Hypotension, hypertension,* **atrial fibrillation, cardiac failure,** *tachycardia*

GI: *Abdominal pain, constipation, diarrhea, dyspepsia, dysphagia, eructation, esophageal edema/bleeding, hematemesis, melena, nausea, vomiting, anorexia*

MISC: Dehydration, weight decrease, anemia, photosensitivity reaction, UTI, moniliasis

RESP: **Pleural effusion,** pneumonia, dyspnea, respiratory insufficiency, **tracheoesophageal fistula**

Contraindications: Porphyria, porphyrin allergy (porfirmer); tracheoesophageal, bronchoesophageal fistula; major blood vessels with eroding tumors (PDT)

G **Precautions:** Elderly, pregnancy
P **C,** lactation, children

Pharmacokinetics

Absorption	Unknown
Distribution	Unknown
Metabolism	Unknown
Excretion	Unknown
Half-life	250 hr

Pharmacodynamics

Unknown

Interactions

Drug classifications

Phenothiazines: ↑ photosensitivity
Sulfonamides: ↑ photosensitivity
Sulfonylureas: ↑ photosensitivity
Thiazides: ↑ photosensitivity

NURSING CONSIDERATIONS

Assessment

- Assess for ocular sensitivity; sensitivity to sun, bright lights, car headlights; patients should wear dark sunglasses with an average white light transmittance of <4%
- Assess for chest pain: may be so severe as to necessitate opiate analgesics
- Assess for extravasation at inj site: take care to protect from light

Nursing diagnoses

✓ Infection, risk for (adverse reactions)
✓ Knowledge deficit (teaching)

Implementation

- Give as a single slow **IV** inj over 3-5 min at 2 mg/kg; reconstitute each vial with 31.8 ml of D_5 or 0.9% NaCl (2.5 mg/ml), shake well, do not mix with other drugs or sol, protect from light, and use immediately
- Laser light is initiated 630 nm wavelength laser light
- Wipe spills with damp cloth, avoid skin/eye contact, use rubber gloves, eye protection; dispose of material in polyethylene bag according to policy

Patient/family education

- Advise patient to report chest pain, eye sensitivity
- Advise patient to wear sunglasses with average white light transmittance of <4%; avoid exposure to sunlight or bright light for 30 days

potassium acetate/potassium bicarbonate (℞)

K+Care ET, K-Electrolyte, K-Ide, Klor-Con/EF, K-Lyte, K-Vescent

potassium bicarbonate/potassium chloride (℞)

Klorvess, Klorvess Effervescent Granules, K-Lyte/Cl, Neo-K ♣

potassium bicarbonate/potassium citrate (℞)

Effer-K, K-Lyte DS

potassium chloride (℞)

Apo-K ♣, Cena-K, Gen-K, K+care, K+10, Kalium Durules ♣, Kaochlor, Kaochlor S-F, Kaon-Cl, Kay Ciel, KCl, K-Dur, K-Lease, K-Long ♣, K-Lor, Klor-Con, Klorvess, Klotrix, K-Lyte/Cl powder, K-med, K-Norm, K-Sol, K-Tab, Micro-K, Micro-LS, Potasalan, Roychlor, Rum-K, Slow-K, Ten-K

potassium chloride/potassium bicarbonate/potassium citrate

Kaochlor Eff

potassium gluconate

Kaon, Kaylixir, K-G Elixir, Potassium-Rougier ♣

potassium gluconate/potassium chloride

Kolyum

potassium gluconate/potassium citrate

Twin-K

Func. class.: Electrolyte
Chem. class.: Potassium

Pregnancy category C

Action: Needed for adequate transmission of nerve impulses and cardiac contraction, renal function, intracellular ion maintenance

➡ **Therapeutic Outcome:** Potassium level 3.0-5.0 mg/dl

Uses: Prevention and treatment of hypokalemia

Dosage and routes

Potassium bicarbonate

Adult: PO dissolve 25-50 mEq in water qd-qid

Potassium acetate—hypokalemia

P ***Adult and child:*** PO 40-100 mEq/day in divided doses × 2-4 days

Hypokalemia (prevention)

P ***Adult and child:*** PO 20 mEq/day in 2-4 divided doses

Potassium chloride

Adult: PO 40-100 mEq in divided doses tid-qid; **IV** 20 mEq/hr when diluted as 40 mEq/1000 ml, max 150 mEq/day

P ***Child:*** PO 2-4 mEq/kg/day

Potassium gluconate

Adult: PO 40-100 mEq in divided doses tid-qid

Potassium phosphate

Adult: **IV** 1 mEq/hr in sol of 60 mEq/L, max 150 mEq/day; PO 40-100 mEq/day in divided doses

P ***Child:*** **IV** max rate of infusion 1 mEq/kg/min

Available forms: Tabs for sol 6.5, 25 mEq; inj for prep of **IV** 2, 4 mEq; ext rel caps 8, 10 mEq; powder for sol 3.3, 5, 6.7, 10, 13.3 mEq/5 ml; tabs 4, 13.4 mEq; ext rel tabs 6.7, 8, 10 mEq; inj for prep of **IV** 1.5, 2, 2.4, 3, 3.2 mEq/ml; elixir 6.7 mEq/5 ml; tabs 2, 5 mEq; oral sol 2.375 mEq/5 ml; inj for prep of **IV** 4.4, 4.7 mEq/ml

Adverse effects

CNS: Confusion

CV: Bradycardia, *cardiac depression,* **dysrhythmias, arrest, peaking T waves, lowered R and depressed RST, prolonged PR interval, widened QRS complex**

GI: Nausea, vomiting, cramps, pain, *diarrhea,* ulceration of small bowel

P

GU: Oliguria
INTEG: Cold extremities, rash

Contraindications: Renal disease (severe), severe hemolytic disease, Addison's disease, hyperkalemia, acute dehydration, extensive tissue breakdown

Precautions: Cardiac disease, potassium-sparing diuretic therapy, systemic acidosis, pregnancy **C**

Pharmacokinetics and pharmacodynamics unavailable.

Interactions

Drug classifications

Angiotensin converting enzyme inhibitors: ↑ hyperkalemia
Potassium-sparing diuretics: ↑ hyperkalemia

NURSING CONSIDERATIONS

Assessment

- Assess ECG for peaking T waves, lowered R, depressed RST, prolonged PR interval, widening QRS complex, hyperkalemia; drug should be reduced or discontinued
- Monitor potassium level during treatment (3.5-5.0 mg/dl is normal level)
- Monitor I&O ratio; watch for decreased urinary output; notify prescriber immediately; check urinary pH in patients receiving the drug as a urinary acidifier
- Assess cardiac status: rate, rhythm, CVP, PWP, PAWP if being monitored directly

Nursing diagnoses

✓ Nutrition, altered: less than body requirements (uses)
✓ Knowledge deficit (teaching)

Implementation

IV IV route

- Give through large-bore needle to decrease vein inflammation; check for extravasation; administer in large vein, **P** avoiding scalp vein in child
- After diluting in large volume of **IV** sol give as an **IV** inf slowly to prevent toxicity; never give **IV** bol or IM

Potassium acetate

Additive compatibilities: Metoclopramide

Potassium chloride

Y-site compatibilities: Acyclovir, aldesleukin, allopurinol, amifostine, aminophylline, amiodarone, ampicillin, amrinone, atropine, aztreonam, betamethasone, calcium gluconate, cefmetazole, cephalothin, cephapirin, chlordiazepoxide, chlorpromazine, ciprofloxacin, cladribine, cyanocobalamin, dexamethasone, digoxin, diltiazem, diphenhydramine, dobutamine, dopamine, droperidol, edrophonium, enalaprilat, epinephrine, esmolol, estrogens, ethacrynate, famotidine, fentanyl, filgrastim, fludarabine, fluorouracil, furosemide, gallium, granisetron, heparin, hydralazine, idarubicin, indomethacin, insulin, regular, isoproterenol, kanamycin, labetalol, lidocaine, lorazepam, magnesium sulfate, melphalan, meperidine, methicillin, methoxamine, methylergonovine, midazolam, minocycline, morphine, neostigmine, norepinephrine, ondansetron, oxacillin, oxytocin, paclitaxel, penicillin G potassium, pentazocine, phytonadione, piperacillin/tazobactam, prednisolone, procainamide, prochlorperazine, propofol, propranolol, pyridostigmine, sargramostim, scopolamine, sodium bicarbonate, succinylcholine, tacrolimus, teniposide, theophylline, thiotepa, trimethaphan, trimethobenzamide, vinorelbine, zidovudine

Additive compatibilities: Aminophylline, amiodarone, atracurium, bretylium, calcium chloride, cefepime, cephalothin, cephapirin, chloramphenicol, cimetidine, ciprofloxacin, clindamycin, cloxacillin, corticotropin, cytarabine, dimenhydrinate, dopamine, enalaprilat, erythromycin, floxacillin, fluconazole, furosemide, heparin, hydrocortisone, isoproterenol, lidocaine, metaraminol, methicillin, methyldopate, metoclopramide, mitoxantrone, nafcillin, netilmicin, norepinephrine, oxacillin, penicillin G potassium or sodium, phenylephrine, piperacillin, ranitidine, sodium bicarbonate, thiopental, vancomycin, verapamil, vit B/C

Potassium chloride
Y-site compatibilities:
Aldesleukin, amifostine, granisetron, lorazepam, midazolam, thiotepa

PO route

- Give with meal or pc; dissolve effervescent tab, powder in 8 oz of cold water or juice; do not give IM, SC
- Store at room temp

Patient/family education

- Teach patient to eat foods rich in potassium after medication is discontinued
- Advise patient to avoid OTC products: antacids, salt substitutes, analgesics, vit preparations, unless specifically directed by prescriber
- Advise patient to report hyperkalemia symptoms or continued hypokalemia symptoms
- Tell patient to take cap with full glass of liq; to dissolve powder or tab completely in at least 120 ml of water or juice; not to chew time rel or ext rel preparations
- Emphasize importance of regular follow-up

Evaluation

Positive therapeutic outcome

- Absence of fatigue, muscle weakness, and decreased thirst and urinary output, cardiac changes
- Potassium level normal

pramipexole (℞)
(pra-mi-pex′ol)
Mirapex
Func. class.: Antiparkinsonian agent
Chem. class.: Dopamine receptor agonist, nonergot
Pregnancy category C

Action: Selective agonist for D_2 receptors (presynaptic/postsynaptic sites); binding at D_3 receptor contributes to antiparkinson effects

Therapeutic Outcome: Decreased symptoms of Parkinson's disease (involuntary movements)

Uses: Parkinsonism

Investigational uses: Restless legs syndrome

Dosage and routes

Initial treatment
Adult: PO from a starting dose of 0.375 mg/day given in 3 divided doses; increase gradually by 0.125 mg/dose at 5-7 day intervals until total daily dose of 4.5 mg is reached

Maintenance treatment
Adult: PO 1.5-4.5 mg qd in 3 divided doses

Renal dose
Adult: PO CrCl 35-59 ml/min 0.125 mg bid, may increase q5-7 days to 1.5 mg bid; CrCl 15-34 ml/min 0.125 mg qd, may increase q5-7 days to 1.5 mg qd

Restless legs syndrome (off-label)
Adult: PO 0.125-0.375 mg 1-2h before bedtime, increase gradually

Available forms: Tabs 0.125, 0.25, 1, 1.5 mg

Adverse effects

CNS: *Agitation, insomnia,* psychosis, hallucinations, depression, dizziness, headache, confusion
CV: *Orthostatic hypotension,* edema, syncope, tachycardia
EENT: Blurred vision

GI: *Nausea, anorexia,* constipation, dysphagia, dry mouth
GU: Impotence, urinary frequency

Contraindications: Hypersensitivity

Precautions: Renal disease, cardiac disease, MI with dysrhythmias, affective disorders, psychosis, pregnancy **C**, preexisting dyskinesias

Pharmacokinetics

Absorption	Well absorbed
Distribution	Widely distributed
Metabolism	Liver, minimally
Excretion	Kidneys, unchanged
G **Half-life**	8 hr, 12 hr in elderly

Pharmacodynamics

Onset	Unknown
Peak	2 hr
Duration	Unknown

Interactions

Individual drugs

Cimetidine: ↑ pramipexole levels
Diltiazem: ↑ pramipexole levels
Levodopa: ↑ pramipexole levels
Metoclopramide: ↓ pramipexole effect
Quinidine: ↑ pramipexole levels
Ranitidine: ↑ pramipexole levels
Triamterene: ↑ pramipexole levels

Drug classifications

Butyrophenones: ↓ pramipexole effect
Dopamine antagonists: ↓ pramipexole levels
Phenothiazines: ↓ pramipexole effect

Herb/drug

Chaste tree fruit: ↓ pramipexole effect

NURSING CONSIDERATIONS

Assessment

- Monitor B/P, respiration during initial treatment; hypotension or hypertension should be reported
- Assess mental status: affect, mood, behavioral changes, depression; complete suicide assessment
- Monitor renal function studies
- Assess for involuntary movements in parkinsonism: akinesia, tremors, staggering gait, muscle rigidity, drooling; these symptoms should improve with therapy

Nursing diagnoses

✓ Mobility, impaired (uses)
✓ Injury, risk for (uses)
✓ Knowledge deficit (teaching)
✓ Noncompliance (teaching)

Implementation

PO route

- Give drug until NPO before surgery
- Adjust dosage to patient response
- Give with meals to decrease GI upset

Patient/family education

- Advise patient that therapeutic effects may take several wk to a few mo
- Caution patient to change positions slowly to prevent orthostatic hypotension
- Instruct patient to use drug exactly as prescribed; if drug is discontinued abruptly, parkinsonian crisis may occur; if treatment is to be discontinued, taper over 1 wk; avoid alcohol, OTC sleeping products

Evaluation

Positive therapeutic outcome

- Decreased akathisia, other involuntary movements
- Improved mood

pravastatin (℞)

(pra'va-sta-tin)
Pravachol
Func. class.: Antilipidemic

Pregnancy category X

Action: Inhibits biosynthesis of VLDL, LDL, which are responsible for cholesterol development, by inhibiting the enzyme HMG-CoA reductase

Therapeutic Outcome: Decreasing cholesterol levels and LDL, increased HDL

Uses: As an adjunct in primary hypercholesterolemia types IIa, IIb, apolipoprotein B (Apo B), artherosclerosis, to reduce the risk of recurrent MI

Dosage and routes

Adult: PO 10-20 mg qd hs (range 10-40 mg qd)

G ***Elderly/renal/hepatic dose:*** PO 10 mg/day

Available forms: Tabs 10, 20, 40 mg

Adverse effects

CNS: Headache, dizziness, psychic disturbances

EENT: Lens opacities, common cold, rhinitis, cough

GI: Nausea, constipation, diarrhea, dyspepsia, flatus, abdominal pain, heartburn, **liver dysfunction, pancreatitis, hepatitis**

INTEG: Rash, pruritus, photosensitivity

MS: Muscle cramps, myalgia, **myositis, rhabdomyolysis**

Contraindications: Hypersensitivity, pregnancy **X,** lactation, active liver disease

Precautions: Past liver disease, alcoholism, severe acute infections, trauma, hypotension, uncontrolled seizure disorders, severe metabolic disorders, electrolyte imbalances, renal disease

Do Not Confuse:
Pravachol/Prevacid

Pharmacokinetics

Absorption	Poorly absorbed, erratic
Distribution	Unknown
Metabolism	Liver, extensively
Excretion	Feces (70%-75%); kidneys, unchanged (10%), breast milk (minimal)
Half-life	2 hr

Pharmacodynamics

Onset	Unknown
Peak	1-1½ hr
Duration	Unknown

Interactions

Individual drugs

Cholestyramine: ↓ action of pravastatin
Clarithromycin: ↑ risk for myopathy
Clofibrate: ↑ risk for myopathy
Colestipol: ↓ action of pravastatin
Cyclosporine: ↑ risk of myopathy, rhabdomyolysis
Erythromycin: ↑ risk of myopathy, rhabdomyolysis
Gemfibrozil: ↑ risk of myopathy, rhabdomyolysis
Itraconazole: ↑ risk for myopathy
Niacin: ↑ risk of myopathy, rhabdomyolysis
Propranolol: ↓ effect of pravastatin
Warfarin: ↑ bleeding

Drug classifications

Protease inhibitors: ↑ risk of myopathy

Lab test interferences

↑ CPK, ↑ liver function tests

NURSING CONSIDERATIONS

Assessment

- Assess nutrition: fat, protein, carbohydrates; nutritional analysis should be completed by dietitian before treatment
- Monitor triglycerides, esterol, cholesterol at baseline and throughout treatment; LDL and HDL should be watched closely; if increased, drug should be discontinued
- Assess for muscle tenderness, pain, obtain CPK; rhabdomyolysis may occur
- Monitor ophthal status qyr

Nursing diagnoses

✓ Knowledge deficit (teaching)
✓ Noncompliance (teaching)

Implementation

- Give hs only; give 1 hr before or 4 hr after bile acid sequestrants

P

• Store in cool environment in airtight, light-resistant container

Patient/family education

• Inform patient that compliance is needed for positive results to occur; not to double doses or skip doses
• Teach patient that risk factors should be decreased: high-fat diet, smoking, alcohol consumption, absence of exercise
• Advise patient to notify prescriber of weakness, tenderness, or limited mobility
• Explain to patient that contraception is necessary, since drug produces teratogenic effects

Evaluation

Positive therapeutic outcome

• Decreased cholesterol, serum triglyceride levels and improved ratio with HDL

prazosin (Rx)

(pra'zoe-sin)

Minipress, prazosin

Func. class.: Antihypertensive

Chem. class.: α_1-Adrenergic blocker

Pregnancy category C

Action: Blocks α-mediated vasoconstriction of adrenergic receptors, inducing peripheral vasodilation

Therapeutic Outcome: Decreased B/P in hypertension; decreased cardiac preload, afterload

Uses: Hypertension

Investigational uses: Benign prostatic hypertrophy to decreased urine outflow obstruction

Dosage and routes

Hypertension

Adult: PO 1 mg bid or tid, increasing to 20 mg qd in divided doses if required, usual range 6-15 mg/day, not to exceed 1 mg initially; max 20-40 mg/day

P ***Child:*** PO 0.5-7 mg bid

Benign prostatic hypertrophy

Adult: PO 1-5 mg bid

Available forms: Caps 1, 2, 5 mg

Adverse effects

CNS: *Dizziness, headache, drowsiness,* anxiety, depression, vertigo, weakness, fatigue

CV: *Palpitations, orthostatic hypotension,* tachycardia, edema, rebound hypertension

EENT: Blurred vision, epistaxis, tinnitus, dry mouth, red sclera

GI: *Nausea,* vomiting, diarrhea, constipation, abdominal pain

GU: Urinary frequency, incontinence, impotence, priapism, water and sodium retention

Contraindications: Hypersensitivity

Precautions: Pregnancy **C**, P children

Pharmacokinetics	
Absorption	60%
Distribution	Widely distributed
Metabolism	Liver, extensively
Excretion	Kidneys, unchanged (10%), bile (90%)
Half-life	2-3 hr

Pharmacodynamics	
Onset	2 hr
Peak	1-3 hr
Duration	6-12 hr

Interactions

Individual drugs

Alcohol: ↑ hypotension
Indomethacin: ↓ effect
Nitroglycerin: ↑ hypotension

Drug classifications

Antihypertensives: ↑ hypotension
β-Adrenergic blockers: ↑ hypotension
Nitrates: ↑ hypotension

Lab test interferences

↑ Urinary norepinephrine, ↑ VMA

NURSING CONSIDERATIONS

Assessment

- Monitor B/P, orthostatic hypotension, syncope; check for edema in feet, legs daily; monitor I&O, weight daily; notify prescriber of changes
- Assess for allergic reactions: rash, fever, pruritus, urticaria; drug should be discontinued if antihistamines fail to help
- Assess for orthostatic hypotension; tell patient to rise slowly from sitting or lying position

Nursing diagnoses

✓ Cardiac output, decreased (uses)
✓ Injury, risk for (adverse reactions)
✓ Knowledge deficit (teaching)
✓ Noncompliance (teaching)

Implementation

- Severe hypotension may occur after 1st dose of this medication; hypotension may be prevented by reducing or discontinuing diuretic therapy 3 days before beginning prazosin therapy
- Store in airtight container at 86° F (30° C) or less

Patient/family education

- Instruct patient not to discontinue drug abruptly; stress the importance of complying with dosage schedule, even if feeling better; if dose is missed, take as soon as remembered; take at same time each day
- Advise patient not to use OTC products (cough, cold, allergy) unless directed by prescriber; also to avoid large amounts of caffeine
- Emphasize the need to rise slowly to sitting or standing position to minimize orthostatic hypotension
- Teach patient to notify prescriber of mouth sores, sore throat, fever, swelling of hands or feet, irregular heartbeat, chest pain
- Caution patient to report excessive perspiration, dehydration, vomiting, diarrhea; may lead to fall in B/P
- Caution patient that drug may cause dizziness, fainting, light-headedness; may occur during 1st few days of therapy; to avoid hazardous activities
- Teach patient how to take B/P and normal readings for age group; instruct to take B/P q7 days

Evaluation

Positive therapeutic outcome

- Decreased B/P in hypertension

Treatment of overdose:

Administer volume expanders or vasopressors, discontinue drug, place in supine position

prednisolone (℞)

(pred-niss'oh-lone)

Articulose-50, Delta-Cortef, prednisolone, Prelone, Key-Pred 25, Key-Pred 50, Predaject-50, Predalone 50, Predcor-25, Predcor-50, Prednisolone Acetate, Hydeltrasol, Key-Pred-SP, Pediapred, Hydeltra-T.B.A., Predalone-T.B.A., Prednisol TBA

Func. class.: Corticosteroid

Chem. class.: Intermediate-acting glucocorticoid

Pregnancy category C

Action: Decreases inflammation by suppressing migration of polymorphonuclear leukocytes, fibroblasts; reversal to increase capillary permeability and lysosomal stabilization, minimal mineralocorticoid

P

➔ **Therapeutic Outcome:** Decreased inflammation, decreased adrenal insufficiency

Uses: Severe inflammation, immunosuppression, neoplasms

Dosage and routes

Adult: PO 2.5-15 mg bid-qid; IM 2-30 mg (acetate, phosphate) q12h; **IV** 2-30 mg (phosphate) q12h, 2-30 mg in joint or soft tissue (phosphate), 4-40 mg in joint of lesion (tebutate)

Asthma/antiinflammatory

P ***Child:*** PO 1-2 mg/kg/day; **IV** 2-4 mg/kg/day

Available forms: *Prednisolone:* tabs 5 mg, syrup 5 mg/5 ml, 15 mg/5 ml; *prednisolone acetate:* inj 25, 50 mg/ml; *prednisolone tebutate:* inj 20 mg/ml; *prednisolone phosphate:* inj 20 mg/ml, oral liq 5 mg/5 ml

Adverse effects

CNS: Depression, flushing, sweating, headache, mood changes

CV: Hypertension, **circulatory collapse, thrombophlebitis, embolism,** tachycardia

EENT: Fungal infections, increased intraocular pressure, blurred vision

GI: Diarrhea, nausea, abdominal distention, **GI hemorrhage,** increased appetite, **pancreatitis**

HEMA: **Thrombocytopenia**

INTEG: Acne, poor wound healing, ecchymosis, petechiae

MS: Fractures, osteoporosis, weakness

Contraindications: Psychosis, hypersensitivity, idiopathic thrombocytopenia, acute glomerulonephritis, amebiasis, fungal infections, nonasthmatic bronchial disease, P child <2 yr

Precautions: Pregnancy **C,** diabetes mellitus, glaucoma, osteoporosis, seizure disorders, ulcerative colitis, CHF, myasthenia gravis

Do Not Confuse:
prednisolone/prednisone

Pharmacokinetics

Absorption	Well absorbed (PO, IM), completely absorbed (**IV**)
Distribution	Widely distributed; crosses placenta
Metabolism	Liver, extensively
Excretion	Kidney, breast milk
Half-life	2-4 hr

Pharmacodynamics

	PO	IM (phosphate)	IV	IA/IL
Onset	1 hr	Rapid	Rapid	Slow
Peak	2 hr	1 hr	Unknown	Unknown
Duration	1½ days	Unknown	Unknown	Up to 1 mo

Interactions

Individual drugs

Alcohol: ↑ GI effects
Amphotericin B: ↑ hypokalemia
Aspirin: ↑ GI effects
Insulin: ↑ need for insulin
Mezlocillin: ↑ hypokalemia
Phenytoin: ↓ action, ↑ metabolism
Piperacillin: ↑ hypokalemia
Rifampin: ↓ action, ↑ metabolism
Ticarcillin: ↑ hypokalemia

Drug classifications

Barbiturates: ↓ action, ↑ metabolism
Diuretics: ↑ hypokalemia
Hypoglycemic agents: ↑ need for hypoglycemic agents

Herb/drug

Aloe: ↑ hypokalemia
Buckthorn: ↑ hypokalemia
Cascara sagrada: ↑ hypokalemia
Senna: ↑ hypokalemia

Lab test interferences

↑ Cholesterol, ↑ sodium, ↑ blood glucose, ↑ uric acid, ↑ calcium, ↑ urine glucose
↓ Calcium, ↓ potassium, ↓ T_4, ↓ T_3, ↓ thyroid ^{131}I uptake test, ↓ urine 17-OHCS, ↓ 17-KS, ↓ PBI
False negative: Skin allergy tests

NURSING CONSIDERATIONS

Assessment

- Monitor potassium, blood glucose, urine glucose while patient is on long-term therapy; hypokalemia and hyperglycemia may occur
- Monitor weight daily; notify prescriber of weekly gain >5 lb; monitor I&O ratio; be alert for decreasing urinary output and increasing edema

- Monitor B/P q4h, pulse; notify prescriber if chest pain occurs
- Monitor plasma cortisol levels during long-term therapy (normal level; 138-635 nmol/L [SI units] when measured at 8 AM)
- Assess adrenal function periodically for hypothalamic-pituitary-adrenal axis suppression
- Assess infection: increased temp, WBC even after withdrawal of medication; drug masks infection symptoms
- Assess for potassium depletion: paresthesias, fatigue, nausea, vomiting, depression, polyuria, dysrhythmias, weakness, edema, hypertension, cardiac symptoms
- Assess mental status: affect, mood, behavioral changes, aggression
- Monitor temp; if fever develops, drug should be discontinued
- Assess for systemic absorption: increased temp, inflammation, irritation (top)

Nursing diagnoses

✓ Infection, risk for (adverse reactions)
✓ Knowledge deficit (teaching)
✓ Noncompliance (teaching)

Implementation

IV IV route

- Give by direct **IV** only sodium phosphate product; give over >1 min; may be given by **IV** inf in D_5W, 0.9% NaCl
- Give after shaking susp (parenteral)
- Give titrated dose; use lowest effective dosage

Y-site compatibilities:
Ciprofloxacin, potassium chloride, vit B/C

Additive compatibilities:
Ascorbic acid, cephalothin, cytarabine, erythromycin, fluorouracil, heparin, methicillin, penicillin G potassium, penicillin G sodium, vit B/C

Additive incompatibilities:
Calcium gluceptate, methotrexate, polymyxin B sulfate

IM route

- Give IM inj deep in large muscle mass; rotate sites; avoid deltoid; use 21-G needle
- Give in one dose in AM to prevent adrenal suppression; avoid SC administration; may damage tissue

PO route

- Give with food or milk to decrease GI symptoms

Patient/family education

- Advise patient that ID as steroid user should be carried
- Advise patient to notify prescriber if therapeutic response decreases; dosage adjustment may be needed
- Caution patient not to discontinue abruptly; adrenal crisis can result
- Caution patient to avoid OTC products: salicylates, alcohol in cough products, cold preparations unless directed by prescriber
- Teach patient all aspects of drug usage including cushingoid symptoms
- Teach patient symptoms of adrenal insufficiency: nausea, anorexia, fatigue, dizziness, dyspnea, weakness, joint pain
- Advise patient that long-term therapy may be needed to clear infection (1-2 mo depending on type of infection)

Evaluation

Positive therapeutic outcome

- Decreased inflammation

P

prednisone 🔑 (℞)

(pred′ni-sone)

Apo-Prednisone 🍁, Deltasone, Liquid Pred, Meticorten, Orasone, Panasol-S, Prednicen-M, prednisone, Sterapred, Winpred

Func. class.: Corticosteroid

Chem. class.: Intermediate-acting glucocorticoid

Pregnancy category C

Action: Decreases inflammation by suppressing migration of polymorphonuclear leukocytes, fibroblasts; reversal to increase capillary permeability and lysosomal stabilization

Therapeutic Outcome: Decreased inflammation, decreased adrenal insufficiency

Uses: Severe inflammation, immunosuppression, neoplasms, multiple sclerosis, collagen disorders, dermatologic disorders

Dosage and routes

Adult: PO 1.5-2.5 mg bid-qid, then qd or qod; maintenance up to 250 mg/day

P ***Child:*** PO 0.05-2 mg/kg/day divided 1-4 ×/day

Nephrosis

P ***Child 18 mo-4 yr:*** 7.5-10 mg qid initially

P ***Child 4-10 yr:*** 15 mg qid initially

P ***Child >10 yr:*** 20 mg qid initially

Multiple sclerosis

Adult: PO 200 mg/day × 1 wk, then 80 mg qod × 1 mo

Available forms: Tabs 1, 2.5, 5, 10, 20, 25, 50 mg; oral sol 5 mg/5 ml; syrup 5 mg/5 ml

Adverse effects

CNS: Depression, flushing, sweating, headache, mood changes

CV: Hypertension, **circulatory collapse, thrombophlebitis, embolism,** tachycardia

EENT: Fungal infections, increased intraocular pressure, blurred vision

GI: Diarrhea, nausea, abdominal distention, **GI hemorrhage,** increased appetite, **pancreatitis**

HEMA: **Thrombocytopenia**

INTEG: Acne, poor wound healing, ecchymosis, petechiae

MS: Fractures, osteoporosis, weakness

Contraindications: Psychosis, hypersensitivity, idiopathic thrombocytopenia, acute glomerulonephritis, amebiasis, fungal infections, nonasthmatic bronchial disease, P child <2 yr, AIDS, TB

Precautions: Pregnancy **C,** diabetes mellitus, glaucoma, osteoporosis, seizure disorders, ulcerative colitis, CHF, myasthenia gravis, renal disease, esophagitis, peptic ulcer

Do Not Confuse:
prednisone/methylprednisolone, prednisone/prednisolone, prednisone/Prilosec

Pharmacokinetics	
Absorption	Well absorbed
Distribution	Widely distributed; crosses placenta
Metabolism	Liver, extensively
Excretion	Kidney, breast milk
Half-life	3-4 hr

Pharmacodynamics	
Onset	Unknown
Peak	1-2 hr
Duration	1½ days

Interactions

Individual drugs

Alcohol: ↑ GI effects

Amphotericin B: ↑ hypokalemia

Aspirin: ↑ GI effects

Insulin: ↑ need for insulin

Mezlocillin: ↑ hypokalemia

Ticarcillin: ↑ hypokalemia

Drug classifications

Diuretics: ↑ hypokalemia

Hypoglycemic agents: ↑ need for hypoglycemic agents

Herb/drug

Aloe: ↑ hypokalemia
Buckthorn: ↑ hypokalemia
Rhubarb: ↑ hypokalemia
Senna: ↑ hypokalemia

Lab test interferences

↑ Cholesterol, ↑ sodium, ↑ blood glucose, ↑ uric acid, ↑ calcium, ↑ urine glucose
↓ Calcium, ↓ potassium, ↓ T_4, ↓ T_3, ↓ thyroid ^{131}I uptake test, ↓ urine 17-OHCS, ↓ 17-KS, ↓ PBI
False negative: Skin allergy tests

NURSING CONSIDERATIONS

Assessment

- Monitor potassium, blood glucose, urine glucose while on long-term therapy; hypokalemia and hyperglycemia may occur
- Monitor weight daily; notify prescriber of weekly gain >5 lb; monitor I&O ratio; be alert for decreasing urinary output and increasing edema
- Monitor B/P q4h, pulse; notify prescriber if chest pain occurs
- Monitor plasma cortisol levels during long-term therapy (normal level 138-635 nmol/L when measured at 8 AM)
- Assess adrenal function periodically for hypothalamic-pituitary-adrenal axis suppression
- Assess infection: increased temp, WBC even after withdrawal of medication; drug masks infection symptoms
- Assess for potassium depletion: paresthesias, fatigue, nausea, vomiting, depression, polyuria, dysrhythmias, weakness, edema, hypertension, cardiac symptoms
- Assess mental status: affect, mood, behavioral changes, aggression
- Monitor temp; if fever develops, drug should be discontinued
- Assess for systemic absorption: increased temp, inflammation, irritation (top)

Nursing diagnoses

✓ Infection, risk for (adverse reactions)
✓ Knowledge deficit (teaching)
✓ Noncompliance (teaching)

Implementation

- Give with food or milk to decrease GI symptoms; use measuring device for liq route

Patient/family education

- Advise patient that ID as steroid user should be carried
- Advise patient to notify prescriber if therapeutic response decreases; dosage adjustment may be needed
- Caution patient not to discontinue abruptly; adrenal crisis can result
- Caution patient to avoid OTC products: salicylates, alcohol in cough products, cold preparations unless directed by prescriber
- Teach patient all aspects of drug usage including cushingoid symptoms
- Teach patient symptoms of adrenal insufficiency: nausea, anorexia, fatigue, dizziness, dyspnea, weakness, joint pain
- Advise patient that long-term therapy may be needed to clear infection (1-2 mo depending on type of infection)

Evaluation

Positive therapeutic outcome

- Decreased inflammation

primidone (℞)

(pri'mi-done)

Apo-Primidone ✤, Mysoline, PMS-Primidone ✤, primidone, Sertan ✤

Func. class.: Anticonvulsant
Chem. class.: Barbiturate derivative

Pregnancy category D

Action: Raises seizure threshold by conversion of drug to phenobarbital; decreases neuron firing

Therapeutic Outcome: Reduction in seizure activity

P

Uses: Generalized tonic-clonic (grand mal), complex-partial, psychomotor seizures

Dosage and routes

P ***Adult and child >8 yr:*** PO 100-125 mg hs on days 1, 2, 3; then 100-125 mg bid on days 4, 5, 6; then 100-125 mg tid on days 7, 8, 9; then maintenance 250 mg tid-qid, max 2 g/day in divided doses

P ***Child <8 yr:*** PO 50 mg hs on days 1, 2, 3; then 50 mg bid on days 4, 5, 6; then 100 mg bid on days 7, 8, 9; maintenance 125-250 mg tid

Available forms: Tabs 50, 250 mg; susp 250 mg/5 ml; chew tabs 125 mg 🍁

Adverse effects

CNS: *Stimulation, drowsiness,* dizziness, confusion, sedation, headache, flushing, hallucinations, **coma,** psychosis, ataxia, *vertigo*
EENT: Diplopia, nystagmus, edema of eyelids
GI: *Nausea, vomiting, anorexia,* **hepatitis**
GU: Impotence
HEMA: **Thrombocytopenia, leukopenia, neutropenia, eosinophilia, megaloblastic anemia,** decreased serum folate level, lymphadenopathy
INTEG: Rash, edema, alopecia, lupus-like syndrome

Contraindications: Hypersensitivity, porphyria, pregnancy **D**

Precautions: COPD, hepatic disease, renal disease, hyperactive P children

Pharmacokinetics

Absorption	60%-80%
Distribution	Widely distributed; crosses placenta
Metabolism	Liver, converted to phenobarbital + PEMA
Excretion	Kidneys, breast milk
Half-life	3-24 hr

Pharmacodynamics

Onset	Unknown
Peak	4 hr
Duration	Unknown

Interactions

Individual drugs

Acebutolol: ↓ effectiveness
Acetazolamide: ↓ primidone levels
Alcohol: ↑ CNS depression
Carbamazepine: ↓ primidone levels
Chloramphenicol: ↓ effectiveness
Doxycycline: ↑ half-life
Griseofulvin: ↓ effectiveness
Isoniazide: ↑ primidone levels
Metoprolol: ↓ effectiveness
Nicotinamide: ↑ primidone levels
Phenobarbital: ↑ toxicity
Propranolol: ↓ effectiveness
Quinidine: ↓ effectiveness
Timolol: ↓ effectiveness

Drug classifications

Antidepressants, tricyclic: ↑ CNS depression
Antihistamines: ↑ CNS depression
Glucocorticoids: ↓ effectiveness
Hydantoins: ↑ primidone levels
Opiates: ↑ CNS depression
Oral contraceptives: ↓ effectiveness
Phenothiazines: ↓ CNS depression
Sedative/hypnotics: ↑ CNS depression
Succinimides: ↓ primidone levels

Lab test interferences

False: ↑ Sulfobromophthalein

NURSING CONSIDERATIONS

Assessment

- Assess mental status: mood, sensorium, affect, memory (long, short), G especially elderly
- Assess for blood dyscrasias: fever, sore throat, bruising, rash, jaundice, epistaxis (long-term treatment only)
- Assess seizure activity including type, location, duration, and character; provide seizure precaution
- Assess renal studies: urinalysis, BUN, urine creatinine
- Monitor blood studies: RBC, Hct,

Hgb, reticulocyte counts weekly for 4 wk then monthly
- Monitor hepatic studies: ALT, AST, bilirubin, creatinine
- Monitor drug levels during initial treatment
- Assess for signs of physical withdrawal if medication is suddenly discontinued
- Assess eye problems: need for ophthal exam before, during, after treatment (slit lamp, funduscopy, tonometry)
- Assess allergic reaction: red raised rash; if this occurs, drug should be discontinued
- Monitor for toxicity: bone marrow depression, nausea, vomiting, ataxia, diplopia, CV collapse

Nursing diagnoses

✓ Injury, risk for (side effects)
✓ Knowledge deficit (teaching)

Implementation

- May give with food to decrease gastric irritation
- May crush tab and mix with food or fluid

Patient/family education

- Teach patient to carry ID card or bracelet stating name, drugs taken, condition, prescriber's name, phone number
- Advise patient to avoid driving and other activities that require alertness
- Caution patient to avoid alcohol and CNS depressants; increased sedation may occur
- Teach patient not to discontinue medication quickly after long-term use; taper off over several wk

Evaluation

Positive therapeutic outcome
- Decreased seizure activity

probenecid (℞)

(proe-ben′e-sid)
Benemid, Benuryl ✱, Probalan, probenecid
Func. class.: Uricosuric; antigout
Chem. class.: Sulfonamide derivative
Pregnancy category B

Action: Inhibits tubular reabsorption of urates, with increased excretion of uric acids

→ **Therapeutic Outcome:** Decreased uric acid levels

Uses: Hyperuricemia in gout, gouty arthritis; adjunct to cephalosporin or penicillin treatment (gonorrhea)

Dosage and routes

Gonorrhea

Adult: PO 1 g with 3.5 g of ampicillin or 1 g 30 min before 4.8 million U of aqueous penicillin G procaine injected into 2 sites IM

Gout/gouty arthritis

Adult: PO 250 mg bid for 1 wk, then 500 mg bid, not to exceed 2 g/day; maintenance 500 mg/day × 6 mo

Adjunct in penicillin/cephalosporin treatment

P ***Adult and child >50 kg:*** PO 500 mg qid

P ***Child <50 kg:*** PO 25 mg/kg, then 40 mg/kg in divided doses qid

Renal dose

CrCl <30 ml/min avoid use

Available forms: Tabs 0.5 g

Adverse effects

CNS: Drowsiness, headache
CV: Bradycardia
GI: *Gastric irritation, nausea, vomiting, anorexia,* **hepatic necrosis**
GU: Glycosuria, thirst, frequency, **nephrotic syndrome**
INTEG: Rash, dermatitis, pruritus, fever

P

META: *Acidosis, hypokalemia, hyperchloremia,* hyperglycemia
RESP: **Apnea,** irregular respirations

Contraindications: Hypersensitivity, severe hepatic disease, severe renal disease, CrCl <50 mg/min, history of uric acid calculus

P **Precautions:** Pregnancy **B,** child <2 yr

Pharmacokinetics

Absorption	Well absorbed
Distribution	Crosses placenta
Metabolism	Liver
Excretion	Kidneys
Half-life	5-8 hr

Pharmacodynamics

Onset	½ hr
Peak	2-4 hr
Duration	8 hr

Interactions

Individual drugs

Acyclovir: ↑ toxicity
Allopurinol: ↑ effect
Aspirin: ↑ uricosuric effect
Clofibrate: ↑ effect
Dapsone: ↑ effect
Dyphylline: ↑ effect
Heparin: ↑ effect
Methotrexate: ↑ toxicity
Nitrofurantoin: ↑ toxicity
Penicillamine: ↑ effect
Zidovudine: ↑ effect

Drug classifications

Barbiturates: ↑ effect
Benzodiazepines: ↑ effect
Cephalosporins: ↑ levels
Fluoroquinolones: ↑ levels
NSAIDs: ↑ toxicity
Penicillins: ↑ levels

Herb/drug

Henbane: ↑ anticholinergic effect

Lab test interferences

↑ BSP/urinary PSP, ↑ theophylline levels
False positive: Urine glucose with copper sulfate test

NURSING CONSIDERATIONS

Assessment

- Monitor I&O ratio; observe for decrease in urinary output; increase fluids to 2-3 L/day; urine may be alkalized with sodium bicarbonate acetazolamide
- Assess mobility, joint pain, and swelling in the joints
- Monitor CBC, urine pH, uric acid and BUN, creatinine before and periodically during treatment

Nursing diagnoses

✓ Pain, chronic (uses)
✓ Mobility, impaired (uses)
✓ Knowledge deficit (teaching)

Implementation

- Give with food or antacid to decrease GI upset
- Reduce dosage gradually if uric acid levels are normal after 6 mo

Patient/family education

- Advise patient to increase fluids to 2-3 L/day, avoid caffeine, alcohol
- Caution patient to avoid salicylates; probenecid levels will be decreased
- Advise patient to report any pain, redness, or hard area, usually in legs
- Instruct patient in importance of complying with medical regimen including weight loss program, diet restrictions, and alcohol intake

Evaluation

Positive therapeutic outcome

- Decreased pain in joints
- Normal serum uric acid levels
- Increased duration of antiinfectives

procainamide (℞)

(proe'kane-ah-mide)

Procan SR, Promine, procainamide, Procanbid, Pronestyl, Pronestyl-SR

Func. class.: Antidysrhythmic (class IA)

Chem. class.: procaine HCl amide analog

Pregnancy category C

Action: Prolongs action potential duration and effective refractory period; reduces disparity in refractory between normal and infarcted myocardium; prevents increased myocardial excitability and conduction contractility

Therapeutic Outcome: Prevention of dysrhythmias

Uses: Premature ventricular contractions (PVCs), atrial fibrillation, paroxysmal atrial tachycardia (PAT), ventricular tachycardia, atrial dysrhythmias, ventricular tachycardia

Dosage and routes

Atrial fibrillation/PAT

Adult: PO 1-1.25 g; may give another 750 mg if needed; if no response, 500 mg-1g q2h until desired response; maintenance 50 mg/kg in divided doses q6h

Ventricular tachycardia

Adult: PO 1 g; maintenance 50 mg/kg/day given in 3-hr intervals; sus rel tab 500 mg-1.25 g q6h

Other dysrhythmias

Adult: **IV** bol 100 mg q5 min, given 25-50 mg/min, max 500 mg; or 17 mg/kg total, then **IV** inf 2-6 mg/min

Available forms: Caps 250, 375, 500 mg; tabs 250, 375, 500 mg; sus rel tabs 250, 500, 750, 1000 mg; inj **IV** 100, 500 mg/ml

Adverse effects

CNS: *Headache, dizziness,* confusion, psychosis, restlessness, irritability, weakness, seizures

CV: *Hypotension,* **heart block, cardiovascular collapse, arrest**

GI: Nausea, vomiting, anorexia, diarrhea, hepatomegaly

HEMA: Systemic lupus erythematosus syndrome, **agranulocytosis, thrombocytopenia, neutropenia, hemolytic anemia**

INTEG: Rash, urticaria, edema, swelling (rare), pruritus

Contraindications: Hypersensitivity, myasthenia gravis, severe heart block

Precautions: Pregnancy **C,** lactation, children, renal disease, liver disease, CHF, respiratory depression

Pharmacokinetics

Absorption	Well absorbed
Distribution	Rapidly distributed
Metabolism	Liver
Excretion	Kidneys, unchanged (50%-70%)
Half-life	2½-4½ hr; increased in renal disease

Pharmacodynamics

	PO	PO–EXT REL	IV
Onset	½ hr	Unknown	Rapid
Peak	1-1½ hr	Unknown	½-1 hr
Duration	3 hr	Up to 8 hr	3-4 hr

Interactions

Individual drugs

Atropine: ↑ anticholinergic effect
Digoxin: ↑ blood levels, toxicity
Disopyramide: ↑ levels, toxicity
Flecainide: ↑ levels, toxicity
Lidocaine: Bradycardia, arrest
Haloperidol: ↑ anticholinergic effect
Mexiletine: ↑ levels, toxicity
Phenytoin: ↑ blood levels
Quinidine: ↑ levels, toxicity
Trimethoprim: ↑ procainamide action
Warfarin: ↑ level, bleeding

Drug classifications

Antidepressants: ↑ antidepressant action

P

Antihistamines: ↑ antihistamine action
β-Adrenergic blockers: ↑ dysrhythmias, arrest
Calcium channel blockers: ↑ dysrhythmias, arrest
Phenothiazines: ↑ anticholinergic effect

Lab test interferences
↑ CPK

NURSING CONSIDERATIONS
Assessment

- Assess for oxygenation or perfusion deficit: decreased B/P, chest pain, dizziness, loss of consciousness
- Assess respiratory status: auscultate lung fields for bibasilar crackles in patients with advanced CHF
- Monitor I&O ratio; electrolytes: potassium, sodium, chloride; watch for decreasing urinary output, possible retention
- Monitor liver function studies: AST, ALT, bilirubin, alkaline phosphatase
- Monitor ECG continuously to determine drug effectiveness; measure PR, QRS, QT intervals; check for PVCs, other dysrhythmias; check B/P continuously for hypotension, hypertension; for rebound hypertension after 1-2 hr; prolonged PR/QT intervals, QRS complex; if QT or QRS increases by 50% or more, withhold next dose, notify prescriber
- Monitor for dehydration or hypovolemia
- Monitor for CNS symptoms: confusion, psychosis, numbness, depression, involuntary movements; if these occur, drug should be discontinued
- Monitor blood levels (therapeutic level 3-10 μg/ml), ANA titer or N-acetylprocainamide levels; notify prescriber of abnormal results
- Assess cardiac rate, respiration: rate, rhythm, character, chest pain, ventricular tachycardia, supraventricular tachycardia or fibrillation

Nursing diagnoses

✓ Cardiac output, decreased (uses)
✓ Impaired gas exchange (adverse reactions)
✓ Knowledge deficit (teaching)

Implementation

PO route

- Give on an empty stomach with a full glass of water
- May be given with meals if GI irritation occurs; absorption will be decreased

⊘ Tab may be crushed and mixed with fluid or foods for patients with swallowing difficulties; do not break, chew, or crush sus rel tab

IV IV route

- Give by direct **IV** after diluting 100 mg/10 ml of D_5W or sterile water for inj; give 50 mg/min or less
- Give by intermittent inf after diluting to a conc of 2-4 mg/ml, 200 mg up to 1 g/50-500 ml of D_5W; give over 30 min (2-6 mg/min maintenance); use infusion pump for correct dosage
- Do not use if sol is dark or if precipitate is present

Y-site compatibilities:
Amiodarone, famotidine, heparin, hydrocortisone, potassium chloride, ranitidine, vit B/C

Y-site incompatibilities:
Milrinone

Additive compatibilities:
Amiodarone, dobutamine, flumazenil, lidocaine, netilmicin, verapamil

Additive incompatibilities:
Esmolol, ethacrynate, milrinone

Solution compatibilities:
D_5W, D_5/0.9% NaCl, 0.45% NaCl, 0.9% NaCl, water for inj

Patient/family education

- Advise patient to report side effects immediately to prescriber; to take exactly as prescribed; if dose is missed take when remembered if within 3-4 hr of next dose, do not double doses
- Caution patient that dark glasses may be needed for photophobia; to use sunscreen or stay out of sun to

prevent burns; avoid temp extremes; impairment of heat-regulating mechanism can occur

- Advise patient to complete follow-up appointment with prescriber including pulmonary function studies, chest x-ray
- Instruct patient that dry mouth may be relieved by frequent sips of water, hard candy, sugarless gum
- Caution patient to make position changes from lying to standing slowly to prevent orthostatic hypotension

Evaluation

Positive therapeutic outcome

- Decreased PVCs, ventricular tachycardia

Treatment of overdose: O_2, artificial ventilation, ECG, administer dopamine for circulatory depression, administer diazepam or thiopental for convulsions, isoproterenol

procarbazine (℞)

(proe-kar'ba-zeen)

Matulane, Natulan ✤

Func. class.: Antineoplastic, alkylating agent

Chem. class.: Hydrazine derivative

Pregnancy category D

Action: Inhibits DNA, RNA, protein synthesis, cell cycle S phase specific; has multiple sites of action; a nonvesicant

Therapeutic Outcome: Prevention of rapidly growing malignant cells

Uses: Lymphoma, Hodgkin's disease, cancers resistant to other therapy

Investigational uses: Brain, lung malignancies, other lymphomas, multiple myeloma, malignant melanoma, polycythemia vera

Dosage and routes

Adult: PO 2-4 mg/kg/day for first wk; maintain dosage of 4-6 mg/kg/day until platelets and WBC fall; after recovery, 1-2 mg/kg/day

P ***Child:*** PO 50 mg/m^2/day for 7 days, then 100 mg/m^2 until desired response, leukopenia, or thrombocytopenia occurs; 50 mg/day is maintenance after bone marrow recovery

Available forms: Caps 50 mg

Adverse effects

CNS: Headache, dizziness, **seizures,** insomnia, hallucinations, confusion, **coma,** pain, chills, fever, sweating, paresthesias

EENT: Retinal hemorrhage, nystagmus, photophobia, diplopia

GI: *Nausea, vomiting,* anorexia, diarrhea, constipation, dry mouth, stomatitis

GU: Azoospermia, cessation of menses

HEMA: **Thrombocytopenia, anemia, leukopenia, myelosuppression, bleeding tendencies,** purpura, petechiae, epistaxis

INTEG: *Rash,* pruritus, dermatitis, alopecia, herpes, hyperpigmentation

MS: Arthralgias, myalgias

RESP: Cough, pneumonitis

Contraindications: Hypersensitivity, thrombocytopenia, bone marrow depression, pregnancy **D**

Precautions: Renal disease, hepatic disease, radiation therapy

Pharmacokinetics

Absorption	Well absorbed
Distribution	Widely distributed; crosses blood-brain barrier
Metabolism	Liver
Excretion	Kidneys
Half-life	1 hr

Pharmacodynamics

Unknown

Interactions

Individual drugs

Alcohol: ↑ CNS depressant, disulfiram reaction

Guanadrel: ↑ hypertensive crisis

P

Guanethidine: ↑ hypertensive crisis
Levodopa: ↑ hypertensive crisis
Meperidine: Avoid use; paradoxic reactions
Radiation: ↑ toxicity, bone marrow suppression
Reserpine: ↑ hypertensive crisis

Drug classifications

Antidepressants: ↑ hypertensive crisis
Antihistamines: ↑ CNS depression
Antineoplastics: ↑ toxicity bone marrow suppression
CNS depressants: ↑ CNS depression
Local anesthetics: ↑ hypertensive crisis
MAOIs: ↑ seizures, temperature
Opiates: ↑ CNS depression
Sedative/hypnotics: ↑ CNS depression
Sympathomimetic amines: Hypertensive crisis
Vasoconstrictors: ↑ hypertensive crisis

NURSING CONSIDERATIONS

Assessment

- Monitor CBC, differential, platelet count weekly; withhold drug if WBC is <4000/mm^3 or platelet count is <75,000/mm^3; notify prescriber of results if WBC <20,000/mm^3, platelets <150,000/mm^3
- Monitor pulmonary function tests, chest x-ray films before, during therapy; chest film should be obtained q2 wk during treatment; check for dyspnea, rales, unproductive cough, chest pain, tachypnea
- Monitor renal function studies: BUN, serum uric acid, urine CrCl before, during therapy; I&O ratio; report fall in urine output of 30 ml/hr; check for decreased hyperuricemia
- Monitor for cold, fever, sore throat (may indicate beginning of infection); identify edema in feet, joint and stomach pain, shaking; prescriber should be notified
- Assess for bleeding: hematuria, guaiac, bruising or petechiae, mucosa or orifices q8h, no rectal temp
- Assess for tyramine-containing foods in the diet; hypertensive crisis can occur

Nursing diagnoses

✓ Injury, risk for (adverse reactions)
✓ Body image disturbance (adverse reactions)
✓ Infection, risk for (adverse reactions)
✓ Knowledge deficit (teaching)

Implementation

- Give with foods, fluids for GI upset; open cap and give with food/fluids for swallowing difficulty; administer as directed

Patient/family education

- Teach patient to avoid use of products containing aspirin or NSAIDs, razors, commercial mouthwash, since bleeding may occur; to report symptoms of bleeding (hematuria, tarry stools)
- Caution patient to report signs of anemia (fatigue, headache, irritability, faintness, shortness of breath)
- Advise patient to report any changes in breathing or coughing even several mo after treatment; to avoid crowds and persons with respiratory tract or other infections
- Inform patient hair loss is common; discuss the use of wigs or hairpieces
- Caution patient not to have any vaccinations without the advice of the prescriber; serious reactions can occur
- Advise patient that contraception is needed during treatment and for several mo after the completion of therapy

Evaluation

Positive therapeutic outcome

- Absence of swelling at night
- Increased appetite, increased weight

prochlorperazine (℞)
(proe-klor-pair'a-zeen)

Chlorpazine, Compa-Z, Compazine, Contranzine, Provazin ♣, Stemetil ♣, Ultrazine

Func. class.: Antiemetic/antipsychotic

Chem. class.: Phenothiazine, piperazine derivative

Pregnancy category C

Action: Depresses cerebral cortex, hypothalamus, limbic system, which control activity aggression; blocks neurotransmission produced by dopamine at synapse; exhibits a strong α-adrenergic, anticholinergic blocking action; mechanism for antipsychotic effects is unclear; acts centrally by blocking chemoreceptor trigger zone, which in turn acts on vomiting center

→ **Therapeutic Outcome:** Decreased nausea, vomiting, decreased signs and symptoms of psychosis

Uses: Nausea, vomiting, psychosis

Dosage and routes

Postoperative nausea/vomiting

Adult: IM 5-10 mg 1-2 hr before anesthesia; may repeat in 30 min; **IV** 5-10 mg 15-30 min before anesthesia; **IV** inf 20 mg/L D_5W or 0.9% NaCl 15-30 min before anesthesia, max 40 mg/day

Severe nausea/vomiting

Adult: PO 5-10 mg tid-qid; sus rel 15 mg qd in AM or 10 mg q12h; rec 25 mg/bid; IM 5-10 mg; may repeat q4h, max 40 mg/day

P ***Child 18-39 kg:*** PO 2.5 mg tid or 5 mg bid; max 15 mg/day; IM 0.132 mg/kg

P ***Child 14-17 kg:*** PO/rec 2.5 mg bid-tid, max 10 mg/day; IM 0.132 mg/kg

P ***Child 9-13 kg:*** PO/rec 2.5 mg qd-bid, max 7.5 mg/day; IM 0.132 mg/kg

Antipsychotic

P ***Adult and child ≥12 yr:*** PO 5-10 mg tid-qid; may increase q2-3 day, max 150 mg/day; IM 10-20 mg q2-4h up to 4 doses, then 10-20 mg q4-6h, max 200 mg/day; rec 10 mg tid-qid may increase by 5-10 mg q2-3 days as needed

P ***Child 2-12 yr:*** PO 2.5 mg bid-tid; IM 132 μg/kg, max 10 mg/dose

Antianxiety

P ***Adult and child ≥12 yr:*** 5 mg tid-qid, max 20 mg/day or >12 wk; IM 5-10 mg q3-4h, max 40 mg/day; **IV** 2.5-10 mg; max 40 mg/day

P ***Child 2-12 yr:*** IM 132 μg/kg

Available forms: Syrup 5 mg/ml; inj 5 mg/ml; tabs 5, 10, 25 mg; sus rel caps 10, 15, 30 mg; supp 2.5, 5, 25 mg

Adverse effects

CNS: Tardive dyskinesia, *euphoria,* **depression, EPS,** restlessness, tremor, dizziness, **neuroleptic malignant syndrome**

CV: **Circulatory failure, tachycardia**

GI: Nausea, vomiting, anorexia, dry mouth, diarrhea, constipation, weight loss, metallic taste, cramps, hepatitis

RESP: **Respiratory depression**

Contraindications: Hypersensitivity to phenothiazines, coma, seizure, encephalopathy, bone marrow depression

P **Precautions:** Children <2 yr,
G pregnancy **C,** elderly

Do Not Confuse:
Compazine/Coumadin, prochlorperazine/chlorpromazine

Pharmacokinetics

Absorption	Variably absorbed (PO); well absorbed (IM)
Distribution	Widely distributed; high concentration in CNS; crosses placenta
Metabolism	Liver, extensively; GI mucosa
Excretion	Kidneys, breast milk
Half-life	Unknown

Pharmacodynamics

	PO	PO–SUS REL	REC	IM	IV
Onset	½ hr	½ hr	1 hr	10-20 min	4-5 min
Peak	Unkn	Unkn	Unkn	Unkn	Unkn
Duration	3-4 hr	10-12 hr	3-4 hr	3-4 hr	3-4 hr

Interactions
Individual drugs
Alcohol: ↑ effects of both drugs, oversedation
Aluminum hydroxide: ↓ absorption
Bromocriptine: ↓ antiparkinsonian activity
Disopyramide: ↑ anticholinergic effects
Epinephrine: ↑ toxicity
Guanethidine: ↓ antihypertensive response
Levodopa: ↓ antiparkinsonian activity
Lithium: ↓ prochlorperazine levels, ↑ EPS, masking of lithium toxicity
Magnesium hydroxide: ↓ absorption
Norepinephrine: ↓ vasoresponse, ↑ toxicity
Phenobarbital: ↓ effectiveness, ↑ metabolism
Drug classifications
Antacids: ↓ absorption
Anticholinergics: ↑ anticholinergic effects
Antidepressants: ↑ CNS depression
Antidiarrheals, adsorbent: ↓ absorption
Antihistamines: ↑ CNS depression
Antihypertensives: ↑ hypotension
Antithyroid agents: ↑ agranulocytosis
Barbiturate anesthetics: ↑ CNS depression
β-Adrenergic blockers: ↑ effects of both drugs
General anesthetics: ↑ CNS depression
MAOIs: ↑ CNS depression
Opiates: ↑ CNS depression
Sedative/hypnotics: ↑ CNS depression
▨ *Herb/drug*
Henbane: ↑ anticholinergic effect
Lab test interferences
↑ Liver function tests, ↑ cardiac enzymes, ↑ cholesterol, ↑ blood glucose, ↑ prolactin, ↑ bilirubin, ↑ PBI, ↑ cholinesterase, ↑ ^{131}I, ↑ alkaline phosphatase, ↑ leukocytes, ↑ granulocytes, ↑ platelets
↓ Hormones (blood and urine)
False positive: Pregnancy tests, PKU, urine bilirubin
False negative: Urinary steroids, 17-OHCS, pregnancy tests

NURSING CONSIDERATIONS
Assessment
- Assess mental status: orientation, mood, behavior, presence and type of hallucinations before initial administration and monthly; this drug should significantly reduce psychotic behavior
- Check for swallowing of PO medication; check for hoarding or giving of medication to other patients
- Monitor I&O ratio; palpate bladder if low urinary output occurs, **G** especially in elderly; urinalysis recommended before, during prolonged therapy
- Monitor bilirubin, CBC, liver function studies monthly
- Assess affect, orientation, LOC, reflexes, gait, coordination, sleep pattern disturbances
- Monitor B/P with patient sitting, standing, and lying; take pulse and respirations q4h during initial treatment; establish baseline before starting treatment; report drops of 30

mm Hg; obtain baseline ECG, Q-wave and T-wave changes
- Check for dizziness, faintness, palpitations, tachycardia on rising; severe orthostatic hypotension is common
- Identify neuroleptic malignant syndrome: hyperpyrexia, muscle rigidity, increased CPK, altered mental status; drug should be discontinued
- Assess for EPS including akathisia (inability to sit still, no pattern to movements), tardive dyskinesia (bizarre movements of the jaw, mouth, tongue, extremities), pseudoparkinsonism (ragged tremors, pill rolling, shuffling gait); an antiparkinsonism drug should be prescribed
- Assess for constipation, urinary retention daily; if these occur, increase bulk, water in diet

Nursing diagnoses

✓ Thought processes, altered (uses)
✓ Coping, ineffective individual (uses)
✓ Knowledge deficit (teaching)
✓ Noncompliance (teaching)

Implementation

PO route
- Give drug in liq form mixed in glass of juice or cola if hoarding is suspected; do not mix in caffeine drinks, tannics, pectins
- G • Give decreased dosage in elderly since metabolism is slowed
- Give PO with full glass of water, milk; or give with food to decrease GI upset
- Store in airtight, light-resistant container; oral sol in amber bottle
- ⊘ • Do not crush or chew sus rel cap

IM route
- Inject slowly in deep muscle mass; do not give SC; aspirate to avoid **IV** administration; do not administer sol with a precipitate; have patient lie down afterward for at least 30 min

IV **IV route**
- Give by direct **IV** after diluting **IV** using 0.9% NaCl to 1 mg/1 ml; administer at 1 mg/min or less
- Administer by intermittent inf after diluting 20 mg/L or less LR, Ringer's, dextrose, saline, or any combination

Syringe compatibilities:
Atropine, butorphanol, chlorpromazine, cimetidine, diamorphine, diphenhydramine, droperidol, fentanyl, glycopyrrolate, hydroxyzine, meperidine, metoclopramide, nalbuphine, pentazocine, perphenazine, promazine, promethazine, ranitidine, scopolamine, sufentanil

Syringe incompatibilities:
Dimenhydrinate, midazolam, pentobarbital, thiopental

Y-site compatibilities:
Amsacrine, calcium gluconate, cisplatin, cladribine, cyclophosphamide, cytarabine, doxorubicin, fluconazole, granisetron, heparin, hydrocortisone, melphalan, methotrexate, ondansetron, paclitaxel, potassium chloride, propofol, sargramostim, sufentanil, teniposide, thiotepa, vinorelbine, vit B/C

Y-site incompatibilities:
Foscarnet

Additive compatibilities:
Amikacin, ascorbic acid, dexamethasone, dimenhydrinate, erythromycin, ethacrynate, lidocaine, nafcillin, netilmicin, sodium bicarbonate, vit B/C

Additive incompatibilities:
Aminophylline, amphotericin B, ampicillin, calcium gluceptate, cefoperazone, cephalothin, chloramphenicol, chlorothiazide, floxacillin, furosemide, hydrocortisone sodium succinate, methohexital sodium, penicillin G sodium, phenobarbital, thiopental

Patient/family education

- Teach patient to use good oral hygiene; frequent rinsing of mouth, sugarless gum for dry mouth
- Caution patient to avoid hazardous activities until drug response is

P

determined; dizziness, blurred vision may occur
- Inform patient that orthostatic hypotension occurs often and to rise from sitting or lying position gradually; to remain lying down after IM inj for at least 30 min; tell patient to avoid hot tubs, hot showers, tub baths, since hypotension may occur; tell patient that in hot weather heat stroke may occur; take extra precautions to stay cool
- Advise patient to avoid abrupt withdrawal of this drug, or EPS may result; drug should be withdrawn slowly
- Teach patient to avoid OTC preparations (cough, hay fever, cold) unless approved by prescriber, since serious drug interactions may occur; avoid use with alcohol, CNS depressants; increased drowsiness may occur; avoid activities requiring mental alertness
- Instruct patient to use a sunscreen and sunglasses to prevent burns
- Teach patient about EPS and necessity of meticulous oral hygiene, since oral candidiasis may occur
- Advise patient to take antacids 2 hr before or after taking this drug
- Advise patient to report sore throat, malaise, fever, bleeding, mouth sores; if these occur, CBC should be done and drug discontinued
- Teach patient not to double or skip doses
- Teach patient urine may turn pink to reddish brown
- Instruct patient to report dark urine, clay-colored stools, bleeding, bruising, rash, blurred vision

Evaluation

Positive therapeutic outcome
- Relief of nausea and vomiting
- Decrease in emotional excitement, hallucinations, delusions, paranoia
- Reorganization of patterns of thought, speech

Treatment of overdose: Lavage if orally ingested; provide airway; *do not induce vomiting or use epinephrine*

progesterone (Key Drug) (℞)

(proe-jess'ter-one)

Crinone, progesterone, Progesterone in Oil, Prometrium

Func. class.: Progestogen

Chem. class.: Progesterone derivative

Pregnancy category D

Action: Inhibits secretion of pituitary gonadotropins, which prevents follicular maturation, ovulation; stimulates growth of mammary tissue; antineoplastic action against endometrial cancer

Therapeutic Outcome: Decreased abnormal uterine bleeding, absence of amenorrhea

Uses: Contraception, amenorrhea, premenstrual syndrome, abnormal uterine bleeding, endometrial hyperplasia prevention

Investigational uses: Corpus luteum dysfunction

Dosage and routes

Infertility

Adult: VAG 90 mg qd

Amenorrhea/uterine bleeding

Adult: IM 5-10 mg qd × 6-8 doses

Endometrial hyperplasia prevention

Adult: PO 200 mg/day

Available forms: Caps 100, 200 mg; inj 50 mg/ml; powder micronized, vag gel 8%

Adverse effects

CNS: Dizziness, headache, migraines, depression, fatigue

CV: Hypotension, thrombophlebitis, edema, **thromboembolism, stroke, pulmonary embolism, MI**

EENT: Diplopia

GI: *Nausea,* vomiting, anorexia, cramps, increased weight, **cholestatic jaundice**
GU: Amenorrhea, cervical erosion, breakthrough bleeding, dysmenorrhea, vaginal candidiasis, breast changes, *gynecomastia, testicular atrophy, impotence,* endometriosis, **spontaneous abortion**
INTEG: Rash, urticaria, acne, hirsutism, alopecia, oily skin, seborrhea, purpura, melasma
META: Hyperglycemia
SYST: **Angioedema, anaphylaxis**

Contraindications: Breast cancer, hypersensitivity, thromboembolic disorders, reproductive cancer, genital bleeding (abnormal, undiagnosed), cerebral hemorrhage, pregnancy **D**

Precautions: Lactation, hypertension, asthma, blood dyscrasias, gallbladder disease, CHF, diabetes mellitus, bone disease, depression, migraine headache, seizure disorders, hepatic disease, renal disease, family history of breast or reproductive tract cancer

Pharmacokinetics

Absorption	Unknown
Distribution	Unknown
Metabolism	Unknown
Excretion	Breast milk
Half-life	Unknown

Pharmacodynamics

	IM	REC	VAG
Onset	Unknown	Unknown	Unknown
Peak	Unknown	Unknown	Unknown
Duration	24 hr	24 hr	24 hr

Interactions

Individual drugs

Bromocriptine: ↓ effectiveness of bromocriptine

Herb/drug

Alfalfa: ↑ hormonal effect

Lab test interferences

↑ Alkaline phosphatase, ↑ nitrogen (urine), ↑ pregnanediol, ↑ amino acids, ↑ factors VII, VIII, IX, X
↓ GTT, ↓ HDL

NURSING CONSIDERATIONS

Assessment

- Monitor B/P at beginning of treatment and periodically; check weight daily; notify prescriber of weekly weight gain >5 lb
- Monitor I&O ratio: be alert for decreasing urinary output, increasing edema, hypertension
- Assess liver function studies: ALT, AST, bilirubin periodically during long-term therapy
- Assess edema, hypertension, cardiac symptoms, jaundice
- Assess mental status: affect, mood, behavioral changes, depression
- Assess for hypercalcemia

Nursing diagnoses

- ✓ Sexual dysfunction (uses)
- ✓ Tissue perfusion, altered (adverse reactions)
- ✓ Injury, risk for (adverse reactions)
- ✓ Knowledge deficit (teaching)

Implementation

IM route

- Store in dark area
- Give titrated dose; use lowest effective dosage; give oil sol deep in large muscle mass; rotate sites; use after warming to dissolve crystals

Patient/family education

- Teach patient to report breast lumps, vaginal bleeding, edema, jaundice, dark urine, clay-colored stools, dyspnea, headache, blurred vision, abdominal pain, numbness or stiffness in legs, chest pain
- Teach patient to report suspected pregnancy

Evaluation

Positive therapeutic outcome

- Decreased abnormal uterine bleeding
- Absence of amenorrhea
- Prevented pregnancy

P

promazine (℞)

(proe'ma-zeen)

promazine, Sparine

Func. class.: Antipsychotic/neuroleptic

Chem. class.: Phenothiazine, aliphatic

Pregnancy category C

Action: Depresses cerebral cortex, hypothalamus, limbic system, which control activity, aggression; blocks neurotransmission produced by dopamine at synapse; exhibits a strong α-adrenergic, anticholinergic blocking action; as antiemetic, inhibits medullary chemoreceptor trigger zone; mechanism for antipsychotic effects is unclear

Therapeutic Outcome: Decreased signs and symptoms of psychosis, absence of nausea, vomiting

Uses: Psychotic disorders, schizophrenia, nausea, vomiting, alcohol withdrawal

Dosage and routes

Psychosis

Adult: PO 10-200 mg q4-6h; max 1000 mg/day; IM 50-150 mg, followed in 30 min with additional dose up to a total dose of 300 mg

G ***Elderly:*** PO 25 mg qd-bid, increase by 25 mg q4-7 days

P ***Child >12 yr:*** PO 10-25 mg q4-6h

Available forms: Tabs 25, 50 mg; inj 25, 50 mg/ml

Adverse effects

CNS: *EPS: (pseudoparkinsonism, akathisia, dystonia, tardive dyskinesia), drowsiness, headache,* **seizures, neuroleptic malignant syndrome**

CV: *Orthostatic hypotension,* **cardiac arrest,** ECG changes, **tachycardia**

EENT: Blurred vision, glaucoma, dry eyes

GI: *Dry mouth, nausea, vomiting, anorexia, constipation,* diarrhea, jaundice, weight gain

GU: Urinary retention, urinary frequency, enuresis, impotence, amenorrhea, gynecomastia

HEMA: Anemia, **leukopenia, leukocytosis, agranulocytosis**

INTEG: *Rash,* photosensitivity, dermatitis

RESP: **Laryngospasm,** dyspnea, **respiratory depression**

Contraindications: Hypersensitivity, blood dyscrasias, coma, P child <12 yr, brain damage, bone marrow depression, glaucoma

Precautions: Pregnancy **C,** lactation, seizure disorders, hypertension, hepatic disease, cardiac disease

Pharmacokinetics

Absorption	Variably absorbed (PO); well absorbed (IM); completely absorbed (**IV**)
Distribution	Widely distributed; high concentration in CNS; crosses placenta
Metabolism	Liver, extensively
Excretion	Kidneys, breast milk
Half-life	Unknown

Pharmacodynamics

	PO	IM
Onset	½ hr	Up to ½ hr
Peak	2-4 hr	Unknown
Duration	4-6 hr	4-6 hr

Interactions

Individual drugs

Alcohol: ↑ effects of both drugs, oversedation

Aluminum hydroxide: ↓ absorption

Bromocriptine: ↓ antiparkinsonian activity

Disopyramide: ↑ anticholinergic effects

Epinephrine: ↑ toxicity

Guanethidine: ↓ antihypertensive response

Levodopa: ↓ antiparkinsonian activity

Lithium: ↓ promazine levels, ↑ EPS, masking of lithium toxicity
Magnesium hydroxide: ↓ absorption
Norepinephrine: ↓ vasoresponse, ↑ toxicity
Phenobarbital: ↓ effectiveness, ↑ metabolism

Drug classifications

Antacids: ↓ absorption
Anticholinergics: ↑ anticholinergic effects
Antidepressants: ↑ CNS depression
Antidiarrheals, adsorbent: ↓ absorption
Antihistamines: ↑ CNS depression
Antihypertensives: ↑ hypotension
Antithyroid agents: ↑ agranulocytosis
Barbiturate anesthetics: ↑ CNS depression
β-Adrenergic blockers: ↑ effects of both drugs
General anesthetics: ↑ CNS depression
MAOIs: ↑ CNS depression
Opiates: ↑ CNS depression
Sedative/hypnotics: ↑ CNS depression

Herb/drug

Henbane: ↑ anticholinergic effect

Lab test interferences

↑ Liver function tests, ↑ cardiac enzymes, ↑ cholesterol, ↑ blood glucose, ↑ prolactin, ↑ bilirubin, ↑ PBI, ↑ cholinesterase, ↑ iodine, ↑ alkaline phosphatase, ↑ leukocytes, ↑ granulocytes, ↑ platelets
↓ Hormones (blood and urine)
False positive: Pregnancy tests, PKU, urine bilirubin
False negative: Urinary steroids, 17-OHCS

NURSING CONSIDERATIONS

Assessment

- Assess mental status: orientation, mood, behavior, presence and type of hallucinations before initial administration and monthly; this drug should significantly reduce psychotic behavior
- Check for swallowing of PO medication; check for hoarding or giving of medication to other patients
- Monitor I&O ratio; palpate bladder if low urinary output occurs, especially in elderly; urinalysis recommended before, during prolonged therapy
- Monitor bilirubin, CBC, liver function studies monthly
- Assess affect, orientation, LOC, reflexes, gait, coordination, sleep pattern disturbances
- Monitor B/P with patient sitting, standing and lying, take pulse and respirations q4h during initial treatment; establish baseline before starting treatment; report drops of 30 mm Hg; obtain baseline ECG, Q- and T-wave changes
- Check for dizziness, faintness, palpitations, tachycardia on rising; severe orthostatic hypotension is common
- Identify for neuroleptic malignant syndrome: hyperpyrexia, muscle rigidity, increased CPK, altered mental status; drug should be discontinued
- Assess for EPS including akathisia (inability to sit still, no pattern to movements), tardive dyskinesia (bizarre movements of the jaw, mouth, tongue, extremities), pseudoparkinsonism (ragged tremors, pill rolling, shuffling gait); an antiparkinsonian drug should be prescribed
- Assess for constipation, urinary retention daily; if these occur, increase bulk, water in diet

Nursing diagnoses

- ✓ Thought processes, altered (uses)
- ✓ Coping, ineffective individual (uses)
- ✓ Knowledge deficit (teaching)
- ✓ Noncompliance (teaching)

Implementation

PO route

- Give decreased dosage in elderly since metabolism is slowed
- Give PO with full glass of water, milk; or give with food to decrease GI upset

• Store in airtight, light-resistant container

IM route

• Inject in deep muscle mass; do not give SC; do not administer sol with a precipitate; patient should remain recumbent for at least 30 min to prevent severe hypotension

Patient/family education

• Teach patient to use good oral hygiene; frequent rinsing of mouth, sugarless gum for dry mouth

• Advise patient to avoid hazardous activities until drug response is determined; dizziness, blurred vision may occur

• Inform patient that orthostatic hypotension occurs often and to rise from sitting or lying position gradually; to remain lying down after IM inj for at least 30 min; tell patient to avoid hot tubs, hot showers, tub baths, since hypotension may occur; tell patient that in hot weather heat stroke may occur; take extra precautions to stay cool

• Caution patient to avoid abrupt withdrawal of this drug, or EPS may result; drug should be withdrawn slowly

• Teach patient to avoid OTC preparations (cough, hay fever, cold) unless approved by prescriber, since serious drug interactions may occur; avoid use with alcohol, CNS depressants; increased drowsiness may occur

• Caution patient to use a sunscreen and sunglasses to prevent burns

• Teach patient about EPS and necessity of meticulous oral hygiene, since oral candidiasis may occur

• Instruct patient to take antacids 2 hr before or after taking this drug

• Teach patient to report sore throat, malaise, fever, bleeding, mouth sores; if these occur, CBC should be performed and drug discontinued

• Teach patient that urine may turn pink or red

Evaluation

Positive therapeutic outcome

• Decrease in emotional excitement, hallucinations, delusions, paranoia

• Reorganization of patterns of thought, speech

Treatment of overdose:

Lavage if orally ingested; provide airway; *do not induce vomiting or use epinephrine*

promethazine (℞)

(proe-meth'a-zeen)

Anergan 50, Phenergan, Phenergan Fortis, Phenergan Plain, promethazine HCl

Func. class.: Antihistamine, H_1-receptor antagonist; antiemetic; sedative/hypnotic

Chem. class.: Phenothiazine derivative

Pregnancy category C

Action: Acts on blood vessels, GI, respiratory system by competing with histamine for H_1-receptor site; decreases allergic response by blocking histamine; also acts on chemoreceptor trigger zone to decrease vomiting; increases CNS stimulation, has anticholinergic response

Therapeutic Outcome: Absence of allergy symptoms and rhinitis, absence of nausea/vomiting, sedation

Uses: Motion sickness, rhinitis, allergy symptoms, sedation, nausea, preoperative and postoperative sedation

Dosage and routes

Nausea

Adult: PO/IM/**IV**/rec 10-25 mg; may repeat 12.5-25 mg q4-6h

P ***Child >2 yr:*** PO/IM/**IV**/rec 0.25-0.5 mg/kg q4-6h

Motion sickness

Adult: PO 25 mg bid; give 30-60 min before departure

P ***Child >2 yr:*** PO/IM/rec 12.5-25 mg bid; give 30-60 min before departure

Allergy/rhinitis

Adult: PO 12.5 mg qid, or 25 mg hs

P ***Child >2 yr:*** PO 6.25-12.5 mg tid or 25 mg hs

Sedation

Adult: PO/IM/**IV**/rec 25-50 mg hs

P ***Child >2 yr:*** PO/IM/rec/**IV** 12.5-25 mg hs

Sedation (preoperative/ postoperative)

Adult: PO/IM/**IV** 25-50 mg

P ***Child >2 yr:*** PO/IM/**IV** 12.5-25 mg

Available forms: Tabs 12.5, 25, 50 mg; supp 12.5, 25, 50 mg; inj 25, 50 mg/ml; syrup 6.25, 10, 25 mg/5 ml

Adverse effects

CNS: Dizziness, drowsiness, poor coordination, fatigue, anxiety, euphoria, confusion, paresthesia, neuritis, EPS, **neuroleptic malignant syndrome**

CV: Hypotension, palpitations, tachycardia

EENT: Blurred vision, dilated pupils, tinnitus, nasal stuffiness, dry nose, throat, mouth, photosensitivity

GI: Constipation, dry mouth, nausea, vomiting, anorexia, diarrhea

GU: Retention, dysuria, frequency

HEMA: **Thrombocytopenia, agranulocytosis, hemolytic anemia**

INTEG: Rash, urticaria, photosensitivity

RESP: Increased thick secretions, **P** wheezing, chest tightness, **apnea in pediatric patients**

Contraindications: Hypersensitivity to H_1-receptor antagonist, acute asthma attack, lower respiratory tract disease

Precautions: Increased intraocular pressure, renal disease, cardiac disease, hypertension, bronchial asthma, seizure disorder, stenosed peptic ulcers, hyperthyroidism, prostatic hypertrophy, bladder neck obstruction, pregnancy **C**

Do Not Confuse:

Phenergan/Theragran

Pharmacokinetics

Absorption	Well absorbed (PO, IM); erratically absorbed (rec)
Distribution	Widely distributed; crosses the blood-brain barrier, placenta
Metabolism	Liver
Excretion	Kidneys, breast milk
Half-life	Unknown

Pharmacodynamics

	PO/IM/REC	IV
Onset	20 min	3-5 min
Peak	Unknown	Unknown
Duration	4-6 hr	4-6 hr

Interactions

Individual drugs

Alcohol: ↑ CNS depression

Atropine: ↑ anticholinergic reactions

Disopyramide: ↑ anticholinergic reactions

Haloperidol: ↑ anticholinergic reactions

Quinidine: ↑ anticholinergic reactions

Drug classifications

Antidepressants: ↑ anticholinergic reactions

Antihistamines: ↑ anticholinergic reactions

CNS depressants: ↑ CNS depression

MAOIs: ↑ anticholinergic effect

Opiates: ↑ CNS depression

Phenothiazines: ↑ anticholinergic reactions

Sedative/hypnotics: ↑ CNS depression

Herb/drug

Henbane: ↑ anticholinergic effect

Lab test interferences

↑ Serum glucose

False negative: Skin allergy tests (discontinue antihistamines 3 days before testing)

NURSING CONSIDERATIONS

Assessment

- Assess respiratory status: rate, rhythm, increase in bronchial secretions, wheezing, chest tightness; provide fluids to 2 L/day to decrease secretion thickness
- Monitor I&O ratio: be alert for urinary retention, frequency, dysuria, G especially elderly; drug should be discontinued if these occur
- Monitor CBC during long-term therapy; blood dyscrasias may occur but are rare

Nursing diagnoses

✓ Airway clearance, ineffective (uses)
✓ Injury, risk for (adverse reactions)
✓ Knowledge deficit (teaching)
✓ Noncompliance (teaching, overuse)

Implementation

PO route

- Give with meals to decrease GI upset
- Store in airtight, light-resistant container

IM route

- Give IM inj in large muscle mass; aspirate to avoid **IV** administration; do not give SC; necrosis may occur

IV **IV route**

- Give **IV** directly; give 25 mg or less over 1 min; rapid drop in B/P may occur with rapid administration

Syringe compatibilities: Atropine, butorphanol, chlorpromazine, cimetidine, diphenhydramine, droperidol, fentanyl, glycopyrrolate, hydromorphone, hydroxyzine, meperidine, metoclopramide, midazolam, pentazocine, perphenazine, prochlorperazine, promazine, ranitidine, scopolamine

Syringe incompatibilities: Dimenhydrinate, heparin, pentobarbital, thiopental

Y-site compatibilities: Amifostine, amsacrine, aztreonam, ciprofloxacin, cisplatin, cladribine, cyclophosphamide, cytarabine, doxorubicin, filgrastim, fluconazole, fludarabine, granisetron, melphalan, ondansetron, sargramostim, teniposide, thiotepa, vinorelbine

Y-site incompatibilities: Cefoperazone, foscarnet, heparin

Additive compatibilities: Amikacin, ascorbic acid, chloroquine, hydromorphone, netilmicin, vit B/C

Additive incompatibilities: Aminophylline, carbenicillin, chloramphenicol, chlorothiazide, floxacillin, furosemide, heparin, hydrocortisone sodium succinate, methicillin, methohexital, penicillin G, pentobarbital, phenobarbital, thiopental

Patient/family education

- Inform patient that a false negative result may occur with skin testing; these procedures should not be scheduled until 3 days after discontinuing use
- Advise patient to take 30 min before departure to prevent motion sickness
- Caution patient to avoid hazardous activities, activities requiring alertness, since dizziness may occur; instruct patient to request assistance with ambulation
- Advise patient to avoid alcohol, other depressants; serious CNS depression may occur
- Teach patient all aspects of drug use; to notify prescriber if confusion, sedation, hypotension occur; to avoid driving and other hazardous activity if drowsiness occurs
- Advise patient to take 1 hr ac or 2 hr pc to facilitate absorption
- Caution patient not to exceed recommended dosage; dysrhythmias may occur
- Inform patient hard candy, gum, frequent rinsing of mouth may be used for dryness

Evaluation

Positive therapeutic outcome

- Absence of motion sickness
- Absence of nausea, vomiting

Treatment of overdose: Administer ipecac syrup or lavage, diazepam, vasopressors, barbiturates (short-acting)

propantheline (℞)

(proe-pan'the-leen)

Pro-Banthine, Propanthel ♣, propantheline bromide

Func. class.: GI anticholinergic; antimuscarinic

Chem. class.: Synthetic quaternary ammonium compound

Pregnancy category C

Action: Inhibits muscarinic actions of acetylcholine at postganglionic parasympathetic neuroeffector sites

→ **Therapeutic Outcome:** Absence of peptic ulcer disease symptoms

Uses: Treatment of peptic ulcer disease, irritable bowel syndrome, duodenography, urinary incontinence

Investigational uses: Antispasmodic uses

Dosage and routes

Adult: PO 15 mg tid ac, 30 mg hs

G ***Elderly:*** PO 7.5 mg tid ac

Antispasmodic

P ***Child:*** PO 2-3 mg/kg/day

Antisecretory

P ***Child:*** PO 1.5 mg/kg/day in 3-4 divided doses

Available forms: Tabs 7.5, 15 mg

Adverse effects

CNS: *Confusion, stimulation in* G *elderly,* headache, insomnia, dizziness, drowsiness, anxiety, weakness, hallucinations

CV: Palpitations, tachycardia, G orthostatic hypotension (elderly)

EENT: *Blurred vision,* photophobia, mydriasis, cycloplegia, increased ocular tension

GI: *Dry mouth, constipation,* **paralytic ileus,** heartburn, nausea, vomiting, dysphagia, absence of taste

GU: Hesitancy, retention, impotence

INTEG: Urticaria, rash, pruritus, anhidrosis, fever, allergic reactions

Contraindications: Hypersensitivity to anticholinergics, narrow-angle glaucoma, GI obstruction, myasthenia gravis, paralytic ileus, GI atony, toxic megacolon

Precautions: Hyperthyroidism, CAD, dysrhythmias, CHF, ulcerative colitis, hypertension, hiatal hernia, hepatic disease, renal disease, pregnancy **C,** urinary retention, prostatic hypertrophy

Pharmacokinetics

Absorption	Moderately absorbed
Distribution	Unknown
Metabolism	Unknown
Excretion	Unknown
Half-life	Unknown

Pharmacodynamics

Onset	½ hr
Peak	2-6 hr
Duration	4-6 hr

Interactions

Individual drugs

Amantadine: ↑ anticholinergic effect
Atropine: ↑ anticholinergic effect
Disopyramide: ↑ anticholinergic effect
Haloperidol: ↑ anticholinergic effect
Potassium chloride, oral: ↑ GI lesions
Quinidine: ↑ anticholinergic effect

Drug classifications

Antacids: ↓ absorption of propantheline
Anticholinergics: ↑ anticholinergic effect
Antidepressants, tricyclic: ↑ anticholinergic effect
Antihistamines: ↑ anticholinergic effect
Phenothiazines: ↑ anticholinergic effect

P

NURSING CONSIDERATIONS

Assessment

- Assess for the pain of peptic ulcer disease before, during, and after treatment

Nursing diagnoses

- ✓ Pain (uses)
- ✓ Constipation (adverse reactions)
- ✓ Thought processes, impaired (adverse reactions)
- ✓ Knowledge deficit (teaching)

Implementation

- Give 30 min ac and hs; do not give with antacids; separate by at least 1 hr

Patient/family education

- Teach patient to report blurred vision, chest pain, allergic reactions
- Advise patient not to perform strenuous activity in high temp; heat stroke may result due to decreased perspiration
- Instruct patient to take as prescribed; not to skip doses
- Instruct patient to report change in vision; blurring or loss of sight; drug should be discontinued
- Advise patient not to operate machinery or drive if dizziness occurs
- Caution patient not to take OTC products without approval of prescriber

Evaluation

Positive therapeutic outcome

- Decreased pain in peptic ulcer disease

HIGH ALERT

propoxyphene (℞)

(proe-pox'i-feen)

Darvon, Darvon-N, Dolene, Novapropoxyn ✱, propoxyphene HCl

Func. class.: Opiate analgesics

Chem. class.: Synthetic opiate

Pregnancy category C

Controlled substance schedule IV

Action: Depresses pain impulse transmission at the spinal cord level by interacting with opioid receptors

➡ **Therapeutic Outcome:** Decreased pain

Uses: Mild to moderate pain

Dosage and routes

Adult: PO 65 mg q4h prn (HCl)

Adult: PO 100 mg q4h prn (napsylate)

Available forms: *Propoxyphene HCl:* caps 32, 65 mg; *propoxyphene napsylate:* tabs 100 mg; oral susp 50 mg/5 ml

Adverse effects

CNS: *Drowsiness, dizziness, confusion, headache, sedation,* euphoria, **seizures, hyperthermia**

CV: Palpitations, bradycardia, change in B/P, **dysrhythmias**

EENT: Tinnitus, blurred vision, miosis, diplopia

GI: *Nausea, vomiting, anorexia, constipation, cramps*

GU: Urinary retention, dysuria

INTEG: *Rash,* urticaria, bruising, flushing, diaphoresis, pruritus

RESP: **Respiratory depression**

Contraindications: Hypersensitivity to acetylsalicylic acid products (some preparations), addiction (narcotic)

Precautions: Addictive personality,

pregnancy **C,** lactation, increased ICP, MI (acute), severe heart disease, respiratory depression, hepatic
P disease, renal disease, child <18 yr,
G elderly

Pharmacokinetics

Absorption	Well absorbed
Distribution	Widely distributed; crosses placenta
Metabolism	Liver, extensively
Excretion	Kidneys, breast milk
Half-life	6-12 hr

Pharmacodynamics

Onset	½-1 hr
Peak	2-2½ hr
Duration	4-6 hr

Interactions

Individual drugs

Alcohol: ↑ respiratory depression, hypotension, sedation
Nalbuphine: ↓ analgesia
Pentazocine: ↓ analgesia

Drug classifications

Antihistamines: ↑ respiratory depression, hypotension
CNS depressants: ↑ respiratory depression, hypotension
MAOIs: Use ↓ dosage; reaction is unpredictable
Sedative/hypnotics: ↑ respiratory depression, hypotension

Smoking

↓ Analgesic effect

Lab test interferences

↑ Amylase

NURSING CONSIDERATIONS

Assessment

- Assess pain: location, duration, intensity before and 1 hr after administration
- Monitor CNS changes: dizziness, drowsiness, euphoria, LOC, pupil reaction
- Monitor allergic reactions: rash, urticaria

Nursing diagnoses

✓ Pain (uses)
✓ Sensory-perceptual alteration: visual, auditory (adverse reactions)
✓ Breathing pattern, ineffective (adverse reactions)
✓ Injury, risk for (adverse reactions)
✓ Knowledge deficit (teaching)

Implementation

- Give with antiemetic if nausea, vomiting occur
- Give when pain is beginning to return; determine dosage interval by patient response; continuous dosing of medication is more effective than when given prn
- Withdraw medication slowly after long-term use to prevent withdrawal symptoms
- Store in light-resistant container at room temp
- May be given with food or milk to lessen GI upset

Patient/family education

- Teach patient to avoid CNS depressants: alcohol, sedative/hypnotics for at least 24 hr after taking this drug
- Discuss with patient that dizziness, drowsiness, and confusion are common; to avoid getting up without assistance
- Discuss in detail all aspects of the drug, including purpose and what to expect after anesthesia
- Advise patient to make position changes slowly to lessen orthostatic hypotension

Evaluation

Positive therapeutic outcome

- Decreased pain

Treatment of overdose:

Naloxone 0.2-0.8 mg **IV**, O_2, **IV** fluids, vasopressors

P

propranolol 🔑 (℞)
(proe-pran′oh-lole)
Apo-Propranolol ✤, Detensol ✤, Inderal, Inderal LA, propranolol HCl, Propranolol Intensol, Novo-pranol ✤
Func. class.: Antihypertensive, antianginal
Chem. class.: β-Adrenergic blocker
Pregnancy category C

Action: Competitively blocks stimulation of β-adrenergic receptor within vascular smooth muscle; produces chronotropic, inotropic activity (decreases rate of SA node discharge, increases recovery time), slows conduction of AV node, decreased heart rate, which decreases O_2 consumption in myocardium; also suppresses renin-aldosterone-angiotensin system at high doses, inhibits β_2-receptors in bronchial system (high doses)

➡ **Therapeutic Outcome:** Decreased B/P, heart rate

Uses: Chronic stable angina pectoris, hypertension, supraventricular dysrhythmias, migraine prophylaxis, MI, pheochromocytoma, essential tremor, tetralogy of Fallot, cyanotic spells related to hypertrophic subaortic stenosis, dysrhythmias associated with thyrotoxicosis

Investigational uses: Hyperthyroidism adjunct therapy, Parkinson's tremor, prevention of variceal bleeding caused by portal hypertension, akathisia, mitral valve prolapse, anxiety

Dosage and routes

Dysrhythmias

Adult: PO 10-30 mg tid-qid; **IV** bol 0.5-3 mg given 1 mg/min; may repeat in 2 min; may repeat q4h thereafter

P ***Child:*** PO 0.5-1 mg/kg/day divided q6-8h, **IV** 0.01-0.1 mg/kg

Hypertension

Adult: PO 40 mg bid or 80 mg qd (ext rel) initially; usual dosage 120-240 mg/day bid-tid or 120-160 mg qd (ext rel)

P ***Child:*** PO 0.5-1 mg/kg/day divided q6-12h

Angina

Adult: PO 80-320 mg in divided doses bid-qid or 80 mg qd (ext rel); usual dosage 160 mg qd (ext rel)

MI prophylaxis

Adult: PO 180-240 mg/day tid-qid starting 5 days to 3 wk after MI

Pheochromocytoma

Adult: PO 60 mg/day × 3 days preoperatively in divided doses or 30 mg/day in divided doses (inoperable tumor)

Migraine

Adult: PO 80 mg/day (ext rel) or in divided doses; may increase to 160-240 mg/day in divided doses

P ***Child:*** PO 0.6-1.5 mg/kg/day divided q8h

Essential tremor

Adult: PO 40 mg bid; usual dosage 120 mg/day

Tetralogy of Fallot

P ***Child:*** PO 1-2 mg/kg/dose q6h

Available forms: Sus rel caps 60, 80, 120, 160 mg; ext rel caps 60 mg; tabs 10, 20, 40, 60, 90 mg; inj 1 mg/ml; oral sol 4 mg, 8 mg/ml; conc oral sol 80 mg/ml

Adverse effects

CNS: Depression, hallucinations, dizziness, fatigue, lethargy, paresthesia, bizarre dreams, disorientation
CV: *Bradycardia, hypotension,* **CHF**, palpitations, AV block, peripheral vascular insufficiency, vasodilatation
EENT: Sore throat, **laryngospasm,** blurred vision, dry eyes
GI: Nausea, vomiting, diarrhea, colitis, constipation, cramps, dry mouth,

hepatomegaly, gastric pain, acute pancreatitis
GU: Impotence, decreased libido, UTIs
HEMA: **Agranulocytosis, thrombocytopenia**
INTEG: Rash, pruritus, fever
META: Hyperglycemia, hypoglycemia
MISC: Facial swelling, weight change, Raynaud's phenomenon
MS: Joint pain, arthralgia, muscle cramps, pain
RESP: Dyspnea, respiratory dysfunction, **bronchospasm**, cough

Contraindications: Hypersensitivity to this drug, cardiac failure, cardiogenic shock, 2nd- or 3rd-degree heart block, bronchospastic disease, sinus bradycardia, CHF

Precautions: Diabetes mellitus, pregnancy **C**, renal disease, lactation, hyperthyroidism, COPD, hepatic P disease, children, myasthenia gravis, peripheral vascular disease, hypotension, CHF

Do Not Confuse:
Inderal/Toradol, Inderal LA/IMDUR

Pharmacokinetics

Absorption	Well absorbed (PO); slowly absorbed (ext rel); completely absorbed (**IV**)
Distribution	Widely distributed; crosses blood-brain barrier, protein binding 90%
Metabolism	Liver, extensively
Excretion	Kidneys
Half-life	3-5 hr; EXT REL 8-11 hr

Pharmacodynamics

	PO	PO–EXT REL	IV
Onset	½ hr	Unknown	Rapid
Peak	1-1½ hr	6 hr	1 min
Duration	6-12 hr	24 hr	4-6 hr

Interactions
Individual drugs
Alcohol: ↑ hypotension (large amounts)
Epinephrine: α-Adrenergic stimulation
Hydralazine: ↑ hypotension, bradycardia
Indomethacin: ↓ antihypertensive effect
Insulin: ↑ hypoglycemia
Methyldopa: ↑ hypotension, bradycardia
Prazosin: ↑ hypotension, bradycardia
Reserpine: ↑ hypotension, bradycardia
Thyroid hormones: ↓ effect of propranolol
Verapamil: ↑ myocardial depression

Drug classifications
Antihypertensives: ↑ hypertension
Cardiac glycosides: ↑ bradycardia
Nitrates: ↑ hypotension
Sulfonylureas: ↓ hypoglycemic effect
Theophyllines: ↓ bronchodilatation

Lab test interferences
False: ↑ Urinary catecholamines

NURSING CONSIDERATIONS
Assessment
- Monitor B/P during beginning treatment, periodically thereafter; pulse q4h; note rate, rhythm, quality; check apical/radial pulse before administration; notify prescriber of any significant changes (pulse <50 bpm)
- Check for baselines in renal, liver function tests before therapy begins and periodically thereafter
- Assess for edema in feet, legs daily; monitor I&O, weight daily; check for jugular vein distention, rales bilaterally; dyspnea (CHF)
- Monitor skin turgor, dryness of mucous membranes for hydration G status, especially elderly

Nursing diagnoses
✓ Cardiac output, decreased (uses)
✓ Injury, potential for (adverse reactions)
✓ Knowledge deficit (teaching)
✓ Noncompliance (teaching)

Implementation
PO route
- Given ac, hs, tab may be crushed or

P

swallowed whole; do not crush or chew ext rel cap; give with food to prevent GI upset; reduce dosage in renal dysfunction

- Store protected from light, moisture; placed in cool environment

IV route

- Give by direct **IV** undiluted or diluted 1 mg/10 ml of D_5W for inj; administer over 1 min or more
- Give by intermittent inf after diluting in 50 ml of D_5W, 0.9% NaCl, D_5/0.45% NaCl, D_5/0.9% NaCl, LR; administer over 15 min

Syringe compatibilities: Amrinone, benzquinamide, milrinone

Y-site compatibilities: Amrinone, heparin, hydrocortisone, meperidine, milrinone, morphine, potassium chloride, tacrolimus, vit B/C

Y-site incompatibilities: Diazoxide

Additive compatibilities: Dobutamine, verapamil

Solution compatibilities: 0.9% NaCl, 0.45% NaCl, Ringer's, D_5W, D_5/0.9% NaCl, D_5/0.45% NaCl

Patient/family education

- Teach patient not to discontinue drug abruptly, taper over 2 wk; may cause precipitate angina if stopped abruptly
- Teach patient not to use OTC products containing α-adrenergic stimulants (such as nasal decongestants, cold preparations); to avoid alcohol, smoking and to limit sodium intake as prescribed
- Teach patient how to take pulse and B/P at home; advise when to notify prescriber
- Instruct patient to comply with weight control, dietary adjustments, modified exercise program
- Instruct patient to carry/wear ID to identify drug being taken, allergies; tell patient drug controls symptoms but does not cure
- Caution patient to avoid hazardous activities if dizziness, drowsiness is present
- Teach patient to report symptoms of CHF: difficult breathing, especially on exertion or when lying down, night cough, swelling of extremities or bradycardia, dizziness, confusion, depression, fever
- Teach patient to take drug as prescribed, not to double doses, skip doses; take any missed doses as soon as remembered if at least 8 hr until next dose

Evaluation

Positive therapeutic outcome

- Decreased B/P in hypertension (after 1-2 wk)
- Decreased tremors
- Absence of dysrhythmias
- Decreased migraine headaches

Treatment of overdose:

Lavage, **IV** atropine for bradycardia, **IV** theophylline for bronchospasm, digitalis, O_2, diuretic for cardiac failure, hemodialysis, **IV** glucose for hyperglycemia, **IV** diazepam (or phenytoin) for seizures

propylthiouracil (℞)

(proe-pill-thye-oh-yoor'a-sill)

propylthiouracil, Propyl-Thyracil ✤, PTU

Func. class.: Thyroid hormone antagonist (antithyroid)

Chem. class.: Thioamide

Pregnancy category D

Action: Blocks synthesis peripherally of T_3, T_4, inhibits organification of iodine

Therapeutic Outcome: Decreased T_3, T_4 levels, hyperthyroid symptoms

Uses: Preparation for thyroidectomy, thyrotoxic crisis, hyperthyroidism, thyroid storm

Dosage and routes
Thyrotoxic crisis
P ***Adult and child:*** PO same as hyperthyroidism with iodine and propranolol
Preparation for thyroidectomy
Adult: PO 600-1200 mg/day
P ***Child:*** PO 10 mg/kg/day in divided doses
Hyperthyroidism
Adult: PO 100 mg tid increasing to 300 mg q8h if condition is severe; continue to euthyroid state, then 100 mg qd-tid
P ***Child >10 yr:*** PO 100 mg tid; continue to euthyroid state, then 25 mg tid to 100 mg bid
P ***Child 6-10 yr:*** PO 50-150 mg in divided doses q8h
P ***Neonates:*** PO 10 mg/kg/day in divided doses

Available forms: Tabs 50, 100 mg

Adverse effects
CNS: *Drowsiness, headache, vertigo, fever,* paresthesias, neuritis
GI: *Nausea, diarrhea, vomiting, jaundice, hepatitis,* loss of taste
GU: **Nephritis**
HEMA: **Agranulocytosis, leukopenia, thrombocytopenia, hypothrombinemia, lymphadenopathy,** bleeding, vasculitis, periarteritis
INTEG: *Rash, urticaria, pruritus, alopecia, hyperpigmentation,* lupus-like syndrome
MS: Myalgia, arthralgia, nocturnal muscle cramps, osteoporosis

Contraindications: Hypersensitivity, pregnancy **D**, lactation

Precautions: Infection, bone marrow depression, hepatic disease

Pharmacokinetics	
Absorption	Rapidly absorbed
Distribution	Crosses placenta; concentration in thyroid gland
Metabolism	Liver
Excretion	Urine, bile, breast milk
Half-life	1-2 hr

Pharmacodynamics	
Onset	30-40 min
Peak	Unknown
Duration	2-4 hr

Interactions
Individual drugs
Heparin: ↑ anticoagulant effect
Lithium: ↑ antithyroid effect
Radiation: ↑ bone marrow depression
Drug classifications
Antineoplastics: ↑ bone marrow depression
Oral anticoagulants: ↑ anticoagulant effect
Phenothiazines: ↑ agranulocytosis
Lab test interferences
↑ Pro-time, ↑ AST, ↑ ALT, ↑ alkaline phosphatase

NURSING CONSIDERATIONS
Assessment
- Monitor pulse, B/P, temp; I&O ratio; check for edema (puffy hands, feet, periorbits); indicates hypothyroidism
- Check weight daily with same clothing, scale, time of day
- Monitor T_3, T_4, which are increased; check serum TSH, which is decreased; assess free thyroxine index, which is increased if dosage is too low; discontinue drug 3-4 wk before radioactive iodine uptake test
- Monitor blood work: CBC for blood dyscrasias (leukopenia, thrombocytopenia, agranulocytosis); liver function tests
- ! Assess overdose (peripheral edema, heat intolerance, diaphoresis, palpitations, dysrhythmias, severe tachycardia, increased temp, delirium, CNS

P

irritability); drug should be discontinued
- Assess for hypersensitivity (rash, enlarged cervical lymph nodes); drug may have to be discontinued
- Assess for hypoprothrombinemia (bleeding, petechiae, ecchymosis)
- Monitor clinical response: after 3 wk should include increased weight, decreased pulse, decreased T_4
- Assess for bone marrow depression: sore throat, fever, fatigue

Nursing diagnoses
✓ Knowledge deficit (teaching)
✓ Noncompliance (teaching)

Implementation
- Give with meals to decrease GI upset
- Give at same time each day to maintain drug level
- Give lowest dosage that relieves symptoms
- Store in light-resistant container
- Increase fluids to 3-4 L/day, unless contraindicated

Patient/family education
- Advise patient to abstain from breast-feeding after delivery; drug appears in breast milk
- Teach patient to take pulse daily and to keep graph of weight, pulse, mood
- Advise patient to report redness, swelling, sore throat, mouth lesions, which indicate blood dyscrasias
- Caution patient to avoid OTC products that contain iodine; that seafood, other iodine-containing foods may be restricted by prescriber
- Caution patient not to discontinue this medication abruptly; thyroid crisis may occur; stress patient compliance
- Teach patient that response may take several mo if thyroid is large
- Teach patient symptoms/signs of overdose: periorbital edema, cold intolerance, mental depression; notify prescriber at once
- Teach patient symptoms of inadequate dose: tachycardia, diarrhea, fever, irritability; prescriber should be notified to adjust dosage
- Teach patient to take medication exactly as prescribed, not to skip or double doses; missed doses should be taken when remembered up to 1 hr before next dose
- Instruct patient to carry identification indicating medication taken and condition being treated

Evaluation
Positive therapeutic outcome
- Weight gain
- Decreased pulse
- Decreased T_4
- Decreased B/P

protamine (℞)
(proe'ta-meen)
Func. class.: Heparin antagonist
Chem. class.: Low-molecular-weight protein
Pregnancy category C

Action: Binds heparin, making it ineffective

➡ **Therapeutic Outcome:** Prevention of heparin overdose

Uses: Heparin overdose; neutralizes heparin in procedures

Dosage and routes
P ***Adult and child:*** **IV** 1 mg of protamine/90-115 U of heparin given; administer slowly over 1-3 min; not to exceed 50 mg/10 min

Available forms: Inj 10 mg/ml

Adverse effects
CNS: Lassitude
CV: Hypotension, bradycardia, **circulatory collapse**
GI: Nausea, vomiting, anorexia
INTEG: *Rash,* dermatitis, urticaria
HEMA: Bleeding, **anaphylaxis**
RESP: Dyspnea, **pulmonary edema, severe respiratory distress**

Contraindication: Hypersensitivity

Precautions: Pregnancy **C**, lactation, children, allergy to salmon

Pharmacokinetics

Absorption	Completely absorbed
Distribution	Unknown
Metabolism	Unknown
Excretion	Unknown
Half-life	Unknown

Pharmacodynamics

Onset	5 min
Peak	Unknown
Duration	2 hr

Interactions: None

NURSING CONSIDERATIONS

Assessment

- Monitor blood studies (Hct, platelets, occult blood stools) q3 mo
- Monitor coagulation tests (APTT, ACT) 15 min after dose, then in several hr
- Monitor VS, B/P, pulse q30 min, plus 3 hr after dose
- Assess for skin rash, urticaria, dermatitis
- Assess for allergy to salmon; use with caution in these patients

Nursing diagnoses

✓ Injury, risk for (uses)
✓ Tissue perfusion, altered (uses)
✓ Knowledge deficit (teaching)

Implementation

- Give by direct **IV** after diluting 50 mg/5 ml of sterile bacteriostatic water for inj; shake; give 20 mg or less over 1-3 min
- Give by intermittent inf after further diluting with equal volume of NaCl or D_5W and run over 2-3 hr; titrate to APTT, ACT; use infusion pump
- Store at 36-46° F (2-8° C)

Additive compatibilities: Cimetidine, ranitidine, verapamil

Additive incompatibilities: Penicillins, cephalosporins

Patient/family education

- Explain reason for medication and expected results
- Caution patient to avoid contact activities that may result in bleeding

Evaluation

Positive therapeutic outcome

- Reversal of heparin overdose

pseudoephedrine (OTC)

(soo-doe-e-fed′rin)

Afrin, Allermed, Canafed, Cenafed, Children's Congestion Relief, Children's Silfedrine, Congestion Relief, Decofed Syrup, DeFed-60, Dorcol Children's Decongestant, Drixoral Non-Drowsy Formula, Dynafed, Eltor ♣, Efidac/24, Genaphed, Halofed, Mini Thin Pseudo, Pedia Care Infant's Decongestant, pseudoephedrine HCl, Pseudogest, Seudotabs, Sinustop Pro, Sudafed, Sudafed 12 hour, Sudex, Triaminic AM Decongestant Formula

Func. class.: Adrenergic

Chem. class.: Substituted phenylethylamine

Pregnancy category B

Action: Primary activity through α-adrenergic effects on respiratory mucosal membranes reducing congestion, hyperemia, edema; minimal bronchodilatation secondary to β-adrenergic effects

Therapeutic Outcome: Decreased nasal congestion, swelling

Uses: Nasal decongestant, otitis media adjustment, adjunct with antihistamines

Dosage and routes

P ***Adult and child >12 yr:*** PO 60 mg q6h; ext rel 60-120 mg q12h or q24h

G ***Elderly:*** PO 30-60 mg q6h prn

P

P ***Child 6-12 yr:*** PO 30 mg q6h, max 120 mg/day

P ***Child 2-6 yr:*** PO 15 mg q6h, max 60 mg/day

Available forms: Ext rel caps 120, 240 mg; oral sol 15 mg, 30 mg/5 ml; drops 7.5 mg/0.8 ml; tabs 30, 60 mg; caps 60 mg; ext rel tabs 120 mg

Adverse effects

CNS: ***Tremors, anxiety,*** insomnia, headache, dizziness, anxiety, hallucinations, **seizures**

CV: Palpitations, tachycardia, hypertension, chest pain, **dysrhythmias, CV collapse**

EENT: Dry nose, irritation of nose and throat

GI: ***Anorexia, nausea, vomiting,*** dry mouth

GU: Dysuria

Contraindications: Hypersensitivity to sympathomimetics, narrow-angle glaucoma

Precautions: Pregnancy **B,** cardiac disorders, hyperthyroidism, diabetes mellitus, prostatic hypertrophy

Pharmacokinetics

Absorption	Well absorbed
Distribution	Enters CSF, crosses placenta
Metabolism	Liver, partially
Excretion	Kidneys, unchanged (75%); breast milk
Half-life	7 hr

Pharmacodynamics

	PO	PO–EXT REL
Onset	15-30 min	1 hr
Peak	Unknown	Unknown
Duration	4-6 hr	12 hr

Interactions

Individual drugs

Methyldopa: ↓ effect of pseudoephedrine

Rauwolfia: ↓ effect of pseudoephedrine

Drug classifications

β-Adrenergic blockers: Hypertensive crisis

MAOIs: Hypertensive crisis

Urinary acidifiers: ↓ effect of pseudoephedrine

Urinary alkalizers: ↑ effect of pseudoephedrine

NURSING CONSIDERATIONS

Assessment

- Assess for CNS side effects in the G elderly: excitation, seizures, hallucinations
- Monitor for nasal congestion; auscultate lung sounds; check for P tenacious bronchial secretions; children with otitis media should be assessed for eustachian tube congestion
- Monitor B/P and pulse throughout treatment

Nursing diagnoses

✓ Airway clearance, ineffective (uses)
✓ Knowledge deficit (teaching)

Implementation

- Give ext rel cap and tab whole
- Do not crush, break or chew
- Give several hr before bedtime if insomnia occurs
- Store at room temp

Patient/family education

- Teach patient reason for drug administration and expected results
- Instruct patient not to use continuously, or more than recommended dose; rebound congestion may occur
- Advise patient to check with prescriber before using other drugs, as drug interactions may occur
- Advise patient to avoid taking near bedtime; stimulation can occur
- Caution patient not to use if stimulation, restlessness, tremors occur
- P Notify parents of possible excessive agitation in children

Evaluation

Positive therapeutic outcome

- Decreased nasal congestion

psyllium (OTC)
(sill'i-um)

Alramucil, Fiberall, Fiberall Natural Flavor and Orange Flavor, Genifiber, Hydrocil Instant, Karacil ✦, Konsyl, Konsyl Orange, Maalox Daily Fiber Therapy, Metamucil, Metamucil Lemon Lime, Metamucil Orange Flavor, Metamucil Sugar Free, Metamucil Sugar Free Orange Flavor, Modane Bulk, Mylanta Natural Fiber Supplement, Natural Fiber Laxative, Natural Fiber Laxative Sugar Free, Natural Vegetable Reguloid, Perdiem, Prodiem Plain ✦, Reguloid Natural, Reguloid Orange, Reguloid Sugar Free Orange, Reguloid Sugar Free Regular, Restore, Restore Sugar Free, Serutan, Syllact, V-Lax

Func. class.: Laxative, bulk-forming

Chem. class.: Psyllium colloid

Pregnancy category C

Action: Promotes peristalsis by combining with water in the intestine to form a gel-like substance that is easily evacuated

Therapeutic Outcome: Decreased constipation, decreased diarrhea in colitis

Uses: Chronic constipation, ulcerative colitis, irritable bowel syndrome

Dosage and routes

Adult: PO 1-2 tsp in 8 oz of water bid or tid, then 8 oz of water or 1 premeasured packet in 8 oz of water bid or tid, then 8 oz of water

Child >6 yr: 1 tsp in 4 oz of water hs

Available forms: Chew pieces 1.7, 3.4 g/piece; powder effervescent 3.4, 3.7 g/packet; granules 2.5, 4.03 g/tsp; powder 3.3, 3.4, 3.5, 4.94 g/tsp; wafers 3.4 g/wafer

Adverse effects

GI: *Nausea, vomiting, anorexia, diarrhea,* cramps, intestinal/esophageal blockage

Contraindications: Hypersensitivity, intestinal obstruction, abdominal pain, nausea/vomiting, fecal impaction

Precautions: Pregnancy **C**

Pharmacokinetics

Absorption	None
Distribution	None
Excretion	Feces
Half-life	Unknown

Pharmacodynamics

Onset	12-24 hr
Peak	2-4 days
Duration	Unknown

Interactions

Drug classifications

Cardiac glycosides: ↓ absorption of cardiac glycosides

Oral anticoagulants: ↓ absorption of oral anticoagulants

Salicylates: ↓ absorption of salicylates

Lab test interferences

↑ Blood glucose

NURSING CONSIDERATIONS

Assessment

- Monitor blood, urine electrolytes if used often by patient; check I&O ratio to identify fluid loss
- Assess for cramping, rectal bleeding, nausea, vomiting; if these symptoms occur, drug should be discontinued; identify cause of constipation; identify whether fluids, bulk, or exercise is missing from lifestyle
- Assess stool for color, consistency, amount, presence of flatulence

Nursing diagnoses

- ✓ Constipation (uses)
- ✓ Knowledge deficit (teaching)
- ✓ Noncompliance (teaching)

Implementation

- Give alone for better absorption;

P

give after mixing with water immediately before use; administer with 8 oz of water or juice followed by another 8 oz of fluid

- Administer in AM or PM (oral dose)

Patient/family education

- Discuss with patient that adequate fluid consumption is necessary
- Teach patient that normal bowel movements do not always occur daily
- Caution patient not to use in presence of abdominal pain, nausea, vomiting; tell patient to notify prescriber if constipation is unrelieved or if symptoms of electrolyte imbalance occur (muscle cramps, pain, weakness, dizziness, excessive thirst)
- Teach patient not to use laxatives for long-term therapy; bowel tone will be lost and will decrease
- Teach patient to shake susp well as needed
- Teach patient not to take hs as a laxative; may interfere with sleep; also problems with lipid pneumonia
- Teach patient not to use with food or vitamin preparations; delays digestion and absorption of fat-soluble vitamins

Evaluation

Positive therapeutic outcome

- Decreased constipation in 12-24 hr

pyrazinamide (℞)

(peer-a-zin′a-mide)

PMS Pyrazinamide ♣, pyrazinamide, Tebrazid ♣

Func. class.: Antitubercular agent

Chem. class.: Pyrazinoic acid amine/nicoturimide analog

Pregnancy category C

Action: Bactericidal interference with lipid; nucleic acid biosynthesis is possible

Therapeutic Outcome: Bactericidal for *Mycobacterium* species

Uses: Tuberculosis, as an adjunct when other drugs are not feasible

Dosage and routes

P ***Adult and child:*** PO 15-30 mg/kg qd, max 2 g/day

Available forms: Tabs 500 mg

Adverse effects

CNS: Headache

GI: **Hepatotoxicity,** abnormal liver function tests, peptic ulcer, nausea, vomiting, anorexia, cramps, diarrhea

GU: Urinary difficulty, increased uric acid

HEMA: **Hemolytic anemia**

INTEG: Photosensitivity, urticaria

Contraindications: Hypersensitivity, severe hepatic damage, acute gout

P **Precautions:** Pregnancy **C,** child <13 yr, renal failure, diabetes, porphyria, chronic gout

Pharmacokinetics	
Absorption	Well absorbed
Distribution	Widely distributed
Metabolism	Liver, extensively
Excretion	Kidneys, breast milk
Half-life	9-10 hr

Pharmacodynamics	
Onset	Unknown
Peak	2 hr
Duration	9½ hr; metabolites 12 hr

Interactions: None

NURSING CONSIDERATIONS

Assessment

- C&S studies should be done before treatment begins, and periodically during treatment
- Monitor serum uric acid, which may be elevated and cause gout symptoms
- Monitor liver studies weekly: ALT, AST, bilirubin; hepatic status: decreased appetite, jaundice, dark urine, fatigue

- Monitor renal status before treatment and monthly thereafter: BUN, creatinine, output, sp gr, urinalysis, uric acid
- Monitor mental status often: affect, mood, behavioral changes; psychosis may occur

Nursing diagnoses

✓ Infection, risk for (uses)
✓ Diarrhea (adverse reactions)
✓ Injury, risk for (adverse reactions)
✓ Knowledge deficit (teaching)
✓ Noncompliance (teaching)

Implementation

- Give with meals to decrease GI symptoms
- Give antiemetic if vomiting occurs
- May be given with other antitubercular drugs

Patient/family education

- Instruct patient that compliance with dosage schedule, duration is necessary; that scheduled appointments must be kept or relapse may occur
- Advise diabetic patient to use blood glucose monitor to obtain correct result
- Advise patient to report weakness, fatigue, loss of appetite, nausea, vomiting, yellowing of skin or eyes, tingling/numbness of hands/feet

Evaluation

Positive therapeutic outcome

- Decreased symptoms of TB
- Sputum culture negative × 3

pyridostigmine (℞)

(peer-id-oh-stig'meen)

Mestinon, Mestinon SR, Mestinon Timespan, Regonol

Func. class.: Cholinergic, anticholinesterase

Chem. class.: Tertiary amine carbamate

Pregnancy category C

Action: Inhibits destruction of acetylcholine, which increases concentration at sites where acetylcholine is released; this facilitates transmission of impulses across myoneural junction

➔ **Therapeutic Outcome:** Decreased action of nondepolarizing muscle relaxant; increased muscle strength in myasthenia gravis

Uses: Nondepolarizing muscle relaxant antagonist, myasthenia gravis

Dosage and routes

Myasthenia gravis

Adult: PO 60-180 mg bid-qid, not to exceed 1.5 g/day; IM/**IV** 1/30 of PO dose; sus rel 180-540 mg qd or bid at intervals of at least 6 hr

P ***Child:*** 7 mg/kg/day in 5-6 divided doses

Nondepolarizing neuromuscular blocker antagonist

Adult: 0.6-1.2 mg **IV** atropine, then 10-30 mg

P ***Child:*** 0.1-0.25 mg/kg/dose

Available forms: Tabs 60 mg; ext rel tabs 180 mg; syrup 60 mg/5 ml; inj 5 mg/ml

Adverse effects

CNS: Dizziness, headache, sweating, weakness, **seizures,** uncoordination, paralysis, drowsiness, LOC

CV: Tachycardia, dysrhythmias, bradycardia, AV block, hypotension, ECG changes, **cardiac arrest,** syncope

EENT: Miosis, blurred vision, lacrimation, visual changes
GI: *Nausea, diarrhea, vomiting, cramps, increased salivary and gastric secretions, peristalsis*
GU: Frequency, incontinence, urgency
INTEG: Rash, urticaria, flushing
RESP: **Respiratory depression, bronchospasm, constriction, laryngospasm, respiratory arrest**

Contraindications: Bradycardia, hypotension, obstruction of intestine, renal system, bromide sensitivity

Precautions: Seizure disorders, bronchial asthma, coronary occlusion, hyperthyroidism, dysrhythmias, peptic ulcer, megacolon, poor GI motility, pregnancy **C**

Pharmacokinetics

Absorption	Poorly absorbed (PO)
Distribution	Widely distributed; crosses placenta
Metabolism	Liver, plasma cholinesterase
Excretion	Kidneys
Half-life	2 hr (**IV**); 4 hr (PO)

Pharmacodynamics

	PO	IM/IV	PO–EXT REL
Onset	20-30 min	2-15 min	½-1 hr
Peak	Unknown	Unknown	Unknown
Duration	3-6 hr	2-4 hr	3-6 hr

Interactions

Individual drugs

Digitalis: Bradycardia
Magnesium: ↓ action of pyridostigmine
Mecamylamine: ↓ action of pyridostigmine
Polymyxin: ↓ action of pyridostigmine
Procainamide: ↓ action of pyridostigmine
Quinidine: ↓ action of pyridostigmine

Drug classifications

Antidepressants: ↑ antagonism
Antihistamines: ↑ antagonism
Cholinesterase inhibitors: ↑ toxicity
Muscle relaxants, depolarizing: ↑ action of muscle relaxants
Phenothiazines: ↑ antagonism

NURSING CONSIDERATIONS

Assessment

- Monitor VS, respiration; increased B/P during test and at baseline
- Monitor diabetic patient carefully, since this drug lowers blood glucose

Nursing diagnoses

✓ Breathing pattern, ineffective (uses)
✓ Knowledge deficit (teaching)

Implementation

IV route

- Give **IV** undiluted, give through Y-tube or 3-way stopcock; give 0.5 mg or less/min
- Give only when atropine sulfate available for cholinergic crisis

Syringe compatibilities:

Glycopyrrolate

Y-site compatibilities:

Heparin, hydrocortisone, potassium chloride, vit B/C

PO route

- Give only after all other cholinergics have been discontinued
- Give increased doses as ordered if tolerance occurs
- Give larger doses as ordered after exercise or fatigue
- Give on empty stomach for better absorption
- Store at room temp

Patient/family education

- Advise patient to wear ID specifying myasthenia gravis, drugs taken

Evaluation

Positive therapeutic outcome

- Increased muscle strength, hand grasp
- Improved gait
- Absence of labored breathing (if severe)

Treatment of overdose: Discontinue drug, atropine 1-4 mg **IV**

pyridoxine (vitamin B_6) (OTC, ℞)

(peer-i-dox'een)

Beesix, Doxine, Nestrex, pyridoxine HCl, Pyri, Rodex, Vitabee 6

Vitamin B_6

Func. class.: Vitamin B_6, water soluble

Pregnancy category A

Action: Needed for fat, protein, carbohydrate metabolism; enhances glycogen release from liver and muscle tissue; needed as coenzyme for metabolic transformations of a variety of amino acids

Therapeutic Outcome: Absence of vitamin B_6 deficiency

Uses: Vitamin B_6 deficiency associated with the following: inborn errors of metabolism, seizures, cycloserine, hydralazine penicillamine, isoniazid therapy, oral contraceptives, alcoholism, polyneuritis

Investigational uses: Palmar-plantar erythrodysesthesia syndrome

Dosage and routes

RDA

Adult: PO male 1.7-2 mg; female 1.4-1.6 mg

Vitamin B_6 deficiency

Adult: PO/IM/**IV** 10-20 mg qd × 3 wk

P ***Child:*** PO/IM/**IV** 100 mg until desired response

Deficiency caused by isoniazid, cycloserine, hydralazine, penicillamine

Adult: PO 6-100 mg qd

P ***Child:*** PO 5-25 mg/day

Prevention of deficiency caused by isoniazid, cycloserine, hydralazine, penicillamine

Adult: PO 6-50 mg qd

P ***Child:*** PO 0.5-1.5 mg qd

P ***Infant:*** PO 0.1-0.5 mg qd

Palmar-plantar erythrodysesthesia syndrome (off-label)

Adult: PO 50-150 mg qd

Available forms: Tabs 10, 25, 50, 100 mg; time rel tabs 100 mg; inj 100 mg/ml; time rel caps 100 mg

Adverse effects

CNS: Paresthesia

INTEG: Pain at inj site

Contraindication: Hypersensitivity

Precautions: Pregnancy **A,** lactation, P children, Parkinson's disease

Pharmacokinetics

Absorption	Well absorbed (PO)
Distribution	Stored in liver, muscle, brain; crosses placenta
Metabolism	Unknown
Excretion	Kidneys, unchanged (not used)
Half-life	Unknown

Pharmacodynamics

Unknown

Interactions

Individual drugs

Chloramphenicol: ↓ effects of pyridoxine

Cycloserine: ↓ effects of pyridoxine

Hydralazine: ↓ effects of pyridoxine

Isoniazid: ↓ effects of pyridoxine

Levodopa: ↓ effects of levodopa

Penicillamine: ↓ effects of pyridoxine

Drug classifications

Immunosuppressants: ↓ effects of pyridoxine

P

Oral contraceptives: ↓ effects of pyridoxine

Lab Test Interferences

False: ↑ urobilinogen

NURSING CONSIDERATIONS

Assessment

- Monitor pyridoxine levels throughout treatment
- Assess nutritional status: yeast, liver, legumes, bananas, green vegetables, whole grains
- Assess for pyridoxine (B_6) deficiency: nausea, vomiting, dermatitis, cheilosis, seizures, irritability, dermatitis before and during treatment

Nursing diagnoses

☑ Nutrition: less then body requirements (uses)

☑ Knowledge deficit (teaching)

☑ Noncompliance (teaching, overuse)

Implementation

IV **IV route**

- Give **IV** undiluted or added to most **IV** sol; give 50 mg or less/1 min if undiluted

IM route

- Rotate sites; burning or stinging at site may occur; give by Z-track to minimize pain
- Store in airtight, light-resistant container

Syringe compatibilities:
Doxapram

Additive incompatibilities:
Erythromycin, iron salts, kanamycin, riboflavin, streptomycin

PO route

- Ext rel cap and tab should be swallowed whole; do not break, crush, or chew

IM/SC route

- Administer in different site each time to avoid pain

Patient/family education

- Teach patient to avoid other vitamin supplements unless directed by prescriber
- Advise patient to increase meat, bananas, potatoes, lima beans, whole grain cereals in diet which are high in vit B_6
- Caution patient not to increase dosage, since serious reactions may occur

Evaluation

Positive therapeutic outcome

- Absence of nausea, vomiting, anorexia, skin lesions, glossitis, stomatitis, edema, convulsions, restlessness, paresthesia

pyrimethamine (℞)

(peer-i-meth′a-meen)

Daraprim, Fansidar (with sulfadoxine)

Func. class.: Antimalarial, antiprotozoal

Chem. class.: Folic acid antagonist

Pregnancy category C

Action: Inhibits folic acid metabolism in parasite; prevents transmission by stopping growth of fertilized gametes

Therapeutic Outcome: Prevention of malaria

Uses: Malaria prophylaxis, antiprotozoal action against *Plasmodium vivax*

Investigational uses: *Pneumocystis carinii* pneumonia as an adjunct

Dosage and routes

Prophylaxis of malaria

P ***Adult and child >10 yr:*** PO 25 mg qwk

P ***Child 4-10 yr:*** PO 12.5 mg qwk

P ***Child <4 yr:*** PO 6.25 mg qwk

Toxoplasmosis

Adult: PO 100 mg, then 25 mg qd × 4-5 wk, with 1 g sulfadiazine q6h

P ***Child:*** PO 1 mg/kg/day in 2 divided doses or 2 mg/kg/day × 3 days, then 1 mg/kg/day or divided twice qd × 4 wk, max 25 mg/day

Toxoplasmosis in AIDS patients

Adult: PO 100-200 mg/day × 1-2 days, then 50-100 mg/day × 3-6 wk, then 25-50 mg/day for life (given with clindamycin or sulfadiazine)

Available forms: Tabs 25 mg; combo tabs 500 mg sulfadoxine/25 mg pyrimethamine

Adverse effects

CNS: Stimulation, irritability, **seizures,** tremors, ataxia, fatigue

CV: **Dysrhythmias**

GI: Nausea, vomiting, cramps, anorexia, diarrhea, atrophic glossitis, gastritis

HEMA: **Thrombocytopenia, leukopenia, pancytopenia, megaloblastic anemia,** decreased folic acid, **agranulocytosis**

INTEG: Skin eruptions, photosensitivity

RESP: **Respiratory failure**

Contraindications: Hypersensitivity, chloroquine-resistant malaria, megaloblastic anemia caused by folate deficiency

Precautions: Blood dyscrasias, seizure disorder, pregnancy **C,** lactation, glucose-6-phosphate dehydrogenase disease, renal/hepatic disease

Pharmacokinetics	
Absorption	Well absorbed
Distribution	Widely; crosses placenta
Metabolism	Liver, extensively
Excretion	Kidneys, unchanged (30%); breast milk
Half-life	4 days

Pharmacodynamics	
Onset	Unknown
Peak	2 hr
Duration	Unknown

Interactions

Individual drugs

Folic acid: ↑ synergistic action

Radiation: ↑ bone marrow suppression

Drug classifications

Antiinfectives: ↑ bone marrow suppression

Bone marrow depressants: ↑ bone marrow suppression

NURSING CONSIDERATIONS

Assessment

- C&S studies should be done before treatment begins and periodically during treatment
- Monitor serum uric acid, which may be elevated and cause gout symptoms
- Monitor liver studies weekly: ALT, AST, bilirubin; hepatic status: decreased appetite, jaundice, dark urine, fatigue
- Monitor renal status before therapy and monthly thereafter: BUN, creatinine, output, sp gr, urinalysis
- Monitor mental status often: affect, mood, behavioral changes; psychosis may occur

Nursing diagnoses

- ✓ Infection, risk for (uses)
- ✓ Diarrhea (adverse reactions)
- ✓ Injury, risk for (adverse reactions)
- ✓ Knowledge deficit (teaching)
- ✓ Noncompliance (teaching)

Implementation

- Give with meals to decrease GI symptoms
- Give antiemetic if vomiting occurs

Patient/family education

- Instruct patient that compliance with dosage schedule, duration is necessary; that scheduled appointments must be kept or relapse may occur
- Advise diabetic patient to use blood glucose monitor to obtain correct result
- Advise patient to report weakness, fatigue, loss of appetite, nausea, vomiting, yellowing of skin or eyes, sore throat, glossitis

P

Evaluation

Positive therapeutic outcome

- Decreased symptoms of toxoplasmosis
- Decreased symptoms of *Pneumocystis carinii* pneumonia

quetiapine (℞)

(kwe-tie′a-peen)

Seroquel

Func. class.: Antipsychotic

Pregnancy category C

Action: Functions as an antagonist at multiple neurotransmitter receptors in the brain including 5-HT_{1A}, 5-HT_2, dopamine D_1, D_2, H_1, adrenergic α_1, α_2 receptors

Therapeutic Outcome: Decreased hallucination and disorganized thought

Uses: Psychotic disorders

Dosage and routes

Adult: PO 25 mg bid, with incremental increases of 25-50 mg bid-tid on days 2 and 3 to a dose of 300-400 mg qd given bid-tid

Available forms: Tabs 25, 100, 200 mg

Adverse effects

CNS: EPS, pseudoparkinsonism, akathisia, dystonia, tardive dyskinesia, drowsiness, insomnia, agitation, anxiety, *headache,* **neuroleptic malignant syndrome,** dizziness

CV: Orthostatic hypotension, **tachycardia**

GI: Nausea, anorexia, constipation, abdominal pain, dry mouth

INTEG: Rash

MISC: Asthenia, back pain, fever, ear pain

RESP: Rhinitis

Contraindications: Hypersensitivity

Precautions: Children, lactation, long-term use, seizures, dementia, pregnancy **C,** hepatic disease, elderly, breast cancer

Pharmacokinetics

Absorption	Rapidly
Distribution	Widely
Metabolism	Liver, extensively
Excretion	Urine, feces
Half-life	≥6 hr

Pharmacodynamics

Onset	Unknown
Peak	1.5 hr
Duration	Up to 12 hr

Interactions

Individual drugs

Carbamazepine: ↑ quetiapine clearance
Cimetidine: ↓ clearance of quetiapine
Fluconazole: ↑ quetiapine action
Itraconazole: ↑ quetiapine action
Ketoconazole: ↑ quetiapine action
Levodopa: ↓ effect of levodopa
Lorazepam: ↓ clearance of lorazepam
Phenytoin: ↑ clearance of quetiapine
Rifampin: ↑ quetiapine clearance
Thioridazine: ↑ clearance of quetiapine

Drug classifications

Barbiturates: ↑ clearance of quetiapine
Dopamine agonists: ↓ effects of dopamine agonists
Glucocorticoids: ↑ clearance of quetiapine

NURSING CONSIDERATIONS

Assessment

- Assess mental status: orientation, mood, behavior, presence and type of hallucinations before initial administration and monthly; this drug should significantly reduce psychotic behavior
- Check that patient swallows all PO medication; check for hoarding or giving of medication to other patients
- Monitor I&O ratio, palpate bladder

if low urinary output occurs, especially in elderly; urinalysis recommended before, during prolonged therapy
• Monitor bilirubin, CBC, liver function studies monthly
• Assess affect, orientation, LOC, reflexes, gait, coordination, sleep pattern disturbances
• Monitor B/P with patient in sitting, standing, and lying positions; take pulse and respirations q4h during initial treatment; establish baseline before starting treatment; report drops of 30 mm Hg; obtain baseline ECG and monitor Q- and T-wave changes
• Check for dizziness, faintness, palpitations, tachycardia on rising; severe orthostatic hypotension is common
• Identify for neuroleptic malignant syndrome: hyperpyrexia, muscle rigidity, increased CPK, altered mental status; drug should be discontinued
• Assess for EPS including akathisia (inability to sit still, no pattern to movements), tardive dyskinesia (bizarre movements of the jaw, mouth, tongue, extremities) pseudoparkinsonism (rigidity, tremors, pill rolling, shuffling gait); an antiparkinson drug should be prescribed
• Assess for constipation, urinary retention daily; if these occur, increase bulk, water in diet

Nursing diagnoses
✓ Thought processes, altered (uses)
✓ Coping, ineffective individual (uses)
✓ Knowledge deficit (teaching)
✓ Noncompliance (teaching)

Implementation
• PO with full glass of water, milk; or give with food to decrease GI upset
• Store in airtight, light-resistant container

Patient/family education
• Teach patient to use good oral hygiene; frequent rinsing of mouth, sugarless gum for dry mouth
• Caution patient to avoid hazardous activities until drug response is determined; dizziness, blurred vision may occur
• Inform patient that orthostatic hypotension occurs often; patient should rise from sitting or lying position gradually
• Instruct patient to avoid hot tubs, hot showers, tub baths; hypotension may occur
• Inform patient that heat stroke may occur in hot weather, and to take extra precautions to stay cool
• Advise patient to avoid abrupt withdrawal of this drug or EPS may result; drug should be withdrawn slowly
• Teach patient to avoid OTC preparations (cough, hayfever, cold) unless approved by prescriber; serious drug interactions may occur; avoid use with alcohol, CNS depressants because increased drowsiness may occur

Evaluation
Positive therapeutic outcome
• Decrease in emotional excitement, hallucinations, delusions, paranoia
• Reorganization of patterns of thought, speech

Treatment of overdose:
Lavage, provide airway

quinapril (℞)
(kwin'a-pril)
Accupril
Func. class.: Antihypertensive
Chem. class.: Angiotensin-converting enzyme (ACE) inhibitor

Pregnancy category
D (2nd/3rd trimesters);
C (1st trimester)

Action: Selectively suppresses renin-angiotensin-aldosterone system; inhibits ACE, prevents conversion of angiotensin I to angiotensin II; results in dilation of arterial, venous vessels

Therapeutic Outcome: Decreased B/P in hypertension

Uses: Hypertension, alone or in combination with thiazide diuretics, systolic CHF

Dosage and routes

Hypertension

Adult: PO 10-20 mg qd initially, then 20-80 mg/day divided bid or qd

G ***Elderly:*** PO 10 mg qd, titrate to desired response

Congestive heart failure

Adult: PO 2.5 mg initially, then 5-40 mg/day maintenance dose given qd or in 2 divided doses

Renal dose

CrCl 30-60 ml/min 5 mg/day initially; CrCl <30 ml/min 2.5 mg/day initially

Available forms: Tabs 5, 10, 20, 40 mg

Adverse effects

CNS: Headache, dizziness, fatigue, somnolence, depression, malaise, nervousness, vertigo

CV: Hypotension, postural hypotension, syncope, palpitations, angina pectoris, MI, tachycardia, vasodilation

GI: Nausea, constipation, vomiting, gastritis, GI hemorrhage, dry mouth

GU: Increased BUN, creatinine, decreased libido, impotence, UTI

HEMA: **Thrombocytopenia, agranulocytosis**

INTEG: **Angioedema,** rash, sweating, photosensitivity, pruritus

META: Hyperkalemia

MISC: Back pain, amblyopia, pharyngitis

MS: Arthralgia, arthritis, myalgia

RESP: Cough, bronchitis

Contraindications: Hypersensitivity to ACE inhibitors, pregnancy **D** (2nd/3rd trimesters), P children

Precautions: Impaired renal and liver function, dialysis patients, hypovolemia, blood dyscrasias, COPD, asthma, G elderly, lactation, pregnancy **C** (1st trimester)

Pharmacokinetics

Absorption	Well absorbed
Distribution	Unknown, crosses placenta
Metabolism	Unknown
Excretion	Unknown
Half-life	2 hr

Pharmacodynamics

Onset	½-1 hr
Peak	2-6 hr
Duration	12-24 hr

Interactions

Individual drugs

Alcohol: ↑ hypotension (large amounts)
Allopurinol: ↑ hypersensitivity
Hydralazine: ↑ toxicity
Indomethacin: ↓ antihypertensive effect
Lithium: ↑ serum levels
Prazosin: ↑ toxicity

Drug classifications

Adrenergic blockers: ↑ hypotension
Antacids: ↓ absorption
Antihypertensives: ↑ hypotension
Diuretics: ↑ hypotension
Diuretics, potassium-sparing: ↑ toxicity
Ganglionic blockers: ↑ hypotension
Nitrates: ↑ hypotension
Potassium supplements: ↑ toxicity
Sympathomimetics: ↑ toxicity

Lab test interferences

False positive: Urine acetone, ANA titer

NURSING CONSIDERATIONS

Assessment

- Monitor blood studies: neutrophils, decreased platelets; WBC with differential baseline and periodically q3 mo; if neutrophils <1000/mm^3 discontinue treatment
- Monitor B/P, check for orthostatic hypotension, syncope; if changes occur dosage change may be required
- Monitor renal studies (protein, BUN, creatinine); and periodically

LFTs, uric acid, also glucose may be elevated; watch for increased levels that may indicate nephrotic syndrome and renal failure; monitor renal symptoms: polyuria, oliguria, frequency, dysuria
- Check potassium levels throughout treatment, although hyperkalemia rarely occurs
- Check for edema in feet, legs daily, weight daily in CHF
- Assess for allergic reactions: rash, fever, pruritus, urticaria; drug should be discontinued if antihistamines fail to help

Nursing diagnoses

✓ Cardiac output, decreased (uses)
✓ Injury, risk for physical (adverse reactions)
✓ Knowledge deficit (teaching)
✓ Noncompliance (teaching)

Implementation

- Store in airtight container at 86° F (30° C) or less
- Severe hypotension may occur after 1st dose of this medication; may be prevented by reducing or discontinuing diuretic therapy 3 days before beginning quinapril therapy

Patient/family education

- Advise patient not to discontinue drug abruptly; advise patient to tell all persons associated with care
- Teach patient not to use OTC products (cough, cold, allergy) unless directed by physician; serious side effects can occur
- Inform patient that xanthines such as coffee, tea, chocolate, cola can prevent action of drug
- Caution patient on the importance of complying with dosage schedule, even if feeling better; to continue with medical regimen to decrease B/P: exercise, cessation of smoking, decreasing stress, diet modifications
- Emphasize the need to rise slowly to sitting or standing position to minimize orthostatic hypotension; not to exercise in hot weather or increased hypotension can occur
- Teach patient to notify prescriber of mouth sores, sore throat, fever, swelling of hands or feet, irregular heartbeat, chest pain, coughing, shortness of breath
- Caution patient to report excessive perspiration, dehydration, vomiting, diarrhea; may lead to fall in B/P
- Caution patient that drug may cause dizziness, fainting, light-headedness; may occur during 1st few days of therapy; to avoid activities that may be hazardous
- Teach patient how to take B/P, and normal readings for age group

Evaluation

Positive therapeutic outcome
- Decreased B/P in hypertension

Treatment of overdose: 0.9% NaCl **IV** inf, hemodialysis

quinidine (℞)

(kwin'i-deen)

Apo-Quinidine ✱, Cin-Quin, Duraquin, Novoquinidin ✱, Quinaglute, Quinalan, quinidine gluconate; Cardioquin; Quinidex Extentabs, quinidine sulfate

Func. class.: Antidysrhythmic (class IA)

Chem. class.: Quinine dextro isomer

Pregnancy category C

Action: Prolongs action potential duration and effective refractory period, thus decreasing myocardial excitability; anticholinergic properties

➔ **Therapeutic Outcome:** Treatment of dysrhythmias

Uses: Premature ventricular contractions (PVCs), atrial fibrillation, flutter; paroxysmal atrial tachycardia, ventricular tachycardia

Investigational uses: Malaria/**IV** quinidine gluconate

Q

Dosage and routes

Quinidine sulfate

Atrial fibrillation/flutter

Adult: PO 200 mg q2-3h × 5-8 doses; may increase qd until sinus rhythm is restored; max 4 g/day given only after digitalization

Paroxysmal supraventricular tachycardia

Adult: PO 400-600 mg q2-3h, then 200-300 mg q6-8h or 300-600 mg q8-12h (sus rel)

Premature atrial/ventricular contraction

Adult: PO 200-300 mg q6-8h or 300-600 mg (sus rel) q8-12h, not to exceed 4 g/day

P ***Child:*** PO 30 mg/kg/day or 900 mg/m^2/day in 5 divided doses

Quinidine gluconate

Adult: PO 324-660 mg q6-12h (sus rel); IM 600 mg, then 400 mg q2h; **IV** give 16 mg/min

Quinidine polygalacteronate

Adult: PO 275-825 mg q3-4h × 4 doses, then increase by 137.5-275 mg; repeat up to 4 × until dysrhythmia decreases

P ***Child:*** PO 8.25 mg/kg (247.5 mg/m^2) 5/day

Pharmacokinetics

Absorption	Well absorbed (PO, IM), slowly absorbed (sus-rel)
Distribution	Widely distributed, crosses placenta
Metabolism	Liver
Excretion	Kidney unchanged, breast milk
Half-life	6-8 hr

Available forms:
Gluconate: sus rel tabs 324, 330 mg; inj gluconate 80 mg/ml; *sulfate:* tabs 200, 300 mg; sus rel tabs 300 mg; *polygalacturonase:* tabs 275 mg

Adverse effects

CNS: *Headache, dizziness,* involuntary movement, confusion, psychosis, restlessness, irritability, syncope, excitement

CV: *Hypotension, bradycardia, PVCs,* **heart block, cardiovascular collapse, arrest, torsade de pointes**

EENT: Cinchonism: tinnitus, blurred vision, hearing loss, mydriasis, disturbed color vision

GI: Nausea, vomiting, anorexia, *diarrhea,* **hepatotoxicity**, abdominal pain

HEMA: **Thrombocytopenia,** hemolytic anemia, agranulocytosis, hypoprothrombinemia

INTEG: Rash, urticaria, angioedema, swelling, photosensitivity

RESP: Dyspnea, **respiratory depression**

Contraindications:
Hypersensitivity, blood dyscrasias, severe heart block, myasthenia gravis

Precautions:
Pregnancy **C**, lactation, P children, renal disease, potassium imbalance, liver disease, CHF, respiratory depression

Interactions

Individual drugs

Amiodarone: ↑ toxicity
Cimetidine: ↑ effects of quinidine
Digoxin: ↑ blood levels, ↑ toxicity
Nifedipine: ↓ effects of quinidine
Phenytoin: ↓ effects of quinidine
Propranolol: ↑ effects of quinidine

Pharmacodynamics

	PO (SULFATE)	PO-SUS REL	PO (GLUCONATE)	PO (POLYGALACTURONASE)	IM	IV
Onset	½ hr	Unknown	Unknown	Unknown	½ hr	5 min
Peak	1-1½ hr	4 hr	4 hr	6 hr	½-1½ hr	Unknown
Duration	6-8 hr	8-12 hr	6-8 hr	8-12 hr	6-8 hr	6-8 hr

Rifampin: ↓ effects of quinidine
Verapamil: ↑ effects of quinidine
Warfarin: ↑ levels of warfarin

Drug classifications
Antacids: ↑ effects of quinidine
Anticholinergics: ↑ vagolytic effects
Anticoagulants, oral: ↑ levels of anticoagulant
Antidysrhythmics: ↑ cardiac depression
Barbiturates: ↓ effects of quinidine
Phenothiazines: ↑ cardiac depression
Thiazide diuretics: ↑ effects of quinidine

Herb/drug
Aloe: ↑ hypokalemia
Buckthorn: ↑ hypokalemia
Cascara sagrada: ↑ hypokalemia
Senna: ↑ hypokalemia

Food/drug
Grapefruit juice: ↓ absorption

Lab test interferences
↑ CPK

NURSING CONSIDERATIONS
Assessment
- Monitor ECG continuously to determine drug effectiveness, measure PR, QRS, QT intervals, check for PVCs, other dysrhythmias; monitor B/P continuously for hypotension, hypertension; for rebound hypertension after 1-2 hr; check for dehydration or hypovolemia
- Monitor I&O ratio, electrolytes (potassium, sodium, chloride); check weight daily; check for signs of CHF or pulmonary toxicity: dyspnea, fatigue, cough, fever, chest pain; if these occur, drug should be discontinued
- Monitor liver function studies: AST, ALT, bilirubin, alkaline phosphatase
- Assess for CNS symptoms: confusion, psychosis, numbness, depression, involuntary movements; if these occur, drug should be discontinued
- Monitor cardiac rate, respiration: rate, rhythm, character, chest pain; watch for ventricular tachycardia, supraventricular tachycardia, or fibrillation that indicates toxicity

Nursing diagnoses
✓ Cardiac output, decreased (uses)
✓ Impaired gas exchange (adverse reactions)
✓ Knowledge deficit (teaching)

Implementation
PO route
- Give on an empty stomach with a full glass of water
- May be given with meals if GI irritation occurs, absorption will be decreased
- Tab may be crushed and mixed with fluid or foods for patients with swallowing difficulties; do not break, chew or crush sus rel tab

IV route
- Give by intermittent inf after diluting 800 mg/50 ml of D_5W; gluconate: (16 mg/ml) give at 1 ml/min or less using an infusion pump for correct dose
- Do not use colored sol or sol with precipitate
- Diluted quinidine is stable for 24 hr at room temp

Y-site compatibilities:
Diazepam, milrinone

Y-site incompatibilities:
Furosemide

Additive compatibilities:
Bretylium, cimetidine, milrinone, ranitidine, verapamil

Additive incompatibilities:
Amiodarone

Patient/family education
- Instruct patient to report adverse effects immediately to prescriber
- Caution patient that sunglasses may be needed for photophobia; to use sunscreen, protective clothing, or stay out of sun to prevent burns
- Instruct patient to complete follow-up appointments with health care provider including pulmonary function studies, chest x-ray, ophth and otoscopic exams

Q

Treatment of overdose: O_2, artificial ventilation, ECG, administer dopamine for circulatory depression, administer diazepam or thiopental for seizures, isoproterenol

rabeprazole (℞)

(rab-ee-pray'zole)

Aciphex

Func. class.: Proton pump inhibitor

Chem. class.: Benzimidazole

Pregnancy category C

Action: Suppresses gastric secretion by inhibiting hydrogen/potassium ATPase enzyme system in the gastric parietal cell; characterized as a gastric acid pump inhibitor, since it blocks the final step of acid production

Therapeutic Outcome: Absence of duodenal ulcers; decreased gastroesophageal reflux

Uses: Gastroesophageal reflux disease (GERD), severe erosive esophagitis, poorly responsive systemic GERD, pathologic hypersecretory conditions (Zollinger-Ellison syndrome, systemic mastocytosis, multiple endocrine adenomas); possibly effective for treatment of duodenal ulcers

Dosage and routes

Healing of duodenal ulcers

Adult: PO 20 mg qd × ≤4 wk, to be taken after breakfast

Erosive esophagitis/GERD

Adult: PO 20 mg qd × 4-8 wk

Pathologic hypersecretory conditions

Adult: PO 60 mg/day; may increase to 120 mg in 2 divided doses

Available forms: Tabs, delayed rel 20 mg

Adverse effects

CNS: *Headache, dizziness, asthenia*

CV: Chest pain, angina, tachycardia, bradycardia, palpitations, peripheral edema

EENT: Tinnitus, taste perversion

GI: *Diarrhea, abdominal pain, vomiting, nausea, constipation, flatulence, acid regurgitation,* abdominal swelling, anorexia, irritable colon, esophageal candidiasis, dry mouth

GU: UTI, frequency, increased creatinine, **proteinuria, hematuria,** testicular pain, glycosuria

HEMA: **Pancytopenia, thrombocytopenia, neutropenia, leukocytosis,** anemia

INTEG: Rash, dry skin, urticaria, pruritus, alopecia

META: Hypoglycemia, increased hepatic enzymes, weight gain

MISC: *Back pain,* fever, fatigue, malaise

RESP: *Upper respiratory tract infections, cough,* epistaxis

Contraindications: Hypersensitivity

Precautions: Pregnancy **C,** lactation, children

Pharmacokinetics

Absorption	Unknown
Distribution	Unknown
Metabolism	Liver, extensively
Excretion	Kidneys, feces
Half-life	Unknown

Pharmacodynamics

Unknown

Interactions

Individual drugs

Clarithromycin: ↑ levels of rapeprazole

Diazepam: ↑ serum levels of rapeprazole

Phenytoin: ↑ serum levels of rapeprazole

Sucralfate: ↓ rapeprazole levels

Drug classifications

Benzodiazepines: ↑ levels of rapeprazole

NURSING CONSIDERATIONS
Assessment
- Assess GI system: bowel sounds q8h, abdomen for pain and swelling, anorexia
- Monitor hepatic enzymes: AST, ALT, increased alkaline phosphatase during treatment

Nursing diagnoses
✓ Pain (uses)
✓ Knowledge deficit (teaching)

Implementation
- Give after breakfast qd; do not crush, break, chew delayed rel tab

Patient/family education
- Advise patient to report severe diarrhea; drug may have to be discontinued
- Caution patient to avoid driving and other hazardous activities until response to drug is known
- Caution patient to avoid alcohol, salicylates, NSAIDs; may cause GI irritation

Evaluation
Positive therapeutic outcome
- Absence of epigastric pain, swelling, fullness

raloxifene (℞)
(ral-ox′ih-feen)
Evista
Func. class.: Bone resorption inhibitor, selective estrogen receptor modulator (SERM)
Chem. class.: Benzthiophene

Pregnancy category X

Action: Reduces resorption of bone and decreases bone turnover; mediated through estrogen receptor binding

➔ Therapeutic Outcome: Absence of osteoporosis in postmenopausal women

Uses: Prevention of osteoporosis in postmenopausal women

Dosage and routes
Hormone replacement
Adult: PO 60 mg qd

Available forms: Tabs 60 mg

Adverse effects
CNS: Insomnia, migraines, depression
CV: Hot flashes
GI: ***Nausea,*** vomiting, diarrhea, anorexia, cramps
GU: Vaginitis, UTI, leukorrhea, endometrial disorder, breast pain
INTEG: Rash, sweating
META: Weight gain, peripheral edema
MS: Arthralgia, myalgia, leg cramps, arthritis
RESP: Sinusitis, pharyngitis, increased cough, pneumonia, laryngitis

Contraindications: Hypersensitivity, pregnancy **X**, lactation

Precautions: Lactation, venous thromboembolic events, hepatic disease

Pharmacokinetics	
Absorption	Unknown
Distribution	Highly protein bound
Metabolism	Unknown
Excretion	Feces, breast milk
Half-life	28-32 hr (elimination)

Pharmacodynamics	
Onset	Unknown
Peak	Unknown
Duration	Unknown

Interactions
Individual drugs
Ampicillin: ↓ action of raloxifene
Cholestyramine: ↓ action of raloxifene
Drug classifications
Anticoagulants: ↓ action of anticoagulants
Highly protein-bound drugs: Administer cautiously
Lab test interferences
↑ Apolipoproteins A_1 and B, ↑ lipoprotein, ↑ fibrinogen, ↑ LDL cholesterol, ↑ total cholesterol, ↑ corticoste-

R

roid-binding globulin, ↑ thyroxine-binding globulin (TBG)
↓ Calcium, ↓ total protein, ↓ albumin, ↓ platelets

NURSING CONSIDERATIONS

Assessment

- Obtain bone density test baseline and periodically throughout treatment
- Monitor blood glucose of diabetic patients
- Monitor weight daily, notify prescriber of weekly weight gain >5 lb
- Monitor B/P q4h, watch for increase caused by H_2O and sodium retention
- Monitor liver function studies: AST, ALT, bilirubin, alkaline phosphatase
- Monitor I&O ratio; decreasing urinary output, increasing edema

Nursing diagnoses

☑ Immobility, risk for (uses)
☑ Knowledge deficit (teaching)

Implementation

PO route

- Administer without regard to meals

Patient/family education

- Teach patient to weigh weekly, report gain >5 lb
- Teach patients to discontinue drug 72 hr before prolonged bedrest
- Advise patient to avoid maintaining one position for long periods
- Advise patient to take calcium supplements, vit D if intake is inadequate
- Advise patient to increase exercise using weights
- Advise patient to stop smoking and to decrease alcohol consumption
- Inform patient that this drug does not help control hot flashes
- Teach patient to report fever, acute migraine, insomnia, emotional distress; UTI or vaginal burning/itching; swelling, warmth, or pain in calves

Evaluation

Positive therapeutic outcome

- Prevention of osteoporosis

ramipril (℞)

(ra-mi'pril)
Altace
Func. class.: Antihypertensive
Chem. class.: Angiotensin-converting enzyme (ACE) inhibitor

Pregnancy category
D (2nd/3rd trimesters), C (1st trimester)

Action: Selectively suppresses renin-angiotensin-aldosterone system; inhibits ACE; prevents conversion of angiotensin I to angiotensin II; results in dilation of arterial, venous vessels

➔ **Therapeutic Outcome:** Decreased B/P in hypertension

Uses: Hypertension, alone or in combination with thiazide diuretics; CHF (after MI), reduction in risk of MI, stroke, death from CV disorders

Dosage and routes

Adult: PO 2.5 mg qd initially, then 2.5-20 mg/day divided bid or qd; renal impairment: 1.25 mg qd with CrCl <40 ml/min/1.73 m^2, increase as needed to max 5 mg/day

CHF

Adult: PO 1.25-2.5 mg bid, may increase to 5 mg bid

Available forms: Caps 1.25, 2.5, 5, 10 mg

Adverse effects

CNS: *Headache, dizziness,* anxiety, insomnia, paresthesia, fatigue, depression, malaise, vertigo, **seizures,** hearing loss
CV: *Hypotension,* chest pain, palpitations, angina, syncope, **dysrhythmia**
GI: Nausea, constipation, vomiting, dyspepsia, dysphagia, anorexia, diarrhea, abdominal pain
GU: **Proteinuria,** increased BUN, creatinine, impotence
HEMA: Decreased Hct, Hgb, **eosinophilia, leukopenia**
INTEG: **Angioedema,** rash, sweating, photosensitivity, pruritus

META: Hyperkalemia
MS: Arthralgia, arthritis, myalgia
RESP: Cough, dyspnea

Contraindications: Hypersensitivity to ACE inhibitors, pregnancy **D** (2nd/3rd trimesters), lactation, P children

Precautions: Impaired renal and liver function, dialysis patients, hypovolemia, blood dyscrasias, COPD, G asthma, elderly, renal artery stenosis, pregnancy **C** (1st trimester)

Do Not Confuse:
Altace/alteplase, Altace/Artane, ramipril/enalapril

Pharmacokinetics

Absorption	Well absorbed
Distribution	Not known, crosses placenta
Metabolism	Liver, extensively
Excretion	Urine
Half-life	Ramipril (5 hr), ramiprilat (24 hr)

Pharmacodynamics

Onset	½-1 hr
Peak	6-8 hr
Duration	24-72 hr

Interactions

Individual drugs

Alcohol: ↑ hypotension (large amounts)
Allopurinol: ↑ hypersensitivity
Digoxin: ↑ serum levels
Hydralazine: ↑ toxicity
Indomethacin: ↓ antihypertensive effect
Lithium: ↑ serum levels
Prazosin: ↑ toxicity

Drug classifications

Adrenergic blockers: ↑ hypotension
Antacids: ↓ absorption
Antihypertensives: ↑ hypotension
Diuretics: ↑ hypotension
Diuretics, potassium sparing: ↑ toxicity
Ganglionic blockers: ↑ hypotension
Nitrates: ↑ hypotension
Potassium supplements: ↑ toxicity
Sympathomimetics: ↑ toxicity

Lab test interferences

False positive: Urine acetone, ANA titer

NURSING CONSIDERATIONS

Assessment

- Monitor blood studies: neutrophils, decreased platelets; WBC with differential baseline and periodically q3mo, if neutrophils <1000/mm^3, discontinue treatment
- Monitor B/P, check for orthostatic hypotension, syncope; if changes occur, dosage may need to be changed
- Monitor renal studies: protein, BUN, creatinine; watch for increased levels that may indicate nephrotic syndrome and renal failure; monitor renal symptoms: polyuria, oliguria, frequency, dysuria
- Establish baselines in renal, liver function tests before therapy begins and monitor periodically; LFTs, uric acid, and glucose may be increased
- Check potassium levels throughout treatment, although hyperkalemia rarely occurs
- Check for edema in feet, legs daily, weight daily in CHF
- Assess for allergic reactions: rash, fever, pruritus, urticaria; drug should be discontinued if antihistamines fail to help

Nursing diagnoses

- ✓ Cardiac output, decreased (uses)
- ✓ Injury, risk for (side effects)
- ✓ Knowledge deficit (teaching)
- ✓ Noncompliance (teaching)

Implementation

- Caps can be opened and added to food
- Store in airtight container at 86° F (30° C) or less
- Severe hypotension may occur after 1st dose of this medication; decreased hypotension may be prevented by reducing or discontinuing diuretic

R

therapy 3 days before beginning benazepril therapy
• Give **IV** inf of 0.9% NaCl (as ordered) to expand fluid volume if severe hypotension occurs

Patient/family education
• Caution patient not to discontinue drug abruptly; advise patient to tell all persons associated with care
• Teach patient not to use OTC products (cough, cold, allergy) unless directed by physician; serious side effects can occur; xanthines such as coffee, tea, chocolate, cola can prevent action of drug
• Instruct patient on the importance of complying with dosage schedule, even if feeling better; to continue with medical regimen to decrease B/P: exercise, cessation of smoking, decreasing stress, diet modifications
• Emphasize the need to rise slowly to sitting or standing position to minimize orthostatic hypotension; not to exercise in hot weather because increased hypotension can occur
• Teach patient to notify prescriber of mouth sores, sore throat, fever, swelling of hands or feet, irregular heartbeat, chest pain, coughing, shortness of breath
• Caution patient to report excessive perspiration, dehydration, vomiting, diarrhea; may lead to fall in B/P
• Caution patient that drug may cause dizziness, fainting, lightheadedness; may occur during 1st few days of therapy; to avoid activities that may be hazardous
• Teach patient how to take B/P, and normal readings for age group

Evaluation
Positive therapeutic outcome
• Decreased B/P in hypertension

Treatment of overdose: 0.9% NaCl **IV** inf, hemodialysis

ranitidine (℞)
(ra-nit′i-deen)
Apo-Ranitidine ♣, Zantac, Zantac-C ♣

ranitidine bismuth citrate
Tritec

Func. class.: H_2 histamine receptor antagonist

Pregnancy category B

Action: Inhibits histamine at H_2 receptor site in the gastric parietal cells, which inhibits gastric acid secretion

➔ **Therapeutic Outcome:** Healing of duodenal ulcers or gastric ulcers; prevention of duodenal ulcers; decreases symptoms of gastroesophageal reflux disease (GERD) or Zollinger-Ellison syndrome

Uses: Short-term treatment of duodenal and gastric ulcers and maintenance; management of GERD, Zollinger-Ellison syndrome, active duodenal ulcers with *Helicobacter pylori* in combination with clarithromycin

Investigational uses: Prevention of aspiration pneumonitis, stress ulcers, upper GI bleeding

Dosage and routes
Renal dose
CrCl <50 ml/min PO q24h, IM/**IV** q8-24h

Adult: PO 150 mg bid, 300 mg hs; IM 50 mg q6-8h; **IV** bol 50 mg diluted to 20 ml over 5 min q6-8h; **IV** intermittent inf 50 mg/100 ml of D_5 over 15-20 min q6-8h

P ***Child:*** PO 4-5 mg/kg/day divided q8-12h, max 6 mg/kg/day or 300 mg; **IV** 2-4 mg/kg/day divided q6-8h

Duodenal ulcer
Adult: PO 150 mg bid, maintenance 150 mg hs

Zollinger-Ellison syndrome
Adult: PO 150 mg bid, may increase if needed
Gastric ulcer
Adult: PO 150 mg bid × 6 wk, then 150 mg hs
GERD
Adult: PO 150 mg bid
Erosive esophagitis
Adult: PO 150 mg qid
Ranitidine bismuth citrate
Adult: PO 400 mg bid × 4 wk with clarithromycin 500 mg tid × 1st 2 wk

Available forms: *Ranitidine:* tabs 75, 150, 300 mg; inj 0.5, 25 mg/ml; caps ✦ 150, 300 mg; syrup 15 mg/ml; sol for inj 25 mg/ml; effervescent tabs 75, 100 mg; effervescent granules 150 mg/packet; *ranitidine bismuth citrate:* tabs 400 mg

Adverse effects
CNS: Headache, sleeplessness, dizziness, confusion, agitation, depression, hallucination
CV: Tachycardia, bradycardia, premature ventricular contractions
EENT: Blurred vision, increased ocular pressure
GI: Constipation, abdominal pain, diarrhea, nausea, vomiting, **hepatotoxicity**
GU: Impotence, gynecomastia
INTEG: Urticaria, rash, fever

Contraindications: Hypersensitivity

Precautions: Pregnancy **B,** lactation, child <12 yr, hepatic disease, renal disease

Do Not Confuse:
ranitidine/amantadine, Zantac/Xanax, Zantac/Zofran

Pharmacokinetics

Absorption	Well absorbed (PO, IM), completely absorbed (**IV**)
Distribution	Widely distributed, crosses placenta
Metabolism	Liver (30%)
Excretion	Kidneys unchanged (70%)
Half-life	2-3 hr, ↑ renal disease

Pharmacodynamics

	PO	IV/IM
Onset	Unknown	Unknown
Peak	2-3 hr	15 min
Duration	8-12 hr	8-12 hr

Interactions
Individual drugs
Ketoconazole: ↓ absorption of ranitidine
Drug classifications
Antacids: ↓ absorption of ranitidine
Smoking
↓ Effectiveness
Lab test interferences
↑ Alkaline phosphatase, ↑ AST, ↑ creatinine
False positive: Gastric bleeding test

NURSING CONSIDERATIONS
Assessment
- Assess patient with ulcers or suspected ulcers: epigastric or abdominal pain, hematemesis, occult blood in stools, blood in gastric aspirate before and throughout treatment, monitor gastric pH (5 should be maintained)
- Monitor I&O ratio, BUN, creatinine, CBC with differential monthly

Nursing diagnoses
✓ Pain (uses)
✓ Knowledge deficit (teaching)

Implementation
PO route
- May be given with or without meals
- Give antacids 1 hr before or 1 hr after this drug

IV **IV route**

Direct **IV**

- Give by direct **IV** after diluting 50 mg/20 ml of 0.9% D_5W, NaCl over 5 min or more

Intermittent infusion

- Give by intermittent inf over 15 min after diluting 50 mg/100 ml of D_5W, 0.9% NaCl

Continuous infusion

- Give by continuous inf for a concentration 150 mg/250 ml, give 6.25 mg/hr
- Give Zollinger-Ellison patients up to a conc of 2.5 mg/ml at 1 mg/kg/hr initially

Syringe compatibilities:
Atropine, cyclizine, dexamethasone, dimenhydrinate, diphenhydramine, dobutamine, dopamine, fentanyl, glycopyrrolate, hydromorphone, meperidine, metoclopramide, morphine, nalbuphine, oxymorphone, pentazocine, perphenazine, prochlorperazine, promethazine, scopolamine

Syringe incompatibilities:
Hydroxyzine, methotrimeprazine, midazolam, pentobarbital, phenobarbital

Y-site compatibilities: Acyclovir, aldesleukin, allopurinol, amifostine, aminophylline, atracurium, aztreonam, bretylium, dobutamine, dopamine, doxorubicin, enalaprilat, epinephrine, esmolol, fentanyl, filgrastim, fluconazole, fludarabine, foscarnet, furosemide, gallium, granisetron, heparin, hydromorphone, idarubicin, labetalol, lorazepam, melphalan, meperidine, methotrexate, midazolam, milrinone, morphine, nicardipine, nitroglycerin, norepinephrine, ondansetron, paclitaxel, pancuronium, piperacillin, piperacillin/tazobactam, procainamide, propofol, sargramostim, vecuronium, zidovudine

Additive compatibilities:
Acetazolamide, amikacin, aminophylline, chloramphenicol, chlorothiazide, ciprofloxacin, colistimethate, dexamethasone, digoxin, dobutamine, dopamine, doxycycline, furosemide, gentamicin, heparin, lidocaine, penicillin G sodium, potassium chloride, ticarcillin, tobramycin, vancomycin

Additive incompatibilities:
Amphotericin B, clindamycin

Patient/family education

- Caution patient that gynecomastia, impotence may occur and are reversible after treatment is discontinued
- Advise patient to avoid driving, other hazardous activities until stabilized on this medication; drowsiness or dizziness may occur
- Caution patient to avoid black pepper, caffeine, alcohol, harsh spices, extremes in temp of food; tell patient to avoid OTC preparations (aspirin, cough, cold preparations) because condition may worsen
- Inform patient that smoking decreases the effectiveness of the drug; that smoking cessation should be considered
- Instruct patient that drug must be continued for prescribed time to be effective and taken exactly as prescribed; doses should not be doubled; a missed dose should be taken when remembered up to 1 hr before next dose
- Advise patient to report bruising, fatigue, malaise; blood dyscrasias may occur
- Inform patient to report diarrhea, black tarry stools, sore throat, rash, dizziness, confusion, rash, or delirium to prescriber immediately

Evaluation

Positive therapeutic outcome

- Decreased pain in abdomen
- Healing of ulcers
- Absence of gastroesophageal reflux

HIGH ALERT

remifentanil (℞)

(re-me-fin'ta-nill)

Ultiva

Func. class.: Opiate agonist analgesic

Chem. class.: µ-Opioid agonist

Pregnancy category C

Controlled substance schedule II

Action: Inhibits ascending pain pathways in limbic system, thalamus, midbrain, hypothalamus

➔ **Therapeutic Outcome:** Maintenance of anesthesia

Uses: In combination with other drugs in general anesthesia, as a primary anesthetic in general surgery

Dosage and routes

Adult: Induction **IV** 0.5-1 µg/kg/min with a hypnotic or volatile agent; maintenance with isoflurane (0.4-1.5 MAC) or propofol (100-200 µg/kg/min) 0.25 µg/kg/min

Available forms: Powder for inj, lyophilized 1 mg/ml after reconstitution

Adverse effects

CNS: Drowsiness, *dizziness,* confusion, *headache,* sedation, euphoria, delirium, agitation, anxiety

CV: Palpitations, **bradycardia,** change in B/P; facial flushing, syncope, **asystole**

EENT: Tinnitus, blurred vision, miosis, diplopia

GI: *Nausea, vomiting,* anorexia, constipation, cramps, dry mouth

GU: Urinary retention, dysuria

INTEG: Rash, urticaria, bruising, flushing, diaphoresis, pruritus

MS: Rigidity

RESP: **Respiratory depression, apnea**

P **Contraindications:** Child <12 yr, hypersensitivity

Precautions: Pregnancy **C,** lactation, increased ICP, acute MI, severe heart disease; renal disease, hepatic disease, asthma, respiratory conditions, seizure disorders, elderly G

Pharmacokinetics

Absorption	Complete
Distribution	Unknown
Metabolism	Unknown
Excretion	Unknown
Half-life	Unknown

Pharmacodynamics

Onset	Immediate
Peak	Unknown
Duration	Unknown

Interactions

Individual drugs

Alcohol: ↑ respiratory depression, hypotension, profound sedation

Drug classifications

Antihistamines: ↑ respiratory depression, hypotension, profound sedation

Phenothiazines: ↑ respiratory depression, hypotension, profound sedation

Sedative/hypnotics: ↑ respiratory depression, hypotension, profound sedative

NURSING CONSIDERATIONS

Assessment

- Monitor I&O ratio, check for decreasing output; may indicate urinary retention, especially in elderly G
- Assess CNS changes: dizziness, drowsiness, hallucinations, euphoria, LOC pupil reaction
- Assess allergic reactions: rash, urticaria
- Assess respiratory dysfunction: respiratory depression, character, rate, rhythm; notify prescriber if respira-

R

tions are <12/min; CV status, bradycardia, syncope

- Use pain scoring to determine pain perception

Nursing diagnoses

✓ Knowledge deficit (teaching)

Implementation

- Give by direct **IV** over 1½-3 min; use tuberculin syringe
- Store in light-resistant area at room temperature

Y-site compatibilities: Acyclovir, alfentanil, amikacin, aminophylline, ampicillin, ampicillin/sulbactam, amrinone, aztreonam, bretylium, bumetanide, buprenorphine, butorphanol, calcium gluconate, cefazolin, cefotaxime, cefotetan, cefoxitin, ceftazidime, ceftizoxime, ceftriaxone, cefuroxime, cimetidine, ciprofloxacin, cisatracurium, clindamycin, dexamethasone, digoxin, diphenhydramine, dobutamine, dopamine, doxycycline, droperidol, enalaprilat, epinephrine, esmolol, famotidine, fentanyl, fluconazole, furosemide, ganciclovir, gentamicin, haloperidol, heparin, hydrocortisone sodium succinate, hydromorphone, hydroxyzine, imipenem/cilastatin, isoproterenol, ketorolac, lidocaine, lorazepam, magnesium sulfate, mannitol, meperidine, methlyprednisolone sodium succinate, metoclopramide, metronidazole, mezlocillin, midazolam, minocycline, morphine, nalbuphine, netilmicin, nitroglycerin, norepinephrine, ofloxacin, ondansetron

Patient/family education

- Advise patient to call for assistance when ambulating or smoking; drowsiness, dizziness may occur
- Advise patient to make position changes slowly to prevent orthostatic hypotension

Evaluation

Positive therapeutic outcome

- Maintenance of anesthesia

repaglinide (℞)

(re-pag′lih-nide)

Prandin

Func. class.: Antidiabetic

Chem. class.: Meglitinides

Pregnancy category C

Action: Causes functioning β-cells in pancreas to release insulin, leading to drop in blood glucose levels; closes ATP-dependent potassium channels in the β-cell membrane; this leads to opening of calcium channels; increased calcium influx induces insulin secretion

➔ **Therapeutic Outcome:** Blood glucose controlled

Uses: Stable adult-onset diabetes mellitus, type II (NIDDM)

Dosage and routes

Adult: PO 1-2 mg with each meal, max 16 mg/day, adjust at weekly intervals

Available forms: Tabs 0.5, 1, 2 mg

Adverse effects

CNS: ***Headache, weakness,*** paresthesia

ENDO: ***Hypoglycemia***

GI: Nausea, vomiting, diarrhea, constipation, dyspepsia

INTEG: Rash, allergic reactions

MS: Back pains, arthralgia

RESP: URI, sinusitis, rhinitis, bronchitis

Contraindications: Hypersensitivity to meglitinides, diabetic ketoacidosis, type I diabetes

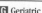

G **Precautions:** Pregnancy **C,** elderly, cardiac disease, severe renal disease, severe hepatic disease, thyroid disease, severe hypoglycemic reactions,
P lactation, children

Pharmacokinetics

Absorption	Complete
Distribution	98% protein binding, crosses placenta
Metabolism	Liver
Excretion	Urine/feces
Half-life	1 hr

Pharmacodynamics

Onset	2-4 hr
Peak	2-8 hr
Duration	24 hr

Interactions
Individual drugs
Carbamazepine: ↑ repaglinide metabolism
Chloramphenicol: ↑ effect of repaglinide
Erythromycin: ↓ repaglinide metabolism
Isoniazid: ↓ action of repaglinide
Phenobarbital: ↓ action of repaglinide
Phenytoin: ↓ action of repaglinide
Probenecid: ↑ effect of repaglinide
Rifampin: ↓ action of repaglinide
Drug classifications
Antifungals: ↓ repaglinide metabolism
Barbiturates: ↑ repaglinide metabolism
β-Adrenergic blockers: ↑ repaglinide effect
Calcium channel blockers: ↓ repaglinide effect
Corticosteroids: ↓ repaglinide effect
Coumarins: ↑ repaglinide effect
Diuretics, thiazide: ↓ repaglinide effect
Estrogens: ↓ repaglinide effect
NSAIDs: ↑ repaglinide effect
Oral contraceptives: ↓ repaglinide effect
Phenothiazines ↓ repaglinide effect
Salicylates: ↑ repaglinide effect
Sulfonamides: ↑ repaglinide effect
Sympathomimetics: ↓ repaglinide effect
Thyroid preparations: ↓ repaglinide effect
Herb/drug
Broom: ↓ hypoglycemia
Buchu: ↓ hypoglycemia
Chromium: ↑ or ↓ hypoglycemia
Dandelion: ↓ hypoglycemia
Fenugreek: ↑ or ↓ hypoglycemia
Ginseng: ↑ or ↓ hypoglycemia
Juniper: ↓ hypoglycemia
Karela: ↑ glucose tolerance

NURSING CONSIDERATIONS
Assessment
- Assess for hypoglycemic or hyperglycemic reaction, which can occur soon after meals

Nursing diagnoses
- ✓ Nutrition, altered (more than body requirements) (uses)
- ✓ Knowledge deficit (teaching)
- ✓ Noncompliance (teaching)

Implementation
PO route
- 15 min before meals: 2, 3, or 4 ×/day preprandially
- Skip dose if meal is skipped; add dose if meal is added
- Store in airtight container in cool environment

Patient/family education
- Advise patient to avoid alcohol; explain disulfiram reaction
- Teach patient to use a capillary blood glucose test while taking this drug
- Teach patient the symptoms of hypoglycemia and hyperglycemia; what to do about each
- Teach patient that drug must be continued on daily basis; explain consequence of discontinuing drug abruptly
- Advise patient to avoid OTC medications unless ordered by prescriber
- Advise patient that diabetes is a lifelong illness; drug will not cure disease
- Advise patient to eat all food included in diet plan to prevent

R

hypoglycemia; to have glucagon emergency kit available
- Instruct patient to carry a ID for emergency purposes

Evaluation
Positive therapeutic outcome
- Decrease in polyuria, polydipsia, polyphagia, clear sensorium, absence of dizziness, stable gait

Treatment of overdose:
Glucose 25 g **IV** via D_{50} sol, 50 ml or 1 mg glucagon

reserpine (℞)
(re-ser'peen)
Novoreserpine ♣, Reserfia ♣, reserpine
Func. class.: Antihypertensive, antiadrenergic agent (peripherally acting)
Chem. class.: Rauwolfia derivative
Pregnancy category D

Action: Inhibits norepinephrine release, depleting norepinephrine stores in adrenergic nerve endings; therapeutic effect is due to peripheral effect

Therapeutic Outcome: Decreased B/P

Uses: Hypertension

Dosage and routes
Hypertension
Adult: PO 0.25-0.5 mg qd × 1-2 wk, then 0.1-0.25 mg qd for maintenance
G ***Elderly:*** PO 0.05 mg qd, increase by 0.05 weekly to desired dose
Psychiatric disorders
Adult: PO 0.5 mg qd, range 0.1-1 mg

Available forms: Tabs 0.1, 0.25 mg

Adverse effects
CNS: *Drowsiness, fatigue, lethargy, dizziness,* depression, anxiety, headache, increased dreaming, nightmares, seizures, parkinsonism, EPS (high doses)
CV: *Bradycardia,* chest pain, dysrhythmias, prolonged bleeding time, **thrombocytopenia,** purpura
EENT: Lacrimation, miosis, blurred vision, ptosis, dry mouth, epistaxis
GI: Nausea, vomiting, cramps, peptic ulcer, dry mouth, increased appetite, anorexia
GU: Impotence, dysuria, nocturia, sodium and H_2O retention, edema, breast engorgement, galactorrhea, gynecomastia
INTEG: Rash, purpura, alopecia, flushing, warm feeling, pruritus, ecchymosis
RESP: **Bronchospasm,** dyspnea, cough, rales

Contraindications: Hypersensitivity, depression, suicidal patients, active peptic ulcer disease, ulcerative colitis, pregnancy **D,** Parkinson's disease

Precautions: Lactation, seizure P disorders, renal disease, children

Do Not Confuse:
reserpine/Risperdal

Pharmacokinetics

Absorption	40%-50%
Distribution	Widely distributed, crosses placenta
Metabolism	Liver
Excretion	Feces 50% unabsorbed drug, kidneys small amounts
Half-life	11 days

Pharmacodynamics

Onset	Unknown
Peak	4 hr
Duration	1-6 wk

Interactions
Individual drugs
Alcohol: ↑ CNS depression
Drug classifications
Amphetamines: ↓ hypotensive effects
Anesthetics: ↑ CNS depression

Antidepressants, tricyclic: ↓ hypotensive effects
β-Adrenergic blockers: ↑ bradycardia
Cardiac glycosides: ↑ bradycardia
Diuretics: ↑ hypotensive effects
MAOIs: avoid use
Nitrates: ↑ hypotensive effects
Opiates: ↑ CNS depression
Sedative/hypnotics: ↑ CNS depression

Lab test interferences
↑ VMA excretion, ↑ 5-HIAA excretion, ↑ prolactin
Interference: 17-OHCS, 17-KS

NURSING CONSIDERATIONS

Assessment

- Monitor B/P, orthostatic hypotension, syncope; check for edema in feet, legs daily; check I&O ratio; monitor weight daily; notify prescriber of changes
- Assess for allergic reactions: rash, fever, pruritus, urticaria; drug should be discontinued if antihistamines fail to help
- Assess for orthostatic hypotension, tell patient to rise slowly from sitting or lying position

Nursing diagnoses

✓ Cardiac output, decreased (uses)
✓ Injury, risk for (adverse reactions)
✓ Knowledge deficit (teaching)
✓ Noncompliance (teaching)

Implementation

- Store in airtight container at 86° F (30° C) or less
- May be used in combination with other antihypertensives
- May be given with food to prevent GI symptoms

Patient/family education

- Caution patient not to discontinue drug abruptly and discuss the importance of complying with dosage schedule, even if feeling better; if dose is missed take as soon as remembered; take dose at same time each day
- Teach patient not to use OTC products (cough, cold, allergy) unless directed by prescriber and to avoid large amounts of caffeine
- Emphasize the need to rise slowly to sitting or standing position to minimize orthostatic hypotension
- Teach patient to notify prescriber of swelling of hands or feet, irregular heartbeat, chest pain
- Caution patient to report excessive perspiration, dehydration, vomiting, diarrhea; may lead to fall in B/P
- Caution patient that drug may cause dizziness, fainting, light-headedness; may occur during 1st few days of therapy; to avoid hazardous activities
- Teach patient how to take B/P, and normal readings for age group; to take B/P q7 days

Evaluation

Positive therapeutic outcome

- Decreased B/P in hypertension, decrease in psychiatric symptoms

Treatment of overdose:

Administer volume expanders or vasopressors; discontinue drug; place patient in supine position

respiratory syncytial virus immune globulin (RSV-IGIV) (℞)

RespiGam
Func. class.: Immune serums
Chem. class.: Immunoglobulin G (IgG)

Pregnancy category C

Action: High titer of neutralizing antibody against respiratory syncytial virus (RSV)

➔ **Therapeutic Outcome:** Resolution of infection

Uses: Prevention of serious lower respiratory tract infection caused by RSV in children <2 yr with broncho-

R

pulmonary dysplasia or premature birth

Dosage and routes

P ***Child <2 yr:*** **IV** inf 1.5 ml/kg/hr × 15 min, then 3 ml/kg/hr 15-30 min; then 6 ml/kg/hr from 30 min to end of inf given monthly

Available forms: Inj 2500 mg

Adverse effects

CNS: Fever

CV: Hypertension, tachycardia, fluid overload

GI: Diarrhea, gastroenteritis, vomiting

OTHER: Rash, overdose effect, inj site inflammation, **anaphylaxis, angioneurotic edema**

RESP: **Respiratory distress, hypoxia,** tachypnea, rales, wheezing

Contraindications: Hypersensitivity to this drug or other human immunoglobulin preparations; IgA deficiency

Precautions: Pregnancy **C**, fluid overload

Pharmacokinetics	
Absorption	Unknown
Distribution	Unknown
Metabolism	Unknown
Excretion	Unknown
Half-life	Unknown

Pharmacodynamics

Unknown

Interactions

Individual drugs

DPT vaccine: ↓ immune response

***Haemophilus* influenza b vaccine:** ↓ immune response

MMR vaccine: ↓ immune response

NURSING CONSIDERATIONS

Assessment

- Monitor VS for increase in heart rate, respiratory rate, retractions, rales; a loop diuretic may be needed for fluid overload
- Assess for aseptic meningitis syndrome (AMS): severe headache, drowsiness, photophobia, fever, painful eye movements, nausea, vomiting, muscle rigidity; discontinue RSV-IGIV if these occur

Nursing diagnoses

✓ Infection, risk for (uses)

✓ Knowledge deficit (teaching)

Implementation

- Give by infusion: do not admix; begin infusion within 6 hr and complete within 12 hr after the single-use vial is entered
- Store refrigerated, do not freeze, do not shake vial; discard after use

Patient/family education

- Teach patient the reason for **IV** inf and expected results

retinoic acid

See tretinoin

Rh_o (D) immune globulin, standard dose IM (℞)

Gamulin Rh, HypoRho-D, RhoGAM

Rh_o (D) Globulin microdose IM

HypoRho-D Mini-Dose, MICRh$_o$GAM, Mini-Gamulin R

Rh_o (D) immune globulin IV (℞)

WinRho SD, WinRho SDF

Func. class.: Immune globulins

Pregnancy category C

Action: Suppresses immune response of nonsensitized Rh_o (D or D^u)-negative patients who are exposed to Rh_o (D or D^u)-positive blood

➡ **Therapeutic Outcome:** Absence of Rh factor and transfusion error

Uses: Prevention of isoimmunization in Rh-negative women exposed to Rh-positive blood given after abortions, miscarriages, amniocentesis

Dosage and routes

After delivery

Adult: IM 1 vial (standard dose) of fetal packed RBCs <15 ml, or 2 vials of fetal packed RBCs >15 ml; given within 72 hr of delivery or miscarriage

Before delivery

Adult: IM 1 vial (standard dose) at 26-28 wk, 1 vial (standard dose) 72 hr after delivery

Pregnancy termination <13 wk

Adult: IM 1 vial (micro dose) within 72 hr

Pregnancy termination >13 wk

Adult: IM 1 vial (standard dose) within 72 hr

Fetal-maternal hemorrhage

Adult: IM packed RBCs volume of hemorrhage/15 = needed vials (standard dose)

Transfusion error

Adult: IM (standard dose—1 vial) give within 72 hr

After 34 wk gestation

Adult: IM/**IV** 120 µg, give within 72 hr (**IV** dose)

Available forms: Inj single-dose vial (50 µg/vial—microdose, 300 µg/vial—standard); inj 120, 300 µg Rh_o(D) immune globulin IV

Adverse effects

CNS: Lethargy

INTEG: Irritation at inj site, fever

MS: Myalgia

Contraindications: Previous immunization with this drug, Rh_o (O)-positive/D^u-positive patient

Precautions: Pregnancy **C**

Do Not Confuse:
Gamulin Rh/MICRh_oGAM

Pharmacokinetics	
Absorption	Well absorbed
Distribution	Unknown
Metabolism	Unknown
Excretion	Unknown
Half-life	Unknown

Pharmacodynamics	
Onset	Rapid
Peak	Unknown
Duration	Unknown

Interactions

Drug classifications

Live virus vaccines: ↓ antibody response to vaccine

NURSING CONSIDERATIONS

Assessment

- Assess for allergies, reactions to immunizations; previous immunization with this drug
- Obtain type and cross-match of mother's blood and of neonate's cord blood; neonate must be Rh_o(D)-positive, mother must be Rh_o(D)-negative and (D^u)-negative, medication should be given if there is a doubt
- Assess for intravascular hemolysis: back pain, chills, hemoglobinuria (idiopathic thrombocytopenic purpura)

Nursing diagnoses

✓ Knowledge deficit (teaching)

Implementation

IM route

- Reconstitute Rh_o (D) immune globulin IV using 1.25 ml of 0.9% NaCl swirl
- Do not use Rh_o (D) immune globulin or Rh_o (D) immune globulin microdose by **IV**
- Give after sending newborn's cord blood to lab after delivery for type, cross-match
- Give IM in deltoid muscle within 3 hr if possible; aspirate to prevent **IV** administration
- Give only equal lot numbers of drug, cross-match

R

• Give only MICRh$_o$GAM for abortions or miscarriages <13 wk unless fetus or father is Rh-negative
• Store in refrigerator

IV **IV direct route**
• Roconstitute Rh$_o$ (D) immune globulin IV using 2.5 ml of 0.9% NaCl, swirl, give over 3-5 min
• Do not use Rh$_o$ (D) immune globulin or Rh$_o$ (D) immune globulin microdose by **IV**

Patient/family education
• Teach patient how drug works; that drug must be given after subsequent deliveries if subsequent babies are Rh-positive

Evaluation
Positive therapeutic outcome
• Prevention of Rh$_o$(D) sensitization in transfusion error
• Prevention of erythroblastosis fetalis in subsequent Rh$_o$(D)-positive neonates

ribavarin (℞)
(rye-ba-vye'rin)
Virazole
Func. class.: Synthetic antiviral
Chem. class.: Tricyclic amine
Pregnancy category X

Action: Prevents replication of DNA and RNA synthesis

➔ **Therapeutic Outcome:** Resolution of severe lower respiratory tract infections

Uses: Severe lower respiratory tract P infections in infants and children

Investigational uses: Influenza A or B (early)

Dosage and routes
P ***Infants and young children:*** INH 20 mg/ml × 12-18 hr/day × 3-7 days

Available forms: Powder for reconstitution for aerosol 6 g/vial

Adverse effects
CNS: Dizziness, faintness
CV: Hypotension, cardiac arrest
EENT: Eye irritation, conjunctivitis, blurred vision, photosensitivity
INTEG: Rash

Contraindications: Hypersensi- P tivity, lactation, child <1 yr, pregnancy **X**

Precautions: Epilepsy, hepatic disease, renal disease

Pharmacokinetics	
Absorption	Inh (systemic)
Distribution	To respiratory tract
Metabolism	Liver
Excretion	Respiratory tract
Half-life	9½ hr

Pharmacodynamics	
Onset	Unknown
Peak	Inh end
Duration	Unknown

Interactions
Individual drugs
Zidovudine: ↓ antiviral action, ↑ toxicity
Drug classification
Cardiac glycosides: ↑ toxicity

NURSING CONSIDERATIONS
Assessment
• Assess allergies before initiation of treatment, reaction of each medication; list allergies on chart in bright red letters
• Monitor respiratory status: rate, character, wheezing, tightness in chest
• Obtain C&S test results before starting treatment

Nursing diagnoses
✓ Infection, risk for (uses)
✓ Gas exchange, impaired (uses)
✓ Knowledge deficit (teaching)

Implementation
• Give by the Viratek small particle aerosol generator (SPAG-2), do not use other inhalation equipment

- May be given by an oxygen hood for infants, or a face mask may be attached to the SPAG-2
- Reconstitute 6 g of sterile water for inj or inh, place sol in the Erlenmeyer flask and dilute further to 20 mg/ml

Patient/family education
- Teach patient and parents aspects of drug therapy

Evaluation
Positive therapeutic outcome
- Absence of respiratory syncytial virus (RSV)

riboflavin (vitamin B_2) (OTC)
(rye'boo-flay-vin)

Func. class.: Vitamin B_2, water soluble

Pregnancy category A

Action: Needed for respiratory reactions (catalyzes proteins) and for normal vision

Therapeutic Outcome: Prevention or treatment of riboflavin deficiency

Uses: Vit B_2 deficiency or polyneuritis; cheilosis adjunct with thiamine

Dosage and routes
Adult and child >12 yr: PO 5-25 mg qd

Child <12 yr: PO 2-10 mg qd, then 0.6 mg/1000 cal ingested

RDA

Adult: Males 1.4-1.8 mg; females 1.2-1.3 mg

Available forms: Tabs 5, 10, 25, 50, 100, 250 mg

Adverse effects
GU: Yellow discoloration of urine (large doses)

Contraindications: Child <12 yr

Precautions: Pregnancy **A**

Pharmacokinetics

Absorption	Well absorbed (by active transport)
Distribution	60% protein bound, widely distributed, crosses placenta
Metabolism	Unknown
Excretion	Kidneys (unchanged), excess amounts
Half-life	1-1½ hr

Pharmacodynamics
Unknown

Interactions
Individual drugs

Alcohol: ↑ riboflavin need

Probenecid: ↑ riboflavin need

Tetracycline: ↓ action of tetracycline

Drug classifications

Antidepressants, tricyclic: ↑ riboflavin need

Phenothiazines: ↑ riboflavin need

Lab test interferences

False: ↑ Urinary catecholamines, ↑ urobilinogen

NURSING CONSIDERATIONS
Assessment
- Assess patient's nutritional status: liver, eggs, dairy products, yeast, whole grain, green vegetables
- Assess for vit B_2 deficiency: photophobia, cheilosis, stomatitis, ocular swelling

Nursing diagnoses
- ✓ Nutrition: less than body requirements (uses)
- ✓ Knowledge deficit (teaching)

Implementation
- Give with food for better absorption
- Store in airtight, light-resistant container

Patient/family education
- Inform patient that urine may turn bright yellow
- Instruct patient about addition of needed foods that are rich in riboflavin

R

Evaluation

Positive therapeutic outcome

- Absence of headache, GI problems, cheilosis, skin lesions, depression, burning, itchy eyes, anemia

rifabutin (℞)

(riff'a-byoo-tin)

Mycobutin

Func. class.: Antimycobacterial

Chem. class.: Rifamycin S derivative

Pregnancy category B

Action: Inhibits DNA-dependent RNA polymerase in susceptible strains

Therapeutic Outcome: Antimycobacterial death of *Escherichia coli, Bacillus subtilis,* and *Mycobacterium avium*

Uses: Prevention of *M. avium* complex (MAC) in patients with advanced HIV infection

Dosage and routes

Adult: PO 300 mg qd (may take as 150 mg bid)

Available forms: Caps 150 mg

Adverse effects

CNS: *Headache,* fatigue, anxiety, confusion, insomnia

GI: *Nausea, vomiting, anorexia, diarrhea,* heartburn, **hepatitis**

GU: Hematuria

HEMA: **Hemolytic anemia, eosinophilia, thrombocytopenia, leukopenia**

INTEG: *Rash*

MISC: Flulike syndrome, shortness of breath, chest pressure

MS: Asthenia, arthralgia, myalgia

Contraindications: Hypersensitivity, active TB, WBC <1000/mm^3, platelets <50,000/mm^3

Precautions: Pregnancy **B,** lactation, hepatic disease, blood dyscrasias, P children

Do Not Confuse:

rifabutin/rifampin

Pharmacokinetics

Absorption	Well absorbed
Distribution	Widely distributed
Metabolism	Liver
Excretion	Kidney
Half-life	45 hr

Pharmacodynamics

Onset	Unknown
Peak	2-3 hr

Interactions

Individual drugs

Alcohol: ↑ toxicity

Carbamazepine: ↑ toxicity

Cycloserine: ↑ toxicity

Ethionamide: ↑ toxicity

Rifampin: ↑ toxicity

Ritonavir: ↑ rifabutin level

Drug classifications

Antacids, aluminum: ↓ absorption

Food/drug

High-fat foods: ↓ absorption

NURSING CONSIDERATIONS

Assessment

- Assess for active TB: chest x-ray, sputum culture, blood culture, biopsy of lymph nodes, obtain PPD test; drug should be given only for MAC and never for TB
- Monitor CBC for neutropenia, thrombocytopenia, eosinophilia

Nursing diagnoses

- ✓ Infection, risk for (uses)
- ✓ Diarrhea (adverse reaction)
- ✓ Injury, risk for (adverse reaction)
- ✓ Knowledge deficit (teaching)
- ✓ Noncompliance (teaching)

Implementation

- Give with meals to decrease GI symptoms; better to take on empty stomach 1 hr ac or 2 hr pc; high-fat food slows absorption
- Give antiemetic if vomiting occurs

Patient/family education

- Caution patient that compliance

with dosage schedule and duration is necessary

- Instruct patient that scheduled appointments must be kept or relapse may occur
- Instruct patient to notify prescriber if hepatitis, neutropenia, or thrombocytopenia occurs: sore throat, fever, bleeding, bruising, yellow sclera, anorexia, nausea, vomiting, fatigue, weakness; myositis: muscle or bone pain
- Advise patient that urine, feces, saliva, sputum, sweat, tears may be colored red-orange; soft contact lens may become permanently stained
- Caution patients using oral contraceptives to use a nonhormonal method of birth control because rifabutin may decrease efficiency of oral contraceptives

Evaluation

Positive therapeutic outcome

- Decreased symptoms of *M. avium* in patients with HIV

rifampin (℞)

(rif'am-pin)

Rifadin, Rimactane, Rofact ✱

Func. class.: Antitubercular

Chem. class.: Rifamycin B derivative

Pregnancy category C

Action: Inhibits DNA-dependent polymerase, decreases replication

➡ **Therapeutic Outcome:** Bactericidal against the following organisms: mycobacteria, *Staphylococcus aureus, Hemophilus influenzae, Neisseria meningitides, Legionella pneumophilia*

Uses: Pulmonary TB, meningococcal carriers (prevention)

Dosage and routes

Tuberculosis

Adult: PO/**IV** max 600 mg/day as single dose 1 hr ac or 2 hr pc or 10 mg/kg/day 2-3 ×/wk

6 mo regimen: 2 mo treatment of isoniazid, rifampin, pyrazinamide, and possibly streptomycin or ethambutol; then rifampin and isoniazid × 4 mo

9 mo regimen: Rifampin and isoniazid supplemented with pyrazinamide, or streptomycin or ethambutol

P ***Child >5 yr:*** PO/**IV** 10-20 mg/kg/day as single dose 1 hr ac or 2 hr pc, max 600 mg/day, with other antitubercular drugs

Meningococcal carriers

Adult: PO/**IV** 600 mg bid × 2 days

P ***Child >5 yr:*** PO/**IV** 10 mg/kg bid × 2 days, max 600 mg/dose

P ***Infant 3 mo-1 yr:*** PO 5 mg/kg bid for 2 days

Available forms: Caps 150, 300 mg; powder for inj 600 mg/vial

Adverse effects

CNS: Headache, fatigue, anxiety, drowsiness, confusion

EENT: Visual disturbances

GI: *Nausea, vomiting, anorexia, diarrhea,* **pseudomembranous colitis,** *heartburn,* sore mouth and tongue, pancreatitis, elevated LFTs

GU: **Hematuria, acute renal failure, hemoglobinuria**

HEMA: **Hemolytic anemia, eosinophilia, thrombocytopenia, leukopenia**

INTEG: Rash, pruritus, urticaria

MISC: Flulike syndrome, menstrual disturbances, edema, shortness of breath

MS: Ataxia, weakness

Contraindications: Hypersensitivity

Precautions: Pregnancy **C,** lactation, hepatic disease, blood dyscrasias

Do Not Confuse:

rifampin/rifabutin

R

Pharmacokinetics

Absorption	Well absorbed (PO), completely absorbed (**IV**)
Distribution	Widely distributed, crosses placenta
Metabolism	Liver—extensively
Excretion	Feces
Half-life	3 hr

Pharmacodynamics

	PO	IV
Onset	Rapid	Rapid
Peak	2-3 hr	Inf end

Interactions

Individual drugs

Alcohol: ↑ toxicity
Chloramphenicol: ↓ effect of chloramphenicol
Disopyramide: ↓ effect of disopyramide
Fluconazole: ↓ effect of fluconazole
Imidazole: ↓ antifungal action
Isoniazid: ↑ toxicity
Ketoconazole: ↑ toxicity
Lithium: ↑ lithium toxicity
Miconazole: ↑ toxicity
Phenytoin: ↓ effect of phenytoin
Quinidine: ↓ effect of quinidine
Theophylline: ↓ effect of theophylline
Tocainide: ↓ effect of tocainide
Verapamil: ↓ effect of verapamil

Drug classifications

Antifungals: ↓ antifungal action
Glucocorticoids: ↓ effect
Opiates: ↓ effect
Oral contraceptives: ↓ effect

NURSING CONSIDERATIONS

Assessment

- Monitor liver studies qwk: ALT, AST, bilirubin
- Monitor renal status: before, qmo: BUN, creatinine, output, sp gr, urinalysis
- Monitor mental status often: affect, mood, behavioral changes; psychosis may occur
- Monitor hepatic status: decreased appetite, jaundice, dark urine, fatigue
- Assess for infection: sputum culture, lung sounds
- C&S should be performed before beginning treatment, during, and after therapy is completed

Nursing diagnoses

- ✓ Infection, risk for (uses)
- ✓ Diarrhea (adverse reactions)
- ✓ Injury, risk for (adverse reactions)
- ✓ Knowledge deficit (teaching)
- ✓ Noncompliance (teaching)

Implementation

PO route

- Administer with meals to decrease GI symptoms; better to take on empty stomach 1 hr ac or 2 hr pc

IV **IV route**

Intermittent **IV**

- Give by intermittent inf after reconstituting 600 mg/10 ml of sterile water for inj, agitate gently; dilute further in 100 or 500 ml of 0.9% NaCl or D_5W; give 100 ml/30 min or 500 ml/3 hr
- Do not mix with other drugs or sols

Patient/family education

- Instruct patient that compliance with dosage schedule, duration is necessary
- Instruct patient that scheduled appointments must be kept or relapse may occur
- Instruct patient to notify prescriber if hepatitis, neutropenia, or thrombocytopenia occurs: sore throat, fever, bleeding, bruising, yellow sclera, anorexia, nausea, vomiting, fatigue, weakness
- Advise patient that urine, feces, saliva, sputum, sweat, tears may be colored red-orange; soft contact lens may be permanently stained
- Caution patients using oral contraceptives to use a nonhormonal method of birth control because rifabutin may decrease the efficiency of oral contraceptives

Evaluation

Positive therapeutic outcome

- Decreased symptoms of TB

rifapentine (℞)

(riff'ah-pen-teen)

Priftin

Func. class.: Antitubercular

Chem. class.: Rifamycin derivative

Pregnancy category C

Action: Inhibits DNA-dependent polymerase, decreases tubercule bacilli replication

Therapeutic Outcome: Resolution of pulmonary TB

Uses: Pulmonary TB; must be used with at least one other antitubercular drug

Dosage and routes

Intensive phase

Adult: PO 600 mg (4 150 mg tabs 2 ×/wk), with an interval of 72 hr between doses × 2 mo; must be given with at least one other antitubercular drug

Continuation phase

Adult: PO continue with 1 ×/wk × 4 mo in combination with isoniazid or other appropriate antitubercular drug

Available forms: Tabs 150 mg

Adverse effects

CNS: Headache, fatigue, anxiety, dizziness

EENT: Visual disturbances

GI: *Nausea, vomiting, anorexia, diarrhea,* bilirubinemia, hepatitis, increased ALT, AST, *heartburn,* **pancreatitis**

GU: **Hematuria,** pyuria, proteinuria, urinary casts, urine discoloration

HEMA: **Thrombocytopenia, leukopenia, neutropenia, lymphopenia,** anemia, **leukocytosis,** purpura, hematoma

INTEG: Rash, pruritis, urticaria, acne

MISC: Edema, aggressive reaction, increased B/P

MS: Gout, arthrosis

Contraindications: Hypersensitivity to rifamycins, porphyria

Precautions: Pregnancy **C,** lactation, hepatic disease, blood dyscrasias, children <12 yr, HIV, elderly

Pharmacokinetics

Absorption	Unknown
Distribution	Unknown
Metabolism	Unknown
Excretion	Unknown
Half-life	Unknown

Pharmacodynamics

Onset	Unknown
Peak	Unknown
Duration	Unknown

Interactions

Individual drugs

Amitriptyline: ↓ action of amitriptyline
Chloramphenicol: ↓ action of chloramphenicol
Clarithromycin: ↓ action of clarithromycin
Clofibrate: ↓ action of clofibrate
Cyclosporine: ↓ action of cyclosporine
Dapsone: ↓ action of dapsone
Delaviridine: ↓ action of delaviridine
Diazepam: ↓ action of diazepam
Digoxin: ↓ action of digoxin
Diltiazam: ↓ action of diltiazem
Disopyramide: ↓ action of disopyramide
Doxycycline: ↓ action of doxycycline
Fentanyl: ↓ action of fentanyl
Fluconazole: ↓ action of fluconazole
Haloperidol: ↓ action of haloperidol
Indinavir: ↓ action of indinavir
Itraconazole: ↓ action of itraconazole
Ketoconazole: ↓ action of ketoconazole
Methadone: ↓ action of methadone
Mexiletine: ↓ action of mexiletine

R

Nelfinavir: ↓ action of nelfinavir
Nifedipine: ↓ action of nifedipine
Nortriptyline: ↓ action of nortriptyline
Phenytoin: ↓ action of phenytoin
Quinidine: ↓ action of quinidine
Quinine: ↓ action of quinine
Ritonavir: ↓ action of ritonavir
Saquinavir: ↓ action of saquinavir
Sildenafil: ↓ action of sildenafil
Tacrolimus: ↓ action of tacrolimus
Theophylline: ↓ action of theophylline
Tocainide: ↓ action of tocainide
Verapamil: ↓ action of verapamil
Warfarin: ↓ action of warfarin
Zidovudine: ↓ action of zidovudine

Drug classifications

Anticoagulants: ↓ action of anticoagulants
Antidiabetics: ↓ action of antidiabetics
Barbiturates: ↓ action of barbiturates
β-Adrenergic blockers: ↓ action of β-blocker
Corticosteroids: ↓ action of corticosteroids
Fluoroquinolones: ↓ action of fluoroquinolones
Oral contraceptives: ↓ action of oral contraceptives
Phenothiazines: ↓ action of phenothiazines
Protease inhibitors: Use extreme caution
Thyroid preparations: ↓ action of thyroid preparations

Food/drug

Food: ↑ drug concentration by 44% with food

Lab test interferences:

Interference: Folate level, vit B_{12}

NURSING CONSIDERATIONS

Assessment

- Obtain baselines in CBC, AST, ALT, bilirubin, platelets
- Assess for infection: sputum culture, lung sounds
- Assess signs of anemia: Hct, Hgb, fatigue
- Monitor liver studies qmo: ALT, AST, bilirubin
- Monitor renal status qmo: BUN, creatinine, output, sp gr, urinalysis
- Assess hepatic status: decreased appetite, jaundice, dark urine, fatigue

Nursing diagnoses

✓ Infection, risk for (uses)
✓ Diarrhea (side effects)
✓ Knowledge deficit (teaching)
✓ Noncompliance (teaching)

Implementation

PO route

- Give PO, may be given with food for GI upset
- Give antiemetic if vomiting occurs
- Administer after C&S is completed; qmo to detect resistance

Patient/family education

- Advise patient that compliance with dosage schedule, duration is necessary
- Instruct patient that scheduled appointments must be kept; relapse may occur
- Teach patient that urine, feces, saliva, sputum, sweat, tears may be colored red-orange; soft contact lenses, dentures may be permanently stained
- Teach patient to use alternate method of contraception, oral contraceptive action may be decreased
- Teach patient to report flulike symptoms: excessive fatigue, anorexia, vomiting, sore throat; unusual bleeding, jaundice of skin, eyes

Evaluation

Positive therapeutic outcome

- Decreased symptoms of TB
- Negative culture

riluzole (℞)
(ri-loo'zole)
Rilutek
Func. class.: Amyotropic lateral sclerosis (ALS) agent
Chem. class.: Benzathiazole
Pregnancy category C

Action: Unknown; may act by inhibiting glutamate, interfering with binding of amino acid receptors, inactivation of voltage-dependent sodium channels

➔ **Therapeutic Outcome:** Decreased symptoms of ALS

Uses: ALS

Dosage and routes
Adult: PO 50 mg q12h, take 1 hr ac or 2 hr pc

Available forms: Tabs 50 mg

Adverse effects
CNS: Hypertonia, depression, dizziness, insomnia, somnolence, vertigo
CV: Hypertension, tachycardia, phlebitis, palpitation, postural hypertension
GI: Nausea, vomiting, dyspepsia, anorexia, diarrhea, flatulence, stomatitis, dry mouth
GU: UTI, dysuria
HEMA: **Neutropenia**
INTEG: Pruritus, eczema, alopecia, **exfoliative dermatitis**
RESP: Decreased lung function; rhinitis, increased cough

Contraindications: Hypersensitivity

Precautions: Neutropenia, renal disease, hepatic disease, G elderly, P pregnancy **C,** lactation, children

Pharmacokinetics

Absorption	Well
Distribution	Unknown
Metabolism	Extensively—live
Excretion	Urine, feces
Half-life	Unknown

Pharmacodynamics
Unknown

Interactions
Individual drugs
Amitriptyline: ↓ elimination of riluzole
Caffeine: ↓ elimination of riluzole
Cigarette smoke: ↑ elimination of riluzole
Omeprazole: ↑ elimination of riluzole
Rifampin: ↑ elimination of riluzole
Theophylline: ↓ elimination of riluzole
Drug classifications
Quinolones: ↓ elimination of riluzole
Food/drug
Charcoal-broiled foods: ↑ elimination of riluzole
High fat meal: ↓ absorption

NURSING CONSIDERATIONS
Assessment
- Monitor LFTs: AST, ALT, bilirubin, GGT, baseline and qmo × 3 mo, then q3 mo
- Assess for neutropenia (neutrophils <500/mm^3)

Nursing diagnoses
- ✓ Physical mobility, impaired (uses)
- ✓ Knowledge deficit (teaching)

Implementation
- Give 1 hr ac or 2 hr pc; a high-fat meal decreases absorption

Patient/family education
- Advise to report febrile illness, may indicate neutropenia
- Teach reason for drug and expected results

R

rimantadine (℞)
(ri-man'ti-deen)
Flumadine
Func. class.: Synthetic antiviral
Chem. class.: Tricyclic amine
Pregnancy category C

Action: Prevents uncoating of nucleic acid in viral cell, preventing penetration of virus to host; causes release of dopamine from neurons

Therapeutic Outcome: Prevention of influenza type A

Uses: Prophylaxis or treatment of influenza type A

Dosage and routes

Renal/hepatic dose

Reduce as needed

Influenza type A prophylaxis

Adult: PO 100 mg bid; in renal or hepatic disease, lower dose to 100 mg/day

P ***Child: <10 yr:*** PO 5 mg/kg/day, max 150 mg

Treatment

P ***Adult and child >10 yr:*** PO 100 mg bid; in renal or hepatic disease, lower dose to 100 mg/day; start treatment at onset of symptoms, continue for at least 1 wk

G ***Elderly:*** PO 100 mg/day

Available forms: Tabs 100 mg; syrup 50 mg/5 ml

Adverse effects

CNS: Headache, dizziness, fatigue, depression, hallucinations, tremors, **seizures**, insomnia, *poor concentration,* asthenia, gait abnormalities
CV: Pallor, palpitations, hypertension
EENT: Tinnitus, taste abnormality, eye pain
GI: Nausea, vomiting, constipation, dry mouth, anorexia, abdominal pain, diarrhea, dyspepsia
INTEG: Rash

Contraindications: Hypersensitivity to drugs of adamantance class (this drug, amantadine), lactation, P child <1 yr

Precautions: Epilepsy, hepatic disease, renal disease, pregnancy **C**

Do Not Confuse: rimantadine/amantadine

Pharmacokinetics

Absorption	Minimally absorbed (PO)
Distribution	Widely distributed, crosses placenta, CSF concentration 50% plasma
Metabolism	Liver
Excretion	95% unchanged—kidneys
Half-life	2-3.5 hr, increased in renal disease

Pharmacodynamics

	PO
Onset	Unknown
Peak	1½-2½

Interactions

Individual drugs

Amphotericin B: ↑ neurotoxicity, nephrotoxicity
Interferon: ↑ neurotoxicity, nephrotoxicity
Methotrexate: ↑ neurotoxicity, nephrotoxicity
Probenecid: ↑ neurotoxicity, nephrotoxicity

Drug classification

Aminoglycosides: ↑ neurotoxicity, nephrotoxicity

NURSING CONSIDERATIONS

Assessment

- Assess for seizures; if seizures occur, drug should be discontinued
- Assess allergies before initiation of treatment, patient's reaction to each medication; list allergies on chart
- Monitor respiratory status: rate, character, wheezing, tightness in chest

Nursing diagnoses

✓ Infection, risk for (uses)
✓ Knowledge deficit (teaching)

Implementation

- Give before exposure to influenza; continue for 10 days after contact
- Give at least 4 hr before bedtime to prevent insomnia
- Administer pc for better absorption,

to decrease GI symptoms; cap may be opened and mixed with food for easy swallowing
- Give in divided doses to prevent CNS disturbances: headache, dizziness, fatigue, drowsiness
- Store in airtight, dry container

Patient/family education
- Instruct patient about aspects of drug therapy: need to report dyspnea, dizziness, poor concentration, behavioral changes
- Advise patient to avoid hazardous activities if dizziness occurs
- Caution patient to consult prescriber before taking OTC medications, alcohol; serious drug interactions may result

Evaluation

Positive therapeutic outcome
- Absence of fever, malaise, cough, dyspnea

Treatment of overdose: Withdraw drug, maintain airway, administer epinephrine, aminophylline, O_2, **IV** corticosteroids, physostigmine

risedronate (℞)

(rih-sed'roh-nate)

Actonel

Func. class: Bone resorption inhibitor

Chem. class.: Biphosphonate

Pregnancy category C

Action: Absorbs calcium phosphate crystal in bone and may directly block dissolution of hydroxyapatite crystals of bone; inhibits bone resorption, apparently without inhibiting bone formation, mineralization

Therapeutic Outcome: Increased bone mass, activity without fractures

Uses: Paget's disease, osteoporosis in postmenopausal women, glucocorticoid-induced osteoporosis

Dosage and routes

Paget's disease

Adult: PO 30 mg qd × 2 mo; give calcium and vit D if dietary intake is lacking; if relapse occurs, retreatment is advised

Treatment/prevention of postmenopausal osteoporosis/glucocorticoid-induced osteoporosis

Adult: PO 5 mg qd

Available forms: Tabs 30 mg

Adverse effects

CNS: Dizziness, headache

CV: Chest pain

GI: *Abdominal pain, anorexia,* diarrhea, *nausea*

MS: *Bone pain,* arthralgia

Contraindications: Hypersensitivity to biphosphonates

P **Precautions:** Children, lactation, pregnancy **C**, renal disease

Pharmacokinetics	
Absorption	Unknown
Distribution	To bones
Metabolism	Unknown
Excretion	Kidneys
Half-life	Unknown

Pharmacodynamics	
Onset	Unknown
Peak	Unknown
Duration	Unknown

Interactions

Drug classifications

Antacids: ↓ absorption of risedronate

Calcium supplement: ↓ absorption of risedronate

Food/drug

Food: ↓ bioavailability: take ½ hr before food or drinks

NURSING CONSIDERATIONS

Assessment
- Assess for symptoms of Paget's disease: headache, bone pain, increased head circumference

R

- Monitor electrolytes; renal function studies (calcium, phosphorus, magnesium, potassium)
- Assess for hypercalcemia: paresthesia, twitching, laryngospasm, Chvostek's/Trousseau's signs

Nursing diagnoses
- ✓ Immobility, impaired (uses)
- ✓ Nutrition, altered, less than body requirements (uses)
- ✓ Knowledge deficit (teaching)

Implementation
- Give PO for 2 months to be effective in Paget's disease
- Give with a full glass of water; patient should be in upright position
- Administer supplemental calcium and vit D in Paget's disease
- Give qd ≥30 min ac
- Store in cool environment, out of direct sunlight

Patient/family education
- Advise patient to sit upright for ½ hr after dose to prevent irritation
- Instruct patient to comply with diet
- Advise patient to notify prescriber if pregnancy is planned or suspected

Evaluation
Positive therapeutic outcome
- Increased bone mass, absence of fractures

risperidone (℞)
(res-pare'a-done)

Risperdal

Func. class.: Antipsychotic

Chem. class.: Benzisoxazole derivative

Pregnancy category C

Action: Unknown; may be mediated through both dopamine type 2 (D_2) and serotinin type 2 ($5\text{-}HT_2$) antagonism

Therapeutic Outcome: Decreased hallucination and disorganized thought

Uses: Psychotic disorders

Dosage and routes
Adult: PO 1 mg bid, with incremental increases of 1 mg bid on days 2 and 3 to a dose of 3 mg bid by day 3; then do not increase dose for at least 1 wk

G ***Elderly:*** PO 0.5 mg qd-bid increase by 1 mg qwk

Hepatic dose

Adult: PO 0.5 mg, increase by 0.5 mg bid, then increase to 1.5 mg bid

Available forms: Tabs 1, 2, 3, 4 mg; oral sol 1 mg/ml

Adverse effects
CNS: *EPS (pseudoparkinsonism, akathisia, dystonia, tardive dyskinesia), drowsiness, insomnia, agitation, anxiety, headache,* **neuroleptic malignant syndrome**

CV: Orthostatic hypotension, **tachycardia**

EENT: Blurred vision

GI: *Nausea,* vomiting, *anorexia, constipation,* jaundice, weight gain

RESP: Rhinitis

Contraindications: Hypersensitivity, lactation, seizure disorders

P **Precautions:** Children, renal disease, pregnancy **C,** hepatic disease, G elderly, breast cancer

Do Not Confuse: Risperdal/reserpine

Pharmacokinetics	
Absorption	Unknown
Distribution	Unknown
Metabolism	Liver, extensively
Excretion	Unknown
Half-life	Unknown

Pharmacodynamics	
Onset	Unknown
Peak	Unknown
Duration	Up to 12 hr

Interactions
Individual drugs
Alcohol: ↑ effects of both drugs, oversedation
Lithium: ↑ EPS, masking of lithium toxicity
Tegretol: ↑ excretion of risperidone
Drug classifications
Antidepressants: ↑ CNS depression
Antihistamines: ↑ CNS depression
Barbiturate anesthetics: ↑ CNS depression
General anesthetics: ↑ CNS depression
MAOIs: ↑ CNS depression
Opiates: ↑ CNS depression
Sedative/hypnotics: ↑ CNS depression
Herb/drug
Kava: ↑ CNS depression
Lab test interferences
↑ LFTs, ↑ cardiac enzymes, ↑ cholesterol, ↑ blood glucose, ↑ prolactin, ↑ bilirubin, ↑ PBI, ↑ cholinesterase, ↑ I, ↑ alkaline phosphatase, ↑ leukocytes, ↑ granulocytes, ↑ platelets
↓ Hormones (blood and urine)
False positive: Pregnancy tests, PKU, urine bilirubin
False negative: Urinary steroids, 17-OCHS

NURSING CONSIDERATIONS
Assessment
- Assess mental status: orientation, mood, behavior, presence and type of hallucinations before initial administration and monthly; this drug should significantly reduce psychotic behavior
- Check that patient swallows all PO medication; check for hoarding or giving of medication to other patients
- Monitor I&O ratio, palpate bladder if low urinary output occurs, especially in elderly; urinalysis recommended before, during prolonged therapy
- Monitor bilirubin, CBC, liver function studies monthly
- Assess affect, orientation, LOC, reflexes, gait, coordination, sleep pattern disturbances
- Monitor B/P with patient in sitting, standing, and lying positions; take pulse and respirations q4h during initial treatment; establish baseline before starting treatment; report drops of 30 mm Hg; obtain baseline ECG and monitor Q- and T-wave changes
- Check for dizziness, faintness, palpitations, tachycardia on rising; severe orthostatic hypotension is common
- Identify for neuroleptic malignant syndrome: hyperpyrexia, muscle rigidity, increased CPK, altered mental status; drug should be discontinued
- Assess for EPS including akathisia (inability to sit still, no pattern to movements), tardive dyskinesia (bizarre movements of the jaw, mouth, tongue, extremities) pseudoparkinsonism (rigidity, tremors, pill rolling, shufling gait); an antiparkinsonian drug should be prescribed
- Assess for constipation, urinary retention daily; if these occur, increase bulk, water in diet

Nursing diagnoses
- ✓ Thought processes, altered (uses)
- ✓ Coping, ineffective individual (uses)
- ✓ Knowledge deficit (teaching)
- ✓ Noncompliance (teaching)

Implementation
- PO with full glass of water, milk; or give with food to decrease GI upset
- Store in airtight, light-resistant container

Patient/family education
- Teach patient to use good oral hygiene; frequent rinsing of mouth, sugarless gum for dry mouth
- Caution patient to avoid hazardous activities until drug response is determined; dizziness, blurred vision may occur
- Inform patient that orthostatic hypotension occurs often; patient should rise from sitting or lying

R

position gradually and remain lying down for at least 30 min after IM inj

- Instruct patient to avoid hot tubs, hot showers, tub baths; hypotension may occur
- Inform patient that heat stroke may occur in hot weather, and to take extra precautions to stay cool
- Advise patient to avoid abrupt withdrawal of this drug, or EPS may result; drug should be withdrawn slowly
- Teach patient to avoid OTC preparations (cough, hay fever, cold) unless approved by prescriber; serious drug interactions may occur; avoid use with alcohol, CNS depressants because increased drowsiness may occur
- Advise patient to use contraception, to inform prescriber if pregnancy is planned or suspected

Evaluation

Positive therapeutic outcome

- Decrease in emotional excitement, hallucinations, delusions, paranoia
- Reorganization of patterns of thought, speech

Treatment of overdose: Lavage, provide airway

ritonavir (℞)

(ri-toe'na-veer)

Norvir

Func. class.: Antiretroviral

Chem. class.: Protease inhibitor

Pregnancy category B

Action: Inhibits HIV protease and prevents maturation of the infectious virus

➔ **Therapeutic Outcome:** Improvement of HIV infection

Uses: HIV in combination with zidovudine, zalcitabine, or alone

Dosage and routes

Adult: PO 600 mg bid; if nausea occurs, begin dose at ½ and gradually increase

P ***Child:*** PO 250 mg/m^2 bid, titrate upward to 400 mg/m^2 bid

Available forms: Caps 100 mg; oral sol 80 mg/ml

Adverse effects

CNS: Paresthesia, headache, **seizures**

GI: Diarrhea, buccal mucosa ulceration, abdominal pain, nausea, taste perversion, dry mouth

INTEG: Rash

MISC: Asthenia, **angioedema, anaphylaxis, Stevens-Johnson syndrome**

MS: Pain

Contraindications: Hypersensitivity

Precautions: Liver disease, P pregnancy **B**, lactation, children

Pharmacokinetics

Absorption	Unknown
Distribution	Unknown
Metabolism	Unknown
Excretion	Unknown
Half-life	Unknown

Pharmacodynamics

Unknown

Interactions

Individual drugs

Clarithromycin: ↑ level of both drugs

Desipramine: ↑ ritonavir level

Disulfiram: ↑ ritonavir level

Fluconazole: ↑ ritonavir level

Metronidazole: ↑ ritonavir level

Phenytoin: ↓ ritonavir level

Sulfamethoxazole: ↓ ritonavir level

Theophylline: ↓ ritonavir level

Zalcitabine: ↑ ritonavir level of both drugs

Zidovudine: ↓ ritonavir level

Drug classifications

Barbiturates: ↓ ritonavir level

Lab test interferences

↑ ALT, ↑ GGT, ↑ prothrombin time, ↑ triglycerides

↓ Hct, ↓ RBC

NURSING CONSIDERATIONS

Assessment

- Assess signs of infection, anemia
- Monitor viral load and CD4 baseline and throughout therapy
- Assess liver function studies: ALT, AST
- Monitor C&S before drug therapy; drug may be taken as soon as culture is done; repeat C&S after treatment; determine the presence of other sexually transmitted disease
- Assess bowel pattern before, during treatment; if severe abdominal pain with bleeding occurs, drug should be discontinued; monitor hydration
- Assess skin eruptions, rash
- Assess allergies before treatment, reaction to each medication; place allergies on chart

Nursing diagnoses

✓ Infection, risk for (uses)
✓ Knowledge deficit (teaching)

Implementation

- Administer with food
- Mix oral powder with high-calorie drink
- Store caps in refrigerator

Patient/family education

- Teach patient to take as prescribed; if dose is missed, take as soon as remembered up to 1 hr before next dose; do not double dose
- Teach patient that drug must be taken in equal intervals around the clock to maintain blood levels for duration of therapy

rituximab (℞)

(rih-tuks'ih-mab)

Rituxan

Func. class.: Misc. antineoplastic
Chem. class.: Murine/human monoclonal antibody

Pregnancy category C

Action: Directed against the CD20 antigen that is found on malignant B lymphocytes; CD20 regulates a portion of cell-cycle initiation/differentiation

➔ **Therapeutic Outcome:** Decreased tumor size, prevention of spread of cancer

Uses: Non-Hodgkin's lymphoma (CD20 positive, B-cell), bulky disease (tumors >10 cm)

Dosage and routes

Adult: **IV** inf 375 mg/m^2 qwk × 4 doses; give at 50 mg/hr for 1st inf; if hypersensitivity does not occur, increase rate by 50 mg/hr q½h, max 400 mg/hr; slow/interrupt inf if hypersensitivity occurs; other inf can be given at 100 mg/hr and increased by 100 mg/hr, max 400 mg/hr

Available forms: Inj 10 mg/ml

Adverse effects

CV: **Cardiac dysrhythmias**
GI: *Nausea, vomiting, anorexia*
GU: **Renal failure**
HEMA: **Leukopenia, neutropenia, thrombocytopenia**
INTEG: *Irritation at inj site, rash,* **fatal mucocutaneous infections (rare)**
MISC: Fever, chills, asthenia, headache, angioedema, hypotension, myalgia, bronchospasm
SYST: **Stevens-Johnson syndrome**

Contraindications: Hypersensitivity, murine proteins, cardiac conditions

P G **Precautions:** Lactation, children, elderly, pregnancy **C**

R

Pharmacokinetics

Absorption	Unknown
Distribution	Unknown
Metabolism	Unknown
Excretion	Unknown
Half-life	42-79 min

Pharmacodynamics

Onset	Unknown
Peak	Unknown
Duration	Unknown

Interactions

Unknown

NURSING CONSIDERATIONS
Assessment
- Assess for signs of fatal infusion reaction: hypoxia, pulmonary infiltrates, acute respiratory distress syndrome, MI, ventricular fibrillation, cardiogenic shock; most fatal infusion reactions occur with 1st inf, discontinue drug
- Assess for signs of severe mucocutaneous reactions: Stevens-Johnson syndrome, lichenoid dermatitis, toxic epidermal lysis; signs occur 1-13 wk after drug was given
- Assess for tumor lysis syndrome: acute renal failure requiring hemodialysis, hyperkalemia, hypocalcemia, hyperuricemia, hyperphosphatasemia
- Monitor CBC, differential, platelet count weekly; withhold drug if WBC is <3500/mm^3, or platelet count <100,000/mm^3; notify prescriber of these results; drug should be discontinued
- Assess food preferences: list likes, dislikes
- Assess GI symptoms: frequency of stools
- Assess signs of dehydration: rapid respirations, poor skin turgor, decreased urine output, dry skin, restlessness, weakness

Nursing diagnoses
✓ Injury, risk for (side effects)
✓ Knowledge deficit (teaching)

Implementation
IV route
- Administer after diluting to a final conc of 1-4 mg/ml; use 0.9% NaCl, D_5W, gently invert bag to mix; do not mix with other drugs
- Increase fluid intake to 2-3 L/day to prevent dehydration, unless contraindicated
- Change **IV** site q48h
- Provide nutritious diet with iron, vitamin supplement, low fiber, few dairy products
- Store vials at 36°-40° F, protect vials from direct sunlight, inf sol is stable at 36°-46° F × 24 hr and room temp for another 12 hr

Patient/family education
- Teach patient to report adverse reactions

Evaluation
Positive therapeutic outcome
- Decrease in tumor size, decrease in spread of cancer

rivastigmine (℞)
(riv-as-tig′mine)
Exelon
Func. class.: Cholinesterase inhibitor

Pregnancy category B

Action: May enhance cholinergic functioning by increasing acetylcholine

Therapeutic Outcome: Decreased signs and symptoms of Alzheimer's dementia

Uses: Alzheimer's dementia

Dosage and routes
Adult: PO 1.5 mg bid for 2 wk or more, may increase to 3 mg bid after 2 wk or more; may increase to 4.5 mg bid and thereafter 6 mg bid

Available forms: Caps 1.5, 3, 4.5, 6 mg; sol 2 mg/ml

Adverse effects
CNS: ***Tremors, confusion, insomnia,*** psychosis, hallucination, depression, dizziness, headache, anxiety, somnolence, fatigue, syncope
GI: ***Nausea, vomiting, anorexia, abdominal distress, flatulence,*** diarrhea, constipation
MISC: UTI, asthenia, increased sweating, hypertension, influenza-like syncope, weight change

Contraindications: Hypersensitivity, narrow-angle glaucoma, undiagnosed skin lesions

Precautions: Renal disease, hepatic disease, respiratory disease, seizure disorder, peptic ulcer, pregnancy **B**, asthma, lactation, children, cardiac disease, urinary obstruction, asthma

Pharmacokinetics

Absorption	Rapidly, completely
Distribution	Not known
Metabolism	To decarbamylated metabolite
Excretion	Kidney—metabolites, clearance lowered in elderly, hepatic disease, ↑ nicotine use
Half-life	1½ hr

Pharmacodynamics

Unknown

Interactions

Drug classifications

Cholinomimetics: ↑ synergistic effect

Food/drug

↓ Rivastigmine absorption

NURSING CONSIDERATIONS

Assessment

- Monitor liver function studies: AST, ALT, alkaline phosphatase, LDH, bilirubin, CBC
- Assess for severe GI effects: nausea, vomiting, anorexia, weight loss
- Monitor B/P, respiration during initial treatment; hypo/hypertension should be reported
- Assess mental status: affect, mood, behavioral changes, depression; complete suicide assessment

Nursing diagnoses

✓ Knowledge deficit (teaching)
✓ Cognitive impairment (uses)

Implementation

- Give with meals; take with AM and PM meal even though absorption may be decreased
- Provide assistance with ambulation during beginning therapy

Patient/family education

- Teach patient procedure for giving oral sol; use instruction sheet provided
- Teach patient to notify prescriber of severe GI effects

Evaluation

Positive therapeutic outcome

- Increased coherence, decreased symptoms of Alzheimer's disease

rizatriptan (℞)

(rye-zah-trip'tan)

Maxalt, Maxalt-MLT

Func. class.: Migraine agent

Chem. class.: 5-HT_1-like receptor agonist

Pregnancy category C

Action: Binds selectively to the vascular serotonin type 1 (5-HT_1) receptor, exerts antimigraine effect; causes vasoconstriction in cranial arteries

Therapeutic Outcome: After treatment, relief of migraine

Uses: Acute treatment of migraine

Dosage and routes

Adult: **PO** 5-10 mg single dose, redosing separate by 2 hr or more; max 30 mg/24 hr

Available forms: *Maxalt:* tabs 5, 10 mg; *Maxalt-MLT:* tabs, orally disintegrating 5, 10 mg

Adverse effects

CNS: *Dizziness, headache, fatigue,* warm/cold sensation, flushing, hot flashes

CV: **MI, ventricular fibrillation, ventricular tachycardia, coronary artery vasospasm**

GI: *Nausea,* dry mouth, diarrhea

RESP: Chest tightness, pressure, dyspnea

Contraindications: Angina pectoris, history of MI, documented silent ischemia, Prinzmetal's angina, ischemic heart disease, concurrent ergotamine-containing preparations, uncontrolled hypertension, hypersensitivity, basilar or hemiplegic migraine

Precautions: Postmenopausal women, men >40 yr, risk factors for CAD, hypercholesterolemia, obesity, diabetes, impaired hepatic or renal function, pregnancy **C**, lactation, children, elderly

Pharmacokinetics	
Absorption	Unknown
Distribution	Unknown
Metabolism	Liver (metabolite)
Excretion	Urine/feces
Half-life	2-3 hr

Pharmacodynamics	
Onset	10 min-2 hr
Peak	Unknown
Duration	Unknown

Interactions

Individual drugs

Cimetidine: ↑ action of rizatriptan
Ergot: ↑ vasospastic effects
Propranolol: ↑ action of rizatriptan

Drug classifications

Ergot derivatives: ↑ vasospastic effects
MAOIs: ↑ action of rizatriptan
5-HT_1 receptor agonists: ↑ vasospastic effects
Selective serotonin reuptake inhibitors: ↑ weakness, hyperreflexia, incoordination

NURSING CONSIDERATIONS

Assessment

- Assess for tingling, hot sensations, burning, feeling of pressure, numbness, flushing, injection site reaction
- Assess for stress level, activity, recreation, coping mechanisms
- Assess neurologic status: LOC, blurring vision, nausea, vomiting, tingling in extremities preceding headache
- Monitor for ingestion of tyramine-containing foods (pickled products, beer, wine, aged cheese), food additives, preservatives, colorings, artificial sweeteners, chocolate, caffeine, which may precipitate these types of headaches

Nursing diagnoses

- ✓ Pain (uses)
- ✓ Knowledge deficit (teaching)

Implementation

- Provide quiet, calm environment with decreased stimulation for noise, bright light, excessive talking

Patient/family education

- Teach patient use of orally disintegrating tab: instruct patient not to open blister until use, to peel blister open with dry hands, to place tab on tongue, where it will dissolve, and to swallow with saliva (contains phenylalanine)
- Advise patient to report any side effects to prescriber
- Advise patient to use alternate contraception while taking drug if oral contraceptives are being used

Evaluation

Positive therapeutic outcome

- Decrease in frequency, severity of headache

rofecoxib (℞)
(roh-feh-cock'sib)

Vioxx

Func. class.: Nonsteroidal antiinflammatory
Chem. class.: COX-2 inhibitor

Pregnancy category C

Action: May inhibit prostaglandin synthesis by decreasing enzyme needed for biosynthesis; analgesic, antiinflammatory, antipyretic properties

Therapeutic Outcome: Decreased pain, inflammation

Uses: Acute, chronic osteoarthritis, pain, primary dysmenorrhea

Dosage and routes
Osteoarthritis
Adult: PO 12.5 mg/day as a single dose, may increase to 25 mg if needed
Primary dysmenorrhea
Adult: PO 50 mg qd, use for <5 days

Available forms: Tabs 12.5, 25 mg; susp 12.5, 25 mg/5 ml

Adverse effects
CNS: *Fatigue, anxiety, depression, nervousness, paresthesia*
CV: **Tachycardia,** angina, **MI,** *palpitations,* **dysrhythmias,** *hypertension, fluid retention*
EENT: *Tinnitus, hearing loss, blurred vision, glaucoma, cataract, conjunctivitis, eye pain*
GI: *Nausea, anorexia, vomiting, constipation, dry mouth, diverticulitis, gastritis, gastroenteritis, hemorrhoids, hiatal hernia, stomatitis,* **GI bleeding**
GU: **Nephrotoxicity: dysuria, hematuria, oliguria, azotemia, cystitis, UTI**
HEMA: **Blood dyscrasias,** *epistaxis, bruising, anemia*
INTEG: Purpura, *rash, pruritus, sweating, erythema, petechiae, photosensitivity, alopecia*
RESP: Pharyngitis, shortness of breath, pneumonia, coughing

Contraindications: Hypersensitivity to aspirin, iodides, other NSAIDs, asthma

Precautions: Pregnancy **C,** lactation, P children, bleeding disorders, GI disorders, cardiac disorders, hypersensitivity to other antiinflammatory agents

Pharmacokinetics

Absorption	Well absorbed (PO)
Distribution	Crosses placenta, bound to plasma proteins
Metabolism	Liver
Excretion	Kidneys
Half-life	Unknown

Pharmacodynamics
Unknown

Interactions
Individual drugs
Aspirin: ↓ effectiveness, ↑ adverse reactions
Lithium: ↑ toxicity
Warfarin: ↑ anticoagulant effects
Drug classifications
Angiotensin-converting enzyme inhibitors: may ↓ effects of ACE inhibitors
Anticoagulants: ↑ risk of bleeding
Antineoplastics: ↑ risk of hematologic toxicity
Diuretics: ↓ effectiveness of diuretics
Glucocorticoids: ↑ adverse reactions
NSAIDs: ↑ adverse reactions

NURSING CONSIDERATIONS
Assessment
- Assess patients with asthma, aspirin allergy, or nasal polyps for hypersensitivity
- Assess for pain of osteoarthritis; check ROM, inflammation of joints, characteristics of pain
- Assess for pain, discomfort of dysmenorrhea
- Monitor blood counts during therapy; watch for decreasing platelets; if low, therapy may need to be discontinued, restarted after hematologic recovery; and for blood dyscrasias (thrombocytopenia): bruising, fatigue, bleeding, poor healing

Nursing diagnoses
✓ Pain (uses)
✓ Mobility, impaired physical (uses)
✓ Injury, risk for (side effects)
✓ Knowledge deficit (teaching)

Implementation
PO route
- Administer with food or milk to decrease gastric symptoms
- ⊘ Do not crush, dissolve, or chew

R

Patient/family education
- Teach patient that drug must be continued for prescribed time to be effective; to avoid other NSAIDs, aspirin, alcohol
- Caution patient to report bleeding, bruising, fatigue, malaise, since blood dyscrasias do occur
- Teach patient to take with a full glass of water to enhance absorption

Evaluation
Positive therapeutic outcome
- Decreased pain and inflammation in arthritic conditions
- Decrease pain in dysmenorrhea

ropinirole (℞)
(roe-pin′e-role)

Requip

Func. class.: Antiparkinsonian agent

Chem. class.: Dopamine-receptor agonist, nonergot

Pregnancy category C

Action: Selective agonist for dopamine D_2 receptors (presynaptic/postsynaptic sites); binding at D_3 receptor contributes to antiparkinson effects

➔ **Therapeutic Outcome:** Decreased symptoms of Parkinson's disease (involuntary movements)

Uses: Parkinsonism

Dosage and routes
Adult: PO 0.25 mg tid, titrate weekly to max of 24 mg/day

Available forms: Tabs 0.25, 0.5, 1, 2, 4, 5 mg

Adverse effects
CNS: Dystonia, *agitation, insomnia,* dizziness, psychosis, hallucinations, depression, somnolence

CV: *Orthostatic hypotension,* hypotension, syncope, palpitations, **tachycardia,** hypertension

EENT: Blurred vision

GI: *Nausea, vomiting, anorexia, dry mouth,* constipation, dyspepsia, flatulence

GU: Impotence, urinary frequency

INTEG: Rash, sweating

RESP: Pharyngitis, rhinitis, sinusitis, bronchitis, dyspnea

Contraindications: Hypersensitivity

Precautions: Renal disease, cardiac disease, dysrhythmias, affective disorders, psychosis, pregnancy **C**, hepatic disease

Pharmacokinetics

Absorption	Well absorbed
Distribution	Widely distributed
Metabolism	Liver, extensively
Excretion	Kidneys
Half-life	6 hr

Pharmacodynamics
Unknown

Interactions
Individual drugs
Cimetidine: ↑ effect of ropinirole
Ciprofloxacin: ↑ ropinirole effect
Digoxin: ↑ ropinirole effect
Diltiazem: ↑ ropinirole effect
Enoxacin: ↑ ropinirole effect
Erythromycin: ↑ ropinirole effect
Estrogen: ↓ oral clearance of ropinirole
Fluvoxamine: ↑ ropinirole effect
Levodopa: ↑ effect of levodopa
Mexiletine: ↑ ropinirole effect
Norfloxacin: ↑ ropinirole effect
Tacrine: ↑ ropinirole effect
Theophylline: ↑ ropinirole effect

Herb/drug
Chaste tree fruit: ↓ ropinirole action

NURSING CONSIDERATIONS
Assessment
- Monitor B/P, respiration during initial treatment; hypotension or hypertension should be reported
- Assess mental status: affect, mood,

behavioral changes, depression; complete suicide assessment
- Assess for involuntary movements in parkinsonism: akinesia, tremors, staggering gait, muscle rigidity, drooling; these symptoms should improve with therapy

Nursing diagnoses

- ✓ Mobility, impaired (uses)
- ✓ Injury, risk for (uses)
- ✓ Knowledge deficit (teaching)
- ✓ Noncompliance (teaching)

Implementation

- Give drug until NPO before surgery
- Adjust dosage to patient response
- Give with meals to decrease GI upset

Patient/family education

- Advise patient that therapeutic effects may take several wk to a few mo
- Caution patient to change positions slowly to prevent orthostatic hypotension
- Instruct patient to use drug exactly as prescribed; if drug is discontinued abruptly, parkinsonian crisis may occur

Evaluation

Positive therapeutic outcome
- Decreased akathisia, other involuntary movements
- Increased mood

ropivacaine (℞)

(roe-pi'va-kane)

Naropin

Func. class.: Local anesthetic

Chem. class.: Amide

Pregnancy category B

Action: Competes with calcium for sites in nerve membrane that control sodium transport across cell membrane; decreases rise of depolarization phase of action potential

→ Therapeutic Outcome: Maintenance of local anesthesia

Uses: Peripheral nerve block, caudal anesthesia, central neural block, vaginal block

Dosage and routes

Varies with route of anesthesia

Available forms: Inj 2, 5, 7.5 mg/ml

Adverse effects

CNS: Anxiety, restlessness, **convulsions, loss of consciousness,** drowsiness, disorientation, tremors, shivering

CV: **Myocardial depression, cardiac arrest, dysrhythmias,** bradycardia, hypotension, hypertension, **fetal bradycardia**

EENT: Blurred vision, tinnitus, pupil constriction

GI: Nausea, vomiting

INTEG: Rash, urticaria, allergic reactions, edema, burning, skin discoloration at injection site, tissue necrosis

RESP: **Status asthmaticus, respiratory arrest, anaphylaxis**

Contraindications: Hypersensitivity, [P] child <12 yr, [G] elderly, severe liver disease

Precautions: Severe drug allergies, pregnancy **B**

Pharmacokinetics

Absorption	Complete
Distribution	Unknown
Metabolism	Liver
Excretion	Kidneys
Half-life	Unknown

Pharmacodynamics

Onset	2-8 min
Peak	Unknown
Duration	3-6 hr

Interactions

Individual drugs

Chloroprocaine: ↓ action of ropivacaine

Enflurane: ↑ dysrhythmias
Epinephrine: ↑ dysrhythmias
Halothane: ↑ dysrhythmias
Drug classifications
Antidepressants, tricyclic: ↑ hypertension
MAOIs: ↑ hypertension
Phenothiazines: ↑ hypertension

NURSING CONSIDERATIONS
Assessment
- Assess B/P, pulse, respiration during treatment
- Assess fetal heart tones during labor
- Assess allergic reactions: rash, urticaria, itching
- Assess cardiac status: ECG for dysrhythmias, pulse, B/P during anesthesia

Nursing diagnoses
✓ Knowledge deficit (teaching)

Implementation
- Give only with resuscitative equipment nearby
- Give only drugs without preservatives for epidural or caudal anesthesia
- Use new sol; discard unused portions

Evaluation
Positive therapeutic outcome
- Anesthesia necessary for procedure

Treatment of overdose: Airway, O_2, vasopressor, **IV** fluids, anticonvulsants for seizures

rosiglitazone (℞)
(roes-i-glye'ta-zone)
Avandia
Func. class.: Antidiabetic, oral
Chem. class.: Thiazolidinedione
Pregnancy category C

Action: Improves insulin resistance by hepatic glucose metabolism, insulin receptor kinase activity, insulin receptor phosphorylation

➡ **Therapeutic Outcome:** Decreased symptoms of diabetes mellitus

Uses: Stable adult-onset diabetes mellitus, type II (NIDDM) alone or in combination with sulfonylureas, metformin, or insulin

Dosage and routes
Monotherapy
Adult: PO 4 mg qd or in 2 divided doses, may increase to 8 mg qd or in 2 divided doses after 12 wk

Combination therapy
Adult: PO this drug should be added to metformin, sulfonylureas at the adult dose

Available forms: Tabs 2, 4, 8 mg

Adverse effects
CNS: *Fatigue, headache*
ENDO: *Hyper/hypoglycemia*
MISC: *Accidental injury, upper respiratory tract infection, sinusitis, anemia, back pain, diarrhea, edema*

Contraindications: Hypersensitivity to thiazolidinediones, children, lactation, diabetic ketoacidosis

Precautions: Pregnancy **C**, elderly, thyroid disease, hepatic, renal disease

Pharmacokinetics	
Absorption	Unknown
Distribution	Protein binding 99.8%
Metabolism	Unknown
Excretion	Urine, feces, breast milk
Half-life	Elimination 3-4 hr

Pharmacodynamics	
Onset	Unknown
Peak	6-12 wk
Duration	Unknown

Interactions
Drug classification
Oral contraceptives: May decrease effect of oral contraceptive, alternate method advised

NURSING CONSIDERATIONS
Assessment
- Assess for hypoglycemic reactions (sweating, weakness, dizziness,

anxiety, tremors, hunger), hyperglycemic reactions soon after meals
- Assess CBC (baseline, q3 mo) during treatment; check LFTs periodically; AST, LDH, FBS, ALT (if ALT >2.5 × ULN, do not use), HbA_{2c}, fasting plasma insulin, plasma lipids, lipoproteins, B/P, body weight during treatment

Nursing diagnoses
- ✓ Nutrition, altered: more than body requirements (uses)
- ✓ Knowledge deficit (teaching)

Implementation
- Convert from other oral hypoglycemic agents if needed; change may be made without gradual dosage change; monitor serum or urine glucose and ketones tid during conversion
- Give once daily or in 2 divided doses
- Give tabs crushed and mixed with meal or fluids for patients with difficulty swallowing
- Store in airtight container in cool environment

Patient/family education
- Teach patient to use capillary blood glucose test or Chemstrip tid
- Teach patient symptoms of hypo/hyperglycemia, what to do about each
- Advise patient that drug must be continued on daily basis; explain consequence of discontinuing drug abruptly
- Advise patient to avoid OTC medications or herbal preparations unless approved by prescriber
- Advise patient that diabetes is life-long illness; that this drug is not a cure, only controls symptoms
- Advise patient that all food included in diet plan must be eaten to prevent hypoglycemia
- Advise patient to carry ID and glucagon emergency kit for emergencies
- Instruct patient to notify prescriber if oral contraceptives are used
- Teach patient not to use if breast-feeding, may be secreted in breast milk

Evaluation
Positive therapeutic outcome
- Decrease in polyuria, polydipsia, polyphagia; clear sensorium; absence of dizziness; stable gait; blood glucose at normal level

salmeterol (℞)
(sal-met′er-ole)
Serevent
Func. class.: Adrenergic β_2 agonist
Pregnancy category C

Action: Causes bronchodilatation by action on β_2 (pulmonary) receptors by increasing levels of cAMP, which relaxes smooth muscle; with very little effect on heart rate, maintains improvement in FEV from 3 to 12 hr; prevents nocturnal asthma symptoms

➔ **Therapeutic Outcome:** Ease of breathing

Uses: Prevention of exercise-induced asthma, bronchospasm, COPD

Dosage and routes
Adult: INH 2 puffs bid (AM and PM)

Available forms: Aerosol 25 µg/actuation; inhalation powder 50 µg

Adverse effects
CNS: *Tremors, anxiety,* insomnia, headache, dizziness, stimulation, restlessness, hallucinations, flushing, irritability
CV: Palpitations, **tachycardia,** hypertension, angina, hypotension, **dysrhythmias**
EENT: Dry nose, irritation of nose and throat
GI: Heartburn, nausea, vomiting
MS: Muscle cramps
RESP: **Bronchospasm**

Contraindications: Hypersensitivity to sympathomimetics, tachydysrhythmias, severe cardiac disease

S

Precautions: Lactation, pregnancy C, cardiac disorders, hyperthyroidism, diabetes mellitus, hypertension, prostatic hypertrophy, narrow-angle glaucoma, seizures

Pharmacokinetics

Absorption	Unknown
Distribution	Unknown
Metabolism	Unknown
Excretion	Unknown
Half-life	Unknown

Pharmacodynamics

Onset	5-15 min
Peak	4 hr
Duration	12 hr

Interactions

Drug classifications

β-Adrenergic blockers: Block therapeutic effect
Bronchodilators, aerosol: ↑ action of bronchodilator
MAOIs: ↑ chance of hypertensive crisis
Sympathomimetics: ↑ adrenergic side effects

NURSING CONSIDERATIONS

Assessment

- Monitor respiratory function: vital capacity, FEV, ABGs, lung sounds, heart rate, rhythm (baseline)

Nursing diagnoses

✓ Airway clearance, ineffective (uses)
✓ Impaired gas exchange (uses)
✓ Knowledge deficit (teaching)

Implementation

- Shake aerosol container, ask patient to exhale, then place mouthpiece in mouth, inhale slowly, hold breath, remove, exhale slowly; allow at least 1 min between inhalations
- P G Use spacing device for pediatric/elderly patients
- Store in light-resistant container, do not expose to temp over 86° F (30° C)

Patient/family education

- Caution patient not to use OTC medications because extra stimulation may occur
- Instruct patient to use this medication before other medications and to allow at least 1 min between each, to prevent overstimulation
- Teach patient how to use inhaler; to avoid getting aerosol in eyes; blurring may result; to wash inhaler in warm water qd and dry; to avoid smoking, smoke-filled rooms, and persons with respiratory infections; review package insert with patient
- Instruct patient on administration of dose, not to use more than prescribed; serious side effects may occur

Evaluation

Positive therapeutic outcome

- Absence of dyspnea, wheezing
- Improved airway exchange
- Improved ABGs

Treatment of overdose:

Administer a β_2-adrenergic blocker

salsalate (℞)

(sal-sa'late)

Amigesic, Argesic-SA, Arthra-G, Disalcid, Marthritic, Mono-Gesic, Salflex, Salsalate, Salsitab

Func. class.: Nonnarcotic analgesic; nonsteroidal antiinflammatory agent

Chem. class.: Salicylate

Pregnancy category C

Action: Blocks formation of peripheral prostaglandins, which cause pain and inflammation; antipyretic action results from inhibition of hypothalamic heat-regulating center; does not inhibit platelet aggregation

➔ **Therapeutic Outcome:** Decreased pain, inflammation

Uses: Mild to moderate pain or fever, P including arthritis, juvenile rheumatoid arthritis

Dosage and routes

Adult: PO 3 g/day in divided doses

Available forms: Caps 500 mg; tabs 500, 750 mg

Adverse effects

CNS: Stimulation, drowsiness, dizziness, confusion, **seizures**, headache, flushing, hallucinations, coma
CV: Rapid pulse, **pulmonary edema**
EENT: Tinnitus, hearing loss
ENDO: Hypoglycemia, hyponatremia, hypokalemia, alteration in acid-base balance
GI: *Nausea, vomiting, GI bleeding, diarrhea, heartburn,* anorexia, **hepatotoxicity**
HEMA: **Thrombocytopenia, agranulocytosis, leukopenia, neutropenia, hemolytic anemia,** increased pro-time
INTEG: *Rash,* urticaria, bruising
RESP: Wheezing, hyperpnea

Contraindications: Hypersensitivity to salicylates, NSAIDs, GI bleeding, bleeding disorders, P children <3 yr, vit K deficiency

Precautions: Anemia, hepatic disease, renal disease, Hodgkin's disease, pregnancy **C,** lactation, G elderly

Pharmacokinetics

Absorption	Absorbed in small intestine
Distribution	Rapidly and widely distributed, crosses placenta
Metabolism	Not metabolized
Excretion	Unchanged—kidneys
Half-life	2-3 hr (low doses), 15-30 hr (high doses)

Pharmacodynamics

Onset	30 min
Peak	1-3 hr
Duration	3-6 hr

Interactions

Individual drugs

Alcohol: ↑ bleeding
Cefamandole: ↑ bleeding
Furosemide: ↑ toxic effects
Heparin: ↑ bleeding
Insulin: ↑ effects
Methotrexate: ↑ effects
***P*-Aminobenzoic acid:** ↑ toxic effects
Phenytoin: ↑ effects
Plicamycin: ↑ bleeding
Probenecid: ↓ effects
Spironolactone: ↓ effects
Sulfinpyrazone: ↓ effects
Valproic acid: ↑ effects, ↑ bleeding
Vancomycin: ↑ ototoxicity

Drug classifications

Antacids: ↓ effects of aspirin
Anticoagulants: ↑ effects
Carbonic anhydrase inhibitors: ↑ toxic effects
NSAIDs: ↑ gastric ulcers
Penicillins: ↑ effects
Salicylates: ↓ blood glucose levels
Steroids: ↓ effects of aspirin, ↑ gastric ulcers
Sulfonylamides: ↓ effects
Urinary acidifiers: ↑ salicylate levels
Urinary alkalizers: ↓ effects of aspirin

Food/drug

Foods causing acidic urine may ↑ level

Herb/drug

Alfalfa: ↑ risk of bleeding
Angelica: ↑ risk of bleeding

Lab test interferences

↑ Coagulation studies, ↑ liver function studies, ↑ serum uric acid, ↑ amylase, ↑ CO_2, ↑ urinary protein
↓ Serum potassium, ↓ PBI, ↓ cholesterol, ↓ blood glucose
Interference: Urine catecholamines, pregnancy test

NURSING CONSIDERATIONS

Assessment

- Monitor liver function studies: AST, ALT, bilirubin, creatinine if patient is on long-term therapy
- Monitor renal function studies: BUN, urine creatinine if patient is on long-term therapy
- Monitor blood studies: CBC, Hct, Hgb, pro-time if patient is on long-term therapy

S

- Check I&O ratio; decreasing output may indicate renal failure if patient is on long-term therapy
- Assess hepatotoxicity: dark urine, clay-colored stools, yellowing of the skin and sclera, itching, abdominal pain, fever, diarrhea if patient is on long-term therapy
- Assess for allergic reactions: rash, urticaria; if these occur, drug may have to be discontinued; assess for asthma, aspirin sensitivity, nasal polyps, may develop hypersensitivity
- Assess for ototoxicity: tinnitus, ringing, roaring in ears; audiometric testing needed before, after long-term therapy
- Assess for visual changes: blurring, halos; corneal, retinal damage
- Check edema in feet, ankles, legs
- Identify prior drug history; many drug interactions are possible
- Monitor pain: location, duration, type, intensity, prior to dose and 1 hr after
- Monitor musculoskeletal status: ROM before dose
- Identify fever, length of time, and related symptoms

Nursing diagnoses

- ✓ Pain (uses)
- ✓ Mobility, impaired physical mobility (uses)
- ✓ Knowledge deficit (teaching)
- ✓ Injury, risk for (side effects)

Implementation

- Administer to patient crushed or whole; chewable tab may be chewed
- Give with food or milk to decrease gastric symptoms; give 30 min ac or 2 hr pc; absorption may be slowed
- Give antacids 1-2 hr after enteric products

Patient/family education

- Advise patient to report any symptoms of hepatotoxicity, renal toxicity, visual changes, ototoxicity, allergic reactions, bleeding (long-term therapy)
- Instruct patient to take with 8 oz of water and sit upright for ½ hr after dose
- Caution patient not to exceed recommended dosage; acute poisoning may result
- Advise patient to read label on other OTC drugs; many contain aspirin
- Inform patient that the therapeutic response takes 2 wk (arthritis)
- Teach patient to report tinnitus, confusion, diarrhea, sweating, hyperventilation
- Caution patient to avoid alcohol ingestion; GI bleeding may occur
- Inform patient that patients who have allergies may develop allergic reactions

Evaluation

Positive therapeutic outcome

- Decreased pain
- Decreased inflammation

Treatment of overdose:

Lavage, activated charcoal, monitor electrolytes, VS

saquinavir (℞)

(sa-quen′a-ver)

Invirase, Fortovase

Func. class.: Antiretroviral

Chem. class.: Protease inhibitor

Pregnancy category B

Action: Inhibits HIV protease

➔ Therapeutic Outcome: Prevents maturation of the infectious virus

Uses: HIV in combination with zidovudine (AZT), zalcitabine

Dosage and routes

Adult: PO 600 mg (hard cap) or 1200 mg (soft cap) tid within 2 hr after a full meal; given with either zalcitabine 0.75 mg tid or AZT 200 mg tid

Available forms: Caps 200 mg (soft); 200 mg (hard)

Adverse effects

CNS: *Paresthesia*, headache

GI: *Diarrhea*, buccal mucosa ulceration, *abdominal pain, nausea*
INTEG: *Rash*
MISC: Asthenia, *hyperglycemia*
MS: Pain

Contraindications: Hypersensitivity

Precautions: Liver disease, pregnancy **B**, lactation, children

Pharmacokinetics

Absorption	↑ with food
Distribution	Protein-binding 98%
Metabolism	Extensively
Excretion	Unknown
Half-life	Unknown

Pharmacodynamics

Unknown

Interactions

Individual drugs

Carbamazepine: ↑ saquinavir level
Clarithromycin: ↑ saquinavir level
Clindamycin: ↑ toxicity
Dapsone: ↑ toxicity
Delavirdine: ↑ saquinavir level
Dexamethasone: ↑ saquinavir level
Indinavir: ↑ saquinavir level
Midazolam: ↑ toxicity
Nelfinavir: ↑ saquinavir level
Nevirapine: ↑ saquinavir level
Phenobarbital: ↑ saquinavir level
Phenytoin: ↑ saquinavir level
Quinidine: ↑ toxicity
Rifamycin: ↓ saquinavir level
Ritonavir: ↑ saquinavir level
Triazolam: ↑ toxicity

Drug classifications

Calcium channel blockers: ↑ toxicity
Ergot derivatives: ↑ vasoconstriction, do not use together
HMG-CoA reductase inhibitors: avoid use with saquinavir

Herb/drug

St. John's wort: ↓ saquinavir level, avoid concurrent use

Lab test interferences

Interference: CPK, glucose (low)

NURSING CONSIDERATIONS

Assessment

- Assess signs of infection, anemia
- Monitor liver function studies: ALT, AST
- Monitor C&S before drug therapy; drug may be taken as soon as culture is done; repeat C&S after treatment; determine the presence of other sexually transmitted diseases
- Assess bowel pattern before, during treatment; if severe abdominal pain with bleeding occurs, drug should be discontinued; monitor hydration
- Assess skin eruptions, rash, urticaria, itching
- Assess allergies before treatment, reaction of each medication; place allergies on chart

Nursing diagnoses

- ✓ Infection, risk for (uses)
- ✓ Knowledge deficit (teaching)

Patient/family education

- Advise patient to take as prescribed within 2 hr of a full meal; if dose is missed, take as soon as remembered up to 1 hr before next dose; do not double dose
- Advise patient that drug must be taken in equal intervals around the clock to maintain blood levels for duration of therapy, that Invirase and Fortovase are not interchangeable

sargramostim (℞)

(sar-gram'oh-stim)
Leukine, rhu GM-CSF recombinant human
Func. class.: Biologic modifier: cytokine
Chem. class.: Granulocyte/macrophage colony stimulating factor

Pregnancy category C

Action: Stimulates proliferation and differentiation of hematopoietic

S

progenitor cells (granulocyte, macrophage)

Uses: Acceleration of myeloid recovery in patients with non-Hodgkin's lymphoma, acute lymphoblastic leukemia, autologous bone marrow transplantation in Hodgkin's disease; bone marrow transplantation failure or engraftment delay; mobilization and transplant of peripheral blood progenitor cells (PBPCs)

Dosage and routes

Myeloid reconstitution after autologous bone marrow transplantation

Adult: **IV** 250 μg/m^2/day × 3 wk; give over 2 hr, 2-4 hr after autologous bone marrow inf, and not less than 24 hr after last dose of antineoplastics and 12 hr after last dose of radiotherapy, bone marrow transplantation failure, or engraftment delay

Acceleration of myeloid recovery

Adult: **IV** 250 μg/m^2/day × 14 days; give over 2 hr; may repeat in 7 days, may repeat 500 μg/m^2/day × 14 days after another 7 days if no improvement

Mobilization of PBPCs

Adult: **IV**/SC 250 μg/m^2/day during collection of PBPCs

After PBPC transplantation

Adult: **IV**/SC 250 μg/m^2/day until ANC >1500/mm^3 × 3 days

Available forms: Powder for inj lyophilized 250, 500 μg; liq 500 μg/ml

Adverse effects

CNS: Fever, malaise, CNS disorder, weakness, chills
CV: Supraventricular tachycardia, peripheral edema, pericardial effusion
GI: Nausea, vomiting, diarrhea, anorexia, **GI hemorrhage,** stomatitis, **liver damage**
GU: Urinary tract disorder, abnormal kidney function
HEMA: **Blood dyscrasias, hemorrhage**
INTEG: Alopecia, rash, peripheral edema
MS: Bone pain
RESP: Dyspnea

Contraindications: Hypersensitivity to GM-CSF, yeast products; excessive leukemic myeloid blast in the bone marrow or peripheral blood

Precautions: Pregnancy **C**, lactation, P children; renal, hepatic, lung disease; cardiac disease; pleural, pericardial effusions

Do Not Confuse:
Leukine/leucovorin, Leukine/Leukeran

Pharmacokinetics

Absorption	Completely absorbed
Distribution	Unknown
Metabolism	Unknown
Excretion	Unknown
Half-life	2 hr

Pharmacodynamics

Onset	Rapid
Peak	2 hr
Duration	Unknown

Interactions

Individual drugs

Lithium: ↑ myeloproliferation

Drug classifications

Antineoplastics: Do not use together
Corticosteroids: ↑ myeloproliferation

NURSING CONSIDERATIONS

Assessment

- Monitor blood studies: CBC, differential count before treatment and twice weekly; leukocytosis may occur (WBC >50,000 cells/mm^3, ANC >20,000 cells/mm^3), platelets; if ANC >20,000/mm^3 or 10,000/mm^3 after nadir has occurred, or platelets >500,000/mm^3 reduce dose by ½ or discontinue; if blast cells occur, discontinue
- Monitor renal and hepatic studies before treatment: BUN, creatinine, urinalysis; AST, ALT, alkaline

phosphatase; monitoring is needed twice a week in renal, hepatic disease

- Assess for hypersensitivity reactions/rashes, and local inj site reactions; usually transient
- Assess for increased fluid retention in cardiac disease
- Assess for myalgia, arthralgia in legs, feet; use analgesics

Nursing diagnoses

✓ Infection, risk for (uses)
✓ Knowledge deficit (teaching)

Implementation

- Reconstitute with 1 ml of sterile water for inj without preservative; do not reenter vial; discard unused portion; direct reconstitution sol at side of vial; rotate contents; do not shake

SC route

- Use reconstituted sol

IV route

- Give by intermittent inf after diluting in 0.9% NaCl inj to prepare **IV** inf; if final conc is <10 μg/ml, add human albumin to make a final conc of 0.1% to the NaCl before adding sargramostim to prevent absorption; for a final conc of 0.1% albumin, add 1 mg of human albumin/1 ml of 0.9% NaCl inj; run over 2 hr (bone marrow transplant or failure of graft); over 4 hr (chemotherapy for acute myeloid leukemia); over 24 hr as cont inf (PBPCs); give within 6 hr after reconstitution
- Store in refrigerator; do not freeze

Y-site compatibilities:

Amikacin, aminophylline, aztreonam, bleomycin, butorphanol, calcium gluconate, carboplatin, carmustine, cefazolin, cefepime, cefotaxime, cefotetan, ceftizoxime, ceftriaxone, cefuroxime, cimetidine, cisplatin, clindamycin, cyclophosphamide, cyclosporine, cytarabine, dacarbazine, dactinomycin, dexamethasone, diphenhydramine, dopamine, doxorubicin, doxycycline, droperidol, etoposide, famotidine, fentanyl, floxuridine, fluconazole, fluorouracil, furosemide, gentamicin, granisetron, heparin, idarubicin, ifosfamide, immune globulin, magnesium sulfate, mannitol, mechlorethamine, meperidine, mesna, methotrexate, metoclopramide, metronidazole, mezlocillin, miconazole, minocycline, mitoxantrone, netilmicin, pentostatin, piperacillin/tazobactam, potassium chloride, prochlorperazine, promethazine, ranitidine, teniposide, ticarcillin, ticarcillin/clavulanate, trimethoprim/sulfamethoxazole, vinblastine, vincristine, zidovudine

Y-site incompatibilities:

Acyclovir, ampicillin, ampicillin/sulbactam, cefonicid, cefoperazine, ceftazidime, chlorpromazine, ganciclovir, haloperidol, hydrocortisone, hydromorphone, hydroxyzine, idarubicin, imipenem/cilastatin, lorazepam, methylprednisolone sodium succinate, mitomycin, morphine, nalbuphine, ondansetron, piperacillin, sodium bicarbonate, tobramycin

Patient/family education

- Teach patient reason for medication and expected results
- Advise patient to notify nurse or prescriber of side effects

Evaluation

Positive therapeutic outcome

- WBC and differential recovery
- Absence of infection

S

scopolamine (℞)

(skoe-pol'a-meen)

Transderm-Scop, Isopoto-Hyoscine, Transderm-V, Triptol

Func. class.: Antiemetic, anticholinergic, mydriatic

Chem. class.: Belladonna alkaloid

Pregnancy category C

Action: Inhibits acetylcholine at receptor sites in autonomic nervous system, which controls secretions, free acids in stomach; blocks central muscarinic receptors, which decreases involuntary movements; blocks response of iris sphincter muscle, muscle of accommodation of ciliary body to cholinergic stimulation, resulting in dilation, paralysis of accommodation

Therapeutic Outcome: Absence of vomiting, secretions (preoperatively), involuntary movements

Uses: Reduction of secretions before surgery, calm delirium, uveitis, iritis, cycloplegia, mydriasis; prevention of motion sickness, parkinson symptoms

Investigational uses: Drooling (TD)

Dosage and routes

Ophthalmic route

Adult: Instill 1-2 gtt before refraction or 1-2 gtt qd-tid for iritis or uveitis

P ***Child:*** Instill 1 gtt bid × 2 days before refraction

Prevention of motion sickness

Adult: TD 1 patch placed behind ear 4-5 hr before travel

P Not recommended for children

Parkinson symptoms

Adult: IM/SC/**IV** 0.3-0.6 mg tid-qid diluted using dilution provided

Preoperatively

Adult: SC 0.4-0.6 mg

P ***Child:*** SC 0.006 mg/kg or 0.2 mg/m^2

Drooling (off-label)

Adult: TD 1.5 mg patch q3 days

Available forms: Sol 0.25%; patch 0.5, 1 mg delivered in 72 hr; inj 0.3, 0.4, 0.86, 1 mg/ml

Adverse effects

CNS: Confusion, anxiety, restlessness, irritability, delusions, hallucinations, headache, sedation, depression, incoherence, dizziness, excitement, delirium, flushing, weakness

CV: Palpitations, **tachycardia,** postural hypotension, paradoxical bradycardia

EENT: Blurred vision, photophobia, dilated pupils, difficulty swallowing, mydriasis, cycloplegia

GI: ***Dryness of mouth, constipation,*** nausea, vomiting, abdominal distress, **paralytic ileus**

GU: Hesitancy, retention

INTEG: Urticaria

MISC: Suppression of lactation, nasal congestion, decreased sweating

Contraindications: Hypersensitivity, narrow-angle glaucoma, myasthenia gravis, GI/GU obstruction, hypersensitivity to belladonna, barbiturates

G **Precautions:** Pregnancy **C**, elderly, lactation, prostatic hypertrophy, CHF,
P hypertension, dysrhythmias, children, gastric ulcer

Pharmacokinetics

Absorption	Well absorbed (IM, SC, TD)
Distribution	Crosses placenta, blood-brain barrier
Metabolism	Liver
Excretion	Unknown
Half-life	8 hr

Pharmacodynamics

	SC/IM	IV	TD	OPHTH
Onset	30-45 min	10-15 min	4-5 hr	Unknown
Peak	1 hr	1 hr	Unknown	20-30 min
Duration	6 hr	4 hr	72 hr	3-7 days

Interactions

Individual drugs

Alcohol: ↑ CNS depression

Quinidine: ↑ anticholinergic effect

Drug classifications

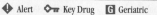

Antidepressants: ↑ anticholinergic effect

Antidepressants, tricyclic: ↑ anticholinergic effect
Antihistamines: ↑ anticholinergic effect
Narcotics: ↑ anticholinergic effect
Phenothiazines: ↑ anticholinergic effect

NURSING CONSIDERATIONS
Assessment
- Assess for eye pain; discontinue use (opticue)
- Monitor I&O ratio; retention commonly causes decreased urinary output
- Assess for parkinsonism, EPS: shuffling gait, muscle rigidity, involuntary movements
- Assess for urinary hesitancy, retention; palpate bladder if retention occurs
- Assess for constipation; increase fluids, bulk, exercise if this occurs
- Assess for tolerance over long-term therapy; dose may have to be increased or changed
- Assess mental status: affect, mood, CNS depression, worsening of mental symptoms during early therapy

Nursing diagnoses
✓ Fluid volume deficit (uses)
✓ Knowledge deficit (teaching)

Implementation
IV SC/IM/IV route
- Administer parenteral dose with patient recumbent to prevent postural hypotension

IV IV route
- Give by direct **IV** after diluting with sterile water; give slowly

Syringe compatibilities:
Atropine, benzquinamide, butorphanol, chlorpromazine, cimetidine, dimenhydrinate, diphenhydramine, droperidol, fentanyl, glycopyrrolate, hydromorphone, hydroxyzine, meperidine, metoclopramide, midazolam, morphine, nalbuphine, pentazocine, pentobarbital, perphenazine, prochlorperazine, promazine, promethazine, ranitidine, sufentanil, thiopental

Y-site compatibilities:
Heparin, hydrocortisone, potassium chloride, propofol, sufentanil, vit B/C

Additive compatibilities:
Floxacillin, furosemide, meperidine, succinylcholine

Patient/family education
- Tell patient to avoid hazardous activities, activities requiring alertness; dizziness may occur

TD route
- Instruct patient to wash, dry hands before and after applying to surface behind ear; to change patch q72h; to apply at least 4 hr before traveling
- Advise patient to discontinue use if blurred vision, severe dizziness, drowsiness occurs; another type of antiemetic may be used or the patch rotated to the other ear
- Instruct patient to read labels of all OTC medications; if any scopolamine is found in product, avoid use
- Advise patient to keep medication out of children's reach
- Caution patient to report change in vision, blurring or loss of sight, trouble breathing, inhibition of sweating, flushing

Ophthalmic route
- Teach patient method of instillation: pressure on lacrimal sac for 1 min; do not touch dropper to eye
- Inform patient that blurred vision will decrease with repeated use of drug
- Advise patient to wait 5 min to use other drops; blink more than usual
- Caution patient not to discontinue this drug abruptly; to taper off over 1 wk

Evaluation
Positive therapeutic outcome
- Decrease in inflammation, cycloplegic refraction
- Decreased secretions
- Absence of motion sickness

S

HIGH ALERT

secobarbital (℞)
(see-koe-bar'bi-tal)
Secogen Sodium ✦, Seconal Sodium Pulvules, Seral ✦
Func. class.: Sedative/hypnotic-barbiturate
Chem. class.: Barbitone (short-acting)

Pregnancy category D

Controlled substance schedule II (USA), schedule G (Canada)

Action: Depresses activity in brain cells primarily in reticular activating system in brainstem; selectively depresses neurons in posterior hypothalamus, limbic structures; decreases seizure activity by inhibition of epileptic activity in CNS

Therapeutic Outcome: Sedation, decreased seizure activity, improved energy

Uses: Insomnia, sedation, preoperative medication, status epilepticus, acute tetanus seizures

Dosage and routes

Insomnia

Adult: PO/IM 100-200 mg hs

P ***Child:*** IM 3-5 mg/kg, max 100 mg, do not inject >5 ml in one site

Sedation/preoperatively

Adult: PO 200-300 mg 1-2 hr preoperatively

P ***Child:*** PO 50-100 mg 1-2 hr preoperatively

Status epilepticus

P ***Adult and child:*** IM/**IV** 250-350 mg

Acute psychotic agitation

P ***Adult and child:*** IM/**IV** 5.5 mg/kg q3-4h

Available forms: Caps 50, 100 mg; tabs 100 mg; inj 50 mg/ml

Adverse effects

CNS: ***Lethargy, drowsiness, hangover,*** dizziness, paradoxical stimulation in the elderly and children, light-headedness, dependency, CNS depression, mental depression, slurred speech

CV: Hypotension, bradycardia

GI: Nausea, vomiting, diarrhea, constipation

HEMA: **Agranulocytosis, thrombocytopenia, megaloblastic anemia** (long-term treatment)

INTEG: ***Rash,*** urticaria, pain, abscesses at inj site, angioedema, thrombophlebitis, **Stevens-Johnson syndrome**

RESP: Depression, **apnea, laryngospasm, bronchospasm**

Contraindications: Hypersensitivity to barbiturates, respiratory depression, pregnancy **D,** addiction to barbiturates, severe liver impairment, porphyria, uncontrolled severe pain

Precautions: Anemia, lactation, hepatic disease, renal disease, hypertension, elderly, acute/chronic pain

Pharmacokinetics

Absorption	Slow (70%-90%) (PO), **IV** complete
Distribution	Not known, crosses placenta
Metabolism	Liver (75%)
Excretion	Kidneys (25% unchanged)
Half-life	2-6 days

Pharmacodynamics

	PO	IM	IV
Onset	30-60 min	10-30 min	5 min
Peak	Unknown	Unknown	30 min
Duration	6-8 hr	4-6 hr	4-6 hr

Interactions

Individual drugs

Alcohol: ↑ CNS depression

Chloramphenicol: ↓ effectiveness

Cyclophosphamide: ↑ hematologic toxicity
Cyclosporine: ↓ effectiveness
Dacarbazine: ↓ effectiveness
Quinidine: ↓ effectiveness
Valproic acid: ↑ sedation

Drug classifications
Anticoagulants: ↓ effectiveness
Antidepressants: ↑ CNS depression
Antidepressants, tricyclic: ↓ effectiveness
Antihistamines: ↑ CNS depression
Glucocorticoids: ↓ effectiveness
MAOIs: ↑ CNS depression
Opiates: ↑ CNS depression
Oral contraceptives: ↓ effectiveness
Sedatives/hypnotics: ↑ CNS depression

Herb/drug
Kava: ↑ CNS depression

NURSING CONSIDERATIONS

Assessment

- Assess patient's mental status: mood, sensorium, affect, memory G (long, short), especially in elderly patients; if using as a hypnotic, assess sleep patterns during therapy; drug suppresses REM sleep with dreaming; withdrawal insomnia may occur after short-term use; do not start using drug again, insomnia will improve in 1-3 nights; patient may experience increased dreaming
- Monitor patient for respiratory dysfunction: respiratory depression, character, rate, rhythm (when using IV **IV**); hold drug if respirations are <10/min or if pupils are dilated. Also check VS q30 min after parenteral route for 2 hr
- Assess patient for barbiturate toxicity: hypotension, pulmonary constriction, cold, clammy skin, cyanosis of lips, CNS depression, nausea, vomiting, hallucinations, delirium, weakness, coma, pupillary constriction; mild symptoms may occur in 8-12 hr without drug
- Assess patient for blood dyscrasias: fever, sore throat, bruising, rash, jaundice, epistaxis (long-term treatment only)
- Assess for pain in postoperative patients; pain threshold is lowered when patients are taking this medication

Nursing diagnoses

- ✓ Sleep pattern disturbance (uses)
- ✓ Injury, risk for (adverse reactions)
- ✓ Knowledge deficit (teaching)

Implementation

- Administer after removal of cigarettes, to prevent fires
- Administer after trying conservative measures for insomnia

PO route

- Tab may be crushed and mixed with food if swallowing is difficult; also may be mixed with other fluids ½-1 hr before bedtime for expected sleeplessness; on empty stomach for best absorption

IM route

- Give in deep muscle mass (gluteal) to minimize irritation to tissues
- Split inj of >5 ml into 2 inj because irritation to tissues may occur

IV **Direct IV route**

- Use large vein to prevent extravasation; if extravasation occurs, use moist heat to the area and procaine sol 5% inj into area
- Give at rate of 65 mg or less/min; titrate to patient response

Syringe incompatibilities:
Benzquinamide, dimenhydrinate, diphenhydramine, erythromycin gluceptate, hydroxyzine, kanamycin, oxytetracycline, phenytoin, prochlorperazine, promazine, promethazine, ranitidine, tetracycline

Additive compatibilities:
Amikacin, aminophylline

Additive incompatibilities:
Cephalothin, chlorpromazine, codeine, ephedrine, hydralazine, hydrocortisone sodium succinate, hydroxyzine, insulin, levorphanol, meperidine, methadone, morphine, norepineph-

S

rine, pentazocine, procaine, prochlorazine mesylate, promazine, promethazine, streptomycin, vancomycin

Solution compatibilities: D_5W, $D_{10}W$, 0.45% NaCl, 0.9% NaCl, Ringer's sol, dextrose/saline combinations, dextrose/Ringer's or dextrose/lactated Ringer's combinations

Patient/family education

- Teach patient that hangover is common
- Instruct patient that drug is indicated only for short-term treatment of insomnia and is probably ineffective after 2 wk
- Inform patient that physical dependency may result when used for extended time (45-90 days depending on dose)
- Caution patient to avoid driving or other activities requiring alertness
- Caution patient to avoid alcohol ingestion or CNS depressants; serious CNS depression may result
- Instruct patient not to discontinue medication quickly after long-term use; drug should be tapered over 1 wk
- Emphasize the need to tell all prescribers that a barbiturate is being taken
- Inform patient that withdrawal insomnia may occur after short-term use; patient should not start using drug again, insomnia will improve in 1-3 nights; patient may experience increased dreaming
- Inform patient that benefits may take 2 nights to be noticed; teach patient alternate measures to improve sleep: reading, exercise several hours before bedtime, warm bath, warm milk, TV, self-hypnosis, deep breathing
- Teach patient to make position changes slowly; orthostatic hypotension may occur
- Instruct patient to notify prescriber immediately if bruising or bleeding occurs; may indicate blood dycrasias

Evaluation

Positive therapeutic outcome

- Improved sleeping patterns
- Decreased seizure activity
- Improved energy

Treatment of overdose: Lavage, activated charcoal, warming blanket, vital signs, hemodialysis, alkalinize urine; give **IV** volume expanders, **IV** fluids

selegiline (℞)

(se-le'ji-leen)

Carbex, Eldepryl, Novo-Selegiline ✱, SD-Deprenyl

Func. class.: Antiparkinson agent

Chem. class.: Levorotatory acetylenic derivative of phenethylamine

Pregnancy category C

Action: Increased dopaminergic activity by inhibition of MAO type B activity; not fully understood

➔ **Therapeutic Outcome:** Decreased symptoms of Parkinson's disease

Uses: Adjunct management of Parkinson's disease in patients being treated with levodopa/carbidopa who have responded poorly to therapy

Investigational use: Alzheimer's disease

Dosage and routes

Adult: PO 10 mg/day in divided doses, 5 mg at breakfast and lunch with levodopa/carbidopa; after 2-3 days begin to reduce the dose of levodopa/carbidopa 10%-30%

Available forms: Tabs 5 mg

Adverse effects

CNS: Increased tremors, chorea, restlessness, blepharospasm, increased bradykinesia, grimacing, tardive dyskinesia, dystonic symptoms, involuntary movements, increased apraxia, hallucinations, dizziness, mood changes, nightmares, delusions,

lethargy, apathy, overstimulation, sleep disturbances, headache, migraine, numbness, muscle cramps, confusion, anxiety, tiredness, vertigo, personality change, back/leg pain
CV: Orthostatic hypotension, hypertension, **dysrhythmia,** palpitations; angina pectoris, hypotension, tachycardia, edema, sinus bradycardia, syncope
EENT: Diploplia, dry mouth, blurred vision, tinnitus
GI: Nausea, vomiting, constipation, weight loss, anorexia, diarrhea, heartburn, rectal bleeding, poor appetite, dysphagia, xerostomia
GU: Slow urination, nocturia, prostatic hypertrophy, hesitation, retention, frequency, sexual dysfunction
INTEG: Increased sweating, alopecia, hematoma, rash, photosensitivity, facial hair
RESP: Asthma, shortness of breath

Contraindications: Hypersensitivity

Precautions: Pregnancy **C,**
P lactation, children

Do Not Confuse:
Eldepryl/enalapril

Pharmacokinetics

Absorption	Well absorbed
Distribution	Widely distributed
Metabolism	Rapidly, liver
Excretion	Metabolites-N-desmethyldeprenyl, amphetamine, methamphetamine
Half-life	9 min

Pharmacodynamics

Onset	Unknown
Peak	½-2 hr
Duration	Unknown

Interactions

Individual drugs

Fluoxetine: ↑ serotonin syndrome (confusion, seizures, fever, hypertension, agitation) discontinue 5 wk before selegiline
Fluvoxamine: ↑ serotonin syndrome (confusion, seizures, fever, hypertension, agitation) discontinue 5 wk before selegiline
Levodopa/carbidopa: ↑ side effects
Meperidine: Do not use— fatal reaction
Paroxetine: ↑ serotonin syndrome (confusion, seizures, fever, hypertension, agitation) discontinue 5 wk before selegiline
Sertraline: ↑ serotonin syndrome (confusion, seizures, fever, hypertension, agitation) discontinue 5 wk before selegiline

Drug classifications

Opioids: Do not use—fatal reaction

Herb/drug

Chaste tree fruit: ↓ selegiline action

Lab test interferences

↓ VMA
False positive: Urine ketones, urine glucose
False negative: Urine glucose (glucose oxidase)
False: ↑ Uric acid, ↑ urine protein

NURSING CONSIDERATIONS

Assessment

- Monitor B/P, respiration throughout treatment
- Assess mental status: affect, mood, behavioral changes, depression; perform suicide assessment
- Assess for decreased Parkinson's symptoms: rigidity, unsteady gait, weakness, tremors; these should decrease in severity

Nursing diagnoses

✓ Physical mobility, impaired (uses)
✓ Knowledge deficit (teaching)

Implementation

- Adjust dosage to patient response
- Give with meals; limit protein taken with drug
- Give at doses <10 mg/day because

S

of risks associated with nonselective inhibition of MAO

Patient/family education

- Caution patient to change positions slowly to prevent orthostatic hypotension
- Advise patient to report side effects: twitching, eye spasms; may indicate overdose
- Caution patient to use drug exactly as prescribed; if drug is discontinued abruptly, parkinsonian crisis may occur
- Instruct patient to avoid foods high in tyramine: cheese, pickled products, wine, beer, large amounts of caffeine
- Instruct patient not to exceed recommended dose of 10 mg; might precipitate a hypertensive crisis; report severe headache or other unusual symptoms

Evaluation

Positive therapeutic outcome

- Decreased symptoms of Parkinson's disease

Treatment of overdose: **IV** fluids for hypertension, **IV** dilute pressure agent for B/P titration

senna, sennasides (OTC)

(sin'na)

Black Draught, Dr. Caldwell Dosalax, Ex-Lax Gentle, Fletcher's Castoria, Gentlax, Senexon, Senna-Gen, Senokot, Senokotxtra, Senolax

Func. class.: Laxative-stimulant

Chem. class.: Anthraquinone

Pregnancy category C

Action: Stimulates peristalsis by action on Auerbach's plexus; softens feces by increasing water and electrolytes in large intestine

Therapeutic Outcome: Decreased constipation

Uses: Acute constipation; bowel preparation for surgery or exam

Dosage and routes

Adult: PO 1-8 tabs (Senokot)/day or 1/2 to 4 tsp of granules added to water or juice; rec supp 1-2 hs; syrup 1-4 tsp hs (1 tsp = 4 ml), 7.5-15 ml; Black Draught: 3/4 oz dissolved in 2.5 oz of liq given between 2-4 PM the day before procedure (X-Prep)

P ***Child >27 kg:*** PO ½ adult dose; do not use Black Draught for children

P ***Child 1 mo-1 yr:*** Syrup 1.25-2.5 ml (Senokot) hs

Available forms: Supp 625 mg, 30 mg sennosides; powder 662 mg/g, 6, 15 mg sennosides/3 g; tabs 8.6 sennosides, 180 mg; oral sol 3 mg senosides/ml

Adverse effects

GI: *Nausea, vomiting, anorexia, abdominal cramps,* diarrhea, flatulence

GU: Pink-red or brown-black discoloration of urine

META: Hypocalcemia, enteropathy, alkalosis, hypokalemia, **tetany**

Contraindications: Hypersensitivity, GI bleeding, intestinal obstruction, CHF, lactation, abdominal pain, nausea/vomiting, appendicitis, acute surgical abdomen

Precautions: Pregnancy **C**

Pharmacokinetics

Absorption	Minimally absorbed (PO)
Distribution	Unknown
Metabolism	Not metabolized
Excretion	Kidneys, feces
Half-life	Unknown

Pharmacodynamics

	PO	REC
Onset	6-24 hr	Unknown
Peak	Unknown	Unknown
Duration	3-4 days	Unknown

Interactions

Individual drugs

Disulfiram: Do not use together

Drug classifications

Oral drugs: ↓ absorption

NURSING CONSIDERATIONS

Assessment

- Monitor blood, urine electrolytes if used often by patient; check I&O ratio to identify fluid loss
- Assess cramping, rectal bleeding, nausea, vomiting; if these symptoms occur, drug should be discontinued; identify cause of constipation; identify whether fluids, bulk, or exercise is missing from lifestyle
- Assess for magnesium toxicity: thirst, confusion, decrease in reflexes
- Monitor blood ammonia level (30-70 mg/100 ml); monitor for clearing of confusion, lethargy, restlessness, irritability (hepatic encephalopathy)

Nursing diagnoses

- ✓ Bowel elimination, altered: constipation (uses)
- ✓ Bowel elimination, altered; diarrhea (side effects)
- ✓ Knowledge deficit (teaching)
- ✓ Noncompliance (teaching)

Implementation

PO route

- Administer on empty stomach for more rapid results
- Give with a full glass of water in AM or PM (oral dose); evacuation occurs 6-12 hr later
- Dissolve granules in water or juice before administration
- Shake oral sol before giving

Patient/family education

- Discuss with patient that adequate fluid consumption is necessary
- Inform patient that normal bowel movements do not always occur daily
- Teach patient not to use in presence of abdominal pain, nausea, vomiting; tell patient to notify prescriber if constipation is unrelieved or if symptoms of electrolyte imbalance occur: muscle cramps, pain, weakness, dizziness, excessive thirst

Evaluation

Positive therapeutic outcome

- Decreased constipation in 8-10 hr

sertraline (℞)

(ser'tra-leen)

Zoloft

Func. class.: Antidepressant

Chem. class.: Selective serotonin reuptake inhibitor (SSRI)

Pregnancy category B

Action: Inhibits serotonin reuptake in CNS, thus increasing action of serotonin; does not affect dopamine, norepinephrine

➡ **Therapeutic Outcome:** Relief of depression, obsessive-compulsive disorder (OCD), posttraumatic stress disorder (PTSD), panic disorder

Uses: Major depression, OCD, posttraumatic stress disorder (PTSD), panic disorder

Investigational uses: Extended interval dosing, premenstrual disorders

Dosage and routes

Adult: PO 50 mg qd; may increase to a maximum of 200 mg/day, do not change dose at intervals of <1 wk; administer qd in AM or PM; or 100 mg 3 ×/wk (off-label)

G ***Elderly:*** PO 25 mg qd, increase by 25 mg q3 days to desired dose

P ***Child 6-12 yr:*** PO 25 mg qd

P ***Child 13-17 yr:*** PO 50 mg qd

Available forms: Tabs 25, 50, 100 mg; liq 20 mg/ml

Adverse effects

CNS: *Insomnia, agitation, somnolence, dizziness, headache, tremor, fatigue,* paresthesia, twitching, confu-

S

sion, ataxia, fever, gait abnormality (elderly)
CV: Palpitations, chest pain
EENT: Vision abnormalities
ENDO: Syndrome of inappropriate antidiuretic hormone (elderly)
GI: Diarrhea, nausea, constipation, anorexia, dry mouth, dyspepsia, *vomiting, flatulence*
GU: Male sexual dysfunction, micturition disorder
INTEG: Increased sweating, rash, hot flashes

Contraindications: Hypersensitivity to this drug or SSRIs

Precautions: Pregnancy **B,** lactation, elderly, hepatic, renal disease, epilepsy

Do Not Confuse:
Zoloft/Zocor

Pharmacokinetics	
Absorption	Well absorbed
Distribution	Unknown, steady state 1 wk
Metabolism	Liver, extensively
Excretion	Feces (14%)
Half-life	1-4 days

Pharmacodynamics	
Onset	Unknown
Peak	4.5-8.4 hr
Duration	Unknown

Interactions
Individual drugs
Cimetidine: ↑ sertraline
Warfarin: ↑ effect of warfarin
Drug classifications
Antidepressants, tricyclic: ↑ effect
Benzodiazepines: ↑ effect
MAOIs: Hypertensive crisis, seizures, do not use together
Herb/drug
St. John's wort: ↑ effect of SSRIs, do not use together
Lab test interferences
↑ AST, ↑ ALT

NURSING CONSIDERATIONS
Assessment
- Assess mental status: mood, sensorium, affect, suicidal tendencies; increase in psychiatric symptoms: depression, panic
- Identify alcohol consumption; if alcohol is consumed, hold dose until AM

Nursing diagnoses
✓ Coping, ineffective individual (uses)
✓ Injury, risk for (adverse reactions)
✓ Knowledge deficit (teaching)
✓ Noncompliance (teaching)

Implementation
- Administer dosage hs if oversedation occurs during day; may take entire dose hs; may crush
- Store at room temp; do not freeze

Patient/family education
- Teach patient that therapeutic effects may take 1 wk
- Instruct patient to use caution in driving or other activities requiring alertness because of drowsiness, dizziness, blurred vision; to avoid rising quickly from sitting to standing, especially elderly
- Advise patient to avoid alcohol ingestion, other CNS depressants
- Teach patient not to discontinue medication quickly after long-term use: may cause nausea, headache, malaise
- Caution patient to wear sunscreen or large hat because photosensitivity can occur
- Teach patient to increase fluids, bulk in diet if constipation, urinary retention occur, especially elderly
- Instruct patient to take gum, hard sugarless candy, or frequent sips of water for dry mouth

Evaluation
Positive therapeutic outcome
- Decrease in depression, OCD
- Absence of suicidal thoughts

Treatment of overdose: ECG monitoring, induce emesis, lavage, activated charcoal, administer anticonvulsant

sibutramine (℞)
(si-byoo'tra-meen)
Meridia
Func. class.: Appetite suppressant
Pregnancy category C
Controlled Substance IV

Action: Inhibits reuptake of serotonin, norepinephrine, dopamine

➔ **Therapeutic Outcome:** Weight loss with B/P in normal range

Uses: Obesity in conjunction with other treatments

Dosage and routes
Adult: PO 10 mg qd; may be increased to 15 mg qd after 4 wk, or lowered to 5 mg qd depending on response

Available forms: Caps 5, 10, 15 mg

Adverse effects
CNS: *Headache,* insomnia, seizures, stimulation, drowsiness, dizziness, nervousness, emotional lability
CV: Hypotension, palpitations, vasodilation, tachycardia
EENT: Laryngitis, pharyngitis, rhinitis, sinusitis
GI: Anorexia, constipation, dry mouth, taste aberration, nausea, increased appetite
GU: Dysmenorrhea
INTEG: Rash, sweating

Contraindications: Hypersensitivity, hypothyroidism, anorexia nervosa, severe hepatic/renal disease, uncontrolled hypertension, history of CAD, CHF, dysrhythmias, lactation

Precautions: History of seizures, G elderly, children <16 yr, narrow-angle P glaucoma, pregnancy **C**

Pharmacokinetics
Absorption	Unknown
Distribution	Widely
Metabolism	Liver (extensively)
Excretion	Unknown
Half-life	14 hr (metabolites)

Pharmacodynamics
Onset	Unknown
Peak	3-4 hr
Duration	Unknown

Interactions
Individual drugs
Dextromethorphan: Fatal serotonin syndrome, do not use together
Dihydroergotamine: Fatal serotonin syndrome, do not use together
Fentanyl: Fatal serotonin syndrome, do not use together
Ketoconazole: ↑ levels of sibutramine
Lithium: Fatal serotonin syndrome, do not use together
Meperidine: Fatal serotonin syndrome, do not use together
Naratriptan: Fatal serotonin syndrome, do not use together
Pentazocine: Fatal serotonin syndrome, do not use together
Sumatriptan: Fatal serotonin syndrome, do not use together
Tryptophan: Fatal serotonin syndrome, do not use together
Zolmitriptan: Fatal serotonin syndrome, do not use together

Drug classifications
Appetite suppressants, centrally acting: Fatal serotonin syndrome, do not use together
Decongestants: Hypertension
MAOIs: Fatal serotonin syndrome, do not use together
Selective serotonin reuptake inhibitors: Fatal serotonin syndrome, do not use together

S

NURSING CONSIDERATIONS
Assessment
- Monitor B/P, pulse during treatment; if B/P or pulse rises or if palpitations, tachycardia occur, drug may need to be discontinued
- Assess patient's current dosage of antihypertensives, antidiabetics; these may need to be adjusted
- Assess need for medication and results when combined with other weight-loss strategies

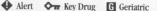

Nursing diagnoses
☑ Knowledge deficit (teaching)
☑ Noncompliance (teaching)

Implementation
- Give PO with or without meals qd

Patient/family education
- Instruct patient to discuss all other medications taken (including OTC) with prescriber; serious, even fatal, interactions can occur
- Advise patient to take exactly as prescribed, not to exceed recommended dose

Evaluation
Positive therapeutic outcome
- Decrease in weight over time

sildenafil (℞)
(sil-den′a-fill)
Viagra
Func. class.: Erectile agent
Chem. class.: Selective inhibitor of cGMP-PDE5

Pregnancy category B

Action: Enhances the effect of nitric oxide (NO) by inhibiting phosphodiesterase type 5 (PDE5), which is necessary for degrading cGMP in the carpus cavernosum

➡ **Therapeutic Outcome:** Ability to achieve and maintain erection

Uses: Treatment of erectile dysfunction

Dosage and routes
Adult: PO 50 mg 1 hr before sexual activity or may be taken ½-4 hr before sexual activity; may be increased to 100 mg or decreased to 25 mg; max once/day

Available forms: Tabs 25, 50, 100 mg

Adverse effects
CNS: *Headache, flushing, dizziness*
CV: **MI, sudden death, CV collapse**
MISC: *Dyspepsia, nasal congestion, UTI, abnormal vision, diarrhea, rash*

Contraindications: Hypersensitivity

Precautions: Anatomical penile deformities, sickle cell anemia, leukemia, multiple myeloma, pregnancy **B**

Pharmacokinetics

Absorption	Rapidly, bioavailability (40%)
Distribution	Unknown
Metabolism	Liver (active metabolites)
Excretion	Feces, urine
Half-life	4 hr

Pharmacodynamics

Onset	Unknown
Peak	½-1½ hr
Duration	Unknown

Interactions
Individual drugs
Amlodipine: ↓ B/P
Cimetidine: ↑ sildenafil levels
Erythromycin: ↑ sildenafil levels
Itraconazole: ↑ sildenafil levels
Ketoconazole: ↑ sildenafil levels
Nitrates: Fatal reaction, do not use together
Rifampin: ↓ sildenafil levels

NURSING CONSIDERATIONS
Assessment
- Identify organic nitrates that should not be used with this drug

Nursing diagnoses
✓ Noncompliance (teaching)
✓ Knowledge deficit (teaching)

Implementation
- Give approximately 1 hr before sexual activity, do not use more than once a day

Patient/family education
- Teach patient that drug does not protect against sexually transmitted diseases, including HIV
- Teach patient that drug absorption is reduced with a high-fat meal
- Teach patient that drug should not be used with nitrates in any form
- Teach patient that tab may be split

Evaluation
Positive therapeutic outcome
- Ability to achieve and maintain an erection

simethicone (OTC)
(si-meth'i-kone)

Extra Strength Gas-X, Extra Strength Maalox Anti-Gas, Extra Strength Maalox GRF Gas Relief Formula ♣, Flatulex, Gas Relief, Gas-X, Genasyme, Maalox Anti-Gas, Maalox GRF Gas Relief Formula, Major-Con, Maximum Strength Gas Relief, Maximum Strength Mylanta Gas Relief, Maximum Strength Phazyme, Mylanta Gas, Mylicon, Ovol ♣, Phazyme, Phazyme-95, Phazyme-125

Func. class.: Antiflatulent

Pregnancy category C

Action: Disperses, prevents gas pockets in GI system; does not decrease gas production

➔ **Therapeutic Outcome:** Belching or flatus

Uses: Flatulence

Dosage and routes
P ***Adult and child >12 yr:*** PO 40-100 mg pc, hs

P ***Child <2 yr:*** PO 20 mg qid

Available forms: Chew tabs 40, 80, 125 mg; tabs 60, 80, 95 mg; drops 40 mg/0.6 ml, 40 mg/ml, 95 mg/1.425 ml; caps 95, 125 mg; caps, soft gel 125 mg

Adverse effects
GI: Belching, rectal flatus

Contraindications: Hypersensitivity

Precautions: Pregnancy **C**

Do Not Confuse:
Mylicon/Mylanta Gas

Pharmacokinetics	
Absorption	None
Distribution	None
Metabolism	None
Excretion	None
Half-life	Unknown

Pharmacodynamics	
Onset	Rapid
Peak	Unknown
Duration	3 hr

Interactions: None

NURSING CONSIDERATIONS
Assessment
- Identify the reason for excess gas production: decreased bowel sounds, recent surgery, other GI conditions

Nursing diagnoses
✓ Pain (uses)
✓ Knowledge deficit (teaching)

Implementation
- Give pc and hs
- Shake susp well before administration
- Chew tab should be chewed and not swallowed whole

Patient/family education
- Caution patient that tab must be

S

chewed; to shake susp well before pouring

Evaluation

Positive therapeutic outcome

- Absence of flatulence

simvastatin (℞)

(sim-va-stat'in)

Zocor

Func. class.: Antilipidemic

Chem. class.: HMG-CoA reductase inhibitor

Pregnancy category X

Action: Inhibits HMG-COA reductase enzyme, which reduces cholesterol synthesis; this enzyme is needed for cholesterol production

Therapeutic Outcome: Decreasing cholesterol levels and LDLs, increased HDLs

Uses: As an adjunct in primary hypercholesterolemia (types IIa, IIb), mixed hyperlipidemia, CAD, isolated hypertriglyceridemia (Frederickson type IV) and type III hyperlipoproteinemia

Dosage and routes

Adult: PO 5-10 mg qd in PM initially, usual range 5-40 mg/day qd in PM, not to exceed 40 mg/day; dosage adjustments may be made at 4-wk intervals or more

G ***Elderly/renal dose***

PO 5 mg/day

Available forms: Tabs 5, 10, 20, 40, 80 mg

Adverse effects

CNS: Headache, tremor, vertigo, peripheral neuropathy

EENT: Lens opacities

GI: Nausea, constipation, diarrhea, dyspepsia, flatus, abdominal pain, heartburn, **liver dysfunction**

INTEG: Rash, pruritus, alopecia, photosensitivity

MS: Muscle cramps, myalgia, **myositis, rhabdomyolysis**

Contraindications: Hypersensitivity, pregnancy **X**, lactation, active liver disease

Precautions: Past liver disease, alcoholism, severe acute infections, trauma, hypotension, uncontrolled seizure disorders, severe metabolic disorders, electrolyte imbalances, G elderly, renal disease

Do Not Confuse:

Zocor/Cozaar, Zocor/Zoloft

Pharmacokinetics	
Absorption	85%
Distribution	Unknown
Metabolism	Liver—extensively
Excretion	70% feces, 20% kidneys
Half-life	3 hr

Pharmacodynamics	
Onset	Unknown
Peak	1-2½ hr
Duration	Unknown

Interactions

Individual drugs

Cholestyramine: ↓ action of simvastatin

Colestipol: ↓ action of simvastatin

Cyclosporine: ↑ risk of myopathy, rhabdomyolysis

Erythromycin: ↑ risk of myopathy

Gemfibrozil: ↑ risk of myopathy, rhabdomyolysis

Niacin: ↑ risk of myopathy

Warfarin: ↑ risk of bleeding

Food/drug

↑ Levels of lovastatin

Lab test interferences

↑ CPK, ↑ LFTs

NURSING CONSIDERATIONS

Assessment

- Assess nutrition: fat, protein, carbohydrates; nutritional analysis should be completed by dietitian before treatment is initiated

- Monitor bowel pattern daily; diarrhea may be a problem
- Monitor triglycerides, cholesterol baseline and throughout treatment; LDL, HDL, triglycerides and cholesterol at 6-8 wk and q6 mo should be watched closely; if increased, drug should be discontinued

Nursing diagnoses

✓ Diarrhea (adverse reactions)
✓ Knowledge deficit (teaching)
✓ Noncompliance (teaching)

Implementation

- Give 30 min before AM and PM meals

Patient/family education

- Inform patient that compliance is needed for positive results to occur; not to double doses
- Advise patient to lower risk factors: high-fat diet, smoking, alcohol consumption, absence of exercise
- Advise patient to notify health care prescriber if the GI symptoms of diarrhea, abdominal or epigastric pain, nausea, vomiting occur; or if chills, fever, sore throat occur

Evaluation

Positive therapeutic outcome

- Decreased cholesterol levels, serum triglycerides and improved ratio with HDLs

sirolimus (℞)

(seer-roe'-li-mus)

Rapamune

Func. class.: Immunosuppressant

Chem. class.: Macrolide

Pregnancy category C

Action: Produces immunosuppression by inhibiting T-lymphocyte activation and proliferation

➔ **Therapeutic Outcome:** Prevention of rejection in organ transplant

Uses: Organ transplants: to prevent rejection, recommended use is with cyclosporine and corticosteroids

Investigational uses: Psoriasis

Dosage and routes

Adult: PO 2 mg qd with 6 mg loading dose, may use 5 mg qd with a 15 mg loading dose

P ***Child >13 yr <40 kg (88 lb):*** PO/mg/m^2/day, 3 mg/m^2/loading dose

Hepatic dose

Reduce by 33% in maintenance dose

Available forms: Oral sol 1 mg/ml

Adverse effects

CNS: *Tremors, headache,* insomnia, paresthesia

CV: Hypertension, **atria fibrillation, CHF,** hypotension, palpitations, **tachycardia**

EENT: Blurred vision, photophobia

GI: Nausea, vomiting, diarrhea, *oral Candida, gum hyperplasia,* **hepatotoxicity,** constipation

GU: UTI, **albuminuria, hematuria, proteinuria, renal failure**

HEMA: Anemia, **thrombocytopenia purpura, leukopenia**

INTEG: Rash, *acne*

META: Creatinine, edema, hypercholesterolemia, hyperlipemia, hypophosphatemia, weight gain, hyperglycemia, hyperkalemia, hyperuricemia, hypokalemia, hypomagnesemia

RESP: **Pleural effusion, atelectasis,** *dyspnea*

SYST: **Lymphoma**

Contraindications: Hypersensitivity to this drug or to components of the drug

Precautions: Severe renal disease, severe hepatic disease, pregnancy **C**, diabetes mellitus, hyperkalemia, hyperuricemia, lymphomas, lactation, P child <13 yr, hypertension

S

Pharmacokinetics

Absorption	Rapidly absorbed
Distribution	92% protein binding
Metabolism	Liver
Excretion	Unknown
Half-life	Unknown

Pharmacodynamics

	PO
Onset	Unknown
Peak	1 hr single dose, 2 hr multiple dosing
Duration	Unknown

Interactions

Individual drugs

Bromocriptine: ↑ blood level
Carbamazepine: ↓ blood levels
Cimetidine: ↑ blood levels
Cyclosporine: ↑ blood levels
Danazol: ↑ blood levels
Erythromycin: ↑ blood levels
Metoclopramide: ↑ blood level
Phenobarbital: ↓ blood levels
Phenytoin: ↓ blood levels
Rifamycin: ↓ blood levels

Drug classifications

Antifungal agents: ↑ sirolimus levels
Calcium channel blockers: ↑ sirolimus levels
HIV protease inhibitors: ↑ blood levels
Live virus vaccines: ↓ effect of vaccines

Food/drug

Food: Alters bioavailability, use consistently with or without food
Grapefruit juice: Do not use with grapefruit juice

NURSING CONSIDERATIONS

Assessment

- Monitor blood studies: Hgb, WBC, platelets monthly during treatment; if leukocytes are <3000/mm^3, or platelets <100,000/mm^3, drug should be discontinued or reduced; decreased Hgb level may indicate bone marrow suppression
- Monitor blood levels in those who may have altered metabolism, trough levels ≥15 ng/ml are associated with increased adverse reactions
- Monitor lipid profile: cholesterol, triglycerides; a lipid-lowering agent may be needed
- Assess for infection and development of lymphoma
- Monitor liver function studies: alkaline phosphatase, AST, ALT, amylase, bilirubin, and for hepatotoxicity: dark urine, jaundice, itching, light-colored stools; drug should be discontinued

Nursing diagnoses

- ☑ Infection, risk for (uses)
- ☑ Knowledge deficit (teaching)

Implementation

- Administer prophylaxis for *Pneumocystis carinii* pneumonia for 1 yr after transplantation; prophylaxis for cytomegalovirus (CMV) is recommended for 90 days after transplantation in those at increased risk for CMV
- Use amber oral dose syringe and withdraw amount of oral sol needed from the bottle, empty correct dose into plastic/glass container holding 60 ml of water/orange juice, stir vigorously and have patient drink at once, refill container with additional 120 ml of water/orange juice, stir vigorously, and have patient drink at once; if using a pouch squeeze entire contents into container and follow above directions
- Give all medications PO if possible; avoid IM inj because bleeding may occur
- Give for 3 days before transplant surgery; patients should be placed in protective isolation
- Store protected from light, refrigerate, stable for 24 months

Patient/family education

- Instruct patient to report fever, rash, severe diarrhea, chills, sore throat, fatigue because serious infections may occur; clay-colored stools, cramping may indicate hepatotoxicity
- Caution patient to avoid crowds or

persons with known infections to reduce risk of infection
- Teach patient to use contraception before, during, and 12 wk after drug has been discontinued

Evaluation

Positive therapeutic outcome
- Absence of graft rejection

sodium bicarbonate (OTC)

Arm and Hammer Pure Baking Soda, Bell/ans, Citrocarbonate, Neut, Soda Mint

Func. class.: Alkalinizer; antacid

Pregnancy category C

Action: Orally neutralizes gastric acid, which forms water, NaCl, CO_2; increases plasma bicarbonate, which buffers H^+ ion concentration; reverses acidosis **IV**

Therapeutic Outcome: Correction of acidosis, gastric acid neutralization

Uses: Acidosis (metabolic), cardiac arrest, alkalinization (systemic/urinary); antacid (PO)

Dosage and routes

Acidosis, metabolic

P ***Adult and child:*** **IV** inf 2-5 mEq/kg over 4-8 hr depending on CO_2, pH

Cardiac arrest

P ***Adult and child:*** **IV** bol 1 mEq/kg of 7.5% or 8.4% sol, then 0.5 mEq/kg q10 min, then doses based on ABGs

P ***Infant:*** **IV** inf not to exceed 8 mEq/kg/day based on ABGs (4.2% sol)

Alkalinization of urine

Adult: PO 325 mg-2 g qid or 48 mEq/kg (4 g), then 12-24 mEq q4h

P ***Child:*** PO 12-120 mg/kg/day (1-10 mEq/kg)

Antacid

Adult: PO 300 mg-2 g chewed, taken with water qd-qid

Available forms: Tabs 300, 325, 600, 650 mg; inj 4.2%, 5%, 7.5%, 8.4%

Adverse effects

CNS: Irritability, headache, confusion, stimulation, tremors, *twitching, hyperreflexia,* **tetany,** weakness, **seizures** caused by alkalosis

CV: Irregular pulse, **cardiac arrest,** water retention, edema, weight gain

GI: Flatulence, *belching, distention,* **paralytic ileus,** acid rebound

GU: Calculi

META: *Alkalosis*

RESP: Shallow, slow respirations, cyanosis, **apnea**

Contraindications: Hypertension, peptic ulcer, renal disease, hypocalcemia

Precautions: CHF, cirrhosis, toxemia, renal disease, pregnancy **C**

Pharmacokinetics

Absorption	Unknown
Distribution	Widely distributed—extracellular fluids
Metabolism	Unknown
Excretion	Kidneys
Half-life	Unknown

Pharmacodynamics

	PO	IV
Onset	2 min	Rapid
Peak	½ hr	Rapid
Duration	1-3 hr	Unknown

Interactions

Individual drugs

Flecainide: ↑ effects
Ketoconazole: ↓ absorption of ketocanazole
Methenamine: ↓ effect of methenamine
Mexiletine: ↑ blood level of mexiletine
Quinidine: ↑ effects

S

Drug classifications
Amphetamines: ↑ effects
Anorexiants: ↑ effects
Barbiturates: ↓ effects of barbiturates
Corticosteroids: ↑ sodium, potassium
Fluoroquinolones: ↑ crystalluria
Salicylates: ↓ effect of salicylates

Herb/drug
Oak bark: ↓ action of sodium bicarbonate

Lab test interferences
↑ Urinary urobilinogen
False positive: Urinary protein, blood lactate

NURSING CONSIDERATIONS

Assessment

- Assess respiratory and pulse rate, rhythm, depth, lung sounds; notify prescriber of abnormalities
- Assess for CO_2 in GI tract; may lead to perforation if ulcer is severe
- Monitor fluid balance (I&O ratio, weight qd, edema); notify prescriber of fluid overload
- Monitor electrolytes, blood pH, PO_2, HCO_3, during beginning treatment; ABGs frequently during emergencies
- Monitor urine pH, urinary output, during beginning treatment
- Monitor extravasation with **IV** administration (tissue sloughing, ulceration, and necrosis)
- Assess for alkalosis: irritability, confusion, twitching, hyperreflexia, stimulation, slow respirations, cyanosis, irregular pulse
- Monitor manifestations of hypokalemia: *RENAL:* acidic urine, reduced urine osmolality, nocturia, polyuria, polydipsia; *CV:* hypotension, broad T wave, U wave, ectopy, tachycardia, weak pulse; *NEURO:* muscle weakness, altered LOC, drowsiness, apathy, lethargy, confusion, depression; *GI:* anorexia, nausea, cramps, constipation, distension, paralytic ileus; *RESP:* hypoventilation, respiratory muscle weakness
- Monitor for manifestations of hyponatremia: *CV:* ↑ B/P, cold, clammy skin, hypo- or hypervolemia; *GI:* anorexia, nausea, vomiting, diarrhea, abdominal cramps; *NEURO:* lethargy, increased ICP, confusion, headache, seizures, coma, fatigue, tremors, hyperreflexia
- Assess for milk-alkali syndrome: confusion, headache, nausea, vomiting, anorexia, urinary stones, hypercalcemia

Nursing diagnoses

- ✓ Gas exchange, impaired (uses)
- ✓ Fluid volume excess (adverse reactions)
- ✓ Knowledge deficit (teaching)

Implementation

PO route

- Tab must be chewed and taken with 8 oz of water
- Dissolve effervescent tab in water
- May be used to neutralize gastric acid in peptic ulcer disease, given 1 and 3 hr pc and hs

IV route

- Give **IV** bol in cardiac arrest, may be repeated q10 min
- Give by intermittent or continuous inf in prepared sol or diluted in an equal amount of any dextrose/saline combination; administer 2-5 mEq/kg over 4-8 hr, not to exceed 50 mEq/hr; **P** slower rate in children

Syringe compatibilities:
Milrinone, pentobarbital

Syringe incompatibilities:
Glycopyrrolate, metoclopramide, thiopental

Y-site compatibilities:
Acyclovir, amifostine, asparaginase, aztreonam, cefepime, cefmetazole, ceftriaxone, cladribine, cyclophosphamide, cytarabine, daunorubicin, dexamethasone, dexchlorpheniramine, doxorubicin, etoposide, famotidine, filgrastim, fludarabine,

gallium, granisetron, heparin, ifosfamide, indomethacin, insulin, melphalan, mesna, methylprednisolone, morphine, paclitaxel, piperacillin/tazobactam, potassium chloride, propofol, tacrolimus, teniposide, thiotepa, tolazoline, vancomycin, vit B/C

Y-site incompatibilities: Amrinone, calcium chloride, idarubicin, sargramostim, verapamil, vinorelbine

Additive compatibilities: Amikacin, aminophylline, amobarbital, amphotericin B, atropine, bretylium, calcium chloride, calcium gluceptate, cefoxitin, ceftazidime, cephalothin, cephapirin, chloramphenicol, chlorothiazide, cimetidine, clindamycin, cytarabine, droperidol/fentanyl, ergonovine, erythromycin, esmolol, floxacillin, furosemide, heparin, hyaluronidase, hydrocortisone, kanamycin, lidocaine, mannitol, metaraminol, methotrexate, methyldopate, multivitamins, nafcillin, nalmefene, netilmicin, nizatidine, ofloxacin, oxacillin, oxytocin, phenobarbital, phenylephrine, phenytoin, phytonadione, potassium chloride, prochlorperazine, thiopental, verapamil

Additive incompatibilities: Amoxicillin, ascorbic acid, carboplatin, carmustine, cefotaxime, cisplatin, codeine, dobutamine, epinephrine, hydromorphone, imipenem/cilastatin, insulin, isoproterenol, labetalol, levorphanol, magnesium sulfate, methadone, morphine, norepinephrine, pentazocine, pentobarbital, procaine, secobarbital, streptomycin, succinylcholine, tetracycline, vit B/C

Patient/family education

- Instruct patient to chew antacid tab and drink 8 oz of water; not to take antacid with milk because milk-alkali syndrome may result; not to use antacid for more than 2 wk
- Advise patient to notify prescriber if indigestion is accompanied by chest pain; dyspnea; diarrhea; dark, tarry stools
- Teach patient about sodium-restricted diet; to avoid use of baking soda for indigestion

Evaluation

Positive therapeutic outcome

- ABGs, electrolytes, blood pH, HCO_3 normal levels
- Decreased gastric pain

sodium biphosphate (OTC)

Fleet Enema, Phospho-soda

Func. class.: Laxative, saline

Pregnancy category C

Action: Increases water absorption in the small intestine by osmotic action; laxative effect occurs by increased peristalsis and water retention

Therapeutic Outcome: Absence of constipation

Uses: Constipation, bowel or rectal preparation for surgery, examination

Dosage and routes

Adult: PO 20-30 ml (Phospho-soda)

P ***Child:*** PO 5-15 ml (Phospho-soda)

P ***Adult and child >12 yr:*** REC enema (118 ml)

P ***Child 2-12 yr:*** REC ½ enema (59 ml)

Available forms: Enema 7 g/phosphate and 19 g/ biphosphate/ 118 ml; oral sol 18 g phosphate/48 g biphosphate/100 ml

Adverse effects

GI: *Nausea, cramps,* diarrhea

META: Electrolyte, fluid imbalances

Contraindications: Hypersensitivity, rectal fissures, abdominal pain, nausea/vomiting, appendicitis, acute surgical abdomen, ulcerated hemor-

S

rhoids, Na-restricted diets (Sal-Hepatica, Phospho-soda)

Precautions: Pregnancy **C**

Pharmacokinetics

Absorption	Up to 20% (rec)
Distribution	Unknown
Metabolism	Unknown
Excretion	Kidneys
Half-life	Unknown

Pharmacodynamics

	PO	REC
Onset	½-3 hr	5 min
Peak	Unknown	Unknown
Duration	Unknown	Unknown

Interactions: None

NURSING CONSIDERATIONS

Assessment

- Assess stools: color, amount, consistency
- Assess for bowel pattern, bowel sounds (frequency, intensity), flatulence, distention, increased temp, dietary patterns (fluid, bulk), exercise
- Assess for cramping, rectal bleeding, nausea, vomiting; if these symptoms occur, drug should be discontinued

Nursing diagnoses

✓ Constipation (uses)
✓ Knowledge deficit (teaching)

Implementation

PO route

- Give on empty stomach
- Mix oral sol in cold water
- Take alone for better absorption; do not take within 1 hr of other drugs

Patient/family education

- Advise patient not to use laxatives or enema for long-term therapy; bowel tone will be lost
- Teach patient that normal bowel movements do not always occur daily
- Caution patient not to use in presence of abdominal pain, nausea, vomiting
- Caution patient to notify prescriber if constipation is unrelieved or if symptoms of electrolyte imbalance occur: muscle cramps, pain, weakness, dizziness, excessive thirst
- Instruct patient to maintain adequate fluid consumption to help prevent constipation

Evaluation

Positive therapeutic outcome

- Decrease in constipation

sodium polystyrene sulfonate (℞)

(po-lee-stye′reen)

Kayexalate, K-Exit ✤, Kionex, PMS Sodium Polystyrene Sulfonate ✤, SPS

Func. class.: Potassium-removing resin

Chem. class.: Cation exchange resin

Pregnancy category C

Action: Removes potassium by exchanging sodium for potassium in body; occurs primarily in large intestine

➔ **Therapeutic Outcome:** Potassium levels within accepted range

Uses: Hyperkalemia in conjunction with other measures

Dosage and routes

Adult: PO 15 g qd-qid; rec enema 30-50 g/100 ml of sorbitol warmed to body temp q6h

P ***Child:*** PO/rec 1 mEq of K exchanged/g of resin, approximate dose 1 g/kg q6h

Available forms: Susp, 15 g polystyrene sulfonate, 21.5 ml sorbitol, 15 g (65 mEq) sodium/60 ml; powder 15 g/4 level tsp

Adverse effects

GI: *Constipation,* anorexia, nausea, vomiting, diarrhea (sorbitol), *fecal impaction,* gastric irritation

META: Hypocalcemia, hypokalemia, hypomagnesemia, sodium retention

Precautions: Pregnancy **C**, renal failure, CHF, severe edema, severe hypertension

Pharmacokinetics

Absorption	None
Distribution	None
Metabolism	None
Excretion	Feces
Half-life	Unknown

Pharmacodynamics

	PO	REC
Onset	2-12 hr	2-12 hr
Peak	Unknown	Unknown
Duration	6-24 hr	4-6 hr

Interactions

Drug classifications

Antacids, calcium or magnesium: ↓ effect of sodium polystyrene

Laxatives: ↓ effect of sodium polystyrene

NURSING CONSIDERATIONS

Assessment

- Assess bowel function daily: amount of stool, color, characteristics
- Assess for hypotension: confusion, irritability, muscular pain, weakness
- Monitor for manifestations of hypokalemia: *RENAL:* acidic urine, reduced urine osmolality, nocturia, polyuria, polydipsia; *CV:* hypotension, broad T wave, U wave, ectopy, tachycardia, weak pulse; *NEURO:* muscle weakness, altered LOC, drowsiness, apathy, lethargy, confusion, depression; *GI:* anorexia, nausea, cramps, constipation, distension, paralytic ileus; *RESP:* hypoventilation, respiratory muscle weakness
- Monitor for manifestations of hyperkalemia: confusion, dyspnea, weakness, dysrhythmias
- Monitor for manifestations of hypocalcemia: *CNS:* personality changes, anxiety, disturbances, depression, psychosis, nausea, vomiting, *GI:* constipation, abdominal pain from muscle spasm; *CV:* decreased contractility, decreased cardiac output, hypotension, lengthened ST segment, prolonged QT interval; *INTEG:* scaling eczema, alopecia, hyperpigmentation; *NEURO:* tetany, muscle twitching, cramping grimacing, seizure, altered deep tendon reflexes, spasm
- Monitor for manifestations of hypomagnesemia; *CNS:* agitation; *NEURO:* muscle twitching, paresthesias, hyperactive reflexes, positive Babinski reflex, dysphagia, nystagmus, seizures, tetany; *GI:* nausea, vomiting, diarrhea, anorexia, abdominal distention; *CV:* ectopy; tachycardia, broad, flat, or inverted T waves; depressed ST segment; prolonged QT interval; decreased cardiac output; hypotension
- Monitor electrolytes: potassium, sodium, calcium, magnesium; I&O ratio, weight qd
- Monitor ECG for spiked T waves, depressed ST segments, prolonged QT interval and widening QRS complex

Nursing diagnoses

✓ Constipation (adverse reactions)
✓ Diarrhea (adverse reactions)
✓ Knowledge deficit (teaching)

Implementation

PO route

- Give oral dose as susp mixed with H_2O or syrup (20-100 ml)
- Give mild laxative as ordered to prevent constipation and fecal impaction; sorbitol as ordered to prevent constipation

Rectal route

- Give by retention enema after mixing with warm water; introduce by gravity, continue stirring, flush with 100 ml of fluid, clamp, and leave in place for at least ½-1 hr
- Complete irrigation of colon after enema with 1-2 qt of nonsodium sol, drain

S

- Store freshly prepared sol for 24 hr at room temp

Patient/family education

- Explain reason for medication and expected results

Evaluation

Positive therapeutic outcome

- Potassium level 3.5-5 mg/dl

somatropin (℞)

(soe-ma-troe'pin)

Genotropin, Humatrope, Norditropin, Nutropin, Nutropin AQ, Nutropin Depot, Saizen, Serostim

Func. class.: Pituitary hormone

Chem. class.: Growth hormone

Pregnancy category C

Action: Stimulates growth; similar to natural growth hormone—both preparations are developed by recombinant DNA technique

Therapeutic Outcome: Increase in height as a result of skeletal growth in pituitary growth hormone deficiency

Uses: Pituitary growth hormone deficiency (hypopituitary dwarfism), children with human growth hormone deficiency, AIDs wasting syndrome, cachexia, adults with somatropin deficiency syndrome (SDS)

Dosage and routes

Genotropin: SC 0.16-0.24 mg/kg 1 wk, divided into 6 or 7 inj, give in abdomen, thigh, buttocks

Humatrope: SC/IM 0.18 mg/kg divided into equal doses either on 3 alternate days or 6 ×/wk, max wk dose is 0.3 mg/kg

Growth hormone deficiency

Nutropin/Nutropin AQ: SC 0.2 mg/kg/wk

Serostim: SC hs >55 kg 6 mg, 45-55 kg 5 mg, 35-45 kg 4 mg

Norditropin: SC 0.024-0.034 mg/kg 6-7 ×/wk

Available forms: Powder for inj (lyophilized) 1.5 mg (4 IU/ml), 4 mg (12 IU/vial), 5 mg (13 IU/vial), 5 mg (15 IU/vial), 5 mg (15 IU/vial) rDNA origin, 5.8 mg (15 IU/ml), 6 mg (18 IU/ml), 8 mg (24 IU/vial), 10 mg (26 IU/vial), inj 10 mg (30 IU/vial); 5, 10, 15 mg/1.5 ml

Adverse effects

CNS: Headache, **growth of intracranial tumor**

ENDO: *Hyperglycemia, ketosis, hypothyroidism*

GU: *Hypercalciuria*

INTEG: Rash, urticaria, pain, inflammation at inj site

MS: Tissue swelling, joint and muscle pain

SYST: *Antibodies to growth hormone*

Contraindications: Hypersensitivity to benzyl alcohol, closed epiphyses, intracranial lesions

Precautions: Diabetes mellitus, hypothyroidism, pregnancy **C**

Pharmacokinetics

Absorption	Well absorbed (SC/IM)
Distribution	Unknown
Metabolism	Unknown
Half-life	15-60 min

Pharmacodynamics

	IM/SC (GROWTH)
Onset	Unknown
Peak	Unknown
Duration	7 days

Interactions

Drug classifications

Androgens: ↑ epiphyseal closure

Glucocorticosteroids: ↓ growth, ↓ somatotropin response

Thyroid hormones: ↑ epiphyseal closure

NURSING CONSIDERATIONS

Assessment

- Identify growth hormone antibodies if patient fails to respond to therapy
- Monitor thyroid function tests: T_3, T_4, T_7, TSH to identify hypothyroidism
- Assess for allergic reaction: rash, itching, fever, nausea, wheezing
- Assess for hypercalciuria: urinary stones; groin, flank pain; nausea, vomiting, frequency, hematuria, chills
- P • Monitor growth rate of child at intervals during treatment

Nursing diagnoses

- ✓ Body image disturbance (uses)
- ✓ Knowledge deficit (teaching)

Implementation

- Store in refrigerator for <1 mo; if reconstituted, <1 wk; do not use discolored or cloudy sol

IM route

- Norditropin: After reconstituting 4-8 mg/2 ml diluent
- Humetrope: 5 mg/1.5-5 ml dilute, do not shake
- Nutropin/Nutropin AQ: Reconstitute 5 mg/1-5 ml or 10 mg/1-10 ml of bacteriostatic water for inj (benzyl alcohol preserved)

Patient/family education

- Explain reason for medication and expected results; that treatment may continue for yr
- Advise patient that routine follow-up is needed to monitor growth rate
- Instruct parents on procedure for medication preparation and inj use; request demonstration, return demonstration; provide written instructions

Evaluation

Positive therapeutic outcome

- Growth in children until epiphyseal plates close

sotalol (℞)

(soe-ta'lole)

Betapace, Betapace AF, Sotacar ✦

Func. class.: Antidysrhythmic, group II, III

Chem. class.: Nonselective β-blocker

Pregnancy category B

Action: Competitively blocks stimulation of β-adrenergic receptor within vascular smooth muscle; produces chronotropic, inotropic activity (decreases rate of SA node discharge, increases recovery time), slows conduction of AV node, decreases heart rate, which decreases O_2 consumption in myocardium; also decreases renin-aldosterone-angiotensin system at high doses, inhibits β_2 receptors in bronchial system (high doses)

→ **Therapeutic Outcome:** Decreased B/P, heart rate, AV conduction

Uses: Life-threatening ventricular dysrhythmias; Betapace AF: to maintain sinus rhythm in symptomatic atrial fibrillation/flutter

Dosage and routes

Adult: PO initial 80 mg bid, may increase to total of 240-320 mg/day

Renal dose

CrCl 30-60 ml/min q24h; CrCl 10-29 ml/min q36-48h; CrCl <10 ml/min individualize dose

Betapace AF

Adult: PO initial 80 mg, titrate upward to 120 mg during initial hospitalization

Renal dose (Betapace AF)

CrCl >60 ml/min q12h; CrCl 40-60 ml/min q24h; CrCl <40 ml/min do not use

Available forms: Tabs 80, 120, 160, 240 mg; Betapace AF 80, 120, 160 mg

Adverse effects

CNS: Dizziness, mental changes, drowsiness, fatigue, headache, catatonia, depression, anxiety, nightmares, paresthesia, lethargy, insomnia, decreased concentration
CV: Orthostatic hypotension, bradycardia, **CHF,** chest pain, **ventricular dysrhythmias,** AV block, peripheral vascular insufficiency, palpitations, **prodysrhythmia, torsade de pointes; Betapace AF: life-threatening ventricular dysrhythmias**
EENT: Tinnitus, visual changes, sore throat, double vision, dry, burning eyes
GI: Nausea, vomiting, diarrhea, dry mouth, flatulence, constipation, anorexia
HEMA: **Agranulocytosis, thrombocytopenic purpura (rare), thrombocytopenia, leukopenia**
INTEG: Rash, alopecia, urticaria, pruritus, fever
MISC: Facial swelling, decreased exercise tolerance, weight change, Raynaud's disease
MS: Joint pain, arthralgia, muscle cramps, pain
RESP: **Bronchospasm,** dyspnea, wheezing, nasal stuffiness, pharyngitis

Contraindications: Hypersensitivity to β-blockers, cardiogenic shock, heart block (2nd or 3rd degree), sinus bradycardia, CHF, bronchial asthma, congenital or acquired long QT syndrome

Precautions: Major surgery, pregnancy **B,** lactation, diabetes mellitus, renal disease, thyroid disease, COPD, well-compensated heart failure, CAD, nonallergic bronchospasm, electrolyte disturbances, bradycardia, cardiac dysrhythmias, peripheral vascular disease

Pharmacokinetics

Absorption	Variable (30%)
Distribution	Crosses placenta, minimal penetration in CNS
Metabolism	Liver, protein binding 0%
Excretion	70% unchanged—kidneys
Half-life	10-24 hr, ↑ in renal disease

Pharmacodynamics

Onset	Several hr
Peak	Unknown
Duration	Unknown

Interactions

Individual drugs

Digoxin: ↑ blood levels, ↑ toxicity
Disopyramide: ↑ levels, ↑ toxicity
Flecainide: ↑ levels, ↑ toxicity
Lidocaine: Bradycardia, arrest
Mexiletine: ↑ levels, ↑ toxicity
Phenytoin: ↑ blood levels
Procainamide: ↑ levels, ↑ toxicity
Quinidine: ↑ levels, ↑ toxicity
Warfarin: ↑ level, ↑ bleeding

Drug classifications

Calcium channel blockers: ↑ dysrhythmias, arrest

Herb/drug

Aloe: ↑ hypokalemia
Buckthorn: ↑ hypokalemia
Cascara sagrada: ↑ hypokalemia
Senna: ↑ hypokalemia

Lab test interferences

False: ↑ Urinary catecholamines

NURSING CONSIDERATIONS

Assessment

- Monitor B/P during beginning treatment, periodically thereafter; pulse q4h; note rate, rhythm, quality: apical/radial pulse before administration; notify prescriber of any significant changes (pulse <50 bpm); monitor ECG continuously (Betapace AF); use QT interval to determine patient eligibility; baseline QT must be ≤450 msec, if prolonged to 500 msec reduce or stop drug
- Check for baselines in renal, liver function tests before therapy begins

- Assess for edema in feet, legs daily, monitor I&O ratio, daily weight; check for jugular vein distention, rales, bilaterally, dyspnea (CHF)
- Monitor skin turgor, dryness of mucous membranes for hydration G status, especially in elderly

Nursing diagnoses

✓ Cardiac output, decreased (uses)
✓ Injury, risk for (adverse reactions)
✓ Knowledge deficit (teaching)
✓ Noncompliance (teaching)

Implementation

- Given ac, hs, tab may be crushed or swallowed whole; give with food to prevent GI upset; reduce dosage in renal dysfunction
- Store protected from light, moisture; place in cool environment

Patient/family education

- Teach patient not to discontinue drug abruptly, taper over 2 wk; may cause precipitate angina if stopped abruptly
- Teach patient not to use OTC products containing α-adrenergic stimulants (such as nasal decongestants, cold preparations); to avoid alcohol and smoking and to limit sodium intake as prescribed
- Teach patient how to take pulse and B/P at home, advise when to notify prescriber
- Instruct patient to comply with weight control, dietary adjustments, modified exercise program
- Caution patient to carry/wear ID to identify drug being taken, allergies
- Inform patient that drug controls symptoms but does not cure
- Caution patient to avoid hazardous activities if dizziness, drowsiness is present
- Teach patient to report symptoms of CHF: difficulty breathing, especially on exertion or when lying down; night cough; swelling of extremities; bradycardia; dizziness; confusion; depression; fever
- Teach patient to take drug as prescribed, not to double or skip doses; take any missed doses as soon as remembered if at least 4 hr until next dose

Evaluation

Positive therapeutic outcome

- Absence of dysrhythmias

Treatment of overdose:

Lavage; **IV** atropine for bradycardia; **IV** theophylline for bronchospasm; digitalis, O_2, diuretic for cardiac failure; hemodialysis; **IV** glucose for hyperglycemia; **IV** diazepam (or phenytoin) for seizures

sparfloxacin (℞)

(spar-floks'a-sin)

Zagam

Func. class.: Antiinfective

Chem. class.: Fluoroquinolone antibacterial

Pregnancy category C

Action: Interferes with conversion of intermediate DNA fragments into high-molecular-weight DNA in bacteria; DNA gyrase inhibitor

➔ **Therapeutic Outcome:** Bactericidal action against the following organisms: *Chlamydia pneumoniae, Haemophilus influenzae, Haemophilus parainfluenzae, Moraxella catarrhalis*

Uses: Adult infections (including complicated): lower respiratory, community-acquired pneumonia, chronic bronchitis

Dosage and routes

Adult: PO 400 mg loading dose, then 200 mg q24h × 10 days

Renal dose

Adult: PO 400 mg on day 1 if CrCl <50 ml/min; then 200 mg qod on days 2-10

Available forms: Tabs 200 mg

S

Adverse effects

CNS: Headache, dizziness, insomnia
CV: QT interval prolongation, vasodilation
GI: Nausea, flatulence, abdominal pain, **pseudomembranous colitis,** *vomiting,* diarrhea
HEMA: **Leukopenia,** eosinophilia, anemia
INTEG: Pruritus, photosensitivity
SYST: **Anaphylaxis, Stevens-Johnson syndrome**

Contraindications: Hypersensitivity to quinolones

Precautions: Pregnancy **C,** P lactation, children, renal disease, seizure disorder

Pharmacokinetics	
Absorption	Slow-erratic
Distribution	Widely distributed
Metabolism	Liver
Excretion	Kidneys, feces
Half-life	20 hr

Pharmacodynamics
Unknown

Interactions

Individual drugs

Amiodarone: ↑ torsade de pointes
Bepridil: ↑ torsade de pointes
Caffeine: ↑ toxicity
Calcium: ↓ sparfloxacin absorption
Cimetidine: ↑ sparfloxacin
Cyclosporine: ↑ neurotoxicity
Disopyramide: ↑ torsade de pointes
Erythromycin: ↑ torsade de pointes
Pentamine: ↑ torsade de pointes
Phenytoin: ↓ effect
Probenecid: ↑ sparfloxacin
Sucralfate: ↓ absorption
Theophylline: ↑ theophylline level, toxicity
Warfarin: ↑ warfarin level
Zinc sulfate: ↓ absorption of sparfloxacin

Drug classifications

Antacids: ↓ absorption of sparfloxacin
Antidepressants, tricyclic: ↑ torsade de pointes
Antidysrhythmics, class IA/III: ↑ torsade de pointes
Phenothiazines: ↑ torsade de pointes

Lab test interferences

↑ AST, ↑ ALT

NURSING CONSIDERATIONS

Assessment

- Assess patient for previous sensitivity reaction
- Assess patient for signs and symptoms of infection including characteristics of wounds, sputum, urine, stool, WBC >10,000/mm^3, fever; obtain baseline information before and monitor during treatment
- Obtain C&S before beginning drug therapy to identify if correct treatment has been initiated
- Assess for allergic reactions, anaphylaxis: rash, urticaria, pruritus, chills, fever, joint pain; may occur a few days after therapy begins; epinephrine and resuscitation equipment should be available for anaphylactic reaction
- Identify urine output; if decreasing, notify prescriber (may indicate nephrotoxicity); also check for increased BUN, creatinine
- Monitor blood studies: AST, ALT, CBC, Hct, bilirubin, LDH, alkaline phosphatase, Coombs' test monthly if patient is on long-term therapy
- Assess bowel pattern qd; if severe diarrhea occurs, drug should be discontinued
- Monitor for bleeding: ecchymosis, bleeding gums, hematuria, stool guaiac daily if on long-term therapy
- Assess for overgrowth of infection: perineal itching, fever, malaise, redness, pain, swelling, drainage, rash, diarrhea, change in cough, sputum

Nursing diagnoses

- ✓ Infection, risk for (uses)
- ✓ Diarrhea (side effects)
- ✓ Injury, risk for (side effects)

☑ Knowledge deficit (teaching)
☑ Noncompliance (teaching)

Implementation

PO route

- Give around the clock to maintain proper blood levels
- Give 4 hr before or after antacids/calcium

IV route

- Check for irritation, extravasation, phlebitis daily
- For intermittent inf, dilute to 1-2 mg/ml of D_5W, 0.9% NaCl; give over 60 min; sol will remain stable under refrigeration for 2 wk

Patient/family education

- Advise patient to contact prescriber if vaginal itching, loose foul-smelling stools, furry tongue occur; may indicate superinfection; report itching, rash, pruritus, urticaria
- Instruct patient to take all medication prescribed for the length of time ordered; drug must be taken around the clock to maintain blood levels; do not give medication to others
- Teach patient to avoid direct sunlight or use sunscreen to prevent phototoxicity
- Advise patient to drink plenty of fluids, take 4 hr before or after antacids/calcium
- Advise patient to notify prescriber of diarrhea with blood or pus
- Advise patient to increase fluid intake to 2 L/day to prevent crystalluria
- Advise patient to avoid hazardous activities until response is known
- Advise patient not to use theophylline with this product unless approved by prescriber
- Instruct patient to rinse mouth frequently, use sugarless candy or gum for dry mouth

Evaluation

Positive therapeutic outcome

- Absence of signs/symptoms of infection (WBC <10,000/mm^3, temp WNL)
- Reported improvement in symptoms of infection

spectinomycin (℞)

(spek-ti-noe-mye'sin)

Trobicin

Func. class.: Antiinfective

Chem. class.: Aminocyclitol

Pregnancy category B

Action: Inhibits bacterial synthesis by binding to 30S subunit on ribosome

Therapeutic Outcome: Treatment and resolution of gonococcal infection

Uses: Gonorrhea, gonococcal urethritis, cervicitis, proctitis, disseminated gonococcal infection

Dosage and routes

Adult and child >45 kg: IM 2-4 g as single dose

Child <45 kg: IM 40 mg/kg as single dose

Gonococcal infections in pregnancy

Adult: IM 2 g, to treat those allergic to cephalosporins

Available forms: Powder for inj 400 mg/ml when reconstituted

Adverse effects

CNS: Dizziness, chills, fever, insomnia, headache, anxiety

GI: *Nausea,* vomiting, increased BUN

GU: Decreased urine output

HEMA: Anemia

INTEG: *Pain at injection site,* urticaria, rash, pruritus, fever

SYST: **Anaphylaxis**

Contraindications: Hypersensitivity, syphilis

Precautions: Pregnancy **B,** infants, children, lactation

S

Pharmacokinetics

Absorption	Well absorbed
Distribution	Unknown
Metabolism	Liver
Excretion	Kidneys
Half-life	1⅕-2½ hr

Pharmacodynamics

Onset	Rapid
Peak	1 hr

Interactions: None

NURSING CONSIDERATIONS

Assessment

- Monitor gonorrhea culture after treatment
- Monitor I&O ratio; report decreased output
- Monitor liver function studies: AST, ALT, serum alkaline phosphatase after multiple doses
- Monitor blood studies: Hct, Hgb, BUN if multiple diagnoses given
- Monitor serologic test for gonorrhea 3 mo after treatment
- Assess for allergies before treatment, reaction of each medication

Nursing diagnoses

✓ Infection, risk for (uses)
✓ Knowledge deficit (teaching)

Implementation

- Give after shaking vial; IM in deep muscle mass (glutens only); with 20-G needle; no more than 5 ml/site
- Store at room temp; reconstituted sol should be discarded after 24 hr

Evaluation

Positive therapeutic outcome

- Negative gonorrhea culture after treatment

spironolactone (℞)

(speer′on-oh-lak′tone)

Aldactone, Novospiroton ♣

Func. class: Potassium-sparing diuretic

Chem. class.: Aldosterone antagonist

Pregnancy category D

Action: Competes with aldosterone at receptor sites in the distal tubule in the renal system, resulting in excretion of sodium, chloride, water, bicarbonate, and calcium; potassium, phosphate, and hydrogen are retained

➔ **Therapeutic Outcome:** Diuretic and antihypertensive effect while retaining potassium; lowered aldosterone levels

Uses: Edema of CHF, hypertension, diuretic-induced hypokalemia, primary hyperaldosteronism (diagnosis, short-term treatment, long-term treatment), edema of nephrotic syndrome, cirrhosis of the liver with ascites

Investigational uses: CHF

Dosage and routes

Edema/hypertension

Adult: PO 25-400 mg/qd in single or divided doses

CHF

Adult: PO 12.5-25 mg/day

Edema

P ***Child:*** PO 3.3 mg/kg/day in single or divided doses

Hypertension

P ***Child:*** PO 1-2 mg/kg bid

Hypokalemia

Adult: PO 25-100 mg/day; if PO, potassium supplements are unable to be used

Primary hyperaldosteronism diagnosis

Adult: PO 400 mg/day × 4 days depending on the test, then 100-400 mg/day maintenance

Available forms: Tabs 25, 50, 100 mg

Adverse effects

CNS: Headache, confusion, drowsiness, lethargy, ataxia
ELECT: Hyperchloremic metabolic acidosis, **hyperkalemia,** hyponatremia
ENDO: Impotence, gynecomastia, irregular menses, amenorrhea, postmenopausal bleeding, hirsutism, deepening voice
GI: Diarrhea, cramps, bleeding, gastritis, vomiting
HEMA: **Agranulocytosis**

Contraindications: Hypersensitivity, anuria, severe renal disease, hyperkalemia, pregnancy **D**

Precautions: Dehydration, hepatic disease, lactation, elderly, renal disease

Pharmacokinetics	
Absorption	GI tract; well absorbed
Distribution	Crosses placenta
Metabolism	Liver to canrenone (active metabolite)
Excretion	Renal; breast milk
Half-life	12-24 hr (canrenone)

Pharmacodynamics	
Onset	24-48 hr
Peak	48-72 hr
Duration	Unknown

Interactions

Individual drugs

Aspirin: ↓ action of spironolactone
Lithium: ↑ action, toxicity

Drug classifications

ACE inhibitors: ↑ hyperkalemia
Anticoagulants: ↓ effects of anticoagulants
Antihypertensives: ↑ action
Diuretics, potassium-sparing: ↑ hyperkalemia
Potassium products: ↑ hyperkalemia
Salt substitutes: ↑ hyperkalemia

Food/drug

Potassium foods: ↑ hyperkalemia

Herb/drug

Licorice: Hypokalemic alkalosis

Lab test interferences

False: ↑ Urinary catecholamines
Interference: Glucose, insulin tolerance tests

NURSING CONSIDERATIONS

Assessment

- Monitor for manifestations of hyperkalemia: *MS:* fatigue, muscle weakness; *CV:* arrhythmias, hypotension, *NEURO:* paresthesias, confusion, *RESP:* dyspnea
- Monitor for manifestations of hyponatremia: *CV:* ↑ B/P, cold, clammy skin, hypo- or hypervolemia; *GI:* anorexia, nausea, vomiting, diarrhea, abdominal cramps; *NEURO:* lethargy, increased ICP, confusion headache, seizures, coma, fatigue, tremors, hyperreflexia
- Monitor for manifestations of hyperchloremia: *NEURO:* weakness, lethargy, coma; *RESP:* deep rapid breathing
- Assess fluid volume status: I&O ratios and record, count or weigh diapers as appropriate, weight, distended red veins, crackles in lung, color, quality, and sp gr of urine, skin turgor, adequacy of pulses, moist mucous membranes, bilateral lung sounds, peripheral pitting edema; dehydration symptoms of decreasing output, thirst, hypotension, dry mouth and mucous membranes should be reported
- Monitor electrolytes: potassium, sodium, calcium, magnesium; also include BUN, ABGs, uric acid, CBC, blood glucose

Nursing diagnoses

- ✓ Urinary elimination, altered (adverse reactions)
- ✓ Fluid volume deficit (adverse reactions)
- ✓ Fluid volume excess (uses)
- ✓ Knowledge deficit (teaching)

S

Implementation

- Give in AM to avoid interference with sleep
- With food, if nausea occurs, absorption may be increased; take at same time each day

Patient/family education

- Teach patient to take medication early in day to prevent nocturia
- Instruct patient to take with food or milk if GI symptoms of nausea and anorexia occur
- Teach patient to maintain a record of weight on a weekly basis and notify prescriber of weight loss of >5 lb
- Caution patient that this drug causes an increase in potassium levels, that foods high in potassium should be avoided; refer to dietitian for assistance planning
- Teach patient not to use alcohol, or any OTC medications without prescriber's approval; serious drug reactions may occur
- Emphasize the need to contact prescriber immediately if muscle cramps, weakness, nausea, dizziness, or numbness occurs
- Teach patient to take own B/P and pulse and record
- Advise patient that dizziness and confusion may occur; avoid driving or other hazardous activities if alertness is decreased
- Teach patient to continue taking medication even if feeling better; this drug controls symptoms but does not cure the condition
- Advise patient with hypertension to continue other treatment (exercise, weight loss, relaxation techniques, cessation of smoking)

Evaluation

Positive therapeutic outcome

- Prevention of hypokalemia (diuretic use)
- Decreased edema
- Decreased B/P
- Decreased aldosterone levels
- Increased diuresis

Treatment of overdose:

- Lavage if taken orally, monitor electrolytes
- Administer sodium bicarbonate
- Monitor hydration, CV, renal status

stavudine (℞)

(sta'vu-deen)

Zerit

Func. class.: Antiretroviral

Chem. class.: Primidone nucleoside

Pregnancy category C

Action: Prevents replication of HIV by the inhibition of the enzyme reverse transcriptase

➔ **Therapeutic Outcome:** Decreasing diarrhea, fatigue, night sweats; increased body weight

Uses: Treatment of advanced HIV infection for patients who have not responded to other antivirals

Dosage and routes

Adult >60 kg: PO 40 mg q12h up to 2 mg/kg/day

Adult <60 kg: 30 mg q12h

P ***Child <30 kg:*** PO 2 mg/kg/day divided q12h

Renal dose

Adult >60 kg: CrCl 26-50 ml/min 20 mg q12h; CrCl 10-25 ml/min 20 mg q24h

Adult <60 kg: CrCl 26-50 ml/min 15 mg q12h; CrCl 10-25 ml/min 15 mg q24h

Available forms: Caps 15, 20, 30, 40 mg; oral powder for sol 1 mg/ml

Adverse effects

CNS: *Peripheral neuropathy,* headache, chills/fever, malaise

GI: **Hepatotoxicity**

HEMA: **Bone marrow suppression,** anemia

INTEG: Rash

MISC: **Lactic acidosis**
MS: Myalgia

Contraindications: Hypersensitivity to this drug or zidovudine, didanosine, zalcitabine; severe peripheral neuropathy

Precautions: Advanced HIV infections, pregnancy **C**, lactation, bone marrow suppression, renal disease, liver disease, folic acid or vit B_{12} deficiency, peripheral neuropathy

Pharmacokinetics

Absorption	Rapidly absorbed, 82% bioavailability
Distribution	Cerebrospinal fluid
Metabolism	Unknown
Excretion	Kidneys, breast milk
Half-life	Elimination: 1-1.6 hr, intracellular: 3-3.5 hr

Pharmacodynamics

Onset	Unknown
Peak	1 hr
Duration	Unknown

Interactions
Individual drugs
Chloramphenicol: ↑ peripheral neuropathy
Dapsone: ↑ peripheral neuropathy
Didanosine: ↑ peripheral neuropathy
Ethambutol: ↑ peripheral neuropathy
Hydralazine: ↑ peripheral neuropathy
Lithium: ↑ peripheral neuropathy
Phenytoin: ↑ peripheral neuropathy
Vincristine: ↑ peripheral neuropathy
Zalcitabine: ↑ peripheral neuropathy

Drug classifications
Myelosuppressants: ↑ myelosuppressor

NURSING CONSIDERATIONS
Assessment
- ❗ Assess for lactic acidosis and severe hepatomegaly with steatosis; death may result
- Monitor viral load and CD4 counts baseline and throughout treatment
- Monitor for peripheral neuropathy: tingling, pain in extremities; if these occur discontinue drug
- Monitor for pancreatitis: severe upper abdominal pain, nausea, vomiting throughout treatment; if these occur discontinue drug
- Monitor blood studies: WBC, differential, RBC, Hct, Hgb, platelets
- Monitor renal studies: urinalysis, protein, blood
- Obtain C&S before drug therapy; drug may be taken as soon as culture is performed; repeat C&S after therapy
- Monitor bowel pattern before, during treatment
- Monitor fluid overload; drug requires large volume to stay in sol
- Assess for weakness, tremors, confusion, dizziness, psychosis; if these occur, drug may have to be decreased or discontinued

Nursing diagnoses
- ☑ Infection, risk for (uses)
- ☑ Knowledge deficit (teaching)

Implementation
- Give with or without meals; absorption does not appear to be lowered when taken with food

Patient/family education
- Teach patient signs of peripheral neuropathy: burning, weakness, pain, pricking feeling in the extremities
- Caution patient that this drug should not be given with antineoplastics
- Inform patient that GI complaints and insomnia resolve after 3-4 wk of treatment
- Inform patient that drug is not a cure for AIDS, but will control symptoms
- Advise patient to call prescriber if sore throat, swollen lymph nodes, malaise, fever occur; may indicate presence of other infections
- Caution patient that even with drug administration, virus is still infective and may be passed on to others

S

- Caution patient that follow-up visits must be continued because serious toxicity may occur; blood counts must be done q2 wk
- Teach patient that drug must be taken q4h around the clock even during night
- Caution patient that serious drug interactions with other medications may occur, check with prescriber first if taking chloramphenicol, dapsone, cisplatin, didanosine, ethambutol, lithium, antifungals, antineoplastics
- Inform patient that other drugs may be necessary to prevent other infections
- Inform patient that drug may cause fainting or dizziness

Evaluation

Positive therapeutic outcome

- Decreased symptoms of HIV infection

HIGH ALERT

streptokinase 🔑 (℞)

(strep-toe-kye'nase)

Kabikinase, Streptase

Func. class.: Thrombolytic enzyme

Chem. class.: β-Hemolytic *Streptococcus* filtrate (purified)

Pregnancy category C

Action: Activates conversion of plasminogen to plasmin (fibrinolysin): plasmin breaks down clots (fibrin), fibrinogen, factors V, VII; occlusion of venous access lines

➔ **Therapeutic Outcome:** Lysis of emboli, or thrombosis in various parts of the body

Uses: Deep vein thrombosis (DVT), pulmonary embolism, arterial thrombosis, arterial embolism, arteriovenous cannula occlusion, lysis of coronary artery thrombi after MI, acute evolving transmural MI

Dosage and routes

Lysis of coronary artery thrombi

Adult: **IV** inf 20,000 IU, then 2000 IU/min over 1 hr

Arteriovenous cannula occlusion

Adult: **IV** inf 250,000 IU/2 ml sol into occluded limb of cannula run over ½ hr; clamp for 2 hr; aspirate contents; flush with NaCl sol and reconnect

Thrombosis/embolism /DVT/ pulmonary embolism

Adult: **IV** inf 250,000 IU over ½ hr, then 100,000 IU/hr for 72 hr for deep thrombosis; 100,000 IU/hr over 24-72 hr for pulmonary embolism; 100,000 IU/hr × 24-72 hr for arterial thrombosis or embolism

Acute evolving transmural MI

Adult: **IV** inf 1,500,000 IU diluted to a volume of 45 ml; give within 1 hr; intracoronary inf 20,000 IU by bol, then 2,000 IU/min × 1 hr, total dose 140,000 IU

Available forms: Powder for inj, lyophilized 250,000, 600,000, 750,000, 1,500,000 IU vial

Adverse effects

CNS: Headache, fever
CV: **Dysrhythmias,** hypotension, noncardiogenic pulmonary edema, **pulmonary embolism**
EENT: Periorbital edema
GI: Nausea
HEMA: Decreased Hct, **bleeding**
INTEG: Rash, urticaria, phlebitis at infusion site, itching, flushing
MS: Low back pain
RESP: Altered respirations, shortness of breath, **bronchospasm**
SYST: **GI, GU, intracranial retroperitoneal bleeding, surface bleeding, anaphylaxis**

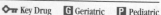

Contraindications: Hypersensitivity, active bleeding, intraspinal surgery, CNS, neoplasms, ulcerative

colitis, enteritis, severe hypertension, severe renal disease, hepatic disease, hypocoagulation, COPD, subacute bacterial endocarditis, rheumatic valvular disease, cerebral embolism/thrombosis/hemorrhage, intraarterial diagnostic procedure or surgery (10 days), recent major surgery

Precautions: Arterial emboli from left side of heart, pregnancy **C**

Pharmacokinetics

Absorption	Completely absorbed
Distribution	Unknown
Metabolism	>80%—liver, rapidly cleared by reticuloendothelial system
Excretion	Kidneys
Half-life	35 min

Pharmacodynamics

Onset	Immediate
Peak	Rapid
Duration	<12 hr

Interaction

Individual drugs

Abciximab: ↑ bleeding risk
Aspirin: ↑ bleeding risk
Clopidogrel: ↑ bleeding risk
Dipyridamole: ↑ bleeding risk
Eptifibatide: ↑ bleeding risk
Heparin: ↑ bleeding risk
Plicamycin: ↑ bleeding risk
Tirofiban: ↑ bleeding risk
Ticlopidine: ↑ bleeding risk
Valproic acid: ↑ bleeding risk

Drug classifications

Anticoagulants, oral: ↑ bleeding risk
Cephalosporins: ↑ bleeding risk
NSAIDs: ↑ bleeding risk

Lab test interferences

↑ Pro-time, ↑ APTT, ↑ TT
↓ Plasminogen, ↓ fibrinogen

NURSING CONSIDERATIONS

Assessment

- Monitor VS, B/P, pulse, respirations (including peripheral), neurologic signs, temp at least q4h; temp >104° F (40° C) indicates internal bleeding; monitor rhythm closely; ventricular dysrhythmias may occur with hyperfusion; monitor heart, breath sounds, neurologic status, peripheral pulses
- ❗ Assess for bleeding during first hr of treatment: hematuria, hematemesis, bleeding from mucous membranes, epistaxis, ecchymosis; guaiac, all body fluids, stools; may require transfusion (rare); blood studies (Hct, platelets, PTT, pro-time, TT, APTT) before starting therapy; pro-time or APTT must be less than 2 × control before starting therapy; TT or pro-time q3-4h during treatment
- Assess allergy: fever, rash, itching, chills; mild reaction may be treated with antihistamines; report to prescriber
- Monitor ECG on monitor, watch for segment changes, changes in rhythm; sinus bradycardia, ventricular tachycardia, accelerated idioventricular rhythm may occur as a result of reperfusion (coronary thrombosis); cardiac enzymes, radionuclide myocardial scanning/coronary angiography
- Monitor ABGs, respiratory rate (depth, characteristics), pulse, B/P, hemodynamics (pulmonary embolism)
- Monitor peripheral pulses, assess Homan's sign, check for redness, swelling qh; notify prescriber of changes; B/P should not be taken in extremities (deep vein thrombosis)
- Check catheter for ability to aspirate blood from port; patient must exhale and hold breath when inserting and removing syringe to prevent air embolism (catheter/cannula occlusion)
- Assess for Guillain-Barré syndrome that may occur after treatment with this drug
- Assess for respiratory depression

S

Nursing diagnoses
- ✓ Tissue perfusion, altered (uses)
- ✓ Injury, risk for (adverse reactions)
- ✓ Impaired gas exchange (uses)
- ✓ Knowledge deficit (teaching)

Implementation
- Give after reconstituting with provided diluent; add appropriate amount of sterile water for inj (no preservatives) 20-mg vial/20 ml or 50 mg-vial/50 ml to make 1 mg/ml, mix by slow inversion or dilute with NaCl, D_5W to a concentration of 0.5 mg/ml; further dilution, 1.5-<0.5 mg/ml may result in precipitation of drug; use 18-G needle; flush line with NaCl after administration; reconstituted **IV** sol within 8 hr; within 6 hr of coronary occlusion for best results
- Give **IV** loading dose over 30 min to avoid hypotension
- Give **IV** over 1 hr after dilution with 4-5 g/250 ml of 0.9% NaCl, D_5W, LR; may give by continuous inf after loading dose(s) of 1 g/hr diluted in 50-100 ml of compatible sol; use infusion pump; do not give by direct **IV**
- Give heparin therapy after thrombolytic therapy is discontinued, TT, ACT, or APTT less than 2 × control (about 3-4 hr); **IV** heparin with loading dose is recommended after discontinuing streptokinase to prevent redevelopment of thrombis
- Avoid invasive procedures, injection, taking temp via rectal route
- Apply pressure for 30 sec to minor bleeding sites; 30 min to sites of atrial puncture, followed by pressure dressing; inform prescriber if this does not attain hemostasis; apply pressure dressing
- Store powder at room temp or refrigerate; protect from excessive light

Y-site compatibilities:
Dobutamine, dopamine, heparin, lidocaine, nitroglycerin

Additive incompatibilities:
Do not mix with other medications

Patient/family education
- Teach patient reason for medication, signs and symptoms of bleeding, allergic reactions, when to notify prescriber
- Explain that patient is to continue bed rest to avoid injury

Evaluation
Positive therapeutic outcome
- Lysis of thrombi or emboli

streptomycin (℞)
(strep-toe-mye'sin)

Func. class.: Antiinfective, antitubercular

Chem. class.: Aminoglycoside

Pregnancy category D

Action: Interferes with protein synthesis in bacterial cell by binding to ribosomal subunit, causing inaccurate peptide sequence to form in protein chain, resulting in bacterial death

➔ **Therapeutic Outcome:** Bactericidal effects for the following organisms: sensitive strains of *Mycobacterium tuberculosis,* nontuberculous infections caused by sensitive strains of *Yersinia pestis, Brucella, Haemophilus influenzae, Klebsiella pneumoniae, Escherichia coli, Enterobacter aerogenes, Streptococcus viridans, Francisella tularensis, Proteus*

Uses: Active TB; used in combination for streptococcal and enterococcal infections; endocarditis, tularemia, plague

Dosage and routes
Tuberculosis
Adult: IM 15 mg/kg (max 1 g) qd × 2-3 mo, then 1 g 2-3 ×/wk given with other antitubercular drugs

P ***Child:*** IM 20-40 mg/kg/day in divided doses given with other antitubercular drugs; max 15 mg/kg/day

Streptococcal endocarditis
Adult: IM 1 g q12h × 1 wk with penicillin, then 500 mg bid × 1 wk
Enterococcal endocarditis
Adult: IM 1 g q12h × 2 wk, then 500 mg q12h × 4 wk with penicillin, max 15 mg/kg/day

Available forms: Inj 500 mg, 1 g/ml

Adverse effects

CNS: Confusion, dizziness, depression, numbness, tremors, **seizures**, muscle twitching, **neurotoxicity**
CV: Hypotension, myocarditis, palpitations
EENT: *Ototoxicity,* tinnitus, deafness, visual disturbances
GI: *Nausea, vomiting, anorexia,* increased ALT, AST, bilirubin, hepatomegaly, **hepatic necrosis,** splenomegaly
GU: **Oliguria, hematuria, renal damage, azotemia, renal failure, nephrotoxicity**
HEMA: **Agranulocytosis, thrombocytopenia, leukopenia, eosinophilia, anemia**
INTEG: *Rash,* burning, urticaria, dermatitis, alopecia

Contraindications: Severe renal disease, hypersensitivity, pregnancy **D**

Precautions: Neonates, mild renal disease, myasthenia gravis, lactation, **G** hearing deficits, elderly, Parkinson's disease

Pharmacokinetics

Absorption:	Well absorbed
Distribution	Widely distributed in extracellular fluids, poorly distributed in CSF; crosses placenta
Metabolism	Minimal—liver
Excretion	Mostly unchanged (>90%) kidneys
Half-life	2-2½ hr, increase in renal disease

Pharmacodynamics

Onset	Rapid
Peak	1-2 hr

Interactions

Individual drugs
Amphotericin B: ↑ Ototoxicity, neurotoxicity, nephrotoxicity
Cisplatin: ↑ Ototoxicity, neurotoxicity, nephrotoxicity
Ethacrynic acid: ↑ Ototoxicity, neurotoxicity, nephrotoxicity
Furosemide: ↑ Ototoxicity, neurotoxicity, nephrotoxicity
Mannitol: ↑ Ototoxicity, neurotoxicity, nephrotoxicity
Methoxyflurane: ↑ Ototoxicity, neurotoxicity, nephrotoxicity
Polymyxin: ↑ Ototoxicity, neurotoxicity, nephrotoxicity
Succinylcholine: ↑ Neuromuscular blockade, respiratory depression
Vancomycin: ↑ Ototoxicity, neurotoxicity, nephrotoxicity
Drug classifications
Aminoglycosides: ↑ Ototoxicity, neurotoxicity, nephrotoxicity
Anesthetics: ↑ Neuromuscular blockade, respiratory depression
Nondepolarizing neuromuscular blockers: ↑ Neuromuscular blockade, respiratory depression
Penicillins: Inactivated in renal disease

NURSING CONSIDERATIONS
Assessment

- Assess patient for previous sensitivity reaction
- Assess patient for signs and symptoms of infection including characteristics of sputum, urine, stool WBC >10,000/mm^3, temp
- Obtain baseline information before and during treatment
- Complete C&S testing before and after drug therapy to identify if correct treatment has been initiated
- Assess for allergic reactions: rash, urticaria, pruritus, chills, fever, joint

S

pain; angioedema may occur a few days after therapy begins; epinephrine, resuscitation equipment should be available for anaphylactic reaction
- Identify urine output; if decreasing, notify prescriber (may indicate nephrotoxicity); also increased BUN, creatinine, urine CrCl <80 ml/min
- Monitor blood studies: AST, ALT, CBC, Hct, bilirubin, LDH, alkaline phosphatase, Coombs' test monthly if patient is on long-term therapy
- Monitor electrolytes: potassium, sodium, chloride, magnesium monthly if patient is on long-term therapy
- Monitor for bleeding: ecchymosis, bleeding gums, hematuria, stool guaiac daily if on long-term therapy
- Assess for overgrowth of infection: perineal itching, fever, malaise, redness, pain, swelling, drainage, rash, diarrhea, change in cough, sputum
- Obtain weight before treatment; calculation of dosage is usually based on ideal body weight, but may be calculated on actual body weight
- Monitor I&O ratio; urinalysis daily for proteinuria, cells, casts; report sudden change in urine output
- Obtain serum peak 60 min after IM inj, trough level obtained just before next dose; blood level should be 2-4 × bacteriostatic level
- Monitor for deafness by audiometric testing, ringing, roaring in ears, vertigo; assess hearing before, during, after treatment
- Monitor for dehydration: high sp gr, decrease in skin turgor, dry mucous membranes, dark urine
- Monitor for overgrowth of infection including increased temp, malaise, redness, pain, swelling, perineal itching, diarrhea, stomatitis, change in cough, sputum

Nursing diagnoses
- ✓ Infection, risk for (uses)
- ✓ Diarrhea (adverse reactions)
- ✓ Injury, risk for (adverse reactions)
- ✓ Knowledge deficit (teaching)
- ✓ Noncompliance (teaching)

Implementation
- Give deeply in large muscle mass
- Reconstitute with 4.2-4.5 ml of sterile water for inj or 0.9% NaCl/1 g (200 mg/ml), 3.2-3.5 ml/1 g (250 mg/ml), 17 ml/5 g (250 mg/ml); give at 500 mg/ml or less

Syringe compatibilities:
Penicillin G sodium

Syringe incompatibilities:
Heparin

Y-site compatibilities:
Esmolol

Additive compatibilities:
Bleomycin

Patient/family education
- Teach patient to report sore throat, bruising, bleeding, joint pain, may indicate blood dyscrasias (rare); ringing, roaring in the ears
- Advise patient to contact prescriber if vaginal itching, loose, foul-smelling stools, furry tongue occur; may indicate superinfection

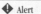

Evaluation
Positive therapeutic outcome
- Absence of signs/symptoms of infection
- Reported improvement in symptoms of infection

Treatment of overdose:
Withdraw drug, hemodialysis, monitor serum levels of drug, may give ticarcillin or carbenicillin

succimer (℞)
(sux'i-mer)
Chemet
Func. class: Heavy metal antagonist
Chem. class.: Chelating agent
Pregnancy category C

Action: Binds with ions of lead to form a water-soluble complex that is excreted by kidneys

Therapeutic Outcome: Removal of lead from the body

Uses: Lead poisoning in children with lead levels above 45 μg/dl; may be beneficial in mercury, arsenic poisoning

Dosage and routes

Child: PO 10 mg/kg or 350 mg/m^2 q8h × 5 days, then 10 mg/kg or 350 mg/m^2 q12h × 2 wk; another course may be required depending on lead levels; allow 2 wk between courses

Available forms: Caps 100 mg

Adverse effects

CNS: Drowsiness, dizziness, paresthesia, sensorimotor neuropathy
EENT: Otitis media, watery eyes, film in eyes, plugged ears
GI: *Nausea, vomiting, diarrhea, metallic taste, anorexia*
GU: **Proteinuria,** decreased urination, voiding difficulties
HEMA: **Increased platelets, intermittent eosinophilia**
INTEG: Rash, urticaria, pruritus
META: Increased AST, ALT, alkaline phosphatase, cholesterol
RESP: Sore throat, rhinorrhea, nasal congestion, cough
SYST: Back, stomach, head, rib, flank pain; abdominal cramps; chills; fever; flulike symptoms, head cold; headache

Contraindications: Hypersensitivity

Precautions: Pregnancy **C,** lactation, children <1 yr

Pharmacokinetics	
Absorption	Rapidly absorbed
Distribution	Unknown
Metabolism	Liver—extensively
Excretion	Kidneys—unchanged
Half-life	2 days

Pharmacodynamics	
Onset	Up to 2 hr
Peak	2-4 hr
Duration	8-12 hr

Interactions

Drug classifications

Heavy metal antagonist, others: Do not use together

NURSING CONSIDERATIONS

Assessment

- Assess VS, B/P, pulse, respirations, weigh daily
- Monitor I&O ratio, kidney function studies, BUN, creatinine, CrCl; watch for decreasing urine output
- Assess neurologic status: watch for paresthesias, beginning of seizures
- Monitor urine: pH, albumin, casts, blood, coproporphyrins, calcium
- Assess for febrile reactions that may occur 4-8 hr after drug therapy
- Monitor for cardiac abnor- malities: dysrhythmias, hypotension, tachycardia
- Assess for allergic reactions (rash, urticaria); if these occur, drug should be discontinued

Nursing diagnoses

✓ Poisoning, risk for (uses)
✓ Injury, risk for (uses, adverse reactions)
✓ Knowledge deficit (teaching)

Implementation

- Give PO whole or cap contents mixed with food or fluid

Patient/family education

- Explain reason for medication and expected results
- Provide a referral to health department to assess lead levels in home or workplace
- Teach patient to increase fluid intake

Evaluation

Positive therapeutic outcome

- Decreased symptoms of lead intoxication
- Decreased lead level <50 μg/dl

S

HIGH ALERT

succinylcholine (℞)

(suk-sin-ill-koe'leen)

Anectine, Anectine Flo-Pack, Quelicin, succinylcholine chloride, Sucostrin, Suxamethonium

Func. class.: Neuromuscular blocker (depolarizing—ultra short)

Pregnancy category C

Action: Inhibits transmission of nerve impulses by binding with cholinergic receptor sites, antagonizing action of acetylcholine; causes release of histamine

➔ **Therapeutic Outcome:** Paralysis of skeletal muscles

Uses: Facilitation of endotracheal intubation, skeletal muscle relaxation during orthopedic manipulations

Dosage and routes

Adult: **IV** 0.6 mg/kg, then 2.5 mg/min as needed; IM 2.5 mg/kg, max 150 mg

P ***Child:*** **IV**/IM 1-2 mg/kg, max 150 mg IM

Available forms: Inj 20, 50, 100 mg/ml; powder for inj 100/vial; powder for inf 500 mg/vial, 1 g/vial

Adverse effects

CV: Bradycardia, tachycardia; increased, decreased B/P, **sinus arrest, dysrhythmias**

EENT: Increased secretions, increased intraocular pressure

HEMA: **Myoglobulinemia**

INTEG: Rash, flushing, pruritus, urticaria

MS: Weakness, muscle pain, fasciculation, prolonged relaxation

RESP: **Prolonged apnea, bronchospasm, cyanosis, respiratory depression**

Contraindications: Hypersensitivity, malignant hyperthermia, decreased plasma pseudocholinesterase, penetrating eye injuries, acute narrow-angle glaucoma

Precautions: Pregnancy **C**, cardiac disease, severe burns, fractures (fasciculation may increase damage), P lactation, children <2 yr, electrolyte imbalances, dehydration, neuromuscular disease, respiratory disease, collagen diseases, glaucoma, eye surgery, penetrating eye wounds, G elderly or debilitated patients

Pharmacokinetics

Absorption	Well absorbed (IM)
Distribution	Widely distributed, crosses placenta
Metabolism	Plasma (90%)
Excretion	Hydrolyzed in urine (active/inactive metabolites)
Half-life	Unknown

Pharmacodynamics

	IV	IM
Onset	1 min	2-3 min
Peak	2-3 min	Unknown
Duration	6-10 min	10-30 min

Interactions

Individual drugs

Clindamycin: ↑ neuromuscular blockade

Enflurane: ↑ neuromuscular blockade

Isofluorophate: ↑ paralysis

Isoflurane: ↑ neuromuscular blockade

Lincomycin: ↑ neuromuscular blockade

Quinidine: ↑ neuromuscular blockade

Drug classifications

Aminoglycosides: ↑ neuromuscular blockade

β-Adrenergic blockers: ↑ neuromuscular blockade

Diuretics, potassium-losing: ↑ neuromuscular blockade

Local anesthetics: ↑ neuromuscular blockade

Magnesium salts: ↑ neuromuscular blockade
Opioids: ↑ neuromuscular blockade
Polymyxin antibiotics: ↑ neuromuscular blockade

Herb/drug
Melatonin: blocks succinylcholine

NURSING CONSIDERATIONS

Assessment

- Assess for electrolyte imbalances (potassium, magnesium); may lead to increased action of this drug
- Monitor VS (B/P, pulse, respirations, airway) until fully recovered; rate, depth, pattern of respirations, strength of hand grip
- Monitor I&O ratio; check for urinary retention, frequency, hesitancy
- Assess for recovery: decreased paralysis of face, diaphragm, leg, arm, rest of body
- Assess for allergic reactions: rash, fever, respiratory distress, pruritus; drug should be discontinued if these occur

Nursing diagnoses

✓ Communication, impaired verbal (adverse reactions)
✓ Breathing pattern, ineffective (uses)

Implementation

IV route

- Use nerve stimulator by anesthesiologist to determine neuromuscular blockade
- Give anticholinesterase to reverse neuromuscular blockade
- Give by **IV** inf; dilute 1-2 mg/ml in D_5, isotonic saline sol, give 0.5-10 mg/min, titrate to patient response; may be given directly over 1 min

Syringe compatibilities:
Heparin

Y-site compatibilities:
Etomidate, heparin, potassium chloride, propofol, vit B/C

Additive compatibilities:
Amikacin, cephapirin, isoproterenol, meperidine, methyldopate, morphine, norepinephrine, scopolamine

Additive incompatibilities:
Barbiturates, nafcillin, sodium bicarbonate

IM route

- Give deep IM, preferably high in deltoid muscle
- Store in refrigerator; store powder at room temp; close container tightly

Patient/family education

- Explain reason for medication and expected results
- Provide reassurance if communication is difficult during recovery from neuromuscular blockade; postoperative stiffness is normal, soon subsides

Evaluation

Positive therapeutic outcome

- Paralysis of jaw, eyelid, head, neck, rest of body

Treatment of overdose:

Edrophonium or neostigmine, atropine, monitor VS; may require mechanical ventilation

sucralfate (℞)

(soo-kral'fate)
Carafate, Sulcrate ♣
Func. class.: Protectant; antiulcer
Chem. class.: Aluminum hydroxide/sulfated sucrose

Pregnancy category B

Action: Forms a complex that adheres to ulcer site, adsorbs pepsin

Therapeutic Outcome: Healing of ulcers

Uses: Duodenal ulcer, oral mucositis, stomatitis after radiation of head and neck

Investigational uses: Gastric ulcers, gastroesophageal reflux

Dosage and routes

Ulcers

Adult: PO 1 g qid 1 hr ac, hs

P *Child:* PO 40-80 mg/kg/day

Prevention of ulcers

Adult: PO 1 g bid, 1 hr ac

Gastroesophageal reflux disease (GERD)

Adult: PO 1 g qid 1 hr ac and hs

P *Child:* PO 500 mg-1g qid, 1 hr ac and hs

Available forms: Tabs 1 g; oral susp 500 mg/5 ml ♣

Adverse effects

CNS: Drowsiness, dizziness

GI: *Dry mouth, constipation,* nausea, gastric pain, vomiting

INTEG: Urticaria, rash, pruritus

Contraindications: Hypersensitivity

Precautions: Pregnancy **B**, lactation, P children, renal failure

Do Not Confuse:
Carafate/Cafergot

Pharmacokinetics	
Absorption	Minimally absorbed
Distribution	Unknown
Metabolism	Not metabolized
Excretion	Feces (90%)
Half-life	6-20 hr

Pharmacodynamics	
Onset	½ hr
Peak	Unknown
Duration	6 hr

Interactions

Individual drugs

Phenytoin: ↓ absorption
Tetracycline: ↓ absorption

Drug classifications

Antacids: ↓ absorption of sucralfate
Fat-soluble vitamins: ↓ absorption
Fluoroquinolones: ↓ absorption

NURSING CONSIDERATIONS

Assessment

- Monitor gastric pH (>5 should be maintained); blood in stools

Nursing diagnoses

- ✓ Pain, chronic (uses)
- ✓ Pain (uses)
- ✓ Constipation (adverse reactions)
- ✓ Knowledge deficit (teaching)

Implementation

- Give on empty stomach 1 hr ac and hs
- Do not crush, chew tabs
- Store at room temp

Patient/family education

- Instruct patient to take medication on empty stomach
- Caution patient to take full course of therapy, not to use over 8 wk, to avoid smoking
- Caution patient to avoid antacids within ½ hr of drug or 1 hr after this drug

Evaluation

Positive therapeutic outcome

- Absence of pain or GI complaints

HIGH ALERT

sufentanil (℞)

(soo-fen'ta-nil)

Sufenta

Func. class.: Opiate analgesic

Pregnancy category C

Controlled substance schedule II

Action: Inhibits ascending pain pathways in CNS, increases pain threshold, alters pain perception

Therapeutic Outcome: Anesthesia, decreased pain

Uses: Primary anesthetic, adjunct to general anesthetic

Dosage and routes

Primary anesthetic

Adult: **IV** 8-30 μg/kg given with 100% O_2, a muscle relaxant

Adjunct

Adult: **IV** 1-8 μg/kg given with nitrous oxide/O_2

Available forms: Inj 50 μg/ml

Adverse effects

CNS: *Drowsiness, dizziness, confusion, headache, sedation, euphoria*

CV: Palpitations, bradycardia, change in B/P

EENT: Tinnitus, blurred vision, miosis, diplopia

GI: *Nausea, vomiting, anorexia, constipation, abdominal cramps*

GU: Increased urinary output, dysuria, urinary retention

INTEG: *Rash,* urticaria, bruising, flushing, diaphoresis, pruritus

RESP: **Respiratory depression**

Contraindications: Hypersensitivity, addiction (opiate)

Precautions: Addictive personality, pregnancy **C,** lactation, increased ICP, MI (acute), severe heart disease, respiratory depression, hepatic disease, renal disease, child <18 yr

Pharmacokinetics

Absorption	Completely absorbed
Distribution	Crosses placenta
Metabolism	Liver—extensively, small intestines—small amount
Excretion	Kidneys, breast milk
Half-life	2½ hr

Pharmacodynamics

Onset	1½-3 hr
Peak	Unknown
Duration	5 min

Interactions

Individual drugs

Alcohol: ↑ respiratory depression, hypotension, ↑ sedation
Cimetidine: ↑ recovery
Erythromycin: ↑ recovery
Nalbuphine: ↓ analgesia
Pentazocine: ↓ analgesia

Drug classifications

Antihistamines: ↑ respiratory depression, hypotension
CNS depressants: ↑ respiratory depression, hypotension
MAOIs: Do not use 2 wk before sufentanil
Phenothiazines: ↑ respiratory depression, hypotension
Sedative/hypnotics: ↑ respiratory depression, hypotension

Herb/drug

Kava: ↑ CNS depression

Lab test interferences

↑ Amylase

NURSING CONSIDERATIONS

Assessment

- Monitor VS after parenteral route; note muscle rigidity, drug history, liver, kidney function tests
- Monitor respiratory dysfunction: respiratory depression, character, rate, rhythm; notify prescriber if respirations are <10/min
- Monitor for CNS changes: dizziness, drowsiness, hallucinations, euphoria, LOC, pupil reaction
- Monitor allergic reactions: rash, urticaria

Nursing diagnoses

- ✓ Pain (uses)
- ✓ Sensory perceptual alteration: visual, auditory (adverse reactions)
- ✓ Breathing pattern, ineffective (adverse reactions)
- ✓ Knowledge deficit (teaching)

Implementation

- Give by inj (IM, **IV**), only with resuscitative equipment available; give slowly to prevent rigidity
- Give **IV** undiluted by anesthesiologist or diluted as an inf in 0.9% NaCl

Y-site compatibilities:

Amphotericin B, cholesteryl, cisatracurium, remifentanil

- Store in light-resistant area at room temp

S

Patient/family education
- Advise patient to report any symptoms of CNS changes, allergic reactions
- Caution patient to avoid CNS depressants: alcohol, sedative/hypnotics for at least 24 hr after this drug
- Discuss with patient that dizziness, drowsiness, and confusion are common, to avoid getting up without assistance
- Discuss in detail all aspects of the drug

Evaluation
Positive therapeutic outcome
- Maintenance of anesthesia

Treatment of overdose:
Naloxone 0.2-0.8 **IV**, O_2, **IV** fluids, vasopressors

sulfamethoxazole
See also trimethoprim/sulfamethoxazole

sulfamethoxazole (℞)
(sul-fa-meth-ox'a-zole)

Apo-Sulfamethoxazole ✦, Gantanol, Urobak

Func. class.: Antiinfective

Chem. class.: Sulfonamide, intermediate-acting

Pregnancy category B

Action: Interferes with bacterial biosynthesis of proteins by competitive antagonism of *p*-aminobenzoic acid (PABA)

➔ **Therapeutic Outcome:** Bactericidal action against susceptible organisms: streptococci and staphylococci, *Clostridium perfringens, Clostridium tetani, Nocardia asteroides;* gram-negative pathogens, including *Enterobacter, Escherichia coli, Klebsiella, Proteus mirabilis, Proteus vulgaris, Salmonella, Shigella*

Uses: UTIs, chancroid, inclusion conjunctivitis, malaria, meningococcal meningitis, nocardiosis, acute otitis media, toxoplasmosis, trachoma

Dosage and routes
Adult: PO 2 g, then 1 g bid or tid for 7-10 days

P ***Child >2 mo:*** PO 50-60 mg/kg then 25-30 mg/kg × 1 dose bid, max 75 mg/kg/day

Lymphogranuloma venereum

Adult: PO 1 g bid × 14 days

Renal dose

CrCl <50 ml/min 50% of dose

Available forms: Tabs 500 mg; oral susp 500 mg/5 ml

Adverse effects
CNS: Headache, insomnia, hallucinations, depression, vertigo, fatigue, anxiety, convulsions, drug fever, chills, drowsiness

CV: **Allergic myocarditis**

GI: *Nausea, vomiting, abdominal pain,* stomatitis, **hepatitis,** glossitis, **pancreatitis,** diarrhea, **enterocolitis,** anorexia

GU: **Renal failure, toxic nephrosis,** increased BUN, creatinine, crystalluria, hematuria, proteinuria

HEMA: **Leukopenia, thrombocytopenia, agranulocytosis, hemolytic anemia, aplastic anemia**

INTEG: Rash, dermatitis, urticaria, erythema, photosensitivity, alopecia

SYST: **Anaphylaxis, Stevens-Johnson syndrome**

Contraindications: Hypersensitivity to sulfonamides, sulfonylureas, thiazide and loop diuretics, salicylates, P sunscreen with PABA, lactation, infants <2 mo (except congenital toxoplasmosis), pregnancy at term, porphyria

Precautions: Pregnancy **B,** lactation, impaired hepatic/renal function, severe allergy, bronchial asthma

Pharmacokinetics

Absorption	Well absorbed
Distribution	Widely distributed, crosses placenta
Metabolism	Liver, large amounts
Excretion	Unchanged kidneys (20%), enters breast milk
Half-life	7-12 hr

Pharmacodynamics

Onset	1 hr
Peak	3-4 hr

Interactions
Individual drugs
Cyclosporine: ↑ nephrotoxicity
Indomethacin: ↑ drug-free concentrations
Methotrexate: ↑ toxicity
Phenytoin: ↑ folic acid deficiency
Probenecid: ↑ drug-free concentrations
Drug classifications
Anticoagulants, oral: ↑ effects of anticoagulant
Barbiturates: ↑ effects
Hypoglycemics, oral: ↑ effects of hypoglycemics
Salicylates: ↑ drug-free concentrations
Thiazide diuretics: ↑ thrombocytopenia
Uricosuric agents: ↑ effect
Lab test interferences
False positive: Urinary glucose test

NURSING CONSIDERATIONS
Assessment
- Assess patient for previous sensitivity reaction
- Assess patient for signs and symptoms of infection including characteristics of wounds, sputum, urine, stool, WBC >10,000/mm^3, elevated temp; obtain baseline information before and during treatment
- Complete C&S studies before beginning drug therapy to identify if correct treatment has been initiated
- Assess for allergic reactions: rash, urticaria, pruritus, chills, fever, joint pain; angioedema may occur a few days after therapy begins; epinephrine, resuscitation equipment should be on unit for anaphylactic reaction; AIDS patients are more susceptible
- Monitor blood studies: CBC, Hct, bilirubin, alkaline phosphatase monthly if patient is on long-term therapy
- Monitor for bleeding: ecchymosis, bleeding gums, hematuria, stool guaiac daily if patient is on long-term therapy
- Assess for overgrowth of infection: perineal itching, fever, malaise, redness, pain, swelling, drainage, rash, diarrhea, change in cough, sputum

Nursing diagnoses
- ✓ Infection, risk for (uses)
- ✓ Diarrhea (adverse reactions)
- ✓ Injury, risk for (adverse reactions)
- ✓ Knowledge deficit (teaching)
- ✓ Noncompliance (teaching)

Implementation
- Give around the clock to maintain proper blood levels; give on empty stomach to increase absorption of drug; do not give within 3 hr of other agents, drug actions may occur
- Give with 8 oz of water to prevent crystalluria

Patient/family education
- Teach patient to report sore throat, bruising, bleeding, joint pain; may indicate blood dyscrasias (rare)
- Advise patient to contact prescriber if vaginal itching, loose, foul-smelling stools, furry tongue occur; may indicate superinfection; report itching, rash, pruritus, urticaria
- Instruct patient to take all medication prescribed for the length of time ordered; drug must be taken around the clock to maintain blood levels; do not give medication to others

Evaluation
Positive therapeutic outcome
- Absence of signs/symptoms of

S

infection (WBC <10,000/mm^3, temp WNL, absence of urinary pain, hematuria)
- Reported improvement in symptoms of infection
- Negative C&S

sulfasalazine (℞)
(sul-fa-sal'a-zeen)
Azulfidine, Azulfidine EN-tabs, PMS-Sulfusalazine ♣, S.A.S. ♣, Salazopyrin ♣, sulfasalazine
Func. class.: Antiinflammatory
Chem. class.: Sulfonamide

Pregnancy category C

Action: Prodrug to deliver sulfapyridine and 5-aminosalicylic acid to colon; antinflammatory in connective tissue

Therapeutic Outcome: Treatment of ulcerative colitis, rheumatoid arthritis

Uses: Ulcerative colitis, rheumatoid arthritis (delayed rel tab) in patients who inadequately respond to or are intolerant of analgesics/NSAIDs, P juvenile rheumatoid arthritis (Azulfidine EN-tabs)

Investigational uses: Ankylosing spondylitis, Crohn's disease, psoriasis

Dosage and routes

Bowel disease

Adult: PO 3-4 g/day in divided doses; maintenance 1.5-2 g/day in divided doses q6h

P ***Child >2 yr:*** PO 40-60 mg/kg/day in 4-6 divided doses, then 20-30 mg/kg/day in 4 doses, max 2 g/day

Rheumatoid arthritis

Adult: PO 2 g/day in evenly divided doses, initiate treatment with a lower dose of enteric-coated tab

P ***Child ≥2 yr:*** PO 30 mg/kg/24 hr, divided into 4 doses

Renal dose

CrCl 10-30 ml/min bid; CrCl <10 ml/min qd

Available forms: Tabs 500 mg; oral susp 250 mg/5 ml; delayed rel tabs 500 mg

Adverse effects

CNS: Headache, confusion, insomnia, hallucinations, depression, vertigo, fatigue, anxiety, **seizures,** drug fever, chills

CV: **Allergic myocarditis**

GI: *Nausea, vomiting, abdominal pain,* stomatitis, **hepatitis,** glossitis, **pancreatitis,** diarrhea, anorexia

GU: **Renal failure, toxic nephrosis,** increased BUN, creatinine, crystalluria

Contraindications: Hypersensitivity to sulfonamides or salicylates, pregnancy at term, P child <2 yr, intestinal, urinary obstruction

Precautions: Pregnancy **C,** lactation, impaired hepatic function, severe allergy, bronchial asthma, impaired renal function

Do Not Confuse:
sulfasalazine/sulfisoxazole

Pharmacokinetics	
Absorption	Partially absorbed
Distribution	Crosses placenta
Metabolism	Liver
Excretion	Kidneys, breast milk
Half-life	6 hr

Pharmacodynamics	
Onset	1 hr
Peak	1½-6 hr
Duration	6-12 hr

Interactions

Individual drugs

Digoxin: ↓ effectiveness
Methotrexate: ↓ renal excretion
Phenytoin: ↓ hepatic clearance

Drug classifications

Anticoagulants, oral: ↑ toxicity
Hypoglycemics, oral: ↑ toxicity

Food/drug
Iron, folic acid will be poorly absorbed
Lab test interferences
False positive: Urinary glucose test

NURSING CONSIDERATIONS
Assessment
- Monitor I&O ratio; note color, amount, character, pH of urine if drug administered for UTIs; output should be 800 ml less than intake; if urine is highly acidic, alkalization may be needed
- Monitor kidney function studies: BUN, creatinine, urinalysis if on long-term therapy
- Monitor blood dyscrasias: skin rash, fever, sore throat, bruising, bleeding, fatigue, joint pain; monitor CBC before, during therapy (q3 mo)
- Assess for allergic reaction: rash, dermatitis, urticaria, pruritus, dyspnea, bronchospasm

Nursing diagnoses
✓ Injury, risk for (uses)
✓ Knowledge deficit (teaching)

Implementation
- Give with full glass of water to maintain adequate hydration; increase fluids to 2 L/day to decrease crystallization in kidneys; contact lens, urine, skin may be yellow-orange
- Give total daily dose in evenly spaced doses and after meals to help minimize GI intolerance
- Store in airtight, light-resistant container at room temp

Patient/family education
- Advise patient to take each oral dose with full glass of water to prevent crystalluria
- Teach patient to avoid sunlight or to use sunscreen to prevent burns
- Teach patient to avoid OTC medication (aspirin, vit C) unless directed by prescriber
- Advise patient to notify prescriber if skin rash, sore throat, fever, mouth sores, unusual bruising, bleeding occur
- Advise patient to use rectal susp hs and retain all night

Evaluation
Positive therapeutic outcome
- Absence of fever, mucus in stools or pain in joints

sulfinpyrazone (℞)
(sul-fin-peer'a-zone)
Anturan ✤, Anturane, sulfinpyrazone
Func. class.: Uricosuric
Chem. class.: Pyrazolone

Pregnancy category C

Action: Inhibits tubular reabsorption of urates, with increased excretion of uric acid; inhibits prostaglandin synthesis, which decreases platelet aggregation

➔ **Therapeutic Outcome:** Decreased uric acid levels, absence of platelet aggregation

Uses: Inhibition of platelet aggregation, gout

Dosage and routes
Inhibition of platelet aggregation
Adult: PO 200 mg qid
Gout/gouty arthritis
Adult: PO 100-200 mg bid × 1 wk, then 200-400 mg bid, not to exceed 800 mg/day

Available forms: Tabs 100 mg; caps 200 mg

Adverse effects
CNS: Dizziness, **seizures, coma**
EENT: Tinnitus
GI: Gastric irritation, nausea, vomiting, anorexia, **hepatic necrosis,** GI bleeding
GU: Renal calculi, hypoglycemia
HEMA: **Agranulocytosis** (rare)

S

INTEG: Rash, dermatitis, pruritus, fever, photosensitivity
RESP: **Apnea,** irregular respirations

Contraindications: Hypersensitivity to pyrazolone derivatives, blood dyscrasias, CrCl <50 ml/min, active peptic ulcer, GI inflammation

Precautions: Pregnancy **C**

Pharmacokinetics

Absorption	Well absorbed
Distribution	Unknown
Metabolism	Liver
Excretion	Feces (metabolites/ active drug)
Half-life	4 hr

Pharmacodynamics

Onset	Unknown
Peak	1-2 hr
Duration	4-6 hr

Interactions

Individual drugs:
Acetaminophen: ↑ toxicity
Aspirin: ↑ risk of bleeding
Cefamandole: ↑ risk of bleeding
Cefoperazone: ↑ risk of bleeding
Cefotetan: ↑ risk of bleeding
Niacin: ↓ effect of sulfinpyrazone
Nitrofurantoin: ↑ effect of sulfinpyrazone
Plicamycin: ↑ risk of bleeding
Theophylline: ↓ effect of sulfinpyrazone
Tolbutamide: ↑ effect of tolbutamide
Valproic acid: ↑ risk of bleeding
Verapamil: ↓ effect of sulfinpyrazone
Warfarin: ↑ effect of warfarin

Drug classifications
Anticoagulants: ↑ risk of bleeding
Antiinflammatory agents: ↑ risk of bleeding
Salicylates: ↓ effect of sulfinpyrazone
Thrombolytics: ↑ risk of bleeding

Lab test interferences
↑ Alkaline phosphatase, ↑ AST/ALT
False positive: RBC, Hgb

NURSING CONSIDERATIONS

Assessment

- Monitor I&O ratio; observe for decrease in urinary output; increase fluids to 2-3 L/day
- Monitor CBC, platelets, reticulocytes before, during therapy (q3 mo)
- Assess mobility, joint pain, and swelling in the joints

Nursing diagnoses

- ✓ Pain, chronic (uses)
- ✓ Immobility, impaired physical (uses)
- ✓ Knowledge deficit (teaching)

Implementation

- Give with food or antacid to decrease GI upset
- Reduce dose gradually if uric acid levels are normal after 6 mo

Patient/family education

- Advise patient to increase fluids to 3-4 L/day
- Caution patient to avoid alcohol, OTC preparations that contain alcohol; skin rashes may occur
- Advise patient to report any pain, redness, or hard area, usually in legs
- Instruct patient on importance of complying with medical regimen; bone marrow depression may occur

Evaluation

Positive therapeutic outcome

- Decreased pain in joints
- Normal serum uric acid levels
- Increased duration of antiinfectives

sulfisoxazole (℞)

(sul-fi-sox′a-zole)

Gantrisin, Gantrisin Pediatric, Novo-Soxazole 🍁, sulfisoxazole

Func. class.: Antiinfective
Chem. class.: Sulfonamide, short-acting

Pregnancy category B

Action: Interferes with bacterial biosynthesis of proteins by competitive antagonism of *p*-aminobenzoic acid (PABA)

Therapeutic Outcome: Bactericidal action against susceptible organisms: gram-positive pathogens, including streptococci and staphylococci, Clostridium perfringens, Clostridium tetani, Nocardia asteroides; gram-negative pathogens, including *Enterobacter, Escherichia coli, Klebsiella, Proteus mirabilis, Proteus vulgaris, Salmonella, Shigella*

Uses: UTIs; chancroid, trachoma, toxoplasmosis, acute otitis media, malaria, *Haemophilus influenzae* meningitis, meningococcal meningitis, nocardiosis

Dosage and routes

UTIs, other systemic infections

Adult: PO 2-4 g loading dose, then 1-2 g qid × 7-10 days

P ***Child >2 mo:*** PO 75 mg/kg or 2 g/m^2 loading dose, then 120-150 mg/kg/day or 4 g/m^2/day in divided doses q6h, max 6 g/day

Chlamydia trachomatis

Adult: PO 500 mg-1 g qid × 3 wk

Renal dose

CrCl 10-50 ml/min q8-12h; CrCl <10 ml/min q12-24h

Available forms: Tabs 500 mg; liq 500 mg/5 ml

Adverse effects

CNS: Headache, insomnia, hallucinations, depression, vertigo, fatigue, anxiety, **seizures,** drug fever, chills, drowsiness

CV: **Allergic myocarditis**

GI: Nausea, vomiting, abdominal pain, stomatitis, **hepatitis,** glossitis, pancreatitis, diarrhea, **enterocolitis,** anorexia

GU: **Renal failure, toxic nephrosis,** increased BUN, creatinine, crystalluria, hematuria, proteinuria

HEMA: **Leukopenia, thrombocytopenia, agranulocytosis, hemolytic anemia, aplastic anemia**

INTEG: Rash, dermatitis, urticaria, erythema, photosensitivity, alopecia

SYST: **Anaphylaxis, Stevens-Johnson syndrome**

Contraindications: Hypersensitivity to sulfonamides and sulfonylureas, thiazide and loop diuretics, salicylates; sunscreen with PABA, P lactation, infants <2 mo (except congenital toxoplas mosis); pregnancy at term, porphyria

Precautions: Pregnancy **B,** lactation, impaired hepatic/renal function, severe allergy, bronchial asthma

Do Not Confuse:
sulfisoxazole/sulfasalazine

Pharmacokinetics	
Absorption	Well absorbed
Distribution	Widely distributed, crosses placenta
Metabolism	Liver, mostly
Excretion	Breast milk
Half-life	4-7 hr

Pharmacodynamics	
Onset	Unknown
Peak	2-4 hr

Interactions

Individual drugs

Cyclosporine: ↑ nephrotoxicity
Indomethacin: ↑ drug-free concentrations
Methotrexate: ↑ toxicity
Phenytoin: ↑ folic acid deficiency
Probenecid: ↑ drug-free concentrations

Drug classifications

Anticoagulants, oral: ↑ effects of anticoagulant
Barbiturates: ↑ effects of barbiturates
Hypoglycemics, oral: ↑ effects of hypoglycemics
Salicylates: ↑ drug-free concentrations
Thiazide diuretics: ↑ thrombocytopenia

S

Uricosuric agents: ↑ effects of uricosurics

Lab test interferences

False positive: Urinary glucose test

NURSING CONSIDERATIONS

Assessment

- Assess patient for previous sensitivity reaction
- Assess patient for signs and symptoms of infection including characteristics of wounds, sputum, urine, stool, WBC >10,000/mm^3, temp; obtain baseline information before and during treatment
- Complete C&S testing before beginning drug therapy to identify if correct treatment has been initiated
- Assess for allergic reactions: rash, urticaria, pruritus, chills, fever, joint pain; angioedema may occur a few days after therapy begins; epinephrine, resuscitation equipment should be available for anaphylactic reaction
- Monitor blood studies: CBC, Hct, bilirubin, alkaline phosphatase monthly if patient is on long-term therapy
- Monitor for bleeding: ecchymosis, bleeding gums, hematuria, stool guaiac daily if on long-term therapy
- Assess for overgrowth of infection: perineal itching, fever, malaise, redness, pain, swelling, drainage, rash, diarrhea, change in cough, sputum

Nursing diagnoses

- ☑ Infection, risk for (uses)
- ☑ Diarrhea (adverse reactions)
- ☑ Injury, risk for (adverse reactions)
- ☑ Knowledge deficit (teaching)
- ☑ Noncompliance (teaching)

Implementation

- Give around the clock to maintain proper blood levels; give on an empty stomach to increase absorption of drug; do not give within 3 hr of other agents; drug interactions may occur
- Give with 8 oz of water

Patient/family education

- Teach patient to report sore throat, bruising, bleeding, joint pain; may indicate blood dyscrasias (rare)
- Advise patient to contact prescriber if vaginal itching; loose, foul-smelling stools; or furry tongue occur; may indicate superinfection; report itching, rash, pruritus, urticaria
- Instruct patient to take all medication prescribed for the length of time ordered; drug must be taken around the clock to maintain blood levels; medication should not be shared with others

Evaluation

Positive therapeutic outcome

- Absence of signs/symptoms of infection (WBC <10,000/mm^3, temp WNL, absence of urinary pain, hematuria)
- Reported improvement in symptoms of infection
- Negative C&S

sulindac (℞)

(sul-in'dak)

Apo-Sulin ✦, Clinoril, Novosundac ✦, sulindac

Func. class.: Nonsteroidal antiinflammatory

Chem. class.: Indeneacetic acid derivative

Pregnancy category C

Action: Inhibits prostaglandin synthesis by decreasing an enzyme needed for biosynthesis; analgesic, antiinflammatory, antipyretic

➔ **Therapeutic Outcome:** Decreased pain, inflammation

Uses: Mild to moderate pain, osteoarthritis, rheumatoid, gouty arthritis, ankylosing spondylitis

Dosage and routes

Arthritis

Adult: PO 150 mg bid, may increase to 200 mg bid

Bursitis/acute arthritis

Adult: PO 200 mg bid × 1-2 wk, then reduce dose

Available forms: Tabs 150, 200 mg

Adverse effects

CNS: Dizziness, drowsiness, fatigue, tremors, confusion, insomnia, anxiety, depression, *headache*

CV: Tachycardia, peripheral edema, palpitations, dysrhythmias

EENT: Tinnitus, hearing loss, blurred vision

GI: *Nausea, anorexia, vomiting, diarrhea,* jaundice, **cholestatic hepatitis,** constipation, flatulence, cramps, dry mouth, peptic ulcer, **bleeding, ulceration, perforation**

GU: **Nephrotoxicity: dysuria, hematuria, oliguria, azotemia**

HEMA: **Blood dyscrasias with prolonged use**

INTEG: Purpura, *rash, pruritus,* sweating, photosensitivity

Contraindications: Hypersensitivity, asthma, severe renal disease, severe hepatic disease, active ulcers

Precautions: Pregnancy **C**, lactation, children, bleeding disorders, GI disorders, cardiac, renal disorders, hypersensitivity to other antiinflammatory agents

Do Not Confuse:
Clinoril/Clozaril, Clinoril/Oruvail

Pharmacokinetics	
Absorption	Well absorbed
Distribution	Not known
Metabolism	Converted to active drug—liver
Excretion	Minimal unchanged kidneys, breast milk
Half-life	7.8 hr; 16.4 hr active metabolite

Pharmacodynamics	
Onset	Unknown
Peak	2 hr
Duration	Unknown

Interactions

Individual drugs

Acetaminophen (long-term use): ↑ renal reactions

Alcohol: ↑ adverse reactions

Aspirin: ↓ effectiveness, ↑ adverse reactions

Cyclosporine: ↑ nephrotoxicity

Diflunisal: ↓ sulindac effect

Digoxin: ↑ toxicity, ↑ levels

Insulin: ↓ insulin effect

Lithium: ↑ toxicity

Methotrexate: ↑ toxicity

Phenytoin: ↑ toxicity

Probenecid: ↑ toxicity

Radiation: ↑ risk of hematologic toxicity

Sulfonylurea: ↑ toxicity

Drug classifications

Anticoagulants: ↑ risk of bleeding

Antihypertensives: ↓ effect of antihypertensives

Antineoplastics: ↑ risk of hematologic toxicity

β-Adrenergic blockers: ↑ antihypertension

Cephalosporins: ↑ risk of bleeding

Diuretics: ↓ effectiveness of diuretics

Glucocorticoids: ↑ adverse reactions

Hypoglycemics: ↓ hypoglycemic effect

NSAIDs: ↑ adverse reactions

Potassium supplements: ↑ adverse reactions

Sulfonamides: ↑ toxicity

Lab test interferences

↑ Liver function studies, ↑ serum potassium, ↑ glucose, ↑ alkaline phosphatase

NURSING CONSIDERATIONS

Assessment

- Monitor blood counts during therapy; watch for decreasing platelets; if low, therapy may need to be discontinued, restarted after hematologic recovery; and for blood dyscrasia (thrombocytopenia): bruising, fatigue, bleeding, poor healing
- Assess pain: frequency, intensity,

S

characteristics, relief 1-2 hr after medication
- Assess for asthma, aspirin hypersensitivity, nasal polyps; hypersensitivity may develop

Nursing diagnoses

- ☑ Pain (uses)
- ☑ Mobility, impaired physical (uses)
- ☑ Knowledge deficit (teaching)
- ☑ Injury, risk for (adverse reactions)

Implementation

- Administer with food or milk to decrease gastric symptoms; food slows absorption slightly, does not decrease absorption

Patient/family education

- Advise patient that drug must be continued for prescribed time to be effective; to avoid aspirin, alcoholic beverages
- Caution patient to report bleeding, bruising, fatigue, malaise because blood dyscrasias do occur
- Instruct patient to use caution when driving; drowsiness, dizziness may occur
- Teach patient to take with a full glass of water to enhance absorption; (Do Not Crush) do not crush, break, or chew

Evaluation

Positive therapeutic outcome

- Decreased pain
- Decreased inflammation
- Increased mobility

sumatriptan (℞)

(soo-ma-trip'tan)

Imitrex

Func. class.: Antimigraine agent

Chem. class.: 5-HT_1 receptor agonist

Pregnancy category C

Action: Binds selectively to the vascular 5-HT_1 receptor subtype and exerts antimigraine effect; causes vasoconstriction in cranial arteries

Therapeutic Outcome: Absence of migraines

Uses: Acute treatment of migraine with or without aura and cluster headache

Dosage and routes

Adult: SC 6 mg or less; may repeat in 1 hr; not to exceed 12 mg/24 hr; PO 25 mg with fluids, max 100 mg; nasal: 1 dose of 5, 10, or 20 mg in one nostril, may repeat in 2 hr, max 40 mg/24 hr

Hepatic dose

Adult: PO 25 mg, if no response after 2 hr, give up to 50 mg

Available forms: Inj 6 mg (12 mg/ml); tabs 25, 50, 100 mg; nasal spray 5 mg/100 mcl-U dose spray device 20 mg/100 mcl-U

Adverse effects

CV: *Flushing,* **MI**

EENT: Throat, mouth, nasal discomfort, vision changes

GI: Abdominal discomfort

INTEG: *Inj site reaction,* sweating

MS: *Weakness, neck stiffness,* myalgia

NEURO: *Tingling, hot sensation, burning, feeling of pressure, tightness, numbness, dizziness, sedation,* headache, anxiety, fatigue

RESP: Chest tightness, pressure

Contraindications: Angina pectoris, history of MI, documented silent ischemia, Prinzmetal's angina, ischemic heart disease, **IV** use, concurrent ergotamine-containing preparations, uncontrolled hypertension, hypersensitivity, basilar or hemiplegic migraine

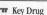

Precautions: Postmenopausal women, men >40 yr, risk factors for CAD, hypercholesterolemia, obesity, diabetes, impaired hepatic or renal function, pregnancy **C**, lactation, [P] children, [G] elderly

Pharmacokinetics

Absorption	Well absorbed (SC)
Distribution	10%-20% plasma protein binding
Metabolism	Liver (metabolite)
Excretion	Urine, feces
Half-life	2 hr

Pharmacodynamics

	SC
Onset	10-20 min
Peak	10 min-2 hr
Duration	Up to 24 hr (pain relief)

Interactions
Individual drugs
Ergotamine: ↑ risk of vasospastic reaction
Drug classifications
MAOIs: ↑ sumatriptan levels
SSRI : ↑ sumatriptan effect

NURSING CONSIDERATIONS
Assessment
- Assess for tingling, hot sensation, burning, feeling of pressure, numbness, flushing, inj site reaction
- Assess B/P; signs/symptoms of coronary vasospasm
- Monitor stress level, activity, reaction, coping mechanisms of patient
- Assess neurologic status: LOC, blurring vision, nausea, vomiting, tingling in extremities preceding headache
- Assess for ingestion of tyramine-containing foods (pickled products, beer, wine, aged cheese), food additives, preservatives, colorings, artificial sweeteners, chocolate, caffeine, which may precipitate these types of headaches

Nursing diagnoses
✓ Pain (uses)
✓ Knowledge deficit (teaching)

Implementation
PO route
- Swallow whole; take with fluids as soon as symptoms appear; may take a second dose >4 hr, max 200 mg/24 hr

SC route
- Give by SC route only, avoid IM or **IV** administration, use only for actual migraine attack

Patient/family education
- Caution patient not to take more than 2 dose/day or 12 mg/day; allow at least 1 hr between doses
- Caution patient to avoid driving or hazardous activities if dizziness or drowsiness occurs
- Teach patient to report chest tightness, heat, flushing, drowsiness, dizziness, fatigue, sudden severe abdominal pain or any allergic reactions that occur to prescriber immediately
- Inform patient to report any side effects to prescriber
- Caution patient to use contraception when taking drug, to notify prescriber if pregnancy is suspected or planned

Nasal spray
- Teach patient to spray once in 1 nostril, may repeat if headache returns, do not repeat if pain continues after 1st dose

Evaluation
Positive therapeutic outcome
- Decrease in frequency, severity of headache

tacrine (℞)
(tack'rin)
Cognex
Func. class.: Reversible cholinesterase inhibitor

Pregnancy category C

Action: Elevates acetylcholine concentrations (cerebral cortex) by slowing degrading of acetylcholine released in cholinergic neurons; does not alter underlying dementia

Therapeutic Outcome: Improvement in symptoms of dementia in Alzheimer's disease

Uses: Treatment of mild to moderate dementia in Alzheimer's disease

Dosage and routes

Adult: PO 10 mg qid × 6 wk, then 20 mg qid × 6 wk, increase at 6-wk intervals if patient tolerates drug well and if transaminase is within normal limits

Available forms: Caps 10, 20, 30, 40 mg

Adverse effects

CNS: *Dizziness, confusion, insomnia,* tremor, *ataxia, somnolence, anxiety, agitation, depression, hallucinations, hostility, abnormal thinking,* chills, fever

CV: Hypotension or hypertension

GI: *Nausea, vomiting, anorexia, abdominal pain, constipation,* dyspepsia, flatulence, **GI bleeding**

GU: *Frequency, UTI, incontinence*

INTEG: *Rash,* flushing

RESP: *Rhinitis, upper respiratory tract infection, cough,* pharyngitis

Contraindications: Hypersensitivity to this drug or acridine derivatives, patients treated with this drug who developed jaundice with a total bilirubin of >3 mg/dl

Precautions: Sick sinus syndrome, history of ulcers, GI bleeding, hepatic disease, bladder obstruction, asthma, P pregnancy **C**, lactation, children, seizure disorder

Do Not Confuse:
Cognex/Corgard

Pharmacokinetics

Absorption	Rapidly absorbed, low
Distribution	55% plasma protein bound
Metabolism	Liver, extensively
Excretion	Unknown
Half-life	2-4 hr

Pharmacodynamics

Unknown

Interactions

Individual drugs

Bethanechol: ↑ effect
Cimetidine: ↑ tacrine level
Succinylcholine: ↑ effect
Theophylline: ↑ toxicity

NURSING CONSIDERATIONS

Assessment

- Monitor ALT qo wk × 4-16 wk, then q3 mo; weekly ALT × 6 wk if dose is increased
- Monitor B/P for hypotension or hypertension
- Assess mental status: affect, mood, behavioral changes, depression, hallucinations, confusion; conduct suicide assessment
- Assess GI status: nausea, vomiting, anorexia, constipation, abdominal pain; add bulk and increase fluids for constipation
- Assess GU status: urinary frequency, incontinence

Nursing diagnoses

- ✓ Injury, risk for (uses)
- ✓ Thought processes, altered (uses)
- ✓ Knowledge deficit (teaching)

Implementation

- Give dosage adjusted to patient's response no more than q6 wk
- Provide assistance with ambulation if needed during beginning therapy; dizziness, ataxia may occur
- Give between meals; if GI symptoms occur, may be given with meals

Patient/family education

- Advise patient to report side effects: twitching, eye spasms; may indicate overdose
- Instruct patient to use drug exactly as prescribed at regular intervals, preferably between meals; may be taken with meals for GI upset; drug is not a cure
- Advise patient to notify prescriber of

nausea, vomiting, diarrhea (dose increased or beginning treatment) or rash, very dark or very light stools, jaundice (delayed onset)
- Caution patient not to increase or abruptly decrease dose; serious consequences may result

Evaluation

Positive therapeutic outcome
- Decrease in confusion, improved mood

Treatment of overdose:
Withdraw drug, administer tertiary anticholinergics, provide supportive care

tacrolimus (℞)
(tak-roe'li-mus)

Prograf

Func. class.: Immunosuppressant

Chem. clas.: Macrolide

Pregnancy category C

Action: Produces immunosuppression by inhibiting lymphocytes (T)

➔ **Therapeutic Outcome:** Prevention of rejection in organ transplant

Uses: Organ transplants, to prevent rejection

Dosage and routes

P ***Adult and child:*** **IV** 0.03-0.05 mg/kg/day × 3 days then PO 0.15 mg/kg bid; adjust dose in renal impairment

Available forms: Inj **IV**

Adverse effects

CNS: *Tremors, headache,* insomnia, paresthesia, anxiety, hyperesthesia, numbness, dizziness, fatigue

CV: Hypertension

EENT: Blurred vision, photophobia

GI: Nausea, vomiting, diarrhea, *oral Candida, gum hyperplasia,* **hepatotoxicity,** constipation, GI bleeding

GU: Urinary tract infections, **albuminuria, hematuria, proteinuria, renal failure**

HEMA: Anemia, **leukocytosis, thrombocytopenia purpura**

INTEG: Rash, flushing, itching, alopecia

META: Hirsutism, hyperglycemia, hyperkalemia, hyperuricemia, hypokalemia, hypomagnesemia

RESP: Pleural effusion, atelectasis, dyspnea

SYST: **Anaphylaxis**

Contraindications: Hypersensitivity

Precautions: Severe renal disease, severe hepatic disease, pregnancy **C,** diabetes mellitus, hyperkalemia, hyperuricemia

Pharmacokinetics

Absorption	Erractically absorbed (PO), completely absorbed (**IV**)
Distribution	Crosses placenta, 75% protein binding
Metabolism	Liver to metabolite
Excretion	Kidney—minimal, breast milk, bile
Half-life	10 hr

Pharmacodynamics

	PO	IV
Onset	Unknown	Unknown
Peak	1-4 hr	Unknown
Duration	12 hr	12 hr

Interactions

Individual drugs

Cyclosporine: ↑ nephrotoxicity, do not use together

Danazol: ↑ toxicity

Erythromycin: ↑ toxicity

Ibuprofen: ↑ oliguria

NURSING CONSIDERATIONS

Assessment

- Monitor blood studies: Hgb, WBC, platelets during treatment monthly; if WBC is <3000/mm^3, or platelet count <100,000/mm^3, drug should be discontinued or reduced; decreased Hgb level may indicate bone marrow suppression

T

- Monitor liver function studies: alkaline phosphatase, AST, ALT, amylase, bilirubin, and for hepatotoxicity: dark urine, jaundice, itching, light-colored stools; drug should be discontinued

Nursing diagnoses

- ✓ Infection, risk for (uses)
- ✓ Knowledge deficit (teaching)

Implementation

PO route

- Give all medications PO if possible; avoid IM inj because bleeding may occur
- Give with meals to reduce GI upset; nausea is common
- Give for several days before transplant surgery; patients should be placed in protective isolation

IV IV route

- Give after diluting in 0.9% NaCl or D_5W to a concentration of 0.004-0.02 mg/ml as a cont inf

Y-site compatibilities:
Acyclovir, aminophylline, amphotericin B, ampicillin, ampicillin/sulbactam, benztropine, calcium gluconate, cefazolin, cefotetan, ceftazidime, ceftriaxone, cefuroxime, chloramphenicol, cimetidine, ciprofloxacin, clindamycin, dexamethasone, digoxin, diphenhydramine, dobutamine, dopamine, doxycycline, erythromycin, esmolol, fluconazole, furosemide, ganciclovir, gentamicin, haloperidol, heparin, hydrocortisone, imipenem/cilastatin, insulin (regular), isoproterenol, leucovorin, lorazepam, methylprednisolone, metoclopramide, metronidazole, mezlocillin, multivitamins, nitroglycerin, nitroprusside, oxacillin, penicillin G potassium, perphenazine, phenytoin, piperacillin, potassium chloride, propranolol, ranitidine, sodium bicarbonate, trimethoprim/sulfamethoxazole, vancomycin

Patient/family education

- Instruct patient to report fever, rash, severe diarrhea, chills, sore throat, fatigue because serious infections may occur; clay-colored stools, cramping may indicate hepatotoxicity
- Caution patient to avoid crowds or persons with known infections to reduce risk of infection

Evaluation

Positive therapeutic outcome

- Absence of graft rejection
- Immunosuppression in autoimmune disorders

tamoxifen (℞)

(ta-mox'i-fen)

Alpha-Tamoxifen ✤, Med Tamoxifen ✤, Nolvadex, Nolvadex-D ✤, Novo-Tamoxifen ✤, Tamofen ✤, Tamone ✤, Tamoplex ✤

Func. class.: Antineoplastic
Chem. class.: Antiestrogen hormone

Pregnancy category D

Action: Inhibits cell division by binding to cytoplasmic estrogen receptors; resembles normal cell complex but inhibits DNA synthesis and estrogen response of target tissue

➔ **Therapeutic Outcome:** Prevention of rapidly growing malignant cells

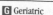

Uses: Advanced breast carcinoma that has not responded to other therapy in estrogen receptor-positive patients (usually postmenopausal), prevention of breast cancer, after breast surgery/radiation in ductal carcinoma in situ

Investigational uses: Mastalgia, pain/size of gynecomastia

Dosage and routes

Breast cancer

Adult: PO 20-40 mg qd, doses >20 mg/day divide AM/PM

High risk for breast cancer

Adult: PO 20 mg qd × 5 yr

Ductal carcinoma in situ
Adult: PO 20 mg qd × 5 yr

Available forms: Tabs 10, 20 mg

Adverse effects

CNS: *Hot flashes, headache, lightheadedness,* depression
CV: Chest pain
EENT: Ocular lesions, retinopathy, corneal opacity, blurred vision (high doses)
GI: *Nausea, vomiting,* altered taste (anorexia)
GU: Vaginal bleeding, pruritus vulvae
HEMA: **Thrombocytopenia, leukopenia,** deep vein thrombosis, pulmonary embolism
INTEG: *Rash,* alopecia
META: Hypercalcemia

Contraindications: Hypersensitivity, pregnancy **D**

Precautions: Leukopenia, thrombocytopenia, lactation, cataracts

Pharmacokinetics

Absorption	Adequately absorbed
Distribution	Unknown
Metabolism	Liver—extensively
Excretion	Feces—slowly, small amounts (kidneys)
Half-life	1 wk

Pharmacodynamics

Onset	Unknown
Peak	4-7 hr
Duration	Unknown

Interactions

Individual drugs
Bromocriptine: ↑ tamoxifen level
Radiation: ↑ myelosuppression

Drug classifications
Anticoagulants: ↑ risk of bleeding
Antineoplastics: ↑ thromboembolic action

Lab test interferences
↑ Serum calcium

NURSING CONSIDERATIONS

Assessment

- Monitor CBC, differential, platelet count weekly; withhold drug if WBC is $<4000/mm^3$ or platelet count is $<75,000/mm^3$; notify prescriber of results; monitor calcium levels (hypercalcemia is common)
- Assess for tumor flare: increase in bone, tumor pain during beginning treatment; give analgesics as ordered to decrease pain
- Assess for bleeding: hematuria, guaiac, bruising or petechiae, mucosa or orifices q8h, no rectal temp

Nursing diagnoses

✓ Injury, risk for (adverse reactions)
✓ Knowledge deficit (teaching)

Implementation

- Give with food or fluids for GI upset; do not break, crush, or chew enteric products; repeat dose may be needed if vomiting occurs
- Store in light-resistant container at room temp

Patient/family education

- Instruct patient to report any complaints, side effects to prescriber; if dose is missed, do not double next dose
- Advise patient that vaginal bleeding, pruritus, hot flashes can occur, and are reversible after discontinuing treatment
- Instruct patient to report immediately decreased visual acuity, which may be irreversible; stress need for routine eye exams
- Inform patient about who should be told about tamoxifen therapy
- Advise patient to report vaginal bleeding immediately; that tumor flare (increase in size or tumor, increased bone pain) may occur and will subside rapidly; may take analgesics for pain; that premenopausal women must use mechanical birth control method because ovulation may be induced (teratogenic drug)
- Caution patient to use sunscreen

T

and protective clothing to prevent burns because photosensitivity is common

- Teach patient that hair loss may occur during treatment; a wig or hairpiece may make patient feel better; new hair may be different in color, texture
- Inform patient rash or lesions are temporary and may become large during beginning therapy
- Advise patient to increase fluids to 2 L/day unless contraindicated

Evaluation

Positive therapeutic outcome

- Decreased spread of malignant cells in breast cancer

tamsulosin (℞)

(tam-sue-lo'sen)

Flomax

Func. class.: Selective α-adrenergic blocker

Chem. class.: Sulfamoyl phenethylamine derivative

Pregnancy category B

Therapeutic Outcome: Decreased symptoms of benign prostatic hyperplasia (BPH)

Uses: Symptoms of BPH

Dosage and routes

Adult: PO 0.4 mg qd, increasing to 0.8 mg qd if required after 2 wk

Available forms: Caps 0.4 mg

Adverse effects

CNS: Dizziness, headache, asthenia

CV: Chest pain

EENT: Amblyopia

GI: Nausea, diarrhea

GU: Decreased libido, abnormal ejaculation

MS: Back pain

RESP: Rhinitis, pharyngitis, cough

Contraindications: Hypersensitivity

Precautions: Pregnancy **B,** P children, lactation, hepatic disease, coronary artery disease, severe renal disease

Pharmacokinetics

Absorption	Well absorbed
Distribution	Not known; 98% plasma protein bound
Metabolism	Liver, extensively
Excretion	Kidneys
Half-life	9-15 hr

Pharmacodynamics

Unknown

Interactions

Drug classifications

α_1-Adrenergic blockers: Do not use together

NURSING CONSIDERATIONS

Assessment

- Monitor CBC with differential and liver function studies; B/P and heart rate
- Monitor urodynamic studies/urinary flow rates, residual volume
- Assess for BPH: change in urinary patterns, baseline and throughout treatment
- Monitor I&O ratios, weight qd, edema, report weight gain or edema

Nursing diagnoses

- ✓ Cardiac output, decreased (uses)
- ✓ Injury, potential for physical (side effects)
- ✓ Knowledge deficit (teaching)
- ✓ Noncompliance (teaching)

Implementation

- Store in airtight container at 86° F (30° C) or less
- May be given with food to prevent GI symptoms

Patient/family education

- Teach patient not to discontinue drug abruptly; emphasize the importance of complying with dosage schedule, even if feeling better; if dose is missed take as soon as remembered; take at same time each day

- Teach patient not to use OTC products (cough, cold, allergy) unless directed by prescriber; also to avoid large amounts of caffeine
- Caution patient that drug may cause dizziness, may occur during 1st few days of therapy; to avoid hazardous activities

Evaluation

Positive therapeutic outcome

- Decreased symptoms of BPH

tazobactam

See piperacillin/tazobactam

telmisartan (℞)

(tel-mih-sar'tan)

Micardis

Func. class.: Antihypertensive

Chem. class.: Angiotensin II receptor (type AT_1)

Pregnancy category

C (1st trimester)

D (2nd/3rd trimesters)

Action: Blocks the vasoconstrictor and aldosterone-secreting effects of angiotensin II; selectively blocks the binding of angiotensin II to the AT_1 receptor found in tissues

Therapeutic Outcome: ↓ B/P

Uses: Hypertension, alone or in combination

Investigational uses: Heart failure

Dosage and routes

Adult: PO 40 mg qd; range 20-80 mg

Available forms: Tabs 40, 80 mg

Adverse effects

CNS: Dizziness, insomnia, anxiety

GI: *Diarrhea,* dypepsia, *anorexia, vomiting*

MS: *Myalgia, pain*

RESP: Cough, *upper respiratory tract infection*

Contraindications: Hypersensitivity, pregnancy **D** (2nd/3rd trimesters)

Precautions: Hypersensitivity to angiotensin-converting enzyme (ACE) inhibitors; pregnancy **C** (1st trimester); lactation, P children, G elderly

Pharmacokinetics

Absorption	Unknown
Distribution	Highly protein bound
Metabolism	Liver (extensively)
Excretion	Urine/feces
Half-life	Terminal 24 hr

Pharmacodynamics

Onset	Unknown
Peak	Unknown
Duration	Unknown

Interactions

Digoxin: ↑ digoxin peak, trough concentrations

Drug classifications

Barbiturates: ↓ antihypertensive action

Diuretics: ↑ antihypertensive action

NSAIDs: ↓ antihypertensive action

NURSING CONSIDERATIONS

Assessment

- Monitor B/P, pulse q4h; note rate, rhythm, quality
- Monitor electrolytes: potassium, sodium, chloride
- Monitor baselines in renal, liver function tests before therapy begins
- Assess edema in feet, legs qd
- Assess skin turgor, dryness of mucous membranes for hydration status

Nursing diagnoses

- ✓ Tissue perfusion, altered (uses)
- ✓ Knowledge deficit (teaching)
- ✓ Noncompliance (teaching)

T

Implementation
- Give without regard to meals
- Give increased dose to black patients, B/P response may be reduced

Patient/family education
- Instruct patient to comply with dosage schedule, even if feeling better
- Advise patient to notify prescriber of mouth sores, fever, swelling of hands or feet, irregular heartbeat, chest pain
- Teach patient that excessive perspiration, dehydration, vomiting, diarrhea may lead to fall in blood pressure; consult prescriber if these occur
- Teach patient that drug may cause dizziness, fainting; light-headedness may occur
- Advise patient to use contraception while taking this drug
- Teach patient to notify prescriber of all prescriptions, OTC preparations, and supplements taken

Evaluation
Positive therapeutic outcome
- Decreased B/P

temazepam (℞)
(tem-az′a-pam)
Razepam, Restoril, Temazepam
Func. class.: Sedative/hypnotic
Chem. class.: Benzodiazepine

Pregnancy category X

Controlled substance schedule IV (USA)
schedule F (Canada)

Action: Produces CNS depression at limbic, thalamic, hypothalamic levels of the CNS; may be mediated by neurotransmitter γ-aminobutyric acid (GABA); results are sedation, hypnosis, skeletal muscle relaxation, anticonvulsant activity, anxiolytic action

➡ **Therapeutic Outcome:** Decreased insomnia

Uses: Insomnia (short-term)

Dosage and routes
Adult: PO 15-30 mg hs
G ***Elderly:*** PO 7.5 mg hs

Available forms: Caps 7.5, 15, 30 mg

Adverse effects
CNS: *Lethargy, drowsiness, daytime sedation,* dizziness, confusion, lightheadedness, headache, anxiety, irritability
CV: Chest pain, pulse changes
GI: Nausea, vomiting, diarrhea, heartburn, abdominal pain, constipation, anorexia
HEMA: **Leukopenia, granulocytopenia** (rare)

Contraindications: Hypersensitivity to benzodiazepines, pregnancy **X**, lactation, intermittent porphyria

Precautions: Anemia, hepatic disease, renal disease, suicidal individuals, drug abuse, G elderly, psychosis, P child <15 yr, acute narrow-angle glaucoma, seizure disorders

Pharmacokinetics

Absorption	Well absorbed
Distribution	Widely distributed, crosses placenta, crosses blood-brain barrier
Metabolism	Liver
Excretion	Kidneys, breast milk
Half-life	10-20 hr

Pharmacodynamics

Onset	½ hr
Peak	2-3 hr
Duration	6-8 hr

Interactions
Individual drugs
Alcohol: ↑ CNS depression
Cimetidine: ↑ action
Disulfiram: ↑ action
Fluoxetine: ↑ action
Isoniazid: ↑ action
Ketoconazole: ↑ action
Levodopa: ↓ action of levodopa
Metoprolol: ↑ action

Propoxyphene: ↑ action
Propranolol: ↑ action
Rifampin: ↓ action of temazepam
Theophylline: ↓ sedative effects
Valproic acid: ↑ action

Drug classifications

Antidepressants: ↑ CNS depression
Antihistamines: ↑ CNS depression
Barbiturates: ↓ effect of temazepam
Opiates: ↑ CNS depression
Oral contraceptives: ↑ effect

Herb/drug

Kava: ↑ CNS depression

Lab test interferences

↑ AST/ALT, ↑ serum bilirubin
↓ Radioactive iodine uptake
False: ↑ 17-OHCS

NURSING CONSIDERATIONS

Assessment

- Assess mental status: mood, sensorium, anxiety, affect, sleeping pattern, drowsiness, dizziness, especially G elderly; physical dependency, withdrawal symptoms: anxiety, panic attacks, agitation, convulsions, headache, nausea, vomiting, muscle pain, weak- ness; suicidal tendencies; for indications of increasing tolerance and abuse
- Monitor B/P (lying, standing), pulse; if systolic B/P drops 20 mm Hg, hold drug, notify prescriber
- Monitor blood studies: CBC during long-term therapy; blood dycrasias have occurred rarely; decreased hematocrit, neutropenia may occur
- Monitor hepatic studies: AST, ALT, bilirubin, creatinine LDH, alkaline phosphatase
- Monitor I&O ratio; indicate renal dysfunction

Nursing diagnoses

- ✓ Anxiety (uses)
- ✓ Depression (uses)
- ✓ Injury, risk for (adverse reactions)
- ✓ Knowledge deficit (teaching)

Implementation

- Give with food or milk to decrease GI symptoms; if patient is unable to swallow medication whole, tab may be crushed and mixed with foods or fluids
- Give sugarless gum, hard candy, frequent sips of water for dry mouth

Patient/family education

- Inform patient that drug may be taken with food, and that fluids and tab may be crushed or swallowed whole
- Advise patient not to use for everyday stress or longer than 3 mo unless directed by prescriber; not to take more than prescribed amount; may be habit forming; not to double or skip doses
- Caution patient to avoid OTC preparations unless approved by prescriber; alcohol and CNS depressants will increase CNS depression
- Advise patient to avoid driving, activities that require alertness, because drowsiness may occur; to avoid alcohol ingestion or other psychotropic medications; to rise slowly or fainting may occur, especially G in elderly; that drowsiness may worsen at beginning of treatment
- Caution patient not to discontinue medication abruptly after long-term use; withdrawal symptoms include vomiting, cramping, tremors, seizures
- Advise patient to use contraception while taking this drug

Evaluation

Positive therapeutic outcome

- Decreased anxiety, restlessness, sleeplessness (short-term treatment only)

Treatment of overdose:

Lavage, VS, supportive care

T

temozolomide (℞)

(tem-oo-zole'oo-mide)

Temodar

Func. class.: Antineoplastic alkylating agents

Chem. class.: Imidazotetrazine derivative

Pregnancy category D

Action: A pro-drug that undergoes conversion to 5-(3-methyl-1-triazeno) imidazole-4-carboxamide (MTIC); MTIC action prevents DNA transcription

Therapeutic Outcome: Prevention of rapidly growing malignant cells

Uses: Anaplastic astrocytoma with relapse

Dosage and routes

Adult: PO adjust dose based on nadir neutrophil and platelet counts 150 mg/m^2/day × 5 days during 28-day cycle

Available forms: Caps 5, 20, 100, 250 mg

Adverse effects

CNS: **Seizures,** *hemiparesis, dizziness, poor coordination, amnesia, insomnia, paresthesia, somnolence, paresis, ataxia, anxiety, dysphagia, depression, confusion*

GI: *Nausea, anorexia, vomiting*

GU: *Urinary incontinence, UTI, frequency*

HEMA: **Thrombocytopenia, leukopenia,** anemia

INTEG: *Rash, pruritus*

MISC: *Headache, fatigue, asthenia, fever, edema, back pain, weight increase, diplopia*

RESP: *Upper respiratory tract infection, pharyngitis, sinusitis, coughing*

Contraindications: Hypersensitivity to this drug or dacarbazine, pregnancy **D**, lactation

Precautions: Radiation therapy, renal, hepatic disease

Pharmacokinetics

Absorption	Rapid, complete
Distribution	Crosses blood-brain barrier
Metabolism	To MTIC and metabolite
Excretion	Urine, feces
Half-life	1.8 hr

Pharmacodynamics

Onset	Unknown
Peak	1 hr
Duration	Unknown

Interactions

Individual drugs

Radiation: ↑ toxicity, bone marrow suppression

Drug classifications

Antineoplastics: ↑ toxicity, bone marrow suppression

Bone marrow-suppressing drugs: ↑ bone marrow suppression

Live virus vaccines: ↑ adverse reactions, ↓ antibody reaction

Food/drug

↓ Absorption

NURSING CONSIDERATIONS

Assessment

- Assess symptoms indicating severe allergic reaction: rash, pruritus, urticaria, purpuric skin lesions, itching, flushing; drug should be discontinued
- Obtain CBC on day 22 (21 days after 1st dose), CBC weekly until recovery if ANC is <1.5 × 10^9/L and platelets <100 × 10^9/L, do not administer to patients that do not tolerate 100 mg/m^2; myelosuppression usually occurs late in the treatment cycle
- Assess for seizures throughout treatment
- Monitor renal function studies: BUN, creatinine, urine CrCl before and during therapy; I&O ratio; report fall in urine output to <30 ml/hr
- Monitor temp q4h (may indicate beginning of infection)
- Monitor liver function tests before

and during therapy (bilirubin, AST, ALT, LDH) as needed or monthly; note jaundice of skin or sclera, dark urine, clay-colored stools, itchy skin, abdominal pain, fever, diarrhea; hepatotoxicity can be serious and fatal
- Assess for bleeding: hematuria, stool guaiac, bruising or petechiae, mucosa or orifices q8h; check for inflammation of mucosa, breaks in skin

Nursing diagnoses
- ✓ Injury, risk for (adverse reactions)
- ✓ Body image disturbance (adverse reactions)
- ✓ Infection, risk for (adverse reactions)
- ✓ Knowledge deficit (teaching)

Implementation
- Give fluids **IV** or PO before chemotherapy to hydrate patient
- Give antiemetic 30-60 min before giving drug to prevent vomiting, and prn; antibiotics for prophylaxis of infection
- Provide liq diet: carbonated beverages; gelatin may be added if patient is not nauseated or vomiting
- Capsules should not be opened, if accidentally damaged, do not allow contact with skin, or inhale; take caps one at a time with 8 oz of water at the same time of day
- Give on empty stomach to prevent nausea/vomiting

Patient/family education
- Teach patient to avoid use of products containing aspirin or NSAIDs, razors, commercial mouthwash, since bleeding may occur; to report symptoms of bleeding (hematuria, tarry stools)
- Instruct patient to report signs of anemia (fatigue, headache, irritability, faintness, shortness of breath)
- Caution patient not to have any vaccinations without the advice of prescriber; serious reactions can occur
- Advise patient contraception is needed during treatment and for several months after completion of therapy; drug has teratogenic properties

Evaluation
Positive therapeutic outcome
- Prevention of rapid division of malignant cells

HIGH ALERT

tenecteplase (℞)
(ten-ek'ta-place)

TNKase

Func. class.: Thrombolytic enzyme

Chem. class.: β-Hemolytic *Streptococcus* filtrate (purified)

Pregnancy category C

Action: Activates conversion of plasminogen to plasmin (fibrinolysin): plasmin breaks down clots (fibrin), fibrinogen, factors V, VII; occlusion of venous access lines

➔ **Therapeutic Outcome:** Resolution of MI

Uses: Acute MI

Dosage and routes
Adult <60 kg: **IV** bol 30 mg, give over 6 sec

Adult ≥60-<70 kg: **IV** bol 35 mg, give over 7 sec

Adult ≥70-<80 kg: **IV** bol 40 mg, give over 8 sec

Adult ≥80-<90 kg: **IV** bol 45 mg, give over 9 sec

Adult ≥90 kg: **IV** bol 50 mg, give over 10 sec

Available forms: Powder for inj, lyophilized 50 mg

Adverse effects
CV: Dysrhythmias, hypotension, pulmonary edema, **pulmonary embolism, cardiogenic shock, cardiac arrest, heart failure, myocardial reinfarction, myocardial rupture, tamponade, pericar-**

T

ditis, pericardial effusion, thrombosis
HEMA: Decreased Hct, **bleeding**
INTEG: Rash, urticaria, phlebitis at **IV** inf site, itching, flushing
SYST: **GI, GU, intracranial, retroperitoneal bleeding, surface bleeding, anaphylaxis**

Contraindications: Hypersensitivity, active bleeding, intraspinal surgery, CNS neoplasms, ulcerative colitis, enteritis, severe hypertension, severe renal disease, hepatic disease, hypocoagulation, COPD, subacute bacterial endocarditis, rheumatic valvular disease, cerebral embolism/thrombosis/hemorrhage, intraarterial diagnostic procedure or surgery (10 days), recent major surgery

Precautions: Arterial emboli from left side of heart, pregnancy **C**, lactation, children [P]

Pharmacokinetics	
Absorption	Unknown
Distribution	Unknown
Metabolism	Liver
Excretion	Unknown
Half-life	20-24 min

Pharmacodynamics	
Onset	Immediate
Peak	Unknown
Duration	Unknown

Interactions
Individual drugs
Aspirin: ↑ bleeding potential
Indomethacin: ↑ bleeding potential
Phenylbutazone: ↑ bleeding potential

Drug classifications
Anticoagulants: ↑ bleeding potential
Antithrombolytics: ↑ bleeding potential

Lab test interferences
↑ Pro-time, ↑ APTT, ↑ TT
↓ Plasminogen, ↓ fibrinogen

NURSING CONSIDERATIONS
Assessment
- Assess for allergy: fever, rash, itching, chills; mild reaction may be treated with antihistamines
- [Alert] Assess for bleeding during 1st hr of treatment; hematuria, hematemesis, bleeding from mucous membranes, epistaxis, ecchymosis; may require transfusion (rare), continue to assess for bleeding for 24 hr
- Monitor blood studies (Hct, platelets, PTT, pro-time, TT, APTT) before starting therapy; pro-time or APTT must be less than 2 × control before starting therapy; PTT or pro-time q3-4h during treatment
- Assess for hypersensitive reactions: fever, rash, dyspnea; drug should be discontinued; for previous reactions to streptokinase
- Monitor VS, B/P, pulse, respirations, neurologic signs, temp at least q4h; temp >104° F (40° C) indicates internal bleeding; cardiac rhythm after intracoronary administration; systolic pressure increase >25 mm Hg should be reported to prescriber
- [Alert] Assess for neurologic changes that may indicate intracranial bleeding
- [Alert] Assess for retroperitoneal bleeding: back pain, leg weakness, diminished pulses
- Assess for respiratory depression

Nursing diagnoses
- ✓ Knowledge deficit (teaching)
- ✓ Decreased cardiac output (uses)

Implementation
IV route
- Give as soon as thrombi identified; not useful for thrombi >1 wk old
- Administer cryoprecipitate or fresh frozen plasma if bleeding occurs
- Administer loading dose at beginning of therapy; may require increased loading doses
- Give heparin after fibrinogen level >100 mg/dl; heparin infusion to increase PTT to 1.5-2 × baseline for 3-7 days; **IV** heparin with loading

dose is recommended after discontinuing streptokinase to prevent redevelopment of thrombi

- Aseptically withdraw 10 ml of sterile H_2O for inj from diluent vial, use red cannula syringe-filling device, inject all contents of syringe into drug vial, direct into powder, swirl, withdraw correct dose, discard any unused solution; stand the shield with dose vertically on flat surface and passively recap the red cannula, remove entire shield assembly by twisting counterclockwise, give by **IV** bol
- About 10% of patients have high streptococcal antibody titers requiring increased loading doses
- **IV** therapy: use upper extremity vessel that is accessible to manual compression

Y-site compatibilities: Dobutamine, dopamine, heparin, lidocaine, nitroglycerin

- Provide bed rest during entire course of treatment
- Avoid venous or arterial puncture, inj, rectal temp; any invasive treatment
- Treat fever with acetaminophen or aspirin
- Apply pressure for 30 sec to minor bleeding sites; inform prescriber if this does not attain hemostasis; apply pressure dressing

Evaluation

Positive therapeutic outcome

- Resolution of myocardial infarction

tenofovir disoproxil fumarate

See Appendix A, Selected New Drugs

terazosin (℞)

(ter-ay'zoe-sin)

Hytrin, terazosin

Func. class.: Antihypertensive

Chem. class.: Adrenergic blocker (peripherally acting)

Pregnancy category C

Action: Peripheral blood vessels are dilated, peripheral resistance lowered; reduction in blood pressure results from α-adrenergic receptors being blocked

➔ **Therapeutic Outcome:** Decreased B/P in hypertension, decreased symptoms of benign prostatic hyperplasia (BPH)

Uses: Hypertension, as a single agent or in combination with diuretics or β-blockers, BPH

Dosage and routes

Adult: PO 1 mg hs, may increase doses slowly to desired response; max 20 mg/day

Available forms: Caps 1, 2, 5, 10 mg

Adverse effects

CNS: *Dizziness, headache, drowsiness,* anxiety, depression, vertigo, weakness, fatigue

CV: Palpitations, orthostatic hypotension, tachycardia, edema, rebound hypertension

EENT: Blurred vision, epistaxis, tinnitus, dry mouth, red sclera, nasal congestion, sinusitis

GI: *Nausea,* vomiting, diarrhea, constipation, abdominal pain

GU: Urinary frequency, incontinence, impotence, priapism

RESP: Dyspnea

Contraindications: Hypersensitivity

Precautions: Pregnancy **C**, P children, lactation

T

Pharmacokinetics

Absorption	Well absorbed
Distribution	Not known
Metabolism	Liver—50%
Excretion	Kidneys unchanged—10%, feces unchanged—20%
Half-life	9-12 hr

Pharmacodynamics

Onset	15 min
Peak	1 hr
Duration	24 hr

Interactions

Individual drugs

Alcohol: ↑ CNS depression

Drug classifications

Antihypertensives: ↑ hypotension
Estrogens: ↓ antihypertensive effect
Nitrates: ↑ hypotensive effects
NSAIDs: ↓ antihypertensive effect
Sympathomimetics: ↓ antihypertensive effect

Herb/drug

Angelica: ↑ terazosin effect

Lab test interferences

↑ VMA excretion, ↑ 5-HIAA excretion
Interference: 17-OHCS, 17-KS

NURSING CONSIDERATIONS

Assessment

- Monitor B/P, orthostatic hypotension, syncope; check for edema in feet, legs daily; I&O ratio; weight daily; notify prescriber of changes
- Assess for allergic reactions: rash, fever, pruritus, urticaria; drug should be discontinued if antihistamines fail to help

Nursing diagnoses

- ✓ Cardiac output, decreased (uses)
- ✓ Injury, risk for (adverse reactions)
- ✓ Knowledge deficit (teaching)
- ✓ Noncompliance (teaching)

Implementation

- Store in airtight container at 86° F (30° C) or less
- May be used in combination with other antihypertensives
- May be given with food to prevent GI symptoms

Patient/family education

- Caution patient not to discontinue drug abruptly; the importance of complying with dosage schedule, even if feeling better; if dose is missed take as soon as remembered; take medication at same time each day
- Teach patient not to use OTC products (cough, cold, allergy) unless directed by prescriber; also to avoid large amounts of caffeine
- Emphasize the need to rise slowly to sitting or standing position to minimize orthostatic hypotension
- Teach patient to notify prescriber of mouth sores, sore throat, fever, swelling of hands or feet, irregular heartbeat, chest pain
- Caution patient to report excessive perspiration, dehydration, vomiting, diarrhea; may lead to fall in B/P
- Caution patient that drug may cause dizziness, fainting, light-headedness; may occur during 1st few days of therapy; to avoid hazardous activities
- Teach patient how to take B/P, and normal readings for age group; to take B/P q7 days

Evaluation

Positive therapeutic outcome

- Decreased B/P in hypertension
- Decreased symptoms of BPH

Treatment of overdose:

Administer volume expanders or vasopressors; discontinue drug; place patient in supine position

terbutaline (℞)

(ter-byoo'te-leen)

Brethaire, Brethine, Bricanyl

Func. class.: Selective β_2-agonist; bronchodilator

Chem. class.: Catecholamine

Pregnancy category B

Action: Relaxes bronchial smooth muscle by direct action on β_2-adrenergic receptors through accumulation of cAMP at β-adrenergic receptor sites; results are bronchodilation, diuresis, and CNS and cardiac stimulation; relaxes uterine smooth muscle

Therapeutic Outcome: Bronchodilation with ease of breathing

Uses: Bronchospasm

Investigational uses: Premature labor, hyperkalemia

Dosage and routes

Bronchospasm

P ***Adult and child >12 yr:*** INH 2 puffs q1 min, then q4-6h; PO 2.5-5 mg q8h; SC 0.25 mg q8h

Bronchodilation

P ***Adult/child >15 yr:*** PO 2.5-5 mg q6h during day, max 15 mg/24 hr

P ***Child 12-15 yr:*** PO 2.5 mg tid

Available forms: Tabs 2.5, 5 mg; aerosol 0.2 mg/actuation; inj 1 mg/ml

Adverse effects

CNS: Tremors, anxiety, insomnia, headache, dizziness, stimulation

CV: Palpitations, tachycardia, hypertension, dysrhythmias, **cardiac arrest**

GI: Nausea, vomiting

Contraindications: Hypersensitivity to sympathomimetics, narrow-angle glaucoma, tachydysrhythmias

Precautions: Pregnancy **B,** cardiac disorders, hyperthyroidism, diabetes mellitus, prostatic hypertension, G lactation, elderly, hypertension, glaucoma

Pharmacokinetics

Absorption	Well absorbed (SC), partially absorbed (PO)
Distribution	Unknown
Metabolism	Liver—partially
Excretion	Unknown
Half-life	Unknown

Pharmacodynamics

	PO	INH	SC	IV
Onset	½ hr	5-15 min	10-15 min	Rapid
Peak	1-2 hr	1-2 hr	½-1 hr	Unknown
Duration	4-8 hr	4-6 hr	1½-4 hr	Unknown

Interactions

Drug classifications

β-Adrenergic blockers: Block therapeutic effect

Bronchodilators, aerosol: ↑ action of bronchodilator

MAOIs: ↑ chance of hypertensive crisis

Sympathomimetics: ↑ adrenergic side effects

NURSING CONSIDERATIONS

Assessment

- Monitor respiratory func- tion: vital capacity, FEV, ABGs, lung sounds, heart rate, rhythm (baseline)
- Determine that patient has not received theophylline therapy before giving dose; assess client's ability to self-medicate
- Monitor for evidence of allergic reactions; withhold dose and notify prescriber
- Assess for paradoxical bronchospasm: dyspnea, wheezing, keep emergency resuscitative equipment nearby
- Assess for labor: maternal heart rate, B/P, contractions, fetal heart rate

Nursing diagnoses

✓ Airway clearance, ineffective (uses)

✓ Impaired gas exchange (uses)

T

✓ Knowledge deficit (teaching)
✓ Noncompliance (teaching)

Implementation

Aerosol route

- Give after shaking; ask patient to exhale, place mouthpiece in mouth, then inhale slowly; hold breath, remove, exhale slowly; allow at least 1 min between inhalations
- Store in light-resistant container, do not expose to temp over 86° F (30° C)

PO route

- Give PO with meals to decrease gastric irritation; tab may be crushed and mixed with foods and fluids

IM route

- Do not give by IM route

SC route

- May give by SC route

IV **IV route**

- Give at 5 μg q10 min until contractions are stopped, use infusion pump for correct dose; after ½-1 hr with no contraction decrease dose by 5 μg; switch to PO dose when possible

Syringe compatibilities:
Doxapram

Y-site compatibilities:
Regular insulin

Additive compatibilities:
Aminophylline

Additive incompatibilities:
Bleomycin

Patient/family education

- Advise patient not to use OTC medications; extra stimulation may occur; to use this medication before other medications and allow at least 5 min between each to prevent overstimulation
- Teach patient how to use inhaler; to avoid getting aerosol in eyes because blurring may result; to wash inhaler in warm water qd and dry; to avoid smoking, smoke-filled rooms, persons with respiratory infections; review package insert with patient
- Teach patient that paradoxical bronchospasm may occur; to stop drug immediately and notify prescriber; to limit caffeine products such as chocolate, coffee, tea, and colas
- Instruct patient on administration of dose, not to use more than prescribed; serious side effects may occur; if taking PO regularly and dose is missed, take when remembered; space other doses on new time schedule

Evaluation

Positive therapeutic outcome

- Absence of dyspnea, wheezing after 1 hr
- Improved airway exchange
- Improved ABGs

Treatment of overdose:
Administer a β_2-adrenergic blocker

testosterone (℞)
(tess-toss'te-rone)
AndroGel

testosterone, long acting

testosterone enanthate
Delatestryl

testosterone cypionate
Depo-Testosterone

testosterone pellets
Testopel

testosterone transdermal
Androderm, Testoderm, Testoderm TTS, Testoderm with Adhesive

testosterone gel
AndroGel 1%

Func. class.: Androgenic anabolic steroid
Chem. class.: Halogenated testosterone derivative

Pregnancy category X
Controlled substance III

Action: Increases weight by building body tissue; increases potassium, phosphorus, chloride, nitrogen levels;

increases bone development; responsible for maintenance of secondary sex characteristics (male)

Therapeutic Outcome: Increased hormone levels in eunuchoidism, decreased tumor growth in female breast cancer, onset of male puberty

Uses: Female breast cancer, eunuchoidism, male climacteric, oligospermia, impotence, osteoporosis, weight loss in AIDS patients, vulvar dystrophies, low testosterone levels

Dosage and routes

Replacement

Adult: **IM** 25-50 mg 2-3 ×/wk (base or propionate) or 50-400 mg q2-4 wk (enanthate or cypionate); TD Testoderm 4-6 mg applied q24h; Androderm 5 mg applied q24h; once qd (gel)

Breast cancer

Adult: IM 50-100 mg 3 ×/wk (propionate) or 200-400 mg q2-4 wk (cypionate or enanthate)

Delayed male puberty

P ***Child >12 yr:*** IM up to 100 mg/mo for up to 6 mo

Available forms: *Enanthate:* inj 200 mg/ml; *cypionate:* inj 100, 200 mg/ml; pellets 75 mg; TD 2.5, 4, 5, 6 mg/24 hr; gel 1%

Adverse effects

CNS: Dizziness, headache, fatigue, tremors, paresthesias, flushing, sweating, anxiety, lability, insomnia, carpal tunnel syndrome

CV: Increased B/P

EENT: Conjunctival edema, nasal congestion

ENDO: Abnormal GTT

GI: Nausea, vomiting, constipation, weight gain, **cholestatic jaundice**

GU: Hematuria, amenorrhea, vaginitis, decreased libido, decreased breast size, clitoral hypertrophy, testicular atrophy

INTEG: Rash, acneiform lesions, oily hair and skin, flushing, sweating, acne vulgaris, alopecia, hirsutism

MS: Cramps, spasms

Contraindications: Severe renal disease, severe cardiac disease, severe hepatic disease, hypersensitivity, pregnancy **X,** lactation, genital bleeding (abnormal)

Precautions: Diabetes mellitus, CV disease, MI

Pharmacokinetics

Absorption	Well but slowly absorbed
Distribution	Crosses placenta
Metabolism	Liver
Excretion	Kidneys, breast milk
Half-life	8 days (cypionate) 10-100 min (base)

Pharmacodynamics

	IM (base)	IM (cypionate)	IM (enanthate)	IM (propionate)
Onset	Unknown	Unknown	Unknown	Unknown
Peak	Unknown	Unknown	Unknown	Unknown
Duration	1-3 days	2-4 wk	2-4 wk	1-3 days

Interactions

Individual drugs

ACTH: ↑ edema

Insulin: ↓ effects of insulin

Oxyphenbutazone: ↑ effects of oxyphenbutazone

Drug classifications

Adrenal steroids: ↑ edema

Anticoagulants: ↑ pro-time

Antidiabetics, oral: ↑ effects of oral antidiabetics

Lab test interferences

↑ Serum cholesterol, ↑ blood glucose, ↑ urine glucose

↓ Serum Ca, ↓ serum K, ↓ T_4, ↓ T_3, ↓ thyroid ^{131}I uptake test, ↓ urine 17-OHCS, ↓ 17-KS, ↓ PBI

T

NURSING CONSIDERATIONS

Assessment

- Monitor patient's weight daily; notify prescriber if weekly weight gain is >5 lb; assess I&O ratio; be alert for decreasing urinary output, increasing edema
- Monitor B/P q4h
- P Assess growth rate in adolescent because growth rate may be uneven (linear/bone growth) if used for extended periods
- Monitor electrolytes: potassium, sodium, chloride, calcium; cholesterol
- Monitor liver function studies: ALT, AST, bilirubin
- Assess edema, hypertension, cardiac symptoms, jaundice
- Assess mental status: affect, mood, behavioral changes, aggression
- Assess signs of masculinization in female: increased libido, deepening of voice, decreased breast tissue, enlarged clitoris, menstrual irregularities; male: gynecomastia, impotence, testicular atrophy
- Assess hypercalcemia: lethargy, polyuria, polydipsia, nausea, vomiting, constipation; drug may have to be decreased
- Assess hypoglycemia in diabetics because oral antidiabetic action is increased

Nursing diagnoses

- ✓ Infection, risk for (adverse reactions)
- ✓ Injury, risk for (adverse reactions)
- ✓ Knowledge deficit (teaching)

Implementation

- Administer diet with increased calories, protein; decreased sodium if edema occurs
- Administer supportive drug if anemia occurs
- Give titrated dose; use lowest effective dose
- Give IM deep into upper outer quadrant of gluteal muscle; route can be painful

Gel route

- Apply qd to clean, dry area on shoulders, upper arms, or abdomen

Patient/family education

- Inform patient that drug needs to be combined with complete health plan: diet, rest, exercise
- Caution patient to notify prescriber if therapeutic response decreases; not to discontinue this medication abruptly
- Inform women patients to report menstrual irregularities; about changes in sex characteristics
- Discuss that 1-3 mo course is necessary for response in breast cancer
- TD patches: testoderm to skin of scrotum, Androderm to skin of back, upper arms, thighs, abdomen; area must be dry and free of hair; may be reapplied after bathing, swimming

Evaluation

Positive therapeutic outcome

- Decrease size of tumor in breast cancer
- Increased androgen levels

tetracycline (℞)

(tet-ra-sye'kleen)

Achromycin V, Alatel, Apo-Tetra ♣, Novotetra ♣, Nu-Tetra ♣, Panmycin, Robitet, Sumycin, Teline, Tetracap, tetracycline HCl, Tetracyn, Tetralan, Tetralean ♣, Tetram

Func. class.: Broad-spectrum antiinfective

Chem. class.: Tetracycline

Pregnancy category D

Action: Inhibits protein synthesis and phosphorylation in microorganisms; bacteriostatic

➔ **Therapeutic Outcome:** Bactericidal action against susceptible organisms: gram-positive pathogens *Bacillus antracis, Clostridium* *perfringens, Clostridium tetani, Listeria monocytogenes, Nocardia, Propionibacterium acnes, Actinomyces isrealii;* gram-negative pathogens *Haemophilus influenzae, Legionella pneumophila, Yersinia entercolitica, Yersinia pestis, Neisseria gonorrhoeae, Neisseria meningitidis*

Uses: Syphilis, *Chlamydia trachomatis,* gonorrhea, lymphogranuloma venereum, uncommon gram-positive, gram-negative organisms, rickettsial infections

Dosage and routes

Adult: PO 250-500 mg q6h

P ***Child >8 yr:*** PO 25-50 mg/kg/day in divided doses q6h

Gonorrhea

Adult: PO 1.5 g, then 500 mg qid for a total of 9 g over 7 days

Chlamydia trachomatis

Adult: PO 500 mg qid × 7 days

Syphilis

Adult: PO 2-3 g in divided doses × 10-15 days; if syphilis duration >1 yr, must treat 30 days

Brucellosis

Adult: PO 500 mg qid × 3 wk with 1 g of streptomycin IM 2 ×/day × 1 wk, and 1 ×/day the 2nd wk

Urethral syndrome in women

Adult: PO 500 mg qid × 7 days

Acne

Adult: 1 g/day in divided doses; maintenance 125-500 mg/day

Available forms: Oral susp 125 mg/5 ml, caps 100, 200, 500 mg; tabs 100, 250, 500 mg

Adverse effects

CNS: Fever, headache, paresthesia
CV: **Pericarditis**
EENT: Dysphagia, glossitis, decreased calcification (permanent discoloration) of deciduous teeth, oral candidiasis
GI: *Nausea,* abdominal pain, *vomiting, diarrhea,* anorexia, enterocolitis, **hepatotoxicity,** flatulence, abdominal cramps, epigastric burning, stomatitis
GU: *Increased BUN*
HEMA: **Eosinophilia, neutropenia, thrombocytopenia, leukocytosis, hemolytic anemia**
INTEG: *Rash, urticaria, photosensitivity, increased pigmentation,* **exfoliative dermatitis,** pruritus, **angioedema**

Contraindications: Hypersensitivity to tetracyclines, P children <8 yr, pregnancy **D**, lactation

Precautions: Renal disease, hepatic disease

Pharmacokinetics

Absorption	60%-80% (PO), lower (IM)
Distribution	Widely distributed, some in CSF; crosses placenta
Metabolism	Not metabolized
Excretion	Unchanged—kidneys
Half-life	6-10 hr

Pharmacodynamics

Onset	1-2 hr
Peak	2-3 hr

Interactions

Individual drugs

Calcium: Forms chelates, ↓ absorption
Carbamazepine: ↑ effect of carbamazepine
Cholestyramine: ↓ absorption of tetracycline
Colestipol: ↓ absorption of tetracycline
Iron: Forms chelates, ↓ absorption
Magnesium: Forms chelates, ↓ absorption
Phenytoin: ↓ effect of tetracycline
Sucralfate: Prevents absorption of tetracycline

Drug classifications

Anticoagulants, oral: ↑ effect of anticoagulants
Barbiturates: ↓ effect of tetracycline

Oral contraceptives: ↓ effect of oral contraception

Food/drug

↓ Absorption with dairy products; forms insoluble chelate

Herb/drug

Dong Quai: ↑ photosensitivity

Lab test interferences

False: ↑ Urinary catecholamines

False negative: Urine glucose with Clinistix, Tes-Tape

NURSING CONSIDERATIONS

Assessment

- Assess patient for previous sensitivity reaction
- Assess patient for signs and symptoms of infection including characteristics of wounds, sputum, urine, stool, WBC >10,000/mm^3, temp; obtain baseline information before and during treatment
- Complete C&S testing before beginning drug therapy to identify if correct treatment has been initiated
- Assess for allergic reactions: rash, urticaria, pruritus, chills, fever, joint pain; angioedema may occur a few days after therapy begins; epinephrine, resuscitation equipment should be available for anaphylactic reaction
- Identify urine output; if decreasing, notify prescriber (may indicate nephrotoxicity); also, increased BUN, creatinine
- Monitor blood studies: AST, ALT, CBC, Hct, bilirubin, LDH, alkaline phosphatase, monthly if patient is on long-term therapy
- Assess bowel pattern qd; if severe diarrhea occurs, drug should be discontinued
- Monitor for bleeding: ecchymosis, bleeding gums, hematuria, stool guaiac daily if on long-term therapy; blood dyscrasias may occur
- Assess for overgrowth of infection: perineal itching, fever, malaise, redness, pain, swelling, drainage, rash, diarrhea, change in cough, sputum

Nursing diagnoses

- ✓ Infection, risk for (uses)
- ✓ Diarrhea (adverse reactions)
- ✓ Injury, risk for (adverse reactions)
- ✓ Knowledge deficit (teaching)
- ✓ Noncompliance (teaching)

Implementation

PO route

- Give around the clock to maintain proper blood levels; give with food to increase absorption of drug; do not give within 3 hr of other agents; drug actions may occur; take on an empty stomach
- Give with 8 oz of water
- Shake liq preparation well before giving; use calibrated device for proper dosing

Patient/family education

- Teach patient to report sore throat, bruising, bleeding, joint pain; may indicate blood dyscrasias (rare)
- Advise patient to use sunscreen when outdoors to decrease photosensitivity reaction
- Advise patient to contact prescriber if vaginal itching; loose, foul-smelling stools, furry tongue occur; may indicate superinfection; report itching, rash, pruritus, urticaria
- Instruct patient to take all medication prescribed for the length of time ordered; drug must be taken around the clock to maintain blood levels; do not give medication to others

Evaluation

Positive therapeutic outcome

- Absence of signs/symptoms of infection (WBC <10,000/mm^3, temp WNL, absence of red, draining wounds)
- Reported improvement in symptoms of infection

theophylline (℞)

(thee-off'i-lin)

Accurbron, Aquaphyllin, Asmalix, Bronkodyl, Elixomin, Elixophyllin, Lanophyllin, Quibron-T Dividose, Quibron-T/SR, Respbid, Slo-bid Gyrocaps, Slo-Phyllin, Sustaire, Theo-24, Theobid Duracaps, Theochron, Theoclear-80, Theoclear L.A., Theo-Dur, Theolair-SR,Theo-Sav, Theospan-SR, Theostat 80, Theovent, Theo-X, T-Phy, Uni-Dur, Uniphyl

Func. class.: Spasmolytic, bronchodilator

Chem. class.: Xanthine, ethylenediamine

Pregnancy category C

Action: Relaxes smooth muscle of respiratory system by blocking phosphodiesterase, which increases cAMP, which increases bronchodilation, diuresis, circulation, CNS stimulation

Therapeutic Outcome: Ability to breathe without difficulty

Uses: Bronchial asthma, bronchospasm of COPD, chronic bronchitis

Dosage and routes

Bronchospasm, bronchial asthma

Adult: PO 100-200 mg q6h; dosage must be individualized; rec 250-500 mg q9-12h

P ***Child:*** PO 50-100 mg q6h, max 12 mg/kg/24 hr

COPD, chronic bronchitis

Adult: PO 30-660 q6-8h pc (sodium glycinate)

P ***Child 1-9 yr:*** PO 5 mg/kg loading dose, then 4 mg/kg q6h

P ***Child 9-16 yr:*** PO 5 mg/kg loading dose, then 3 mg/kg q6h

Apnea of prematurity

P ***Neonate:*** 2-10 mg/kg/day divided q8-12h (usual loading dose is 4 mg/kg)

Available forms: Caps 50, 100, 200, 250 mg; tabs 100, 125, 200, 225, 250, 300 mg; time rel tabs 100, 200, 250, 300, 400, 500 mg; time rel caps 50, 65, 100, 125, 130, 200, 250, 260, 300, 400, 500 mg; elixir 80, 11.25 mg/15 mg; sol 80 mg/15 ml; liq 80, 150, 160 mg/15 ml; susp 300 mg/15 ml

Adverse effects

CNS: *Anxiety, restlessness, insomnia, dizziness, seizures,* headache, light-headedness, muscle twitching, tremors

CV: *Palpitations, sinus tachycardia,* hypotension, other dysrhythmias, fluid retention with tachycardia

ENDO: Hyperglycemia

GI: *Nausea, vomiting, anorexia,* diarrhea, bitter taste, dyspepsia, gastric distress

INTEG: Flushing, urticaria

RESP: Increased rate

Contraindications: Hypersensitivity to xanthines, tachydysrhythmias

G **Precautions:** Elderly, CHF, cor pulmonale, hepatic disease, active peptic ulcer disease, diabetes mellitus, hyperthyroidism, hypertension,
P children, pregnancy **C**

Pharmacokinetics

Absorption	Well absorbed (PO), slowly absorbed (ext rel)
Distribution	Crosses placenta, widely distributed
Metabolism	Liver
Excretion	Kidneys, breast milk
Half-life	3-13, increased in liver disease, CHF, elderly

Pharmacodynamics

	PO	POTIME REL	IV
Onset	Rapid	Slow	Immediate
Peak	1 hr	4-8 hr	Inf end
Duration	6 hr	12-24 hr	6-8 hr

T

Interactions

Individual drugs

Carbamazepine: ↓ theophylline level
Cimetidine: ↑ action of theophylline
Ciprofloxacin: ↑ theophylline action
Erythromycin: ↑ action of theophylline
Lithium: ↓ effect of lithium
Phenobarbital: ↓ theophylline
Phenytoin: ↓ theophylline
Propranolol: ↑ action of theophylline
Rifampin: ↓ theophylline

Drug classifications

β-Adrenergic blockers: cardiotoxicity
Oral contraceptives: ↑ theophylline action

Herb/drug

Ma Huang: ↑ toxicity

NURSING CONSIDERATIONS

Assessment

- Monitor theophylline blood levels (therapeutic level is 5-15 μg/ml); toxicity may occur with small increase above 15 μg/ml
- Monitor I&O; diuresis occurs; dehydration may result in elderly or children
- Assess for signs of toxicity: irritability, insomnia, restlessness, tremors, nausea, vomiting
- Monitor respiratory rate, rhythm, depth; auscultate lung fields bilaterally; notify prescriber of abnormalities
- Assess for allergic reactions: rash, urticaria; if these occur, drug should be discontinued

Nursing diagnoses

✓ Airway clearance, ineffective (uses)
✓ Knowledge deficit (teaching)

Implementation

PO route

- Give PO pc to decrease GI symptoms; absorption may be affected

IV route

Y-site compatibilities:

Acyclovir, ampicillin, aztreonam, cefazolin, cefotetan, ceftazidime, ceftriaxone, cimetidine, clindamycin, dexamethasone, diltiazem, dobutamine, dopamine, doxycycline, erythromycin, famotidine, fluconazole, gentamicin, haloperidol, heparin, hydrocortisone, lidocaine, methyldopate, methylprednisolone, metronidazole, midazolam, nafcillin, nitroglycerin, nitroprusside, penicillin G potassium, piperacillin, potassium chloride, ranitidine, ticarcillin, ticarcillin/clavulanate, tobramycin, vancomycin

Additive compatibilities:

Cefepime, chlorpromazine, fluconazole, methylprednisolone, verapamil

Patient/family education

- Advise patient to check OTC medications, current prescription medications for ephedrine, which will increase stimulation, and to avoid alcohol, caffeine
- Caution patient to avoid hazardous activities; dizziness may occur
- Inform patient that if GI upset occurs, to take drug with 8 oz of water; avoid food; absorption may be decreased
- Teach patient not to crush, dissolve, or chew slow-release products
- Teach patient that contents of bead-filled cap may be sprinkled over food for children's use
- Advise patient to notify prescriber of toxicity: nausea, vomiting, anxiety, insomnia, convulsions
- Advise patient to notify prescriber of change in smoking habit; dosage may have to be changed

Evaluation

Positive therapeutic outcome

- Ability to breathe more easily

thiamine (vitamin B_1) (PO, OTC; IV ℞)

Betaxin ✱, Betalin S, Biamine, Revitonus, Thiamilate, thiamine HCl, vitamin B_1

Func. class.: Vitamin B_1

Chem. class.: Water soluble

Pregnancy category A

Action: Needed for pyruvate metabolism, carbohydrate metabolism

Therapeutic Outcome: Prevention and treatment of thiamine deficiency

Uses: Vit B_1 deficiency or polyneuritis, cheilosis adjunct with thiamine beriberi, Wernicke-Korsakoff syndrome, pellagra, metabolic disorders

Dosage and routes

RDA

Adult: Male 1.2-1.5 mg; females 1.1 mg; pregnancy 1.5 mg; lactation 1.6 mg

P ***Child 7-10 yr:*** 1.3 mg

P ***Child 4-6 yr:*** 0.9 mg

P ***Child 1-3 yr:*** 0.7 mg

P ***Infants 6 mo-1 yr:*** 0.4 mg

P ***Neonates and infants to 6 mo:*** 0.3 mg

Beriberi

Adult: IM 10-20 mg tid × 2 wk, then 5-10 mg qd × 1 mo

Beriberi with cardiac failure

P ***Adult and child:*** **IV** 10-30 mg tid

Available forms: Tabs 50, 100, 250, 500 mg; inj 100 mg/ml; enteric-coated tabs 20 mg

Adverse effects

CNS: Weakness, restlessness

CV: **Collapse, pulmonary edema,** hypotension

EENT: Tightness of throat

GI: Hemorrhage, *nausea, diarrhea*

INTEG: **Angioneurotic edema,** cyanosis, sweating, warmth

SYST: **Anaphylaxis**

Contraindications: Hypersensitivity

Precautions: Pregnancy **A**

Do Not Confuse:
thiamine/Tenormin

Pharmacokinetics

Absorption	Well absorbed (PO, IM), completely absorbed (**IV**)
Distribution	Widely distributed
Metabolism	Liver
Excretion	Kidneys (unchanged—excess amounts)
Half-life	Unknown

Pharmacodynamics

Unknown

Interactions

Drug classifications

Neuromuscular blockers: ↑ effect

NURSING CONSIDERATIONS

Assessment

- Monitor thiamine levels throughout treatment
- Assess nutritional status: yeast, beef, liver, whole or enriched grains, legumes

Nursing diagnoses

- ✓ Nutrition: less than body requirements (uses)
- ✓ Knowledge deficit (teaching)

Implementation

IV route

- **IV** undiluted given over 5 min or diluted with **IV** sol and given as an inf at a rate of 100 mg or less/5 min or more

Syringe compatibilities: Doxapram

Y-site compatibilities: Famotidine

Additive incompatibilities: Barbiturates; sol with neutral or alkaline pH, such as carbonates, bicarbonates, citrates and acetates;

T

erythromycin, kanamycin, or streptomycin

IM route

- Give by IM inj; rotate sites if pain and inflammation occur; do not mix with alkaline sol; Z-track to minimize pain
- Application of cold may decrease pain
- Store in airtight, light-resistant container

Patient/family education

- Teach patient necessary foods to be included in diet: yeast, beef, liver, legumes, whole grains

Evaluation

Positive therapeutic outcome

- Absence of nausea, vomiting, anorexia, insomnia, tachycardia, paresthesias, depression, muscle weakness

thiethylperazine (℞)

(thye-eth-il-per′a-zeen)

Norzine, Torecan

Func. class.: Antiemetic

Chem. class.: Phenothiazine, piperazine derivative

Pregnancy category X

Action: Acts centrally by blocking chemoreceptor trigger zone, which in turn acts on vomiting center

Therapeutic Outcome: Control of nausea, vomiting

Uses: Nausea, vomiting

Dosage and routes

Adult: PO/IM 10 mg/qd-tid

Available forms: Tabs 10 mg; inj 5 mg/ml

Adverse effects

CNS: *Euphoria, depression,* restlessness, tremor, EPS, **seizures,** drowsiness, confusion

CV: **Circulatory failure, tachycardia,** postural hypotension, ECG changes

GI: Nausea, vomiting, anorexia, dry mouth, diarrhea, constipation, weight loss, metallic taste, cramps

GU: Urinary retention, dark urine

RESP: **Respiratory depression**

Contraindications: Hypersensitivity to phenothiazines, coma, seizure, encephalopathy, bone marrow depression, pregnancy **X**

Precautions: Children <2 yr, elderly

Do Not Confuse: Torecan/Toradol

Pharmacokinetics

Absorption	Readily absorbed
Distribution	Crosses placenta
Metabolism	Liver
Excretion	Kidneys, breast milk
Half-life	Unknown

Pharmacodynamics

	PO	IM
Onset	45-60 min	Unknown
Peak	Unknown	Unknown
Duration	4 hr	Unknown

Interactions

Drug classifications

Antacids: ↓ absorption

Anticholinergics: ↑ anticholinergic effects

Antidepressants: ↑ CNS depression

Antidiarrheals, adsorbent: ↓ absorption

Antihistamines: ↑ CNS depression

Antihypertensives: ↑ hypotension

Antithyroid agents: ↑ agranulocytosis

Barbiturate anesthetics: ↑ CNS depression

β-Adrenergic blockers: ↑ effects of both drugs

General anesthetics: ↑ CNS depression

MAOIs: ↑ CNS depression

Opiates: ↑ CNS depression

Sedative/hypnotics: ↑ CNS depression

NURSING CONSIDERATIONS
Assessment
- Monitor I&O ratio, palpate bladder if low urinary output occurs, especially G in elderly; urinalysis recommended before, during prolonged therapy
- Monitor bilirubin, CBC, liver function studies monthly
- Assess affect, orientation, LOC, reflexes, gait, coordination, sleep pattern disturbances
- Monitor B/P with patient in sitting, standing, and lying positions; take pulse and respirations q4h during initial treatment; establish baseline before starting treatment; report drops of 30 mm Hg
- Check for dizziness, faintness, palpitations, tachycardia on rising; severe orthostatic hypotension is common
- ❗ Identify for neuroleptic malignant syndrome: hyperpyrexia, muscle rigidity, increased CPK, altered mental status; drug should be discontinued
- Assess for EPS including akathisia (inability to sit still, no pattern to movements), tardive dyskinesia (bizarre movements of the jaw, mouth, tongue, extremities), pseudoparkinsonism (tremors, pill rolling, shuffling gait); antiparkinsonian drug should be prescribed
- Assess for constipation, urinary retention daily; if these occur, increase bulk, water in diet

Nursing diagnoses
- ✓ Thought processes, altered (uses)
- ✓ Coping, ineffective individual (uses)
- ✓ Knowledge deficit (teaching)
- ✓ Noncompliance (teaching)

Implementation
IM route
- Give IM inj in large muscle mass; aspirate to avoid **IV** administration; give slowly; have patient remain supine for 1 hr after administration

Syringe compatibilities:
Butorphanol, hydromorphone, midazolam, ranitidine

Y-site compatibilities:
Aldesleukin

Patient/family education
- Teach patient to use good oral hygiene; frequent rinsing of mouth, sugarless gum for dry mouth
- Caution patient to avoid hazardous activities until drug response is determined; dizziness, blurred vision may occur
- Inform patient that orthostatic hypotension occurs often and to rise from sitting or lying position gradually
- Instruct patient to remain lying down after IM inj for at least 30 min
- Advise patient to avoid hot tubs, hot showers, tub baths, since hypotension may occur
- Inform patient that heat stroke may occur in hot weather, and to take extra precautions to stay cool
- Teach patient to avoid OTC preparations (cough, hay fever, cold) unless approved by prescriber because serious drug interactions may occur; avoid use with alcohol, CNS depressants because increased drowsiness may occur
- Inform patient to use sunglasses and sunscreen to prevent burns
- Teach patient about EPS
- Instruct patient to report sore throat, malaise, fever, bleeding, mouth sores; if these occur, CBC should be performed and drug discontinued

Evaluation
Positive therapeutic outcome
- Absence of nausea, vomiting

thioguanine (6-TG) (℞)

(thye-oh-gwah'neen)

thioguanine, Lanvis ✦

Func. class.: Antineoplastic-antimetabolite

Chem. class.: Purine analog

Pregnancy category D

Action: Interferes with synthesis, utilization of purine nucleotides; specific for S phase of cell cycle

➔ **Therapeutic Outcome:** Prevention of rapidly growing malignant cells

Uses: Acute leukemias, chronic granulocytic leukemia, lymphomas, multiple myeloma, solid tumors

Dosage and routes

P ***Adult and child:*** PO 2 mg/kg/day, then increase slowly to 3 mg/kg/day after 4 wk

Available forms: Tabs 40 mg

Adverse effects

GI: *Nausea, vomiting, anorexia, diarrhea, stomatitis,* **hepatotoxicity,** gastritis, jaundice

GU: **Renal failure,** hyperuricemia, oliguria

HEMA: **Thrombocytopenia, leukopenia, myelosuppression, anemia**

INTEG: *Rash,* dermatitis, dry skin

Contraindications: Prior drug resistance, leukopenia (WBC 2500/mm^3), thrombocytopenia (platelets <100,000/mm^3), anemia, pregnancy **D**

Precautions: Liver disease

Pharmacokinetics

Absorption	Variably absorbed, 30%
Distribution	Crosses placenta
Metabolism	Liver—extensively
Excretion	Kidneys
Half-life	11 hr

Pharmacodynamics

Unknown

Interactions

Individual drugs

Radiation: ↑ toxicity, bone marrow suppression

Drug classifications

Antineoplastics: ↑ toxicity, bone marrow suppression

Lab test interferences

↑ Uric acid (blood, urine)

NURSING CONSIDERATIONS

Assessment

- Assess buccal cavity q8h for dryness, sores or ulceration, white patches, oral pain, bleeding, dysphagia; obtain prescription for viscous lidocaine (Xylocaine)
- ◆ Assess symptoms indicating severe allergic reaction: rash, pruritus, urticaria, purpuric skin lesions, itching, flushing
- Monitor CBC, differential, platelet count weekly; withhold drug if WBC is <4000/mm^3 or platelet count is <100,000/mm^3, notify prescriber of results if WBC <20,000/mm^3, platelets </50,000/mm^3
- Assess for increased uric acid levels, swelling, joint pain (primarily in extremities); patient should be well hydrated to prevent urate deposits
- Monitor renal function studies: BUN, creatinine, serum uric acid, urine CrCl before and during therapy; I&O ratio; report fall in urine output to <30 ml/hr
- Monitor temp q4h (may indicate beginning of infection)
- Monitor liver function tests before and during therapy (bilirubin, AST, ALT, LDH) as needed or monthly; jaundice, sclera, dark urine, clay-colored stools, itchy skin, abdominal pain, fever, diarrhea
- Assess for bleeding: hematuria, stool guaiac, bruising or petechiae, mucosa or orifices q8h; inflammation of mucosa, breaks in skin
- Identify edema in feet, joint pain, stomach pain, shaking; prescriber should be notified

Nursing diagnoses

- ✓ Injury, risk for (adverse reactions)
- ✓ Body image disturbance (adverse reactions)
- ✓ Infection, risk for (adverse reactions)
- ✓ Knowledge deficit (teaching)

Implementation

- Avoid contact with skin (very irritating), wash completely to remove
- Give fluids **IV** or PO before chemotherapy to hydrate patient
- Give antiemetic 30-60 min before giving drug to prevent vomiting, and prn; antibiotics for prophylaxis of infection
- Give top or systemic analgesics for pain
- Provide liq diet: carbonated beverages; gelatin may be added if patient is not nauseated or vomiting
- Provide rinsing of mouth tid-qid with water, club soda; brushing of teeth bid-qid with soft brush or cotton-tipped applicators for stomatitis; use unwaxed dental floss
- Give 1 hr ac or 2 hr pc to prevent vomiting

Patient/family education

- Inform patient that contraceptive measures are recommended during therapy
- Caution patient to avoid use of products containing aspirin or NSAIDs, razors, commercial mouthwash, bleeding may occur; to report symptoms of bleeding (hematuria, tarry stools)
- Advise patient to report signs of anemia (fatigue, headache, irritability, faintness, shortness of breath)
- Caution patient not to have any vaccinations without advice of prescriber; serious reactions can occur

Evaluation

Positive therapeutic outcome

- Prevention of rapid division of malignant cells

thioridazine (℞)

(thye-or-rid'a-zeen)

Apo-Thioridazine ✦, Mellaril, Mellaril Concentrate, Mellaril-5, Novo-Ridazine ✦, PMS-Thioridazine ✦, thioridazine HCl

Func. class.: Antipsychotic/neuroleptic

Chem. class.: Phenothiazine, piperidine

Pregnancy category C

Action: Depresses cerebral cortex, hypothalamus, limbic system, which control activity, aggression; blocks neurotransmission produced by dopamine at synapse; exhibits strong α-adrenergic, anticholinergic blocking action; mechanism for antipsychotic effects is unclear

➔ **Therapeutic Outcome:** Decreased signs and symptoms of psychosis

Uses: Psychotic disorders, schizophrenia, behavioral problems in children, alcohol withdrawal as adjunct, anxiety, major depressive disorders, organic brain syndrome

Dosage and routes

Psychosis

Adult: PO 25-100 mg tid, max dose 800 mg/day; dose is gradually increased to desired response, then reduced to minimum maintenance

Depression/behavioral problems/organic brain syndrome

Adult: PO 25 tid, range from 10 mg bid-qid to 50 mg tid-qid

G ***Geriatric:*** PO 10-25 mg qd-bid, increase 4-7 days by 10-25 mg to desired dose

P ***Child 2-12 yr:*** PO 0.5-3 mg/kg/day in divided doses

Available forms: Tabs 10, 15, 25, 50, 100, 150, 200 mg; conc 30,

T

100 mg/ml; susp 25, 100 mg/5 ml; syrup 10 mg/15 ml

Adverse effects

CNS: *EPS (rare) (pseudoparkinsonism, akathisia, dystonia, tardive dyskinesia),* **seizures,** *headache,* confusion, **neuroleptic malignant syndrome**
CV: Orthostatic hypotension, **cardiac arrest,** ECG changes, **tachycardia**
EENT: Blurred vision, glaucoma, dry eyes
GI: *Dry mouth, nausea, vomiting, anorexia, constipation,* diarrhea, jaundice, weight gain
GU: Urinary retention, urinary frequency, enuresis, impotence, amenorrhea, gynecomastia
HEMA: Anemia, **leukopenia, leukocytosis, agranulocytosis**
INTEG: *Rash,* photosensitivity, dermatitis
RESP: **Laryngospasm,** dyspnea, **respiratory depression**

Contraindications: Hypersensitivity, blood dyscrasias, coma, P child <2 yr, brain damage, bone marrow depression

Precautions: Pregnancy **C,** lactation, seizure disorders, hypertension, hepatic disease, cardiac disease

Do Not Confuse:

Mellaril/Elavil

Pharmacokinetics

Absorption	Variably absorbed (tab)
Distribution	Widely distributed, high concentrations in CNS, crosses placenta
Metabolism	Liver, extensively, GI mucosa
Excretion	Kidneys, breast milk
Half-life	26-36 hr

Pharmacodynamics

Onset	Erratic
Peak	2-4 hr
Duration	8-12 hr

Interactions

Individual drugs

Alcohol: ↑ effects of both drugs, oversedation
Aluminum hydroxide: ↓ absorption
Bromocriptine: ↓ antiparkinson activity
Disopyramide: ↑ anticholinergic effects
Epinephrine: ↑ toxicity
Guanethidine: ↓ antihypertensive response
Levodopa: ↓ antiparkinson activity
Lithium: ↓ thioridazine levels, ↑ EPS, masking of lithium toxicity
Magnesium hydroxide: ↓ absorption
Norepinephrine: ↓ vasoresponse, ↑ toxicity
Phenobarbital: ↓ effectiveness, ↑ metabolism

Drug classifications

Antacids: ↓ absorption
Anticholinergics: ↑ anticholinergic effects
Antidepressants: ↑ CNS depression
Antidiarrheals, adsorbent: ↓ absorption
Antihistamines: ↑ CNS depression
Antihypertensives: ↑ hypotension
Antithyroid agents: ↑ agranulocytosis
Barbiturate anesthetics: ↑ CNS depression
β-Adrenergic blockers: ↑ effects of both drugs
General anesthetics: ↑ CNS depression
MAOIs: ↑ CNS depression
Opiates: ↑ CNS depression
Sedative/hypnotics: ↑ CNS depression

Herb/drug

Kava: ↑ CNS depression

Lab test interferences

↑ LFTs, ↑ cardiac enzymes, ↑ cholesterol, ↑ blood glucose, ↑ prolactin, ↑ bilirubin, ↑ PBI, ↑ cholinesterase, ↑ ^{131}I, ↑ alkaline phosphatase,

↑ leukocytes, ↑ granulocytes, ↑ platelets
↓ Hormones (blood and urine)
False positive: Pregnancy tests, PKU, urine bilirubin
False negative: Urinary steroids, 17-OHCS

NURSING CONSIDERATIONS
Assessment

- Assess mental status: orientation, mood, behavior, presence of hallucinations, and type before initial administration and monthly; this drug should significantly reduce psychotic behavior
- Check for swallowing of PO medication; check for hoarding or giving of medication to other patients
- Monitor I&O ratio, palpate bladder if low urinary output occurs, especially in elderly; urinalysis recommended before, during prolonged therapy (G)
- Monitor bilirubin, CBC, liver function studies monthly
- Assess affect, orientation, LOC, reflexes, gait, coordination, sleep pattern disturbances
- Monitor B/P sitting, standing, and lying, take pulse and respirations q4h during initial treatment; establish baseline before starting treatment; report drops of 30 mm Hg; obtain baseline ECG, monitor Q- and T-wave changes
- Check for dizziness, faintness, palpitations, tachycardia on rising; severe orthostatic hypotension is common
- (!) Identify for neuroleptic malignant syndrome: hyperpyrexia, muscle rigidity, increased CPK, altered mental status; drug should be discontinued
- Assess for EPS including akathisia (inability to sit still, no pattern to movements), tardive dyskinesia (bizarre movements of the jaw, mouth, tongue, extremities), pseudoparkinsonism (ragged tremors, pill rolling, shuffling gate); an antiparkinsonian drug should be prescribed
- Assess for constipation, urinary retention daily; if these occur, increase bulk, water in diet

Nursing diagnoses

- ✓ Thought processes, altered (uses)
- ✓ Coping, ineffective individual (uses)
- ✓ Knowledge deficit (teaching)
- ✓ Noncompliance (teaching)

Implementation

- Administer drug in liq form mixed in glass of juice or cola if hoarding is suspected; do not mix in caffeine drinks, tannics, pectins
- (G) Decrease dose in elderly because metabolism is slowed
- Administer PO with full glass of water, milk; or give with food to decrease GI upset
- Store in airtight, light-resistant container, oral sol in amber bottle

Patient/family education

- Teach patient to use good oral hygiene; frequent rinsing of mouth, sugarless gum for dry mouth
- Advise patient to avoid hazardous activities until drug response is determined; dizziness, blurred vision are common
- Inform patient that orthostatic hypotension occurs often and to rise from sitting or lying position gradually; to avoid hot tubs, hot showers, tub baths because hypotension may occur
- Instruct patient that in hot weather, heat stroke may occur; take extra precautions to stay cool
- Caution patient to avoid abrupt withdrawal of this drug, or EPS may result; drug should be withdrawn slowly
- Teach patient to avoid OTC preparations (cough, hay fever, cold) unless approved by prescriber; serious drug interactions may occur; avoid use with alcohol, CNS depressants; increased drowsiness may occur
- Advise patient to use sunglasses and sunscreen to prevent burns
- Teach patient about EPS and necessity for meticulous oral hygiene because oral candidiasis may occur

T

- Advise patient to take antacids 2 hr before or after this drug
- Instruct patient to report sore throat, malaise, fever, bleeding, mouth sores; if these occur, CBC should be performed and drug discontinued

Evaluation
Positive therapeutic outcome
- Decrease in emotional excitement, hallucinations, delusions, paranoia
- Reorganization of patterns of thought, speech

Treatment of overdose:
Lavage if orally ingested; provide airway; *do not induce vomiting or use epinephrine,* CV monitoring, continuous ECG

thiotepa (℞)
(thye-oh-tep'a)
Thioplex
Func. class.: Antineoplastic
Chem. class.: Alkylating agent
Pregnancy category D

Action: Responsible for cross-linking DNA strands leading to cell death; activity is not cell cycle–specific

Therapeutic Outcome: Prevention of rapidly growing malignant cells

Uses: Hodgkin's disease, lymphomas; breast, ovarian, lung, bladder cancer; neoplastic effusions

Dosage and routes
Adult: **IV** 0.3-0.4 mg/kg at 1-4 wk intervals

Neoplastic effusions
Adult: Intracavity 0.6-0.8 mg/kg

Bladder cancer
Adult: Instill 60 mg/30-60 ml water for inj in bladder for 2 hr once weekly × 4 wk

Available forms: Powder for inj 15 mg

Adverse effects
CNS: Dizziness, headache
GI: *Nausea, vomiting, anorexia*
GU: *Hyperuricemia,* **hematuria, amenorrhea, azoospermia**
HEMA: **Thrombocytopenia, leukopenia, pancytopenia**
INTEG: Rash, pruritus

Contraindications: Hypersensitivity, pregnancy **D**

Precautions: Radiation therapy, bone marrow suppression, impaired renal or hepatic function

Pharmacokinetics

Absorption	Variably absorbed
Distribution	Unknown
Metabolism	Liver—extensively
Excretion	Kidneys
Half-life	Unknown

Pharmacodynamics
Unknown

Interactions
Individual drugs
Radiation: ↑ toxicity, bone marrow suppression
Succinylcholine: ↑ apnea
Drug classifications
Antineoplastics: ↑ toxicity, bone marrow suppression

NURSING CONSIDERATIONS
Assessment
- ❗ Assess symptoms indicating severe allergic reaction: rash, pruritus, urticaria, itching, flushing
- Monitor CBC, differential, platelet count weekly; withhold drug if WBC is <4000/mm^3 or platelet count is <100,000/mm^3; notify prescriber of results if WBC <20,000/mm^3, platelets <150,000/mm^3
- Monitor renal function studies: BUN, creatinine, serum uric acid, urine CrCl before and during therapy; I&O ratio; report fall in urine output to <30 ml/hr
- Monitor temp q4h (may indicate beginning of infection)
- Monitor liver function tests (biliru-

bin, AST, ALT, LDH) before and during therapy as needed or monthly; jaundice, sclera, dark urine, clay-colored stools, itchy skin, abdominal pain, fever, diarrhea

- Assess for bleeding: hematuria, stool guaiac, bruising or petechiae, mucosa or orifices q8h; inflammation of mucosa, breaks in skin
- Identify dyspnea, rales, unproductive cough, chest pain, tachypnea
- Identify effects of alopecia on body image; discuss feelings about body changes

Nursing diagnoses

✓ Injury, risk for (adverse reactions)
✓ Body image disturbance (adverse reactions)
✓ Infection, risk for (adverse reactions)
✓ Knowledge deficit (teaching)

Implementation

- Give fluids **IV** or PO before chemotherapy to hydrate patient
- Give antacid before oral agent, give drug after evening meal, before bedtime; antiemetic 30-60 min before drug to prevent vomiting, and prn; antibiotics for prophylaxis of infection
- Give top or systemic analgesics for pain
- Give liq diet: carbonated beverages; gelatin may be added if patient is not nauseated or vomiting
- Provide rinsing of mouth tid-qid with water, club soda; brushing of teeth bid-qid with soft brush or cotton-tipped applicators for stomatitis; use unwaxed dental floss

IV **IV route**

Direct route

- Give **IV** after diluting 15 mg/1.5 ml of sterile H_2O for inj; give over 1-3 min, use a 0.22 µ filter

Intermittent infusion

- May be further diluted in 50-100 ml of D_5W, 0.9% NaCl, Ringer's, LR

Syringe compatibilities:

Procaine HCl, (2%), epinephrine 1:1000

Y-site compatibilities:

Acyclovir, allopurinol, amifostine, amikacin, aminophylline, amphotericin B, ampicillin, ampicillin/sulbactam, aztreonam, bleomycin, bumetanide, buprenorphine, butorphanol, calcium gluconate, carboplatin, carmustine, cefazolin, cefepime, cefonicid, cefoperazone, cefotaxime, cefotetan, cefoxitin, ceftazidime, ceftizoxime, ceftriaxone, cefuroxime, chlorpromazine, cimetidine, ciprofloxacin, clindamycin, cyclophosphamide, cytarabine, dacarbazine, dactinomycin, daunorubicin, diphenhydramine, dobutamine, dopamine, doxorubicin, doxycycline, droperidol, enalaprilat, etoposide, famotidine, floxuridine, fluconazole, fludarabine, fluorouracil, furosemide, gallium, ganciclovir, gentamicin, granisetron, haloperidol, heparin, hydrocortisone, hydromorphone, hydroxyzine, idarubicin, ifosfamide, imipenem/cilastatin, leucovorin, lorazepam, magnesium sulfate, mannitol, melphalan, meperidine, mesna, methotrexate, methylprednisolone, metoclopramide, metronidazole, mezlocillin, miconazole, mitomycin, mitoxantrone, morphine, nalbuphine, netilmicin, ofloxacin, ondansetron, paclitaxel, piperacillin, piperacillin/tazobactam, plicamycin, potassium chloride, prochlorperazine, promethazine, ranitidine, sodium bicarbonate, streptozocin, teniposide, ticarcillin, ticarcillin/clavulanate, tobramycin, trimethoprim-sulfamethoxazole, vancomycin, vinblastine, vincristine, zidovudine

Instillation route

- Reconstitute sol, then mix 60 mg/30-60 ml of sterile water; instill by Foley catheter; patient's position may be changed every few min; the patient must retain sol for 2 hr to provide for cell death

Intracavity route

- Reconstitute sol and administer by effusion tube as directed

T

Patient/family education

- Caution patient to avoid use of products containing aspirin or NSAIDs, razors, commercial mouthwash because bleeding may occur; to report symptoms of bleeding (hematuria, tarry stools)
- Advise patient to report signs of anemia (fatigue, headache, irritability, faintness, shortness of breath)
- Advise patient to report any changes in breathing or coughing even several mo after treatment; to avoid crowds or persons with respiratory or other infections
- Inform patient that hair may be lost during treatment; a wig or hairpiece may make patient feel better; new hair may be different in color, texture
- Caution patient not to have any vaccinations without the advice of the prescriber because serious reactions can occur
- Advise patient that contraception is needed during treatment and for several mo after the completion of therapy

Evaluation

Positive therapeutic outcome

- Prevention of rapid division of malignant cells

thiothixene (℞)

(thye-oh-thix'een)

Navane, thiothixene

Func. class.: Antipsychotic/neuroleptic

Chem. class.: Thioxanthene

Pregnancy category C

Action: Depresses cerebral cortex, hypothalamus, limbic system, which control activity, aggression; blocks neurotransmission produced by dopamine at synapse; exhibits strong α-adrenergic blocking action; mechanism for antipsychotic effects is unclear

➔ **Therapeutic Outcome:** Decreased signs and symptoms of psychosis

Uses: Psychotic disorders, schizophrenia, acute agitation

Dosage and routes

Adult: PO 2-5 mg bid-qid depending on severity of con- dition; dose gradually increased to 15-30 mg if needed; IM 4 mg bid-qid; max dose 30 mg qd; administer PO dose as soon as possible

G ***Elderly:*** PO 1-2 mg qd-bid, increase by 1-2 mg q4-7 days to desired dose

Available forms: Caps 1, 2, 5, 10, 20 mg; conc 5 mg/ml; inj 2 mg/ml; powder for inj 5 mg/ml

Adverse effects

CNS: *EPS (pseudoparkinsonism, akathisia, dystonia, tardive dyskinesia),* seizures, *headache*

CV: *Orthostatic hypotension,* hypertension, **cardiac arrest,** ECG changes, **tachycardia**

EENT: Blurred vision, glaucoma

GI: *Dry mouth, nausea, vomiting, anorexia, constipation,* diarrhea, jaundice, weight gain

GU: Urinary retention, urinary frequency, enuresis, impotence, amenorrhea, gynecomastia

HEMA: Anemia, **leukopenia, leukocytosis, agranulocytosis**

INTEG: *Rash,* photosensitivity, dermatitis

RESP: **Laryngospasm,** dyspnea, **respiratory depression**

Contraindications: Hypersensitivity, blood dyscrasias, P child <12 yr, bone marrow depression, circulatory collapse, CNS depression, coma, alcoholism, CV disease, hepatic disease, Reye's syndrome, narrow-angle glaucoma

Precautions: Pregnancy **C,** lactation, seizure disorders, hypertension, hepatic disease, G elderly

Do Not Confuse:
Navane/Norvasc

Pharmacokinetics

Absorption	Well absorbed (PO, IM)
Distribution	Widely distributed, crosses placenta
Metabolism	Liver
Excretion	Kidneys, breast milk
Half-life	34 hr

Pharmacodynamics

	PO	IM
Onset	Slow	15-30 min
Peak	2-8 hr	1-6 hr
Duration	Up to 12 hr	Up to 12 hr

Interactions
Individual drugs
Alcohol: ↑ effects of both drugs, oversedation
Aluminum hydroxide: ↓ absorption
Bromocriptine: ↓ antiparkinson activity
Disopyramide: ↑ anticholinergic effects
Guanethidine: ↓ antihypertensive response
Levodopa: ↓ antiparkinson activity
Lithium: ↓ chlorpromazine levels, ↑ EPS, masking of lithium toxicity
Magnesium hydroxide: ↓ absorption
Norepinephrine: ↓ vasoresponse, ↑ toxicity
Phenobarbital: ↓ effectiveness, ↑ metabolism
Drug classifications
Antacids: ↓ absorption
Anticholinergics: ↑ anticholinergic effects
Antidepressants: ↑ CNS depression
Antidiarrheals, adsorbent: ↓ absorption
Antihistamines: ↑ CNS depression
Antihypertensives: ↑ hypo- tension
Antithyroid agents: ↑ agranulocytosis
Barbiturate anesthetics: ↑ CNS depression
β-Adrenergic blockers: ↑ effects of both drugs
General anesthetics: ↑ CNS depression
MAOIs: ↑ CNS depression
Opiates: ↑ CNS depression
Sedative/hypnotics: ↑ CNS depression
Herb/drug
Kava: ↑ CNS depression
Lab test interferences
↑ LFTs, ↑ cardiac enzymes, ↑ cholesterol, ↑ blood glucose, ↑ prolactin, ↑ bilirubin, ↑ PBI, ↑ cholinesterase, ↑ ^{131}I, ↑ alkaline phosphatase, ↑ leukocytes, ↑ granulocytes, ↑ platelets
↓ Hormones (blood and urine)
False positive: Pregnancy tests, PKU, urine bilirubin
False negative: Urinary steroids, 17-OHCS

NURSING CONSIDERATIONS
Assessment
- Assess mental status: orientation, mood, behavior, presence of hallucinations (and type) before initial administration and monthly; this drug should significantly reduce psychotic behavior
- Check for swallowing of PO medication; check for hoarding or giving of medication to other patients
- Monitor I&O ratio, palpate bladder if low urinary output occurs, especially G in elderly; urinalysis recommended before, during prolonged therapy
- Monitor bilirubin, CBC, liver function studies monthly
- Assess affect, orientation, LOC, reflexes, gait, coordination, sleep pattern disturbances
- Monitor B/P sitting, standing, and lying, take pulse and respirations q4h during initial treatment; establish baseline before starting treatment; report drops of 30 mm Hg; obtain baseline ECG, check for Q- and T-wave changes
- Check for dizziness, faintness,

T

palpitations, tachycardia on rising; severe orthostatic hypotension is common

- Identify for neuroleptic malignant syndrome: hyperpyrexia, muscle rigidity, increased CPK, altered mental status; drug should be discontinued
- Assess for EPS including akathisia (inability to sit still, no pattern to movements), tardive dyskinesia (bizarre movements of the jaw, mouth, tongue, extremities), pseudoparkinsonism (ragged tremors, pill rolling, shuffling gait); an antiparkinson drug should be prescribed
- Assess for constipation, urinary retention daily; if these occur, increase bulk, water in diet

Nursing diagnoses

- ✓ Thought processes, altered (uses)
- ✓ Coping, ineffective individual (uses)
- ✓ Knowledge deficit (teaching)
- ✓ Noncompliance (teaching)

Implementation

PO route

- Give drug in liq form mixed in glass of juice or cola if hoarding is suspected; do not mix in caffeine drinks, tannics, pectins
- G Give decreased dose to elderly because metabolism is slowed
- Give PO with full glass of water, milk; or give with food to decrease GI upset
- Store in tight, light-resistant container; store oral sol in amber bottle

IM route

- Dilute 10-mg vial/2.2 ml of sterile water for inj to 5 mg/ml
- Inj in deep muscle mass, do not give SC; do not administer sol with a precipitate

Syringe compatibilities: Benztropine, diphenhydramine, hydroxyzine

Patient/family education

- Teach patient to use good oral hygiene; frequent rinsing of mouth, sugarless gum for dry mouth
- Advise patient to avoid hazardous activities until drug response is determined; dizziness, blurred vision is common
- Inform patient that orthostatic hypotension occurs often and to rise from sitting or lying position gradually and to remain lying down after IM inj for at least 30 min; tell patient to avoid hot tubs, hot showers, tub baths because hypotension may occur; tell patient that in hot weather, heat stroke may occur, so to take extra precautions to stay cool
- Caution patient to avoid abrupt withdrawal of this drug, or EPS may result; drug should be withdrawn slowly
- Teach patient to avoid OTC preparations (cough, hayfever, cold) unless approved by prescriber, because serious drug interactions may occur; avoid use with alcohol, CNS depressants because increased drowsiness may occur
- Caution patient to use sunglasses and sunscreen to prevent burns
- Teach patient about EPS and necessity of meticulous oral hygiene because oral candidiasis may occur
- Tell patient to take antacids 2 hr before or after this drug
- Advise patient to report sore throat, malaise, fever, bleeding, mouth sores; if these occur, CBC should be performed and drug discontinued

Evaluation

Positive therapeutic outcome

- Decrease in emotional excitement, hallucinations, delusions, paranoia
- Reorganization of patterns of thought, speech

Treatment of overdose: Lavage if orally ingested; provide airway; *do not induce vomiting or use epinephrine*

thyroid USP (desiccated) (℞)

(thye'roid)

Armour Thyroid, Cholaxin ♣, S-P-T, Thyrar, Thyroid Strong, thyroid USP

Func. class.: Thyroid hormone

Chem. class.: Active thyroid hormone in natural state and ratio

Pregnancy category A

Action: Increases metabolic rates; controls protein synthesis; increases cardiac output, renal blood flow, O_2 consumption, body temp, blood volume, growth, development at cellular level

→ **Therapeutic Outcome:** Correction of lack of thyroid hormone

Uses: Hypothyroidism, cretinism P (juvenile hypothyroidism), myxedema

Dosage and routes

Hypothyroidism

Adult: PO 65 mg qd, increased by 65 mg q30 days until desired response; maintenance dose 65-195 mg qd

G ***Elderly:*** PO 7.5-15 mg qd, double dose q6-8 wk until desired response

Cretinism/juvenile hypothyroidism

P ***Child over 1 yr:*** PO up to 180 mg qd titrated to response

P ***Child 4-12 mo:*** PO 30-60 mg qd

P ***Child 1-4 mo:*** PO 15-30 mg qd; may increase q2 wk; titrated to response; maintenance dose 30-45 mg qd

Myxedema

Adult: PO 16 mg qd, double dose q2 wk, maintenance 65-195 mg/day

Available forms: Tabs 15, 30, 60, 90, 120 mg; enteric-coated tabs 30, 60, 120 mg; sugar-coated tabs 30, 60, 120, 180 mg; caps pork 60, 90, 120, 180 mg; tabs bovine 30, 60, 120 mg

Adverse effects

CNS: *Insomnia, tremors,* headache, thyroid storm

CV: *Tachycardia, palpitations, angina,* **dysrhythmias,** hypertension, **cardiac arrest**

GI: Nausea, diarrhea, increased or decreased appetite, cramps

MISC: Menstrual irregularities, weight loss, sweating, heat intolerance, fever

Contraindications: Adrenal insufficiency, MI, thyrotoxicosis

G **Precautions:** Elderly, angina pectoris, hypertension, ischemia, cardiac disease, pregnancy **A,** lactation

Do Not Confuse:

Thyrar/Thyrolar

Pharmacokinetics

Absorption	Well absorbed
Distribution	Widely distributed, does not cross placenta
Metabolism	Liver, tissues
Excretion	Feces via bile, breast milk
Half-life	T_3—2 days; T_4—1 wk

Pharmacodynamics

Onset	1 hr
Peak	12-48 hr
Duration	Unknown

Interactions

Individual drugs

Cholestyramine: ↓ absorption of thyroid hormone

Colestipol: ↓ absorption of thyroid hormone

Digitalis: ↓ effect of digitalis

Insulin: ↑ requirement for insulin

Phenytoin (IV): ↑ release of thyroid hormone

Drug classifications

Amphetamines: ↑ CNS, cardiac stimulation

Anticoagulants, oral: ↑ requirements for anticoagulants

β-Adrenergic blockers: ↓ effect of β-blockers

T

Decongestants: ↑ CNS, cardiac stimulation
Vasopressors: ↑ CNS, cardiac stimulation

Herb/drug

Bugleweed: Do not use together

Lab test interferences

↑ CPK, ↑ LDH, ↑ AST, ↑ PBI, ↑ blood glucose
↓ Thyroid function tests

NURSING CONSIDERATIONS

Assessment

- Identify if the patient is taking anticoagulants, antidiabetic agents; document on chart
- Take B/P, pulse before each dose; monitor I&O ratio and weight every day in same clothing, using same scale, at same time of day
- Monitor height, weight, psychomotor development, and growth rate if **P** given to a child
- Monitor T_3, T_4, FTIs, which are decreased; radioimmunoassay of TSH, which is increased; radioactive iodine uptake (RAIU), which is increased if patient's dose of medication is too low
- Monitor pro-time; patient may require decreased dosage of anticoagulant; check for bleeding, bruising
- Assess for increased nervousness, excitability, irritability, which may indicate that dose of medication is too high, usually after 1-3 wk of treatment
- Assess cardiac status: angina, palpitation, chest pain, change in VS; **G** the elderly patient may have undetected cardiac problems and baseline ECG should be completed before treatment

Nursing diagnoses

✓ Knowledge deficit (teaching)
✓ Noncompliance (teaching)

Implementation

- Give in AM if possible as a single dose to decrease sleeplessness; at same time each day to maintain drug level
- Give only for hormone imbalances; not to be used for obesity, male infertility, menstrual conditions, lethargy; give lowest dose that relieves **G** symptoms; lower dose to the elderly and in cardiac diseases
- Store in airtight, light-resistant container
- Wean patient off medication 4 wk before RAIU test

Patient/family education

- Teach patient that drug is not a cure but controls symptoms and that treatment is long-term
- Instruct patient to report excitability, irritability, anxiety, sweating, heat intolerance, chest pain, palpitations, which indicate overdose
- Advise patient not to switch brands unless approved by prescriber; bioavailability may differ; do not take with food; absorption will be decreased
- Teach patient that drug may be discontinued after giving birth; thyroid panel will be evaluated after 1-2 mo
- Teach patient that hyperthyroid **P** child will show almost immediate behavior/personality change; that hair **P** loss will occur in child and is temporary
- Caution patient that drug is not to be taken to reduce weight
- Caution patient to avoid OTC preparations containing iodine; read labels; other medications should not be used unless approved by prescriber
- Teach patient to avoid iodine-containing food: iodized salt, soybeans, tofu, turnips, certain kinds of seafood and bread

Evaluation

Positive therapeutic outcome

- Absence of depression
- Weight loss, increased diuresis, pulse, appetite
- Absence of constipation, peripheral edema, cold intolerance, pale, cool dry skin, brittle nails, alopecia, coarse hair, menorrhagia, night blindness,

paresthesias, syncope, stupor, coma, rosy cheeks

- Improved levels of T_3, T_4 by laboratory tests
- P • Child: Age-appropriate weight, height, and psychomotor development

Treatment of overdose: Withhold dose for up to 1 wk, acute overdose—gastric lavage or induce emesis, then activated charcoal; provide supportive treatment to control symptoms

thyrotropin alfa

See Appendix B, Recent FDA Drug Approvals

tiagabine (℞)

(tie-ah-ga'been)

Gabatril

Func. class.: Anticonvulsant

Pregnancy category C

Action: Mechanism unknown; may increase seizure threshold

Uses: Adjunct treatment of partial seizures

Dosage and routes

Adult: PO 4 mg qd, may increase by 4-8 mg qwk until desired response, max 56 mg/day

P ***Child 12-18 yr:*** PO 4 mg qd, may increase by 4 mg at beginning of wk 2, may increase by 4-8 mg qwk until desired response, max 32 mg/day

Available forms: Tabs 2, 4, 12, 16, 20 mg

Adverse effects

CNS: Dizziness, anxiety, somnolence, ataxia, amnesia, unsteady gait, depression

CV: Vasodilation

GI: Nausea, diarrhea, vomiting

INTEG: Pruritus, rash

RESP: Pharyngitis, coughing

Contraindications: Hypersensitivity to this drug

Precautions: Hepatic disease, P renal disease, pregnancy **C**, lactation, G child <12 yr, elderly

Pharmacokinetics

Absorption	>95%
Distribution	Unknown
Metabolism	Liver
Excretion	Kidneys
Half-life	7-9 hr

Pharmacodynamics

Unknown

Interactions: Unknown

NURSING CONSIDERATIONS

Assessment

- Monitor renal studies: urinalysis, BUN, urine creatinine q3 mo
- Monitor hepatic studies: ALT, AST, bilirubin
- Assess description of seizures: location, duration, presence of aura
- Assess mental status: mood, sensorium, affect, behavioral changes; if mental status changes, notify prescriber
- Assess eye problems, need for ophth exams before, during, after treatment (slit lamp, funduscopy, tonometry)
- Assess allergic reaction: purpura, red raised rash; if these occur, drug should be discontinued

Implementation

- Store at room temp away from heat and light
- Provide hard candy, frequent rinsing of mouth, gum for dry mouth
- Provide assistance with ambulation during early part of treatment; dizziness occurs
- Provide seizure precautions: padded side rails; move objects that may harm patient
- Provide increased fluids, bulk in diet for constipation

T

Patient/family education

- Advise patient to carry ID stating patient's name, drugs taken, condition, prescriber's name and phone number
- Advise patient to avoid driving, other activities that require alertness
- Teach patient not to discontinue medication quickly after long-term use

Evaluation

Positive therapeutic outcome

- Decreased seizure activity; document on patient's chart

Treatment of overdose:

Lavage, VS

ticarcillin (℞)

(tye-kar-sill'in)

ticar

Func. class.: Broad-spectrum antiinfective

Chem. class.: Extended-spectrum penicillin

Pregnancy category B

Action: Interferes with cell wall replication of susceptible organisms; osmotically unstable cell wall swells, bursts from osmotic pressure

➔ **Therapeutic Outcome:** Decreased symptoms of infection

Uses: Respiratory, soft tissue, urinary tract infections, bacterial septicemia; effective for gram-positive cocci *(Staphylococcus aureus, Streptococcus faecalis, Streptococcus pneumoniae)*, gram-negative cocci *(Neisseria gonorrhoeae)*, gram-positive bacilli *(Clostridium perfringens, Clostridium tetani)*, gram-negative bacilli *(Bacteroides, Fusobacterium nucleatum, Escherichia coli, Proteus mirabilis, Salmonella, Morganella morganii, Proteus rettgeri, Enterobacter, Pseudomonas aeruginosa, Serratia, Peptococcus, Peptostreptococcus, Eubacterium)*

Dosage and routes

Adult: **IV**/IM 4-24 g/day in divided doses q4-6h; infuse over ½-2 hr

P ***Child:*** **IV**/IM 50-300 mg/kg/day in divided doses q4-8h

P ***Neonate:*** **IV** inf 75-100 mg/kg/8-12 hr

Renal dose

CrCl <30 ml/min reduce dose

Available forms: Inj 1, 3, 6, 20, 30 g

Adverse effects

CNS: Lethargy, hallucinations, anxiety, depression, twitching, **coma, seizures**

GI: *Nausea, vomiting, diarrhea;* increased AST, ALT, abdominal pain, glossitis, colitis

GU: Oliguria, proteinuria, hematuria, *vaginitis, moniliasis,* **glomerulonephritis**

HEMA: Anemia, increased bleeding time, **bone marrow depression, granulocytopenia**

INTEG: Rash

META: Hypokalemia

Contraindications: Hypersensitivity to penicillins

Precautions: Hypersensitivity to cephalosporins, pregnancy **B,** lactation, renal disease

Pharmacokinetics

Absorption	Unknown
Distribution	Widely, breast milk
Metabolism	Liver, small amount
Excretion	Kidneys
Half-life	70 min

Pharmacodynamics

	IM	IV
Onset	Unknown	Unknown
Peak	1 hr	30-45 min
Duration	4-6 hr	4 hr

Interactions

Individual drugs

Aspirin: ↑ ticarcillin concentration

Heparin: ↑ effect of heparin
Probenecid: ↑ ticarcillin concentrations

Drug classifications

Aminoglycosides, IV: ↓ effect of ticarcillin
Erythromycins: ↓ effect of ticarcillin
Neuromuscular blockers: ↑ effect of neuromuscular blockers
Oral contraceptives: ↓ effect of oral contraceptives
Tetracyclines: ↓ effect of ticarcillin

Herb/drug

Khat: ↓ absorption

Lab test interferences

False positive: Urine glucose, urine protein

NURSING CONSIDERATIONS

Assessment

- Monitor I&O ratio; report hematuria, oliguria, since penicillin in high doses is nephrotoxic
- Monitor any patient with compromised renal system, since drug is excreted slowly in poor renal system function; toxicity may occur rapidly
- Monitor LFTs: AST, ALT
- Monitor blood studies: WBC, RBC, Hgb, Hct, bleeding time
- Monitor renal function studies: urinalysis, protein, blood, BUN, creatinine
- Monitor C&S before drug therapy; drug may be given as soon as culture is performed
- Assess bowel pattern before, during treatment
- Check for skin eruptions after administration of penicillin to 1 wk after discontinuing drug
- Assess respiratory status: rate, character, wheezing, tightness in chest
- Assess allergies before initiation of treatment, reaction of each medication; highlight allergies on chart

Implementation

- Give **IV** after diluting 1 g or less/4 ml of sterile H_2O for inj; dilute further with 10-20 ml or more D_5W, 0.9% NaCl, or sterile H_2O for inj sol; give 1 g or less/5 min or more or by intermittent inf over ½-2 hr or by continuous inf at prescribed rate

Y-site compatibilities: Acyclovir, allopurinol, amifostine, aztreonam, cyclophosphamide, diltiazem, famotidine, filgrastim, fludarabine, granisetron, hydromorphone, heparin, IL-2, insulin (regular), magnesium sulfate, melphalan, meperidine, morphine, ondansetron, perphenazine, propofol, sargramostim, teniposide, theophylline, thiotepa, verapamil, vinorelbine

Additive compatibilities: Ranitidine, verapamil

- Give drug after C&S has been completed
- Have adrenalin, suction, tracheostomy set, endotracheal intubation equipment
- Provide adequate fluid intake (2 L) during diarrhea episodes
- Provide scratch test to assess allergy on order from prescriber; usually done when penicillin is only drug of choice
- Store at room temp, reconstituted sol 72 hr at room temp

Evaluation

Positive therapeutic outcome

- Absence of fever, purulent drainage, redness, inflammation

Patient/family education

- Advise patient that culture may be done after completed course of medication
- Teach patient to report sore throat, fever, fatigue (may indicate superinfection)
- Teach patient to wear or carry ID if allergic to penicillins
- Advise patient to notify nurse of diarrhea

Treatment of overdose:

Withdraw drug, maintain airway, administer epinephrine, aminophylline, O_2, **IV** corticosteroids for anaphylaxis

ticarcillin/clavulanate (℞)

(tye-kar-sill'in)

Chem. class: Broad-spectrum antibiotic

Func. class.: Extended-spectrum penicillin

Pregnancy category B

Action: Interferes with cell wall replication of susceptible organisms; osmotically unstable cell wall swells, bursts from osmotic pressure

Therapeutic Outcome: Resolution of infection

Uses: Respiratory, soft tissue, urinary tract infections; bacterial septicemia; effective for gram-positive cocci *(Staphylococcus aureus, Streptococcus faecalis, Streptococcus pneumoniae)*, gram-negative cocci *(Neisseria gonorrhoeae)*, gram-positive bacilli *(Clostridium perfringens, Clostridium tetani)*, gram-negative bacilli *(Bacteroides, Fusobacterium nucleatum, Escherichia coli, Proteus mirabilis, Salmonella, Morganella morganii, Proteus rettgeri, Enterobacter, Pseudomonas aeruginosa, Serratia, Peptococcus, Peptostreptococcus, Eubacterium)*

Dosage and routes

Adult: **IV** inf 1 vial containing ticarcillin 3 g, clavulanate 0.1 g q4-6h, infuse over 30 min

P ***Child <60 kg:*** **IV** 200-300 mg ticarcillin/kg/day in divided doses q4-6h

Available forms: Inj IM, **IV** 3 g ticarcillin and 0.1 g clavulanate; **IV** inf 3 g ticarcillin and 0.1 g clavulanate; discs 75 μg ticarcillin, 10 μg clavulanate; powder for inj 3 g ticarcillin, 0.1 g clavulanate, 30 g ticarcillin, 1 g clavulanate

Adverse effects

CNS: Lethargy, hallucinations, anxiety, depression, twitching, **coma, seizures**

GI: Nausea, vomiting, diarrhea, increased AST, ALT, abdominal pain, glossitis, colitis

GU: Oliguria, proteinuria, hematuria, *vaginitis, moniliasis,* **glomerulonephritis**

HEMA: Anemia, increased bleeding time, **bone marrow depression, granulocytopenia**

META: Hypokalemia, hypokalemia, alkalosis, hypernatremia

Contraindications: Hypersensitivity to penicillins

Precautions: Hypersensitivity to cephalosporins, pregnancy **B**

Pharmacokinetics

Absorption	Completely absorbed (**IV**)
Distribution	Widely distributed, crosses blood-brain barrier
Metabolism	Liver
Excretion	Kidneys
Half-life	64-68 min

Pharmacodynamics

	IV
Onset	Unknown
Peak	30-45 min
Duration	4 hr

Interactions

Individual drugs

Cholestyramine: ↓ absorption of thyroid hormone

Colestipol: ↓ absorption of thyroid hormone

Digitalis: ↓ effect of digitalis

Insulin: ↑ requirement for insulin

Phenytoin (IV): ↑ release of thyroid hormone

Drug classifications

Amphetamines: ↑ CNS, cardiac stimulation

Anticoagulants, oral: ↑ requirements for anticoagulants

β-Adrenergic blockers: ↓ effect of β-blockers

Decongestants: ↑ CNS, cardiac stimulation
Oral contraceptives: ↓ effect of oral contraceptives
Vasopressors: ↑ CNS, cardiac stimulation

Herb/drug
Khat: ↓ absorption

Lab test interferences
False positive: Urine glucose, urine protein Coombs' test

NURSING CONSIDERATIONS
Assessment
- Monitor I&O ratio; report hematuria, oliguria because penicillin in high doses is nephrotoxic
- Monitor any patient with compromised renal system because drug is excreted slowly in poor renal system function; toxicity may occur rapidly
- Monitor LFTs: AST, ALT
- Monitor blood studies: WBC, RBC, Hgb, Hct, bleeding time
- Monitor renal function studies: urinalysis, protein, blood
- Obtain C&S test results before initiating drug therapy; drug may be given as soon as culture is performed
- Assess bowel pattern before, during treatment
- Assess skin eruptions after administration of penicillin to 1 wk after discontinuing drug
- Assess respiratory status: rate, character, wheezing, and tightness in chest
- Assess allergies before initiation of treatment, reaction of each medication

Nursing diagnoses
✓ Infection, risk for (uses)
✓ Knowledge deficit (teaching)

Implementation
IV route
- Give **IV** after diluting 3.1 g or less/13 ml of sterile H_2O or NaCl (200 mg/ml), shake; may further dilute in 50-100 ml or more 0.9% NaCl, D_5W, or LR sol and run over ½ hr

Y-site compatibilities:
Allopurinol, aztreonam, cefepime, cyclophosphamide, diltiazem, famotidine, filgrastim, fluconazole, fludarabine, foscarnet, heparin, insulin (regular), melphalan, meperidine, morphine, ondansetron, perphenazine, sargramostim, teniposide, theophylline, vinorelbine
- Give drug after C&S has been completed
- Have adrenalin, suction, tracheostomy set, endotracheal intubation equipment available
- Give adequate fluid intake (2 L) during diarrhea episodes
- Obtain scratch test results to assess allergy after securing order from prescriber; usually done when penicillin is only drug of choice
- Store at room temp, reconstituted sol for 12-24 hr or 3-7 days refrigerated

Patient/family education
- Advise patient that C&S may be performed after completed course of medication
- Instruct patient to report sore throat, fever, fatigue (may indicate superinfection)
- Advise patient to wear or carry ID if allergic to penicillins

Evaluation
Positive therapeutic outcome
- Absence of fever, purulent drainage, redness, inflammation

Treatment of overdose:
Withdraw drug, maintain airway, administer epinephrine, aminophylline, O_2, **IV** corticosteroids for anaphylaxis

T

ticlopidine (℞)
(tye-cloe′pi-deen)
Ticlid
Func. class.: Platelet aggregation inhibitor

Pregnancy category B

Action: Inhibits first and second phases of ADP-induced effects in platelet aggregation

➔ **Therapeutic Outcome:** Decreased stroke by decreasing platelet aggregation

Uses: Reducing the risk of stroke in high-risk patients

Investigational uses: Intermittent claudication, chronic arterial occlusion, subarachnoid hemorrhage, uremic patients with AV shunts/fistulas, open heart surgery, coronary artery bypass grafts, primary glomerulonephritis

Dosage and routes
Adult: PO 250 mg bid with food

Available forms: Tabs 250 mg

Adverse effects
CNS: Dizziness
GI: Nausea, vomiting, diarrhea, GI discomfort, **cholestatic jaundice, hepatitis,** increased cholesterol LDL, VLDL
HEMA: **Bleeding (epistaxis, hematuria, conjunctival hemorrhage, GI bleeding), agranulocytosis, neutropenia, thrombocytopenia**
INTEG: Rash, pruritus

Contraindications: Hypersensitivity, active liver disease, blood dyscrasias, active bleeding

Precautions: Past liver disease, renal disease, elderly **G**, pregnancy **B**, lactation, children **P**, increased bleeding risk

Pharmacokinetics
Absorption	Well absorbed
Distribution	Unknown
Metabolism	Liver—extensively
Excretion	Kidneys—unchanged drug
Half-life	Increased with repeat dosing; 4-5 days (multiple doses)

Pharmacodynamics
Onset	Unknown
Peak	1-3 hr
Duration	Unknown

Interactions
Individual drugs
Aspirin: ↑ bleeding tendencies
Cimetidine: ↑ effects of ticlopidine
Digoxin: ↓ plasma levels of ticlopidine
Theophylline: ↑ effects of theophylline
Drug classifications
Antacids: ↓ plasma levels of ticlopidine
Anticoagulants: ↑ bleeding tendencies

NURSING CONSIDERATIONS
Assessment
- Monitor liver function studies: AST, ALT, bilirubin, creatinine if patient is on long-term therapy (4 mo or more)
- Monitor blood studies: CBC, Hct, Hgb, pro-time if patient is on long-term therapy; CBC q2 wk × 3 mo therapy; thrombocytopenia, neutropenia may occur
- Monitor bleeding time baseline and throughout therapy, levels may be 2-5 × normal limit

Nursing diagnoses
✓ Injury, risk for (uses)
✓ Knowledge deficit (teaching)

Implementation
- Give with food to decrease gastric symptoms

Patient/family education
- Advise patient that blood studies will be necessary during treatment

• Advise patient to report any unusual bleeding to prescriber
• Instruct patient to take with food or just after eating to minimize GI discomfort
• Caution patient to report side effects such as diarrhea, skin rashes, subcutaneous bleeding, signs of cholestasis (yellow skin and sclera, dark urine, light-colored stools)

Evaluation

Positive therapeutic outcome
• Absence of stroke

tiludronate (℞)

(till-oo'droe-nate)

Skelid

Func. class.: Bone resorption inhibitor

Chem. class.: Bisphosphonate

Pregnancy category C

Action: Decreases bone reabsorption and new bone development

Therapeutic Outcome: Decreased bone reabsorption and reduced calcium levels WNL

Uses: Paget's disease

Dosage and routes

Adult: PO 400 mg qd, with 8 oz of water × 3 mo

Available forms: Tabs 400 mg

Adverse effects

CNS: Headache, somnolence, dizziness, anxiety, vertigo, nervousness, involuntary movements
ENDO: Hyperparathyroidism
GI: *Nausea, diarrhea,* dry mouth, gastritis, vomiting, flatulence, gastric ulcers
GU: **Nephrotoxicity,** UTI
INTEG: Rash, epidermal necrosis, pruritus, sweating
MS: *Bone pain,* decreased mineralization of nonaffected bones, pathologic fractures
RESP: Rhinitis, rales, sinusitis, upper respiratory tract infection

Contraindications: Hypersensitivity to bisphosphonates, pathologic fractures, children, colitis, severe renal disease with creatinine >5 mg/dl

Precautions: Pregnancy **C,** renal disease, lactation, restricted vit D/Ca, GI disease

Pharmacokinetics	
Absorption	Rapid
Distribution	Unknown, steady state 10 days
Metabolism	None
Excretion	Feces (unabsorbed), kidney (unchanged)
Half-life	150 hr

Pharmacodynamics	
Onset	Unknown
Peak	Unknown
Duration	6 mo

Interactions

Individual drugs

Aspirin: ↓ effect of tiludronate
Indomethacin: ↑ effect of tiludronate

Drug classifications

Antacids: ↓ absorption of tiludronate
Mineral supplements with magnesium, calcium, or aluminum: ↓ absorption of tiludronate

NURSING CONSIDERATIONS

Assessment

• Assess for GI symptoms, polyuria, flushing, head swelling, tingling, headache; may indicate hypercalcemia; nervousness, irritability, twitching, seizures, spasm, paresthesia indicates hypocalcemia at start of treatment
• Identify nutritional status; evaluate diet for sources of vit D (milk, some seafood), calcium (dairy products, dark green vegetables), phosphates
• Monitor BUN, creatinine, uric acid, chloride, electrolytes, urine pH,

T

urinary calcium, magnesium, phosphate, urinalysis (calcium should be kept at 9-10 mg/dl), albumin, alkaline phosphatase baseline and q3-6 mo; check urine sediment for casts throughout treatment

- Assess for increased drug level; toxic reactions occur rapidly; have calcium chloride or gluconate on hand if calcium level drops too low; check for tetany

Nursing diagnoses

- ✓ Injury, risk for (adverse reactions)
- ✓ Pain, chronic (uses)
- ✓ Knowledge deficit (teaching)

Implementation

- Administer on empty stomach to improve absorption (2 hr ac), with 6-8 oz of water

Patient/family education

- Caution patient to notify prescriber of hypercalcemic relapse: renal calculi, nausea, vomiting, thirst, lethargy, deep bone or flank pain
- Teach patient to follow a low-calcium diet as prescribed (Paget's disease, hypercalcemia)
- Advise patient to notify prescriber of diarrhea, nausea; dose may be divided to lessen these symptoms

Evaluation

Positive therapeutic outcome

- Calcium levels 9-10 mg/dl
- Decreasing symptoms of Paget's disease including pain

timolol (℞)

(tye'moe-lole)

Apo-Timol ✤, Blocadren, Novo-Timol ✤, timolol maleate, Timoptic

Func. class.: Antihypertensive; antiglaucoma

Chem. class.: Nonselective β-blocker

Pregnancy category C

Action: Competitively blocks stimulation of β-adrenergic receptor within vascular smooth muscle; (decreases rate of SA node discharge, increases recovery time), slows conduction of AV node, decreases heart rate, which decreases O_2 consumption in myocardium; also decreases renin-aldosterone-angiotensin system; at high doses inhibits $β_2$ receptors in bronchial system

➔ **Therapeutic Outcome:** Decreased B/P, decreased arrhythmias, absence of death from MI, decreased aqueous humor in the eye, absence of migraine headaches

Uses: Mild to moderate hypertension, sinus tachycardia, persistent atrial extrasystoles, tachydysrhythmias, prophylaxis of angina pectoris, reduction of mortality after MI

Investigational uses: Mitral valve prolapse, hypertrophic cardiomyopathy, thyrotoxicosis, tremors, anxiety, pheochromocytoma, tachyarrhythmias, angina pectoris

Dosage and routes

Hypertension

Adult: PO 10 mg bid, or 20 mg qd, may increase by 10 mg q2-3 days, not to exceed 60 mg/day

MI

Adult: 10 mg bid beginning 1-4 wk after MI

Glaucoma

Adult: Ophth i gtt qd or bid

P **Child:** Ophth i gtt qd or bid (0.25% sol only)

Migraine headache prevention

Adult: PO 10 mg bid, or 20 mg qd, may increase to 30 mg/day, 20 mg in AM, 10 mg in PM

Available forms: Tabs 5, 10, 20 mg; ophth sol 0.25%, 0.5%

Adverse effects

CNS: *Insomnia, dizziness,* hallucinations, anxiety

CV: Hypotension, bradycardia, **CHF,** edema, chest pain, bradycardia, claudication

EENT: *Visual changes,* sore throat, *double vision,* dry burning eyes

GI: *Nausea,* vomiting, **ischemic colitis,** diarrhea, *abdominal pain,* **mesenteric arterial thrombosis**

GU: Impotence, urinary frequency

HEMA: **Agranulocytosis, thrombocytopenia, purpura**

INTEG: Rash, alopecia, pruritus, fever

META: Hypoglycemia

MUSC: *Joint pain, muscle pain*

RESP: **Bronchospasm,** dyspnea, cough, rales

Contraindications: Hypersensitivity to β-blockers, cardiogenic shock, heart block (2nd or 3rd degree), sinus bradycardia, CHF, cardiac failure

Precautions: Major surgery, pregnancy **C,** lactation, diabetes mellitus, renal disease, thyroid disease, COPD, well-compensated heart failure, CAD, nonallergic bronchospasm

Do Not Confuse:
Timoptic/Viroptic

Pharmacokinetics

Absorption	Well absorbed (PO), ophth (minimal)
Distribution	Protein binding <10%
Metabolism	Liver—extensively
Excretion	Breast milk
Half-life	3 hr

Pharmacodynamics

	PO
Onset	Unknown
Peak	2-4 hr
Duration	12-24 hr

Interactions

Individual drugs

Alcohol: ↑ hypotension (large amounts)
Epinephrine: α-Adrenergic stimulation
Hydralazine: ↑ hypotension, bradycardia
Indomethacin: ↓ antihypertensive effect
Insulin: ↑ hypoglycemia
Methyldopa: ↑ hypotension, bradycardia
Prazosin: ↑ hypotension, bradycardia
Reserpine: ↑ hypotension, bradycardia
Thyroid hormones: ↓ effect of timolol
Verapamil: ↑ myocardial depression

Drug classifications

Antihypertensives: ↑ hypotension
β_2-Adrenergic agonists: ↓ bronchodilatation
Cardiac glycosides: ↑ bradycardia
Nitrates: ↑ hypotension
Sulfonylureas: ↓ hypoglycemic effect
Theophyllines: ↓ bronchodilatation

Lab test interferences

False: ↑ Urinary catecholamines

NURSING CONSIDERATIONS

Assessment

- Assess for headaches: location, severity, duration, frequency baseline and throughout treatment
- Monitor B/P during beginning treatment, periodically thereafter; pulse q4h; note rate, rhythm, quality: apical/radial pulse before administration; notify prescriber of any significant changes (pulse <50 bpm)
- Check for baselines in renal, liver function tests before therapy begins
- Assess for edema in feet, legs daily,

T

monitor I&O ratio, daily weight; check for jugular vein distention, rales, bilaterally, dyspnea (CHF)

• Monitor skin turgor, dryness of mucous membranes for hydration status, especially elderly

Nursing diagnoses

✓ Cardiac output, decreased (uses)
✓ Injury, risk for physical (side effects)
✓ Knowledge deficit (teaching)
✓ Noncompliance (teaching)

Implementation

PO route

• Given ac, hs, tab may be crushed or swallowed whole; give with food to prevent GI upset; reduced dosage in renal dysfunction

• Store protected from light, moisture; place in cool environment

Patient/family education

• Teach patient not to discontinue drug abruptly; taper over 2 wk; may cause precipitate angina if stopped abruptly

• Advise patient not to use OTC products containing α-adrenergic stimulants (such as nasal decongestants, cold preparations); to avoid alcohol, smoking and to limit sodium intake as prescribed

• Teach patient how to take pulse and B/P at home; advise patient when to notify prescriber

• Instruct patient to comply with weight control, dietary adjustments, modified exercise program

• Advise patient to carry/wear ID to identify drug being taken, any allergies; tell patient drug controls symptoms but does not cure

• Caution patient to avoid hazardous activities if dizziness, drowsiness is present

• Teach patient to report symptoms of CHF; difficult breathing, especially on exertion or when lying down; night cough; swelling of extremities or bradycardia; dizziness; confusion; depression; fever

• Teach patient to take drug as prescribed, not to double doses, skip doses; take any missed doses as soon as remembered if at least 4 hr until next dose

Evaluation

Positive therapeutic outcome

• Decreased B/P in hypertension (after 1-2 wk)

• Absence of dysrhythmias

Treatment of overdose:

Lavage, **IV** atropine for bradycardia, **IV** theophylline for bronchospasm, digitalis, O_2, diuretic for cardiac failure, hemodialysis, **IV** glucose for hyperglycemia, **IV** diazepam (or phenytoin) for seizures

---

HIGH ALERT

tinzaparin (℞)

(tin-zay-par′in)

Innohep

Func. class.: Anticoagulant

Chem. class.: Unfractionated porcine heparin

Pregnancy category C

Action: Prevents conversion of fibrinogen to fibrin and prothrombin to thrombin by enhancing inhibitory effects of antithrombin III; produces higher ratio of antifactor Xa to antifactor IIa

➔ **Therapeutic Outcome:** Resolution of deep vein thrombosis

Uses: Treatment of deep vein thrombosis, pulmonary emboli when given with warfarin

Dosage and routes

Adult: SC 175 anti-Xa IU/kg qd ≥6 days and until adequate anticoagulation with warfarin (INR ≥2 for 2 consecutive days)

Available forms: Inj 40,000 IU/2 ml

Adverse effects

CNS: Fever, confusion

GI: Nausea
GU: Edema, peripheral edema
***HEMA:* Hypochromic anemia, thrombocytopenia**, bleeding
INTEG: Ecchymosis

Contraindications: Hypersensitivity to this drug, heparin, or pork; hemophilia, leukemia with bleeding, peptic ulcer disease, thrombocytopenic purpura, heparin-induced thrombocytopenia

G **Precautions:** Alcoholism, elderly, pregnancy **C**, hepatic disease (severe), renal disease (severe), blood dyscrasias, severe hypertension, subacute bacterial endocarditis, acute nephritis, P lactation, children

Pharmacokinetics

Absorption	Unknown
Distribution	Unknown
Metabolism	Unknown
Excretion	Unknown
Half-life	4.5 hr

Pharmacodynamics

Onset	Unknown
Peak	3-5 hr (max antithrombin activity)
Duration	Unknown

Interactions
Drug classifications
Anticoagulants, oral: ↑ tinzaparin action
Salicylates: ↑ tinzaparin action
Herb/drug
Bromelain: ↑ risk of bleeding
Cinchona bark: ↑ risk of bleeding

NURSING CONSIDERATIONS
Assessment
- Monitor blood studies (Hct, platelets, occult blood in stools), anti-Xa; thrombocytopenia may occur
- Assess for bleeding gums, petechiae, ecchymosis, black tarry stools, hematuria

Nursing diagnoses
- ✓ Cardiac output, decreased (uses)
- ✓ Knowledge deficit (teaching)

Implementation
- Give only after screening patient for bleeding disorders
- Give SC only; do not give IM
- Give SC to recumbent patient; rotate inj sites (left/right anterolateral, left/right posterolateral abdominal wall)
- Insert whole length of needle into skin fold held with thumb and forefinger
- ! Use only this drug when ordered; not interchangeable with heparin
- Give at same time each day to maintain steady blood levels
- Do not massage area or aspirate when giving SC injection
- Avoid all IM injections that may cause bleeding
- Store at 77° F (25° C); do not freeze

Patient/family education
- Advise patient to use soft-bristle toothbrush to avoid bleeding gums, to use electric razor
- Instruct patient to report any signs of bleeding: gums, under skin, urine, stools

Evaluation
Positive therapeutic outcome
- Resolution of deep vein thrombosis

Treatment of overdose: Protamine SO_4 1% sol; dose should equal dose of tinzaparin

T

tirofiban (℞)
(tie-roh-fee'ban)
Aggrastat
Func. class.: Antiplatelet
Chem. class.: Nonpeptide antagonist
Pregnancy category B

Action: Activation of platelet glycoprotein (GP) IIb/IIIa receptor that leads to binding of fibrinogen and von

Willebrand's factor, which causes platelet aggregation

Therapeutic Outcome: Increased platelet count

Uses: Acute coronary syndrome

Dosage and routes

Adult: **IV** 0.4 μg/kg/min × 30 min, then 0.1 μg/kg/min

Renal dose

Adult: **IV** CrCl <30 ml/min 0.2 μg/kg/min × 30 min, then 0.05 μg/kg/min, during angiography and for up to 24 hr after angioplasty

Available forms: Inj for sol 250 μg/ml, inj 50 μg/ml

Adverse effects

CNS: Dizziness
CV: Bradycardia
HEMA: Bleeding, **thrombocytopenia**
INTEG: Rash
MISC: Dissection, coronary artery edema, pain in legs/pelvis, sweating

Contraindications: Hypersensitivity, active internal bleeding, stroke, major surgery, severe trauma, intracranial neoplasm, aneurysm, hemorrhage

Precautions: Pregnancy **B,** lactation, G elderly, renal disease, bleeding tendencies

Pharmacokinetics	
Absorption	Unknown
Distribution	Plasma clearance 20%-25%
Metabolism	Liver
Excretion	Urine/feces
Half-life	2 hr

Pharmacodynamics	
Onset	Unknown
Peak	Unknown
Duration	Unknown

Interactions

Individual drugs

Abciximab: ↑ risk of bleeding
Aspirin: ↑ bleeding
Cefamandole: ↑ risk of bleeding
Cefoperazone: ↑ risk of bleeding
Cefotetan: ↑ risk of bleeding
Clopidogrel: ↑ risk of bleeding
Dipyridamole: ↑ risk of bleeding
Heparin: ↑ bleeding
Plicamycin: ↑ risk of bleeding
Valproic acid: ↑ risk of bleeding

NURSING CONSIDERATIONS

Assessment

- Monitor B/P pulse during treatment until stable; take B/P lying, standing; orthostatic hypotension is common
- Monitor platelet counts, Hct, Hgb, before treatment, within 6 hr of loading dose and at least qd thereafter; watch for bleeding from puncture sites, catheters or in stools, urine

Nursing diagnoses

✓ Tissue perfusion, altered (uses)

Implementation

- **IV:** Give ½ dose in renal disease
- Dilute inj: withdraw and discard 100 ml from a 500 ml bag of sterile 0.9% NaCl or D_5 and replace this vol with 50 ml of tirofiban inj from one vial
- Tirofiban inj for sol is premixed in containers of 500 ml 0.9% NaCl (50 mg/ml)
- Minimize other arterial/venous punctures IM inj, catheter use, intubation, to reduce bleeding risks

Patient/family education

- Advise patient that it is necessary to quit smoking to prevent excessive vasoconstriction
- Teach patient to avoid hazardous activities; dizziness may occur

Evaluation

Positive therapeutic outcome

- Decreased platelet count

tizanidine (℞)

(tye-za'na-deen)

Zanaflex

Func. class.: Skeletal muscle relaxant, central acting

Chem. class.: Imidazole

Pregnancy category C

Action: Unknown; possesses central α_2-adrenergic agonist properties; reduces excitation of spinal cord interneurons; also acts on the basal ganglia, producing muscle relaxation

Therapeutic Outcome: Decreased spasticity of muscles

Uses: Spinal cord injury, spasticity in multiple sclerosis, tension headache

Dosage and routes

Adult: PO Reduce dose in renal failure; 4-36 mg qd in 3 divided doses

Spasticity:

Adult: PO 4-8 mg as a single dose; may increase in 2-4 mg increments until desired response, may repeat q6-8h up to 3 doses/24 hr, max 36 mg/day

Tension headache:

Adult: PO 2 mg tid, may increase by 4-6 mg tid after 2 wk interval

Available forms: Tabs 4 mg

Adverse effects

CNS: *Dizziness,* asthenia, somnolence, *fatigue, insomnia,* severe sedation

CV: *Hypotension*

GI: *Nausea, constipation, vomiting,* diarrhea, **hepatotoxicity,** *dry mouth,* anorexia

GU: Urinary frequency, UTI

INTEG: Rash, pruritus, sweating, skin ulcer

Contraindications: Hypersensitivity

Precautions: Renal disease, hepatic disease, stroke, cardiac disease, pregnancy **C,** elderly

Pharmacokinetics

Absorption	Complete
Distribution	Widely
Metabolism	Liver, extensively
Excretion	Kidneys, feces
Half-life	2½ hr

Pharmacodynamics

Onset	Unknown
Peak	1-2 hr
Duration	3-6 hr

Interactions

Individual drugs

Alcohol: CNS depression

Drug classifications

Antidepressants, tricyclic: ↑ CNS depression

Barbiturates: ↑ CNS depression

Diuretics: ↑ hypotensive effects

Opiates: ↑ CNS depression

Oral contraceptives: ↑ adverse reactions of tizanidine

Sedative/hypnotics: ↑ CNS depression

Lab test interferences

↑ AST, ↑ alkaline phosphatase

NURSING CONSIDERATIONS

Assessment

- Assess for muscle spasticity baseline and throughout treatment
- Monitor B/P, heart rate
- Perform neurologic exam in spasticity: deep tendon reflexes, muscle tone, clonus, sensory function
- Monitor liver, renal function tests, electrolytes, CBC with differential during long-term treatment
- Assess for allergic reactions: rash, fever, respiratory distress; severe weakness, numbness in extremities
- Assess CNS depression: dizziness, drowsiness, psychiatric symptoms
- Check dosage, as individual titration is required

Nursing diagnoses

✓ Mobility, impaired uses
✓ Injury, risk for (adverse reactions)
✓ Knowledge deficit (teaching)

T

Implementation
- Give with meals for GI symptoms; gum, frequent sips of water for dry mouth
- Store in airtight container at room temp

Patient/family education
- Advise patient not to discontinue medication quickly; spasticity, will occur; drug should be tapered off over 1-2 wk
- Advise patient not to take with alcohol, other CNS depressants, take as directed, if dose is missed, take as soon as remembered, unless it is almost time for next dose
- Caution patient to avoid altering activities while taking this drug; to avoid hazardous activities if drowsiness or dizziness occurs; to rise from sitting or lying slowly to prevent fainting
- Advise patient to avoid using OTC medications (cough preparations, antihistamines) unless directed by prescriber
- Notify prescriber if fainting, hallucinations, dark urine, stomach pain, yellowing of skin/eyes occur

Evaluation
Positive therapeutic outcome
- Decreased pain, spasticity

tobramycin (℞)
(toe-bra-mye'sin)

Nebcin, tobramycin sulfate, Tobrex, TOBI

Func. class.: Antiinfective

Chem. class.: Aminoglycoside

Pregnancy category D

Action: Interferes with protein synthesis in bacterial cell by binding to ribosomal subunit, causing inaccurate peptide sequence to form in protein chain, causing bacterial death

➡ **Therapeutic Outcome:** Bactericidal effects for the following organisms: *Pseudomonas aeruginosa, Enterobacter, Escherichia coli, Providencia, Citrobacter, Staphylococcus, Proteus, Klebsiella, Serratia*

Uses: Severe systemic infections of CNS, respiratory, GI, urinary tract, bone, skin, soft tissues, eye, cystic fibrosis (nebulizer) for *P. aeruginosa*

Dosage and routes
Adult: IM/**IV** 3 mg/kg/day in divided doses q8h; may give up to 5 mg/kg/day in divided doses q6-8h; once qd dosing is an option

P ***Child:*** IM/**IV** 6-7.5 mg/kg/ day in 3-4 equal divided doses

P ***Child ≥6 yr:*** NEB 300 mg bid in repeating cycles of 28 days on/28 days off; give inh over 10-15 min using a hand-held PARI LC PLUS reusable nebulizer with a DeVilbiss Pulmo-Aid compressor

P ***Neonates <1 wk:*** IM up to 4 mg/kg/day in divided doses q12h; **IV** up to 4 mg/kg/day in divided doses q12h diluted in 50-100 mg NS or D_5W; give over 30-60 min

Available forms: Inj 10, 40 mg/ml; powder for inj 1.2 g; inj 20 mg/2 ml; 0.3% ophth, neb sol 300 mg/5 ml

Adverse effects
CNS: Confusion, depression, numbness, tremors, **convulsions,** muscle twitching, **neurotoxicity,** dizziness, vertigo

CV: Hypotension, hypertension, palpitations

EENT: *Ototoxicity,* deafness, visual disturbances, tinnitus

GI: *Nausea, vomiting, anorexia,* increased ALT, AST, bilirubin, hepatomegaly, **hepatic necrosis,** splenomegaly

GU: **Oliguria, hematuria, renal damage, azotemia, renal failure, nephrotoxicity**

HEMA: **Agranulocytosis, thrombocytopenia, leukopenia, eosinophilia,** anemia

INTEG: *Rash,* burning, urticaria, dermatitis, alopecia

Contraindications: Severe renal disease, hypersensitivity to aminoglycosides, pregnancy **D**

P **Precautions:** Neonates, mild renal disease, myasthenia gravis, lactation, hearing deficits, Parkinson's disease

Do Not Confuse:
Tobrex/Tobra Dex

Pharmacokinetics

Absorption	Well absorbed (IM), completely absorbed (**IV**)
Distribution	Widely distributed in extracellular fluids
Metabolism	Minimal—liver
Excretion	Mostly unchanged (>90%) kidneys
P **Half-life**	2-3 hr, increased in renal disease, neonates

Pharmacodynamics

	IM	IV	OPHTH
Onset	Rapid	Rapid	Rapid
Peak	1 hr	Inf end	Unknown

Interactions

Individual drugs

Amphotericin B: ↑ ototoxicity, neurotoxicity, nephrotoxicity
Cisplatin: ↑ ototoxicity, neurotoxicity, nephrotoxicity
Ethacrynic acid: ↑ ototoxicity, neurotoxicity, nephrotoxicity
Furosemide: ↑ ototoxicity, neurotoxicity, nephrotoxicity
Mannitol: ↑ ototoxicity, neurotoxicity, nephrotoxicity
Methoxyflurane: ↑ ototoxicity, neurotoxicity, nephrotoxicity
Polymyxin: ↑ ototoxicity, neurotoxicity, nephrotoxicity
Succinylcholine: ↑ neuromuscular blockade, respiratory depression
Vancomycin: ↑ ototoxicity, neurotoxicity, nephrotoxicity

Drug classifications

Aminoglycosides: ↑ otoxicity, neurotoxicity, nephrotoxicity
Anesthetics: ↑ neuromuscular blockade, respiratory depression
Nondepolarizing neuromuscular blockers: ↑ neuromuscular blockade, respiratory depression
Penicillins: ↑ ototoxicity, neurotoxicity, nephrotoxicity

NURSING CONSIDERATIONS

Assessment

- Assess patient for previous sensitivity reaction

Systemic route

- Assess patient for signs and symptoms of infection including characteristics of wounds, sputum, urine, stool WBC >10,000/mm^3, temp; baseline and during treatment
- Complete C&S testing before beginning drug therapy to identify if correct treatment has been initiated
- Assess for allergic reactions: rash, urticaria, pruritus, chills, fever, joint pain
- Identify urine output; if decreasing, notify prescriber (may indicate nephrotoxicity); also, obtain BUN, creatinine, urine CrCl (<80 ml/min) values; urinalysis daily for proteinuria, cells, casts; report sudden change in urine output
- Monitor blood studies: AST, ALT, CBC, Hct, bilirubin, LDH, alkaline phosphatase, Coombs' test monthly if patient is on long-term therapy
- Monitor electrolytes: potassium, sodium, chloride, magnesium monthly if patient is on long-term therapy
- Monitor for bleeding: ecchymosis, bleeding gums, hematuria, stool guaiac daily if patient is on long-term therapy
- Assess for overgrowth of infection: perineal itching, fever, malaise, redness, pain, swelling, drainage, rash, diarrhea, change in cough, sputum
- Obtain weight before treatment; calculation of dosage is usually based on ideal body weight, but may be calculated on actual body weight

T

- Monitor VS during inf, watch for hypotension, change in pulse
- Assess **IV** site for thrombophlebitis including pain, redness, swelling q30 min, change site if needed; apply warm compresses to discontinued site
- Obtain serum peak, drawn at 30-60 min after **IV** inf or 60 min after IM inj, trough level drawn just before next dose; peak 4-12 µg/ml, trough 1-2 µg/ml
- Monitor for deafness by audiometric testing, ringing, roaring in ears, vertigo; assess hearing before, during, after treatment
- Monitor for dehydration: high sp gr, decrease in skin turgor, dry mucous membranes, dark urine
- Monitor for overgrowth of infection including increased temp, malaise, redness, pain, swelling, perineal itching, diarrhea, stomatitis, change in cough, sputum

Nursing diagnoses

✓ Infection, risk for (uses)
✓ Diarrhea (adverse reactions)
✓ Injury, risk for (adverse reactions)
✓ Knowledge deficit (teaching)
✓ Noncompliance (teaching)

Implementation

IM route

- Give deeply in large muscle mass

IV **IV route**

- Give **IV** diluted in 50-100 ml of 0.9% NaCl, $D_{10}W$, D_5/0.9% NaCl, 0.9% NaCl, Ringer's, LR, D_5W (adult), infuse over 20-60 min
- Flush after inf with D_5W, 0.9% NaCl
- Separate aminoglycosides and penicillins by ≥1 hr

Syringe compatibilities:
Doxapram

Syringe incompatibilities:
Cefamandole, clindamycin, heparin, sargramostim

Y-site compatibilities:
Acyclovir, amifostine, amiodarone, amsacrine, aztreonam, ciprofloxacin, cyclophosphamide, diltiazem, enalaprilat, esmolol, filgrastim, fluconazole, fludarabine, foscarnet, furosemide, granisetron, hydromorphone, IL-2, insulin (regular), labetalol, magnesium sulfate, melphalan, meperidine, midazolam, morphine, perphenazine, tacrolimus, teniposide, theophylline, thiotepa, tolazoline, vinorelbine, zidovudine

Additive compatibilities:
Aztreonam, bleomycin, calcium gluconate, cefoxitin, ciprofloxacin, clindamycin, furosemide, metronidazole, ofloxacin, ranitidine, verapamil

Additive incompatibilities:
Cefamandole, floxacillin

Nebulizer route

- Give as close to q12h apart as possible; do not use <6 hr apart
- Do not mix with dornase alfa in the nebulizer

Patient/family education

Nebulizer

- Have patient inhale sitting or standing, breathe normally through the mouthpiece, may use nose clips
- Advise patient to use multiple therapies first, then tobramycin

Systemic route

- Teach patient to report sore throat, bruising, bleeding, joint pain; may indicate blood dyscrasias (rare)
- Advise patient to contact prescriber if vaginal itching, loose, foul-smelling stools, furry tongue occur; may indicate superinfection
- Advise patient to notify prescriber of diarrhea with blood or pus; may indicate pseudomembranous colitis

Evaluation

Positive therapeutic outcome

- Absence of signs/symptoms of infection (WBC <10,000/mm^3, temp WNL, absence of red, draining wounds)
- Reported improvement in symptoms of infection

Treatment of overdose:

Withdraw drug, hemodialysis, exchange transfusion in the newborn, monitor serum levels of drug, may give ticarcillin or carbenicillin

tocainide (℞)
(toe-kay'nide)
Tonocard
Func. class.: Antidysrhythmic (class IB)
Chem. class.: Lidocaine analog
Pregnancy category C

Action: Increases electrical stimulation threshold of ventricle, His-Purkinje system, which stabilizes cardiac membrane and decreases automaticity

➔ **Therapeutic Outcome:** Decreased ventricular dysrhythmia

Uses: Life-threatening ventricular dysrhythmias (multifocal/unifocal premature ventricular contractions [PVCs]), ventricular tachycardia

Dosage and routes
Adult: PO 400 mg q8h, may increase to 1.2-1.8 g/day in divided doses q8-12h

Available forms: Tabs 400, 600 mg

Adverse effects
CNS: *Headache, dizziness,* involuntary movement, confusion, psychosis, restlessness, irritability, paresthesias, tremors, **seizures**
CV: *Hypotension, bradycardia,* angina, PVCs, **heart block, CV collapse, cardiac arrest, CHF,** chest pain, tachycardia, prodysrhythmias
EENT: Tinnitus, blurred vision, hearing loss
GI: Nausea, vomiting, anorexia, diarrhea, hepatitis
HEMA: **Blood dyscrasias: leukopenia, agranulocytosis, hypoplastic anemia, thrombocytopenia**
INTEG: Rash, urticaria, edema, swelling
RESP: Dyspnea, **respiratory depression, pulmonary fibrosis**

Contraindications: Hypersensitivity to amides, severe heart block

Precautions: Pregnancy **C**, lactation, children, renal disease, liver disease, CHF, respiratory depression, myasthenia gravis, blood dyscrasias

Pharmacokinetics
Absorption	Well absorbed
Distribution	Widely distributed, crossed blood-brain barrier
Metabolism	Liver
Excretion	Kidney (up to 50% unchanged)
Half-life	10-17 hr

Pharmacodynamics
Onset	1 hr
Peak	½-2 hr
Duration	8-12 hr

Interactions
Individual drugs
Cimetidine: ↓ levels of tocainide
Digoxin: ↑ blood levels, ↑ toxicity
Disopyramide: ↑ levels, ↑ toxicity
Flecainide: ↑ levels, ↑ toxicity
Lidocaine: ↑ effect
Mexiletine: ↑ levels, ↑ toxicity
Phenytoin: ↑ blood levels
Procainamide: ↑ levels, ↑ toxicity
Quinidine: ↑ levels, ↑ toxicity
Rifampin: ↓ tocainide levels
Warfarin: ↑ levels, ↑ bleeding
Drug classifications
β-Adrenergic blockers: ↑ dysrhythmias, arrest
Calcium channel blockers: ↑ dysrhythmias, arrest
Herb/drug
Aloe: ↑ hypokalemia
Buckthorn: ↑ hypokalemia
Cascara sagrada: ↑ hypokalemia
Senna: ↑ hypokalemia
Lab test interferences
↑ CPK

T

NURSING CONSIDERATIONS

Assessment

- Assess for oxygenation or perfusion deficit: decreased B/P, chest pain, dizziness, loss of consciousness
- Assess respiratory status: auscultate lung fields for bibasilar crackles in patients with advanced CHF
- Assess for urinary retention: check for pain, abdominal absorption, palpate bladder; check males with benign prostatic hypertrophy; anticholinergic reaction may cause retention
- Monitor I&O ratio; electro- lytes: (potassium, sodium, chloride); watch for decreasing urinary output, possible retention
- Monitor liver function studies: AST, ALT, bilirubin, alkaline phosphatase
- Monitor ECG to determine drug effectiveness; measure PR, QRS, QT intervals; check for PVCs, other dysrhythmias; monitor B/P for hypotension, hypertension; for rebound hypertension after 1-2 hr
- Monitor patient for CNS symptoms: confusion, psychosis, numbness, depression, involuntary movements; if these occur, drug should be discontinued
- Assess pulmonary toxicity: dyspnea, fatigue, cough, fever, chest pain; drug should be discontinued if these occur
- Assess cardiac rate, respiration (rate, rhythm, character), chest pain, ventricular tachycardia, supraventricular tachycardia or fibrillation

Nursing diagnoses

✓ Cardiac output, decreased (uses)
✓ Impaired gas exchange (adverse reactions)
✓ Knowledge deficit (teaching)

Implementation

- Give with meals to decrease GI upset

Patient/family education

- Inform patient or family of reason for medication and expected results
- Teach patient method for taking pulse at home and what to report to prescriber
- Advise patient to avoid hazardous activities until drug response is known; dizziness, confusion, sedation may occur
- Advise patient to use a bracelet or other ID indicating medications taken, condition, and prescriber's name and phone number
- Instruct patient to report bleeding, bruising, respiratory symptoms, chills, fever, sore throat to prescriber

Evaluation

Positive therapeutic outcome

- Decreased dysrhythmias

Treatment of overdose: Defibrillation, vasopressor for hypotension

tolcapone (℞)

(toll'cah-pone)

Tasmar

Func. class.: Antiparkinson agent

Chem. class.: Catecholamine inhibitor (COMT)

Pregnancy category C

Action: Selective, reversible inhibitor of catecholamine; used as adjunct to levodopa/carbidopa therapy

➔ Therapeutic Outcome: Increased ability to move and speak

Uses: Parkinsonism

Dosage and routes

Adult: PO 100-200 mg tid, with levodopa/carbidopa therapy; max 600 mg/day; discontinue if no benefit in 3 wk

Renal dose

Adult: PO 100 mg tid or less

Available forms: Tabs 100, 200 mg

Adverse effects

CNS: Dystonia, dyskinesia, dreaming, *fatigue, headache, confusion,* psychosis, hallucination, dizziness

CV: ***Orthostatic hypotension,*** chest pain, hypotension
EENT: Cataract, eye inflammation
GI: ***Nausea, vomiting, abdominal distress,*** diarrhea, constipation, **fatal liver failure,** elevated LFTs
GU: UTI, urine discoloration, uterine tumor, micturition disorder, hematuria
HEMA: **Hemolytic anemia, leukopenia, agranulocytosis**
INTEG: Sweating, alopecia

Contraindications: Hypersensitivity, hepatic disease

Precautions: Renal disease, cardiac disease, hepatic disease, hypertension, pregnancy **C,** asthma, lactation

Pharmacokinetics

Absorption	Rapidly
Distribution	Protein binding 99%
Metabolism	Liver (extensively)
Excretion	Urine (60%), feces (40%)
Half-life	2-3 hr

Pharmacodynamics

Onset	Unknown
Peak	2 hr
Duration	Unknown

Interactions

Individual drugs

Apomorphine: May influence pharmacokinetics
Dobutamine: May influence pharmacokinetics
Isoproterenol: May influence pharmacokinetics
α-Methyldopa: May influence pharmacokinetics

Drug classifications

MAOIs: ↓ normal catecholamine metabolism; MAO-B inhibitor may be used

NURSING CONSIDERATIONS

Assessment

- Monitor liver function enzymes: AST, ALT, alkaline phosphatase, LDH, bilirubin, CBC
- Assess involuntary movements in parkinsonism: akinesia, tremors, staggering gait, muscle rigidity, drooling
- Monitor B/P, respiration during initial treatment; hypo/hypertension should be reported
- Monitor mental status: affect, mood, behavioral changes

Nursing diagnoses

✓ Physical mobility, impaired (uses)
✓ Injury, risk for (uses)
✓ Knowledge deficit (teaching)

Implementation

PO route

- Administer tid with levodopa/carbidopa therapy
- Provide assistance with ambulation during beginning therapy

Patient/family education

- Advise patient to change positions slowly to prevent orthostatic hypotension
- Advise patient that urine, sweat may change color
- Teach patient that food taken within 1 hr ac or 2 hr pc increases action of drug by 20%
- Teach patient to report nausea, vomiting, anorexia

Evaluation

Positive therapeutic outcome

- Decrease in akathisia, increased mood

tolmetin (℞)

(tole'met-in)

Tolectin, Tolectin DS, Tolectin 200, Tolectin 600, tolmetin sodium

Func. class.: Nonsteroidal antiinflammatory

Chem. class.: Pyrrole acetic acid derivative

Pregnancy category B

Action: Inhibits prostaglandin synthesis by decreasing an enzyme

T

needed for biosynthesis; analgesic, antiinflammatory, antipyretic

➔ **Therapeutic Outcome:** Decreased pain, inflammatory

Uses: Mild to moderate pain, osteoarthritis, rheumatoid arthritis

Dosage and routes

Adult: PO 400 mg tid-qid, max 2 g/day

P ***Child >2 yr:*** PO 15-30 mg/kg/day in 3 or 4 divided doses

Available forms: Caps 400 mg; tabs 200, 600 mg

Adverse effects

CNS: Dizziness, drowsiness, fatigue, tremors, confusion, insomnia, anxiety, depression, headache

CV: Tachycardia, peripheral edema, palpitations, dysrhythmias, hypertension

EENT: Tinnitus, hearing loss, blurred vision

GI: Nausea, anorexia, vomiting, diarrhea, jaundice, **cholestatic hepatitis,** constipation, flatulence, cramps, dry mouth, peptic ulcer, ulceration, bleeding, perforation

GU: **Nephrotoxicity: dysuria, hematuria, oliguria, azotemia, pseudoproteinuria**

HEMA: **Blood dyscrasias**

INTEG: Purpura, rash, pruritus, sweating

Contraindications: Hypersensitivity, asthma, severe renal disease, severe hepatic disease, ulcer disease

Precautions: Pregnancy **B**, lactation, children, bleeding disorders, GI disorders, cardiac disorders, hypersensitivity to other antiinflammatory agents, peptic ulcer disease

Pharmacokinetics

Absorption	Well absorbed
Distribution	Not known
Metabolism	Extensively
Excretion	Unchanged kidneys—20%
Half-life	3-3½ hr

Pharmacodynamics

Onset	Unknown
Peak	2 hr
Duration	Unknown

Interactions

Individual drugs

Acetaminophen (long-term use): ↑ renal reactions
Alcohol: ↑ adverse reactions
Aspirin: ↓ effectiveness, ↑ adverse reactions
Digoxin: ↑ toxicity, ↑ levels
Insulin: ↓ insulin effect
Lithium: ↑ toxicity
Methotrexate: ↑ toxicity
Phenytoin: ↑ toxicity
Probenecid: ↑ toxicity
Radiation: ↑ risk of hematologic toxicity
Sulfonylurea: ↑ toxicity

Drug classifications

Anticoagulants: ↑ risk of bleeding
Antihypertensives: ↓ effect of antihypertensives
Antineoplastics: ↑ risk of hematologic toxicity
β-Adrenergic blockers: ↑ antihypertension
Cephalosporins: ↑ risk of bleeding
Diuretics: ↓ effectiveness of diuretics
Glucocorticoids: ↑ adverse reactions
Hypoglycemics: ↓ hypoglycemic effect
NSAIDs: ↑ adverse reactions
Potassium supplements: ↑ adverse reactions
Sulfonamides: ↑ toxicity

Lab test interferences

↑ Serum potassium, ↑ liver function studies, ↑ BUN
False positive: Urine protein

NURSING CONSIDERATIONS

Assessment

- Monitor blood counts during therapy; watch for decreasing platelets; if low, therapy may need to be discontinued, restarted after

hematologic recovery; and for blood dyscrasia (thrombocytopenia): bruising, fatigue, bleeding, poor healing
- Assess for asthma, nasal polyps, or aspirin allergy; may indicate hypersensitivity to this product

Nursing diagnoses
- ✓ Pain (uses)
- ✓ Mobility, impaired physical (uses)
- ✓ Injury, risk for (adverse reactions)
- ✓ Knowledge deficit (teaching)

Implementation
- Administer with food or milk to decrease gastric symptoms; food will slow absorption slightly, but will not decrease absorption

Patient/family education
- Inform patient that drug must be continued for prescribed time to be effective; to avoid aspirin, alcoholic beverages
- Caution patient to report bleeding, bruising, fatigue, malaise because blood dyscrasias do occur
- Instruct patient to use caution when driving; drowsiness, dizziness may occur
- Teach patient to take with a full glass of water to enhance absorption; do not crush, break or chew

Evaluation
Positive therapeutic outcome
- Decreased pain
- Decreased inflammation
- Increased mobility

tolterodine (℞)
(tol-tehr'oh-deen)

Detrol

Func. class.: Overactive bladder product

Chem. class.: Muscarinic receptor antagonist

Pregnancy category C

Action: Relaxes smooth muscles in urinary tract by inhibiting acetylcholine at postganglionic sites

➔ **Therapeutic Outcome:** Decreased symptoms of overactive bladder

Uses: Overactive bladder, (frequency, urgency)

Dosage and routes
Adult: **PO** 2 mg bid, hepatic disease 1 mg bid; 4 mg qd, may decrease to 2 mg if needed

Available forms: Tabs 1, 2 mg; ext rel caps 2, 4 mg

Adverse effects
CNS: *Anxiety,* paresthesia, fatigue, *dizziness,* headache

CV: Chest pain, hypertension

EENT: Vision abnormalities, xerophthalmia

GI: *Nausea, vomiting, anorexia,* abdominal pain constipation, dry mouth, dyspepsia

GU: Dysuria, retention, frequency, UTI

INTEG: Rash, pruritis

RESP: Bronchitis, cough, pharyngitis, upper respiratory tract infection

Contraindications: Hypersensitivity, uncontrolled narrow-angle glaucoma, urinary retention, gastric retention

Precautions: Pregnancy **C**, lactation, children, renal/hepatic disease, controlled narrow-angle glaucoma

Pharmacokinetics	
Absorption	Rapidly
Distribution	Highly protein bound
Metabolism	Liver (extensively)
Excretion	Urine/feces
Half-life	Unknown

Pharmacodynamics	
Onset	Unknown
Peak	Unknown
Duration	Unknown

Interactions
Drug classifications

Antibiotics, macrolide: ↑ action of tolterodine

Antifungal agents: ↑ action of tolterodine

Food/drug

↑ Bioavailability of tolterodine

NURSING CONSIDERATIONS

Assessment

- Assess urinary patterns: distension, nocturia, frequency, urgency, incontinence
- Assess allergic reactions: rash; if this occurs, drug should be discontinued

Nursing diagnoses

- ✓ Urinary elimination, altered (uses)
- ✓ Incontinence, functional (uses)
- ✓ Knowledge deficit (teaching)
- ✓ Activity intolerance (uses)

Patient/family education

- Advise patient to avoid hazardous activities; dizziness may occur

Evaluation

Positive therapeutic outcome

- Decreased urinary frequency, urgency

topiramate (℞)

(to-pi-ra′mate)

Topamax

Func. class.: Anticonvulsant, misc

Chem. class.: Carbamate derivative

Pregnancy category C

Action: Mechanism of action unknown; may prevent seizure spread as opposed to an elevation of seizure threshold

➔ **Therapeutic Outcome:** Absence of seizures

Uses: Partial seizures, with or without generalization in adults; tonic-clonic seizures; seizures in Lennox-Gastaut syndrome

Investigational uses: Bipolar disorder, cluster headache, infantile spasms

Dosage and routes

Adjunctive therapy

Adult: PO add 400 mg in 2 divided doses

Renal dose

CrCl <70 ml/min ½ dose

Bipolar disorder (off-label)

Adult: PO 50-200 mg/day, max 400 mg/day

Available forms: Tabs 25, 100, 200 mg; sprinkle caps 15, 25, 50 mg

Adverse effects

CNS: Dizziness, fatigue, cognitive disorder, *insomnia,* anxiety, depression, paresthesia

EENT: Diplopia, vision abnormality

ENDO: Weight loss

GI: *Diarrhea, anorexia,* nausea, dyspepsia, abdominal pain, constipation, dry mouth

GU: Breast pain, dysmenorrhea, menstrual disorder

INTEG: Rash

MISC: Weight loss, leukopenia

RESP: Upper respiratory tract infection, pharyngitis, sinusitis

Contraindications: Hypersensitivity

Precautions: Hepatic disease, renal disease, cardiac disease, elderly (G), lactation, children (P), pregnancy **C**

Pharmacokinetics	
Absorption	Well absorbed
Distribution	Crosses placenta, plasma protein binding (9%-17%); steady state 4 days
Metabolism	Unknown
Excretion	Kidneys unchanged 55%-97%
Half-life	21 hr

Pharmacodynamics	
Onset	Unknown
Peak	2-4 hr
Duration	Unknown

Interactions
Individual drugs
Alcohol: ↑ levels of alcohol
Carbamazepine: ↓ levels of topiramate
Digoxin: ↓ levels of digoxin
Phenytoin: ↓ levels of topiramate
Valproic acid: ↓ levels of topiramate
Drug classifications
Carbonic anhydrase inhibitors: ↑ levels of carbonic anhydrase inhibitors
CNS depressants: ↑ CNS depression
Oral contraceptives: ↓ level of oral contraceptives
Food/drug
↓ Levels of topiramate

NURSING CONSIDERATIONS
Assessment
- Assess mental status: mood, sensorium, affect, memory (long, short), G especially in elderly
- Assess for blood dyscrasias: fever, sore throat, bruising, rash, jaundice, epistaxis (long-term treatment only)
- Assess seizure activity including type, location, duration, and character; provide seizure precaution
- Monitor CBC during long-term therapy
- Assess body weight and evidence of cognitive disorder

Nursing diagnoses
✓ Injury, risk for (side effects)
✓ Knowledge deficit (teaching)

Implementation
- May take with food
- Do not crush, or break tabs; very bitter
- Sprinkle cap can be given whole or opened and sprinkled on soft food; do not chew

Patient/family education
- Teach patient to carry ID stating name, drugs taken, condition, prescriber's name and phone number
- Advise patient to avoid driving, other activities that require alertness
- Teach patient not to discontinue medication abruptly after long-term use

Evaluation
Positive therapeutic outcome
- Decreased seizure activity

Treatment of overdose:
Lavage, VS

HIGH ALERT

topotecan (℞)
(to-poe′ti-kan)
Hycamtin
Func. class: Antineoplastic hormone
Chem. class: Semi-synthetic derivative of camptothecin (topoisomerase inhibitor)

Pregnancy category D

Action: Antitumor drug with topoisomerase I–inhibitory activity; topoisomerase I relieves torsional strain in DNA by causing single-strand breaks; causes double-strand DNA damage

➔ **Therapeutic Outcome:** Decreased tumor size

Uses: Metastatic carcinoma of the ovary after failure of traditional chemotherapy

Dosage and routes
Adult: **IV** inf 1.5 mg/m^2 over 30 min qd × 5 days starting on day 1 of a 2-day course × 4 courses; may be reduced to 0.25 mg/m^2 for subsequent courses if severe neutropenia occurs

Renal dose
Adult: **IV** CrCl 20-39 ml/min 0.75 mg/m^2/day × 5 days on day 1 of a 21-day course

Available forms: Lyophilized powder for inj 4 mg

Adverse effects
CNS: Arthralgia, asthenia, headache, myalgia, pain
GI: Abdominal pain, constipation,

T

diarrhea, obstruction, nausea, stomatitis, vomiting, increased ALT, AST, anorexia
HEMA: **Neutropenia, leukopenia, thrombocytopenia, anemia, sepsis**
INTEG: Total alopecia
RESP: Dyspnea

Contraindications: Hypersensitivity, lactation, severe bone marrow depression, pregnancy **D**

P **Precautions:** Children

Pharmacokinetics

Absorption	Rapidly/completely
Distribution	Unknown
Metabolism	Liver
Excretion	Urine, feces to metabolites
Half-life	8 hr

Pharmacodynamics

Unknown

Interactions
Individual drugs
Cisplatin: ↑ myelosuppression
Granulocyte colony-stimulating factor: ↑ duration of neutropenia

NURSING CONSIDERATIONS
Assessment
- Monitor liver function studies: AST, ALT, alkaline phosphatase, which may be elevated
- Monitor for CNS symptoms: drowsiness, confusion, depression, anxiety
- Monitor CBC, differential, platelet count weekly; withhold drug if WBC is <3500/mm^3 or platelet count is <100,000/mm^3; notify prescriber of these results; drug should be discontinued
- Assess buccal cavity q8h for dryness, sores or ulceration, white patches, oral pain, bleeding, dysphagia
- Assess GI symptoms: frequency of stools, cramping
- Assess signs of dehydration: rapid respiration, poor skin turgor, decreased urine output, dry skin, restlessness, weakness

Nursing diagnoses
- ✓ Infection, risk for (adverse reactions)
- ✓ Knowledge deficit (teaching)

Implementation
- Provide increased fluid intake to 2-3 L/day to prevent dehydration, unless contraindicated
- Change **IV** site q48h
- Rinse mouth tid-qid with water, club soda; brush teeth bid-tid with soft brush or cotton-tipped applicator for stomatitis; use unwaxed dental floss
- Provide nutritious diet with iron, vit K supplements, low fiber, few dairy products

Patient/family education
- Advise patient to avoid foods with citric acid or hot or rough texture if stomatitis is present; to drink adequate fluids
- Advise patient to report stomatitis; any bleeding, white spots, ulcerations in mouth; tell patient to examine mouth qd; report symptoms
- Assess patient to report signs of anemia; fatigue, headache, faintness, shortness of breath, irritability
- Teach patient to use contraception during therapy

Evaluation
Positive therapeutic outcome
- Decreased tumor size, spread of malignancy

toremifene (℞)
(tore′me-feen)
Fareston
Func. class.: Antineoplastic
Chem. class.: Antiestrogen hormone
Pregnancy category D

Action: Inhibits cell division by binding to cytoplasmic estrogen receptors; resembles normal cell complex but inhibits DNA synthesis and estrogen response of target tissue

Therapeutic Outcome: Prevention of rapidly growing malignant cells

Uses: Advanced breast carcinoma that has not responded to other therapy in estrogen-receptor-positive patients (usually postmenopausal)

Dosage and routes

Adult: PO 60 mg qd

Available forms: Tabs 60 mg

Adverse effects

CNS: *Hot flashes, headache, lightheadedness,* depression

CV: Chest pain, **CHF, MI, pulmonary embolism**

EENT: Ocular lesions, retinopathy, corneal opacity, blurred vision (high doses)

GI: *Nausea, vomiting,* altered taste (anorexia)

GU: Vaginal bleeding, pruritus vulvae

HEMA: **Thrombocytopenia, leukopenia**

INTEG: *Rash,* alopecia

META: Hypercalcemia

Contraindications: Hypersensitivity, pregnancy **D**

Precautions: Leukopenia, thrombocytopenia, lactation, cataracts

Pharmacokinetics	
Absorption	Adequately absorbed
Distribution	Unknown
Metabolism	Liver, extensively
Excretion	Feces, slowly, small amounts (kidneys)
Half-life	Unknown

Pharmacodynamics	
Onset	Unknown
Peak	3 hr
Duration	Unknown

Interactions

Individual drugs

Warfarin: ↑ warfarin effect

Lab test interferences

↑ Serum Ca

NURSING CONSIDERATIONS

Assessment

- Monitor CBC, differential, platelet count weekly; withhold drug if WBC is <4000/mm³ or platelet count is <75,000/mm³; notify prescriber of results; monitor calcium levels (hypercalcemia is common)
- Assess for tumor flare: increase in bone, tumor pain during beginning treatment; give analgesics as ordered to decrease pain
- Assess for bleeding: hematuria, guaiac, bruising or petechiae, mucosa or orifices q8h, no rectal temp

Nursing diagnoses

✓ Injury, risk for (adverse reactions)

✓ Knowledge deficit (teaching)

Implementation

- Give with food or fluids to decrease GI upset; do not break, crush, or chew enteric products; repeat dose may be needed if vomiting occurs
- Store in light-resistant container at room temp

Patient/family education

- Instruct patient to report any complaints, side effects to prescriber; if dose is missed, do not double next dose
- Advise patient that vaginal bleeding, pruritus, hot flashes, can occur, and are reversible after discontinuing treatment
- Instruct patient to report immediately decreased visual acuity, which may be irreversible; stress need for routine eye exams
- Inform patient about who should be told about toremifene therapy
- Advise patient to report vaginal bleeding immediately; that tumor flare (increase in size or tumor, increased bone pain) may occur and will subside rapidly; may take analgesics for pain; that premenopausal women must use mechanical birth control method because ovulation may be induced (teratogenic drug)
- Caution patient to use sunscreen

T

and protective clothing to prevent burns because photosensitivity is common
- Teach patient that hair loss may occur during treatment; a wig or hairpiece may make patient feel better; new hair may be different in color, texture
- Inform patient rash or lesions are temporary and may become large during beginning therapy

Evaluation

Positive therapeutic outcome
- Decreased spread of malignant cells in breast cancer

trace elements (chromium, copper, iodide, manganese, selenium, zinc) (℞)

Concentrated Multiple Trace Elements, ConTE-PAK-4, M.T.E.-4 Concentrated, M.T.E.-5, M.T.E.-5 Concentrated, M.T.E.-6, M.T.E.-6 Concentrated, M.T.E.-7, MulTE-PAK-4, MulTE-PAK-5, Multiple Trace Element, Multiple Trace Element Neonatal, Multiple Trace Element Pediatric, Neotrace 4, Ped TE-PAK-4, Pedtrice-4, P.T.E.-4, P.T.E.-5

Func. class.: Mineral supplement

Pregnancy category C

Action: Needed for adequate absorption and synthesis of amino acids

➔ **Therapeutic Outcome:** Replacement for mineral deficiencies

Uses: Prevention of trace element deficiency, a component of TPN

Dosage and routes

Usual dosage may be given in TPN sol

Chromium
Adult: **IV** 10-15 μg qd
P ***Child:*** **IV** 0.14-0.20 μg/ kg/day

Copper
Adult: **IV** 0.5-1.5 mg/day
P ***Child:*** **IV** .05-0.2 mg/kg/day

Iodide
Adult: **IV** 1 μg/kg/day

Manganese
Adult: **IV** 1-3 mg/day

Selenium
Adult: 40-120 μg/day
P ***Child:*** 3 μg/kg/day

Zinc
Adult: **IV** 2-4 mg/day
P ***Child:*** **IV** 0.05 mg/kg/day

Available forms: Many forms available; see particular elements

Adverse effects

CHROMIUM: **Seizures, coma,** nausea, vomiting, ulcers, **renal/hepatic toxicity**
COPPER: Personality changes, diarrhea, weakness, photophobia, muscle weakness
IODINE: Headache, edema of eyelids, acne, metallic taste, sore mouth, running nose
MANGANESE: Incoordination, headache, irritability, lability, slurred speech, impotence
SELENIUM: Alopecia, depression, vomiting, GI cramping, nervousness, garlic smell
ZINC: Vomiting, oliguria, **hypothermia,** vision changes, **tachycardia,** jaundice, **coma**

Precautions: Liver, biliary disease, pregnancy **C,** lactation, severe vomiting or diarrhea

Pharmacokinetics

Absorption	Completely absorbed
Distribution	Widely distributed
Metabolism	Unknown
Excretion	Depends on element
Half-life	Unknown

Pharmacodynamics

Unknown

Interactions: None

NURSING CONSIDERATIONS

Assessment

- Assess trace element levels; notify prescriber if low copper 0.07-0.15 mg/ml, zinc 0.05-0.15 mg/100 ml, manganese 4-20 µg/100 ml, selenium 0.1-0.19 µg/ml
- Assess trace element deficiency if patient is receiving TPN for extended period
- Obtain calorie count to identify nutritional deficiencies
- Assess for toxicity to individual element (see Adverse effects)

Nursing diagnoses

✓ Nutrition: less than body requirements (uses)
✓ Knowledge deficit (teaching)

Implementation

- Give by **IV** inf, often mixed with TPN sol
- Discard unused portions
- Give by continuous inf diluted in 1 L or more **IV** sol; give at prescribed rate

Patient/family education

- Explain reason for and expected results of medication

Evaluation

Positive therapeutic outcome

- Absence of element deficiency

tramadol (℞)

(trah'mah-dol)

Ultram

Func. class.: Central analgesic

Pregnancy category C

Action: Not completely understood, binds to opioid receptors and inhibits reuptake of norepinephrine, serotonin; does not cause histamine release or affect heart rate

Therapeutic Outcome: Relief of pain

Uses: Management of moderate to severe pain

Dosage and routes

Adult: PO 50-100 mg prn q4-6h, max 400 mg/day

G ***Elderly >75 yr:*** PO <300 mg/day in divided dose

Hepatic dose

PO 50 mg q12h

Renal dose

CrCl <30 ml/min q12h, max 200 mg/day

Available forms: Tabs 50 mg

Adverse effects

CNS: Dizziness, CNS stimulation, somnolence, headache, anxiety, confusion, euphoria, **seizures,** hallucinations

CV: Vasodilation, orthostatic hypotension, tachycardia, hypertension, abnormal ECG

GI: Nausea, constipation, vomiting, dry mouth, diarrhea, abdominal pain, anorexia, flatulence, GI bleeding

GU: Urinary retention/frequency, menopausal symptoms, dysuria, menstrual disorder

INTEG: Pruritus, rash, urticaria, vesicles

Contraindications: Hypersensitivity, acute intoxication with any CNS depressant

Precautions: Seizure disorder, P pregnancy **C**, lactation, children, G elderly, renal, hepatic disease, respiratory depression, head trauma, increased ICP, acute abdominal condition, drug abuse

Do Not Confuse:
tramadol/Toradol

T

Pharmacokinetics

Absorption	Rapidly, almost completely absorbed
Distribution	Steady state 2 days
Metabolism	Extensively in liver, may cross blood-brain barrier
Excretion	Unchanged drug 30% in urine
Half-life	Unknown

Pharmacodynamics

Unknown

Interactions

Individual drugs

Carbamazepine: ↓ of tramadol

Drug classifications

MAOIs: Inhibition of norepinephrine and serotonin reuptake; use together with caution

Sedative/hypnotics: ↑ CNS depression

Herb/drug

Kava: ↑ CNS depression

Lab test interferences

↑ Creatinine, ↑ liver enzymes

↓ Hgb

NURSING CONSIDERATIONS

Assessment

- Assess pain: location, type, character; give before pain becomes extreme
- Monitor I&O ratio: check for decreasing output; may indicate urinary retention
- Assess need for drug
- Assess for constipation and bowel pattern; increase fluids, bulk in diet
- Monitor CNS changes: dizziness, drowsiness, hallucinations, euphoria, LOC, pupil reaction
- Determine allergic reactions: rash, urticaria

Nursing diagnoses

- ✓ Pain (uses)
- ✓ Sensory, perceptual alteration: visual, auditory (adverse reactions)
- ✓ Injury, risk for (adverse reactions)
- ✓ Knowledge deficit (teaching)

Implementation

- Give with antiemetic for nausea, vomiting
- Administer when pain is beginning to return; determine dosage interval by patient response
- Store in cool environment, protect from sunlight

Patient/family education

- Teach patient to report any symptoms of CNS changes, allergic reactions
- Teach patient that drowsiness, dizziness, and confusion may occur; to call for assistance
- Instruct patient to make position changes slowly; orthostatic hypotension may occur
- Tell patient to avoid OTC medication and alcohol unless approved by prescriber

Evaluation

Positive therapeutic outcome

- Decreased pain

trandolapril (℞)

(tran-doe'la-prill)

Mavik

Func. class.: Antihypertensive

Chem. class.: Angiotensin-converting enzyme (ACE) inhibitor

Pregnancy category
D (2nd/3rd trimesters); C (1st trimester)

Action: Selectively suppresses renin-angiotensin-aldosterone system; inhibits ACE; prevents conversion of angiotensin I to angiotensin II, resulting in dilatation of arterial and venous vessels and lowered B/P

Therapeutic Outcome: Decreased B/P in hypertension

Uses: Hypertension alone or in combination, heart failure, after MI/left ventricular dysfunction after MI

Dosage and routes

Hypertension

Adult: PO 1 mg/day, 2 mg/day in African Americans, make dosage adjustment ≥wk; up to 8 mg/day

Heart failure (after MI/left ventricular dysfunction)

Adult: PO 1 mg/day, titrate upward to 4 mg/day if tolerated

Renal dose

CrCl <30 ml/min 0.5 mg/day, may increase gradually up to 4 mg/day

Available forms: Tabs 1, 2, 4 mg

Adverse effects

CNS: *Dizziness,* paresthesias, headache, fatigue, drowsiness, depression, sleep disturbances

CV: *Hypotension,* MI, palpitations, angina, TIAs, stroke, bradycardia, dysrhythmias

GI: Nausea, vomiting, cramps, diarrhea, constipation, ileus, pancreatitis, hepatitis, *dyspepsia*

GU: **Proteinuria, renal failure**

HEMA: **Agranulocytosis, neutropenia, leukopenia,** anemia

INTEG: Rash, purpura

MISC: Hyperkalemia, hyponatremia, impotence, *myalgia*

RESP: Dyspnea, cough

Contraindications: Hypersensitivity, history of angioedema, pregnancy **D** (2nd/3rd trimesters)

Precautions: Renal disease, hyperkalemia, hepatic disease, bilateral renal stenosis, post kidney transplant, aortal/mitral valve stenosis, cirrhosis, severe renal disease, untreated CHF, autoimmune diseases, severe hypertension, pregnancy **C** (1st trimester)

Pharmacokinetics

Absorption	40-60%
Distribution	Unknown
Metabolism	Liver
Excretion	Kidneys, feces
Half-life	0.6-1.1 hr, 16-24 hr

Pharmacodynamics

Onset	½ hr
Peak	4-10 hr
Duration	>8 days

Interactions

Individual drugs

Alcohol: ↑ hypotension (large amounts)
Allopurinol: ↑ hypersensitivity
Capsaicin: ↑ coughing
Digoxin: ↑ serum levels of digoxin
Hydralazine: ↑ toxicity
Indomethacin: ↓ antihypertensive effect
Lithium: ↑ serum levels of lithium
Prazosin: ↑ toxicity

Drug classifications

Adrenergic blockers: ↑ hypotension
Antacids: ↓ absorption
Antihypertensives: ↑ hypotension
Diuretics: ↑ hypotension
Diuretics, potassium-sparing: ↑ toxicity
Ganglionic blockers: ↑ hypotension
Phenothiazines: ↑ antihypertensive effects
Potassium supplements: ↑ toxicity of potassium
Sympathomimetics: ↑ toxicity

NURSING CONSIDERATIONS

Assessment

- Monitor blood studies: neutrophils, decreased platelets
- Monitor B/P, orthostatic hypotension, syncope; if changes occur dosage change may be required
- Monitor renal studies: protein, BUN, creatinine; increased levels may indicate nephrotic syndrome and renal failure
- Monitor renal symptoms: polyuria, oliguria, frequency, dysuria
- Establish baselines in renal, liver function tests before therapy begins
- Check potassium levels throughout treatment, although hyperkalemia rarely occurs
- Check for edema in feet, legs daily

T

• Assess for allergic reactions: rash, fever, pruritus, urticaria; drug should be discontinued if antihistamines fail to help

Nursing diagnoses

- ✓ Cardiac output, decreased (uses)
- ✓ Injury, potential for (adverse reactions)
- ✓ Knowledge deficit (teaching)
- ✓ Noncompliance (teaching)

Implementation

• Store in airtight container at 86° F (36° C) or less

Patient/family education

• Advise patient not to discontinue drug abruptly; advise patient to tell all persons associated with health care

• Teach patient not to use OTC products (cough, cold, allergy medications) unless directed by physician; serious side effects can occur; xanthines, such as coffee, tea, chocolate, cola, can prevent action of drug

• Instruct patient on the importance of complying with dosage schedule, even if feeling better; to continue with medical regimen to decrease B/P: exercise, cessation of smoking, decreasing stress, diet modifications

• Emphasize the need to rise slowly to sitting or standing position to minimize orthostatic hypotension; not to exercise in hot weather, which can cause increased hypotension

• Advise patient to notify prescriber of mouth sores, sore throat, fever, swelling of hands or feet, irregular heartbeat, chest pain, coughing, shortness of breath

• Caution patient to report excessive perspiration, dehydration, vomiting, diarrhea; may lead to fall in B/P

• Caution patient that drug may cause dizziness, fainting, light-headedness; may occur during 1st few days of therapy; to avoid activities that may be hazardous

• Teach patient how to take B/P, and normal readings for age group

Evaluation

Positive therapeutic outcome

• Decreased B/P in hypertension

Treatment of overdose:

Lavage, **IV** atropine for bradycardia, **IV** theophylline for bronchospasm, digitalis, O_2, diuretic for cardiac failure, hemodialysis

tranylcypromine (℞)

(tran-ill-sip'roe-meen)

Parnate

Func. class: Antidepressant—MAOI

Chem. class: Nonhydrazine

Pregnancy category C

Action: Increases concentrations of endogenous epinephrine, norepinephrine, serotonin, dopamine in storage sites in CNS by inhibition of MAO; increased concentration reduces depression

→ **Therapeutic Outcome:** Decreased symptoms of depression after 2-3 wk

Uses: Depression, when uncontrolled by other means

Investigational uses: Bulimia, cocaine addiction, migraines, seasonal affective disorder, panic disorder

Dosages and routes

Adult: PO 10 mg bid; may increase to 30 mg/ day after 2 wk

Available forms: Tabs 10 mg

Adverse effects

CNS: *Dizziness, drowsiness,* confusion, headache, anxiety, tremors, stimulation, weakness, hyperreflexia, mania, insomnia, fatigue, weight gain

CV: *Orthostatic hypotension, hypertension,* **dysrhythmias, hypertensive crisis**

EENT: Blurred vision

ENDO: **Syndrome of inappropriate antidiuretic hormone-like symptoms**

GI: Constipation, dry mouth, nausea,

vomiting, *anorexia,* diarrhea, weight gain
GU: Change in libido, frequency
HEMA: Anemia
INTEG: Rash, flushing, increased perspiration

Contraindications: Hypersensitivity to MAOIs, elderly, hypertension, CHF, severe hepatic disease, pheochromocytoma, severe renal disease, severe cardiac disease

Precautions: Suicidal patients, convulsive disorders, severe depression, schizophrenia, hyperactivity, diabetes mellitus, pregnancy **C**

Pharmacokinetics

Absorption	Well absorbed
Distribution	Crosses placenta
Metabolism	Liver, extensively
Excretion	Kidneys, breast milk
Half-life	Unknown

Pharmacodynamics

Unknown

Interactions

Individual drugs
Alcohol: ↑ CNS depression
Buspirone: ↑ pressor effect
Dextromethorphan: ↑ hypertensive crisis
Fluoxetine: Serotonin syndrome, do not use together
Fluvoxame: Serotonin syndrome, do not use together
Guanethidine: ↓ hypertensive crisis
Methylphenidate: ↑ hypertensive crisis
Paroxetine: Serotonin syndrome, do not use together
Sertraline: Serotonin syndrome, do not use together
Sumatriptan: ↑ effects
Drug classifications
Antidepressants, tricyclic: ↑ hypertensive crisis
Antidiabetics: ↑ effects
Antihypertensives: ↑ hypotension
β-Adrenergic blockers: ↑ effects
Diuretics, thiazide: ↑ effects
Opiates: ↑ CNS depression
Rauwolfia alkaloids: ↑ effects
Sulfonamides: ↑ effects
Food/drug
Foods containing tyramine: ↑ hypertensive crisis
Herb/drug
Ephedra: ↑ sympathomimetic action
L-Tryptophan: ↑ effects

NURSING CONSIDERATIONS

Assessment

- Monitor B/P (lying, standing), pulse q4h; if systolic B/P drops 20 mm Hg hold drug, notify prescriber; take vital signs q4h in patients with CV disease
- Monitor hepatic studies: AST, ALT, bilirubin
- Check weight qwk; appetite may increase with drug
- Assess mental status: mood, sensorium, affect, suicidal tendencies; increase in psychiatric symptoms: depression, panic
- Monitor urinary retention, constipation; constipation is more likely to occur in children or elderly
- Assess for withdrawal symptoms: headache, nausea, vomiting, muscle pain, weakness; do not usually occur unless drug was discontinued abruptly
- Identify alcohol consumption; if alcohol is consumed, hold dose until AM

Nursing diagnoses

- ✓ Coping, ineffective individual (uses)
- ✓ Injury, risk for (side effects)
- ✓ Knowledge deficit (teaching)
- ✓ Noncompliance (teaching)

Implementation

- Give with food or milk for GI symptoms; crush if patient is unable to swallow medication whole
- Store at room temp; do not freeze

Patient/family education

- Advise patient that therapeutic effects may take 48 hr-3 wk
- Teach patient to use caution in driving or other activities requiring

alertness because of drowsiness, dizziness, blurred vision; to avoid rising quickly from sitting to standing, G especially elderly
- Caution patient to avoid alcohol ingestion, other CNS depressants
- Advise patient not to discontinue medication quickly after long-term use: may cause nausea, headache, malaise
- Advise patient to increase fluids, bulk in diet if constipation, urinary G retention occur, especially elderly
- Teach patient to take gum, hard sugarless candy, or frequent sips of water for dry mouth
- Teach patient to avoid high-tyramine foods; cheese (aged), sour cream, beer, wine, pickled products, liver, raisins, bananas, figs, avocados, meat tenderizers, chocolate, yogurt; increased caffeine, ginseng
- Teach patient to report headache, palpitation, neck stiffness
- Instruct patient to wear or carry ID with medications taken, condition treated, and prescriber's name and phone number

Evaluation

Positive therapeutic outcome
- Decrease in depression
- Absence of suicidal thoughts

Treatment of overdose: Lavage, activated charcoal, monitor electrolytes, VS, diazepam **IV**, $NaHCO_3$

HIGH ALERT

trastuzumab (℞)

(tras-tuz'uh-mab)

Herceptin

Func. class.: Miscellaneous antineoplastic

Chem. class.: Humanized monoclonal antibody

Pregnancy category B

Action: DNA-derived monoclonal antibody selectively binds to extracellular portion of human epidermal growth factor receptor 2 (HER2); it inhibits proliferation of cancer cells

➔ **Therapeutic Outcome:** Decreasing symptoms of breast cancer

Uses: Breast cancer; metastatic with overexpression of HER2

Dosage and routes

Adult: **IV** 4 mg/kg given over 90 min, then maintenance 2 mg/kg given over 30 min; do not give as **IV** push or bol

Available forms: Lyophilized powder 440 mg

Adverse effects

CNS: *Dizziness, numbness, paresthesias,* depression, insomnia, neuropathy, peripheral neuritis

CV: **Tachycardia, CHF**

GI: Nausea, vomiting, anorexia, diarrhea

HEMA: Anemia, **leukopenia**

INTEG: *Rash,* acne, herpes simplex

META: Edema, peripheral edema

MISC: *Flulike syndrome; fever, headache, chills*

MS: Arthralgia, bone pain

RESP: Cough, dyspnea, pharyngitis, rhinitis, sinusitis

SYST: **Anaphylaxis, angioedema**

Contraindications: Hypersensitivity to this drug, Chinese hamster ovary cell protein

P G **Precautions:** Pregnancy **B**, lactation, children, elderly, cardiac disease, anemia, leukopenia

Pharmacokinetics	
Absorption	Unknown
Distribution	Unknown
Metabolism	Unknown
Excretion	Unknown
Half-life	1.7-12 days

Pharmacodynamics	
Onset	Unknown
Peak	Unknown
Duration	Unknown

Interactions
Individual drugs
Cyclophosphamide: ↑ cardiomyopathy risk

Drug classifications
↑ cardiomyopathy risk

NURSING CONSIDERATIONS
Assessment
- Assess for symptoms of infection; may be masked by drug
- Assess CNS reaction: LOC, mental status, dizziness, confusion
- Assess for CHF and other cardiac symptoms: dyspnea, coughing, gallop; obtain a full cardiac workup including ECG, echocardiogram, multigated angiogram
- Assess for hypersensitivity reactions, anaphylaxis
- Monitor for potentially fatal infusion reactions: fever, chills, nausea, vomiting, pain, headache, dizziness, hypotension; discontinue drug

Nursing diagnoses
✓ Infection, risk for (side effects)
✓ Nutrition, altered, less than body requirements (side effects)
✓ Knowledge deficit (teaching)

Implementation
- Give acetaminophen as ordered to alleviate fever and headache
- Increase fluid intake to 2-3 L/day

IV **IV route**
- Administer after reconstituting vial with 20 ml of bacteriostatic water for inj, 1.1% benzyl alcohol preserved (supplied) to yield 21 mg/ml, mark date on vial 28 days from reconstitution date, if patient is allergic to benzyl alcohol, reconstitute with sterile water for inj; use immediately
- Do not mix or dilute with other drugs or dextrose sol

Patient/family education
- Advise patient to take acetaminophen for fever
- Teach patient to avoid hazardous tasks, since confusion, dizziness may occur
- Teach patient to report signs of infection: sore throat, fever, diarrhea, vomiting
- Inform patient that emotional lability is common; instruct patient to notify prescriber if severe or incapacitating

Evaluation
Positive therapeutic outcome
- Decrease in size of tumors

trazodone (℞)
(tray'zoe-done)
Desyrel, Desyrel Dividose, trazodone HCl, Trazon, Trialodine
Func. class.: Antidepressant, miscellaneous
Chem. class.: Triazolopyridine
Pregnancy category C

Action: Selectively inhibits serotonin uptake by brain, potentiates behavioral changes

➔ **Therapeutic Outcome:** Decreased symptoms of depression after 2-3 wk

Uses: Depression

Investigational uses: Chronic pain syndromes

Dosage and routes:
Adult: PO 150 mg/day in divided doses; may increase by 50 mg/day q3-4d, not to exceed 600 mg/day

G ***Elderly:*** PO 25-50 hs, increase by 25-50 mg q3-7 days, to desired dose

P ***Child 16-18 yr:*** PO 1.5-2 mg/kg/day in divided doses, may increase q3-4 days up to 6 mg/kg/day

Available forms: Tabs 50, 100, 150, 300 mg

Adverse effects
CNS: Dizziness, drowsiness, confusion, headache, anxiety, tremors, stimulation, weakness, insomnia, G nightmares, EPS (elderly), increase in psychiatric symptoms
CV: Orthostatic hypotension, ECG changes, tachycardia, **hypertension,** palpitations
EENT: Blurred vision, tinnitus, mydriasis
GI: Diarrhea, dry mouth, nausea, vomiting, **paralytic ileus,** increased appetite, cramps, epigastric distress, jaundice, **hepatitis,** stomatitis
GU: Retention, **acute renal failure, priapism**
HEMA: **Agranulocytosis, thrombocytopenia, eosinophilia, leukopenia**
INTEG: Rash, urticaria, sweating, pruritus, photosensitivity

Contraindications: Hypersensitivity to tricyclic antidepressants, recovery phase of MI, seizure disorders, prostatic hypertrophy

Precautions: Suicidal patients, severe depression, increased intraocular pressure, narrow-angle glaucoma, urinary retention, cardiac disease, hepatic disease, hyperthyroidism, electroshock therapy, elective surgery, pregnancy **C**

Pharmacokinetics	
Absorption	Well absorbed
Distribution	Widely distributed
Metabolism	Liver, extensively
Excretion	Kidneys—unchanged minimally
Half-life	4½-7½ hr

Pharmacodynamics
Unknown

Interactions
Individual drugs
Alcohol: ↑ CNS depression
Cimetidine: ↑ levels, ↑ toxicity
Clonidine: Severe hypotension, avoid use
Disulfiram: Organic brain syndrome
Fluoxetine: ↑ levels, ↑ toxicity
Guanethidine: ↓ effects
Drug classifications
Analgesics: ↑ CNS depression
Anticholinergics: ↑ side effects
Antihistamines: ↑ CNS depression
Antihypertensives: may block antihypertensive effect
Barbiturates: ↑ effects
Benzodiazepines: ↑ effects
CNS depressants: ↑ effects
MAOIs: ↑ hypertensive crisis, convulsions
Oral contraceptives: effects, toxicity
Phenothiazines: ↑ toxicity
Sedative/hypnotics: ↑ CNS depression
Sympathomimetics, indirect-acting: ↓ effects
Smoking
↑ Metabolism, ↓ effects
Herb/drug
Kava: ↑ CNS depression
Lab test interferences
↑ Serum bilirubin, ↑ blood glucose, ↑ alkaline phosphatase
↓ VMA, ↓ 5-HIAA, ↓ blood glucose
False: ↑ urinary catecholamines

NURSING CONSIDERATIONS

Assessment

- Assess for pain: location, duration, intensity before and 1-2 hr after medication
- Monitor B/P (lying, standing), pulse q4h; if systolic B/P drops 20 mm Hg hold drug, notify prescriber; take vital signs q4h in patients with CV disease
- Monitor blood studies: CBC, leukocytes, differential, cardiac enzymes if patient is receiving long-term therapy
- Monitor hepatic function studies: AST, ALT, bilirubin
- Check weight qwk; appetite may increase with drug
- Assess ECG for flattening of T wave, bundle branch block, AV block, dysrhythmias in cardiac patients
- G Assess for EPS primarily in elderly: rigidity, dystonia, akathisia
- Assess mental status: mood, sensorium, affect, suicidal tendencies; increase in psychiatric symptoms: depression, panic
- Monitor urinary retention, P constipation; constipation is more G likely to occur in children or elderly
- Assess for withdrawal symptoms: headache, nausea, vomiting, muscle pain, weakness; do not usually occur unless drug was discontinued abruptly
- Identify alcohol consumption; if alcohol is consumed, hold dose until AM

Nursing diagnoses

✓ Coping, ineffective individual (uses)
✓ Injury, risk for (adverse reactions)
✓ Knowledge deficit (teaching)
✓ Noncompliance (teaching)

Implementation

- Give with food or milk for GI symptoms; crush if patient is unable to swallow medication whole
- Give dosage hs if oversedation occurs during day; may take entire G dose hs; elderly may not tolerate once/day dosing
- Store at room temp; do not freeze

Patient/family education

- Teach patient that therapeutic effects may take 2-3 wk
- Teach patient to use caution in driving or other activities requiring alertness because of drowsiness, dizziness, blurred vision; to avoid rising quickly from sitting to standing, G especially elderly
- Caution patient to avoid alcohol ingestion, other CNS depressants
- Teach patient not to discontinue medication quickly after long-term use: may cause nausea, headache, malaise
- Advise patient to wear sunscreen or large hat because photosensitivity occurs
- Teach patient to increase fluids, bulk in diet if constipation, urinary G retention occur, especially elderly
- Advise patient to take gum, hard sugarless candy, or frequent sips of water for dry mouth
- Teach family to watch for suicidal ideation or tendencies

Evaluation

Positive therapeutic outcome

- Decrease in depression
- Absence of suicidal thoughts

Treatment of overdose: ECG monitoring, induce emesis, lavage, activated charcoal, administer anticonvulsant

tretinoin (vitamin A acid, retinoic acid) (℞)

(tret'i-noyn)

Retin-A, Stievaa ♣, Tretinoin LF IV, Vesanoid

Func. class.: Vitamin A acid/acne product, antineoplastic—misc.
Chem. class.: Tretinoin derivative

Pregnancy category C (top), D (PO)

Action: Decreases cohesiveness of follicular epithelium, decreases microcomedone formation (top);

induces maturation of acute promyelocytic leukemia, exact action is unknown (PO)

Therapeutic Outcome: Decreased signs/symptoms of leukemia

Uses: Acne vulgaris (grades 1-3) (top); acute promylocytic leukemia (PO)

Investigational uses: Skin cancer

Dosage and routes

P ***Adult and child:*** Top cleanse area, apply hs; cover lightly

Promyelocytic leukemia

Adult: PO 45 mg/m^2/day given as 2 evenly divided doses until remission, discontinue treatment 30 days after remission or after 90 days of treatment, whichever is first

Available forms: Top cream 0.05%, 0.01%; top gel 0.025%, 0.01%; top liq 0.05%; caps 10 mg

Adverse effects

Topical route

INTEG: Rash, stinging, warmth, redness, erythema, blistering, crusting, peeling, contact dermatitis, hypopigmentation, hyperpigmentation

PO route

CNS: Headache, fever, sweating

GI: Nausea, vomiting, **hemorrhage,** abdominal pain, diarrhea, constipation, dyspepsia, distention, **hepatitis**

Contraindications: Hypersensitivity to retinoids or sensitive to parabens, pregnancy **D** (PO)

Precautions: Pregnancy **C** (top), lactation, eczema, sunburn

Pharmacokinetics	
Absorption	Small amounts
Distribution	Unknown
Metabolism	Unknown
Excretion	Kidneys
Half-life	Unknown

Pharmacodynamics
Unknown

Interactions

Individual drugs

Benzoyl peroxide: ↑ peeling
Resorcinol: ↑ peeling
Salicylic acid: ↑ peeling
Sulfur: ↑ peeling

Drug classifications

Abrasive soaps: ↑ peeling
Alcohol astringents: ↑ peeling

NURSING CONSIDERATIONS

Assessment

Topical route

- Assess part of body involved, including time involved, what helps or aggravates condition, cysts, dryness, itching; lesions may become worse at beginning of treatment

Nursing diagnoses

- ✓ Skin integrity, impaired (uses)
- ✓ Body image disturbances (uses)
- ✓ Knowledge deficit (teaching)

Implementation

Topical route

- Apply using gloves, once daily before bedtime; cover area lightly using gauze
- Store at room temp
- Wash hands after application

Liquid

- Apply with gloves or cotton; apply only to affected areas

Patient/family education

Topical route

- Instruct patient to avoid application on normal skin, and to avoid getting cream in eyes, nose, other mucous membranes
- Advise patient to avoid sunlight, sunlamps or to use protective clothing or sunscreen to prevent burns
- Advise patient that treatment may cause warmth, stinging; dryness; peeling will occur
- Inform patient that cosmetics may

be used over drug; not to use shaving lotions

- Inform patient that rash may occur during first 1-3 wk of therapy
- Caution patient that drug does not cure condition; only relieves symptoms; that therapeutic results may be seen in 2-3 wk but may not be optimal until after 6 wk

Evaluation

Positive therapeutic outcome

- Decrease in size and number of lesions

triamcinolone (℞)

(trye-am-sin'oh-lone)

Amcort, Aristocort, Aristocort Forte, Aristocort Intralesional, Aristospan Intra-Articular, Aristospan Intralesional, Articulose L.A., Atolone, Azmacort, Cenocort A-40, Cenocort Forte, Kenacort, Kenaject-40, Kenalog, Kenalog-10, Kenalog-40, Tac-3, Tac-40, Triam-A, triamcinolone, triamcinolone acetonide, Triam Forte, Triamolone 40, Triamonide 40, Tri-Kort, Trilog, Trilone, Trisoject

Func. class.: Corticosteroid; antiinflammatory

Chem. class.: Glucocorticoid, intermediate-acting

Pregnancy category C

Action: Decreases inflammation by suppression of migration of polymorphonuclear leukocytes, fibroblasts, reversal to increase capillary permeability and lysosomal stabilization

➔ **Therapeutic Outcome:** Decreased inflammation, normal immune response

Uses: Severe inflammation, immunosuppression, neoplasms, asthma (steroid dependent), collagen, respiratory, dermatologic disorders

Dosage and routes

Adult: PO 4-12 mg/day in divided doses qd-qid; IM 40 mg qwk (acetonide, or diacetate), 5-48 mg into neoplasms (diacetate, acetonide), 2-40 mg into joint or soft tissue (diacetate, acetonide), 0.5 mg/sq in of affected intralesional skin (hexacetonide), 2-20 mg into joint or soft tissue (hexacetonide)

P ***Child:*** PO 117 μg/kg/day as a single dose or divided doses

Asthma

Adult: INH 2 tid-qid, max 16 inh/day

P ***Child 6-12 yr:*** INH 1-2 tid-qid, max 12 inh/day

Available forms: Tabs 1, 2, 4, 8 mg; syrup 2, 4.85 mg/5 ml; inj 25, 40 mg/ml diacetate; inj 3, 10, 40 mg/ml acetonide; inj 5, 20 mg/ml hexacetonide; inh 100 μg/spray; intranasal 55 μg/spray

Adverse effects

CNS: *Depression, flushing, sweating,* headache, mood changes

CV: *Hypertension,* **circulatory collapse, thrombophlebitis, embolism,** tachycardia, edema

EENT: Fungal infections, increased intraocular pressure, blurred vision

GI: *Diarrhea, nausea, abdominal distention,* **GI hemorrhage,** *increased appetite,* **pancreatitis**

HEMA: **Thrombocytopenia**

INTEG: Acne, poor wound healing, ecchymosis, petechiae

MS: Fractures, osteoporosis, weakness

Contraindications: Psychosis, hypersensitivity, idiopathic thrombocytopenia, acute glomerulonephritis, amebiasis, fungal infections, nonasthmatic bronchial disease, P child <2 yr, AIDS, TB, adrenal insufficiency

Precautions: Pregnancy **C,** diabetes mellitus, glaucoma, osteoporosis, seizure disorders, ulcerative colitis,

CHF, myasthenia gravis, renal disease, esophagitis, peptic ulcer

Interactions

Individual drugs

Amphotericin B: ↑ hypokalemia
Azlocillin: ↑ hypokalemia
Insulin: ↑ need for insulin
Mezlocillin: ↑ hypokalemia
Phenytoin: ↓ action, ↑ metabolism
Piperacillin: ↑ hypokalemia
Rifampin: ↓ action, ↑ metabolism
Ticarcillin: ↑ hypokalemia

Drug classifications

Barbiturates: ↓ action, ↑ metabolism
Diuretics: ↑ hypokalemia
Hypoglycemic agents: ↑ need for hypoglycemic agents

Herb/drug

Aloe: ↑ hypokalemia
Buckthorn: ↑ hypokalemia
Rhubarb: ↑ hypokalemia
Senna: ↑ hypokalemia

Lab test interferences

↑ Cholesterol, ↑ sodium, ↑ blood glucose, ↑ uric acid, ↑ calcium, ↑ urine glucose
↓ Calcium, ↓ potassium, ↓ T_4, ↓ T_3, ↓ thyroid ^{131}I uptake test, ↓ urine 17-OHCS, ↓ 17-KS, ↓ PBI
False negative: Skin allergy tests

Pharmacokinetics

Absorption	Well absorbed (PO, IM)
Distribution	Crosses placenta, widely distributed
Metabolism	Liver—extensively
Excretion	Kidney, breast milk
Half-life	2-5 hr, adrenal suppression 3-4 days

NURSING CONSIDERATIONS

Assessment

- Monitor potassium, blood glucose, urine glucose while on long-term therapy; hypokalemia and hyperglycemia
- Monitor weight daily; notify prescriber of weekly gain >5 lb; I&O ratio; be alert for decreasing urinary output and increasing edema
- Monitor B/P q4h, pulse; notify prescriber if chest pain occurs
- Monitor plasma cortisol levels during long-term therapy (normal level; 138-635 nmol/L [SI units] when measured at 8 AM); adrenal function periodically for hypothalamic-pituitary-adrenal axis suppression
- Assess for infection: increase temp, WBC even after withdrawal of medication; drug masks infection symptoms
- Assess for potassium depletion: paresthesias, fatigue, nausea, vomiting, depression, polyuria, dysrhythmias, weakness
- Assess mental status: affect, mood, behavioral changes, aggression
- Assess nasal passages during long-term treatment for changes in mucus (nasal)
- Monitor temp; if fever develops, drug should be discontinued
- Assess for systemic absorption: increased temp, inflammation, irritation (top)

Nursing diagnoses

- ✓ Infection, risk for (adverse reactions)
- ✓ Knowledge deficit (teaching)
- ✓ Noncompliance (teaching)

Pharmacodynamics

	PO	IM	TOP	INH	INTRANASAL
Onset	Unknown	Unknown	Min to hr	1-2 wk	Unknown
Peak	1-2 hr	1-2 hr	Hr to days	Unknown	2-3 wk
Duration	3 days	Unknown	Hr to days	Unknown	Unknown

Implementation

IM route

- Give IM inj deeply in large muscle mass, rotate sites, avoid deltoid, use 21-G needle
- Give in one dose in AM to prevent adrenal suppression; avoid SC administration; may damage tissue

PO route

- Give with food or milk to decrease GI symptoms

Inhalation route

- G Use spacer device for elderly
- Give inh with water to decrease possibility of fungal infections; titrated dose, use lowest effective dose
- Give after cleaning aerosol top daily with warm water, dry thoroughly
- Store in cool environment; do not puncture or incinerate container

Topical route

- Apply only to affected areas; do not get in eyes
- Apply medication, then cover with occlusive dressing (only if prescribed), seal to normal skin, change q12h; systemic absorption may occur
- Apply only to dermatoses; do not use on weeping, denuded, or infected areas
- Cleanse skin before applying drug
- Continue treatment for a few days after area has cleared
- Store at room temp

Nasal route

- Have patient clear nasal passages before administration; use decongestant if needed; shake inhaler, invert, tilt head backward, insert nozzle into nostril, away from septum; hold other nostril closed and depress activator, inhale through nose, exhale through mouth

Patient/family education

- Advise patient that ID as steroid user should be carried
- Instruct patient to notify patient if therapeutic response decreases; dosage adjustment may be needed; not to discontinue abruptly; adrenal crisis can result
- Caution patient to avoid OTC products: salicylates, alcohol in cough products, cold preparations unless directed by prescriber
- Advise patient on all aspects of drug usage including cushingoid symptoms
- Teach patient symptoms of adrenal insufficiency: nausea, anorexia, fatigue, dizziness, dyspnea, weakness, joint pain
- Teach patient that long-term therapy may be needed to clear infection (1-2 mo depending on type of infection)

Nasal route

- Instruct patient to clear nasal passages if sneezing attack occurs, repeat dose
- Advise patient to continue using product even if mild nasal bleeding occurs; is usually transient
- Teach patient method of instillation after providing written instruction from manufacturer

Inhalation route

- Teach patient proper administration technique; to wash inhaler with warm water and dry after each use
- Teach patient all aspects of drug usage including cushingoid symptoms

Topical route

- Instruct patient to avoid sunlight on affected area; burns may occur

Evaluation

Positive therapeutic outcome

- Decrease in runny nose (nasal)
- Decreased dyspnea, wheezing, dry rales on auscultation (inh)
- Ease of respirations, decreased inflammation
- Absence of severe itching, patches on skin, flaking (top)

T

triamterene (℞)

(try-am'ter-een)

Dyrenium

Func. class.: Potassium-sparing diuretic

Chem. class.: Pteridine derivative

Pregnancy category B

Action: Acts primarily on distal tubule to inhibit reabsorption of sodium, chloride; increase potassium retention and conserve hydrogen ions

→ Therapeutic Outcome: Diuretic and antihypertensive effect while retaining potassium

Uses: Edema, hypertension, diuretic-induced hypokalemia

Dosage and routes

Adult: PO 100 mg bid pc, max 300 mg/day

G ***Elderly:*** PO 50 mg qd, max 100 mg/day

Available forms: Caps 50, 100 mg

Adverse effects

CNS: Weakness, headache, dizziness, fatigue

ELECT: Hyperkalemia, hyponatremia, hypochloremia

GI: Nausea, diarrhea, vomiting, dry mouth, jaundice, liver disease

GU: **Azotemia, interstitial nephritis,** increased BUN, creatinine, renal stones, bluish discoloration of urine

HEMA: **Thrombocytopenia, megaloblastic anemia,** low folic acid levels

INTEG: Photosensitivity, rash

Contraindications: Hypersensitivity, anuria, severe renal, hepatic disease; hyperkalemia

Precautions: Dehydration, hepatic disease, lactation, CHF, renal disease, cirrhosis, pregnancy **B,** lactation

Pharmacokinetics

Absorption	GI tract; well absorbed
Distribution	Crosses placenta
Metabolism	Liver
Excretion	Renal; breast milk
Half-life	3 hr

Pharmacodynamics

Onset	2 hr
Peak	6-8 hr
Duration	12-16 hr

Interactions

Individual drugs

Amantadine: ↑ toxicity of amantadine

Cimetidine: ↓ renal clearance of triamterene

Indomethacin: ↑ nephrotoxicity

Drug classifications

Angiotensin-converting enzyme inhibitors: ↑ hyperkalemia

Antihypertensives: ↑ action

Diuretics, potassium-sparing: ↑ hyperkalemia

NSAIDs: ↓ nephrotoxicity

Potassium products: ↑ hyperkalemia

Salt substitutes: ↑ hyperkalemia

Food/drug

Potassium-containing foods: ↑ hyperkalemia

Lab test interferences

Interference: Quinidine serum levels, LDH

NURSING CONSIDERATIONS

Assessment

- Monitor for manifestations of hyperkalemia: *RENAL:* acidic urine, reduced urine osmolality, nocturia, polyuria, polydipsia; *CV:* hypotension, broad T wave, U wave, ectopy, tachycardia, weak pulse; *NEURO* muscle weakness, altered LOC, drowsiness, apathy, lethargy, confusion, depression, anorexia, nausea, cramps, constipation, distension, paralytic ileus, hypoventilation, respiratory muscle weakness

• Monitor for manifestations of hyponatremia: *CV:* ↑ B/P, cold, clammy skin, hypo- or hypervolemia; *GI:* anorexia, nausea, vomiting, diarrhea, abdominal cramps; *NEURO:* lethargy, increased ICP, confusion, headache, seizures, coma, fatigue, tremors, hyperreflexia
• Monitor for manifestations of hyperchloremia: *NEURO:* weakness, lethargy, coma; *RESP:* deep rapid breathing
• Assess fluid volume status: I&O ratios and record, weight, distended red veins, crackles in lung, color, quality, and sp gr of urine, skin turgor, adequacy of pulses, moist mucous membranes, bilateral lung sounds, peripheral pitting edema; dehydration symptoms of decreasing output, thirst, hypotension, dry mouth and mucous membranes should be reported
• Monitor electrolytes: potassium, sodium, calcium, magnesium; also include BUN, ABGs, uric acid, CBC, blood glucose

Nursing diagnoses

✓ Urinary elmination, altered (adverse reactions)
✓ Fluid volume deficit (adverse reactions)
✓ Fluid volume excess (uses)
✓ Knowledge deficit (teaching)

Implementation

• Give in AM to avoid interference with sleep
• With food, if nausea occurs

Patient/family education

• Teach patient to take medication early in the day to prevent nocturia
• Instruct the patient to take with food or milk if GI symptoms of nausea and anorexia occur
• Teach patient to maintain a record of weight on a weekly basis and notify prescriber of weight loss of 5 lb
• Caution the patient that this drug causes an increase in potassium levels, that foods high in potassium should be avoided; refer to dietitian for assistance planning
• Caution the patient not to exercise in hot weather, and stand for prolonged periods of time because orthostatic hypotension will be enhanced
• Advise patient to wear protective clothing and sunscreen in the sun to prevent photosensitivity
• Teach patient not to use alcohol, or any OTC medications without prescriber's approval because serious drug reactions may occur
• Emphasize the need to contact prescriber immediately if muscle cramps, weakness, nausea, dizziness, or numbness occur
• Teach patient to take own B/P and pulse and record
• Advise patient that dizziness and confusion may occur; avoid driving or other hazardous activities if alertness is decreased
• Teach patient to continue taking medication even if feeling better; this drug controls symptoms but does not cure the condition
• Advise the patient with hypertension to continue other medical treatment (exercise, weight loss, relaxation techniques, cessation of smoking)

Evaluation

Positive therapeutic outcome

• Prevention of hypokalemia (diuretic use)
• Decreased edema
• Decreased B/P
• Increased diuresis

Treatment of overdose:

Lavage if taken orally; monitor electrolytes; administer sodium bicarbonate for potassium 6.5 mEq/L; monitor hydration, CV, renal status

T

triazolam (℞)

(trye-az'oh-lam)

Apo-Triazo ✦, Gen-Triazolam ✦, Halcion, Novotriolam ✦, Nu-Triazol ✦

Func. class.: Sedative-hypnotic, antianxiety

Chem. class.: Benzodiazepine

Pregnancy category X

Controlled substance schedule IV (USA), schedule F (Canada)

Action: Produces CNS depression at limbic, thalamic, hypothalamic levels of CNS; may be mediated by neurotransmitter; γ-aminobutyric acid (GABA); results are sedation, hypnosis, skeletal muscle relaxation, anticonvulsant activity, anxiolytic action

Therapeutic Outcome: Decreased anxiety, insomnia

Uses: Insomnia (short-term), sedative/hypnotic

Dosage and routes

Adult: PO 0.125-0.5 mg hs

G ***Elderly:*** PO 0.625-0.125 mg hs

Available forms: Tabs 0.125, 0.25 mg

Adverse effects

CNS: *Headache, lethargy, drowsiness, daytime sedation,* dizziness, confusion, light-headedness, anxiety, irritability, amnesia, poor coordination

CV: Chest pain, pulse changes

GI: Nausea, vomiting, diarrhea, heartburn, abdominal pain, constipation

HEMA: **Leukopenia, granulocytopenia** (rare)

Contraindications: Hypersensitivity to benzodiazepines, pregnancy **X**, lactation, intermittent porphyria

Precautions: Anemia, hepatic disease, renal disease, suicidal individuals, drug abuse, G elderly, psychosis, P child <15 yr, acute narrow-angle glaucoma, seizure disorders

Pharmacokinetics

Absorption	Well absorbed
Distribution	Widely distributed, crosses placenta, crosses blood-brain barrier
Metabolism	Liver
Excretion	Kidneys, breast milk
Half-life	2-3 hr

Pharmacodynamics

Onset	½ hr
Peak	Unknown
Duration	6-8 hr

Interactions

Individual drugs

Alcohol: ↑ CNS depression
Cimetidine: ↑ action
Disulfiram: ↑ action
Fluoxetine: ↑ action
Isoniazid: ↑ action
Ketoconazole: ↑ action
Levodopa: ↓ action of levodopa
Metoprolol: ↑ action
Propoxyphene: ↑ action
Propranolol: ↑ action
Rifampin: ↓ action of triazolam
Theophylline: ↓ sedative effects
Valproic acid: ↑ action

Drug classifications

Antidepressants: ↑ CNS depression
Antihistamines: ↑ CNS depression
Barbiturates: ↓ effect of triazolam
Opiates: ↑ CNS depression
Oral contraceptives: ↑ effect

Herb/drug

Kava: ↑ CNS depression

Lab test interferences

↑ AST/ALT, ↑ serum bilirubin
False: ↑ 17-OHCS
↓ radioactive iodine uptake

NURSING CONSIDERATIONS

Assessment

- Assess patient's mental status: mood, sensorium, anxiety, affect, sleeping pattern, drowsiness, dizziness, especially G elderly; physical

dependency, withdrawal symptoms: anxiety, panic attacks, agitation, seizures, headache, nausea, vomiting, muscle pain, weakness; suicidal tendencies; for indications of increasing tolerance and abuse
- Monitor patient's B/P (lying, standing), pulse; if systolic B/P drops 20 mm Hg, hold drug, notify prescriber
- Monitor blood studies: CBC during long-term therapy; blood dycrasias have occurred rarely; decreased hematocrit, neutropenia may occur
- Monitor hepatic function studies: AST, ALT, bilirubin, creatinine LDH, alkaline phosphatase
- Monitor I&O ratio; indicate renal dysfunction

Nursing diagnoses
- ✓ Anxiety (uses)
- ✓ Depression (uses)
- ✓ Injury, risk for (adverse reactions)
- ✓ Knowledge deficit (teaching)

Implementation
- Give with food or milk to decrease GI symptoms; if patient is unable to swallow medication whole, tab may be crushed and mixed with foods or fluids
- Give sugarless gum, hard candy, frequent sips of water for dry mouth

Patient/family education
- Advise patient that drug may be taken with food or fluids, and tab may be crushed or swallowed whole
- Caution patient not to use for everyday stress or longer than 3 mo unless directed by prescriber; not to take more than prescribed amount; may be habit forming; not to double doses or skip doses
- Instruct patient to avoid OTC preparations unless approved by prescriber; alcohol and CNS depressants will increase CNS depression
- Caution patient to avoid driving, activities that require alertness because drowsiness may occur; to avoid alcohol ingestion or other psychotropic medications; to rise slowly or G fainting may occur, especially elderly; that drowsiness may worsen at beginning of treatment
- Advise patient not to discontinue medication abruptly after long-term use; withdrawal symptoms include vomiting, cramping, tremors, seizures

Evaluation
Positive therapeutic outcome
- Decreased anxiety, restlessness, sleeplessness (short-term treatment only)

Treatment of overdose:
Lavage, VS, supportive care

trifluoperazine (℞)
(trye-floo-oh-per'a-zeen)

Apo-Trifluoperazine ♣, Novoflurazine ♣, Solazine ♣, Stelazine, Suprazine, Terfluzine, trifluoperazine HCl, Triflurin

Func. class.: Antipsychotic/neuroleptic

Chem. class.: Phenothiazine, piperazine

Pregnancy category C

Action: Depresses cerebral cortex, hypothalamus, limbic system, which control activity, aggression; blocks neurotransmission produced by dopamine at synapse; exhibits strong α-adrenergic, anticholinergic blocking action; mechanism for antipsychotic effects is unclear

➡ **Therapeutic Outcome:** Decreased signs and symptoms of psychosis

Uses: Psychotic disorders, nonpsychotic anxiety, schizophrenia

Dosage and routes
Adult: PO 2-5 mg bid, usual range 15-20 mg/day, may require 40 mg/day or more; IM 1-2 mg q4-6h

G ***Elderly:*** PO 0.5-1 mg qd-bid, q4-7 days by 0.5-1 mg/day to desired dose

P ***Child >6 yr:*** PO 1 mg qd or bid;

IM *not recommended for children,* but 1 mg may be given qd or bid

Nonpsychotic anxiety

Adult: PO 1-2 mg bid, not to exceed 5 mg/day; do not give longer than 12 wk

Available forms: Tabs 1, 2, 5, 10 mg; conc 10 mg/ml; inj 2 mg/ml

Adverse effects

CNS: *EPS (pseudoparkinsonism, akathisia, dystonia, tardive dyskinesia),* **seizures,** *headache,* **neuroleptic malignant syndrome**

CV: *Orthostatic hypotension,* hypertension, **cardiac arrest,** ECG changes, **tachycardia**

EENT: Blurred vision, glaucoma, dry eyes

GI: *Dry mouth, nausea, vomiting, anorexia, constipation,* diarrhea, jaundice, weight gain

GU: Urinary retention, urinary frequency, enuresis, impotence, amenorrhea, gynecomastia

HEMA: Anemia, **leukopenia, leukocytosis, agranulocytosis**

INTEG: *Rash,* photosensitivity, dermatitis

RESP: **Laryngospasm,** dyspnea, **respiratory depression**

Contraindications: Hypersensitivity, CV disease, coma, blood dyscrasias, severe hepatic disease, P child <6 yr, glaucoma

Precautions: Breast cancer, seizure disorders, pregnancy **C,** lactation, diabetes mellitus, respiratory conditions, prostatic hypertrophy, G elderly

Do Not Confuse:
trifluoperazine/trihexyphenidyl

Pharmacokinetics

Absorption	Variably absorbed (PO), well absorbed (IM)
Distribution	Widely distributed, high concentrations in CNS, crosses placenta
Metabolism	Liver—extensively
Excretion	Kidneys, breast milk
Half-life	Unknown

Pharmacodynamics

	PO	IM
Onset	Rapid	Immediate
Peak	2-3 hr	1 hr
Duration	12 hr	12 hr

Interactions

Individual drugs

Alcohol: ↑ effects of both drugs, oversedation
Aluminum hydroxide: ↓ absorption
Bromocriptine: ↓ antiparkinson activity
Disopyramide: ↑ anticholinergic effects
Guanethidine: ↓ antihypertensive response
Levodopa: ↓ antiparkinson activity
Lithium: ↓ chlorpromazine levels, ↑ EPS, masking of lithium toxicity
Magnesium hydroxide: ↓ absorption
Norepinephrine: ↓ vasoresponse, ↑ toxicity
Phenobarbital: ↓ effectiveness, ↑ metabolism

Drug classifications

Antacids: ↓ absorption
Anticholinergics: ↑ anticholinergic effects
Antidepressants: ↑ CNS depression
Antidiarrheals, adsorbent: ↓ absorption
Antihistamines: ↑ CNS depression
Antihypertensives: ↑ hypotension
Antithyroid agents: ↑ agranulocytosis
Barbiturate anesthetics: ↑ CNS depression

β-Adrenergic blockers: ↑ effects of both drugs
General anesthetics: ↑ CNS depression
MAOIs: ↑ CNS depression
Opiates: ↑ CNS depression
Sedative/hypnotics: ↑ CNS depression

Herb/drug

Kava: ↑ CNS depression

Lab test interferences

↑ Liver function tests, ↑ cardiac enzymes, ↑ cholesterol, ↑ blood glucose, ↑ prolactin, ↑ bilirubin, ↑ PBI, ↑ cholinesterase, ↑ alkaline phosphatase, ↑ leukocytes, ↑ granulocytes, ↑ platelets
↓ Hormones (blood and urine)
False positive: Pregnancy tests, PKU, urine bilirubin
False negative: Urinary steroids, 17-OHCS

NURSING CONSIDERATIONS

Assessment

- Assess mental status: orientation, mood, behavior, presence of hallucinations and type before initial administration and monthly; drug should significantly reduce psychotic behavior
- Check for swallowing of PO medication; check for hoarding or giving of medication to other patients
- Monitor I&O ratio, palpate bladder if low urinary output occurs, especially in elderly; urinalysis recommended before, during prolonged therapy
- Monitor bilirubin, CBC, liver function studies monthly
- Assess affect, orientation, LOC, reflexes, gait, coordination, sleep pattern disturbances
- Monitor B/P sitting, standing, and lying, take pulse and respirations q4h during initial treatment; establish baseline before starting treatment; report drops of 30 mm Hg; obtain baseline ECG, monitor Q- and T-wave changes
- Check for dizziness, faintness, palpitations, tachycardia on rising; severe orthostatic hypotension is common
- Identify for neuroleptic malignant syndrome: hyperpyrexia, muscle rigidity, increased CPK, altered mental status; drug should be discontinued
- Assess for EPS including akathisia (inability to sit still, no pattern to movements), tardive dyskinesia (bizarre movements of the jaw, mouth, tongue, extremities), pseudoparkinsonism (ragged tremors, pill rolling, shuffling gait); an antiparkinson drug should be prescribed
- Assess for constipation, urinary retention daily; if these occur, increase bulk, water in diet
- Assess for hypo/hyperglycemia; appetite patterns

Nursing diagnoses

✓ Thought processes, altered (uses)
✓ Coping, ineffective individual (uses)
✓ Knowledge deficit (teaching)
✓ Noncompliance (teaching)

Implementation

PO route

- Give drug in liq form mixed in glass of juice if hoarding is suspected; do not mix in caffeine drinks, tannics, pectins
- Give decreased dose in elderly; metabolism is slowed in the elderly
- Give PO with full glass of water, milk; or give with food to decrease GI upset
- Store in airtight, light-resistant container, oral sol in amber bottle

IM route

- Inj in deep muscle mass, do not give SC; do not administer sol with a precipitate

IV route

- Give **IV** after diluting 10 mg/9 ml of 0.9% NaCl; give 1 mg or less/2 min

T

Syringe compatibilities:
Glycopyrrolate

Additive compatibilities:
Meperidine, netilmicin

Patient/family education

- Teach patient to use good oral hygiene; frequent rinsing of mouth, sugarless gum for dry mouth
- Caution patient to avoid hazardous activities until drug response is determined; dizziness, blurred vision is common
- Inform patient that orthostatic hypotension occurs often; to rise from sitting or lying position gradually and to remain lying down after IM inj for at least 30 min
- Caution patient to avoid tubs, hot showers, tub baths because hypotension may occur
- Instruct patient that heat stroke may occur in hot weather, so take extra precautions to stay cool
- Advise patient to avoid abrupt withdrawal of this drug, or EPS may result; drug should be withdrawn slowly
- Teach patient to avoid OTC preparations (cough, hay fever, cold) unless approved by prescriber because serious drug interactions may occur; avoid use with alcohol, CNS depressants because increased drowsiness may occur
- Advise patient to use sunglasses and sunscreen to prevent burns
- Teach patient about EPS and necessity of meticulous oral hygiene because oral candidiasis may occur
- Advise patient to take antacids 2 hr before or after this drug
- Instruct patient to report sore throat, malaise, fever, bleeding, mouth sores; if these occur, CBC should be performed and drug discontinued

Evaluation

Positive therapeutic outcome

- Decrease in emotional excitement, hallucinations, delusions, paranoia
- Reorganization of patterns of thought, speech

Treatment of overdose:
Lavage if orally ingested; provide airway; *do not induce vomiting or use epinephrine*

trihexyphenidyl (℞)

(trye-hex-ee-fen′i-dill)

Apo-Trihex ✤, Artane, Artane Sequels, Novohexidyl ✤, PMS-Trihexyphenidyl ✤, Trihexy-2, Trihexy-5, trihexyphenidyl HCl, Trihexane

Func. class.: Cholinergic blocker; antiparkinson

Chem. class.: Synthetic tertiary amine

Pregnancy category C

Action: Blocks central muscarinic receptors, which decreases involuntary movements, sweating, salivation

➔ **Therapeutic Outcome:** Decreased involuntary movements

Uses: parkinsonian symptoms, drug-induced EPS

Dosage and routes

Parkinsonian symptoms

Adult: PO 1 mg, increased by 2 mg q3-5 days to a total of 6-10 mg/day; give ext rel cap q12h

Drug-induced EPS

Adult: PO 1 mg/day; usual dose 5-15 mg/day

Available forms: Tabs 2, 5 mg; ext rel caps 5 mg; elixir 2 mg/5 ml

Adverse effects

CNS: Confusion, anxiety, restlessness, irritability, delusions, hallucinations, headache, sedation, depression, incoherence, dizziness, flushing, weakness

CV: Palpitations, tachycardia, postural hypotension

EENT: Blurred vision, photophobia, dilated pupils, difficulty swallowing,

dry eyes, increased intraocular tension, angle-closure glaucoma
GI: Dryness of mouth, constipation, nausea, vomiting, abdominal distress, **paralytic ileus**
GU: Urinary hesitancy, urinary retention, dysuria
INTEG: Urticaria, rash
MISC: Suppression of lactation, nasal congestion, decreased sweating, increased temp, hyperthermia, heat stroke, numbness of fingers
MS: Weakness, cramping

Contraindications: Hypersensitivity, narrow-angle glaucoma, myasthenia gravis, GI/ GU obstruction, tachycardia, myocardial ischemia, unstable CV disease, prostatic hypertrophy

G **Precautions:** Pregnancy **C,** elderly, lactation, tachycardia, abdominal P obstruction, infection, children, gastric ulcer

Do Not Confuse:
Artane/Altace, trihexyphenidyl/ trifluoperazine

Pharmacokinetics

Absorption	Well absorbed
Distribution	Unknown
Metabolism	Unknown
Excretion	Unknown
Half-life	5-10 hr

Pharmacodynamics

	PO	PO-EXT REL
Onset	1 hr	Unknown
Peak	2-3 hr	Unknown
Duration	6-12 hr	Up to 24 hr

Interactions
Individual drugs
Alcohol: ↑ CNS depression
Disopyramide: ↑ anticholinergic effects
Quinidine: ↑ anticholinergic effects
Drug classifications
Analgesics: ↑ CNS depression
Antacids: ↓ absorption
Antidepressants, tricyclic: ↑ anticholinergic effects
Antihistamines: ↑ anticholinergic effects
Opioids: ↑ CNS depression
Phenothiazines: ↑ anticholinergic effects
Sedative/hypnotics: ↑ CNS depression

NURSING CONSIDERATIONS
Assessment
- Monitor I&O ratio; retention commonly causes decreased urinary output, distention, frequency, incontinence
- Assess for parkinsonism, EPS: shuffling gait, muscle rigidity, involuntary movements, pill rolling, muscle spasms, drooling before and during treatment
- Monitor for urinary hesitancy, retention; palpate bladder if retention occurs
- Monitor for constipation, cramping, pain in abdomen, abdominal distention; increase fluids, bulk, exercise if this occurs
- Assess for tolerance over long-term therapy; dose may have to be increased or changed
- Assess for mental status: affect, mood, CNS depression, worsening of mental symptoms during early therapy

Nursing diagnoses
✓ Physical mobility, impaired (uses)
✓ Knowledge deficit (teaching)

Implementation
- Give with or after meals to prevent GI upset; may give with fluids other than water; offer hard candy, frequent drinks, gum to relieve dry mouth
- Give hs to avoid daytime drowsiness in patient with parkinsonism
- Store at room temp

Patient/family education
- Teach patient to use caution in hot weather; drug may increase susceptibility to stroke because perspiration is

T

decreased; patient should remain indoors

- Teach patient not to discontinue this drug abruptly; to taper off over 1 wk to prevent withdrawal symptoms (insomnia, involuntary movements, anxiety, tachycardias)
- Caution patient to avoid driving or other hazardous activities; drowsiness, dizziness may occur
- Advise patient to avoid OTC medications (cough, cold preparations with alcohol, antihistamines) unless directed by prescriber; increased CNS depression may occur
- Instruct patient to rise from sitting or recumbent position slowly to minimize orthostatic hypotension
- Advise patient to use gum, hard candy, frequent sips of water to decrease dry mouth; if dry mouth continues, saliva substitutes may be prescribed
- Instruct patient that doses should not be doubled, but missed dose may be taken up to 2 hr before next dose

Evaluation

Positive therapeutic outcome

- Absence of involuntary movements (pill rolling, tremors, muscle spasms)

trimethobenzamide (℞)

(trye-meth-oh-ben'za-mide)

Arrestin, Benzacot, Brogan, Stemetic, T-Gen, Tebamide, Ticon, Tigan, Tijet-20, Tribun, Trimazide, trimethobenzamide, trimethobenzamide HCl

Func. class.: Antiemetic, anticholinergic

Chem. class.: Ethanolamine derivative

Pregnancy category C

Action: Acts centrally by blocking chemoreceptor trigger zone, which in turn acts on vomiting center

Therapeutic Outcome: Absence of nausea and vomiting

Uses: Nausea, vomiting, prevention of postoperative vomiting

Dosage and routes

Postoperative vomiting

Adult: IM/rec 200 mg before or during surgery; may repeat 3 hr after

Discontinuing anesthesia

P ***Child 13-40 kg:*** PO/rec 100-200 mg tid-qid

P ***Child <13 kg:*** PO/rec 100 mg tid-qid

Nausea/vomiting

Adult: PO 250 mg tid-qid; IM/rec 200 mg tid-qid

Available forms: Caps 100, 250, mg; supp 100, 200 mg; inj 100 mg/ml

Adverse effects

CNS: *Drowsiness,* restlessness, headache, dizziness, insomnia, confusion, nervousness, tingling, *vertigo,* EPS

CV: Hypertension, hypotension, palpitations

EENT: Dry mouth, blurred vision, diplopia, nasal congestion, photosensitivity

GI: Nausea, anorexia, diarrhea, vomiting, constipation

INTEG: Rash, urticaria, fever, chills, flushing

Contraindications: Hypersensitivity to narcotics, shock, children (parenterally) P

P G **Precautions:** Children, cardiac dysrhythmias, elderly, asthma, pregnancy **C,** prostatic hypertrophy, bladder-neck obstruction, narrow-angle glaucoma, stenosing peptic ulcer, pyloroduodenal obstruction

Pharmacokinetics	
Absorption	Unknown
Distribution	Unknown
Metabolism	Liver, extensively
Excretion	Kidneys
Half-life	Unknown

Pharmacodynamics

	PO	IM	REC
Onset	20-40 min	15 min	10-40 min
Peak	Unknown	Unknown	Unknown
Duration	3-4 hr	2-3 hr	3-4 hr

Interactions
Individual drugs
Alcohol: ↑ CNS depression
Drug classifications
Analgesics: ↑ CNS effect
Antidepressants: ↑ CNS effect
Antihistamines: ↑ CNS effect
CNS depressants: ↑ CNS effect
Sedative/hypnotics: ↑ CNS effect

NURSING CONSIDERATIONS
Assessment
- Monitor VS, B/P; check patients with cardiac disease more often
- Assess for signs of toxicity of other drugs or masking of symptoms of disease: brain tumor, intestinal obstructions
- Observe for drowsiness, dizziness
- Assess for nausea, vomiting before and after treatment

Nursing diagnoses
✓ Knowledge deficit (teaching)

Implementation
IM route
- Administer IM inj in large muscle mass; aspirate to avoid **IV** administration

Syringe compatibilities:
Glycopyrrolate, hydromorphone, midazolam, nalbuphine

Y-site compatibilities:
Heparin, hydrocortisone, potassium chloride, vit B/C

PO route
- Cap may be swallowed whole or opened and mixed with food or fluids

Patient/family education
- Teach patient to use good oral hygiene; frequent rinsing of mouth, sugarless gum for dry mouth
- Caution patient to avoid hazardous activities until drug response is determined, drowsiness may occur
- Inform patient that orthostatic hypotension occurs often and to rise from sitting or lying position gradually and to remain lying down after IM inj for at least 30 min
- Advise patient to avoid hot tubs, hot showers, tub baths because hypotension may occur
- Inform patient that in hot weather, heat stroke may occur; take extra precautions to stay cool
- Teach patient to avoid OTC preparations (cough, hayfever, cold) unless approved by prescriber because serious drug interactions may occur; avoid use with alcohol, CNS depressants because increased drowsiness may occur
- Teach patient about EPS
- Instruct patient to report sore throat, malaise, fever, bleeding, mouth sores; if these occur, CBC should be performed and drug discontinued

Evaluation
Positive therapeutic outcome
- Decreased nausea, vomiting

T

trimethoprim/ sulfamethoxazole (cotrimoxazole) (℞)

(trye-meth'oh-prim/sul-fa-meth-ox'a-zole [ko-trye-mox'a-zole])

Apo-Sulfatrim*, Apo-Sulfatrim DS ♣, Bactrim, Bactrim IV, Bethaprim, Comoxol, Cotrim, Novo-Trimel ♣, Novo-Trimel DS ♣, Nu-Cotrimox ♣, Nu-Cotrimox DS ♣, Roubac ♣, Septra, Septra DS, SMZ/TMP, Sulfatrim

Func. class.: Antiinfective

Chem. class.: Miscellaneous sulfonamide

Pregnancy category C

Action: Sulfamethoxazole (SMZ) interferes with bacterial biosynthesis of proteins by competitive antagonism of PABA when adequate levels are maintained; trimethoprim (TMP) blocks synthesis of tetrahydrofolic acid; combination blocks 2 consecutive steps in bacterial synthesis of essential nucleic acids, protein

➡ **Therapeutic Outcome:** Absence of infection, based on C&S

Uses: UTI, otitis media, acute and chronic prostatitis, shigellosis, *Pneumocystis carinii* pneumonitis, chronic bronchitis, chancroid, traveler's diarrhea

Dosage and routes

UTI

Adult: PO 160 mg TMP/800 mg SMZ q12h × 10-14 days

P ***Child:*** PO 8 mg/kg TMP/40 mg/kg SMZ qd in 2 divided doses q12h

Otitis media

P ***Child:*** PO 8 mg/kg TMP/40 mg/kg SMZ qd in 2 divided doses q12h × 10 days

Bacterial infections

P ***Adult and child ≥40 kg:*** 160 mg TMP/800 mg SMZ q12h

P ***Adult and child >2 mo:*** 4-6 mg/kg TMP/20-30 mg/kg SMZ q12h; **IV** 2-2.5 mg/kg TMP/10-12.5 mg/kg SMZ q6h or 4-5 mg/kg TMP/20-25 mg/kg SMZ q12h

Chronic bronchitis

Adult: PO 160 mg TMP/800 mg SMZ q12h × 14 days

Pneumocystis carinii pneumonitis

P ***Adult and child >2 mo:*** PO 3.75-5 mg/kg TMP/18.75-25 mg SMZ q6h × 14 days; **IV** 3.75-5 mg/kg TMP/18.5-25 mg SMZ q6h or 5-6.7 mg/kg TMP/25-33.3 mg SMZ q8h divided doses for up to 14 days

Renal dose

- Dosage reduction necessary in moderate to severe renal impairment (CrCl <30 ml/min)

Available forms: Tabs 80 mg trimethoprim (TMP)/400 mg sulfamethoxazole (SMZ), 160 mg TMP/800 mg SMZ; susp 40 mg/200 mg/5 ml; **IV** 16 mg/80 mg/ml

Adverse effects

CNS: Headache, insomnia, hallucinations, depression, vertigo, fatigue, anxiety, convulsions, drug fever, chills, aseptic meningitis

CV: **Allergic myocarditis**

GI: Nausea, vomiting, abdominal pain, stomatitis, **hepatitis,** glossitis, pancreatitis, diarrhea, **enterocolitis,** anorexia

GU: **Renal failure, toxic nephrosis;** increased BUN, creatinine; crystalluria

HEMA: **Leukopenia, neutropenia, thrombocytopenia, agranulocytosis, hemolytic anemia, hypoprothrombinemia, Henoch-Schönlein purpura, methemoglobinemia, eosinophilia I**

INTEG: Rash, dermatitis, urticaria, erythema, photosensitivity, pain,

inflammation at injection site, **toxic epidermal necrolysis, erythema multiforme**
RESP: Cough, shortness of breath
SYST: **Anaphylaxis, systemic lupus erythematosus, Stevens-Johnson syndrome**

Contraindications: Hypersensitivity to trimethoprim or sulfonamides, pregnancy at term, megaloblastic anemia, infants <2 mo, CrCl <15 ml/min, lactation, porphyria

Precautions: Pregnancy **C**, renal disease, elderly, glucose-6-phosphate dehydrogenase deficiency, impaired hepatic/renal function, possible folate deficiency, severe allergy, bronchial asthma

Pharmacokinetics	
Absorption	Rapid
Distribution	Breast milk, crosses placenta, 68% protein bound
Metabolism	Liver
Excretion	Kidneys
Half-life	8-13 hr

Pharmacodynamics	
Onset	Unknown
Peak	1-4 hr
Duration	Unknown

Interactions

Individual drugs

Cyclosporine: ↓ response
Methotrexate: ↑ bone marrow depression
Phenytoin: ↓ hepatic clearance of phenytoin

Drug classifications

Anticoagulants, oral: ↑ anticoagulant effect
Diuretics, thiazide: ↑ thrombocytopenia
Oral contraceptives: ↓ effectiveness of oral contraceptives
Sulfonylureas: ↑ hypoglycemic response

Lab test interferences

↑ Alkaline phosphatase, ↑ creatinine, ↑ bilirubin
False positive: Urinary glucose test

NURSING CONSIDERATIONS

Assessment

- Assess allergic reactions: rash, fever (AIDS patients more susceptible)
- Monitor I&O ratio; note color, character, pH of urine if drug administered for UTI; output should be 800 ml less than intake; if urine is highly acidic, alkalization may be needed
- Monitor kidney function studies: BUN, creatinine, urinalysis (long-term therapy)
- Assess type of infection; obtain C&S before starting therapy
- Assess blood dyscrasias, skin rash, fever, sore throat, bruising, bleeding, fatigue, joint pain
- Assess allergic reaction: rash, dermatitis, urticaria, pruritus, dyspnea, bronchospasm

Nursing diagnoses

✓ Infection, risk for (uses)
✓ Knowledge deficit (teaching)
✓ Noncompliance (teaching)

Implementation

- Give with full glass of water to maintain adequate hydration; increase fluids to 2 L/day to decrease crystallization in kidneys
- Give medication after C&S; repeat C&S after full course of medication
- Store in airtight, light-resistant container at room temp
- Dilute 5 ml ampule/100-125 ml of D_5W, stable for 6 hr, give over 1-½ hr, do not refrigerate

IV route

Syringe compatibilities:

Heparin

Y-site compatibilities:

Acyclovir, aldesleukin, allopurinol, amifostine, atracurium, aztreonam, cefepime, cyclophosphamide, diltiazem, enalaprilat, esmolol, filgrastim, fludarabine, gallium, granisetron, hydromorphone, labetalol, lorazepam, magnesium sulfate, melphalan, meperidine, morphine, pancuronium, perphenazine, piperacillin/tazobactam, sargramostim, tacrolimus, teniposide, thiotepa, vecuronium, zidovudine

Patient family education

- Teach patient to take each oral dose with full glass of water to prevent crystalluria; drink 8-10 glasses of water/day
- Teach patient to complete course of full treatment to prevent superinfection
- Teach patient to avoid sunlight or use sunscreen to prevent burns
- Teach patient to avoid OTC medications (aspirin, vit C) unless directed by prescriber
- If diabetic, teach patient to use Clinistix or Tes-Tape
- Teach patient to use alternative contraceptive measures; decreased effectiveness of oral contraceptives may result
- Teach patient to notify prescriber if skin rash, sore throat, fever, mouth sores, unusual bruising, bleeding occur

Evaluation

Positive therapeutic outcome
Absence of pain, fever, C&S negative

triprolidine (℞)

(trye-proe'li-deen)
Actidil, Myidil, triprolidine HCl
Func. class.: Antihistamine
Chem. class.: Alkylamine, H_1-receptor antagonist

Pregnancy category C

Action: Acts on blood vessels, GI, respiratory systems by competing with histamine for H_1-receptor site; decreases allergic response by blocking histamine

➔ **Therapeutic Outcome:** Absence of allergy symptoms and rhinitis

Uses: Rhinitis, allergy symptoms

Dosage and routes

Adult: PO 2.5 mg tid-qid
P ***Child >6 yr:*** PO 1.25 mg tid-qid
P ***Child 4-6 yr:*** PO 0.9 mg tid-qid
P ***Child 2-4 yr:*** PO 0.6 mg tid-qid
P ***Child 4 mo-2 yr:*** PO 0.3 mg tid-qid

Available forms: Tabs 2.5 mg; syrup 1.25 mg/5 ml

Adverse effects

CNS: *Dizziness, drowsiness,* poor coordination, fatigue, anxiety, euphoria, confusion, paresthesia, neuritis
CV: Hypotension, palpitations, tachycardia
EENT: Blurred vision, dilated pupils, tinnitus, nasal stuffiness, dry nose, throat, mouth
GI: *Constipation,* dry mouth, nausea, vomiting, anorexia, diarrhea
GU: *Retention,* dysuria, frequency
HEMA: **Thrombocytopenia, agranulocytosis, hemolytic anemia**
INTEG: Rash, urticaria, photosensitivity
RESP: Increased thick secretions, wheezing, chest tightness

Contraindications: Hypersensitivity to H_1-receptor antagonist, acute asthma attack, lower respiratory tract disease

Precautions: Increased intraocular pressure, renal disease, cardiac disease, hypertension, bronchial asthma, seizure disorder, stenosed peptic ulcers, hyperthyroidism, prostatic hypertrophy, bladder neck obstruction, pregnancy **C**

Pharmacokinetics

Absorption	Well absorbed
Distribution	Widely distributed, crosses blood-brain barrier
Metabolism	Liver—extensively
Excretion	Kidneys
Half-life	5 hr

Pharmacodynamics

Onset	15-60 min
Peak	1-2 hr
Duration	6-8 hr

Interactions

Individual drugs

Alcohol: ↑ CNS depression
Atropine: ↑ anticholinergic reactions
Disopyramide: ↑ anticholinergic reactions
Haloperidol: ↑ anticholinergic reactions
Quinidine: ↑ anticholinergic reactions

Drug classifications

Antidepressants: ↑ anticholinergic reactions
Antihistamines: ↑ anticholinergic reactions
CNS depressants: ↑ CNS depression
MAOIs: ↑ anticholinergic effect
Opiates: ↑ CNS depression
Phenothiazines: ↑ anticholinergic reactions
Sedative/hypnotics: ↑ CNS depression

Herb/drug

Henbane: ↑ anticholinergic effect

Lab test interferences

False negative: Skin allergy tests (discontinue antihistamines 3 days before testing)

NURSING CONSIDERATIONS

Assessment

- Assess respiratory status: rate, rhythm, increase in bronchial secretions, wheezing, chest tightness; provide fluids to 2 L/day to decrease thickness of secretions
- Monitor I&O ratio: be alert for urinary retention, frequency, dysuria, G especially in elderly; drug should be discontinued if these occur
- Monitor CBC during long-term therapy; blood dyscrasias may occur but are rare

Nursing diagnoses

- ✓ Airway clearance, ineffective (uses)
- ✓ Injury, risk for (adverse reactions)
- ✓ Knowledge deficit (teaching)
- ✓ Noncompliance (teaching—overuse)

Implementation

- Give on an empty stomach, 1 hr ac or 2 hr pc to facilitate absorption
- Store in airtight, light-resistant container

Patient/family education

- Teach patient all aspects of drug use; to notify prescriber if confusion, sedation, hypotension occur; to avoid driving or other hazardous activity if drowsiness occurs; to avoid alcohol or other CNS depressants that may potentiate effect
- Advise patient to take medication 1 hr ac or 2 hr pc to facilitate absorption
- Caution patient not to exceed recommended dose because dysrhythmias may occur
- Inform patient that hard candy, gum, frequent rinsing of mouth may be used for dryness

Evaluation

Positive therapeutic outcome

- Absence of running or congested nose, rashes

Treatment of overdose:

Administer ipecac syrup or lavage, diazepam, vasopressors, barbiturates (short-acting)

triptorelin (℞)

(trip-toe′rel-in)

Trelstar Depot

Func. class.: Gonadotropin-releasing hormone antagonist

Chem. class.: Synthetic decapeptide analog of LHRH

Pregnancy category X

Action: Inhibitor of pituitary gonadotropin secretion; initially increases LH and FSH, with increases in testosterone, reduction in sex steroid levels

T

Therapeutic Outcome: Decreased signs/symptoms of advanced prostate cancer

Uses: Advanced prostate cancer

Dosage and routes

Adult: IM 3.75 mg qmo

Available forms: Microgranules, depot inj 3.75 mg

Adverse effects

CNS: Headache, insomnia, dizziness, lability, fatigue
CV: *Hypertension*
ENDO: Gynecomastia
GI: Nausea, vomiting, diarrhea
GU: Impotence, urinary retention, UTI
INTEG: Rash, pain on injection, pruritus, hypersensitivity
MS: Osteoneuralgia

Contraindications: Hypersensitivity to this product or other LHRH agonists or LHRH, pregnancy **X**, lactation

Pharmacokinetics

Absorption	Unknown
Distribution	Unknown
Metabolism	CYP/450
Excretion	Liver, kidneys
Half-life	3 hr

Pharmacodynamics

Unknown

Interactions: None known

Lab test interferences

↑ Alkaline phosphatase, ↑ estradiol, ↑ FSH, ↑ LH, ↑ testosterone levels
↓ Testosterone levels, ↓ progesterone

NURSING CONSIDERATIONS

Assessment

- Assess for severe hypersensitivity: discontinue drug and give antihistamines, have emergency equipment nearby
- Monitor I&O ratios; palpate bladder for distention in urinary obstruction
- Monitor for relief of bone pain (back pain)
- Assess levels of testosterone and prostate-specific antigen (PSA)

Nursing diagnoses

☑ Diarrhea (adverse reactions)
☑ Knowledge deficit (teaching)

Implementation

- Give IM using implant, inserted by qualified person
- Use syringe with 20-G needle, withdraw 2 ml of sterile water for inj, inject into vial, shake well, withdraw vial contents, inject immediately

Patient/family education

- Teach patient that gynecomastia may occur but will decrease after treatment is dicontinued

Evaluation

Positive therapeutic outcome

- More normal levels of PSA, acid phosphatase, alkaline phosphatase; testosterone level of <25 ng/dl

HIGH ALERT

tubocurarine (℞)

(too-boh-cure'a-reen)

Tubarine ✦, Tubocuraine

Func. class.: Neuromuscular blocker

Chem. class.: Synthetic curariform

Pregnancy category C

Action: Inhibits transmission of nerve impulses by binding with cholinergic receptor sites, antagonizing action of acetylcholine; no analgesic response

Therapeutic Outcome: Skeletal muscle paralysis during anesthesia

Uses: Facilitation of endotracheal intubation, skeletal muscle relaxation during mechanical ventilation, surgery, or general anesthesia

Dosage and routes

Adult: **IV** bol 0.4-0.5 mg/kg, then 0.08-0.10 mg/kg 20-45 min after 1st dose if needed for prolonged procedures

Available forms: Inj 3 mg/ml (20 U/ml)

Adverse effects

CV: Bradycardia, tachycardia, increased, decreased B/P

EENT: Increased secretions

INTEG: Rash, flushing, pruritus, urticaria

RESP: **Prolonged apnea, bronchospasm, cyanosis, respiratory depression**

Contraindications: Hypersensitivity

Precautions: Pregnancy **C**, cardiac disease, lactation, children <2 yr, electrolyte imbalances, dehydration, neuromuscular disease, respiratory disease

P

Pharmacokinetics

Absorption	Complete bioavailability
Distribution	Extensive, crosses placenta
Metabolism	Liver, small amount
Excretion	Kidneys—unchanged (30%-75%), bile (11%)
Half-life	2 hr

Pharmacodynamics

	IV	IM
Onset	1 min	15-30 min
Peak	5 min	Unknown
Duration	½-1½ hr	Unknown

Interactions

Individual drugs

Clindamycin: ↑ paralysis, length and intensity

Colistin: ↑ paralysis, length and intensity

Lidocaine: ↑ paralysis, length and intensity

Lithium: ↑ paralysis, length and intensity

Magnesium: ↑ paralysis, length and intensity

Polymyxin B: ↑ paralysis, length and intensity

Procainamide: ↑ paralysis, length and intensity

Quinidine: ↑ paralysis, length and intensity

Succinylcholine: ↑ paralysis, length and intensity

Drug classifications

Aminoglycosides: ↑ paralysis, length and intensity

β-Adrenergic blockers: ↑ paralysis, length and intensity

Diuretics, potassium-losing: ↑ paralysis, length and intensity

General anesthetics: ↑ paralysis, length and intensity

NURSING CONSIDERATIONS

Assessment

- Monitor for electrolyte imbalances (potassium, magnesium) before drug is used; electrolyte imbalances may lead to increased action of this drug
- Monitor VS (B/P, pulse, respirations, airway) until fully recovered; rate, depth, pattern of respirations, strength of hand grip; patient should be intubated before use
- Monitor recovery: decreased paralysis of face, diaphragm, leg, arm, rest of body; residual weakness and respiratory problems may occur during recovery period
- Monitor allergic reactions: rash, fever, respiratory distress, pruritus; drug should be discontinued

Nursing diagnoses

- ✓ Breathing pattern, ineffective (uses)
- ✓ Communication, impaired verbal (adverse reactions)
- ✓ Fear (adverse reactions)
- ✓ Knowledge deficit (teaching)

Implementation

- Use peripheral nerve stimulator by anesthesiologist to determine neuromuscular blockade; deep tendon reflexes should be monitored during extended periods
- Give **IV** undiluted by direct **IV** over 1-1½ min (only by qualified person, usually an anesthesiologist)

T

Syringe compatibilities: Pentobarbital, thiopental

Additive incompatibilities: Barbiturates, sodium bicarbonate

Solution compatibilities: D_5, $D_{10}W$, 0.9% NaCl, 0.45% NaCl, Ringer's, LR, dextrose/Ringer's or dextrose/LR combinations

Patient/family education

- Provide reassurance if communication is difficult during recovery from neuromuscular blockade
- Provide explanation to patient regarding all procedures or treatments; patient will remain conscious if anesthesia is not given also

Evaluation

Positive therapeutic outcome

- Paralysis of jaw, eyelid, head, neck, rest of body as evaluated by peripheral nerve stimulator

Treatment of overdose: Edrophonium or neostigmine, atropine, monitor VS; patient may require mechanical ventilation

---

HIGH ALERT

urokinase (℞)

(yoor-oh-kin'ase)

Abbokinase, Abbokinase Open-Cath

Func. class.: Thrombolytic enzyme

Chem. class.: β-Hemolytic *Streptococcus* filtrate (purified)

Pregnancy category B

Action: Promotes thrombolysis by directly converting plasminogen to plasmin

➔ **Therapeutic Outcome:** Lysis of emboli, or thrombosis in various parts of the body

Uses: Venous thrombosis, pulmonary embolism, arterial thrombosis, arterial embolism, arteriovenous cannula occlusion, lysis of coronary artery thrombi after MI

Dosage and routes

Lysis of pulmonary emboli

P ***Adult and child:*** **IV** 4400 IU/kg/hr × 12-24 hr, not to exceed 200 ml; then **IV** heparin, then anticoagulants

Coronary artery thrombosis

Adult: Instill 6000 IU/min into occluded artery for 1-2 hr after giving **IV** bol of heparin 2500-10,000 U; may also give as **IV** inf of 2-3 million U over 45-90 min

Venous catheter occlusion

P ***Adult and child:*** Instill 5000 IU into line, wait 5 min, then aspirate; repeat aspiration attempts q5 min × ½ hr; if occlusion has not been removed, then cap line and wait ½-1 hr, then aspirate; may need 2nd dose if still occluded

Available forms: Powder for inj, 250,000 IU/vial; powder for catheter clearance

Adverse effects

CNS: *Headache,* fever

CV: Hypertension, dysrhythmias, hypertension

EENT: Periorbital edema

GI: *Nausea,* vomiting

HEMA: *Decreased Hct,* **bleeding**

INTEG: *Rash, urticaria,* phlebitis at **IV** inf site, itching, flushing

MS: Low back pain

RESP: Altered respirations, cyanosis, shortness of breath, **bronchospasm**

SYST: **GI, GU, intracranial, retroperitoneal bleeding;** surface bleeding; **anaphylaxis** (rare)

Contraindications: Hypersensitivity, active bleeding, intraspinal surgery, neoplasms of CNS, ulcerative colitis/enteritis, severe hypertension, renal disease, hepatic disease, hypocoagulation, COPD, subacute bacterial endocarditis, rheumatic valvular disease, cerebral embolism/thrombosis/hemorrhage, intraarterial diagnostic procedure or surgery (10 days), recent major surgery

Precautions: Arterial emboli from left side of heart, pregnancy **B**

Pharmacokinetics

Absorption	Completely
Distribution	Unknown
Metabolism	Liver
Excretion	Kidneys
Half-life	10-20 min

Pharmacodynamics

Onset	Rapid
Peak	Rapid
Duration	12 hr

Interactions

Individual drugs

Abciximab: ↑ bleeding potential
Aspirin: ↑ bleeding potential
Clopidogrel: ↑ bleeding potential
Dipyridamole: ↑ bleeding potential
Eptifibatide: ↑ bleeding potential
Heparin: ↑ bleeding potential
Plicamycin: ↑ bleeding potential
Ticlopidine: ↑ bleeding potential
Tirofiban: ↑ bleeding potential
Valproic acid: ↑ bleeding potential

Drug classifications

Anticoagulants, oral: ↑ bleeding potential
Cephalosporins, some: ↑ bleeding potential
NSAIDs: ↑ bleeding potential

Lab test interferences

↑ Pro-time, ↑ APTT, ↑ TT

NURSING CONSIDERATIONS

Assessment

- Monitor VS, B/P, pulse, respirations (including peripheral), neurologic signs, temp at least q4h; temp >104° F (40° C) indicates internal bleeding; monitor rhythm closely; ventricular dysrhythmias may occur with hyperfusion; monitor heart, breath sounds, neurologic status, peripheral pulses
- Assess for bleeding during 1st hr of treatment: hematuria, hematemesis, bleeding from mucous membranes, epistaxis, ecchymosis; guaiac, all body fluids, stools; blood studies (Hct, platelets, PTT, pro-time, TT, APTT) before starting therapy (pro-time or APTT must be less than 2 × control); TT or PT q3-4h during treatment
- Assess hypersensitivity: fever, rash, itching, chills, facial swelling, dyspnea; mild reaction may be treated with antihistamines; notify prescriber of severe reactions, stop drug, keep resuscitative equipment nearby
- Monitor ECG on monitor, watch for segment changes, changes in rhythm; sinus bradycardia, ventricular tachycardia, accelerated idioventricular rhythm may occur because of reperfusion

Nursing diagnoses

- ✓ Tissue perfusion, altered (uses)
- ✓ Injury, high risk for (adverse reactions)
- ✓ Impaired gas exchange (uses)

Implementation

IV Intermittent IV route

- Give **IV** loading dose over 30 min to avoid hypotension
- **IV** after dilution with 4-5 g/250 ml of 0.9% NaCl, D_5W, LR, give over 1 hr; may give by continuous inf after loading dose(s) of 1 g/hr diluted in 50-100 ml of compatible sol; use infusion pump; do not give by direct **IV**
- Give heparin therapy after thrombolytic therapy is discontinued, TT, ACT, or APTT less than 2 × control (about 3-4 hr)
- Avoid invasive procedures, inj, rectal temp
- Apply pressure for 30 sec to minor bleeding sites, 30 min to sites of atrial puncture, followed by pressure dressing; inform prescriber if this does not attain hemostasis
- Store powder at room temp or refrigerate; protect from excessive light

U

Additive incompatibilities: Do not mix with other medications

Patient/family education

- Teach patient reason for medication, signs and symptoms of bleeding, allergic reactions, when to notify health care prescriber

Evaluation

Positive therapeutic outcome

- Lysis of thrombi or emboli

valacyclovir (℞)

(val-a-sye'kloh-vir)

Valtrex

Func. class.: Antiviral

Chem. class.: Acyclic purine nucleoside analog

Pregnancy category B

Action: Interferes with DNA synthesis by conversion to acyclovir, causing decreased viral replication, time of lesional healing

➔ **Therapeutic Outcome:** Absence of itching, painful lesions; crusting and healing of lesions

Uses: Treatment or suppression of herpes zoster, recurrent genital herpes

Investigational uses: Prevention of cytomegalovirus infection, in advanced HIV posttransplant patients

Dosage and routes

Genital herpes

Adult: PO 1 g bid × 10 days initially; 1 g qd or 500 mg bid in those with <10 recurrences/yr

Herpes zoster

Adult: PO 1 g tid × 1 wk

Recurrent episodes

Adult: PO 500 mg bid ×3 days

Suppressive therapy

Adult: PO 1 g qd if ≤10 recurrences/yr

Renal dose

Adult: PO CrCl 30-49 ml/min 1g q12h (herpes zoster); CrCl 10-29 ml/min 1 g q24h (genital herpes); 500 mg q24h (recurrent genital herpes); CrCl <10 ml/min 500 mg q24h (genital herpes), 500 mg q24h (recurrent genital herpes)

Available forms: Tabs 500, 1000 mg

Adverse effects

CNS: Tremors, lethargy, *dizziness, headache, weakness*

GI: *Nausea, vomiting, diarrhea, abdominal pain, constipation*

INTEG: *Rash*

Contraindications: Hypersensitivity to this drug or acyclovir

Precautions: Lactation, hepatic disease, renal disease, electrolyte imbalance, dehydration, pregnancy **B**

Pharmacokinetics	
Absorption	Unknown
Distribution	Crosses placenta, enters breast milk
Metabolism	Converts to acyclovir
Excretion	Unknown
Half-life	2½-3½ hr

Pharmacodynamics	
Onset	Unknown
Peak	Unknown
Duration	Unknown

Interactions

Individual drugs

Cimetidine: Increased blood levels of valacyclovir

Probenecid: Increased blood levels of valacyclovir

NURSING CONSIDERATIONS

Assessment

- Assess for signs of infection; characteristics of lesions
- Assess C&S before drug therapy; drug may be performed as soon as culture is performed; repeat C&S after treatment; determine the presence of other sexually transmitted diseases
- Assess bowel pattern before, during treatment

- Assess for skin eruptions: rash
- Assess allergies before treatment, reaction of each medication; place allergies on chart in bright red letters

Nursing diagnoses

✓ Potential infection (uses)

Patient/family education

- Advise patient to take as prescribed; if dose is missed, take as soon as remembered up to 1 hr before next dose; do not double dose
- Instruct patient to take drug orally before infection occurs; drug should be taken when itching or pain occurs, usually before eruptions
- Inform patient that partners need to be told that patient has herpes; they can become infected; condoms must be worn to prevent reinfections
- Tell patient that drug does not cure infection, just controls symptoms and does not prevent infection to others

Evaluation

Positive therapeutic outcome

- Absence of itching, painful lesions; crusting and healed lesions

Treatment of overdose:

- Discontinue drug
- Provide hemodialysis, resuscitation if needed

valdecoxib

See Appendix A, Selected New Drugs

valganciclovir

See Appendix A, Selected New Drugs

valproate (℞)

(val-proh'ate)

Depacon

valproic acid (℞)

Depakene, Myproic acid

divalproex sodium (℞)

Depakote, Depakote ER, Epival

Func. class.: Anticonvulsant

Chem. class.: Carboxylic acid derivative

Pregnancy category D

Action: Increases levels of γ-aminobutyric acid (GABA) in brain, which decreases seizure activity

➔ **Therapeutic Outcome:** Decreased symptoms of epilepsy, bipolar disorder

Uses: Simple (petit mal), complex (petit mal), absence, mixed seizures, manic episode associated with bipolar disorder, prophylaxis of migraine

Investigational uses: Tonic-clonic (grand mal), myoclonic seizures; rectal (valproic acid) for seizures

Dosage and routes

P ***Adult and child:*** PO 15 mg/kg/day divided in 2-3 doses, may increase by 5-10 mg/kg/day qwk, max 60 mg/kg/day in 2-3 divided doses

Available forms: *Valproic acid:* caps 250, 500 mg; syrup 250 mg/5 ml; *divalproex:* delayed rel tabs 125, 250, 500 mg; *sprinkle caps:* 125 mg; *valproate:* inj 100 mg/ml

Adverse effects

CNS: *Sedation, drowsiness,* dizziness, headache, incoordination, paresthesia, depression, hallucinations, behavioral changes, tremors, aggression, weakness

EENT: Visual disturbances

GI: *Nausea, vomiting, constipation, diarrhea, heartburn,* anorexia, cramps, **hepatic failure, pancreatitis, toxic hepatitis,** stomatitis

V

GU: Enuresis, irregular menses
HEMA: **Thrombocytopenia, leukopenia, lymphocytosis,** increased pro-time
INTEG: *Rash,* alopecia, bruising

Contraindications: Hypersensitivity, pregnancy **D**, hepatic disease

P **Precautions:** Lactation, child <2 yr

Pharmacokinetics	
Absorption	Unknown
Distribution	Breast milk, crosses placenta, widely distributed
Metabolism	Liver
Excretion	Kidneys
Half-life	9-16 hr

Pharmacodynamics	
Onset	15-30 min
Peak	1-4 hr
Duration	4-6 hr

Interactions

Individual drugs

Abciximab: ↑ bleeding risk
Alcohol: ↑ CNS depression
Cefamandole: ↑ bleeding risk
Cefoperazone: ↑ bleeding risk
Cefotetan: ↑ bleeding risk
Cimetidine: ↑ metabolism of valproic acid
Eptifibatide: ↑ bleeding risk
Heparin: ↑ bleeding risk
Phenytoin: ↑ action of phenytoin
Tirofiban: ↑ bleeding risk
Warfarin: ↑ toxicity of warfarin

Drug classifications

Barbiturates: ↑ CNS depression
Benzodiazepines: ↑ sedation
MAOIs: ↑ CNS depression
NSAIDs: ↑ bleeding risk
Salicylates: ↑ toxicity of valproic acid
Thrombolytics: ↑ bleeding risk

Lab test interferences

False positive: Ketones

NURSING CONSIDERATIONS

Assessment

- Monitor blood studies: Hct, Hgb, RBC, serum folate, platelets, pro-time, vit D if on long-term therapy
- Monitor hepatic studies: AST, ALT, bilirubin, creatinine, failure
- Monitor blood levels: therapeutic level 50-100 μg/ml
- Assess mental status: mood, sensorium, affect, memory (long, short)
- Assess respiratory dysfunction: respiratory depression, character, rate, rhythm; hold drug if respirations are <12/min or if pupils are dilated

Implementation

- ⊘ Give tablets or capsules whole
- Give elixir alone; do not dilute with carbonated beverage; do not give syrup to patients on sodium restriction
- Give with food or milk to decrease GI symptoms

Patient/family education

- Teach patient that physical dependency may result from extended use
- Instruct patient to avoid driving, other activities that require alertness
- Advise patient not to discontinue medication quickly after long-term use; seizures may result
- Advise patient to report visual disturbances, rash, diarrhea, light-colored stools, jaundice, protracted vomiting to prescriber

Evaluation

Positive therapeutic outcome

- Decreased seizures

valrubicin (℞)

(val-roo′bih-sin)
Valstar
Func. class.: Antineoplastic, antibiotic
Chem. class.: Anthracycline glycoside
Pregnancy category C

Action: A semisynthetic analog of doxorubicin that inhibits DNA synthesis primarily; replication is decreased by binding to DNA, which causes strand splitting; active throughout entire cell cycle; a vesicant

Therapeutic Outcome: Decreased symptoms of breast cancer

Uses: Bladder cancer

Dosage and routes

Adult: Intravesically 800 mg qwk × 6 wk, delay administration ≥2 wk after transurethral resection or fulguration

Available forms: Sol for intravesical instillation 40 mg/ml

Adverse effects

CV: *Chest pain*

GI: *Nausea, vomiting, anorexia, diarrhea*

GU: *UTI, urinary retention, hematuria*

HEMA: **Thrombocytopenia, leukopenia,** *anemia*

INTEG: *Rash*

Contraindications: Hypersensitivity to anthracyclines or Cremophor EL, urinary tract infection, small bladder

Precautions: Pregnancy **C**, lactation, children

Pharmacokinetics	
Absorption	Unknown
Distribution	Penetrates bladder wall
Metabolism	Unknown
Excretion	Unknown
Half-life	Unknown

Pharmacodynamics	
Onset	Unknown
Peak	Unknown
Duration	Unknown

Interactions: Unknown

NURSING CONSIDERATIONS

Assessment

- Monitor I&O ratio; report fall in urine output of <30 ml/hr
- Monitor temperature q4h; fever may indicate beginning of infection
- Monitor local irritation, pain, burning at injection site

Nursing diagnoses

- Infection, risk for (side effects)
- Nutrition, altered, less than body requirements (side effects)
- Knowledge deficit (teaching)

Implementation

- Administer after urinary catheter is inserted under aseptic conditions, drain bladder and instill the diluted 75 ml of valrubicin by gravity for several min, withdraw catheter; drug should be retained for 2 hr, then void
- Use procedure for handling and disposal of cytotoxic agents
- Do not use polyvinyl chloride (PVC) **IV** tubing
- Prepare/store valrubicin sol in glass, polypropylene, or polyolefin tubing/containers
- For instillation, 5-ml vials (200 mg valrubicin/5-ml vial) should be warmed to room temp, withdraw 20 ml from the 4 vials and dilute with 55 ml of 0.9% NaCl inj to 75 ml of diluted valrubicin sol
- Valrubicin sol is clear red, at lower temps a waxy precipitate may form, warm in hand until sol is clear
- Perform strict hand-washing technique; use gloves, protective clothing
- Provide increased fluid intake to 2-3 L/day to prevent urate, calculi formation
- Store at room temp for 12 hr after reconstituting

Patient/family education

- Advise patient to report any complaints, side effects to nurse or prescriber
- Advise patient to consume fluids to 2 L/day unless contraindicated
- Teach patient that urine and other body fluids may be red-orange for 48 hr
- Teach patient that contraceptive measures are recommended during therapy

V

Evaluation

Positive therapeutic outcome

- Decreased tumor size, spread of malignancy

valsartan (℞)

(val-zar'tan)

Diovan

Func. class.: Antihypertensive

Chem. class.: Angiotensin II receptor antagonist (type AT_1)

Pregnancy category UK

Action: Blocks the vasoconstrictor and aldosterone-secreting effects of angiotensin II; selectively blocks the binding of angiotensin II to the AT_1 receptor found in tissues

Therapeutic Outcome: Decreased B/P

Uses: Hypertension, alone or in combination

Dosage and routes

Adult: PO 80-160 mg qd alone or when used in combination

Available forms: Tabs 80, 160 mg

Adverse effects

CNS: *Dizziness, insomnia,* depression, drowsiness, vertigo

CV: Angina pectoris, 2nd-degree AV block, **cerebrovascular accident,** hypotension, **MI, dysrhythmias**

EENT: Conjunctivitis

GI: Diarrhea, abdominal pain, nausea, **hepatotoxicity**

GU: Impotence, nephrotoxicity

HEMA: *Anemia,* neutropenia

MS: Cramps, myalgia, pain, stiffness

RESP: *Cough*

Contraindications: Hypersensitivity, pregnancy **UK,** severe hepatic disease, bilateral renal artery stenosis

Precautions: Hypersensitivity to angiotensin-converting enzyme inhibitors, CHF, hypertrophic cardiomyopathy, aortic/mitral valve stenosis, CAD; lactation, children, elderly

Pharmacokinetics

Absorption	Well
Distribution	Bound to plasma proteins
Metabolism	Extensive
Excretion	Feces, urine, breast milk
Half-life	9 hr

Pharmacodynamics

Onset	Unknown
Peak	2 hr
Duration	24 hr

Interactions: None significant

NURSING CONSIDERATIONS

Assessment

- Assess B/P, pulse q4h; note rate, rhythm, quality
- Monitor electrolytes: potassium, sodium, chloride; total CO_2
- Obtain baselines in renal, liver function tests before therapy begins
- Assess blood studies: BUN, creatinine, before treatment
- Monitor for edema in feet, legs daily
- Assess for skin turgor, dryness of mucous membranes for hydration status

Nursing diagnoses

- ✓ Fluid volume deficit (side effects)
- ✓ Noncompliance (teaching)
- ✓ Knowledge deficit (teaching)

Implementation

- Administer without regard to meals

Patient/family education

- Teach patient not to take this drug if breast-feeding or pregnant, or have had an allergic reaction to this drug
- If a dose is missed, instruct patient to take as soon as possible, unless it is within an hour before next dose
- Advise patient to comply with dosage schedule, even if feeling better
- Teach patient to notify prescriber of fever, swelling of hands or feet, irregular heartbeat, chest pain

• Advise patient excessive perspiration, dehydration, diarrhea may lead to fall in blood pressure; consult prescriber if these occur
• Inform patient that drug may cause dizziness, fainting; light-headedness may occur
• Caution patient to rise slowly to sitting or standing position to minimize orthostatic hypotension

Evaluation

Positive therapeutic outcome
• Decreased B/P

vancomycin

(van-koe-mye'sin)

Lyphocin, Vancocin, vancomycin HCl

Func. clas.: Antiinfective, misc.
Chem. class.: Tricyclic glycopeptide

Pregnancy category C

Action: Inhibits bacterial cell wall synthesis

➔ **Therapeutic Outcome:** Bactericidal for the following organisms: staphylococci, streptococci, *Corynebacterium, Clostridium*

Uses: Resistant staphylococcal infections, pseudomembranous colitis, staphylococcal enterocolitis, group A β-hemolytic streptococci, endocarditis prophylaxis for dental procedures, diphtheroid endocarditis

Dosage and routes

Serious staphylococcal infections

Adult: **IV** 500 mg (7.5 mg/kg) q6-8h or 1 g (15 mg/kg) q12h, max 4 g/day

P ***Child:*** **IV** 40 mg/kg/day divided q6-12h

P ***Neonates:*** **IV** 15 mg/kg initially followed by 10 mg/kg q8-24h

Pseudomembranous/staphylococcal enterocolitis

Adult: PO 500 mg-2 g/day in 3-4 divided doses for 7-10 days

P ***Child:*** PO 40 mg/kg/day divided q6h, max 2 g/day

P ***Neonates:*** PO 10 mg/kg/day in divided doses

Endocarditis prophylaxis

Adult: **IV** 1 g over 1 hr, 1 hr before dental procedure

P ***Child:*** 20 mg/kg over 1 hr, 1 hr before procedure

Available forms: Pulvules 125, 250 mg; powder for oral sol 1, 10 g; powder for inj **IV** 500 mg; vials 1, 5, 10 g

Adverse effects

CV: **Cardiac arrest, vascular collapse** (rare)
EENT: Ototoxicity, permanent deafness, tinnitus
GI: **Nausea, pseudomembranous colitis**
GU: **Nephrotoxicity, increased BUN, creatinine, albumin, fatal uremia**
HEMA: **Leukopenia, eosinophilia, neutropenia**
INTEG: Chills, fever, rash, thrombophlebitis at inj site, urticaria, pruritus, necrosis (Redman's syndrome)
RESP: Wheezing, dyspnea
SYST: **Anaphylaxis**

Contraindications: Hypersensitivity, previous hearing loss

Precautions: Renal disease, G pregnancy **C**, lactation, elderly, P neonates

Pharmacokinetics	
Absorption	Poorly absorbed (PO), completely absorbed (**IV**)
Distribution	Widely distributed, crosses placenta
Metabolism	Liver
Excretion	PO—feces, IV—kidneys
Half-life	4-8 hr

V

Pharmacodynamics

	IV
Onset	Immediate
Peak	Inf end

Interactions

Individual drugs

Amphotericin B: ↑ toxicity
Bacitracin: ↑ toxicity
Cisplatin: ↑ toxicity
Polymyxin B:↑ toxicity

Drug classifications

Aminoglycosides: ↑ toxicity
Cephalosporins: ↑ toxicity
Nondepolarizing muscle relaxants: ↑ toxicity

NURSING CONSIDERATIONS

Assessment

- Monitor I&O ratio; report hematuria, oliguria because nephrotoxicity may occur
- Monitor any patient with compromised renal system (BUN, creatinine); drug is excreted slowly in poor renal system function; toxicity may occur rapidly
- Monitor blood studies: WBC; serum levels; peak 1 hr after 1 hr inf 25-40 mg/ml; trough before next dose 5-10 mg/ml
- Obtain C&S before drug therapy; drug may be given as soon as culture is performed
- Assess auditory function during, after treatment; hearing loss, ringing, roaring in ears; drug should be discontinued
- Monitor B/P during administration; sudden drop may indicate red man's syndrome
- Assess for signs of infection
- Assess respiratory status: rate, character, wheezing, tightness in chest
- Identify allergies before treatment, reaction of each medication

Nursing diagnoses

✓ Infection, risk for (uses)
✓ Knowledge deficit (teaching)

Implementation

IV IV route

- Give after reconstitution with 10 ml of sterile water for inj (500 mg/10 ml); further dilution is needed for **IV**, 500 mg/100 ml of 0.9% NaCl, D_5W given as intermittent inf over 1 hr; decrease rate of infusion if Red Man's syndrome occurs

Y-site compatibilities:
Acyclovir, allopurinol, amiodarone, amsacrine, atracurium, cyclophosphamide, diltiazem, enalaprilat, esmolol, filgrastim, fluconazole, fludarabine, gallium, granisetron, hydromorphone, insulin (regular), labetalol, lorazepam, magnesium sulfate, melphalan, meperidine, meropenem, midazolam, morphine, ondansetron, paclitaxel, pancuronium, perphenazine, propofol, sodium bicarbonate, tacrolimus, teniposide, theophylline, thiotepa, tolazoline, vecuronium, vinorelbine, warfarin, zidovudine

Additive compatibilities:
Amikacin, atracurium, calcium gluconate, cefepime, cimetidine, corticotropin, dimenhydrinate, hydrocortisone, meropenem, ofloxacin, potassium chloride, ranitidine, verapamil, vit B/C

- Give antihistamine if red man's syndrome occurs: decreased B/P, flushing of neck, face
- Give dose based on serum concentration
- Store at room temp for up to 2 wk after reconstitution
- Have adrenalin, suction, tracheostomy set, endotracheal intubation equipment on unit; anaphylaxis may occur
- Provide adequate intake of fluids (2 L) to prevent nephrotoxicity

Patient/family education

- Teach patient aspects of drug therapy: need to complete entire course of medication to ensure organism death (7-10 days); culture may be performed after completed course of medication

- Advise patient to report sore throat, fever, fatigue; could indicate superinfection
- Instruct patient that drug must be taken in equal intervals around clock to maintain blood levels

Evaluation

Positive therapeutic outcome

- Absence of fever, sore throat
- Negative culture after treatment

HIGH ALERT

vecuronium (℞)

(ve-kure-oh′nee-yum)

Norcuron

Func. class.: Neuromuscular blocker

Chem. class.: Synthetic curariform

Pregnancy category C

Action: Inhibits transmission of nerve impulses by binding with cholinergic receptor sites, antagonizing action of acetylcholine; no analgesic response

Therapeutic Outcome: Skeletal muscle paralysis during anesthesia

Uses: Facilitation of endotracheal intubation; skeletal muscle relaxation during mechanical ventilation, surgery, or general anesthesia

Dosage and routes

P ***Adult and child >9 yr:*** **IV** bol 0.08-0.10 mg/kg, then 0.010-0.015 mg/kg for prolonged procedures

Available forms: 10 mg/5 ml vial

Adverse effects

CNS: Skeletal muscle weakness or paralysis (rarely)

RESP: **Prolonged apnea, possible respiratory paralysis**

Contraindications: Hypersensitivity

Precautions: Pregnancy **C**, cardiac disease, lactation, children <2 yr, electrolyte imbalances, dehydration, neuromuscular disease, respiratory, hepatic disease

Do Not Confuse:

Nocuron/Narcan

Pharmacokinetics

Absorption	Completely absorbed
Distribution	Rapid—to extracellular fluids
Metabolism	Liver (20%)
Excretion	Kidneys—unchanged (35%)
Half-life	1½ hr, increased in liver disease

Pharmacodynamics

Onset	1 min
Peak	5 min
Duration	15-25 min

Interactions

Individual drugs

Clindamycin: ↑ paralysis, length and intensity
Colistin: ↑ paralysis, length and intensity
Lidocaine: ↑ paralysis, length and intensity
Lithium: ↑ paralysis, length and intensity
Magnesium: ↑ paralysis, length and intensity
Polymyxin B: ↑ paralysis, length and intensity
Procainamide: ↑ paralysis, length and intensity
Quinidine: ↑ paralysis, length and intensity
Succinylcholine: ↑ paralysis, length and intensity

Drug classifications

Aminoglycosides: ↑ paralysis, length and intensity
β-Adrenergic blockers: ↑ paralysis, length and intensity
Diuretics, potassium-losing: ↑ paralysis, length and intensity
General anesthetics: ↑ paralysis, length and intensity

NURSING CONSIDERATIONS

Assessment

- Monitor for electrolyte imbalances (potassium, magnesium) before drug is used; electrolyte imbalances may lead to increased action of this drug
- Monitor patient's vital signs (B/P, pulse, respirations, airway) until fully recovered; rate, depth, pattern of respirations, strength of hand grip; patient should be intubated before use
- Monitor patient's recovery: decreased paralysis of face, diaphragm, leg, arm, rest of body; residual weakness and respiratory problems may occur during recovery period
- Monitor allergic reactions: rash, fever, respiratory distress, pruritus; drug should be discontinued

Nursing diagnoses

- ✓ Breathing pattern, ineffective (uses)
- ✓ Communication, impaired verbal (adverse reactions)
- ✓ Fear (adverse reactions)
- ✓ Knowledge deficit (teaching)

Implementation

- Use peripheral nerve stimulator by anesthesiologist to determine neuromuscular blockade; deep tendon reflexes should be monitored during extended periods
- Give by direct **IV** after reconstituting with bacteriostatic water, over 5 min, D_5W, 0.9% NaCl or LR
- Give by direct **IV** after reconstituting dose in 5-10 ml; give by titrating to patient response
- Give by continuous inf after diluting to 10-20 mg/100 ml and by titrating to patient response (only by qualified person, usually an anesthesiologist); do not administer IM
- Store in light-resistant area

Syringe incompatibilities: Barbiturates

Y-site compatibilities: Aminophylline, cefazolin, cefuroxime, cimetidine, diltiazem, dobutamine, dopamine, epinephrine, esmolol, fentanyl, fluconazole, gentamicin, heparin, hydrocortisone, hydromorphone, isoproterenol, labetalol, lorazepam, midazolam, milrinone, morphine, nicardipine, nitroglycerin, nitroprusside, norepinephrine, propofol, ranitidine, trimethoprim/sulfamethoxazole, vancomycin

Y-site incompatibilities: Barbiturates

Patient/family education

- Provide reassurance if communication is difficult during recovery from neuromuscular blockade
- Provide explanation to patients regarding all procedures or treatments; patient will remain conscious if anesthesia is not given also

Evaluation

Positive therapeutic outcome

- Paralysis of jaw, eyelid, head, neck, rest of body as evaluated by peripheral nerve stimulator

Treatment of overdose: Edrophonium or neostigmine, atropine, monitor VS; may require mechanical ventilation

venlafaxine (℞)

(ven-la-fax'een)

Effexor, Effexor XR

Func. class.: Second-generation antidepressant- misc

Pregnancy category C

Action: Potent inhibitor of neuronal serotinin and norepinephrine uptake, weak inhibitor of dopamine; no muscarinic, histaminergic, or α-adrenergic receptors in vitro

➔ **Therapeutic Outcome:** Relief of depression

Uses: Prevention/treatment of depression, long-term treatment of generalized anxiety disorder (Effexor XR)

Investigational uses: Hot flashes

Dosage and routes
Depression
Adult: PO 75 mg/day in 2 or 3 divided doses; taken with food, may be increased to 150 mg/day; if needed may be further increased to 225 mg/day; increments of 75 mg/day should be made at intervals of no less than 4 days; some hospitalized patients may require up to 375 mg/day in 3 divided doses; ext rel 37.5-75 mg PO qd, max 225 mg/day; give Effexor XR qd
Hepatic dose
Moderate impairment 50% of dose
Renal dose
Mild to moderate impairment 75% of dose
Hot flashes (off-label)
Adult: PO 12.5 mg bid × 4 wk or ext rel cap 37.5 mg × 4 wk

Available forms: Tabs scored 25, 37.5, 50, 75, 100 mg; ext rel caps 37.5, 75, 150 mg

Adverse effects
CNS: *Emotional lability, vertigo,* apathy, ataxia, CNS stimulation, euphoria, hallucinations, hostility, increased libido, hypertonia, hypotonia, psychosis
CV: *Migraine,* angina pectoris, extrasystoles, postural hypotension, syncope, thrombophlebitis, hypertension
EENT: *Abnormal vision, ear pain,* cataract, conjunctivitis, corneal lesions, dry eyes, otitis media, photophobia
GI: *Dysphagia, eructation,* colitis, gastritis, gingivitis, **rectal hemorrhage,** stomatitis, stomach and mouth ulceration
GU: *Anorgasmia, dysuria, hematuria, metrorrhagia, vaginitis, impaired urination,* albuminaria, amenorrhea, kidney calculus, cystitis, nocturia, breast and bladder pain, polyuria, **uterine hemorrhage, vaginal hemorrhage,** moniliasis
INTEG: Ecchymosis, acne, alopecia, brittle nails, dry skin, photosensitivity
META: *Peripheral edema, weight loss or gain,* diabetes mellitus, edema, glycosuria, hyperlipemia, hypokalemia
MS: Arthritis, bone pain, bursitis, myasthenia tenosynovitis
RESP: *Bronchitis, dyspnea,* asthma, chest congestion, epistaxis, hyperventilation, laryngitis
SYST: *Accidental injury, malaise, neck pain,* enlarged abdomen, cyst, facial edema, hangover effect, hernia

Contraindications: Hypersensitivity

P G **Precautions:** Mania, pregnancy **C,** lactation, children, elderly

Pharmacokinetics

Absorption	Well absorbed
Distribution	Widely distributed, 27% protein binding
Metabolism	Liver—extensively
Excretion	Kidneys, 87%
Half-life	5-7 hr, 11-13 hr (active metabolite)

Pharmacodynamics
Unknown

Interactions
Individual drugs
Alcohol: ↑ CNS depression
Lithium: ↑ serotonin effect
Drug classifications
Antihistamines: ↑ CNS depression
MAOIs: Hypertensive crisis, convulsions
Opioids: ↑ CNS depression
Sedative/hypnotics: ↑ CNS depression
Lab test interferences
↑ Serum bilirubin, ↑ blood glucose, ↑ alkaline phosphatase
↓ VMA, ↓ 5-HIAA
False: ↑ Urinary catecholamines

NURSING CONSIDERATIONS
Assessment
- Monitor B/P (lying, standing), pulse q4h; if systolic B/P drops 20 mm Hg

V

hold drug, notify prescriber; take vital signs q4h in patients with CV disease
- Monitor blood studies: CBC, leukocytes, differential, cardiac enzymes if patient is receiving long-term therapy
- Monitor hepatic studies: AST, ALT, bilirubin
- Check weight qwk; weight loss or gain; appetite may increase
- Assess mental status: mood, sensorium, affect, suicidal tendencies; increase in psychiatric symptoms: depression, panic
- Monitor urinary retention, constipation; constipation is more likely to occur in children or elderly
- Assess for withdrawal symptoms: headache, nausea, vomiting, muscle pain, weakness; do not usually occur unless drug was discontinued abruptly
- Identify alcohol consumption; if alcohol is consumed, hold dose

Nursing diagnoses

- ✓ Coping, ineffective individual (uses)
- ✓ Injury, risk for physical (side effects)
- ✓ Knowledge deficit (teaching)
- ✓ Noncompliance (teaching)

Implementation

- Give with food or milk for GI symptoms
- Crush if patient is unable to swallow medication whole
- Store at room temp; do not freeze

Patient/family education

- Teach patient that therapeutic effects may take 2-3 wk
- Teach patient to use caution in driving or other activities requiring alertness because of drowsiness, dizziness, blurred vision; to avoid rising quickly from sitting to standing, especially elderly
- Teach patient to avoid alcohol ingestion, other CNS depressants

Evaluation

Positive therapeutic outcome

- Decreased depression
- Absence of suicidal thoughts

Treatment of overdose: ECG monitoring, induce emesis, lavage, activated charcoal, administer anticonvulsant

verapamil (℞)

(ver-ap'a-mil)

Apo-Verap, Calan, Calan SR, Isoptin, Isoptin SR, verapamil HCl, verapamil HCl SR, Verelan

Func. class.: Calcium-channel blocker; antihypertensive; antianginal

Chem. class.: Phenylalkylamine

Pregnancy category C

Action: Inhibits calcium ion influx across cell membrane during cardiac depolarization; produces relaxation of coronary vascular smooth muscle; peripheral vascular smooth muscle; dilates coronary vascular arteries; increases myocardial oxygen delivery in patients with vasospastic angina

Therapeutic Outcome: Decreased angina pectoris, dysrhythmias, B/P

Uses: Chronic stable angina pectoris, vasospastic angina, dysrhythmias, hypertension

Investigational uses: Prevention of migraine headaches, ventricular outflow obstruction in hypertrophic cardiomyopathy

Dosage and routes

Adult: PO 80 mg tid or qid, increase qwk; **IV** bol 5-10 mg >2 min, repeat if necessary in 30 min

Child 1-15 yr: **IV** bol 0.1-0.3 mg/kg over >2 min, repeat in 30 min, not to exceed 10 mg in a single dose

Available forms: Tabs 40, 80, 120 mg; sus rel tabs, 120, 180, 240 mg; inj 5 mg/ml; sus rel caps 120, 180, 240, 360 mg

Adverse effects

CNS: Headache, drowsiness, dizzi-

ness, anxiety, depression, weakness, insomnia, confusion, light-headedness
CV: *Edema,* **CHF**, bradycardia, hypotension, palpitations, AV block
GI: *Nausea,* diarrhea, gastric upset, *constipation,* elevated liver function studies
GU: Nocturia, polyuria
SYST: **Stevens-Johnson syndrome**

Contraindications: Sick sinus syndrome, 2nd- or 3rd-degree heart block, hypotension <90 mm Hg systolic, cardiogenic shock, severe CHF

Precautions: CHF, hypotension, hepatic injury, pregnancy **C**, lactation, P children, renal disease, concomitant β-blocker therapy

Pharmacokinetics

Absorption	Well absorbed (PO)
Distribution	Not known
Metabolism	Liver—extensively
Excretion	Kidneys
Half-life	Biphasic 4 min, 3-7 hr

Pharmacodynamics

	PO	PO-SUS REL	IV
Onset	1-2 hr	Unknown	1-5 min
Peak	½-1½ hr	5-7 hr	3-5 min
Duration	3-7 hr	24 hr	2 hr

Interactions

Individual drugs

Alcohol: ↑ hypotension
Carbamazepine: ↑ toxicity
Digoxin: ↑ digoxin levels, ↑ bradycardia, CHF
Phenobarbital: ↓ effectiveness
Phenytoin: ↓ effectiveness
Propranolol: ↑ toxicity

Drug classifications

Antihypertensives: ↑ hypotension
β-Adrenergic blockers: ↑ bradycardia, CHF
Nitrates: ↑ nitrates

Food/drug

Grapefruit juice: ↑ hypotension

NURSING CONSIDERATIONS

Assessment

- Assess fluid volume status: I&O ratio and record; weight; distended red veins; crackles in lung; color; quality, sp gr of urine; skin turgor; adequacy of pulses; moist mucous membranes; bilateral lung sounds; peripheral pitting edema; dehydration symptoms of decreasing output, thirst, hypotension, dry mouth, and mucous membranes should be reported
- Monitor B/P and pulse, pulmonary capillary wedge pressure (PCWP), central venous pressure, index, often during inf; if B/P drops 30 mm Hg, stop inf and call prescriber
- Monitor ALT, AST, bilirubin daily; if these are elevated, hepatotoxicity is suspected
- Monitor if platelets are <150,000/ mm^3, if so, drug is usually discontinued and another drug started
- Assess for extravasation; change site q48h
- Monitor cardiac status: B/P, pulse, respiration, ECG

Nursing diagnoses

✓ Cardiac output, decreased (uses)
✓ Knowledge deficit (teaching)

Implementation

PO route

- Give once a day, with food to decrease GI symptoms

IV **IV route**

- Give by direct **IV** undiluted (Y-site, 3-way stopcock) over at least 2 min; to prevent serious hypotension, patient should be recumbent for 1 hr or more

Syringe compatibilities:
Amrinone, heparin, milrinone

Y-site compatibilities:
Amrinone, aprofloxacin, dobutamine, dopamine, famotidine, hydralazine, meperidine, methicillin, milrinone, penicillin G potassium, piperacillin, propofol, ticarcillin

Y-site incompatibilities:
Albumin, ampicillin, mezlocillin,

nafcillin, oxacillin, sodium bicarbonate

Additive compatibilities: Amikacin, amiodarone, ascorbic acid, atropine, bretylium, calcium chloride, calcium gluconate, cefamandole, cefazolin, cefotaxime, cefoxitin, cephapirin, chloramphenicol, cimetidine, clindamycin, dexamethasone, diazepam, digoxin, dopamine, epinephrine, erythromycin, gentamicin, heparin, hydrocortisone, hydromorphone, hydrocortisone sodium phosphate, insulin (regular), isoproterenol, lidocaine, magnesium sulfate, mannitol, meperidine, metaraminol, methicillin, methyldopate, methylprednisolone, metoclopramide, mezlocillin, morphine, moxalactam, multivitamins, naloxone, nitroglycerin, norepinephrine, oxytocin, pancuronium, penicillin G potassium, penicillin G sodium, pentobarbital, phenobarbital, phentolamine, phenytoin, piperacillin, potassium chloride, potassium phosphates, procainamide, propranolol, protamine, quinidine, sodium bicarbonate, sodium nitroprusside, theophylline, ticarcillin, tobramycin, tolazoline, vancomycin, vasopressin, vit B/C

Patient/family education

- Advise patient to increase fluids/fiber to counteract constipation
- Caution patient to avoid hazardous activities until stabilized on drug and dizziness is no longer a problem
- Instruct patient to limit caffeine consumption; to avoid alcohol and OTC drugs unless directed by prescriber
- Advise patient to comply with medical regimen: diet, exercise, stress reduction, drug therapy; to notify prescriber of irregular heart beat, shortness of breath, swelling of feet and hands, pronounced dizziness, constipation, nausea, hypotension
- Teach patient to use as directed even if feeling better; may be taken with other CV drugs (nitrates, β-blockers)

Evaluation

Positive therapeutic outcome

- Decreased anginal pain
- Decreased dysrhythmias
- Decreased B/P

Treatment of overdose: Defibrillation, atropine for AV block, vasopressor for hypotension

verteporfin (℞)

(ver-tee-poor'fin)

Visudyne

Func. class.: Ophthalmic phototherapy

Pregnancy category C

Action: A light-activated drug for photodynamic therapy, using a 2-step process with this drug and nonthermal red light

➔ **Therapeutic Outcome:** Improved vision

Uses: Predominantly classic subfoveal choroidal neovascularization (CNV) associated with age-related macular degeneration

Dosage and routes

Adults: Initiate 689 nm wavelength laser light for 83 sec, 15 min after start of the 10 min infusion of verteporfin

Investigtional uses: Psoriasis, psoriatic arthritis, rheumatoid arthritis

Available forms: Lyophilized cake 15 mg

Adverse effects

CNS: Hypesthesia, vertigo, *insomnia*
CV: Hypertension, **atrial fibrillation,** *peripheral vascular disorder, varicose veins*
EENT: Cataracts, diplopia, dry eyes, ocular itching, severe vision loss
GI: Constipation, **GI cancers,** *nausea*
MS: Arthralgia, arthrosis, myesthenia

RESP: Pharyngitis, pneumonia
MISC: Asthenia, back pain, elevated LFTs, photosensitivity

Contraindications: Porphyria, hypersensitivity

G P **Precautions:** Elderly, pregnancy **C**, lactation, children, hepatic disease

Pharmacokinetics	
Absorption	Unknown
Distribution	Unknown
Metabolism	Unknown
Excretion	Feces
Half-life	5-6 hr

Pharmacodynamics
Unknown

Interactions
Drug classifications
Anticoagulants: ↓ action of verteporfin
Antiplatelet agents: ↓ action of verteporfin
Phenothiazines: ↑ photosensitivity
Sulfonamides: ↑ photosensitivity
Sulfonylureas: ↑ photosensitivity
Tetracyclines: ↑ photosensitivity
Thiazides: ↑ photosensitivity

NURSING CONSIDERATIONS
Assessment
- Assess for ocular sensitivity: sensitivity to sun, bright lights, car headlights; patients should wear dark sunglasses with an average light transmittance of <4%
- Assess for extravasation at inj site: take care to protect from light

Nursing diagnoses
✓ Knowledge deficit (teaching)

Implementation
- Give after reconstitution of each vial with 7 ml of sterile water for inj for 2 mg/ml; protect from light and use within 4 hr; solution is dark green
- Wipe spills with damp cloth, avoid skin/eye areas, dispose of material in polyethylene bag according to policy
- Store between 68-77° F

Patient/family education
- Advise patient to report eye sensitivity
- Advise patient to wear sunglasses with average white light transmittance of <4% for 5 days after treatment; also to use protective clothing

Evaluation
Positive therapeutic outcome
- Improved vision

HIGH ALERT

vinblastine (VLB) (℞)
(vin-blast'een)
Alkaban-AQ, Velban, Velbe ✤, Velsar, vinblastine sulfate
Func. class.: Antineoplastic
Chem. class.: Vinca rosea alkaloid
Pregnancy category D

Action: Inhibits mitotic activity, arrests cell cycle at metaphase; inhibits RNA synthesis, blocks cellular use of glutamic acid needed for purine synthesis; a vesicant

➔ **Therapeutic Outcome:** Prevention of rapid growth of malignant cells, immunosuppressive

Uses: Breast, testicular cancer; lymphomas; neuroblastoma; Hodgkin's, non-Hodgkin's lymphomas; mycosis fungoides; histiocytosis; Kaposi's sarcoma

Dosage and routes
Adult: **IV** 0.1 mg/kg or 3.7 mg/m^2 qwk or q2 wk, max 0.5 mg/kg or 18.5 mg/m^2 qwk

P ***Child:*** 2.5 mg/m^2 then dose of 3.75, 5.0, 6.25, and 7.5 at 7-day intervals

Available forms: Inj powder 10 mg for 10 ml **IV** inj

Adverse effects

CNS: Paresthesias, peripheral neuropathy, depression, headache, **seizures**
CV: Tachycardia, orthostatic hypotension
GI: *Nausea, vomiting,* ileus, *anorexia, stomatitis,* constipation, abdominal pain, GI and rectal bleeding, **hepatotoxicity,** pharyngitis
GU: Urinary retention, **renal failure**
HEMA: **Thrombocytopenia, leukopenia, myelosuppression**
INTEG: *Rash,* alopecia, photosensitivity
META: syndrome of inappropriate diuretic hormone
RESP: **Fibrosis, pulmonary infiltrate, bronchospasm**

Contraindications: Hypersensitivity, infants, pregnancy **D**

Precautions: Renal disease, hepatic disease

Do Not Confuse:
vinblastine/vincristine

Pharmacokinetics

Absorption	Complete bioavailability
Distribution	Crosses blood-brain barrier slightly
Metabolism	Liver—active antineoplastic
Excretion	Biliary, kidneys
Half-life	Triphasic—35 min, 53 min, 19 hr

Pharmacodynamics

Unknown

Interactions

Individual drugs

Mitomycin: ↑ bronchospasm
Radiation: ↑ toxicity, bone marrow suppression

Drug classifications

Antineoplastics: ↑ toxicity, bone marrow suppression
Live virus vaccines: ↑ adverse reactions

NURSING CONSIDERATIONS

Assessment

- Monitor B/P (baseline and q15 min) during administration
- Monitor CBC, differential, platelet count weekly; withhold drug if WBC is <2000/mm^3 or platelet count is <75,000/mm^3; notify prescriber of results, recovery will take 3 wk
- Assess for dyspnea, rales, unproductive cough, chest pain, tachypnea
- Monitor renal function studies: BUN, serum uric acid, urine CrCl before, during therapy; I&O ratio; report fall in urine output of 30 ml/hr; for decreased hyperuricemia
- Monitor for cold, fever, sore throat (may indicate beginning of infection); notify prescriber if these occur
- Assess for bleeding: hematuria, guaiac, bruising or petechiae, mucosa or orifices q8h, no rectal temp; avoid IM inj; use pressure to venipuncture sites
- Identify nutritional status: an antiemetic may need to be prescribed
- Assess for symptoms indicating severe allergic reactions: rash, pruritus, urticaria, itching, flushing, bronchospasm, hypotension; epinephrine and resuscitative equipment should be nearby

Nursing diagnoses

✓ Injury, risk for (adverse reactions)
✓ Body image disturbance (adverse reactions)
✓ Infection, risk for (adverse reactions)
✓ Knowledge deficit (teaching)

Implementation

- Give by intermittent inf
- Sol should be prepared by qualified personnel only under controlled conditions
- Use Luer-Loc tubing to prevent leakage; do not let sol come in contact with skin; if contact occurs, wash well with soap and water
- Administer **IV** after diluting 10 mg/10 ml NaCl; give through Y-tube

or 3-way stopcock or directly over 1 min
- Give hyaluronidase 150 U/ml in 1 ml of NaCl, warm compress for extravasation for vesicant activity treatment

Syringe compatibilities: Bleomycin, cisplatin, cyclophosphamide, droperidol, fluorouracil, leucovorin, methotrexate, metoclopramide, mitomycin, vincristine

Y-site compatibilities: Allopurinol, amifostine, aztreonam, bleomycin, cisplatin, cyclophosphamide, doxorubicin, droperidol, filgrastim, fludarabine, fluorouracil, granisetron, heparin, leucovorin, melphalan, methotrexate, metoclopramide, mitomycin, ondansetron, paclitaxel, piperacillin/tazobactam, sargramostim, teniposide, thiotepa, vincristine, vinorelbine

Y-site incompatibilities: Furosemide

Additive compatibilities: Bleomycin

Patient/family education
- Teach patient to avoid use of products containing aspirin or NSAIDs, razors, commercial mouthwash because bleeding may occur; to report symptoms of bleeding (hematuria, tarry stools)
- Instruct patient to report signs of anemia, (fatigue, headache, irritability, faintness, shortness of breath)
- Caution patient to report any changes in breathing or coughing even several mo after treatment
- Advise patient that contraception will be necessary during treatment; teratogenesis may occur
- Advise patient to use sunscreen, wear protective clothing, and sunglasses
- Inform patient that hair may be lost during treatment; a wig or hairpiece may make patient feel better; new hair will be different in color, texture
- Advise patient to avoid vaccinations during treatment; serious reactions may occur
- Teach patient to report signs/symptoms of infection: fever, chills, sore throat; patient should avoid crowds and persons with known infections

Evaluation
Positive therapeutic outcome
- Decreased spread of malignant cells

HIGH ALERT

vincristine (VCR)
(℞)

(vin-kris'teen)

Oncovin, Vincasar PFS, vincristine sulfate

Func. class.: Antineoplastic—misc
Chem. class.: Vinca alkaloid

Pregnancy category D

Action: Inhibits mitotic activity, arrests cell cycle at metaphase; inhibits RNA synthesis, blocks cellular use of glutamic acid needed for purine synthesis; a vesicant

Therapeutic Outcome: Prevention of rapid growth of malignant cells, immunosuppression

Uses: Breast, lung cancer; lymphomas; neuroblastomas; Hodgkin's disease; acute lymphoblastic and other leukemias; rhabdomyosarcoma, Wilms' tumor; osteogenic and other sarcomas

Dosage and routes
Adult: **IV** 1-2 mg/m^2/wk, max 2 mg

P ***Child:*** **IV** 1.5-2 mg/m^2/wk, max 2 mg

Available forms: Inj 1 mg/ml; powder for inj 5 mg/vial

Adverse effects
CNS: *Decreased reflexes, numbness, weakness, motor difficulties,* CNS

depression, cranial nerve paralysis, **seizures**
CV: Orthostatic hypotension
GI: Nausea, vomiting, anorexia, stomatitis, constipation, **paralytic ileus, abdominal pain, hepatotoxicity**
HEMA: **Thrombocytopenia, leukopenia, myelosuppression, anemia**
INTEG: Alopecia

Contraindications: Hypersensitivity, P infants, pregnancy **D**

Precautions: Renal disease, hepatic disease, hypertension, neuromuscular disease

Do Not Confuse:
vincristine/vinblastine

Pharmacokinetics

Absorption	Complete bioavailability
Distribution	Rapidly, widely distributed; blood-brain barrier
Metabolism	Liver
Excretion	Biliary, in feces, crosses placenta
Half-life	Triphasic 0.85 min, 7.4 min, 1.64 min

Pharmacodynamics

Onset	Unknown
Peak	Unknown
Duration	1 wk

Interactions
Individual drugs
L-Asparaginase: ↓ metabolism of vincristine
Mitomycin: ↑ bronchospasm
Radiation: ↑ toxicity, bone marrow suppression
Drug classifications
Antineoplastics: ↑ toxicity, bone marrow suppression
Live virus vaccines: ↓ antibody response

NURSING CONSIDERATIONS
Assessment
• Monitor CBC, differential, platelet count weekly; withhold drug if WBC is <4000/mm^3 or platelet count is <75,000/mm^3; notify prescriber of results; platelets may increase or decrease
• Assess neurologic status: paresthesia, weakness, cranial nerve palsies, orthostatic hypotension, lethargy, agitation, psychosis; notify prescriber
• Monitor renal function studies: BUN, serum uric acid, urine CrCl before, during therapy; I&O ratio; report fall in urine output of 30 ml/hr; for decreased hyperuricemia, hyponatremia, and increased fluid retention (syndrome of inappropriate antidiuretic hormone)
• Monitor for cold, fever, sore throat (may indicate beginning of infection)
• Identify for increased uric acid levels, joint pain in extremities; increase fluid intake to 2-3 L/day unless contraindicated

Nursing diagnoses
✓ Injury, risk for (adverse reactions)
✓ Body image disturbance (adverse reactions)
✓ Infection, risk for (adverse reactions)
✓ Knowledge deficit (teaching)

Implementation
• Administer **IV** after diluting with diluent provided or 1 mg/10 ml of sterile water or 0.9% NaCl; give through Y-tube or 3-way stopcock or directly over 1 min
• Hyaluronidase 150 U/ml in 1 ml of NaCl; apply warm compress for extravasation

Syringe compatibilities:
Bleomycin, cisplatin, cyclophosphamide, doxapram, doxorubicin, droperidol, fluorouracil, heparin, leucovorin, methotrexate, metoclopramide, mitomycin, ondansetron, vincristine

Syringe incompatibilities:
Furosemide

Y-site compatibilities:
Allopurinol, amifostine, aztreonam, bleomycin, cisplatin, cladribine, cyclophosphamide, doxorubicin,

droperidol, filgrastim, fludarabine, fluorouracil, granisetron, heparin, leucovorin, methotrexate, metoclopramide, mitomycin, ondansetron, paclitaxel, sargramostim, teniposide, thiotepa, vincristine, vinorelbine

Y-site incompatibilities:
Furosemide

Patient/family education

- Teach patient to avoid use of products containing aspirin or NSAIDs, razors, commercial mouthwash because bleeding may occur; to report symptoms of bleeding (hematuria, tarry stools)
- Instruct patient to report signs of anemia (fatigue, headache, irritability, faintness, shortness of breath)
- Caution patient to report any changes in breathing or coughing, even several mo after treatment
- Advise patient that contraception will be necessary during treatment; teratogenesis may occur
- Inform patient that hair may be lost during treatment; a wig or hairpiece may make patient feel better; new hair will be different in color, texture
- Advise patient to avoid vaccinations during treatment; serious reactions may occur
- Teach patient to report signs/symptoms of infection: fever, chills, sore throat; patient should avoid crowds or persons with known infections
- Advise patient to increase fluids, bulk in diet, exercise to prevent constipation

Evaluation

Positive therapeutic outcome

- Decreased spread of malignancies

HIGH ALERT

vinorelbine (℞)

(vi-nor′el-bine)

Navelbine

Func. class.: Antineoplastic—misc

Chem. class.: Semi-synthetic vinca alkaloid

Pregnancy category D

Action: Inhibits mitotic activity, arrests cell cycle at metaphase; inhibits RNA synthesis, blocks cellular use of glutamic acid needed for purine synthesis; a vesicant

➔ **Therapeutic Outcome:** Decreased spread of malignancy

Uses: Breast cancer; unresectable, advanced non–small-cell lung cancer (NSCLC) stage IV; may be used alone or in combination with cisplatin for stage III or IV NSCLC

Dosage and routes

Adult: **IV** 30 mg/m^2 qwk

Breast cancer

Adult: **IV** 30 mg/m^2 qwk

Hepatic dose

Adult: **IV** total bilirubin 2.1-3 mg/dl 15 mg/m^2 qwk; total bilirubin ≥3 mg/dl 7.5 mg/m^2 qd

Available forms: Inj 10 mg/ml

Adverse effects

CNS: Paresthesias, peripheral neuropathy, depression, headache, **seizures,** weakness, jaw pain

GI: *Nausea, vomiting,* ileus, *anorexia, stomatitis,* constipation, abdominal pain, GI, diarrhea, **hepatotoxicity**

HEMA: **Neutropenia, anemia, thrombocytopenia**

INTEG: *Rash,* alopecia, photosensitivity

META: syndrome of inappropriate diuretic hormone

MS: Myalgia

V

Contraindications: Hypersensitivity, infants, pregnancy **D**

Precautions: Renal disease, hepatic disease

Pharmacokinetics

Absorption	Poor bioavailability (<50%)
Distribution	Unknown
Metabolism	Liver—to metabolite
Excretion	Bile
Half-life	43 hr

Pharmacodynamics

Onset	Unknown
Peak	1-2 hr
Duration	Unknown

Interactions
Individual drugs
Fluorouracil: ↑ toxicity a possibility

NURSING CONSIDERATIONS
Assessment
- Monitor B/P, (baseline and q15 min) during administration
- Monitor CBC, differential, platelet count weekly; withhold drug if WBC is <4000/mm³ or platelet count is <75,000/mm³; notify prescriber of results, recovery will take 3 wk
- Assess for dyspnea, rales, unproductive cough, chest pain, tachypnea
- Monitor renal function studies: BUN, serum uric acid, urine CrCl before, during therapy, I&O ratio; report fall in urine output of 30 ml/hr; for decreased hyperuricemia
- Monitor for cold, fever, sore throat (may indicate beginning infection); notify health care prescriber if these occur
- Assess for bleeding: hematuria, guaiac, bruising or petechiae, mucosa or orifices q8h: no rectal temp; avoid IM inj; use pressure on venipuncture sites
- Identify nutritional status: an antiemetic may need to be prescribed
- Assess for symptoms indicating severe allergic reactions: rash, pruritus, urticaria, itching, flushing, bronchospasm, hypotension; epinephrine and resuscitative equipment should be nearby

Nursing diagnoses
- ✓ Injury, risk for (adverse reactions)
- ✓ Body image disturbance (adverse reactions)
- ✓ Infection, risk for (adverse reactions)
- ✓ Knowledge deficit (teaching)

Implementation
- Hyaluronidase 150 U/ml in 1 ml of NaCl, warm compress for extravasation for vesicant activity treatment
- Antacid before oral agent; give drug after evening meal before bedtime
- Antiemetic 30-60 min before giving drug and prn to prevent vomiting

Continuous infusion
- Give 40 mg/m² q3 wk after **IV** bol of 8 mg/m²; may be given in combination with doxorubicin, fluorouracil, cisplatin

Y-site compatibilities:
Amikacin, aztreonam, bleomycin, buprenorphine, butorphanol, calcium gluconate, carboplatin, cefotaxime, cisplatin, cimetidine, clindamycin, dexamethasone, enalaprilat, etoposide, famotidine, filgrastim, fluconazole, fludarabine, gentamicin, hydrocortisone, lorazepam, meperidine, morphine, netilmicin, ondansetron, plicamycin, streptozocin, teniposide, ticarcillin, tobramycin, vancomycin, vinblastine, vincristine, zidovudine

Patient/family education
- Teach patient to use liq diet: cola, Jell-O; dry toast or crackers may be added if patient is not nauseated or vomiting
- Advise patient to rinse mouth 3-4 ×/day with water and brush teeth 2-3 ×/day with soft brush or cotton-tipped applicators for stomatitis; use unwaxed dental floss
- Inform patient that a nutritious diet

with iron, vitamin supplements is necessary
- Advise patient to avoid crowds, people with infections, vaccinations

Evaluation

Positive therapeutic outcome
- Decreased spread of malignant cells

vitamin A (PO, OTC; IM, ℞)

Aquasol A, Del-Vi-A, Vitamin A
Func. class.: Vitamin, fat-soluble
Chem. class.: Retinol

Pregnancy category C

Action: Needed for normal bone and tooth development, visual dark adaptation, skin disease, mucosa tissue repair, assists in production of adrenal steroids, cholesterol, RNA

➔ **Therapeutic Outcome:** Prevention, absence of vit A deficiency

Uses: Vit A deficiency

Dosage and routes

P ***Adult and child >8 yr:*** PO 100,000-500,000 IU qd × 3 days, then 50,000 qd × 2 wk; dose based on severity of deficiency; maintenance 10,000-20,000 IU for 2 mo

P ***Child 1-8 yr:*** IM 5,000-15,000 IU qd × 10 days

P ***Infants <1 yr:*** IM 5,000-15,000 IU × 10 days

Maintenance

P ***Child 4-8 yr:*** IM 15,000 IU qd × 2 mo

P ***Child <4 yr:*** IM 10,000 IU qd × 2 mo

Available forms: Caps 10,000, 25,000, 50,000 IU; drops 5000 IU; inj 50,000 IU/ml; tabs 10,000, 25,000, 50,000 IU

Adverse effects

CNS: Headache, increased ICP, intracranial hypertension, lethargy, malaise

EENT: Gingivitis, papilledema, exophthalmos, inflammation of tongue and lips

GI: Nausea, vomiting, anorexia, abdominal pain, *jaundice*

INTEG: Drying of skin, pruritus, increased pigmentation, night sweats, alopecia

MS: Arthralgia, retarded growth, hard areas on bone

META: Hypomenorrhea, hypercalcemia

Contraindications: Hypersensitivity to vit A, malabsorption syndrome (PO)

Precautions: Lactation, impaired renal function, pregnancy **C**

Pharmacokinetics

Absorption	Rapidly absorbed
Distribution	Stored in liver, kidneys, lungs
Metabolism	Liver
Excretion	Breast milk
Half-life	Unknown

Pharmacodynamics

Unknown

Interactions

Individual drugs

Cholestyramine: ↓ absorption of vitamin A

Colestipol: ↓ absorption of vitamin A

Mineral oil: ↓ absorption of vitamin A

Drug classifications

Corticosteroids: ↑ levels of vitamin A

Oral contraceptives: ↑ level of vitamin A

Lab test interferences

False: ↑ Bilirubin, ↑ serum cholesterol

V

NURSING CONSIDERATIONS

Assessment

- Assess nutritional status: increase intake of yellow and dark green vegetables, yellow/orange fruits, vitamin A-fortified foods, liver, egg yolks

- Assess vitamin A deficiency: decreased growth; night blindness; dry, brittle nails; hair loss; urinary stones; increased infection; hyperkeratosis of skin; drying of cornea
- Identify vit A deficiency by plasma vit A, carotene level
- Assess for chronic vit A toxicity: increased calcium, BUN, glucose, cholesterol, triglyceride level

Nursing diagnoses

✓ Nutrition: less than body requirements (uses)
✓ Knowledge deficit (teaching)

Implementation

PO route

- Give with food (PO) for better absorption; do not give **IV** because anaphylaxis may occur
- Store in airtight, light-resistant container

Patient/family education

- Instruct patient that if dose is missed, it should be omitted
- Inform patient that ophth exams may be required periodically throughout therapy
- Instruct patient not to use mineral oil while taking this drug because absorption will be decreased
- Advise patient to notify prescriber of nausea, vomiting, lip cracking, loss of hair, headache
- Caution patient not to take more than the prescribed amount

Evaluation

Positive therapeutic outcome

- Increase in growth rate, weight
- Absence of dry skin and mucous membranes, night blindness

Treatment of overdose: Discontinue drug

vitamin A acid

See tretinoin

vitamin B_1

See thiamine

(vitamin B_{12}) cyanocobalamin/ (vitamin $B_{12}a$) hydroxocobalamin

(PO, OTC; IM/SC, ℞)
(sye-an-oh-koe-bal'a-min)

Acti-B_{12} ♣, Alphamine, Anacobin ♣, Bedoz ♣, B_{12}, Resin, Cobex, Crystamine, Crysti-12, Cyanoject, Cyomin, Hydrobexan, Hydro Cobex, Rubesol-1000, Rubion ♣, Rubramin PC, Vitamin B_{12}

Func. class.: Vitamin B_{12}, water-soluble vitamin

Pregnancy category A

Action: Needed for adequate nerve functioning, protein and carbohydrate metabolism, normal growth, RBC development and cell reproduction

Therapeutic Outcome: Prevention, correction of vit B_{12} deficiency

Uses: Vit B_{12} deficiency; pernicious anemia; vit B_{12} malabsorption syndrome; Schilling test; increased requirements with pregnancy, thyrotoxicosis, hemolytic anemia, hemorrhage, renal and hepatic disease

Dosage and routes

Adult: PO 25 μg qd × 5-10 days, maintenance 100-200 mg IM qmo; IM/SC 30-100 μg qd × 5-10 days, maintenance 100-200 μg IM qmo

P ***Child:*** PO 1 μg qd × 5-10 days, maintenance 60 μg IM qmo or more; IM/SC 1-30 μg qd × 5-10 days, maintenance 60 μg IM qmo or more

Pernicious anemia/ malabsorption syndrome

Adult: IM 100-1000 μg qd × 2 wk, then 100-1000 μg IM qmo

P ***Child:*** IM 100-500 μg over 2 wk or

more given in 100-500 μg doses, then 60 μg IM/SC monthly

Schilling test

P ***Adult and child:*** IM 1000 μg in one dose

Available forms: Tabs 25, 50, 100, 250, 500, 1000 μg; inj 100, 120, 1000 μg/ml

Adverse effects

CNS: Flushing, optic nerve atrophy
CV: **CHF,** peripheral vascular thrombosis, **pulmonary edema**
GI: *Diarrhea*
INTEG: Itching, rash, pain at site
META: Hypokalemia
SYST: **Anaphylactic shock**

Contraindications: Hypersensitivity, optic nerve atrophy

Precautions: Pregnancy **A,**
P lactation, children, cardiac disease, uremia, iron deficiency, folic acid deficiency

Pharmacokinetics

Absorption	Well absorbed (IM, SC)
Distribution	Crosses placenta
Metabolism	Stored in liver, kidney, stomach
Excretion	50%-90% (urine), breast milk
Half-life	Unknown

Pharmacodynamics

Unknown

Interactions

Individual drugs

Alcohol: ↓ absorption
Aminosalicylic acid: ↓ absorption
Chloramphenicol: ↓ absorption
Cimetidine: ↓ absorption
Colchicine: ↓ absorption

Drug classifications

Aminoglycosides: ↓ absorption
Anticonvulsants: ↓ absorption
Potassium products: ↓ absorption

Lab test interferences

False positive: Intrinsic factor

NURSING CONSIDERATIONS

Assessment

- Assess for deficiency: anorexia, dyspepsia on exertion, palpitations, paresthesias, psychosis, visual disturbances, pallor, red inflamed tongue, neuropathy, edema of legs
- Monitor potassium levels during beginning treatment in patients with megaloblastic anemia
- Monitor CBC for increase in reticulocyte count during 1st wk of therapy, then increase in RBC and hemoglobin; folic acid levels, vit B_{12} levels
- Assess nutritional status: egg yolks, fish, organ meats, dairy products, clams, oysters, which are good sources for vit B_{12}
- Monitor for pulmonary edema or worsening of CHF in cardiac patients

Nursing diagnoses

✓ Nutrition; less than body requirements (uses)
✓ Knowledge deficit (teaching)
✓ Noncompliance (teaching) (overuse)

Implementation

PO route

- Give with fruit juice to disguise taste; administer immediately after mixing
- Give with meals if possible for better absorption

IM route

- Give by IM inj for pernicious anemia for life unless contraindicated

IV **IV route**

- May be mixed with TPN sol, but **IV** route is not recommended

Y-site compatibilities:

Heparin, hydrocortisone sodium succinate, potassium chloride

Solution compatibilities:

Dextrose/Ringer's or lactated Ringer's combinations, dextrose/saline combinations, D_5W, $D_{10}W$, 0.45% NaCl, Ringer's or lactated Ringer's sol, ascorbic acid

Patient/family education

- Instruct patient that treatment must

V

continue for life if diagnosed as having pernicious anemia
- Advise patient to eat well-balanced diet from the food pyramid and comply with dietary recommendation
- Caution patient not to exceed the RDA of vit B_{12} because adverse reactions may occur

Evaluation

Positive therapeutic outcome
- Decreased anorexia, dyspnea on exertion, palpitations, paresthesias, psychosis, visual disturbances, edema of legs
- Prevention or correction of vit B_{12} deficiency

Treatment of overdose:
Discontinue drug

vitamin D (cholecalciferol, vitamin D_3 or ergocalciferol, vitamin D_2) (℞, OTC)

Calciferol, Delta-D, Drisdol, Radiostol ✤, Radiostol Forte ✤, vitamin D, vitamin D_3

Func. class.: Vitamin D

Chem. class: Fat soluble vitamin

Pregnancy category C

Action: Needed for regulation of calcium, phosphate levels; normal bone development; parathyroid activity; neuromuscular functioning

Therapeutic Outcome: Prevention of rickets, osteomalacia, normal calcium/phosphate levels

Uses: Vit D deficiency, rickets, renal osteodystrophy, hypoparathyroidism, hypophosphatemia, psoriasis, rheumatoid arthritis

Dosage and routes

Deficiency

Adult: PO/IM 12,000 IU qd, then increased to 500,000 IU/day

P ***Child:*** PO/IM 1500/5000 IU qd × 2-4 wk, may repeat after 2 wk or 600,000 IU as single dose

Hypoparathyroidism

P ***Adult and child:*** PO/IM 200,000 IU given with 4 g calcium tab

Available forms: Tabs 400, 1000, 50,000 IU; caps 25,000, 50,000; oral sol 8000 IU/ml; inj 500,000 IU/ml, 500,000 IU/5 ml

Adverse effects

CNS: Fatigue, weakness, drowsiness, **seizures,** headache, psychosis

CV: Hypertension, dysrhythmias

GI: Nausea, vomiting, anorexia, cramps, diarrhea, constipation, metallic taste, dry mouth, decreased libido

GU: Polyuria, nocturia, **hematuria, albuminuria, renal failure**

INTEG: Pruritus, photophobia

MS: Decreased bone growth, early joint pain, early muscle pain

Contraindications: Hypersensitivity, hypercalcemia, renal dysfunction, hyperphosphatemia

Precautions: CV disease, renal calculi, pregnancy **C**

Do Not Confuse:
Calciferol/calcitriol

Pharmacokinetics

Absorption	Well absorbed
Distribution	Stored in liver
Metabolism	Liver, sun
Excretion	Bile, kidney
Half-life	12-22 hr

Pharmacodynamics

	PO	IM
Onset	Unknown	Unknown
Peak	4 hr	Unknown
Duration	15-20 days	Unknown

Interactions

Individual drugs

Cholestyramine: ↓ absorption of vit D

Colestipol: ↓ absorption of vit D
Mineral oil: ↓ absorption of vit D
Drug classifications
Cardiac glycosides: ↑ dysrhythmias
Corticosteroids: ↓ effects
Diuretics, thiazide: ↑ hypercalciuria
Lab test interferences
False: ↑ Cholesterol

NURSING CONSIDERATIONS
Assessment
- Monitor BUN, urinary calcium, AST, ALT, cholesterol, creatinine, uric acid, chloride, magnesium, electrolytes, urine pH, phosphate—may increase; calcium should be kept at 9-10 mg/dl; vit D at 50-135 IU/dl, phosphate at 70 mg/dl; alkaline phosphatase may be decreased
- Monitor for increased blood level; toxic reactions may occur rapidly
- Assess for dry mouth, metallic taste, polyuria, bone pain, muscle weakness, headache, fatigue, tinnitus, change in LOC, irregular pulse, dysrhythmias, increased respirations, anorexia, nausea, vomiting, cramps, diarrhea, constipation; may indicate hypercalcemia
- Assess renal status: decreased urinary output (oliguria, anuria), edema in extremities, weight gain 5 lb, periorbital edema
- Assess nutritional status, diet for sources of vit D (milk, cod, halibut, salmon, sardines, egg yolk) calcium (dairy products, dark green vegetables), phosphates (dairy products)

Nursing diagnoses
✓ Nutrition, less than body requirements (uses)
✓ Knowledge deficit (teaching)

Implementation
PO route
- PO may be increased q4 wk depending on blood level
- Store in airtight, light-resistant container at room temp

IM route
- Give deeply in large muscle mass, administer slowly, aspirate to avoid **IV** administration, rotate inj site

Patient/family education
- Advise patient to omit dose if missed; to avoid vitamin supplements unless directed by prescriber
- Inform patient of necessary foods to be included in diet
- Advise patient to keep appointments for evaluation because therapeutic and toxic levels are narrow
- Instruct patient to report weakness, lethargy, headache, anorexia, loss of weight; to report nausea, vomiting, abdominal cramps, diarrhea, constipation, excessive thirst, polyuria, muscle and bone pain
- Caution patient to decrease intake of antacids and laxatives containing magnesium

Evaluation
Positive therapeutic outcome
- Calcium levels 9-10 ml/dl
- Decreasing symptoms of bone disease

vitamin E (OTC)
Amino-Opti-E, Aquasol E, Daltose ♣, E-Complex-600, E-Ferol, E-Vitamin Succinate, E-200 I.U. Softgels, Gordo-Vite E, Tocopherol, vitamin E, Vita-Plus E Softgells, Vitec
Func. class.: Vitamin E
Chem. class.: Fat soluble vitamin
Pregnancy category A

Action: Needed for digestion and metabolism of polyunsaturated fats, decreases platelet aggregation, decreases blood clot formation, promotes normal growth and development of muscle tissue, prostaglandin synthesis

➔ **Therapeutic Outcome:** Prevention and treatment of vit E deficiency

Uses: Vit E deficiency, impaired fat absorption, hemolytic anemia in premature neonates, prevention of retrolental fibroplasia, sickle cell anemia, supplement in malabsorption syndrome

Dosage and routes

Deficiency

Adult: PO 60-75 IU qd

P ***Child:*** PO 1 mg/0.6 g of dietary fat

Prevention of deficiency

Adult: PO 30 U/day

P ***Infant:*** PO 5 IU/day

Topical route

P ***Adult and child:*** TOP apply to affected areas as needed

Available forms: Caps 100, 200, 400, 500, 600, 800 ✦, 1000 IU; tabs 100, 200, 400 IU; drops 50 mg/ml; chew tabs 400 U; ointment, cream, lotion, oil

Adverse effects

CNS: Headache, fatigue
CV: Increased risk of thrombophlebitis
EENT: Blurred vision
GI: Nausea, cramps, diarrhea
GU: Gonadal dysfunction
INTEG: Sterile abscess, contact dermatitis
META: Altered metabolism of hormones, thyroid, pituitary, adrenal, altered immunity
MS: Weakness

Contraindications: None significant

Precautions: Pregnancy **A**

Pharmacokinetics

Absorption	20%-80% (PO)
Distribution	Widely distributed, stored in fat
Metabolism	Liver
Excretion	Bile
Half-life	Unknown

Pharmacodynamics

Unknown

Interactions

Individual drugs

Cholestyramine: ↓ absorption
Colestipol: ↓ absorption
Mineral oil: ↓ absorption
Sucralfate: ↓ absorption

Drug classification

Anticoagulants, oral: ↑ action of anticoagulants

NURSING CONSIDERATIONS

Assessment

- Monitor vit E levels during treatment
- Assess nutritional status: intake of wheat germ, dark green leafy vegetables, nuts, eggs, liver, vegetable oils, dairy products, cereals
- Assess for vit E deficiency (usually in neonates): irritability, restlessness, hemolytic anemia

Nursing diagnoses

✓ Nutrition: less than body requirements (uses)
✓ Knowledge deficit (teaching)

Implementation

PO route

- Chewable tab: chew well
- Sol: may be dropped in mouth or mixed with food
- Store in airtight, light-resistant container

Topical route

- Apply top to moisturize dry skin

Patient/family education

- Inform patient necessary foods to be included in diet high in vit E
- Instruct patient to omit if dose missed
- Instruct patient to avoid vit supplements unless directed by prescriber because overdose may occur

Evaluation

Positive therapeutic outcome

- Absence of hemolytic anemia
- Adequate vit E levels

- Improvement in skin lesions
- Decrease in edema

HIGH ALERT

warfarin (℞)

(war'far-in)

Coumadin, Sofarin, warfarin sodium, Warfilone Sodium ✤

Func. class.: Anticoagulant

Pregnancy category X

Action: Interferes with blood clotting by indirect means; depresses hepatic synthesis of vit K-dependent coagulation factors (II, VII, IX, X)

Therapeutic Outcome: Prevention of clotting

Uses: Pulmonary emboli, deep vein thrombosis, MI, atrial dysrhythmias, postcardiac valve replacement

Dosage and routes

Adult: PO 2.5-10 mg/day × 3 days, then titrated to pro-time or INR qd

G ***Elderly:*** PO/**IV** 2-10 mg/day

P ***Child:*** PO 0.1 mg/kg/day titrated to INR

Available forms: Tabs 1, 2, 2.5, 5, 6, 7.5, 10 mg; inj 50 mg/2 ml

Adverse effects

CNS: *Fever*

GI: *Diarrhea,* nausea, vomiting, anorexia, stomatitis, cramps, **hepatitis**

GU: **Hematuria**

HEMA: **Hemorrhage, agranulocytosis, leukopenia, eosinophilia**

INTEG: *Rash,* dermatitis, urticaria, alopecia, pruritus

Contraindications: Hypersensitivity, hemophilia, leukemia with bleeding, peptic ulcer disease, thrombocytopenic purpura, hepatic disease (severe), severe hypertension, subacute bacterial endocarditis, acute nephritis, blood dyscrasias, pregnancy **X**, eclampsia, preeclampsia, lactation

G **Precautions:** Alcoholism, elderly

Do Not Confuse: Coumadin/Cardura, Coumadin/Compazine

Pharmacokinetics

Absorption	Well absorbed (PO), completely absorbed
Distribution	Crosses placenta, 99% plasma protein binding
Metabolism	Liver
Excretion	Kidney, feces (active, inactive metabolites)
Half-life	½-2½ days

Pharmacodynamics

	PO
Onset	12-24 hr
Peak	½-3 days
Duration	3-5 days

Interactions

Individual drugs

Allopurinol: ↑ warfarin action
Amiodarone: ↑ warfarin action
Carbamazepine: ↓ warfarin action
Cefamandole: ↑ warfarin action
Chloramphenicol: ↑ warfarin action
Cimetidine: ↑ warfarin action
Clofibrate: ↑ warfarin action
Cotrimoxazole: ↑ warfarin action
Diflunisal: ↑ warfarin action
Erythromycin: ↑ warfarin action
Heparin: ↑ warfarin action
Isoniazid: ↑ warfarin action
Phenytoin: ↓ warfarin action
Rifampin: ↓ warfarin action
Sucralfate: ↓ warfarin action

Drug classifications

Antidepressants, tricyclic: ↑ warfarin action
Barbiturates: ↓ warfarin action
Corticosteroids: ↓ warfarin action
Estrogens: ↓ warfarin action
NSAIDs: ↑ warfarin action
Oral contraceptives: ↓ warfarin action
Quinolones: ↑ warfarin action
Salicylates: ↑ warfarin action
Thrombolytics: ↑ warfarin action

Food/drug
Grapefruit juice: ↑ action of oral warfarin

Herb/drug
Alfalfa: ↓ anticoagulation
Beet root/greens: ↓ anticoagulation
Broccoli flower buds: ↓ anticoagulation
Bromelain: ↑ risk of bleeding
Brussels sprout buds: ↓ anticoagulation
Cabbage leaves: ↓ anticoagulation
Cayenne: ↑ risk of bleeding
Chinese cabbage leaves: ↓ anticoagulation
Cinchona: ↑ risk of bleeding
Collard leaves: ↓ anticoagulation
Corn silk: ↓ anticoagulation
Crucifer: ↑ metabolism of warfarin
Danshen: ↑ risk of bleeding
Feverfew: ↑ risk of bleeding
Garlic: ↑ risk of bleeding
Ginger: ↑ risk of bleeding
Ginkgo biloba: ↑ risk of bleeding
Ginseng: ↓ anticoagulation
Horse chestnut: ↑ risk of bleeding
Parsley: ↓ anticoagulation
Plantain: ↓ anticoagulation
Quinine: ↑ risk of bleeding
Shepherd's purse: ↓ anticoagulation
Smartweed: ↓ anticoagulation
Stigmas: ↓ anticoagulation
Stinging nettle: ↓ anticoagulation

Lab test interferences
↑ T_3 uptake
↓ Uric acid

NURSING CONSIDERATIONS

Assessment

- Monitor blood studies (Hct, occult blood in stools) q3 mo; partial pro-time, which should be 1½-2 × control, PTT; often done qd, APTT, ACT; platelet count q2-3 days; thrombocytopenia may occur
- Monitor B/P, watch for increasing signs of hypertension
- Assess for bleeding: bleeding gums, petechiae, ecchymosis, black tarry stools, hematuria, epistaxis; decreased B/P may indicate bleeding and possible hemorrhage
- Assess for fever, skin rash, urticaria
- Assess for needed dosage change q1-2 wk

Assess patients carefully for symptoms of Churg-Strauss syndrome (rare): eosinophilia, vasculitis, rash, worsening pulmonary symptoms, cardiac complications, neuropathy

Nursing diagnoses

✓ Injury, risk for (uses, adverse reactions)
✓ Tissue perfusion, altered (uses)
✓ Knowledge deficit (teaching)

Implementation

PO route

- Warfarin is usually given with **IV** heparin for 3 or more days, warfarin blood level may take several days

IV route

- Protect from light, **IV** form is in short supply

Additive compatibilities: Cephapirin

Patient/family education

- Caution patient to avoid OTC preparations unless directed by prescriber; may cause serious drug interactions
- Advise patient that drug may be withheld during active bleeding (menstruation), depending on condition
- Advise patient to use soft-bristle toothbrush to avoid bleeding gums, avoid contact sports, use electric razor, avoid IM inj
- Instruct patient to carry a ID identifying drug taken
- Advise patient to report any signs of bleeding: gums, under skin, urine, stools
- Teach patient to read food labels; limited intake of vit K foods is necessary to maintain consistent prothrombin levels

Evaluation
Positive therapeutic outcome
- Decrease of deep vein thrombosis
- Pro-time (1.3-2.0 × control)

zafirlukast (℞)
(za-feer'loo-cast)
Accolate
Func. class.: Bronchodilator
Chem. class: Leukotriene receptor antagonist

Pregnancy category UK

Action: Antagonizes the contractile action of leukotrienes (LTC_4, LTD_4, LTE_4) in airway smooth muscle; inhibits bronchoconstriction caused by antigens

➔ **Therapeutic Outcome:** Ability to breathe more easily

Uses: Prophylaxis and chronic P treatment of asthma in adults/children >12 yr

Dosage and routes
Adult: PO 20 mg bid, take 1 hr ac or 2 hr pc

Available forms: Tabs 20 mg

Adverse effects
CNS: Headache, dizziness
GI: Nausea, diarrhea, abdominal pain, vomiting
MISC: Infections, pain, asthenia, myalgia, fever, dyspepsia, increased ALT

Contraindications: Hypersensitivity

Precautions: Pregnancy **UK,** G elderly, lactation, children, hepatic P disease

Pharmacokinetics
Unknown

Pharmacodynamics
Unknown

Interactions
Individual drugs
Aspirin: ↑ plasma levels of zafirlukast
Erythromycin: ↓ plasma levels of zafirlukast
Theophylline: ↓ plasma levels of zafirlukast
Warfarin: ↑ pro-time
Food/drug
↓ Bioavailability of zafirlukast

NURSING CONSIDERATIONS
Assessment
- Assess respiratory rate, rhythm, depth; auscultate lung fields bilaterally; notify prescriber of abnormalities

Nursing diagnoses
- ✓ Breathing pattern, ineffective (uses)
- ✓ Knowledge deficit (teaching)
- ✓ Noncompliance (teaching)

Implementation
- Give after meals to decrease GI symptoms; absorption may be affected

Patient/family education
- Advise patient to check OTC medications, current prescription medications, which will increase stimulation
- Advise patient to avoid hazardous activities; dizziness may occur
- Advise patient that if GI upset occurs, to take drug with 8 oz of water; avoid food if possible, absorption may be decreased
- Advise patient to notify prescriber of nausea, vomiting, diarrhea, abdominal pain

Evaluation
Positive therapeutic outcome
- Ability to breathe more easily

zalcitabine (℞)

(zal-sit'a-bin)

ddC, dideoxycitidine, HIVID

Func. class.: Antiretroviral

Chem. class.: Synthetic pyrimidine nucleoside analog of 2′-deoxycytidine

Pregnancy category C

Action: Inhibits HIV replication by the conversion of this drug by cellular enzymes to an active antiviral metabolite

Therapeutic Outcome: Improved symptoms of HIV infection

Uses: Advanced HIV infections in combination in adults and children >13 yr who have been unable to use zidovudine or who have not responded to treatment

Dosage and routes

Adult: PO combined with other antiretrovirals in advanced HIV infection: 0.75 mg administered concomitantly with other antiretrovirals; dosage reduction not necessary for patients weighing >30 kg; in presence of peripheral neuropathy initiate dose at 0.375 mg q8h of zalcitabine

Renal dose

Adult: PO CrCl 10-40 ml/min 0.75 mg q12h; CrCl <10 ml/min 0.75 mg q24h

Available forms: Tabs 0.375, 0.75 mg

Adverse effects

CNS: *Headache, peripheral neuropathy,* **seizures,** confusion, anxiety, hypertonia, abnormal thinking, asthenia, insomnia, CNS depression, pain, *dizziness,* chills, *fever*

CV: Hypertension, vasodilation, dysrhythmia, syncope, palpitation, tachycardia

EENT: Ear pain, otitis, photophobia, visual impairment

ENDO: Hypoglycemia, hyponatremia, hyperbilirubinemia, hyperglycemia

GI: **Pancreatitis,** *diarrhea, nausea, vomiting,* abdominal pain, constipation, stomatitis, dysplasia, liver abnormalities, *oral ulcers,* flatulence, taste perversion, dry mouth, oral thrush, melena, *increased ALT, AST, alkaline phosphatase, amylase,* increased bilirubin

GU: Uric acid, **toxic nephropathy,** polyuria

HEMA: **Leukopenia, granulocytopenia, thrombocytopenia,** anemia

INTEG: *Rash, pruritus,* alopecia, sweating, acne

MS: *Myalgia,* arthritis, myopathy, muscular atrophy

RESP: *Cough,* pneumonia, dyspnea, asthma, hypoventilation

SYST: **Lactic acidosis**

Contraindications: Hypersensitivity

Precautions: Renal, hepatic, cardiac disease, pregnancy **C,** lactation, children (<13 yr), patients with peripheral neuropathy

Pharmacokinetics	
Absorption	Minimally absorbed
Distribution	Unknown
Metabolism	Liver
Excretion	Unknown
Half-life	1.62 hr, increased in renal disease

Pharmacodynamics	
Onset	Unknown
Peak	1½-2½
Duration	Unknown

Interactions

Individual drugs

Amphotericin B: ↑ neurotoxicity, nephrotoxicity

Cimetidine: ↑ neurotoxicity, nephrotoxicity

Foscarnet: ↑ neurotoxicity, nephrotoxicity

Interferon: ↑ neurotoxicity, nephrotoxicity
Methotrexate: ↑ neurotoxicity, nephrotoxicity
Probenecid: ↑ neurotoxicity, nephrotoxicity

Drug classifications

Aminoglycosides: ↑ neurotoxicity, nephrotoxicity
Antacids: ↓ absorption
Nucleoside analogs: ↑ peripheral neuropathy risk

NURSING CONSIDERATIONS

Assessment

- Assess for peripheral neuropathy: tingling or pain in hands and feet, distal numbness; if these occur during therapy, drug may be decreased or discontinued
- Assess for lactic acidosis; severe hepatomegaly with steatosis, which can be fatal; drug should be discontinued
- Assess for pancreatitis: abdominal pain, nausea, vomiting, elevated liver enzymes; drug should be discontinued because condition can be fatal
- P Assess children by dilated retinal examination q6 mo to rule out retinal depigmentation
- Monitor CBC, differential, platelet count qmo; withhold drug if WBC is <4000/mm^3 or platelet count is <75,000/mm^3; notify prescriber of results
- Monitor renal function studies (BUN, serum uric acid, urine CrCl) before, during therapy; these may be elevated throughout treatment
- Monitor temp q4h, may indicate beginning of infection
- Monitor liver function tests (bilirubin, AST, ALT, amylase, alkaline phosphatase, triglycerides) before, during therapy as needed or qmo
- Monitor viral load, CD4 baseline and throughout treatment

Nursing diagnoses

✓ Infection, risk for (uses)
✓ Injury, risk for (adverse reactions)
✓ Knowledge deficit (teaching)

Implementation

- Give on empty stomach, q8h around the clock

Patient/family education

- Advise patient to take on empty stomach; not to take dapsone at same time as ddC; to use exactly as prescribed
- Instruct patient to report signs of infection: increased temp, sore throat, flu symptoms; to avoid crowds and those with known infections
- Caution patient to report signs of anemia: fatigue, headache, faintness, shortness of breath, irritability
- Advise patient to report bleeding; avoid use of razors or commercial mouthwash
- Inform patient that hair may be lost during therapy (rare); a wig or hairpiece may make patient feel better
- Caution patient to avoid OTC products or other medications without approval of prescriber
- Caution patient not to have any sexual contact without use of a condom, that needles should not be shared, that blood from infected individual should not come in contact with another's mucus membranes

Evaluation

Positive therapeutic outcome

- Absence of infection; symptoms of HIV infection

zaleplon (℞)
(zale'plon)
Sonata
Func. class.: Sedative-hypnotic, antianxiety
Chem. class.: Pyrazolopyrimidine
Pregnancy category C

Action: Binds selectively to ω-1 receptor of the γ-aminobutyric acid type A ($GABA_A$) receptor complex; results are sedation, hypnosis, skeletal muscle relaxation, anticonvulsant activity, anxiolytic action

Therapeutic Outcome: Ability to sleep

Uses: Insomnia

Dosage and routes
Adult: PO 10 mg hs; may increase dose to 20 mg hs if needed; 5 mg may be used in low weight persons

G ***Elderly:*** PO 15 mg hs; may increase if needed

Available forms: Caps 5, 10 mg

Adverse effects
CNS: *Drowsiness,* amnesia, depersonalization, hallucinations, hypesthesia, paresthesia, somnolence, tremor, vertigo, dizziness, anxiety
EENT: Vision changes, ear/eye pain, hyperacusis, parosmia
GI: Nausea, anorexia, colitis, dyspepsia, dry mouth, constipation
MISC: Abdominal pain, asthenia, fever, headache, myalgia, dysmenorrhea

Contraindications: Hypersensitivity

Precautions: Hepatic disease, renal disease, elderly, psychosis, child <15 yr, pregnancy **C**, lactation (G, P)

Pharmacokinetics

Absorption	Rapidly absorbed
Distribution	Extravascular tissues crosses blood-brain barrier; crosses placenta
Metabolism	Extensively, liver to inactive metabolites
Excretion	Kidneys
Half-life	1 hr

Pharmacodynamics

Onset	Rapid
Peak	1 hr
Duration	Unknown

Interactions
Individual drugs
Cimetidine: ↑ action of zaleplon
Rifampin: ↓ zaleplon levels
Food/drug
Prolonged absorption
High-fat/heavy meal: Sleep onset reduced

NURSING CONSIDERATIONS
Assessment
- Assess for previous drug dependence or tolerance; if drug dependent or tolerant, amount of medication should be restricted
- Monitor patient's mental status: mood, sensorium, affect, sleeping patterns, drowsiness, dizziness, suicidal tendencies

Nursing diagnoses
✓ Sleep pattern disturbance (uses)
✓ Knowledge deficit (teaching)
✓ Noncompliance (teaching)

Implementation
- Give ½-1 hr before bedtime for sleeplessness; give on empty stomach
- Advise patient that drug may cause memory problems, dependence (if used for longer periods of time), changes in behavior/thinking

Patient/family education
- Inform patient that drug is for short-term use only
- Teach patient to take immediately before going to bed

• Advise patient not to ingest a high-fat/heavy meal before taking
• Advise patient to avoid OTC preparations unless approved by a physician, to avoid alcohol ingestion or other psychotropic medications unless prescribed by a health care provider, that 1-2 wk of therapy may be required before therapeutic effects occur
• Caution patient to avoid driving, activities requiring alertness; drowsiness may occur; until medication response is known, tell patient that drowsiness may worsen at beginning of treatment
• Instruct patient not to discontinue medication abruptly after long-term use

Evaluation

Positive therapeutic outcome
• Decreased sleeplessness

zanamivir (℞)

(zan-a-mee'veer)
Relenza
Func. class.: Antiviral
Chem class.: Nevramidase inhibitor

Pregnancy category B

Action: Inhibits the enzyme needed for influenza virus replication

➔ **Therapeutic Outcome:** Decreased symptoms of influenza type A for those who have been symptomatic for no more than 2 days

Uses: Treatment of influenza type A

Dosage and routes

P ***Adult and child >12 yr:*** INH 2 inhalations (two 5 mg blisters) q12h × 5 days, on the 1st day 2 doses should be taken with at least 2 hr between doses

Available forms: Blisters of powder for inhalation 5 mg

Adverse effects

CNS: *Headache, dizziness,* fatigue
EENT: Ear, nose, throat infections
GI: *Nausea, vomiting, diarrhea*
RESP: Nasal symptoms, cough, sinusitis, bronchitis

Contraindications: Hypersensitivity

G P **Precautions:** Elderly, lactation, children <12 yr, respiratory disease, pregnancy **B**

Pharmacokinetics

Absorption	4%-17% absorbed
Distribution	<10% protein binding
Metabolism	Not metabolized
Excretion	Kidneys unchanged
Half-life	2½-5 hr

Pharmacodynamics

Unknown

Interactions: None known

NURSING CONSIDERATIONS

Assessment

• Assess for symptoms of influenza A: increased temperature, malaise, aches and pains
• Assess for skin eruptions, photosensitivity after administration of drug
• Monitor respiratory status: rate, character, wheezing, tightness in chest
• Assess for allergies before initiation of treatment, reaction of each medication

Nursing diagnoses

✓ Infection, risk for (uses)
✓ Knowledge deficit (teaching)

Implementation

• Give before exposure to influenza; continue for 5 days after contact
• Store in airtight, dry container

Patient/family education

• Give patient "Patient's instruction for use" and review all points before using delivery system
• Teach patient to avoid hazardous activities if dizziness occurs
• Teach patient to take drug exactly as prescribed; to use for the entire 5 days

- Inform patient that this drug does not reduce transmission risk of influenza to others
- Advise patients with asthma or COPD to carry a fast-acting inhaled bronchodilator since bronchospasm may occur; to use scheduled inhaled bronchodilators before using this drug

Evaluation

Positive therapeutic outcome

- Absence of fever, malaise, cough, dyspnea in influenza A

zidovudine (℞)

(zye-doe'vue-deen)

Apo-Zidovudine ✱, Azidothymidine, AZT, Novo-AZT ✱, Retrovir

Func. class.: Antiviral

Chem. class.: Thymidine analog

Pregnancy category C

Action: Inhibits replication of HIV by incorporating into cellular DNA by viral reverse transcriptase, thereby terminating the cellular DNA chain

Therapeutic Outcome: Decreased symptoms of HIV infection

Uses: Symptomatic/asymptomatic HIV infections (AIDS, ARC), confirmed *Pneumocystis carinii* pneumonia, or absolute CD4 lymphocytes <200/mm^3, prevention of maternal-fetal HIV transmission

Dosage and routes

Adult: PO 200 mg q4h; may have to stop treatment if severe bone marrow depression occurs, and restart after bone marrow recovery; **IV** 1-2 mg/kg q4h, initiate PO as soon as possible

P ***Child:*** PO 90-180 mg/m^2/dose q6h; **IV** same as adult

P ***Neonates:*** PO 2-3 mg/kg/dose q6h; **IV** same as adult

Prevention of maternal-fetal HIV transmission

P ***Neonatal:*** PO 2 mg/kg/dose q6h × 6 wk beginning 8-12 hr after birth; **IV** 1.5 mg/kg/dose over 30 min q6h until able to take PO

Maternal (>14 wk gestation): PO 100 mg 5 ×/day until start of labor, then **IV** 2 mg/kg over 1 hr followed by **IV** inf 1 mg/kg/hr until umbilical cord clamped

Asymptomatic HIV infection

P ***Child 3 mo-12 yr:*** PO 90-180 mg/m^2 q6h, max 200 mg q6h; **IV** 1-2 mg/kg over 1 hr q4h

Adult: PO 100 mg q4h while awake (5 ×/day)

Symptomatic HIV infection

P ***Child 3 mo-12 yr:*** PO 90-180 mg/m^2 q6h, max 200 ng q6h; **IV** 1-2 mg/kg over 1 hr q4h

Adult: PO 100 mg q4h; **IV** 1-2 mg/kg over 1 hr q4h

Prevention of HIV after needlestick

Adult: PO 200 mg tid plus lamivudine 150 mg bid, plus a protease inhibitor for high-risk exposure; begin within 2 hr of exposure

Available forms: Caps 100, 300 mg; inj 200 mg/20 ml; oral syrup 50 mg/5 ml

Adverse effects

CNS: *Fever, headache, malaise,* diaphoresis, *dizziness, insomnia,* paresthesia, somnolence, chills, tremor, twitching, anxiety, confusion, depression, lability, vertigo, loss of mental acuity

EENT: Taste change, hearing loss, photophobia

GI: *Nausea, vomiting, diarrhea,* anorexia, cramps, *dyspepsia,* constipation, dysphagia, *flatulence,* rectal bleeding, mouth ulcer

GU: Dysuria, polyuria, frequency, hesitancy

HEMA: **Granulocytopenia, anemia**

INTEG: *Rash,* acne, pruritus, urticaria

MS: Myalgia, arthralgia, muscle spasm

RESP: Dyspnea

Contraindications: Hypersensitivity

Precautions: Granulocyte count <1000/mm^3 or Hgb <9.5 g/dl, pregnancy **C**, lactation, children, severe renal disease, severe hepatic func-tion

Pharmacokinetics

Absorption	Well absorbed (PO), completely absorbed (**IV**)
Distribution	Widely distributed—crosses placenta, CSF
Metabolism	Liver—mostly
Excretion	Kidneys
Half-life	1 hr

Pharmacodynamics

	PO	IV
Onset	Unknown	Rapid
Peak	½-1½ hr	Inf end
Duration	Unknown	Unknown

Interactions

Individual drugs

Amphotericin B: ↑ neurotoxicity, nephrotoxicity
Interferon: ↑ neurotoxicity, nephrotoxicity
Methotrexate: ↑ neurotoxicity, nephrotoxicity
Probenecid: ↑ neurotoxicity, nephrotoxicity

Drug classifications

Aminoglycosides: ↑ neurotoxicity, nephrotoxicity

NURSING CONSIDERATIONS

Assessment

- Assess for peripheral neuropathy: tingling or pain in hands and feet, distal numbness; if these occur, drug may be decreased or discontinued
- Assess for pancreatitis: abdominal pain, nausea, vomiting, elevated liver enzymes; drug should be discontinued because condition can be fatal
- P Assess children by dilated retinal examination q6 mo to rule out retinal depigmentation
- Monitor CBC, differential, platelet count qmo; withhold drug if WBC is <4000/mm^3 or platelet count is <75,000/mm^3; notify prescriber of results; monitor viral load, CD4 counts baseline and throughout treatment
- Monitor renal function studies: BUN, serum uric acid, urine CrCl before, during therapy; these may be elevated throughout treatment
- Monitor temp q4h, may indicate beginning of infection
- Monitor liver function tests before, during therapy (bilirubin, AST, ALT amylase, alkaline phosphatase) prn or qmo

Nursing diagnoses

✓ Infection, risk for (uses)
✓ Injury, risk for physical injury (adverse reactions)
✓ Knowledge deficit (teaching)

Implementation

PO route

- Give on empty stomach, q4h around the clock

IV IV route

- Give by intermittent inf after diluting with D_5W; give over 1 hr (<4 mg/ml), do not give by direct **IV**

Y-site compatibilities:

Acyclovir, allopurinol, amikacin, amphotericin B, aztreonam, ceftazidime, ceftriaxone, cimetidine, clindamycin, dexamethasone, dobutamine, dopamine, erythromycin, fluconazole, fludarabine, gentamicin, heparin, imipenem/cilastatin, lorazepam, metoclopramide, morphine, nafcillin, ondansetron, oxacillin, pentamidine, phenylephrine, piperacillin, potassium chloride, ranitidine, sargramostim, tobramycin, trimethoprim-sulfamethoxazole, vancomycin

Additive incompatibilities:

Blood products or protein solutions

Patient/family education

- Caution patient to take on empty stomach; not to take dapsone at same time as didanosine; to use exactly as prescribed

- Advise patient to report signs of infection: increased temp, sore throat, flu symptoms; to avoid crowds and those with known infections
- Instruct patient to report signs of anemia: fatigue, headache, faintness, shortness of breath, irritability
- Advise patient to report bleeding; avoid use of razors or commercial mouthwash
- Inform patient that hair may be lost during therapy (rare); a wig or hairpiece may make patient feel better
- Caution patient to avoid OTC products or other medications without approval of prescriber
- Caution patient not to have any sexual contact without use of a condom, needles should not be shared, blood from infected individual should not come in contact with another's mucus membranes

Evaluation

Positive therapeutic outcome

- Decreased infection; symptoms of HIV infection

zileuton (℞)

(zye-loo'tahn)

Zyflo

Func. class.: Bronchodilator

Chem. class.: 5-lipoxygenase inhibitor, leukotriene pathway inhibitor

Pregnancy category C

Action: Inhibits leukotriene (LT) formation; leukotrienes exert their effects by increasing neutrophil, eosinophil migration; aggregation of neutrophils, monocytes; smooth muscle contraction, capillary permeability; these actions further lead to bronchoconstriction, inflammation, edema

➡ **Therapeutic Outcome:** Ability to breathe more easily

Uses: Allergic rhinitis, asthma

Investigational uses: Ulcerative colitis, rheumatoid arthritis

Dosage and routes

Asthma

P ***Adult and child >12 yr:*** PO 600 mg qid, may be given with meal and hs

Ulcerative colitis

Adult: PO 600 mg bid

Available forms: Tabs 600 mg

Adverse effects

CNS: Dizziness, insomnia, fatigue, paresthesias, headache

GI: Nausea, abdominal pain, dyspepsia, diarrhea, LFT abnormalities

INTEG: Hives

MS: Myalgia, asthenia

Contraindications: Hepatic disease, elevations in LFTs 3× upper limits, hypersensitivity

Precautions: Acute attacks of asthma, alcohol consumption, pregnancy **C**

Pharmacokinetics	
Absorption	Rapid
Distribution	Protein-binding 93%
Metabolism	Liver
Excretion	Urine
Half-life	2.1-2.5 hr

Pharmacodynamics	
Onset	Unknown
Peak	1-3 hr
Duration	Unknown

Interactions

Individual drugs

Propranolol: ↑ action of zilenton

Theophylline: ↑ action of zilenton

Drug classifications

Anticoagulants: ↑ effects

NURSING CONSIDERATIONS

Assessment

- Assess CBC, blood chemistry, during treatment
- Assess LFTs before and qmo × 3 mo, then q2-3 mo during treatment

- Assess respiratory rate, rhythm, depth; auscultate lung fields bilaterally; notify prescriber of abnormalities
- Assess allergic reactions: rash, urticaria; drug should be discontinued

Nursing diagnoses
✓ Breathing pattern, ineffective (uses)
✓ Knowledge deficit (teaching)
✓ Noncompliance (teaching)

Implementation
- Give PO after meals to decrease GI symptoms; absorption may be affected

Patient/family education
- Advise patient to check OTC medications, current prescription medications for ephedrine, which will increase stimulation; to avoid alcohol
- Advise patient to avoid hazardous activities; dizziness may occur
- Advise patient that if GI upset occurs, to take drug with 8 oz of water or food; absorption may be decreased slightly
- Advise patient to notify prescriber of nausea, vomiting, anxiety, insomnia

Evaluation
Positive therapeutic outcome
- Ability to breathe more easily

zinc sulfate
(PO, OTC; IV, ℞)
(zink sul'fate)

Orazinc, PMS Egozine ♣, Verazinc, Zinca-Pak, Zincate, Zinc 15, Zinc-220, zinc sulfate

Func. class.: Trace element; nutritional supplement

Pregnancy category A

Action: Needed for adequate healing, bone and joint development, taste and smell (23% zinc)

➔ **Therapeutic Outcome:** Replacement of zinc

Uses: Prevention of zinc deficiency, adjunct to vit A therapy

Investigational uses: Wound healing

Dosage and routes
Dietary supplement

Adult: PO 25-50 mg/day

***Nutritional supplement* (IV)**

Adult: 2.5-4 mg/day, may increase by 2 mg/day if needed

P ***Child to 5 yr:*** **IV** 100 µg/kg/day

P ***Infants: <1500 g-3 kg;*** **IV** 300 µg/kg/day

Available forms: Tabs 66, 110 mg; caps 220 mg; inj 1, 5 mg/ml

Adverse effects
GI: Nausea, vomiting, cramps, heartburn, ulcer formation

OVERDOSE: Diarrhea, rash, dehydration, restlessness

Precautions: Pregnancy **A**

Pharmacokinetics	
Absorption	Poorly absorbed (PO), completely absorbed (**IV**)
Distribution	Widely distributed
Metabolism	Liver
Excretion	90%—feces, 10%—kidneys
Half-life	Unknown

Pharmacodynamics

Unknown

Interactions
Individual drugs

Tetracycline: ↓ absorption of tetracycline

NURSING CONSIDERATIONS
Assessment
- Monitor zinc levels during treatment

Nursing diagnoses
✓ Nutrition: less than body requirements (uses)
✓ Knowledge deficit (teaching)

Implementation
PO route
- Give with meals to decrease gastric

upset; restrict dairy products, caffeine, which decrease absorption

IV **IV route**
- Part of TPN

Patient/family education
- Inform patient that element must be taken for 2 mo to be effective
- Advise patient to report immediately nausea, diarrhea, rash, severe vomiting, restlessness, abdominal pain, tarry stools

Evaluation
Positive therapeutic outcome
- Absence of zinc deficiency
- Improved wound healing

ziprasidone (℞)
(zi-praz′ih-dohn)

Geodon

Func. class.: Antipsychotic/neuroleptic

Chem. class.: Benzisoxazole derivative

Pregnancy category C

Action: Unknown; may be mediated through both dopamine type 2 (D_2) and serotonin type 2 ($5\text{-}HT_2$) antagonism

Therapeutic Outcome: Decreased signs/symptoms of psychosis

Uses: Schizophrenia

Dosage and routes
Adult: PO 20 mg bid with food, adjust dosage every 2 days upward to max of 80 mg bid

Available forms: Tabs 20, 40, 60, 80 mg

Adverse effects
CNS: *EPS (pseudoparkinsonism, akathisia, dystonia, tardive dyskinesia), drowsiness, insomnia, agitation, anxiety, headache,* **seizures, neuroleptic malignant syndrome**

CV: Orthostatic hypotension, ***tachycardia, prolonged QT/QTc, sudden death***

EENT: Blurred vision

GI: *Nausea,* vomiting, *anorexia, constipation,* jaundice, weight gain

RESP: Rhinitis

Contraindications: Hypersensitivity, lactation, seizure disorders

P **Precautions:** Children, renal disease, pregnancy **C,** hepatic disease,
G elderly, breast cancer

Pharmacokinetics

Absorption	Unknown
Distribution	Protein binding 90%
Metabolism	Liver—extensively to metabolite
Excretion	Unknown
Half-life	Unknown

Pharmacodynamics
Unknown

Interactions
Individual drugs

Alcohol: ↑ sedation

Carbamazepine: ↑ excretion of ziprasidone

Lithium: ↑ EPS

Drug classifications

Antipsychotics: ↑ EPS

CNS depressants: ↑ sedation

Herb/drug

Kava: ↑ CNS depression

NURSING CONSIDERATIONS
Assessment
- Assess mental status before initial administration
- Check swallowing of PO medication; check for hoarding or giving of medication to other patients
- Monitor I&O ratio; palpate bladder if urinary output is low
- Monitor bilirubin, CBC, liver function studies qmo
- Monitor urinalysis before, during prolonged therapy

- Assess affect, orientation, LOC, reflexes, gait, coordination, sleep pattern disturbances
- Monitor B/P standing and lying; also pulse, respirations; take these q4h during initial treatment; establish baseline before starting treatment; report drops of 30 mm Hg; watch for ECG changes
- Assess dizziness, faintness, palpitations, tachycardia on rising
- Assess EPS, including akathisia (inability to sit still, no pattern to movements), tardive dyskinesia (bizarre movements of the jaw, mouth, tongue, extremities), pseudoparkinsonism (rigidity, tremors, pill rolling, shuffling gait)

❗ Assess for neuroleptic malignant syndrome: hyperthermia, increased CPK, altered mental status, muscle rigidity

- Assess skin turgor qd
- Assess constipation, urinary retention qd; if these occur, increase bulk and water in diet

Nursing diagnoses

✓ Thought processes, altered (uses)
✓ Coping, ineffective individual (uses)
✓ Knowledge deficit (teaching)
✓ Noncompliance (teaching)

Implementation

- [G] Give reduced dose in elderly
- Give antiparkinsonian agent on order from prescriber, to be used for EPS
- Provide decreased stimulus by dimming lights, avoiding loud noises
- Provide supervised ambulation until patient is stabilized on medication; do not involve in strenuous exercise program because fainting is possible; patient should not stand still for a long time
- Provide increased fluids to prevent constipation
- Provide sips of water, candy, gum for dry mouth
- Store in airtight, light-resistant container

Patient/family education

- Advise patient that orthostatic hypotension may occur and to rise from sitting or lying position gradually
- Advise patient to avoid hot tubs, hot showers, tub baths; hypotension may occur
- Advise patient to avoid abrupt withdrawal of this drug; EPS may result; drug should be withdrawn slowly
- Advise patient to avoid OTC preparations (cough, hay fever, cold) unless approved by prescriber, since serious drug interactions may occur; avoid use with alcohol, CNS depressants; increased drowsiness may occur
- Teach patient to avoid hazardous activities if drowsy or dizzy
- Teach patient compliance with drug regimen
- Teach patient to report impaired vision, tremors, muscle twitching
- Teach patient that in hot weather, heat stroke may occur; take extra precautions to stay cool

Evaluation

Positive therapeutic outcome

- Decrease in emotional excitement, hallucinations, delusions, paranoia; reorganization of patterns of thought, speech

Treatment of overdose:

Lavage if orally ingested; provide airway; *do not induce vomiting*

zoledronic acid

See Appendix A, Selected New Drugs

zolmitriptan (℞)

(zole-mih-trip′tan)
Zomig, Zomig-ZMT
Func. class.: Migraine agent
Chem. class.: 5-HT_1 receptor agonist

Pregnancy category C

Action: Binds selectively to the vascular serotonin type 1 (5-HT_1) receptor subtype, exerts antimigraine effect; causes vasoconstriction in cranial arteries

➡ **Therapeutic Outcome:** Decreased severity, frequency of headache

Uses: Acute treatment of migraine with or without aura

Dosage and routes:

Adult: PO Start at 2.5 mg or lower (tab may be broken), may repeat after 2 hr, max 10 mg/24 hr

Available forms: Tabs 2.5, 5 mg; orally disintegrating tabs 2.5 mg

Adverse effects

CV: Palpitations
GI: Abdominal discomfort, nausea
MS: ***Weakness, neck stiffness,*** myalgia
NEURO: ***Tingling, hot sensation, burning, feeling of pressure, tightness, numbness, dizziness, sedation***
RESP: Chest tightness, pressure

Contraindications: Angina pectoris, history of MI, documented silent ischemia, ischemic heart disease, concurrent ergotamine-containing preparations, uncontrolled hypertension, hypersensitivity, basilar or hemiplegic migraine, risk of CV events

Precautions: Postmenopausal women, men >40 yr, risk factors for CAD, hypercholesterolemia, obesity, diabetes, impaired hepatic or renal function, pregnancy **C**, lactation, [P] children, [G] elderly

Pharmacokinetics

Absorption	Unknown
Distribution	25% protein binding
Metabolism	Unknown
Excretion	Unknown
Half-life	3-3½ hr

Pharmacodynamics

Onset	Unknown
Peak	Unknown
Duration	2-3½ hr

Interactions

Individual drugs
Cimetidine: ↑ half-life of zolmitriptan
Ergot: ↑ vasospastic effects

Drug classifications
Ergot derivatives: ↑ vasospastic effects
MAOIs: Do not use within 2 wk
Oral contraceptives: ↑ half-life of zolmitriptan
Selective serotonin reuptake inhibitors (SSRIs): ↑ weakness, hyperreflexia, incoordination

NURSING CONSIDERATIONS

Assessment

- Assess tingling, hot sensation, burning, feeling of pressure, numbness, flushing
- Assess for stress level, activity, recreation, coping mechanisms
- Assess neurologic status: LOC, blurring vision, nausea, vomiting, tingling in extremities preceding headache
- Monitor ingestion of tyramine foods (pickled products, beer, wine, aged cheese), food additives, preservatives, colorings, artifical sweeteners, chocolate, caffeine, which may precipitate these types of headaches
- Assess for serotonin syndrome, if also taking an SSRI

Nursing diagnoses

✓ Pain (uses)
✓ Noncompliance (teaching)
✓ Knowledge deficit (teaching)

Implementation
- Give with fluids as soon as symptoms of migraine occur
- Provide quiet, calm environment with decreased stimulation for noise, bright light, excessive talking

Patient/family education
- Teach patient to report any side effects to prescriber
- Advise patient to use contraception while taking drug

Evaluation
Positive therapeutic outcome
- Decrease in frequency, severity of headache

zolpidem (℞)
(zole-pi'dem)

Ambien

Func. class.: Sedative-hypnotic

Chem. class.: Nonbenzodiazepine of imidazopyridine class

Pregnancy category B

Controlled substance schedule IV

Action: Produces CNS depression at limbic, thalamic, hypothalamic levels of CNS; may be mediated by neurotransmitter γ-aminobutyric acid (GABA); results are sedation, hypnosis, skeletal muscle relaxation, anticonvulsant activity, anxiolytic action

➔ **Therapeutic Outcome:** Ability to sleep, sedation

Uses: Insomnia, short-term treatment

Dosage and routes
Adult: PO 10 mg hs × 7-10 days only; total dose should not exceed 10 mg

G ***Elderly:*** PO 5 mg hs

Available forms: Tabs 5, 10 mg

Adverse effects
CNS: *Headache, lethargy, drowsiness, daytime sedation, dizziness, confusion, light-headedness, anxiety, irritability, amnesia, poor coordination*

CV: *Chest pain, palpitation*

GI: *Nausea, vomiting, diarrhea, heartburn, abdominal pain, constipation*

Contraindications: Hypersensitivity to benzodiazepines

Precautions: Anemia, hepatic disease, renal disease, suicidal individuals, drug abuse, elderly, G psychosis, child <18 yr, P seizure disorders, pregnancy **B**, lactation

Pharmacokinetics

Absorption	Rapidly absorbed
Distribution	Unknown
Metabolism	Liver—inactive metabolite
Excretion	Kidneys, breast milk
G **Half-life**	2½ hr, increased in elderly

Pharmacodynamics
Unknown

Interactions
Individual drugs

Alcohol: ↑ CNS depression

Fluoxetine: ↑ action

Propoxyphene: ↑ action

Drug classifications

Antidepressants: ↑ CNS depression

Antihistamines: ↑ CNS depression

Opiates: ↑ CNS depression

Sedative/hypnotics: ↑ CNS depression

Food/drug

↓ Absorption

Herb/drug

Kava: ↑ CNS depression

Lab test interferences

↑ ALT, ↑ AST, ↑ serum bilirubin

↓ Radioactive iodine uptake

False: ↑ Urinary 17-OHCS

NURSING CONSIDERATIONS
Assessment
- Assess mental status: mood, sensorium, anxiety, affect, sleeping pattern, drowsiness, dizziness, especially G elderly; physical dependency, withdrawal symptoms: anxiety, panic attacks, agitation, seizures, headache, nausea, vomiting, muscle pain, weakness; suicidal tendencies; for indications of increasing tolerance and abuse
- Monitor B/P (lying, standing), pulse; if systolic B/P drops 20 mm Hg, hold drug, notify prescriber
- Monitor blood studies: CBC during long-term therapy; blood dycrasias have occurred rarely; decreased hematocrit, neutropenia may occur
- Monitor hepatic studies: AST, ALT, bilirubin, creatinine LDH, alkaline phosphatase
- Monitor I&O ratio for renal dysfunction

Nursing diagnoses
✓ Anxiety (uses)
✓ Depression (uses)
✓ Injury, risk for (adverse reactions)
✓ Knowledge deficit (teaching)

Implementation
- Give ½-1 hr before bedtime for sleeplessness; give several hr before patient is to arise (to avoid hangover)
- Store in airtight container in cool environment

Patient/family education
- Instruct patient that drug may be taken with food, or fluids and tab may be crushed or swallowed whole
- Caution patient not to use for everyday stress or longer than 3 mo unless directed by prescriber; not to take more than prescribed amount; may be habit forming; not to double or skip doses
- Caution patient to avoid OTC preparations unless approved by prescriber; alcohol and CNS depressants will increase CNS depression
- Advise patient to avoid driving, activities that require alertness, because drowsiness may occur; to avoid alcohol ingestion or other psychotropic medications; to rise slowly or fainting may occur, especially G elderly; that drowsiness may worsen at beginning of treatment
- Instruct patient not to discontinue medication abruptly after long-term use; withdrawal symptoms include vomiting, cramping, tremors, seizures

Evaluation
Positive therapeutic outcome
- Ability to sleep at night
- Decreased amount of early morning awakening if taking drug for insomnia

Treatment of overdose:
Lavage, VS, supportive care

zonisamide (℞)
(zone-is′a-mide)

Zonegran

Func. class.: Anticonvulsant

Chem. class.: Sulfonamides

Pregnancy category C

Action: May act through at sodium and calcium channels, but exact action is unknown

➔ **Therapeutic Outcome:** Decreased seizures

Uses: Epilepsy, adjunctive therapy of partial seizures

Dosage and routes
P ***Adults and child >16 yr:*** PO 100 mg qd, may increase after 2 wk to 200 mg/day, may increase q2 wk, max dose >600 mg/day

Available forms: Caps 100 mg

Adverse effects
CNS: Dizziness, insomnia, paresthesias, depression, fatigue, headache, confusion

EENT: Diplopia, verbal difficulty, speech abnormalities, taste perversion

GI: Nausea, constipation, anorexia, weight loss, diarrhea, dyspepsia
INTEG: Rash

Contraindications:
Hypersensitivity to this drug or sulfonamides, psychiatric condition, hepatic failure

Precautions:
Allergies, hepatic disease, renal disease, G elderly, P pregnancy **C**, lactation, child <16 yr

Pharmacokinetics

Absorption	Unknown
Distribution	Unknown
Metabolism	Liver
Excretion	Kidneys
Half-life	63 hr

Pharmacodynamics

Onset	Unknown
Peak	2-6 hr
Duration	Unknown

Interactions
Drugs inducing CYP 450 enzyme: ↑ half-life of zonisamide

NURSING CONSIDERATIONS
Assessment
- Assess for seizures: duration, type, intensity, precipitating factors
- Monitor blood studies: CBC, platelets q2 wk until stabilized, then qmo × 12, then q3 mo; discontinue drug if neutrophils <1600/mm^3; renal function: albumin conc
- Assess mental status: mood, sensorium, affect, memory (long, short)

Nursing diagnoses
- ✓ Injury, risk for (uses, adverse reactions)
- ✓ Knowledge deficit (teaching)
- ✓ Noncompliance (teaching)

Patient/family education
- Advise patient not to discontinue drug abruptly; seizures may occur
- Advise patient to avoid hazardous activities until stabilized on drug
- Advise patient to carry ID stating drug use

Evaluation
Positive therapeutic outcome
- Decrease in severity of seizures

ALPHA-ADRENERGIC BLOCKERS

Action: Binds to α-adrenergic receptors, causing dilatation of peripheral blood vessels; lowers peripheral resistance, resulting in decreased blood pressure.
Uses: Used for pheochromocytoma, prevention of tissue necrosis, and sloughing associated with extravasation of IV vasopressors.
Adverse effects: The most common side effects are hypotension, tachycardia, nasal stuffiness, nausea, vomiting, and diarrhea.
Contraindications: Hypersensitive reactions may occur, and allergies should be identified before these products are given. Patients with myocardial infarction, coronary insufficiency, angina, or other evidence of coronary artery disease should not use these products.
Pharmacokinetics: Onset, peak, and duration vary among products.
Interactions: Vasoconstrictive and hypertensive effects of epinephrine are antagonized by α-adrenergic blockers.

NURSING CONSIDERATIONS

Assessment

- Monitor electrolytes: potassium, sodium chloride, carbon dioxide
- Monitor weight daily, I&O
- Monitor B/P with patient lying, standing before starting treatment, q4h thereafter
- Assess for nausea, vomiting, diarrhea
- Assess for skin turgor, dryness of mucous membranes for hydration status

Nursing diagnoses

✓ Altered tissue perfusion (uses)
✓ Risk for injury (adverse reactions)
✓ Sleep pattern disturbance (adverse reactions)

Implementation

PO Route

- Start with low dose, gradually increasing to prevent side effects
- Give with food or milk for GI symptoms

Evaluation

- Therapeutic response: decreased B/P, increased peripheral pulses

Patient/family education

- Caution patient to avoid alcoholic beverages
- Advise patient to report dizziness, palpitations, fainting
- Instruct patient to change position slowly or fainting may occur
- Teach patient to take drug exactly as prescribed; to avoid all OTC products (cough, cold, allergy) unless directed by prescriber

Selected Generic Names

phentolamine

ANESTHETICS—GENERAL/LOCAL

Action: Anesthetics (general) act on the CNS to produce tranquilization and sleep before invasive procedures. Anesthetics (local) inhibit conduction of nerve impulses from sensory nerves.

Uses: General anesthetics are used to premedicate for surgery, and for induction and maintenance in general anesthesia. For local anesthetics, refer to individual product listing for indications.

Adverse effects: The most common side effects are dystonia, akathisia, flexion of arms, fine tremors, drowsiness, restlessness, and hypotension. Also common are chills, respiratory depression, and laryngospasm.

Contraindications: Persons with CVA, increased intracranial pressure, severe hypertension, cardiac decompensation should not use these products, since severe adverse reactions can occur.

G **Precautions:** Anesthetics (general) should be used with caution in the elderly, cardiovascular disease (hypotension, bradydysrhythmias), renal disease, liver P disease, Parkinson's disease, children <2 yr. The precaution for anesthetics (local) is pregnancy.

Pharmacokinetics: Onset, peak, and duration vary widely among products. Most products are metabolized in the liver and excreted in urine.

Interactions: MAOIs, tricyclics, phenothiazines may cause severe hypotension or hypertension when used with local anesthetics. CNS depressants will potentiate general and local anesthetics.

NURSING CONSIDERATIONS

Assessment

- Monitor VS q10 min during **IV** administration, q30 min after IM dose

Nursing diagnoses

General

✓ Risk for injury (adverse reactions)
✓ Knowledge deficit (teaching)

Local

✓ Pain (uses)
✓ Knowledge deficit (teaching)

Implementation

- Give anticholinergic preoperatively to decrease secretions
- Administer only with resuscitative equipment nearby
- Provide quiet environment for recovery to decrease psychotic symptoms

Evaluation

- Therapeutic response: maintenance of anesthesia, decreased pain

Selected Generic Names

General anesthetics:
droperidol
etomidate
fentanyl citrate (high alert)
fentanyl citrate/droperidol (high alert)
ketamine (high alert)
methohexital
midazolam
procaine
thiopental (high alert)

Local anesthetics:
🔑 **lidocaine HCl** (high alert)
propofol (high alert)
ropivacaine
tetracaine

ANTACIDS

Action: Antacids are basic compounds that neutralize gastric acidity and decrease the rate of gastric emptying. Products are divided into those containing aluminum, magnesium, calcium, or a combination of these.

Uses: Hyperacidity is decreased by antacids in conditions such as peptic ulcer disease, reflux esophagitis, gastritis, or hiatal hernia.

Adverse effects: The most common side effect caused by aluminum-containing antacids is constipation, which may lead to fecal impaction and bowel obstruction. Diarrhea occurs often when magnesium products are given. Alkalosis may occur when systemic products are used. Constipation occurs more frequently than laxation with calcium carbonate. The release of CO_2 from carbonate-containing antacids causes belching, abdominal distention, and flatulence. Sodium bicarbonate may act as a systemic antacid and produce systemic electrolyte disturbances and alkalosis. Calcium carbonate and sodium bicarbonate may cause rebound hyperacidity and milk-alkali syndrome. Alkaluria may occur when products are used on a long-term basis, particularly in persons with abnormal renal function.

Contraindications: Sensitivity to aluminum or magnesium products may cause hypersensitive reactions. Aluminum products should not be used by persons sensitive to aluminum; magnesium products should not be used by persons sensitive to magnesium. Check for sensitivity before administering.

Precautions: Magnesium products should be given cautiously to patients with renal insufficiency, during pregnancy, or lactation. Sodium content of antacids may be significant; use with caution for patients with hypertension, CHF, or those on a low-sodium diet.

Pharmacokinetics: Duration is 20-40 min. If ingested 1 hr pc, acidity is reduced for at least 3 hr.

Interactions: Drugs whose effects may be increased by some antacids: quinidine, amphetamines, pseudoephedrine, levodopa, valproic acid, dicumarol. Drugs whose effects may be decreased by some antacids: cimetidine, corticosteroids, ranitidine, iron salts, phenothiazines, phenytoin, digoxin, tetracyclines, ketoconazole, salicylates, isoniazid.

NURSING CONSIDERATIONS

Assessment

- Assess for aggravating and alleviating factors of epigastric pain or hyperacidity; identify the location, duration, and characteristics of epigastric pain
- Assess GI symptoms, including constipation, diarrhea, abdominal pain; if severe abdominal pain with fever occurs, these drugs should not be given
- Assess renal symptoms, including increasing urinary pH, electrolytes

Nursing diagnoses

✓ Pain (uses)
✓ Constipation (adverse reactions)
✓ Diarrhea (adverse reactions)

Implementation

- Give all products with an 8-oz glass of water to ensure absorption in the stomach
- Give another antacid if constipation occurs with aluminum products

Evaluation

- Therapeutic response: absence of epigastric pain, decreased acidity

Patient/family education

- Advise patient not to take other drugs within 1-2 hr of antacid administration, since antacids may impair absorption of other drugs

Selected Generic Names

aluminum hydroxide
bismuth subsalicylate
calcium carbonate
magaldrate
magnesium oxide
sodium bicarbonate

ANTIANGINALS

Action: The antianginals are divided into the nitrates, calcium channel blockers, and β-adrenergic blockers. The nitrates dilate coronary arteries, causing decreased preload, and dilate systemic arteries, causing decreased afterload. Calcium channel blockers dilate coronary arteries, decrease SA/AV node conduction. β-Adrenergic blockers decrease heart rate so that myocardial O_2 use is decreased. Dipyridamole selectively dilates coronary arteries to increase coronary blood flow.

Uses: Antianginals are used in chronic stable angina pectoris, unstable angina, vasospastic angina. Some (i.e., calcium channel blockers and β- blockers) may be used as dysrhythmias and in hypertension.

Adverse effects: The most common side effects are postural hypotension, headache, flushing, dizziness, nausea, edema, and drowsiness. Also common are rash, dysrhythmias, and fatigue.

Contraindications: Persons with known hypersensitivity, increased intracranial pressure, or cerebral hemorrhage should not use some of these products.

Precautions: Antianginals should be used with caution in postural hypotension, P pregnancy, lactation, children, renal disease, and hepatic injury.

Pharmacokinetics: Onset, peak, and duration vary widely among coronary products. Most products are metabolized in the liver and excreted in urine.

Interactions: Please check individual monographs, since interactions vary widely among products.

NURSING CONSIDERATIONS

Assessment

- Orthostatic B/P, pulse
- Assess for pain: duration, time started, activity being performed, character
- Assess for tolerance if taken over long period
- Assess for headache, lightheadedness, decreased B/P; may indicate a need for decreased dosage

Nursing diagnoses

- ✓ Altered tissue perfusion: cardiopulmonary (uses)
- ✓ Pain (uses)
- ✓ Risk for injury (uses)
- ✓ Knowledge deficit (teaching)
- ✓ Decreased cardiac output (adverse reactions)

Implementation

- Store protected from light, moisture; place in cool environment

Evaluation

- Therapeutic response: decreased, prevention of anginal pain

Patient/family education

- Instruct patient to keep tabs in original container
- Instruct patient not to use OTC products unless directed by prescriber
- Advise patient to report bradycardia, dizziness, confusion, depression, fever
- Teach patient to take pulse at home; advise when to notify prescriber
- Advise patient to avoid alcohol, smoking, sodium intake
- Advise patient to comply with weight control, dietary adjustments, modified exercise program

- Teach patient to carry ID to identify drug being taken, allergies
- Caution patient to make position changes slowly to prevent fainting

Selected Generic Names

Nitrates:
amyl nitrite
isosorbide
nitroglycerin

β-adrenergic blockers:
atenolol
metoprolol
nadolol
propranolol

Calcium channel blockers:
amlodipine
bepridil
diltiazem (high alert)
nicardipine
nifedipine
verapamil

ANTICHOLINERGICS

Action: Anticholinergics inhibit the muscarinic actions of acetylcholine at receptor sites in the autonomic nervous system; anticholinergics are also known as antimuscarinic drugs.

Uses: Anticholinergics are used for a variety of conditions: gastrointestinal anticholinergics are used to decrease motility (smooth muscle tone) in the GI, biliary, and urinary tracts and for their ability to decrease gastric secretions (propantheline, glycopyrrolate); decreasing involuntary movements in parkinsonism (benztropine, trihexyphenidyl); bradydysrhythmias (atropine); nausea and vomiting (scopolamine); and as cycloplegic mydriatics (atropine, hematropine, scopalamine, cyclopentolate, tropicamide).

Adverse effects: The most common side effects are dry mouth, constipation, urinary retention, urinary hesitancy, headache, and dizziness. Also common is paralytic ileus.

Contraindications: Persons with narrow-angle glaucoma, myasthenia gravis, or GI/GU obstruction should not use some of these products.

Precautions: Anticholinergics should be used with caution in patients who are G elderly, pregnant, or lactating or in those with prostatic hypertrophy, CHF, or hypertension; use with caution in presence of high environmental temp.

Pharmacokinetics: Onset, peak, and duration vary widely among products. Most products are metabolized in the liver and excreted in urine.

Interactions: Increased anticholinergic effects may occur when used with MAOIs and tricyclic antidepressants and amantadine. Anticholinergics may cause a decreased effect of phenothiazines and levodopa.

NURSING CONSIDERATIONS

Assessment

- Assess I&O ratio; retention commonly causes decreased urinary output

- Assess for urinary hesitancy, retention; palpate bladder if retention occurs
- Assess for constipation; increase fluids, bulk, exercise if this occurs
- Identify tolerance over long-term therapy; dosage may need to be increased or changed
- Assess mental status: affect, mood, CNS depression, worsening of mental symptoms during early therapy

Nursing diagnoses

✓ Decreased cardiac output (uses)
✓ Constipation (adverse reactions)
✓ Knowledge deficit (teaching)

Implementation

IV IM/IV Routes

- Give parenteral dose with patient recumbent to prevent postural hypotension
- Give parenteral dose slowly; keep in bed for at least 1 hr after dose; monitor VS
- Give after checking dose carefully; even slight overdose could lead to toxicity

PO Route

- Give with or after meals to prevent GI upset; may give with fluids other than water
- Store at room temp
- Give hard candy, frequent drinks, sugarless gum to relieve dry mouth

Evaluation

- Therapeutic response: decreased secretions, absence of nausea and vomiting

Patient/family education

- Caution patient to avoid driving and other hazardous activities; drowsiness may occur
- Advise patient to avoid OTC medication: cough, cold preparations with alcohol, antihistamines unless directed by prescriber

---

Selected Generic Names

atropine (high alert)
benztropine
biperiden
glycopyrrolate
propantheline
scopolamine (transdermal)
trihexyphenidyl

ANTICOAGULANTS

Action: Anticoagulants interfere with blood clotting by preventing clot formation.
Uses: Anticoagulants are used for deep vein thrombosis, pulmonary emboli, myocardial infarction, open heart surgery, disseminated intravascular clotting syndrome, atrial fibrillation with embolization, and in transfusion and dialysis.

Adverse effects: The most serious adverse reactions are hemorrhage, agranulocytosis, leukopenia, eosinophilia, and thrombocytopenia, depending on the specific product. The most common side effects are diarrhea, rash, and fever.
Contraindications: Persons with hemophilia, leukemia with bleeding, peptic ulcer disease, thrombocytopenic purpura, blood dyscrasias, acute nephritis, and subacute bacterial endocarditis should not use these products.
G **Precautions:** Anticoagulants should be used with caution in alcoholism, elderly, and pregnancy.
Pharmacokinetics: Onset, peak, and duration vary widely among products. Most products are metabolized in the liver and excreted in urine.
Interactions: Salicylates, steroids, and nonsteroidal antiinflammatories will potentiate the action of anticoagulants. Anticoagulants may cause serious effects; please check individual monographs.

NURSING CONSIDERATIONS

Assessment

- Monitor blood studies (Hct, platelets, occult blood in stools) q3 mo
- Monitor partial prothrombin time, which should be 1½-2 × control, PPT; often qd, APTT, ACT, INR
- Monitor B/P; watch for increasing signs of hypertension
- Monitor for bleeding gums, petechiae, ecchymosis, black tarry stools, hematuria
- Monitor for fever, skin rash, urticaria
- Monitor for needed dosage change q1-2 wk

Nursing diagnoses

✓ Altered tissue perfusion (uses)
✓ Risk for injury (side effects)
✓ Knowledge deficit (teaching)

Implementation

SC Route

- Give at same time each day to maintain steady blood levels
- Do not massage area or aspirate when giving SC inj; give in abdomen between pelvic bones; rotate sites; do not pull back on plunger, leave in for 10 sec; apply gentle pressure for 1 min
- Do not change needles
- Avoid all IM inj that may cause bleeding
- Store in tight container (PO dose)

Evaluation

- Therapeutic response: decrease of deep vein thrombosis

Patient/family education

- Advise patient to avoid OTC preparations that may cause serious drug interactions unless directed by prescriber

- Inform patient that drug may be held during active bleeding (menstruation), depending on condition
- Caution patient to use soft-bristle toothbrush to avoid bleeding gums; avoid contact sports; use electric razor
- Instruct patient to carry an ID identifying drug taken
- Instruct patient to report any signs of bleeding: gums, under skin, urine, stools

Selected Generic Names

ardeparin (high alert)
argatroban
dalteparin (high alert)
danaparoid (high alert)
enoxaparin (high alert)
fondaparinux (Appx A)
heparin (high alert)
lepirudin (high alert)
tinzaparin (high alert)
warfarin (high alert)

ANTICONVULSANTS

Action: Anticonvulsants are divided into the barbiturates (p. 1188), benzodiazepines (p. 1190), hydantoins, succinimides, and miscellaneous products. Barbiturates and benzodiazepines are discussed in separate sections. Hydantoins act by inhibiting the spread of seizure activity in the motor cortex. Succinimides act by inhibiting spike and wave formation; they also decrease amplitude, frequency, duration, and spread of discharge in seizures.

Uses: Hydantoins are used in generalized tonic-clonic seizures, status epilepticus, and psychomotor seizures. Succinimides are used for absence of (petit mal) seizures. Barbiturates are used in generalized tonic-clonic and cortical focal seizures.

Adverse effects: Bone marrow depression is the most life-threatening adverse reaction associated with hydantoins or succinimides. The most common side effects are GI symptoms. Other common side effects for hydantoins are gingival hyperplasia and CNS effects such as nystagmus, ataxia, slurred speech, and confusion.

Contraindications: Hypersensitive reactions may occur, and allergies should be identified before these products are given.

Precautions: Persons with renal or hepatic disease should be watched closely.

Pharmacokinetics: Onset, peak, and duration vary widely among products. Most products are metabolized in the liver and excreted in urine, bile, and feces.

Interactions: Decreased effects of estrogens, oral contraceptives (hydantoins).

NURSING CONSIDERATIONS

Assessment

- Monitor renal function studies, including BUN, creatinine, serum uric acid, urine creatinine clearance before and during therapy

- Monitor blood studies: RBC, Hct, Hgb, reticulocyte counts weekly for 4 wk then monthly
- Monitor hepatic studies: AST, ALT, bilirubin, creatinine
- Assess mental status, including mood, sensorium, affect, behavioral changes; if mental status changes, notify prescriber
- Assess for eye problems, including need for ophth examinations before, during, and after treatment (slit lamp, fundoscopy, tonometry)
- Assess for allergic reaction, including red, raised rash; if this occurs, drug should be discontinued
- Assess for blood dyscrasias, including fever, sore throat, bruising, rash, jaundice
- Monitor toxicity, including bone marrow depression, nausea, vomiting, ataxia, diplopia, cardiovascular collapse, Stevens-Johnson syndrome

Nursing diagnoses

- ✓ Risk for injury (uses)
- ✓ Noncompliance (teaching)
- ✓ Sleep pattern disturbance (adverse reactions)

Implementation

PO Route

- Give with food, milk to decrease GI symptoms
- Good oral hygiene is important for patients taking hydantoins

Evaluation

- Therapeutic response, including decreased seizure activity; document on patient's chart

Patient/family education

- Advise patient to carry ID card stating drugs taken, condition, prescriber's name, phone number
- Advise patient to avoid driving, other activities that require alertness

Selected Generic Names

Hydantoins:
fosphenytoin
🔑 phenytoin

Miscellaneous:
acetazolamide
carbamazepine
clonazepam
🔑 diazepam
felbamate
gabapentin
lamotrigine
magnesium sulfate (high alert)
tiagabine
topiramate
valproate/valproic acid/ divalproex sodium
zonisamide

Barbiturates:
amobarbital
🔑 **phenobarbital** (high alert)
primidone
thiopental (high alert)

ANTIDEPRESSANTS

Action: Antidepressants are divided into the tricyclics, MAOIs, and miscellaneous antidepressants. The tricyclics work by blocking reuptake of norepinephrine and serotonin into nerve endings and increasing action of norepinephrine and serotonin in nerve cells. MAOIs act by increasing concentrations of endogenous epinephrine, norepinephrine, serotonin, dopamine in storage sites in CNS by inhibition of MAO; increased concentration reduces depression.

Uses: Antidepressants are used for depression and in some cases enuresis in P children.

Adverse effects: The most serious adverse reactions are paralytic ileus, acute renal failure, hypertension, and hypertensive crisis, depending on the specific product. Common side effects are dizziness, drowsiness, diarrhea, dry mouth, urinary retention, and orthostatic hypotension.

Contraindications: The contraindications for antidepressants are convulsive disorders, prostatic hypertrophy, severe renal, hepatic, cardiac disease depending on the type of medication.

Precautions: Antidepressants should be used cautiously in suicidal patients, severe depression, schizophrenia, hyperactivity, diabetes mellitus, pregnancy, and G the elderly.

Pharmacokinetics: Onset, peak, and duration vary widely among products. Most products are metabolized in the liver and excreted in urine.

Interactions: Please check individual monographs, since interactions vary widely among products.

NURSING CONSIDERATIONS

Assessment

- Monitor B/P (lying, standing), pulse q4h; if systolic B/P drops 20 mm Hg, hold drug, notify prescriber; take VS q4h in patients with cardiovascular disease
- Monitor blood studies: CBC, leukocytes, differential, cardiac enzymes if patient is receiving long-term therapy
- Monitor hepatic studies: AST, ALT, bilirubin, creatinine
- Monitor weight weekly; appetite may increase with drug
- G Monitor for extrapyramidal symptoms (EPS) primarily in elderly: rigidity, dystonia, akathisia
- Assess mental status: mood, sensorium, affect, suicidal tendencies, increase in psychiatric symptoms (depression, panic)
- P G Check for urinary retention, constipation; constipation is more likely to occur in children, elderly
- Assess for withdrawal symptoms: headache, nausea, vomiting, muscle pain, weakness; do not usually occur unless drug was discontinued abruptly
- Identify alcohol consumption; if alcohol is consumed, hold dose until AM

Nursing diagnoses

- ✓ Ineffective individual coping (uses)
- ✓ Risk for injury (uses/adverse reactions)
- ✓ Knowledge deficit (teaching)

Implementation

PO Route

- Give increased fluids, bulk in diet if constipation, urinary retention occur
- Give with food or milk for GI symptoms
- Give gum, hard candy, or frequent sips of water for dry mouth
- Store in airtight container at room temp; do not refreeze
- Provide assistance with ambulation during beginning therapy, since drowsiness/dizziness occurs

Evaluation

- Therapeutic response: decreased depression

Patient/family education

- Teach patient that therapeutic effects may take 2-3 wk
- Advise patient to use caution in driving or other activities requiring alertness because of drowsiness, dizziness, blurred vision
- Caution patient to avoid alcohol ingestion, other CNS depressants
- Instruct patient not to discontinue medication quickly after long-term use; may cause nausea, headache, malaise
- Instruct patient to wear sunscreen or large hat, since photosensitivity may occur

---

Selected Generic Names

Tetracyclic:
mirtazapine

Tricyclics:
amitriptyline
amoxapine
clomipramine
desipramine
doxepin
(Key Drug) imipramine
nortriptyline
trimipramine

Miscellaneous:
bupropion
maprotiline
nefazodone
trazodone
venlafaxine

MAOIs:
phenelzine
tranylcypromine

SSRIs
citalopram
fluoxetine
paroxetine
sertraline

ANTIDIABETICS

Action: Antidiabetics are divided into the insulins that decrease blood sugar, phosphate, and potassium and increase blood pyruvate and lactate; and oral antidiabetics that cause functioning β-cells in the pancreas to release insulin, improves the effect of endogenous and exogenous insulin.

Uses: Insulins are used for ketoacidosis and diabetes mellitus types I (IDDM) and II (NIDDM); oral antidiabetics are used for stable adult-onset diabetes mellitus type II (NIDDM).

Adverse effects: The most common side effect of insulin and oral antidiabetics is hypoglycemia. Other adverse reactions for oral antidiabetics include blood dyscrasias, hepatotoxicity, and, rarely, cholestatic jaundice. Adverse reactions for insulin products include allergic responses and, more rarely, anaphylaxis.

Contraindications: Hypersensitive reactions may occur, and allergies should be identified before these products are given. Oral antidiabetics should not be used in juvenile or brittle diabetes, diabetic ketoacidosis, severe renal disease, or severe hepatic disease.

G **Precautions:** Oral antidiabetics should be used with caution in the elderly, in cardiac disease, pregnancy, lactation, and in the presence of alcohol.

Pharmacokinetics: Onset, peak, and duration vary widely among products. Oral antidiabetics are metabolized in the liver, with metabolites excreted in urine, bile, and feces.

Interactions: Interactions vary widely among products. Check individual monograph for specific information.

NURSING CONSIDERATIONS

Assessment

- Monitor blood, urine glucose levels during treatment to determine diabetes control (oral products)
- Monitor fasting blood glucose, 2 hr PP (60-100 mg/dl normal fasting level) (70-130 mg/dl—normal 2-hr level)
- Assess for hypoglycemic reaction that can occur during peak time

Nursing diagnoses

✓ Altered nutrition: more than body requirements (uses)

Implementation

SC Route

- Give insulin after warming to room temp by rotating in palms to prevent lipodystrophy from injecting cold insulin
- Give human insulin to those allergic to beef or pork
- Rotate inj sites when giving insulin; use abdomen, upper back, thighs, upper arm, buttocks; keep a record of sites

PO Route

- Give oral antidiabetic 30 min ac

Evaluation

- Therapeutic response, including decrease in polyuria, polydipsia, polyphagia, clear sensorium, absence of dizziness, stable gait

Patient/family education

- Advise patient to avoid alcohol and salicylates except on advice of prescriber
- Teach patient symptoms of ketoacidosis: nausea, thirst, polyuria, dry mouth, decreased B/P, dry, flushed skin, acetone breath, drowsiness, Kussmaul respirations
- Teach patient symptoms of hypoglycemia: headache, tremors, fatigue, weakness; and that candy or sugar should be carried to treat hypoglycemia
- Advise patient to test urine for glucose/ketones tid if this drug is replacing insulin
- Advise patient to continue weight control, dietary restrictions, exercise, hygiene

---

Selected Generic Names

acetohexamide
chlorpropamide
glipizide
glyburide
insulin aspart
insulin glargine
(Key Drug) **insulin, isophane suspension** (high alert)
insulin, lispro (high alert)
(Key Drug) **insulin, regular** (high alert)
(Key Drug) **insulin, regular concentrated** (high alert)
insulin, zinc suspension (Ultralente) (high alert)
insulin, zinc suspension (Lente) (high alert)
metformin
miglitol
pioglitazone
repaglinide
rosiglitazone
tolazamide
tolbutamide

ANTIDIARRHEALS

Action: Antidiarrheals work by various actions including direct action on intestinal muscles to decrease GI peristalsis; or by inhibiting prostaglandin synthesis responsible for GI hypermotility; acting on mucosal receptors responsible for peristalsis; or decreasing water content of stools.

Uses: Antidiarrheals are used for diarrhea of undetermined causes.

Adverse effects: The most serious adverse reactions of some products are paralytic ileus, toxic megacolon, and angioneurotic edema. The most common side effects are constipation, nausea, dry mouth, and abdominal pain.

Contraindications: Persons with severe ulcerative colitis, pseudomembranous colitis with some products.

G P **Precautions:** Antidiarrheal should be used with caution in the elderly, pregnancy, lactation, children, dehydration.

Pharmacokinetics: Onset, peak, and duration vary widely among products. Most products are metabolized in the liver and excreted in urine.

Interactions: Please check individual monographs, since interactions vary widely among products.

NURSING CONSIDERATIONS

Assessment

- Monitor electrolytes (potassium, sodium, chloride) if on long-term therapy
- Monitor bowel pattern before; for rebound constipation after termination of medication
- Assess response after 48 hr; if no response, drug should be discontinued
- P Identify dehydration in children

Nursing diagnoses

✓ Diarrhea (uses)
✓ Constipation (adverse reactions)
✓ Fluid volume deficit (adverse reactions)
✓ Knowledge deficit (teaching)

Implementation

PO Route

- Give for 48 hr only

Evaluation

- Therapeutic response: decreased diarrhea

Patient/family education

- Advise patient to avoid OTC products
- Caution patient not to exceed recommended dose

Selected Generic Names

bismuth subsalicylate
difenoxin
kaolin/pectin
loperamide

ANTIDYSRHYTHMICS

Action: Antidysrhythmics are divided into four classes and miscellaneous antidysrhythmics:

- Class I increases the action potential duration and the effective refractory period and reduces disparity in the refractory period between a normal and infarcted myocardium; further subclasses include Ia, Ib, Ic

- Class II decreases the rate of SA node discharge, increases recovery time, slows conduction through the AV node, and decreases heart rate, which decreases O_2 consumption in the myocardium
- Class III increases the action potential duration and the effective refractory period
- Class IV inhibits calcium ion influx across the cell membrane during cardiac depolarization; decreases SA node discharge, decreases conduction velocity through the AV node
- Miscellaneous antidysrhythmics include those such as adenosine, which slows conduction through the AV node, and digoxin, which decreases conduction velocity and prolongs the effective refractory period in the AV node

Uses: These products are used for PVCs, tachycardia, hypertension, atrial fibrillation, angina pectoris.

Adverse effects: Side effects and adverse reactions vary widely among products.

Contraindications: Contraindications vary widely among products.

Precautions: Precautions vary widely among products.

Pharmacokinetics: Onset, peak, and duration vary widely among products.

Interactions: Interactions vary widely among products; check individual monograph for specific information.

NURSING CONSIDERATIONS

Assessment

- Monitor ECG continuously to determine drug effectiveness, PVCs, or other dysrhythmias
- Assess for dehydration or hypovolemia
- Monitor B/P continuously for hypotension, hypertension
- Monitor I&O ratio
- Monitor serum potassium
- Assess for edema in feet and legs daily

Nursing diagnoses

✓ Altered tissue perfusion: cardiopulmonary (uses)
✓ Decreased cardiac output (uses)
✓ Diarrhea (adverse reactions)
✓ Impaired gas exchange (adverse reactions)

Evaluation

- Therapeutic response, including decrease in B/P in hypertension, decreased B/P, edema, moist rales in CHF

Patient/family education

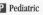

- Advise patient to comply with dosage schedule, even if patient is feeling better
- Instruct patient to report bradycardia, dizziness, confusion, depression, fever

Selected Generic Names

Class I:
moricizine

Class Ia:
disopyramide
🔑 procainamide
🔑 quinidine

Class Ib:
lidocaine (high alert)
mexiletine
🔑 phenytoin
tocainide

Class Ic:
flecainide
indecainide

Class II:
acebutolol
esmolol
🔑 propranolol
sotalol

Class III:
amiodarone (high alert)
🔑 **bretylium** (high alert)
ibutilide (high alert)

Class IV:
🔑 verapamil

Miscellaneous:
adenosine (high alert)
atropine (high alert)
🔑 **digoxin** (high alert)

ANTIFUNGALS (SYSTEMIC)

Action: Antifungals act by increasing cell membrane permeability in susceptible organisms by binding sterols and decreasing potassium, sodium, and nutrients in the cell.

Uses: Antifungals are used for infections of histoplasmosis, blastomycosis, coccidioidomycosis, cryptococcosis, aspergillosis, phycomycosis, candidiasis, sporotrichosis causing severe meningitis, septicemia, and skin infections.

Adverse effects: The most serious adverse reactions include renal tubular acidosis, permanent renal impairment, anuria, oliguria, hemorrhagic gastroenteritis, acute liver failure, and blood dyscrasias. Some common side effects include hypokalemia, nausea, vomiting, anorexia, headache, fever, and chills.

Contraindications: Persons with severe bone depression or hypersensitivity should not use these products.

Precautions: Antifungals should be used with caution in renal disease, pregnancy, and hepatic disease.

Pharmacokinetics: Onset, peak, and duration vary widely among products. Most products are metabolized in the liver and excreted in urine.

Interactions: Please check individual monographs, since interactions vary widely among products.

NURSING CONSIDERATIONS

Assessment

- Monitor VS q15-30 min during first inf; note changes in pulse, B/P
- Monitor I&O ratio; watch for decreasing urinary output, change in sp gr; discontinue drug to prevent permanent damage to renal tubules
- Monitor blood studies; CBC, potassium, sodium, calcium, magnesium q2 wk
- Monitor weight weekly; if weight increases over 2 lb/wk, edema is present; renal damage should be considered
- Assess for renal toxicity: increasing BUN, is >40 mg/dl or if serum creatinine >3 mg/dl; drug may be discontinued or dosage reduced
- Assess for hepatotoxicity: increasing AST, ALT, alkaline phosphatase, bilirubin
- Assess for allergic reaction: dermatitis, rash; drug should be discontinued; antihistamines (mild reaction) or epinephrine (severe reaction) administered
- Assess for hypokalemia: anorexia, drowsiness, weakness, decreased reflexes, dizziness, increased urinary output, increased thirst, paresthesias
- Assess for ototoxicity: tinnitus (ringing, roaring in ears), vertigo, loss of hearing (rare)

Nursing diagnoses

✓ Risk for infection (uses)
✓ Risk for injury (adverse reactions)
✓ Knowledge deficit (teaching)

Implementation

IV IV Route

- Give by **IV** using in-line filter (mean pore diameter >1 µm) using distal veins; check for extravasation, necrosis q8h
- Give drug only after C&S confirms organism, drug needed to treat condition; make sure drug is used in life-threatening infections
- Provide protection from light during inf; cover with foil
- Give symptomatic treatment as ordered for adverse reactions: aspirin, antihistamines, antiemetics, antispasmodics
- Store protected from moisture and light; diluted sol is stable for 24 hr

Evaluation

- Therapeutic response: decreased fever, malaise, rash, negative C&S for infecting organism

Patient/family education

- Teach patient that long-term therapy may be needed to clear infection (2 wk-3 mo depending on type of infection)

Selected Generic Names

amphotericin B
fluconazole
griseofulvin
itraconazole
ketoconazole
nystatin

ANTIHISTAMINES

Action: Antihistamines compete with histamines for H_1 receptor sites. They antagonize in varying degrees most of the pharmacologic effects of histamines.
Uses: Products are used to control the symptoms of allergies, rhinitis, and pruritus.
Adverse effects: Most products cause drowsiness; however, two of the newer products, loratadine and fexofenadine, produce little, if any, drowsiness. Other common side effects are headache and thickening of bronchial secretions. Serious blood dyscrasias may occur, but are rare. Urinary retention, GI effects occur with many of these products.
Contraindications: Hypersensitivity to H_1-receptor antagonists occurs rarely. Patients with acute asthma and lower respiratory tract disease should not use these products, since thick secretions may result. Other contraindications include narrow-angle glaucoma, bladder neck obstruction, stenosing peptic ulcer, symptomatic prostatic hypertrophy, newborn, lactation.
Precautions: These products must be used cautiously in conjunction with intraocular pressure, since they increase intraocular pressure. Caution should also be used in patients with renal and cardiac disease, hypertension, and seizure disorders, pregnancy, lactation and in the elderly.
Pharmacokinetics: Onset varies from 20-60 min, with duration lasting 4-12 hr. In general, pharmacokinetics vary widely among products.
Interactions: Barbiturates, narcotics, hypnotics, tricyclic antidepressants, and alcohol can increase CNS depression when taken with antihistamines.

NURSING CONSIDERATIONS

Assessment

- Check I&O ratio; be alert for urinary retention, frequency, dysuria; drug should be discontinued if these occur
- Assess for blood dyscrasias: thrombocytopenia, agranulocytosis (rare)
- Assess for respiratory status, including rate rhythm, increase in bronchial secretions, wheezing, chest tightness
- Assess for cardiac status, including palpitations, increased pulse, hypotension
- Assess CBC during long-term therapy, since hemolytic anemia, although rare, may occur
- Administer with food or milk to decrease GI symptoms; absorption may be decreased slightly
- Administer whole (sus rel tab)
- Provide hard candy, gum, frequent rinsing of mouth for dryness

Nursing diagnoses

☑ Ineffective airway clearance (uses)

Evaluation

- Therapeutic response: absence of allergy symptoms, itching

Patient/family education

- Advise patient to notify prescriber if confusion, sedation, hypotension occur
- Caution patient to avoid driving and other hazardous activity if drowsiness occurs
- Instruct patient to avoid concurrent use of alcohol and other CNS depressants
- Inform patient to discontinue a few days before skin testing

---

Selected Generic Names

azatadine
brompheniramine
cetirizine
chlorpheniramine
cyproheptadine
desloratadine (Appx A)
⚷ diphenhydramine
fexofenadine
loratadine
promethazine
triprolidine

ANTIHYPERTENSIVES

Action: Antihypertensives are divided into angiotensin converting enzyme (ACE) inhibitors, β-adrenergic blockers, calcium channel blockers, centrally acting adrenergics, diuretics, peripherally acting antiadrenergics, and vasodilators. β-Blockers, calcium channel blockers, and diuretics are discussed in separate sections. ACE inhibitors selectively suppress conversion of renin-angiotensin I to angiotensin II; dilatation of arterial and venous vessels occurs. Centrally acting adrenergics act by inhibiting the sympathetic vasomotor center in the CNS, which reduces impulses in the sympathetic nervous system; blood pressure, pulse rate, and cardiac output decrease. Peripherally acting anti-adrenergics inhibit sympathetic vasoconstriction by inhibiting release of norepinephrine and/or depleting norepinephrine stores in adrenergic nerve endings. Vasodilators act on arteriolar smooth muscle by producing direct relaxation or vasodilatation; a reduction in blood pressure, with concomitant increases in heart rate and cardiac output, occurs.

Uses: Used for hypertension and for heart failure not responsive to conventional therapy. Some products are used in hypertensive crisis, angina, and for some cardiac dysrhythmias.

Adverse effects: The most common side effects are marked hypotension, bradycardia, tachycardia, headache, nausea, and vomiting. Side effects and adverse reactions may vary widely between classes and specific products.

Contraindications: Hypersensitive reactions may occur, and allergies should

be identified before these products are given. Antihypertensives should not be used
P in patients with heart block or in children.

G **Precautions:** Antihypertensives should be used with caution in the elderly, in dialysis patients, and in the presence of hypovolemia, leukemia, and electrolyte imbalances.

Pharmacokinetics: Onset, peak, and duration vary widely among products. Most products are metabolized in the liver, with metabolites excreted in urine, bile, and feces.

Interactions: Interactions vary widely among products; check individual monograph for specific information.

NURSING CONSIDERATIONS

Assessment

- Monitor blood studies: neutrophil; decreased platelets occur with many of the products
- Monitor renal studies: protein, BUN, creatinine; watch for increased levels, which may indicate nephrotic syndrome; obtain baselines in renal and liver function studies before beginning treatment
- Assess for edema in feet and legs daily
- Identify allergic reaction, including rash, fever, pruritus, urticaria: drug should be discontinued if antihistamines fail to help
- Identify symptoms of CHF: edema, dyspnea, wet rales, B/P
- Assess for renal symptoms: polyuria, oliguria, frequency

Nursing diagnoses

✓ Altered tissue perfusion (uses)
✓ Decreased cardiac output (uses)
✓ Diarrhea (adverse reactions)
✓ Impaired gas exchange (adverse reactions)

Implementation

- Place patient in supine or Trendelenburg position for severe hypotension

Evaluation

- Therapeutic response: decrease in B/P in hypotension; decreased B/P, edema, moist rales in CHF

Patient/family education

- Instruct patient to comply with dosage schedule, even if feeling better
- Advise patient to rise slowly to sitting or standing position to minimize orthostatic hypotension

Selected Generic Names

ACE inhibitors:
benazepril
captopril
enalapril
esoprostenol
fosinopril
lisinopril
quinapril
ramipril
spirapril
trandolapril

Angiotension II receptors
candesartan
eprosartan (Appx A)
irbesartan
losartan
telmisartan
valsartan

Centrally acting adrenergics:
🔑 clonidine
methyldopa

Peripherally acting antiadrenergics:
doxazosin
🔑 prazosin
reserpine
terazosin

Vasodilators:
diazoxide
fenoldopam
hydralazine
minoxidil
nitroprusside (high alert)

Antidrenergic:
Combined α-/β-blocker: labetalol

ANTIINFECTIVES

Action: Antiinfectives are divided into several groups, which include but are not limited to penicillins, cephalosporins, aminoglycosides, sulfonamides, tetracyclines, monobactam, erythromycins, and quinolones. These drugs inhibit the growth and replication of susceptible bacterial organisms.

Uses: Used for infections of susceptible organisms. These products are effective against bacterial, rickettsial, and spirochete infections.

Adverse effects: The most common side effects are nausea, vomiting, and diarrhea. Adverse reactions include bone marrow depression and anaphylaxis.

Contraindications: Hypersensitive reactions may occur, and allergies should be identified before these products are given. Cross-sensitivity can occur between products of different classes (penicillins or cephalosporins). Often persons allergic to penicillins are also allergic to cephalosporins.

Precautions: Antiinfectives should be used with caution in persons with renal and liver disease.

Pharmacokinetics: Onset, peak, and duration vary widely among products. Most products are metabolized in the liver, and metabolites are excreted in urine, bile, and feces.

Interactions: Interactions vary widely among products; check individual monograph for specific information.

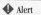

NURSING CONSIDERATIONS
Assessment
- Assess for nephrotoxicity, including increased BUN, creatinine
- Monitor blood studies: AST, ALT, CBC, Hct, bilirubin; test monthly if patient is on long-term therapy
- Monitor bowel pattern qd; if severe diarrhea occurs, drug should be discontinued
- Monitor urine output; if decreasing, notify prescriber; may indicate nephrotoxicity
- Assess for allergic reaction, including rash, fever, pruritus, urticaria; drug should be discontinued
- Assess for bleeding: ecchymosis, bleeding gums, hematuria, stool guaiac daily
- Assess for overgrowth of infection: perineal itching, fever, malaise, redness, pain, swelling, drainage, rash, diarrhea, change in cough, sputum

Nursing diagnoses
✓ Risk for infection (uses)
✓ Diarrhea (adverse reactions)

Implementation
- Give for 10-14 days to ensure organism death, prevention of superinfection
- Give after C&S completed; drug may be taken as soon as culture is obtained

Evaluation
- Therapeutic response: absence of fever, fatigue, malaise, draining wounds

Patient/family education
- Teach patient to comply with dosage schedule, even if feeling better
- Advise patient to report sore throat, bruising, bleeding, joint pain; may indicate blood dyscrasias (rare)

Selected Generic Names

Aminoglycosides:
amikacin
gentamicin
kanamycin
neomycin
netilmicin
streptomycin
tobramycin

Cephalosporins:
cefaclor
cefadroxil
cefamandole
cefazolin
cefdinir
cefditoren (Appx A)
cefepime
cefixime
cefmetazole
cefonicid
cefoperazone
ceforanide
cefotaxime
cefprozil
ceftibuten
cefuroximine
cephalexin (Key Drug)
cephalothin
cephapirin
cephradine
moxalactam

Fluoroquinolones:
alatrofloxacin
ciprofloxacin
levofloxacin
lomefloxacin
norfloxacin
ofloxacin
sparfloxacin
trovafloxacin

Macrolides:
azithromycin
clarithromycin
erythromycin

Miscellaneous:
ertapenem (Appx A)
meropenem

Penicillins:
amoxicillin/clavulanate
ampicillin/sulbactam
cloxacillin
dicloxacillin
imipenem/cilastatin
methicillin
mezlocillin
nafcillin
oxacillin
penicillin G benzathine
penicillin G potassium
penicillin G procaine
penicillin G sodium (Key Drug)
penicillin V
piperacillin
ticarcillin/clavulanate

Sulfonamides:
sulfasalazine
sulfisoxazole

Tetracyclines:
doxycycline
minocycline
tetracycline

ANTINEOPLASTICS

Action: Antineoplastics are divided into alkylating agents, antimetabolites, antibiotic agents, hormonal agents, and miscellaneous agents. Alkylating agents act by cross-linking strands of DNA. Antimetabolites act by inhibiting DNA synthesis. Antibiotic agents act by inhibiting RNA synthesis and by delaying or inhibiting mitosis. Hormones alter the effect of androgens, luteinizing hormone, follicle-stimulating hormone, or estrogen by changing the hormonal environment.

Uses: Uses vary widely among products and classes of drugs. They are used to treat leukemia, Hodgkin's disease, lymphomas, and other tumors throughout the body.

Adverse effects: Most products cause thrombocytopenia, leukopenia, and anemia, and, if these reactions occur, the drug may need to be stopped until the problem is corrected. Other side effects include nausea, vomiting, glossitis, and hair loss. Some products also cause hepatotoxicity, nephrotoxicity, and cardiotoxicity.

Contraindications: Hypersensitive reactions may occur, and allergies should be identified before these products are given. Also, persons with severe liver and kidney disease should not use these products unless the benefits outweigh the risks.

Precautions: Persons with bleeding, severe bone marrow depression, or renal or hepatic disease should be watched closely.

Pharmacokinetics: Onset, peak, and duration vary widely among products. Most products cross the placenta and are excreted in breast milk and in urine.

Interactions: Toxicity may occur when used with other antineoplastics or radiation.

NURSING CONSIDERATIONS

Assessment

- Monitor CBC, differential, platelet count weekly; withhold drug if WBC is <4000 or platelet count is <75,000; notify prescriber of results
- Monitor renal function studies, including BUN, creatinine, serum uric acid, and urine creatinine clearance before and during therapy
- Monitor I&O ratio; report fall in urine output of 30 ml/hr
- Monitor temp q4h (may indicate beginning infection)
- Monitor liver function tests before and during therapy (bilirubin, AST, ALT, LDH) prn or monthly
- Assess for bleeding, including hematuria, guaiac, bruising or petechiae, mucosa, or orifices q8h; obtain prescription for viscous lidocaine (Xylocaine)
- Identify jaundice of skin, sclera, dark urine, clay-colored stools, itchy skin, abdominal pain, fever, diarrhea
- Assess for edema in feet, joint pain, stomach pain, shaking
- Assess for inflammation of mucosa, breaks in skin

Nursing diagnoses

✓ Risk for infection (adverse reactions)
✓ Altered nutrition: less than body requirements (adverse reactions)
✓ Altered oral mucous membrane (adverse reactions)

Implementation

- Check **IV** site for irritation; phlebitis
- Have epinephrine available for hypersensitivity reaction
- Give antibiotics for prophylaxis of infection
- Provide strict medical asepsis, protective isolation if WBC levels are low
- Provide comprehensive oral hygiene, using careful technique and soft-bristle brush

Evaluation

- Therapeutic response: decreased tumor size

Patient/family education

- Advise patient to report signs of infection, including increased temp, sore throat, malaise
- Instruct patient to report signs of anemia, including fatigue, headache, faintness, shortness of breath, irritability
- Instruct patient to report bleeding and to avoid use of razors and commercial mouthwash

---

Selected Generic Names

Alkylating agents:
busulfan (high alert)
carboplatin (high alert)
carmustine (high alert)
chlorambucil
cisplatin (high alert)
(Key Drug) **cyclophosphamide** (high alert)
dacarbazine (high alert)
lomustine
mechlorethamine
melphalan (high alert)
thiotepa

Antimetabolites:
capecitabine
cytarabine (high alert)
(Key Drug) **doxorubicin** (high alert)
etoposide (high alert)
fludarabine
fluorouracil (high alert)
mercaptopurine
thioguanine (6-TG)

Antibiotic agents:
(Key Drug) **bleomycin** (high alert)
dactinomycin (high alert)
daunorubicin (high alert)
epirubicin (high alert)
(Key Drug) **methotrexate** (high alert)
mitomycin (high alert)
mitoxantrone (high alert)
plicamycin (high alert)

Hormonal agents:
flutamide
goserelin acetate
irinotecan (high alert)
leuprolide (high alert)
megestrol
mitotane
nilutamide
tamoxifen
testolactone
topotecan (high alert)

Miscellaneous agents:
alemtuzumab (Appx A)
altretamine
anastrozole
arsenic trioxide
asparaginase (high alert)
cladribine
gemcitabine
imatinib (Appx A)
interferon alfa-2A, interferon alfa-2B
irinotecan (high alert)
pentostatin (high alert)
porfimer
procarbazine
rituximab
vinblastine (high alert)
vincristine (high alert)

ANTIPARKINSONIAN AGENTS

Action: Antiparkinsonian agents are divided into cholinergics and dopamine agonists. Cholinergics work by the blocking or competing at central acetylcholine receptors; dopamine agonists work by decarboxylation to dopamine or by activation of dopamine receptors; monoamine oxidase type B inhibitors increase dopamine activity by inhibiting MAO type B activity.
Uses: These agents are used alone or in combination for patients with Parkinson's disease.
Adverse effects: Side effects and adverse reactions vary widely among products. The most common side effects include involuntary movements, headache, numbness, insomnia, nightmares, nausea, vomiting, dry mouth, and orthostatic hypotension.
Contraindications: Persons with hypersensitivity, narrow-angle glaucoma, and undiagnosed skin lesions should not use these products.
Precautions: Antiparkinsonian agents should be used with caution in pregnancy, P lactation, children, renal, cardiac, hepatic disease, and affective disorder.
Pharmacokinetics: Onset, peak, and duration vary widely among products. Most products are metabolized in the liver and excreted in urine.
Interactions: Please check individual monographs, since interactions vary widely among products.

NURSING CONSIDERATIONS
Assessment
- Monitor B/P, respiration
- Assess mental status: affect, behavioral changes, depression, complete suicide assessment

Nursing diagnoses
✓ Risk for injury (uses)
✓ Risk for impaired mobility (uses)
✓ Knowledge deficit (teaching)

Implementation

- Give drug up until NPO before surgery
- Adjust dosage depending on patient response
- Give with meals; limit protein taken with drug
- Give only after MAOIs have been discontinued for 2 wk
- Assist with ambulation, during beginning therapy if needed
- Test for diabetes mellitus and acromegaly if on long-term therapy

Evaluation

- Therapeutic response: decrease in akathisia, improvement in mood

Patient/family education

- Advise patient to change positions slowly to prevent orthostatic hypotension
- Instruct patient to report side effects: twitching, eye spasm; indicate overdose
- Advise patient to use drug exactly as prescribed; if drug is discontinued abruptly, parkinsonian crisis may occur

Selected Generic Names

🔑 benztropine
biperiden
bromocriptine
cabergoline
carbidopa-levodopa
🔑 levodopa
pramipexole
procyclidine
selegiline
tolcapone
trihexyphenidyl

ANTIPSYCHOTICS

Action: Antipsychotics/neuroleptics are divided into several subgroups: phenothiazines, thioxanthenes, butyrophenones, dibenzoxazepines, dibenzodiazepines, and indolones and other heterocyclic compounds. Although chemically different, these subgroups share many pharmacologic and clinical properties. All antipsychotics work to block postsynaptic dopamine receptors in the brain that are responsible for psychotic behavior, including hallucinations, delusions, and paranoia.

Uses: Antipsychotic behavior is decreased in conditions such as schizophrenia, paranoia, and mania. These agents are also effective for severe anxiety, intractable **P** hiccups, nausea, vomiting, behavioral problems in children, and before surgery for relaxation.

Adverse effects: The most common side effects include extrapyramidal symptoms such as pseudoparkinsonism, akathisia, dystonia, and tardive dyskinesia, which may be controlled by use of antiparkinsonian agents. Serious adverse reactions such as hypotension, agranulocytosis, cardiac arrest, and laryngospasm have occurred. Other common side effects include dry mouth and photosensitivity.

Contraindications: Persons with liver damage, severe hypertension or coronary disease, cerebral arteriosclerosis, blood dyscrasias, bone marrow depression, parkinsonism, severe depression, or narrow angle glaucoma, **P** children <12 yr, or persons withdrawing from alcohol or barbiturates should not use antipsychotics until these conditions are corrected.

G **Precautions:** Caution must be used when antipsychotics are given to the elderly, since metabolism is slowed and adverse reactions can occur rapidly. Hepatic and renal disease may cause poor metabolism and excretion of the drug. Seizure threshold is decreased with these products; increases in the dose of anticonvulsants may be required. Persons with diabetes mellitus, prostatic hypertrophy, chronic respiratory disease, and peptic ulcer disease should be monitored closely.

Pharmacokinetics: Onset, peak, and duration vary widely with different products and routes. Products are metabolized by the liver, are excreted in urine as metabolites, are highly bound to plasma proteins, cross the placenta, and enter breast milk. Half-life can be extended over 3 days.

Interactions: Because other CNS depressants can cause oversedation, these combinations should be used carefully. Anticholinergics may decrease the therapeutic actions of phenothiazines and also cause increased anticholinergic effects.

NURSING CONSIDERATIONS

Assessment

- Monitor bilirubin, CBC, liver function studies monthly, since these drugs are metabolized in the liver and excreted in urine
- Monitor I&O ratio: palpate bladder if low urinary output occurs, since urinary retention occurs with many of these products
- Assess affect, orientation, LOC, reflexes, gait, coordination, sleep pattern disturbances
- Assess dizziness, faintness, palpitations, tachycardia on rising
- Check B/P with patient lying and standing; wide fluctuations between lying and standing B/P may require dosage or product change, since orthostatic hypotension is occurring
- Assess for EPS, including akathisia, tardive dyskinesia, pseudoparkinsonism

Nursing diagnoses

✓ Altered thought processes (uses)
✓ Sensory-perceptual alterations (uses)

Implementation

- Give antiparkinsonian agent if EPS occur
- Administer liq conc mixed in glass of juice or cola, since taste is unpleasant; avoid contact with skin when preparing liq conc or parenteral medications
- Supervise ambulation until stabilized on medication; do not involve in strenuous exercise program, since fainting is possible; patient should not stand still for long periods
- Increase fluids to prevent constipation
- Give sips of water, candy, gum for dry mouth

Evaluation

- Therapeutic response: decrease in excitement, hallucinations, delusions, paranoia, reorganization of thought patterns, speech

Patient/family education

- Advise patient to rise from sitting or lying position gradually, since fainting may occur
- Instruct patient to remain lying down for at least 30 min after IM inj
- Caution patient to avoid hot tubs, hot showers, or tub baths, since hypotension may occur
- Advise patient to wear a sunscreen or protective clothing to prevent burns
- Advise patient to take extra precautions during hot weather to stay cool; heat stroke can occur
- Caution patient to avoid driving and other activities requiring alertness until response to medication is known
- Inform patient that drowsiness or impaired mental/motor activity is evident the first 2 wk, but tends to decrease over time

---

Selected Generic Names

Phenothiazines:
🔑 chlorpromazine
fluphenazine
mesoridazine
perphenazine
prochlorperazine
thioridazine
thiothixene
trifluoperazine

Butyrophenone:
🔑 haloperidol

Miscellaneous:
loxapine
molindone
olanzapine
quetiapine
risperidone

ANTITUBERCULARS

Action: Antituberculars act by inhibiting RNA or DNA, or interfering with lipid and protein synthesis, thereby decreasing tubercle bacilli replication.
Uses: Antituberculars are used for pulmonary tuberculosis.
Adverse effects: They vary widely among products. Most products can cause nausea, vomiting, anorexia, and rash. Serious adverse reactions include renal failure, nephrotoxicity, ototoxicity, and hepatic necrosis.
Contraindications: Persons with severe renal disease or hypersensitivity should not use these products.
Precautions: Antituberculars should be used with caution in pregnancy, lactation, and hepatic disease.
Pharmacokinetics: Onset, peak, and duration vary widely among products. Most products are metabolized in the liver and excreted in urine.

Interactions: Please check individual monographs, since interactions vary widely among products.

NURSING CONSIDERATIONS

Assessment

- Assess for signs of anemia: Hct, Hgb, fatigue
- Monitor liver studies weekly: ALT, AST, bilirubin
- Monitor renal status before treatment and monthly thereafter: BUN, creatinine, output, sp gr, urinalysis
- Monitor hepatic status: decreased appetite, jaundice, dark urine, fatigue

Nursing diagnoses

✓ Risk for infection (uses)
✓ Risk for injury (adverse reactions)
✓ Knowledge deficit (teaching)
✓ Noncompliance (teaching)

Implementation

- Give some of these agents on empty stomach, 1 hr ac (only for isoniazid and rifampin) or 2 hr pc
- Give antiemetic if vomiting occurs
- Give after C&S is completed; monthly to detect resistance

Evaluation

- Therapeutic response: decreased symptoms of TB, culture negative

Patient/family education

- Teach patient that compliance with dosage schedule, duration is necessary
- Teach patient that scheduled appointments must be kept; relapse may occur
- Advise patient to avoid alcohol while taking drug
- Advise patient to report flulike symptoms: excessive fatigue, anorexia, vomiting, sore throat; unusual bleeding, yellowish discoloration of skin/eyes

---

Selected Generic Names

ethambutol
isoniazid
pyrazinamide
rifabutin
rifampin
streptomycin

ANTITUSSIVES/EXPECTORANTS

Action: Antitussives suppress the cough reflex by direct action on the cough center in the medulla. Expectorants act by liquefying and reducing the viscosity of thick, tenacious secretions.

Uses: Antitussives/expectorants are used to treat cough occurring in pneumonia, bronchitis, TB, cystic fibrosis, and emphysema; as an adjunct in atelectasis (expectorants); and for nonproductive cough (antitussives).

Adverse effects: The most common side effects are drowsiness, dizziness, and nausea.

Contraindications: Some products are contraindicated in hypothyroidism, iodine sensitivity, pregnancy, and lactation.

G **Precautions:** Some products should be used cautiously in asthma, elderly, and debilitated patients.

Pharmacokinetics: Onset, peak, and duration vary widely among products. Some products are metabolized in the liver and excreted in urine.

Interactions: Please check individual monographs, since interactions vary widely among products.

NURSING CONSIDERATIONS

Assessment

- Assess cough: type, frequency, character including sputum

Nursing diagnoses:

✓ Ineffective breathing pattern (uses)
✓ Ineffective airway clearance (uses)
✓ Knowledge deficit (teaching)

Implementation

- G Give decreased dosage to elderly patients; their metabolism may be slowed
- Increase fluids to liquefy secretions
- Humidify patient's room

Evaluation

- Therapeutic response: absence of cough

Patient/family education

- Advise patient to avoid driving and other hazardous activities until stabilized on this medication
- Caution patient to avoid smoking, smoke-filled rooms, perfumes, dust, environmental pollutants, cleaners that increase cough

---

Selected Generic Names

Key Drug: acetylcysteine
Key Drug: codeine
dextromethorphan
Key Drug: diphenhydramine
guaifenesin
hydrocodone
potassium iodide

ANTIVIRALS/ANTIRETROVIRALS

Action: Antivirals/antiretrovirals act by interfering with DNA synthesis that is needed for viral replication.

Uses: Antivirals/antiretrovirals are used for mucocutaneous herpes simplex virus, herpes genitalis (HSV_1, HSV_2), advanced HIV infections, herpes simplex virus encephalitis, varicella-zoster encephalomyelitis.

Adverse effects: Serious adverse reactions are fatal metabolic encephalopathy, blood dyscrasias, and acute renal failure. Common side effects are nausea, vomiting, anorexia, diarrhea, headache, vaginitis, and moniliasis.

Contraindications: Persons with hypersensitivity and immunosuppressed individuals with herpes zoster should not use these products.

Precautions: Antivirals/antiretrovirals should be used with caution in renal disease, liver disease, lactation, pregnancy, and dehydration.

Pharmacokinetics: Onset, peak, and duration vary widely among products. Most products are metabolized in the liver and excreted in urine.

Interactions: Please check individual monographs, since interactions vary widely among products.

NURSING CONSIDERATIONS

Assessment

- Assess for signs of infection, anemia
- Monitor I&O ratio; report hematuria, oliguria, fatigue, weakness; may indicate nephrotoxicity; check for protein in urine during treatment
- Monitor any patient with compromised renal system, since drug is excreted slowly in poor renal system function; toxicity may occur rapidly
- Check liver studies: AST, ALT
- Check blood studies: WBC, RBC, Hct, Hgb, bleeding time; blood dyscrasias may occur; drug should be discontinued
- Check renal studies: urinalysis, protein, BUN, creatinine, CrCl
- Obtain C&S before drug therapy; drug may be taken as soon as culture is obtained; repeat C&S after treatment
- Assess bowel pattern before, during treatment; if severe abdominal pain with bleeding occurs, drug should be discontinued
- Identify skin eruptions: rash, urticaria, itching
- Assess for allergies before treatment, reaction of each medication; place allergies on chart

Nursing diagnoses

✓ Risk for infection (uses)
✓ Risk for injury (adverse reactions)
✓ Knowledge deficit (teaching)

Implementation

- Give increased fluids to 3 L/day to decrease crystalluria when given IB
- Store at room temp for up to 12 hr after reconstitution
- Give adequate intake of fluids (2000 ml) to prevent deposit in kidneys

Evaluation

- Therapeutic response: absence of or control of infection

Patient/family education

- Inform patient that drug does not cure infection, just controls symptoms
- Instruct patient to report sore throat, fever, fatigue; could indicate superinfection
- Advise patient that drug must be taken in equal intervals around the clock to maintain blood levels for duration of therapy
- Advise patient to notify prescriber of side effects of bruising, bleeding, fatigue, malaise; may indicate blood dyscrasias

Selected Generic Names

abacavir
(Key Drug) acyclovir
cidofovir
delavirdine
didanosine
famciclovir
foscarnet
ganciclovir
idoxuridine
indinavir
nelfinavir
nevirapine
rimantadine
ritonavir
saquinavir
stavudine
tenofovir (Appx A)
valganciclovir (Appx A)
vidarabine
zalcitabine
(Key Drug) zidovudine

BARBITURATES

Action: Barbiturates act by decreasing impulse transmission to the cerebral cortex.

Uses: All forms of epilepsy can be controlled, since the seizure threshold is increased. (Pediatric) Uses also include febrile seizures in children, sedation, insomnia, hyperbilirubinemia, chronic cholestasis with some of these products. Ultra-short acting barbiturates are used as anesthetics.

Adverse effects: The most common side effects are drowsiness and nausea. Serious adverse reactions such as Stevens-Johnson syndrome and blood dyscrasias may occur with high doses and long-term treatment.

Contraindications: Hypersensitivity may occur, and allergies should be identified before administering. Barbiturates are identified as pregnancy category

D and should not be used in pregnancy. Other contraindications include porphyria and marked impairment of liver function.

G **Precautions:** Caution must be used when these products are given to the elderly or debilitated; usually smaller doses are needed, since metabolism is slowed. Persons with renal and hepatic disease may show delayed excretion. Barbiturates P may produce excitability in children.

Pharmacokinetics: Onset of action can be slow, up to 1 hr, with a peak of 8 hr and a duration of 3-10 hr. These drugs are metabolized by the liver, excreted by the kidneys, cross the placenta, and enter breast milk.

Interactions: Increased CNS depressant effect may occur with alcohol, MAOIs, sedatives, or narcotics. These products should be used together cautiously. Oral anticoagulants, corticosteroids, griseofulvin, quinidine, oral contraceptives, and theophylline may show a decreased effect when used with barbiturates.

NURSING CONSIDERATIONS

Assessment

- Monitor hepatic and renal studies: AST, ALT, bilirubin, creatinine, LDH, alkaline phosphatase, BUN if patient is on long-term therapy, since these products are metabolized and excreted by the liver and kidney
- Monitor blood studies: CBC, hematocrit, hemoglobin, and prothrombin time if patient is on long-term therapy, since these products increase the possibility of bleeding and blood dyscrasias
- Identify barbiturate toxicity: hypotension, pulmonary constriction, cold, clammy skin, cyanosis of lips, insomnia, nausea, vomiting, hallucinations, delirium, weakness

Nursing diagnoses

✓ Sleep pattern disturbance (uses)
✓ Risk for injury (adverse reactions)

Evaluation

- Therapeutic response: appropriate sedation or seizure control

Patient/family education

- Inform patient that physical dependency may result when used for extended periods (45-90 days, depending on dosage)
- Advise patient to avoid driving and activities that require alertness, since drowsiness and dizziness may occur
- Caution patient to abstain from alcohol and other psychotropic medications unless prescribed by prescriber
- Instruct patient not to discontinue medication abruptly after long-term use; withdrawal symptoms will occur

Selected Generic Names

amobarbital
pentobarbital (high alert)
phenobarbital (Key Drug)
secobarbital (high alert)
thiopental (high alert)

BENZODIAZEPINES

Action: Benzodiazepines potentiate the effects of GABA, including any other inhibitory transmitters in the CNS, resulting in decreased anxiety.
Uses: Anxiety is relieved in conditions such as phobic disorders. Benzodiazepines are also used for acute alcohol withdrawal to relieve the possibility of delirium tremens, and some products are used before surgery for relaxation.
Adverse effects: The most common side effects are dizziness, drowsiness, blurred vision, and orthostatic hypotension. Most adverse effects are mediated through the CNS. There is a risk for physical dependence and abuse.
P **Contraindications:** Hypersensitivity, acute narrow-angle glaucoma, children <6 months, liver disease (clonazepam), lactation (diazepam).
G **Precautions:** Caution must be used when these products are given to the elderly or debilitated; usually smaller dosages are needed, since metabolism is slowed. Persons with renal and hepatic disease may show delayed excretion. Clonazepam may increase incidence of seizures.
Pharmacokinetics: Onset of action is ½-1 hr, with a peak of 1-2 hr and a duration of 4-6 hr. These drugs are metabolized by the liver, excreted by the kidneys, cross the placenta, and enter breast milk.
Interactions: Increased CNS depressant effect may occur with other CNS depressants. These products should be used together cautiously. Alcohol should not be used; fatal reactions can occur. The serum concentration and toxicity of digoxin may be increased.

NURSING CONSIDERATIONS

Assessment

- Monitor B/P (with patient lying, standing), pulse; if systolic B/P drops 20 mm Hg, hold drug, notify prescriber; orthostatic hypotension is severe
- Monitor hepatic and renal studies: AST, ALT, bilirubin, creatinine, LDH, alkaline phosphatase
- Assess for physical dependency, withdrawal symptoms, including headache, nausea, vomiting, muscle pain, weakness after long-term use

Nursing diagnoses

- ✓ Anxiety (uses)
- ✓ Risk for injury (adverse reactions)

Implementation
- Give with food or milk for GI symptoms; may give crushed if patient is unable to swallow medication whole

Evaluation
- Therapeutic response: relaxation or decreased anxiety

Patient/family education
- Teach patient that drug should not be used for everyday stress or long term; not to take more than prescribed amount, since drug is habit forming
- Caution patient to avoid driving and activities that require alertness, since drowsiness and dizziness occur
- Caution patient to abstain from alcohol and other psychotropic medications except on advice of prescriber
- Advise patient not to discontinue medication abruptly after long-term use; withdrawal symptoms will occur

---

Selected Generic Names
alprazolam
chlordiazepoxide
clonazepam
diazepam
flurazepam
halazepam
lorazepam
midazolam
oxazepam
prazepam
quazepam
temazepam
triazolam

β-ADRENERGIC BLOCKERS

Action: β-Blockers are divided into selective and nonselective blockers. Nonselective blockers produce a fall in blood pressure without reflex tachycardia or reduction in heart rate through a mixture of β-blocking effects; elevated plasma renins are reduced. Selective β-blockers competitively block stimulation of β_1-receptors in cardiac smooth muscle; these drugs produce chronotropic and inotropic effects.
Uses: β-Blockers are used for hypertension, ventricular dysrhythmias, and prophylaxis of angina pectoris.
Adverse effects: The most common side effects are orthostatic hypotension, bradycardia, diarrhea, nausea, vomiting. Serious adverse reactions include blood dyscrasias, bronchospasm, and CHF.
Contraindications: Hypersensitive reactions may occur, and allergies should be identified before these products are given. β-Adrenergic blockers should not be used in heart block, CHF, or cardiogenic shock.
G **Precautions:** β-Blockers should be used with caution in the elderly or in renal and thyroid disease, COPD, CAD, diabetes mellitus, pregnancy, or asthma.

Pharmacokinetics: Onset, peak, and duration vary widely among products. Most products are metabolized in the liver, with metabolites excreted in urine, bile, and feces.

Interactions: Interactions vary widely among products; check individual monograph for specific information.

NURSING CONSIDERATIONS

Assessment

- Monitor renal studies, including protein, BUN, creatinine; watch for increased levels that may indicate nephrotic syndrome; obtain baselines in renal and liver function studies before beginning treatment
- Monitor I&O ratio, weight daily
- Monitor B/P during beginning treatment and periodically thereafter, pulse q4h; note rate, rhythm, quality
- Monitor apical/radial pulse before administration; notify prescriber of significant changes
- Check for edema in feet and legs daily

Nursing diagnoses

✓ Altered tissue perfusion (uses)
✓ Decreased cardiac output (uses)
✓ Diarrhea (adverse reactions)
✓ Impaired gas exchange (adverse reactions)

Implementation

- Give PO ac, hs; tab may be crushed or swallowed whole
- Give reduced dosage in renal dysfunction

Evaluation

- Therapeutic response: decrease in B/P in hypertension; decreased B/P, edema, moist rales in CHF

Patient/family education

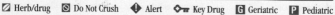

- Instruct patient to comply with dosage schedule, even if feeling better
- Caution patient to rise slowly to sitting or standing position to minimize orthostatic hypotension
- Advise patient to report bradycardia, dizziness, confusion, depression, fever
- Teach patient to take pulse at home; advise when to notify prescriber
- Instruct patient to comply with weight control, dietary adjustment, modified exercise program
- Advise patient to wear support hose to minimize effects of orthostatic hypotension
- Advise patient not to discontinue drug abruptly; taper over 2 wk; may precipitate angina

Selected Generic Names

Selective β_1-receptor blockers:
acebutolol
atenolol
esmolol
metoprolol

Nonselective β_1 and β_2-blockers:
carteolol
nadolol
pindolol
propranolol
timolol

Combined α_1, β_1, and β_2-receptor blocker:
labetalol

BRONCHODILATORS

Action: Bronchodilators are divided into anticholinergics, α/β-adrenergics agonists, β-adrenergic agonists, and phosphodiesterase inhibitors. Anticholinergics act by inhibiting interaction of acetylcholine at receptor sites on bronchial smooth muscle; α/β-adrenergic agonists by relaxing bronchial smooth muscle and increasing diameter of nasal passages; β-adrenergic agonists by action on β_2-receptors, which relaxes bronchial smooth muscle; phosphodiesterase inhibitors by blocking phosphodiesterase and increasing cAMP, which mediates smooth muscle relaxation in the respiratory system.
Uses: Bronchodilators are used for bronchial asthma, bronchospasm associated with bronchitis, emphysema, other obstructive pulmonary diseases, and Cheyne-Stokes respirations, as well as prevention of exercise-induced asthma.
Adverse effects: The most common side effects are tremors, anxiety, nausea, vomiting, and irritation in the throat. The most serious adverse reactions include bronchospasm and dyspnea.
Contraindications: Persons with hypersensitivity, narrow-angle glaucoma, tachydysrhythmias, and severe cardiac disease should not use some of these products.
Precautions: Bronchodilators should be used with caution in lactation, pregnancy, hyperthyroidism, hypertension, prostatic hypertrophy, and seizure disorders.
Pharmacokinetics: Onset, peak, and duration vary widely among products. Most products are metabolized in the liver and excreted in urine.
Interactions: Please check individual monographs, since interactions vary widely among products.

NURSING CONSIDERATIONS

Assessment

- Monitor respiratory function: vital capacity, FEV, ABGs, lung sounds, heart rate and rhythm

Nursing diagnoses
✓ Ineffective airway clearance (uses)
✓ Activity intolerance (uses)
✓ Risk for injury (adverse reactions)
✓ Knowledge deficit (teaching)

Implementation
- Give after shaking; exhale, place mouthpiece in mouth, inhale slowly, hold breath, remove, exhale slowly
- Give gum, sips of water for dry mouth
- Give PO with meals to decrease gastric irritation
- Store in light-resistant container; do not expose to temp over 86° F

Evaluation
- Therapeutic response: absence of dyspnea, wheezing

Patient/family education
- Advise patient not to use OTC medications; extra stimulation may occur
- Teach patient use of inhaler; review package insert with patient; to wash inhaler in warm water qd and dry
- Advise patient to avoid getting aerosol in eyes
- Caution patient to avoid smoking, smoke-filled rooms, persons with respiratory tract infections

---

Selected Generic Names
- albuterol (Key Drug)
- aminophylline
- atropine (Key Drug)
- dyphylline
- **ephedrine** (high alert)
- **epinephrine** (high alert) (Key Drug)
- formoterol (Appx A)
- ipratropium
- isoproterenol
- levalbuterol
- metaproterenol
- mibefradil
- oxtriphylline
- pirbuterol
- terbutaline
- theophylline (Key Drug)

CALCIUM CHANNEL BLOCKERS

Action: These products inhibit calcium ion influx across the cell membrane in cardiac and vascular smooth muscle. This action produces relaxation of coronary vascular smooth muscle, dilates coronary arteries, slows SA/AV node conduction, and dilates peripheral arteries.

Uses: These products are used for chronic stable angina pectoris, vasospastic angina, dysrhythmias, hypertension, and unstable angina.

Adverse effects: The most common side effects are dysrhythmias and edema. Also common are headache, fatigue, drowsiness, and flushing.
Contraindications: Persons with 2nd- or 3rd-degree heart block, sick sinus syndrome, hypotension of <90 mm Hg systolic, Wolff-Parkinson-White syndrome, or cardiogenic shock should not use these products, since worsening of those conditions may occur.
Precautions: CHF may worsen, since edema may be increased. Hypotension may worsen, since B/P is decreased. Patients with renal and liver disease should use these products cautiously, since they are metabolized in the liver and excreted by the kidneys.
Pharmacokinetics: Onset, peak, and duration vary widely with route of administration. Drugs are metabolized by the liver and excreted in the urine primarily as metabolites.
Interactions: Increased levels of digoxin and theophylline may occur when used with these products. Increased effects of β-blockers and antihypertensives may occur with calcium channel blockers.

NURSING CONSIDERATIONS
Assessment
- Monitor cardiac system, including B/P, pulse, respirations, ECG intervals (PR, QRS, QT)

Nursing diagnoses
✓ Altered tissue perfusion: cardiopulmonary (uses)
✓ Decreased cardiac output (adverse reactions)

Implementation
- Give PO ac and hs

Evaluation
- Therapeutic response: decreased anginal pain, decreased B/P, dysrhythmias

Patient/family education
- Teach patient how to take pulse before taking drug; patient should record or graph pulses to identify changes
- Advise patient to avoid hazardous activities until stabilized on this drug, since dizziness occurs frequently
- Inform patient of need for compliance to all areas of medical regimen, including diet, exercise, stress reduction, drug therapy

Selected Generic Names
amlodipine
bepridil
diltiazem (high alert)
felodipine
isradipine
nicardipine
nifedipine
🔑 verapamil

CARDIAC GLYCOSIDES

Action: Products act by inhibiting sodium and potassium ATPase and then making more calcium available to activate contracted proteins. Cardiac contractility and cardiac output are increased.

Uses: These products are used for CHF, atrial fibrillation, atrial flutter, atrial tachycardia, and rapid digitalization in these disorders.

Adverse effects: The most common side effects are cardiac disturbances, headache, hypotension, GI symptoms. Also common are blurred vision and yellow-green halos.

Contraindications: Hypersensitive reactions may occur, and allergies should be identified before these products are given. Also, persons with ventricular tachycardia, ventricular fibrillation, and carotid sinus syndrome should not use these products.

Precautions: Persons with acute MI and those who have or may develop serum potassium, calcium, or magnesium imbalances should use these products cautiously. Also, persons with AV block, severe respiratory disease, hypothyroidism, G renal and liver disease, and the elderly should exercise caution when these drugs are prescribed.

Pharmacokinetics: Onset, peak, and duration vary widely with the route of administration. Digitoxin is inactivated by the liver, and inactive metabolites are excreted in urine. Digoxin is excreted in urine mainly as the parent drug and metabolites.

Interactions: Toxicity may occur when used with diuretics, succinylcholine, quinidine, and thioamines. Increased blood levels may occur with propantheline bromide, spironolactone, quinidine, verapamil, aminoglycosides (PO), amiodarone, anticholinergics, and quinine. Diuretics may increase toxicity.

NURSING CONSIDERATIONS

Assessment

- Montior cardiac system, including B/P, pulse, respirations, and increased urine output
- Monitor apical pulse for 1 min before giving drug; if pulse <60, take again in 1 hr; if <60 notify prescriber
- Monitor electrolytes, including potassium, sodium, chloride, calcium, magnesium; renal function studies, including BUN and creatinine; and blood studies, including AST, ALT, bilirubin
- Monitor I&O ratio, daily weights
- Monitor therapeutic drug levels

Nursing diagnoses

✓ Altered tissue perfusion: cardiopulmonary (uses)
✓ Decreased cardiac output (adverse reactions)

Implementation

- Give potassium supplements if ordered for potassium levels <3

Evaluation

- Therapeutic response: decreased weight, edema, pulse, respiration, and increased urine output

Patient/family education

- Teach patient how to take pulse before taking drug; patient should record or graph pulse to identify changes
- Advise patient to avoid hazardous activities until stabilized on this drug, since dizziness occurs frequently
- Inform patient of need for compliance to all areas of medical regimen, including diet, exercise, stress reduction, drug therapy

---

Selected Generic Names

🔑 **digoxin** (high alert)

CHOLINERGICS

Action: Cholinergics act by preventing destruction of acetylcholine, which increases concentration at sites where acetylcholine is released; this exaggerates the effects of acetylcholine and facilitates transmission of impulses across myoneural junction. Cholinergics may also act by stimulating receptors for acetylcholine.

Uses: Cholinergics are used for myasthenia gravis, as antagonists of nondepolarizing neuromuscular blockade, postoperative bladder distention and urinary distention, postoperative ileus.

Adverse effects: The most serious adverse reactions are respiratory depression, bronchospasm, constriction, laryngospasm, respiratory arrest, convulsions, and paralysis. The most common side effects are nausea, diarrhea, and vomiting.

Contraindications: Persons with obstruction of the intestine or renal system should not use these products.

Precautions: Caution should be used in patients with bradycardia, hypotension, seizure disorders, bronchial asthma, coronary occlusion, hyperthyroidism, and in
P lactation and children.

Pharmacokinetics: Onset, peak, and duration vary widely among products. Most products are metabolized in the liver and excreted in urine.

Interactions: Please check individual monographs since interactions vary widely among products.

NURSING CONSIDERATIONS

Assessment

- Monitor VS, respiration q8h
- Monitor I&O ratio; check for urinary retention of incontinence

- Assess for bradycardia, hypotension, bronchospasm, headache, dizziness, convulsions, respiratory depression; drug should be discontinued if toxicity occurs

Nursing diagnoses

- ✓ Altered urinary elimination (uses)
- ✓ Ineffective breathing pattern (uses)
- ✓ Knowledge deficit (teaching)
- ✓ Noncompliance (teaching)

Implementation

- Give only with atropine sulfate available for cholinergic crisis
- Give only after all other cholinergics have been discontinued
- Give increased dosages if tolerance occurs
- Give larger doses after exercise or fatigue
- Give on empty stomach for better absorption
- Store at room temp

Evaluation

- Therapeutic response: increased muscle strength, hand grasp, improved muscle gait, absence of labored breathing (if severe)

Patient/family education

- Inform patient that drug is not a cure; it only relieves symptoms (myasthenia gravis)
- Advise patient to wear ID specifying myasthenia gravis, drugs taken

---

Selected Generic Names

🔑 bethanechol
edrophonium
neostigmine
physostigmine
pyridostigmine

CHOLINERGIC BLOCKERS

Action: Cholinergic blockers inhibit or block acetylcholine at receptor sites in the autonomic nervous system.

Uses: Many products are used to decrease secretions before surgery, to reverse neuromuscular blockade, and to decrease motility of GI, biliary, urinary tracts. Other products are used for parkinsonian symptoms, including dystonia associated with neuroleptic drugs.

Adverse effects: The most common side effects are dryness of the mouth and constipation, which can be prevented by frequent rinsing of the mouth and increasing water and bulk in the diet.

Contraindications: Hypersensitivity can occur, and allergies should be identified before administering these products. Persons with GI and GU obstruction should not use these products, since constipation and urinary retention may occur. They are also contraindicated in angle closure glaucoma and myasthenia gravis.

G **Precautions:** Caution must be used when these products are given to the elderly, since metabolism is slowed. Also, persons with tachycardia or prostatic hypertrophy should use these products with caution.

Pharmacokinetics: Onset, peak, and duration vary with route.

Interactions: Increase in anticholinergic effect occurs when used with narcotics, barbiturates, antihistamines, MAOIs, phenothiazines, amantadine.

NURSING CONSIDERATIONS

Assessment

- Assess I&O ratio; be alert for urinary retention, frequency, dysuria; drug should be discontinued if these occur
- Assess urinary hesitancy, retention; palpate bladder if retention occurs
- Assess constipation; increase fluids, bulk, exercise
- Assess for tolerance over long-term therapy; dosage may need to be changed
- Assess mental status: affect, mood, CNS depression, worsening of mental symptoms during early therapy

Nursing diagnoses

✓ Impaired physical mobility (uses)
✓ Pain (uses)

Implementation

- Give with food or milk to decrease GI symptoms
- Give parenteral dose with patient recumbent to prevent postural hypotension; give dose slowly, monitoring VS
- Give hard candy, gum, frequent rinsing of mouth for dryness

Evaluation

- Therapeutic response: absence of cramps, absence of EPS

Patient/family education

- Caution patient to avoid driving and other hazardous activity if drowsiness occurs
- Advise patient to avoid concurrent use of cough, cold preparations with alcohol, antihistamines unless directed by prescriber
- Caution patient to use with caution in hot weather, since medication may increase susceptibility to heat stroke

Selected Generic Names

- **atropine** (high alert) (Key Drug)
- benztropine (Key Drug)
- biperiden
- glycopyrrolate
- scopolamine
- trihexyphenidyl

CORTICOSTEROIDS

Action: Corticosteroids are divided into glucocorticoids and mineralocorticoids. Glucocorticoids decrease inflammation by the suppression of migration of polymorphonuclear leukocytes, fibroblasts, increased capillary permeability, and lysosomal stabilization. They also have varied metabolic effects and modify the body's immune responses to many different stimuli. Mineralocorticoids act by increasing resorption of sodium by increasing hydrogen and potassium excretion in the distal tubule.

Uses: Glucocorticoids are used to decrease inflammation and for immunosuppression. In addition, some products may be given for allergy, adrenal insufficiency, or cerebral edema. Mineralocorticoids are given for adrenal insufficiency or adrenogenital syndrome.

Adverse effects: The most common side effects include change in behavior, including insomnia and euphoria; GI irritation, including peptic ulcer; metabolic reactions, including hypokalemia, hyperglycemia, and carbohydrate intolerance; and sodium and fluid retention. Most adverse reactions are dose dependent.

Contraindications: Hypersensitivity may occur and should be identified before administering. Since these products mask infection, they should not be used in systemic fungal infections or amebiasis. Mothers taking pharmacologic doses of corticosteroids should not nurse.

Precautions: Caution must be used when these products are prescribed for diabetic patients, since hyperglycemia may occur. Also, patients with glaucoma, seizure disorders, peptic ulcer, impaired renal function, CHF, hypertension, ulcerative colitis, or myasthenia gravis should be monitored closely if corticosteroids are given. Use with caution in children and the elderly and during pregnancy. (P) (G)

Pharmacokinetics: For oral preparations the onset of action occurs between 1-2 hr, and duration can be up to 2 days, with a half-life of 2-4 days. Pharmacokinetics vary widely among products. These products cross the placenta and appear in breast milk.

Interactions: Decreased corticosteroid effect may occur with barbiturates, rifampin, phenytoin; corticosteroid dosage may need to be increased. There is a possibility of GI bleeding when used with salicylates, indomethacin. Steroids may reduce salicylate levels. When using with digitalis glycosides, potassium-depleting diuretics, and amphotericin, serum potassium levels should be monitored.

NURSING CONSIDERATIONS

Assessment

- Monitor potassium, blood sugar, urine glucose while on long-term therapy; hypokalemia and hyperglycemia are common
- Monitor weight daily; notify prescriber if weekly gain of >5 lb, since these products alter fluid and electrolyte balance
- Assess for potassium depletion, including paresthesias, fatigue, nausea, vomiting, depression, polyuria, dysrhythmias, weakness
- Assess for mental status, including affect, mood, behavioral changes, aggression; if severe personality changes occur, including depression, drug may need to be tapered and then discontinued
- Monitor I&O ratio; be alert for decreasing urinary output and increasing edema
- Monitor plasma cortisol levels during long-term therapy (normal level is 138-635 nmol/L when drawn at 8 AM)
- Assess for infection, including increased temp, WBC, even after withdrawal of medication; drug masks symptoms of infection
- Assess for adrenal insufficiency: nausea, anorexia, fatigue, dizziness, dyspnea, weakness, joint pain

Nursing diagnoses

✓ Risk for infection (adverse reactions)
✓ Body image disturbance (adverse reactions)
✓ Risk for violence: self-directed (suicide) (adverse reactions)

Implementation

- Give with food or milk to decrease GI symptoms

Evaluation

- Therapeutic response: decreased inflammation

Patient/family education

- Advise patient that ID as steroid user should be carried
- Advise patient not to discontinue this medication abruptly or adrenal crisis can result
- Teach patient all aspects of drug use, including cushingoid symptoms
- Instruct patient that single daily or alternate-day doses should be taken in the morning before 9 AM (for replacement therapy)
- Instruct patient to take with meals or a snack

Selected Generic Names

Glucocorticoids:
beclomethasone
betamethasone
🔑 cortisone
hydrocortisone
methylprednisolone
prednisolone
🔑 prednisone
triamcinolone

Mineralocorticoid:
fludrocortisone

DIURETICS

Action: Diuretics are divided into subgroups: thiazides and thiazide-like diuretics, loop diuretics, carbonic anhydrase inhibitors, osmotic diuretics, and potassium-sparing diuretics. Each one of these subgroups differs in its mechanism of action. Thiazides and thiazide-like diuretics increase excretion of water and sodium by inhibiting resorption in the early distal tubule. Loop diuretics inhibit resorption of sodium and chloride in the thick ascending limb of the loop of Henle. Carbonic anhydrase inhibitors increase sodium excretion by decreasing sodium-hydrogen ion exchange throughout the renal tubule. Carbonic anhydrase inhibitors also decrease secretion of aqueous humor in the eye and thus decrease intraocular pressure. Osmotic diuretics increase the osmotic pressure of glomerular filtrate, thus decreasing net absorption of sodium. The potassium-sparing diuretics interfere with sodium resorption at the distal tubule, thus decreasing potassium excretion.

Uses: Blood pressure is reduced in hypertension; edema is reduced in CHF; intraocular pressure is decreased in glaucoma.

Adverse effects: Hypokalemia, hyperuricemia, and hyperglycemia occur most frequently with thiazide diuretics. Aplastic anemia, blood dyscrasias, volume depletion, and dehydration may occur when thiazide-like diuretics, loop diuretics, or carbonic anhydrase inhibitors are given. Side effects and adverse reactions vary widely for the miscellaneous products.

Contraindications: Persons with electrolyte imbalances (sodium, chloride, potassium), dehydration, or anuria should not be given these products until the problem is corrected.

G **Precautions:** Caution must be used when diuretics are given to the elderly, since electrolyte disturbances and dehydration can occur rapidly. Hepatic and renal disorders may cause poor metabolism and excretion of the drug.

Pharmacokinetics: Onset, peak, and duration vary widely among the different subgroups of these drugs.

Interactions: Cholestyramine and colestipol decrease the absorption of thiazide diuretics. Concurrent use of thiazides with diazoxide may increase hyperuricemia, hyperglycemia, and antihypertensive effects of thiazides. Ototoxicity may occur when loop diuretics are used with aminoglycosides. Thiazide and loop diuretics may increase therapeutic and toxic effects of lithium.

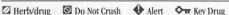

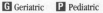

NURSING CONSIDERATIONS

Assessment

- Monitor weight, I&O ratio daily to determine fluid loss; check skin turgor for dehydration
- Monitor electrolytes: potassium, sodium, chloride: include BUN, blood glucose, CBC, serum creatinine, blood pH, ABGs, uric acid, calcium; electrolyte imbalances may occur quickly
- Monitor B/P with patient lying, standing; postural hypotension may occur, since fluid loss occurs from intravascular spaces first
- Assess for signs of metabolic alkalosis, including drowsiness and restlessness
- Assess for signs of hypokalemia with some products, including postural hypotension, malaise, fatigue, tachycardia, leg cramps, weakness

Nursing diagnoses

✓ Fluid volume excess (uses)
✓ Decreased cardiac output (adverse reactions)

Implementation

- Give in AM to avoid interference with sleep if using drug as a diuretic
- Give potassium replacement if potassium is less than 3 mg/dl

Evaluation

- Therapeutic reponse: improvement in edema of feet, legs, sacral area daily if medication is being used in CHF; improvement in B/P if medication is being used as a diuretic; improvement in intraocular pressure if medication is being used to decrease aqueous humor in the eye

Patient/family education

- Teach patient to take drug early in the day (diuretic) to prevent nocturia

---

Selected Generic Names

Thiazides:
hydrochlorothiazide

Thiazide-like:
chlorthalidone
indapamide
metolazone

Loop:
bumetanide
furosemide
torsemide

Carbonic anhydrase inhibitors:
acetazolamide

Potassium-sparing:
amiloride
spironolactone
triamterene

Osmotic:
mannitol

HISTAMINE H_2 ANTAGONISTS

Action: Histamine H_2 antagonists act by inhibiting histamine at H_2 receptor site in parietal cells, which inhibits gastric acid secretion.

Uses: Histamine H_2 antagonists are used for short-term treatment of duodenal and gastric ulcers and maintenance therapy for duodenal ulcer; and for gastroesophageal reflux disease.

Adverse effects: The most serious adverse reactions are agranulocytosis, thrombocytopenia, neutropenia, aplastic anemia, and exfoliative dermatitis. The most common side effects are confusion (not with rantidine), headache and diarrhea.

Contraindications: Persons with hypersensitivity should not use these products.

P **Precautions:** Caution should be used in pregnancy, lactation, children <16 yr, organic brain syndrome, hepatic disease, renal disease.

Pharmacokinetics: Onset, peak, and duration vary widely among products. Most products are metabolized in the liver and excreted in urine.

Interactions: Antacids interfere with absorption of histamine H_2 antagonists. Check individual monographs for other interactions.

NURSING CONSIDERATIONS

Assessment

- Monitor gastric pH (>5 should be maintained)
- Monitor I&O ratio, BUN, creatinine

Nursing diagnoses

✓ Pain (uses)
✓ Risk for injury (bleeding)
✓ Knowledge deficit (teaching)

Implementation

- Give with meals for prolonged drug effect
- Give antacids 1 hr before or 1 hr after cimetidine
- Give **IV** slowly; bradycardia may occur; give over 30 min
- Store diluted sol at room temp for up to 48 hr

Evaluation

- Therapeutic response: decreased pain in abdomen

Patient/family education

- Advise patient that gynecomastia, impotence may occur, but is reversible
- Caution patient to avoid driving and other hazardous activities until patient is stabilized on this medication
- Caution patient to avoid black pepper, caffeine, alcohol, harsh spices, extremes in temp of food
- Caution patient to avoid OTC preparations: aspirin, cough, cold preparations

- Inform patient that drug must be continued for prescribed time to be effective
- Advise patient to report bruising, fatigue, malaise; blood dyscrasias may occur

Selected Generic Names

cimetidine	ranitidine
famotidine	

IMMUNOSUPPRESSANTS

Action: Immunosuppressants produce immunosuppression by inhibiting T lymphocytes.
Uses: Most products are used for organ transplants to prevent rejection.
Adverse effects: The most serious adverse reactions are albuminuria, hematuria, proteinuria, renal failure, and hepatotoxicity. The most common side effects are oral *Candida* infection, gum hyperplasia, tremors, and headache. The most serious adverse reactions for azathioprine are hematologic (leukopenia and thrombocytopenia) and GI (nausea and vomiting). There is a risk of secondary infection.
Contraindications: Products are contraindicated in hypersensitivity.
Precautions: Caution should be used in severe renal disease, severe hepatic disease, and pregnancy.
Pharmacokinetics: Onset, peak, and duration vary widely among products. Most products are metabolized in the liver and excreted in urine.
Interactions: Please check individual monographs, since interactions vary widely among products.

NURSING CONSIDERATIONS

Assessment

- Monitor renal studies: BUN, creatinine at least monthly during treatment, 3 mo after treatment
- Monitor liver function studies: alkaline phosphatase, AST, ALT, bilirubin
- Monitor drug blood levels during treatment
- Assess for hepatotoxicity: dark urine, jaundice, itching, light-colored stools; drug should be discontinued

Nursing diagnoses

✓ Risk for infection (adverse reactions)
✓ Risk for injury (uses)
✓ Knowledge deficit (teaching)

Implementation

- Give for several days before transplant surgery
- Give with meals for GI upset or place drug in chocolate milk
- Give with oral antifungal for *Candida* infections

Evaluation

- Therapeutic response: absence of rejection

Patient/family education

- Advise patient to report fever, chills, sore throat, fatigue, since serious infections may occur
- Caution patient to use contraceptive measures during treatment and for 12 wk after ending therapy

Selected Generic Names

azathioprine
basiliximab (high alert)
cyclosporine
muromonab-CD3
sirolimus
tacrolimus

LAXATIVES

Action: Laxatives are divided into bulk products, lubricants, osmotics, saline laxative stimulants, and stool softeners. Bulks work by absorbing water and expanding to increase moisture content and bulk in the stool. Lubricants increase water retention in the stool, causing reabsorption of water in the bowel. Stimulants act by increasing peristalsis by direct effect on the intestine. Saline draws water into the intestinal lumen. Osmotics increase distention and promote peristalsis. Stool softeners reduce surface tension of liq in the bowel.
Uses: Laxatives are used as a preparation for bowel, rectal examination, constipation, or as stool softeners.
Adverse effects: The most common side effects are nausea, abdominal cramps, and diarrhea.
Contraindications: Persons with GI obstruction, perforation, gastric retention, toxic colitis, megacolon, abdominal pain, nausea, vomiting, and fecal impaction should not use these products.
Precautions: Caution should be used in rectal bleeding, large hemorrhoids, and anal excoriation.
Pharmacokinetics: Onset, peak, and duration vary among products.
Interactions: Please check individual monographs, since interactions vary widely among products.

NURSING CONSIDERATIONS

Assessment

- Monitor blood, urine electrolytes if drug is used often by patient
- Monitor I&O ratio to identify fluid loss
- Determine cause of constipation; identify whether fluids, bulk, or exercise is missing from lifestyle
- Assess for cramping, rectal bleeding, nausea, vomiting; if these symptoms occur, drug should be discontinued

Nursing diagnoses

✓ Constipation (uses)
✓ Diarrhea (adverse reactions)
✓ Knowledge deficit (teaching)

Implementation

- Give alone only with water for better absorption; do not take within 1 hr of antacids, milk, or cimetidine

Evaluation

- Therapeutic response: decrease in constipation

Patient/family education

- Teach patient to swallow tab whole; do not chew
- Caution patient not to use laxatives for long-term therapy; bowel tone will be lost; that normal bowel movements do not always occur daily
- Caution patient not to use in presence of abdominal pain, nausea, vomiting
- Advise patient to notify prescriber of abdominal pain, nausea, vomiting
- Advise patient to notify prescriber if constipation is unrelieved or if symptoms of electrolyte imbalance occur: muscle cramps, pain, weakness, dizziness

---

Selected Generic Names

Bulk laxative:
psyllium

Osmotic agents:
glycerin
lactulose

Saline:
magnesium salts
sodium phosphate/biphosphate

Stimulants:
bisacodyl
cascara
phenolphthalein
senna

Stool softeners:
docusate

NEUROMUSCULAR BLOCKING AGENTS

Action: Neuromuscular blocking agents are divided into depolarizing and nondepolarizing blockers. They act by inhibiting transmission of nerve impulses by binding with cholinergic receptor sites.

Uses: Neuromuscular blocking agents are used to facilitate endotracheal intubation and skeletal muscle relaxation during mechanical ventilation, surgery, or general anesthesia.

Adverse effects: The most serious adverse reactions are prolonged apnea, bronchospasm, cyanosis, respiratory depression, and malignant hyperthermia. The most common side effects are bradycardia and decreased motility.

Contraindications: Persons that are hypersensitive should not be given this product.

Precautions: Caution should be used in pregnancy, thyroid disease, collagen P disease, cardiac disease, lactation, children <2 yr, electrolyte imbalances, dehydration, neuromuscular disease (myasthenia gravis), and respiratory disease.
Pharmacokinetics: Onset, peak, and duration vary widely among products. Most products are metabolized in the liver and excreted in urine.
Interactions: Aminoglycosides potentiate neuromuscular blockade. See individual monographs.

NURSING CONSIDERATIONS

Assessment

- Monitor for electrolyte imbalances (potassium, magnesium); may lead to increased action of this drug
- Monitor VS (B/P, pulse, respirations, airway) q15 min until fully recovered; rate, depth, pattern of respirations, strength of hand grip
- Monitor I&O ratio; check for urinary retention, frequency, hesitancy
- Assess for recovery: decreased paralysis of face, diaphragm, leg, arm, rest of body
- Assess for allergic reactions: rash, fever, respiratory distress, pruritus; drug should be discontinued

Nursing diagnoses

✓ Ineffective breathing pattern (uses)
✓ Risk for injury (adverse reactions)
✓ Knowledge deficit (teaching)

Implementation

- Administer using nerve stimulator by anesthesiologist to determine neuromuscular blockade
- Administer anticholinesterase to reverse neuromuscular blockade
- Administer **IV** undiluted over 1-2 min (only by qualified person, usually an anesthesiologist)
- Store in light-resistant, cool area
- Reassure if communication is difficult during recovery from neuromuscular blockade

Evaluation

- Therapeutic response: paralysis of jaw, eyelid, head, neck, rest of body

---

Selected Generic Names

atracurium
doxacurium (high alert)
gallamine (high alert)
metocurine
mivacurium (high alert)
pancuronium (high alert)
pipecuronium (high alert)
succinylcholine (high alert)
Key Drug **tubocurarine** (high alert)
vecuronium (high alert)

NONSTEROIDAL ANTIINFLAMMATORIES

Action: Nonsteroidal antiinflammatories decrease prostaglandin synthesis by inhibiting an enzyme needed for biosynthesis.

Uses: Nonsteroidal antiinflammatories are used to treat mild to moderate pain, osteoarthritis, rheumatoid arthritis, and dysmenorrhea.

Adverse effects: The most serious adverse reactions are nephrotoxicity (dysuria, hematuria, oliguria, azotemia), blood dyscrasias, and cholestatic hepatitis. The most common side effects are nausea, abdominal pain, anorexia, dizziness, and drowsiness.

Contraindications: Persons with hypersensitivity, asthma, severe renal disease, and severe hepatic disease should not use these products.

P **Precautions:** Caution should be used in pregnancy, lactation, children, bleeding disorders, GI disorders, cardiac disorders, hypersensitivity to other antiinflammatory agents, and the elderly. G

Pharmacokinetics: Onset, peak, and duration vary widely among products. Most products are metabolized in the liver and excreted in urine.

Interactions: Please check individual monographs, since interactions vary widely among products.

NURSING CONSIDERATIONS

Assessment

- Monitor renal, liver, blood studies: BUN, creatinine, AST, ALT, Hgb, before treatment, periodically thereafter
- Monitor audiometric, ophth examination before, during, and after treatment.
- Check for eye, ear problems: blurred vision, tinnitus, may indicate toxicity

Nursing diagnoses

✓ Chronic pain (uses)
✓ Impaired physical mobility (uses)
✓ Knowledge deficit (teaching)
✓ Noncompliance (teaching)

Implementation

- Give with food to decrease GI symptoms; however, best to take on empty stomach to facilitate absorption
- Store at room temp

Evaluation

- Therapeutic response: decreased pain, stiffness in joints, decreased swelling in joints, ability to move more easily

Patient/family education

- Advise patient to report blurred vision, ringing, roaring in ears; may indicate toxicity

- Caution patient to avoid driving, other hazardous activities if dizziness, drowsiness occurs, especially elderly
- Advise patient to report change in urine pattern, increased weight, edema, increased pain in joints, fever, blood in urine; indicate nephrotoxicity
- Inform patient that therapeutic effects may take up to 1 mo

Selected Generic Names

celecoxib
diclofenac
etodolac
flurbiprofen
ibuprofen
indomethacin
ketoprofen
ketorolac
meclofenamate
nabumetone
naproxen
piroxicam
rofecoxib
sulindac
tolmetin
valdecoxib (Appx A)

OPIOID ANALGESICS

Action: These agents depress pain impulse transmission at the spinal cord level by interacting with opioid receptors. Products are divided into opiates and nonopiates.

Uses: Most products are used to control moderate to severe pain and are used before and after surgery.

Adverse effects: GI symptoms, including nausea, vomiting, anorexia, constipation, and cramps are the most common side effects. Other common side effects include lightheadedness, dizziness, sedation. Serious adverse reactions such as respiratory depression, respiratory arrest, circulatory depression, and increased intracranial pressure may result, but are less common and usually dose dependent.

Contraindications: Hypersensitive reactions occur frequently. Check for sensitivity before administering. These drugs should not be used if narcotic addiction is suspected, and they are also contraindicated in acute bronchial asthma and upper airway obstruction.

Precautions: Caution must be used when these products are given to persons with an addictive personality, since the possibility of addiction is so great. Also, persons with increased intracranial pressure may experience an even greater increase in intracranial pressure. Persons with severe heart disease, hepatic or renal disease, respiratory conditions, and seizure disorders should be monitored closely for worsening condition.

Pharmacokinetics: Onset of action is immediate by **IV** route and rapid by IM and PO routes. Peak occurs from 1-2 hr, depending on route, with a duration of 2-8 hr. These agents cross the placenta and appear in breast milk.

Interactions: Barbiturates, other narcotics, hypnotics, antipsychotics, or alcohol can increase CNS depression when taken with narcotics.

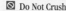

NURSING CONSIDERATIONS

Assessment

- Monitor I&O ratio; be alert for urinary retention, frequency, dysuria; drug should be discontinued if these occur
- Assess for respiratory dysfunction, including respiratory depression, rate, rhythm, character; notify prescriber if respirations are <12/min
- Assess for CNS changes: dizziness, drowsiness, hallucinations, euphoria, LOC, pupil reaction
- Assess for allergic reactions: rash, urticaria
- Assess for need for pain medication, use pain scoring

Nursing diagnoses

✓ Pain (uses)
✓ Impaired gas exchange (adverse reactions)

Implementation

- Give with antiemetic if nausea or vomiting occurs
- Give when pain is beginning to return; determine dosage interval by patient response
- Provide assistance with ambulation; patient should not be ambulating during drug peak

Evaluation

- Therapeutic response: decrease in pain

Patient/family education

- Advise patient to report any symptoms of CNS changes, allergic reactions, or shortness of breath
- Caution patient that physical dependency may result when used for extended periods
- Teach patient that withdrawal symptoms may occur, including nausea, vomiting, cramps, fever, faintness, anorexia
- Advise patient to avoid alcohol and other CNS depressants

Selected Generic Names

buprenorphine
butorphanol
🔑 codeine
fentanyl (high alert)
fentanyl transdermal
hydromorphone (high alert)
🔑 **meperidine** (high alert)
methadone HCl (high alert)
🔑 **morphine** (high alert)
oxycodone (high alert)
oxymorphone (high alert)
pentazocine (high alert)
propoxyphene (high alert)
remifentanil (high alert)
sufentanil (high alert)

SALICYLATES

Action: Salicylates have analgesic, antipyretic, and antiinflammatory effects. The antiinflammatory and analgesic activities may be mediated through the inhibition of prostaglandin synthesis. Antipyretic action results from inhibition of the hypothalamic heat-regulating center.

Uses: The primary uses of salicylates are relief of mild to moderate pain and fever and in inflammatory conditions such as arthritis, thromboembolic disorders, and rheumatic fever.

Adverse effects: The most common side effects are GI symptoms and rash. Serious blood dyscrasias and hepatotoxicity may result when used for long periods at high doses. Tinnitus or impaired hearing may indicate that blood salicylate levels are reaching or exceeding the upper limit of the therapeutic range.

Contraindications: Hypersensitivity to salicylates is common. Check for sensitivity before administering. Persons with bleeding disorders, GI bleeding, and vit K deficiency should not use these products, since salicylates increase prothrombin time. P Children should not use these products, since salicylates have been associated with Reye's syndrome.

Precautions: Caution is needed when salicylates are given to patients with anemia, hepatic or renal disease, or Hodgkin's disease. Caution should also be exercised in pregnancy and lactation.

Pharmacokinetics: Onset of action occurs in 15-30 min, with a peak of 1-2 hr and a duration up to 6 hr. These drugs are metabolized by the liver and excreted by the kidneys.

Interactions: Increased effects of anticoagulants, insulin, methotrexate, heparin, valproic acid, and oral sulfonylureas may occur when used with salicylates. Aspirin may decrease serum concentrations of nonsteroidal antiinflammatory agents.

NURSING CONSIDERATIONS

Assessment

- Monitor hepatic and renal studies: AST, ALT, bilirubin, creatinine, LDH, alkaline phosphatase, BUN if patient is on long-term therapy, since these products are metabolized and excreted by the liver and kidney
- Monitor blood studies: CBC, Hct, Hgb, and prothrombin time if patient is on long-term therapy, since these products increase the possibility of bleeding and blood dyscrasias
- Assess for hepatotoxicity: dark urine, clay-colored stools, jaundice skin and sclera, itching, abdominal pain, fever, diarrhea, which may occur with long-term use
- Assess for ototoxicity: tinnitus, ringing, roaring in ears; audiometric testing is needed before and after long-term therapy

Nursing diagnoses

✓ Pain (uses)
✓ Impaired physical mobility (uses)

- ✓ Activity intolerance (uses)
- ✓ Sensory-perceptual alteration: auditory (adverse reactions)
- ✓ Thermoregulation (uses)

Implementation

- Give with food or milk to decrease gastric irritation; give 30 min ac or 1 hr pc with a full glass of water

Evaluation

- Therapeutic response: decreased pain, fever

Patient/family education

- Advise patient that blood sugar levels should be monitored closely, if patient is diabetic
- Caution patient not to exceed recommended dosage; acute poisoning may result
- Inform patient that therapeutic response takes 2 wk in arthritis
- Caution patient to avoid use of alcohol, since GI bleeding may result
- Advise patient to notify prescriber if ringing in the ears or persistent GI pain occurs
- Advise patient to take with full glass of water to reduce risk of lodging in esophagus

---

Selected Generic Names

aspirin (key drug)
choline salicylate
magnesium salicylate
salsalate

THROMBOLYTICS

Action: Thrombolytics activate conversion of plasminogen to plasmin (fibrinolysin): plasmin is able to break down clots (fibrin).
Uses: Thrombolytics are used to treat deep vein thrombosis, pulmonary embolism, arterial thrombosis, arterial embolism, arteriovenous cannula occlusion, lysis of coronary artery thrombi after MI, acute evolving transmural MI.
Adverse effects: Serious adverse reactions include GI, GU, intracranial, and retroperitoneal bleeding, and anaphylaxis. The most common side effects are decreased Hct, urticaria, headache, and nausea.
Contraindications: Persons with hypersensitivity, active bleeding, intraspinal surgery, neoplasms of the CNS, ulcerative colitis/enteritis, severe hypertension, renal disease, hepatic disease, hypocoagulation, COPD, subacute bacterial endocarditis, rheumatic valvular disease, cerebral embolism/thrombosis/hemorrhage, intraarterial diagnostic procedure or surgery (10 days), and recent major surgery should not use these products.

Precautions: Caution should be used in arterial emboli from left side of heart and pregnancy.
Pharmacokinetics: Onset, peak, and duration vary widely among products. Most products are metabolized in the liver and excreted in urine.
Interactions: Please check individual monographs, since interactions vary widely among products.

NURSING CONSIDERATIONS
Assessment
- Monitor VS, B/P, pulse, respirations, neurologic signs, temp at least q4h, temp is an indicator of internal bleeding, cardiac rhythm following intracoronary administration; systolic pressure increase of >25 mm Hg should be reported to prescriber
- Assess for neurologic changes that may indicate intracranial bleeding
- Assess retroperitoneal bleeding: back pain, leg weakness, diminished pulses
- Assess for allergy: fever, rash, itching, chill; mild reaction may be treated with antihistamines
- Assess for bleeding during 1st hr of treatment: hematuria, hematemesis, bleeding from mucous membranes, epistaxis, ecchymosis
- Monitor blood studies (Hct, platelets, PTT, PT, TT, APTT) before starting therapy; PT or APTT must be less than 2 times control before starting therapy TT or PT q3-4h during treatment

Nursing diagnoses
✓ Risk for injury (uses)

Implementation
- Administer as soon as thrombi identified; not useful for thrombi over 1 wk old
- Administer cryoprecipitate or fresh, frozen plasma if bleeding occurs
- Administer loading dose at beginning of therapy; may require increased loading doses
- Give heparin after fibrinogen level is over 100 mg/dl; heparin inf to increase PTT to 1.5-2 times baseline for 3-7 days
- About 10% of patients have high streptococcal antibody titers requiring increased loading doses
- Give **IV** therapy using 0.8-μm filter
- Store reconstituted sol in refrigerator; discard after 24 hr
- Provide bed rest during entire course of treatment
- Avoid venous or arterial puncture, injection, rec temp
- Provide treatment of fever with acetaminophen or aspirin
- Apply pressure for 30 sec to minor bleeding sites; inform prescriber if this does not attain hemostasis; apply pressure dressing

Evaluation
- Therapeutic response: resolution of thrombosis, embolism

Selected Generic Names

alteplase (high alert)
anistreplase (high alert)
drotrecogin alfa (Appx A)
streptokinase (high alert)
tenecteplase
urokinase (high alert)

THYROID HORMONES

Action: Increase metabolic rates, resulting in increased cardiac output, O_2 consumption, body temp, blood volume, growth, development at cellular level, respiratory rate, enzyme system activity

Uses: Products are used for thyroid replacement.

Adverse effects: The most common side effects include insomnia, tremors, tachycardia, palpitations, angina, dysrhythmias, weight loss, and changes in appetite. Serious adverse reactions include thyroid storm.

Contraindications: Persons with adrenal insufficiency, myocardial infarction, or thyrotoxicosis should not use these products.

G **Precautions:** The elderly and patients with angina pectoris, hypertension, ischemia, cardiac disease, or diabetes mellitus or insipidus should be watched closely when using these products. Caution should be used in pregnancy and lactation.

Pharmacokinetics: Pharmacokinetics vary widely among products; check specific monographs.

Interactions

- Impaired absorption of thyroid products may occur when administered with cholestyramine (separate by 4-5 hr)
- Increased effects of anticoagulants, sympathomimetics, tricyclic antidepressants, catecholamines may occur
- Decreased effects of digitalis, glycosides, insulin, hypoglycemics may occur
- Decreased effects of thyroid products may occur with estrogens

NURSING CONSIDERATIONS

Assessment

- Monitor B/P, pulse before each dose
- Monitor I&O ratio
- Monitor weight qd in same clothing, using same scale, at same time of day
- P Monitor height, growth rate if given to a child
- Monitor T_3, T_4, which are decreased; radioimmunoassay of TSH, which is increased; ratio uptake, which is decreased if patient is on too low a dosage of medication
- Assess for increased nervousness, excitability, irritability; may indicate too high a dosage of medication usually after 1-3 wk of treatment
- Assess for cardiac status: angina, palpitation, chest pain, change in VS

Nursing diagnoses
- ✓ Knowledge deficit (teaching)
- ✓ Noncompliance (teaching)
- ✓ Body image disturbance (adverse reactions)

Implementation
- Give at same time each day to maintain drug level
- Give only for hormone imbalances; not to be used for obesity, male infertility, menstrual conditions, lethargy
- Remove medication 4 wk before RAIU test

Evaluation
- Therapeutic response: absence of depression; increased weight loss, diuresis, pulse, appetite; absence of constipation, peripheral edema, cold intolerance, pale, cool, dry skin, brittle nails, alopecia, coarse hair, menorrhagia, night blindness, paresthesias, syncope, stupor, coma, rosy cheeks

Patient/family education
- P Advise patient that hair loss will occur in child and is temporary
- Advise patient to report excitability, irritability, anxiety; indicates overdose
- Caution patient not to switch brands unless directed by prescriber
- P Caution patient that hypothyroid child will show almost immediate behavior/personality change
- Advise patient that treatment drug is not to be taken to reduce weight
- Advise patient to avoid OTC preparations with iodine; read labels; to avoid iodine-containing food, iodinized salt, soybeans, tofu, turnips, some seafood, some bread

---

Selected Generic Names
Key Drug: levothyroxine (T_4)
liothyronine (T_3)
liotrix
thyroid USP

VASODILATORS

Action: Vasodilators act in various ways. Please check individual monograph for specific action.

Uses: Vasodilators are used to treat intermittent claudication, arteriosclerosis obliterans, vasospasm and muscular ischemia, ischemic cerebral vascular disease, hypertension, and angina.

Adverse effects: The most common side effects are headache, nausea, hypotension or hypertension, and ECG changes.

Contraindications: Some drugs are contraindicated in acute MI, paroxysmal tachycardia, and thyrotoxicosis.

Precautions: Caution should be used in uncompensated heart disease or peptic ulcer disease.
Pharmacokinetics: Onset, peak, and duration vary widely among products. Most products are metabolized in the liver and excreted in urine.
Interactions: Please check individual monographs, since interactions vary widely among products.

NURSING CONSIDERATIONS

Assessment

- Assess bleeding time in individuals with bleeding disorders
- Assess cardiac status: B/P, pulse, rate, rhythm, character; watch for increasing pulse

Nursing diagnoses

✓ Decreased cardiac output (uses)
✓ Altered tissue perfusion: cardiovascular/pulmonary (uses)
✓ Knowledge deficit (teaching)

Implementation

- Give with meals to reduce GI symptoms
- Store in tight container at room temp

Evaluation

- Therapeutic response: ability to walk without pain, increased temp in extremities, increased pulse volume

Patient/family education

- Inform patient that medication is not cure, may need to be taken continuously
- Advise patient that it is necessary to quit smoking to prevent excessive vasoconstriction
- Advise patient that improvement may be sudden, but usually occurs gradually over several wk
- Instruct patient to report headache, weakness, increased pulse, since drug may need to be decreased or discontinued
- Instruct patient to avoid hazardous activities until stabilized on medication; dizziness may occur

---

Selected Generic Names

amyl nitrite
bosentan (Appx A)
dipyridamole
hydralazine
minoxidil
nesiritide (Appx A)
papaverine

VITAMINS

Action: Action varies widely among products and classes; check specific monographs.
Uses: Vitamins are used to correct and prevent vitamin deficiencies.
Adverse effects: There is an absence of side effects or adverse reactions with the water-soluble vitamins (C, B). However, fat-soluble vitamins (A, D, E, K) may accumulate in the body and cause adverse reactions (refer to specific monographs).
Contraindications: Hypersensitive reactions may occur, and allergies should be identified before these products are given.
Pharmacokinetics: Onset, peak, and duration vary widely among products; check individual monograph for specific information.

NURSING CONSIDERATIONS

Nursing diagnoses

✓ Altered nutrition, less than body requirements (uses)

Implementation

- Give PO with food for better absorption
- Store in tight, light-resistant container

Evaluation

- Therapeutic response: absence of vitamin deficiency

Patient/family education

- Advise patient not to take more than prescribed amount

Selected Generic Names

Fat-soluble:
phytonadione
vit A
vit D
vit E

Water-soluble:
ascorbic acid (C)
pyridoxine (B_6)
riboflavin (B_2)
thiamine (B_1)

Miscellaneous:
multivitamins

Appendix A

Selected New Drugs

alemtuzumab (℞)

(al-em-tuz'uh-mab)

Campath

Func. class.: Misc. antineoplastic

Chem. class.: Monoclonal antibody

Pregnancy category C

Action: Composed of recombinant DNA-derived humanized monoclonal antibody (campath-1H), binds to CD52 antigen that is present on surface of B and T lymphocytes, causes lysis of leukemic cells

Therapeutic Outcome: Decrease in number of white blood cells

Uses: B-cell chronic lymphocytic leukemia that has been treated with alkylating agents

Dosage and routes

Adult: **IV** 3 mg over 2 hr daily; when tolerated, increase to 10 mg; when 10 mg tolerated, increase to 30 mg qd; maintenance is 30 mg/day 3x/wk on alternate days

Available forms: Sol for inj 30 mg/3 ml

Adverse effects

CNS: *Dizziness,* insomnia, depression, headache, tremor, somnolence, fatigue

CV: Hypotension, tachycardia, hypertension

GI: Anorexia, diarrhea, constipation, nausea, stomatitis, vomiting, abdominal pain, dyspepsia

HEMA: Anemia, neutropenia, thrombocytopenia, pancytopenia, purpura, epistaxis

INTEG: *Rash,* local reaction, pruritus

META: Hypokalemia, hypomagnesemia

MISC: Rigors, fever

RESP: Cough, pneumonia, rhinitis, bronchospasm, dyspnea, pharyngitis

Contraindications: Hypersensitivity, active systemic infection, immunodeficiency

Precautions: Pregnancy **C**, lactation, children

Pharmacokinetics

Absorption	Unknown
Distribution	Unknown; steady state 6 wk
Metabolism	Unknown
Excretion	Unknown
Half-life	12 days

Pharmacodynamics

Onset	Unknown
Peak	Unknown
Duration	Unknown

Interactions

Drug classifications

Live virus vaccines: Do not administer

Lab test interferences

Diagnostic tests using antibodies

NURSING CONSIDERATIONS

Assessment

- Assess CBC, platelets qwk or more often if myelosuppression occurs; assess $CD4^+$ after therapy until recovery of >200 cells μ/L
- Assess for symptoms of infection; chills, fever, headache, may be masked by drug fever
- Assess CNS reaction: LOC, mental status, dizziness, confusion
- Assess cardiac status: lung sounds;

ECG before and during treatment, especially in those with cardiac disease

- Assess for bone marrow depression: bruising, bleeding, blood in stools, urine, sputum, emesis

Nursing diagnoses

- ✓ Infection, risk for (adverse reactions)
- ✓ Injury, risk for (adverse reactions)
- ✓ Nutrition, altered, less than body requirements (side effects)
- ✓ Body image disturbance (adverse reactions)
- ✓ Knowledge deficit (teaching)

Implementation

IV IV route

- Do not give **IV** push or bolus
- Withdraw amount needed, use 5 μm filter prior to dilution, check for particulate matter and discoloration; inject into 100 ml sterile 0.9% NaCl or D_5W, invert to mix, do not add other drugs or infuse in same **IV** tubing
- Store reconstituted sol for ≤8 hr at room temp, do not freeze; protect from light

Patient/family education

- Instruct patient to take acetaminophen for fever
- Advise patient to avoid hazardous tasks, since confusion, dizziness may occur
- Instruct patient to report signs of infection: sore throat, fever, diarrhea, vomiting

Evaluation

Positive therapeutic outcome

- Decrease in production of malignant lymphocytes

almotriptan (℞)

(al-moh-trip'tan)

Axert

Func. class.: Antimigraine agent

Chem. class.: 5-HT_1 receptor agonist

Pregnancy category C

Action: Binds selectively to the vascular 5-HT_1 receptor subtype, exerts antimigraine effect; causes vasoconstriction in cranial arteries

➔ **Therapeutic Outcome:** Absence of migraines

Uses: Acute treatment of migraine with or without aura

Dosage and routes

Adult: PO may use 6.25 mg dose initially, but 12.5 mg is more effective; may repeat dose after 2 hr; do not give more than 2 doses/24 hr

Available forms: Tabs 6.25, 12.5 mg

Adverse effects

CV: *Flushing,* palpitations, tachycardia, coronary artery vasospasm

EENT: Throat, mouth, nasal discomfort; vision changes

GI: Abdominal discomfort

INTEG: Sweating

MS: *Weakness, neck stiffness,* myalgia

NEURO: *Tingling, hot sensation, burning, feeling of pressure, tightness, numbness, dizziness, sedation,* headache, anxiety, fatigue, cold sensation

RESP: Chest tightness, pressure

Contraindications: Concurrent use of ergotamine-containing preparations, uncontrolled hypertension, hypersensitivity, basilar or hemiplegic migraine; concurrent MAOI therapy or within 2 wk

Precautions: Postmenopausal women, men >40 yr, risk factors for coronary artery disease, hypercholesterolemia, obesity, diabetes, impaired

P hepatic or renal function, pregnancy
G **C**, lactation, children, elderly

Pharmacokinetics

Absorption	Well absorbed (~70%)
Distribution	35% protein bound
Metabolism	Liver (metabolite)
Excretion	Urine, feces
Half-life	3-4 hr

Pharmacodynamics

Onset	Unknown
Peak	1-3 hr
Duration	Unknown

Interactions

Individual drugs

Ergot: ↑ vasospastic effects
Ketoconazole: ↑ plasma concentration of almotriptan

Drug classifications

5-HT$_1$ agonists: ↑ vasospastic effects
Ergot derivatives: ↑ vasospastic effects
MAOIs: ↑ almotriptan effect

NURSING CONSIDERATIONS

Assessment

- Assess B/P, signs/symptoms of coronary vasospasms
- Assess for tingling, hot sensation, burning, feeling of pressure, numbness, flushing
- Assess for stress level, activity, recreation, coping mechanisms
- Assess neurologic status: LOC, blurring vision, nausea, vomiting, tingling in extremities preceding headache
- Assess for ingestion of tyramine-containing foods (pickled products, beer, wine, aged cheese), food additives, preservatives, colorings, artificial sweeteners, chocolate, caffeine, which may precipitate these types of headaches

Nursing diagnoses

✓ Pain (uses)
✓ Knowledge deficit (teaching)

Implementation

- PO, swallow whole
- Provide quiet, calm environment with decreased stimulation from noise, bright light, excessive talking

Patient/family education

- Advise patient to report any side effects to prescriber
- Instruct patient to use contraception while taking drug
- Advise patient to have dark, quiet environment available
- Inform patient that drug does not prevent or reduce number of migraine attacks

Evaluation

Positive therapeutic outcome

- Decrease in severity of migraine

Treatment of overdose:

Gastric lavage followed by activated charcoal; clinical and ECG monitoring for ≥20 hr after overdose

anakinra (℞)

(an-ah-kin'rah)

Kineret

Func. class.: Antirheumatic agent (disease modifying), immunomodulator

Chem. class.: Recombinant form of human interleukin-1 receptor antagonist (IL-1Ra)

Pregnancy category B

Action: A form of human interleukin-1 receptor antagonist (IL-1Ra) produced by DNA technology; blocks activity of IL-1, resulting in decreased cartilage degradation and decreased bone resorption

➔ **Therapeutic Outcome:** Decreased pain, inflammation

Uses: Reduction in signs and symptoms of moderate to severe active rheumatoid arthritis in patients 18 years of age or older who have not responded to other disease-modifying agents

Dosage and routes

Adult: SC 100 mg qd

Available forms: Sol for inj, 100 mg

Adverse effects

CNS: Headache
EENT: Sinusitis
GI: Abdominal pain, nausea, diarrhea
INTEG: Rash, *inj site reaction*
MISC: Flu-like symptoms
RESP: *URI*

Contraindications: Hypersensitivity to *Escherichia coli*-derived proteins or this product, sepsis

Precautions: Pregnancy **B,** lactation, P children, renal impairment, G elderly

Pharmacokinetics	
Absorption	Well absorbed (SC)
Distribution	Unknown
Metabolism	Unknown
Excretion	Unknown
Half-life	4-6 hr

Pharmacodynamics	
Onset	Unknown
Peak	3-7 hr
Duration	Unknown

Interactions

Drug classifications

Vaccines: Do not coadminister; immunizations should be brought up to date before treatment

NURSING CONSIDERATIONS

Assessment

- Assess pain, stiffness, ROM, swelling of joints during treatment
- Assess for injection site pain, swelling; usually occur after 2 injections (4-5 days)
- Assess for infections, stop treatment if present

Nursing diagnoses

✓ Pain (uses)
✓ Mobility, impaired physical (uses)
✓ Injury, risk for (side effects)
✓ Knowledge deficit (teaching)

Implementation

- Do not use if cloudy or discolored or if particulate is present
- Do not admix with other sol or medications, do not use filter

Patient/family education

Teach patient about self-administration if appropriate: inj should be made in thigh, abdomen, upper arm; rotate sites at least 1 in from old site

Evaluation

Positive therapeutic outcome

- Decreased inflammation, pain in joints

bosentan (℞)

(boh-sen-tan)

Tracleer

Func. class.: Vasodilator
Chem. class.: Endothelin receptor antagonist

Pregnancy category X

Action: Peripheral vasodilation occurs via antagonism of the effect of endothelin on endothelium and vascular smooth muscle

→ **Therapeutic Outcome:** Decreased pulmonary arterial hypertension

Uses: Pulmonary arterial hypertension with class III, IV symptoms

Dosage and routes

Adult >40 kg and>12 yr: PO 62.5 mg bid x 4 wk, then 125 mg bid

Adult <40 kg and >12 yr: PO 62.5 mg bid

Available forms: Tabs 62.5, 125 mg

Adverse effects

CNS: Headache, flushing, fatigue
CV: *Hypotension,* palpitations, edema of lower limbs

GI: Abnormal liver function, dyspepsia
INTEG: Pruritus

Contraindications: Pregnancy **X**, hypersensitivity, CVA, CAD

Precautions: Mitral stenosis, G elderly, lactation, impaired hepatic function

Pharmacokinetics

Absorption	50% absorbed
Distribution	Protein binding >98%
Metabolism	Liver (metabolites); induces CYP2C9, CYP3A4, and possibly CYP2C19; steady state 3-5 days
Excretion	Biliary
Half-life	5 hr

Pharmacodynamics

Onset	Unknown
Peak	Unknown
Duration	Unknown

Interactions

Individual drugs

Cyclosporine A: Do not coadminister; bosentan level ↑, cyclosporine level ↓
Glyburide: Do not coadminister; glyburide level ↓ significantly, bosentan also ↓
Ketoconazole: ↑ bosentan level
Simvastatin: ↓ effects

Drug classifications

Contraceptives, hormonal: ↓ effects
Statins: ↓ effects

NURSING CONSIDERATIONS

Assessment

- Assess B/P, pulse during treatment until stable
- Assess hepatic tests: AST, ALT, bilirubin; liver enzymes may increase; if ALT/AST >3 and ≤5 × ULN, confirm lab value, decrease dose or interrupt treatment and monitor AST/ALT q2 wk; if >8 × ULN, stop treatment
- Assess blood studies: Hct, Hgb may be decreased
- Assess hepatic involvement: vomiting, jaundice; drug should be discontinued

Nursing diagnoses

✓ Tissue perfusion, altered (uses)
✓ Knowledge deficit (teaching)

Implementation

- Store at room temp

Patient/family education

- Instruct patient to report jaundice, dark urine, joint pain, fatigue, malaise, bruising, easy bleeding; may indicate blood dyscrasias
- Caution patient to avoid pregnancy; to use nonhormonal form of contraception

Evaluation

Positive therapeutic outcome

- Decrease in pulmonary hypertension

cefditoren pivoxil (℞)

(sef-dih-tor'en pih-vox'il)
Spectracef
Func. class.: Antiinfective
Chem. class.: Cephalosporin (2nd generation)

Pregnancy category B

Action: Inhibits bacterial cell wall synthesis, rendering cell wall osmotically unstable, leading to cell death by binding to cell wall membrane

➔ **Therapeutic Outcome:** Bactericidal effects for *Haemophilus influenzae, Haemophilus parainfluenzae, Streptococcus pneumoniae, Moraxella catarrhalis, Streptococcus pyogenes, Staphylococcus aureus, Staphylococcus pyogenes*

Uses: Acute bacterial exacerbation of chronic bronchitis cause by *Haemophilus influenzae, Haemophilus parainfluenzae, Streptococcus pneumoniae, Moraxella catarrhalis*; pharyngitis/tonsillitis caused by *Streptococcus pyogenes*; uncomplicated skin and skin structure infections caused by *Staphylococcus aureus, Staphylococcus pyogenes*

Dosage and routes

Acute bacterial exacerbation of chronic bronchitis

Adult: PO 400 mg bid × 10 days

Pharyngitis/tonsillitis

Adult: PO 200 mg bid × 10 days

Uncomplicated skin and skin structure infections

Adult: PO 200 mg bid × 10 days

Renal dose

CrCl 30-49 ml/min give ≤200 mg bid × 10 days

CrCl <30 ml/min give 200 mg qd × 10 days

Available forms: Tabs 200 mg

Adverse effects

CNS: Dizziness, headache, fatigue, paresthesia, fever, chills, confusion

GI: *Diarrhea*, nausea, vomiting, anorexia, dysgeusia, glossitis, bleeding; increased AST, ALT, bilirubin, LDH, alkaline phosphatase, abdominal pain, loose stools, flatulence, heartburn, stomach cramps, colitis, jaundice

GU: Vaginitis, pruritus, candidiasis, increased BUN, **nephrotoxicity, renal failure**, pyuria, dysuria, reversible interstitial nephritis

HEMA: **Leukopenia, thrombocytopenia, agranulocytosis,** anemia, *neutropenia, lymphocytosis,* **eosinophilia, pancytopenia, hemolytic anemia, leukocytosis, granulocytopenia**

INTEG: Rash, urticaria, dermatitis, **Stevens-Johnson syndrome,** diaphoresis, flushing

RESP: Dyspnea

SYST: **Anaphylaxis, serum sickness**

Contraindications: Hypersensitivity to cephalosporins or related antibiotics, carnitine deficiency, inborn errors of metabolism, milk protein hypersensitivity

Precautions: Pregnancy **B**, lactation, [P] children, renal disease

Pharmacokinetics

Absorption	GI tract
Distribution	60%-75% bound by plasma proteins, crosses placenta, poor penetration into CSF
Metabolism	Not appreciably metabolized
Excretion	Urine, breast milk
Half-life	½-1 hr

Pharmacodynamics

Onset	Unknown
Peak	1-1 ½ hr
Duration	Unknown

Interactions

Individual drugs

Probenecid: ↑ plasma level of cefditoren

Drug classifications

Aminoglycosides: ↑ renal toxicity

Antacids: ↓ plasma level of cefditoren

H_2-receptor antagonists: ↓ plasma level of cefditoren

NURSING CONSIDERATIONS

Assessment

- [Alert] Assess for nephrotoxicity: increased BUN, creatinine
- Assess I&O ratio
- Assess blood studies: AST, ALT, CBC, Hct, bilirubin, LDH, alkaline phosphatase, Coombs' test qmo if patient is on long-term therapy
- Assess electrolyte status (K, Na, Cl) qmo if patient is on long-term therapy
- Assess bowel pattern qd; if severe diarrhea occurs, discontinue drug; may indicate pseudomembranous colitis
- Assess urine output; if decreasing, notify prescriber; may indicate nephrotoxicity
- [Alert] Assess for anaphylaxis: rash, flushing, urticaria, pruritus, dyspnea

- Assess for bleeding: ecchymosis, bleeding gums, hematuria, stool guaiac daily
- Assess for overgrowth of infection: perineal itching, fever, malaise, redness, pain, swelling, drainage, rash, diarrhea, change in cough, sputum

Nursing diagnoses

- ✓ Infection, risk for (uses)
- ✓ Diarrhea (side effects)
- ✓ Fluid volume deficit, risk for (side effects)
- ✓ Injury, risk for (side effects)
- ✓ Knowledge deficit (teaching)
- ✓ Noncompliance (teaching)

Implementation

- Administer for 10 days to ensure organism death, prevent superinfection
- Give with food if needed for GI symptoms
- Administer after C&S completed

Patient/family education

- Advise patient not to drink alcohol or take medications containing alcohol; reaction may occur
- Instruct patient to complete full course of drug therapy
- Instruct patient to report persistent diarrhea or any side effects
- Advise patient to notify prescriber if breastfeeding

Evaluation

Positive therapeutic outcome

- Decreased symptoms of infection
- Negative C&S

Treatment of anaphylaxis: Epinephrine, antihistamines; resuscitate if needed

darbepoetin alfa (℞)

(dar'bee-poh'-eh-tin al'fah)

Aranesp

Func. class.: Hematopoietic agent

Chem. class.: Recombinant human erythropoietin

Pregnancy category C

Action: Stimulates erythropoiesis by the same mechanism as endogenous erythropoietin; in response to hypoxia, erythropoietin is produced in the kidney and released into the bloodstream, where it interacts with progenitor stem cells to increase red cell production

➔ Therapeutic Outcome: Decreased anemia with increased RBCs

Uses: Anemia associated with chronic renal failure in patients on and not on dialysis

Dosage and routes

Correction of anemia

Adult: SC/**IV** 0.45 μg/kg as a single inj, titrate not to exceed a target Hgb of 12 g/dl

Conversion from epoetin alfa to darbepoetin

Adult: SC/**IV** estimate starting dose based on weekly epoetin alfa dose; because of longer serum half-life, darbepoetin must be administered less frequently than epoetin alfa; if epoetin was given 2-3×/wk, give darbepoetin 1×/wk; if epoetin was given 1×/wk, give darbepoetin 1× q2 wk; do not increase doses more often than 1×/mo

Available forms: Sol 25, 40, 60, 100, 200 μg/ml

Adverse effects

CNS: **Seizures**, sweating, headache, dizziness

CV: *Hypertension*, hypotension, **cardiac arrest**, angina pectoris, **thrombosis, CHF**

GI: Diarrhea, vomiting, nausea, abdominal pain, constipation

MISC: Infection, fatigue, fever, **death**,

chest pain, fluid overload, vascular access hemorrhage
MS: Bone pain, myalgia, limb pain
RESP: Upper respiratory infection, dyspnea, cough, bronchitis

Contraindications: Hypersensitivity to mammalian cell-derived products or human albumin, uncontrolled hypertension

Precautions: Seizure disorder, porphyria, pregnancy **C**, hypertension

Pharmacokinetics	
Absorption	Slow, rate-limiting (SC)
Distribution	Vascular space
Metabolism	Metabolized in body (**IV**), extent unknown
Excretion	Unknown
Half-life	49 hr

Pharmacodynamics	
Onset	Onset of increased reticulocyte count 1-6 wk
Peak	34 hr
Duration	Unknown

Interactions

Drug classifications

Anticoagulants: ↑ anticoagulants needed during hemodialysis

NURSING CONSIDERATIONS

Assessment

- Assess blood studies: ferritin, transferrin monthly; transferrin sat ≥20%, ferritin ≥100 ng/ml; Hgb 2×/wk until stabilized in target range (30%-33%) then at regular intervals; those with endogenous erythropoietin levels of <500 U/L respond to this agent
- Assess renal studies: urinalysis, protein, blood, BUN, creatinine
- Assess B/P; check for rising B/P as Hct rises, antihypertensives may be needed
- Assess CV status: hypertension may occur rapidly leading to hypertensive encephalopathy
- Assess I&O ratio; report drop in output to <50 ml/hr
- Assess for seizures if Hgb is increased within 2 wk by 4 pts
- Assess CNS symptoms: cold sensation, sweating, pain in long bones
- Assess dialysis patients for thrill, bruit of shunts; monitor for circulation impairment

Nursing diagnoses

- ✓ Fatigue (uses)
- ✓ Activity intolerance (uses)
- ✓ Knowledge deficit (teaching)

Implementation

IV IV/SC

- Do not shake, do not dilute, do not mix with other drugs or solutions
- Check for discoloration, particulate matter; do not use if present

Patient/family education

- Caution patient to avoid driving or hazardous activity during beginning of treatment
- Advise patient to monitor B/P
- Advise patient to take iron supplements, vit B_{12}, folic acid as directed

Evaluation

Positive therapeutic outcome

- Increased reticulocyte count, Hgb/Hct
- Increased appetite
- Enhanced sense of well-being

Treatment of overdose: If polycythemia occurs, discontinue drug temporarily; perform phlebotomy if clinically indicated

desloratadine (℞)

(des-lor-at'ah-deen)

Clarinex

Func. class.: Antihistamine, 2nd generation

Chem. class.: Selective histamine (H_1-) receptor antagonist

Pregnancy category C

Action: Binds to peripheral histamine receptors, providing antihistamine action without sedation

➔ **Therapeutic Outcome:** Decreased nasal stuffiness, itching, swollen eyes

Uses: Seasonal allergic rhinitis

Dosage and routes

P ***Adult and child ≥12 yr:*** PO 5 mg qd

Hepatic/renal dose

Adult: PO 5 mg qod

Available forms: Tabs 5 mg

Adverse effects

CNS: Sedation (more common with increased doses), headache

Contraindications: Hypersensitivity, acute asthma attacks, lower respiratory tract disease

Precautions: Pregnancy **C**, bronchial asthma, liver or renal impairment

Pharmacokinetics	
Absorption	Unknown
Distribution	Bound to plasma proteins (82%-87%)
Metabolism	Liver (active metabolites)
Excretion	Urine, feces (metabolites)
Half-life	8 ½-28 hr

Pharmacodynamics	
Onset	1 hr
Peak	1 ½ hr
Duration	24 hr

Interactions

None significant

NURSING CONSIDERATIONS

Assessment

- Assess for allergy: hives, rash, rhinitis; monitor respiratory status

Nursing diagnoses

✓ Airway clearance, ineffective (uses)
✓ Knowledge deficit (teaching)
✓ Noncompliance (teaching, overuse)

Implementation

- May administer without regard to meals
- Store in airtight container at room temp

Patient/family education

- Advise patient to avoid driving, other hazardous activities if drowsiness occurs; to observe caution until drug's effects are known
- Advise patient that drug may cause photosensitivity; use sunscreen or stay out of the sun to prevent burns
- Caution patient to avoid use of other CNS depressants

Evaluation

Positive therapeutic outcome

- Absence of running or congested nose, other allergy symptoms

dexmethylphenidate (℞)

(dex'meth-ul-fen'ih-dayt)

Focalin

Func. class.: Central nervous system (CNS) stimulant

Pregnancy category C

Controlled Substance Schedule II

Action: Increases release of norepinephrine and dopamine into the extraneuronal space, also blocks reuptake of norepinephrine and dopamine into the presynaptic neuron; mode of action in treating attention deficit hyperactivity disorder (ADHD) is unknown

Therapeutic Outcome: Increased alertness, decreased fatigue, ability to stay awake (narcolepsy), increased attention span, decreased hyperactivity (ADHD)

Uses: ADHD

Dosage and routes

P *Child >6 yr:* PO 2.5 mg bid with doses at least 4 hr apart, gradually increase to a maximum of 20 mg/day (10 mg bid); for those taking methylphenidate, use ½ of methylphenidate dose initially, then increase as needed to a maximum of 20 mg/day

Available forms: Tabs 2.5, 5, 10 mg

Adverse effects

CNS: Dizziness, headache, drowsiness, **toxic psychosis, neuroleptic malignant syndrome (rare)**, Gilles de la Tourette's syndrome
CV: Palpitations, B/P changes, angina, **dysrhythmias**
GI: Nausea, anorexia, abnormal liver function, **hepatic coma**, abdominal pain
HEMA: **Leukopenia, anemia, thrombocytopenic purpura**
INTEG: **Exfoliative dermatitis**, urticaria, rash, erythema multiforme
MISC: Fever, arthralgia, scalp hair loss

Contraindications: Hypersensitivity to methylphenidate, anxiety, history of Gilles de la Tourette's P syndrome; children <6 yr, glaucoma, concurrent treatment with MAOIs or within 14 days of discontinuing treatment with MAOIs

Precautions: Hypertension, depression, pregnancy **C**, seizures, lactation, drug abuse, psychosis, cardiovascular disorders

Pharmacokinetics

Absorption	Readily absorbed
Distribution	Unknown
Metabolism	Liver
Excretion	Kidneys
Half-life	2.2 hr

Pharmacodynamics

Onset	½-1 hr
Peak	1-1 ½ hr
Duration	4 hr

Interactions

Drug classifications

Anticoagulants, coumarin (e.g., warfarin): ↑ effects
Anticonvulsants: ↑ effects
Antihypertensives: ↓ effects
Decongestants: ↑ sympathomimetic effect
MAOIs: Hypertensive crisis if coadministered or given within 14 days
SSRIs: ↑ effects
Tricyclics: ↑ effects
Vasoconstrictors: ↑ sympathomimetic effect
Vasopressors: Hypertensive crisis

NURSING CONSIDERATIONS

Assessment

- Assess VS, B/P; may reverse antihypertensives; check patients with cardiac disease more often for increased B/P
- Assess CBC, urinalysis in diabetes; blood sugar, urine sugar; insulin changes may have to be made, since eating will decrease
- P Assess height, growth rate q3 mo in children; growthrate may be decreased
- Assess mental status: mood, sensorium, affect, stimulation, insomnia, aggressiveness
- ❗ Assess withdrawal symptoms: headache, nausea, vomiting, muscle pain, weakness
- Assess appetite, sleep, speech patterns
- Assess for attention span, decreased hyperactivity in persons with ADHD

Nursing diagnoses

- ✓ Thought processes, altered (uses, adverse reactions)
- ✓ Coping, ineffective individual (uses)
- ✓ Knowledge deficit (teaching)
- ✓ Family coping, impaired (uses)

Implementation

Administer:

- Twice daily at least 4 hr apart
- Without regard to meals

Patient/family education

- Advise patient to decrease caffeine consumption (coffee, tea, cola, chocolate); may increase irritability, stimulation
- Caution patient not to break, crush, or chew time rel medication
- Advise patient to avoid OTC preparations unless approved by prescriber
- Caution patient to taper off drug over several wk to avoid depression, increased sleeping, lethargy
- Caution patient to avoid alcohol ingestion
- Caution patient to avoid hazardous activities until stabilized on medication
- Advise patient to get needed rest; patients will feel more tired at end of day

Evaluation

Positive therapeutic outcome

- Decreased hyperactivity or ability to stay awake

Treatment of overdose:

Administer fluids; hemodialysis or peritoneal dialysis; antihypertensive for increased B/P; administer short-acting barbiturate before lavage

drotrecogin alfa (℞)

(droh'treh-koh-jin al'fah)

Xigris

Func. class.: Thrombolytic agent

Chem. class.: Recombinant human activated protein C

Pregnancy category C

Action: Activated protein C exerts an antithrombotic effect by inhibiting Factor Va/VIIIa

Therapeutic Outcome: Reduction of mortality in adult patients with severe sepsis who have a high risk of death

Uses: Severe sepsis (sepsis associated with acute organ dysfunction)

Dosage and routes

***Adult:* IV** inf 24 μg/kg/hr x 96 hr

Available forms: Powder for inj, lyophilized, 5 mg, 20 mg

Adverse effects

HEMA: Decreased Hct, **bleeding**

SYST: **GI, GU, intracranial, intraabdominal, intrathoracic, retroperitoneal bleeding; surface bleeding**

Contraindications: Hypersensitivity, active bleeding, intraspinal surgery, CNS neoplasms, ulcerative colitis, enteritis, hepatic disease, hypocoagulation, hemorrhagic stroke, epidural catheter in place, cerebral embolism/thrombosis/hemorrhage, recent major surgery

Precautions: Recent GI bleeding, prothrombin time –INR >3, pregnancy **C**, lactation, children

Pharmacokinetics	
Absorption	Rapid
Distribution	Plasma
Metabolism	Unknown
Excretion	Unknown
Half-life	Unknown

Pharmacodynamics	
Onset	Within 2 hr of beginning infusion
Peak	96 hr
Duration	2 hr postinfusion

Interactions Formal drug interaction studies not yet conducted; use caution when coadministering drotrecogin alfa with drugs that affect hemostasis

Lab test interferences

Possible variably prolonged APTT, possible altered one-stage coagulation assays based on APTT (factor VIII, IX, XI assays)

NURSING CONSIDERATIONS

Assessment

- Alert: Assess for bleeding during treatment; hematuria, hematemesis, bleeding from mucous membranes, epistaxis, ecchymosis; may require transfusion (rare), continue to assess for bleeding
- Assess blood studies (Hct, platelets, PTT, PT, TT, APTT) before starting therapy; PT or APTT must be less than 2× control before starting therapy; PTT or PT q3-4h during treatment
- Assess VS, B/P, pulse, respirations, neurologic signs, temp at least q4h; temp >104° F (40° C) indicates internal bleeding; cardiac rhythm following intracoronary administration; systolic pressure increase >25 mm Hg should be reported to prescriber
- Alert: Assess for neurologic changes that may indicate intracranial bleeding
- Alert: Assess for retroperitoneal bleeding: back pain, leg weakness, diminished pulses

Nursing diagnoses

✓ Knowledge deficit (teaching)

Implementation

- Store in refrigerator at 2° to 8° C (36° to 46° F); do not freeze
- Protect unreconstituted vials from light; keep in carton until time of use

IV route

- Reconstitute 5 mg vial/2.5 ml; 20 mg vial/10 ml sterile water for inj to a concentration of 2 mg/ml; slowly add sterile water for inj; do not shake or invert, gently swirl until dissolved
- Further dilute with 0.9% NaCl, slowly withdraw prescribed amount and add to bag of 0.9% NaCl, direct stream to side of bag, gently invert bag; do not transport infusion bag between locations using mechanical delivery systems
- Use immediately after reconstituting, may be held for only 3 hr at controlled room temp 59°-86° F and must complete inf within 12 hr after preparation
- Do not use if discolored or if particulate is present
- If using an infusion pump, usual concentration is 100-200 μg/ml; if using a syringe pump, usual concentration is 100-1000 μg/ml
- Use a dedicated **IV** line, or dedicated lumen of central venous catheter, may use only 0.9% NaCl, LR, dextrose, or dextrose/saline mixtures through same line
- Do not expose to heat or direct sunlight

Evaluation

Positive therapeutic outcome

- Decreasing symptoms of sepsis, lack of mortality

dutasteride (℞)

(doo-tass'ter-ide)

Duagen

Func. class.: 5α-reductase inhibitor

Chem. class.: Synthetic 4-azasteroid compound

Pregnancy category X

Action: Inhibits both type 1 and 2 forms of a steroid enzyme that converts testosterone to 5 μ-dihydrotestosterone (DHT), which is responsible for the initial growth of prostatic tissue

Therapeutic Outcome: Decreased symptoms of benign prostatic hyperplasia (BPH)

Uses: Treatment of symptomatic BPH in men with an enlarged prostate gland

Dosage and routes

Adult: PO 0.5 mg qd

Available forms: Cap 0.5 mg

Adverse effects

GU: Decreased libido, impotence, gynecomastia, ejaculation disorders (rare)

Contraindications: Hypersensitivity, pregnancy **X**, lactation, women, children

Precautions: Hepatic disease

Pharmacokinetics

Absorption	Absolute bioavailability ~60%
Distribution	Protein binding 99%
Metabolism	Liver (CYP3A4)
Excretion	Feces
Half-life	5 wk at steady state

Pharmacodynamics

Onset	Rapid
Peak	2-3 hr
Duration	Levels detectable 4-6 mo posttreatment

Interactions

Individual drugs

Cimetidine: ↑ dutasteride concentrations
Ciprofloxacin: ↑ dutasteride concentrations
Diltiazem: ↑ dutasteride concentrations
Ketoconazole: ↑ dutasteride concentrations
Ritonavir: ↑ dutasteride concentrations
Verapamil: ↑ dutasteride concentrations

Drug classifications

CYP3A4-metabolized drugs: ↑ dutasteride concentrations

Lab test interferences

Increase: TSH
Decrease: Prostate-specific antigen (PSA)

NURSING CONSIDERATIONS

Assessment

- Assess for decreasing symptoms in BPH: decreasing urinary retention, frequency, urgency, nocturia
- Assess PSA levels, urinary obstruction; determine the absence of urinary cancer before starting treatment
- Assess liver function studies: ALT, AST, bilirubin

Nursing diagnoses

✓ Knowledge deficit (teaching)
✓ Body image disturbance (adverse reactions)

Implementation

- May be given without regard to meals
- Administer caps whole; do not break, open, or chew

Patient/family education

- Advise patient to notify prescriber if therapeutic response decreases, if edema occurs
- Caution patient not to discontinue drug abruptly
- Inform patient about changes in sex characteristics
- Caution patient not to donate blood for at least 6 mo after last dose to prevent possible blood administration to pregnant female
- Advise patient and family that caps should not be handled by pregnant women since this drug can be absorbed through the skin
- Inform patient that ejaculate volume may decrease during treatment, that drug rarely interferes with sexual function

Evaluation

Positive therapeutic outcome

- Decreased levels of DHT (5 α-dihydrotestosterone)
- Decreased urinary frequency
- Decreased urinary retention
- Decreased urinary urgency
- Decreased nocturia

eprosartan mesylate/ hydrochlorothiazide (℞)

(ep-roh-sar'tan)

Teveten HCT

Func. class.: Antihypertensive

Chem. class.: Angiotensin II receptor antagonist (Subtype AT_1)

Pregnancy category C (1st trimester), D (2nd/3rd trimesters)

Action: Blocks the vasoconstrictor and aldosterone-secreting effects of angiotensin II; selectively blocks the binding of angiotensin II to the AT_1 receptor found in tissues

➔ **Therapeutic Outcome:** Decreased B/P

Uses: Hypertension, alone or in combination with other antihypertensives

Dosage and routes

Adult: PO 600 mg qd; dose may be divided and given bid with total daily doses ranging from 400-800 mg

Available forms: Tabs 600 mg eprosartan/12.5 mg hydrochlorothiazide, 600 mg eprosartan/25 mg hydrochlorothiazide

Adverse effects

CNS: *Dizziness*, depression, fatigue, headache

CV: Chest pain

EENT: Sinusitis

GI: *Diarrhea, dyspepsia,* abdominal pain

GU: UTI

META: Hypertriglyceridemia

MS: Myalgia, arthralgia

RESP: *Cough, upper respiratory infection,* rhinitis, pharyngitis, viral infection

Contraindications: Hypersensitivity, pregnancy **D** 2nd and 3rd trimesters

Precautions: Hypersensitivity to ACE inhibitors; pregnancy **C** 1st trimester, lactation, [P] children, [G] elderly; renal, hepatic disease

Pharmacokinetics

Absorption	Absolute bioavailability ~13%; food delays absorption
Distribution	Protein binding 98%
Metabolism	Moderate renal impairment increases drug levels by 30%,hepatic impairment increases levels by 40%
Excretion	Urine, feces
Half-life	5-9 hr

Pharmacodynamics

Onset	Unknown
Peak	1-2 hr
Duration	Unknown

Interactions

Unknown

Lab test interferences

Decrease: Hgb

Increase: Alanine aminotransferase, aspartate aminotransferase, alkaline phosphatase

NURSING CONSIDERATIONS

Assessment

- Assess B/P with position changes, pulse q4h; note rate, rhythm, quality
- Assess electrolytes: K, Na, Cl
- Assess baselines in renal, LF tests before therapy begins
- Assess for edema in feet, legs qd
- Assess skin turgor, dryness of mucous membranes for hydration status

Nursing diagnoses

✓ Fluid volume deficit (adverse reactions)
✓ Noncompliance (teaching)
✓ Knowledge deficit (teaching)
✓ Injury, risk for (adverse reactions)

Implementation

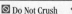

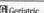

- May be given without regard to meals

Patient/family education

- Advise patient to comply with dosage schedule, even if feeling better
- Advise patient to notify prescriber of fever, swelling of hands or feet, chest pain
- Inform patient that excessive perspiration, dehydration, diarrhea may lead to fall in blood pressure; consult prescriber if these occur
- Inform patient that drug may cause dizziness; advise to avoid hazardous activities until effect is known
- Advise patient not to take this medication if pregnant or breastfeeding, or if allergic reaction to this drug has occurred
- Advise patient to take missed dose as soon as possible, unless within 1 hr of next dose

Evaluation

Positive therapeutic outcome

- Decreased B/P

ertapenem (℞)

(er-tah-pen'em)

Invanz

Func. class.: Antiinfective-misc.
Chem. class.: Carbapenem

Pregnancy category B

Action: Interferes with cell wall replication of susceptible organisms; osmotically unstable cell wall swells, bursts from osmotic pressure

➔ **Therapeutic Outcome:** Bactericidal action against the following organisms: *Bacteroides fragilis, Bacteroides distasonis, Bacteroides ovatus, Bacteroides thetaiotaomicron, Bacteroides uniformis; Clostridium clostridioforme, Escherichia coli, Eubacterium lentum, Haemophilus influenzae* (beta-lactamase-negative), *Klebsiella pneumoniae, Moraxella catarrhalis, Peptostreptococcus* sp., *Porphyromonas asaccharolytica, Prevotella bivia, Staphylococcus aureus* (methicillin-susceptible); *Streptococcus agalactiae, Streptococcus pneumoniae* (penicillin-susceptible), *Streptococcus pyogenes*

Uses: Adult patients with moderate to severe intraabdominal infections, complicated skin/skin structure infections, community-acquired pneumonia, complicated UTI, acute pelvic infections

Dosage and routes

Complicated intraabdominal infections

Adult: **IV**/IM 1 gm qd × 5-14 days

Complicated skin/skin structure infections

Adult: **IV**/IM 1 gm qd × 7-14 days

Community-acquired pneumonia

Adult: **IV**/IM 1 gm qd × 10-14 days

Complicated UTI

Adult: **IV**/IM 1 gm qd × 10-14 days

Acute pelvic infections

Adult: **IV**/IM 1 gm qd × 3-10 days

Available forms: Powder, lyophilized, 1 gm

Adverse effects

CNS: Insomnia, **seizures**, dizziness, *headache*

GI: *Diarrhea, nausea, vomiting,* **pseudomembranous colitis**

GU: *Vaginitis*

INTEG: *Rash,* urticaria, *pruritus,* pain at injection site, *infused vein complication, phlebitis/thrombophlebitis,* erythema at injection site

RESP: Dyspnea, cough, pharyngitis, rales, respiratory distress

SYST: **Anaphylaxis**

Contraindications: Hypersensitivity to this drug or its components, to amide-type local anesthetics (IM only); anaphylactic reactions to beta-lactams

P G **Precautions:** Pregnancy **B,** lactation, elderly, children, renal disease

Pharmacokinetics

Absorption	Almost completely absorbed (IM); completely (**IV**)
Distribution	85%-95% plasma protein bound
Metabolism	Liver (IM, **IV**)
Excretion	Urine (80%), feces (10%), breast milk (IM, **IV**)
Half-life	4 hr (**IV**)

Pharmacodynamics

	IM	IV
Onset	Unknown	Immediate
Peak	2.3 hr	Dose-dependent
Duration	Unknown	Unknown

Interactions
Individual drugs
Probenecid: ↑ ertapenem plasma levels; do not coadminister

NURSING CONSIDERATIONS
Assessment
- Assess for sensitivity to carbapenem antibiotics, other beta-lactam antibiotics, penicillins
- Assess for renal disease: lower dose may be required
- Assess bowel pattern qd: if severe diarrhea occurs, drug should be discontinued; may indicate pseudomembranous colitis
- Assess for infection: temperature, sputum, characteristics of wound before, during, after treatment
- (Alert) Assess for allergic reactions, anaphylaxis: rash, urticaria, pruritus; may occur a few days after therapy begins
- Assess for overgrowth of infection: perineal itching, fever, malaise, redness, pain, swelling, drainage, rash, diarrhea, change in cough or sputum

Nursing diagnoses
- ✓ Infection, risk for (uses)
- ✓ Diarrhea (adverse reaction)
- ✓ Injury, risk for (adverse reactions)
- ✓ Knowledge deficit (teaching)
- ✓ Noncompliance (teaching)

Implementation
- Administer by **IV** or IM
- Give after C&S is taken

IM route
- Reconstitute 1 gm vial of ertapenem with 3.2 ml of 1% lidocaine HCl without epinephrine, shake well
- Withdraw contents, administer deep IM in large muscle mass, use within 1 hr

IV route
- Do not co-infuse or mix with other medications; do not use diluents containing dextrose
- Reconstitute 1 gm vial of ertapenem with either 10 ml of water for inj, 0.9% NaCl, or bacteriostatic water for inj
- Shake well to dissolve, transfer contents of reconstituted vial to 50 ml 0.9% NaCl inj
- Complete inf within 6 hr

Patient/family education
- Advise patient to report severe diarrhea; may indicate pseudomembranous colitis
- Advise patient to report overgrowth of infection: black, furry tongue, vaginal itching, foul-smelling stools
- Caution patient to avoid breastfeeding; drug is excreted in breast milk

Evaluation
Positive therapeutic outcome
- Negative C&S, absence of signs and symptoms of infection

Treatment of overdose:
Administer epinephrine, antihistamines; resuscitate if needed (anaphylaxis)

esomeprazole (℞)
(es'oh-mep'rah-zohl)

Nexium

Func. class.: Anti-ulcer, proton pump inhibitor

Chem. class.: Benzimidazole

Pregnancy category B

Action: Suppresses gastric secretion by inhibiting hydrogen/potassium ATPase enzyme system in the gastric parietal cell; characterized as gastric acid pump inhibitor, since it blocks final step of acid production

Therapeutic Outcome: Absence of duodenal ulcers; decreased gastroesophageal reflux

Uses: Gastroesophageal reflux disease (GERD), severe erosive esophagitis; treatment of active duodenal ulcers in combination with antiinfectives for *Helicobacter pylori* infection

Dosage and routes
***Active duodenal ulcers associated with* H. pylori**

Adult: PO 40 mg qd × 10 days in combination with clarithromycin 500 mg bid × 10 days and amoxicillin 1000 mg bid × 10 days

GERD

Adult: PO 20 or 40 mg qd × 4-8 wk

Available forms: Caps 20, 40 mg

Adverse effects
CNS: *Headache, dizziness*

GI: *Diarrhea, flatulence,* anorexia, dry mouth

GU: UTI, urinary frequency

INTEG: *Rash,* dry skin

MISC: Fatigue

RESP: *Cough*

Contraindications: Hypersensitivity

Precautions: Pregnancy **B,** lactation, children, elderly

Pharmacokinetics

Absorption	Unknown
Distribution	97% plasma protein bound
Metabolism	Liver (metabolites)
Excretion	Urine (metabolites), feces (metabolites); in elderly, elimination rate ↓, bioavailability ↑
Half-life	1-1 ½ hr

Pharmacodynamics

Onset	Unknown
Peak	1 ½ hr
Duration	Unknown

Interactions
Individual drugs

Diazepam: Possible ↓ diazepam clearance resulting in ↑ diazepam serum concentrations

Flurazepam: ↑ serum levels of esomeprazole

Triazolam: ↑ serum levels of esomeprazole

Warfarin: Possible ↑ bleeding

NURSING CONSIDERATIONS
Assessment
- Assess GI system: bowel sounds q8h, abdomen for pain, swelling, anorexia
- Assess hepatic enzymes: AST, ALT, alkaline phosphatase during treatment

Nursing diagnoses
- ✓ Pain (uses)
- ✓ Knowledge deficit (teaching)

Implementation
- Administer at least 1 hr before eating
- Make sure capsule is swallowed whole; do not break, crush, or chew

Patient/family education
- Instruct patient to report severe diarrhea; drug may have to be discontinued
- Advise diabetic patients that hypoglycemia may occur
- Advise patient to avoid hazardous activities; dizziness may occur
- Advise patient to avoid alcohol,

salicylates, ibuprofen; may cause GI irritation

Evaluation
Positive therapeutic outcome
- Absence of epigastric pain, swelling, fullness

fondaparinux (℞)
(fon-dah-pair'ih-nux)
Arixtra
Func. class.: Anticoagulant, antithrombotic
Chem. class.: Synthetic, selective factor Xa inhibitor
Pregnancy category B

Action: Acts by antithrombin III (ATIII)-mediated selective inhibition of Factor Xa; neutralization of Factor Xa interrupts blood coagulation and inhibits thrombin formation; does not inactivate thrombin (activated Factor II) or affect platelets

Therapeutic Outcome: Prevention of deep vein thrombosis

Uses: Prevention of deep-vein thrombosis, pulmonary emboli in hip and knee replacement, hip fracture surgery

Dosage and routes
Adult: SC 2.5 mg qd; after hemostasis established, initial dose is given 6-8 hr after surgery

Available forms: Inj 2.5 mg/0.5 ml single-dose syringe

Adverse effects
CNS: *Fever*, confusion, headache, dizziness, *insomnia*
GI: *Nausea, vomiting*, diarrhea, dyspepsia, *constipation*, increased AST, ALT
GU: UTI, urinary retention
HEMA: *Anemia*, minor bleeding, purpura, hematoma, **thrombocytopenia, major bleeding (intracranial, cerebral, retroperitoneal hemorrhage), postoperative hemorrhage**
INTEG: Local reaction—*rash*, pruritus, inj site bleeding, increased wound drainage, bullous eruption
META: Hypokalemia
MISC: Hypotension, pain, *edema*

Contraindications: Hypersensitivity to this drug, heparin, or pork; hemophilia, leukemia with bleeding, peptic ulcer disease, hemorrhagic stroke, surgery, thrombocytopenic purpura, weight <50 kg, severe renal disease (CrCl <30 ml/min), **P** children

Precautions: Alcoholism, hepatic disease (severe), blood dyscrasias, heparin-induced thrombocytopenia, severe hypertension, subacute bacterial endocarditis, acute nephritis, lactation, pregnancy **B**, **G** elderly

Pharmacokinetics	
Absorption	Rapidly, completely absorbed
Distribution	Blood; does not bind to plasma proteins except 94% to ATIII
Metabolism	Unknown
Excretion	Eliminated unchanged in 72 hr in normal renal function
Half-life	17-21 hr

Pharmacodynamics	
Onset	Unknown
Peak	3 hr
Duration	Unknown

Interactions
- Do not mix with other drugs or infusion fluids
- Before starting fondaparinux, discontinue use of other drugs that may increase the risk of hemorrhage; monitor closely if coadministration is essential

NURSING CONSIDERATIONS
Assessment
- Assess blood studies (Hct, CBC, coagulation studies, platelets, occult

blood in stools), anti-Xa; thrombocytopenia may occur

- Assess for bleeding: gums, petechiae, ecchymosis, black tarry stools, hematuria; notify prescriber
- Assess for neurologic symptoms in patients who have received spinal anesthesia

Nursing diagnoses

- ✓ Injury, risk for (uses, adverse reactions)
- ✓ Tissue perfusion, altered (uses)
- ✓ Knowledge deficit (teaching)

Implementation

- Do not mix with other drugs or solutions
- Administer for 5-9 days
- Give only after screening patient for bleeding disorders
- Administer SC only; do not give IM
- Store at 77° F (25° C); do not freeze

SC route

- Check for discolored sol or sol with particulate; if present, do not give
- Begin 2 hr prior to surgery
- Administer to recumbent patient, rotate inj sites (left/right anterolateral, left/right posterolateral abdominal wall)
- Wipe surface of inj site with alcohol swab, twist plunger cap and remove, remove rigid needle guard by pulling straight off needle, do not aspirate, do not expel air bubble from surface
- Insert whole length of needle into skin fold held with thumb and forefinger
- When drug is injected, a soft click may be felt or heard
- Give at same time each day to maintain steady blood levels
- Avoid all IM injections that may cause bleeding
- ⚠ Administer only this drug when ordered; not interchangeable with heparin

Patient/family education

- Advise patient to use soft-bristle toothbrush to avoid bleeding gums, to use electric razor
- Advise patient to report any signs of bleeding: gums, under skin, urine, stools
- Caution patient to avoid OTC drugs containing aspirin

Evaluation

Positive therapeutic outcome

- Absence of deep vein thrombosis

formoterol fumarate (℞)

(for-moh'ter-ahl fyoo'mah-rayt)

Foradil Aerolizer

Func. class.: β-adrenergic agonist

Chem. class.: Sympathomimetic catecholamine

Pregnancy category C

Action: Has β_1 and β_2 action; relaxes bronchial smooth muscle and dilates the trachea and main bronchi by increasing levels of cAMP, which relaxes smooth muscles; causes increased contractility and heart rate by acting on β-receptors in the heart

➔ **Therapeutic Outcome:** Bronchodilation, increased heart rate and cardiac output from action on β-receptors in heart

Uses: Maintenance treatment of asthma, prevention of exercise-induced bronchospasm

Dosage and routes

Maintenance treatment of asthma

P ***Adult/child ≥5 yr:*** INH AM and PM, 1 cap q12h using aerolizer inhaler

Prevention of exercise-induced bronchospasm

P ***Adult/child ≥12 yr:*** PRN occasionally 1 cap at least 15 min before exercise

Available forms: INH powder in cap 12 μg

Adverse effects

CNS: Tremors, *anxiety*, insomnia, headache, dizziness, stimulation
CV: Palpitations, tachycardia, hypertension
GI: Nausea, vomiting
RESP: Bronchial irritation, dryness of oropharynx, **bronchospasms** (overuse)

Contraindications: Hypersensitivity to sympathomimetics, narrow-angle glaucoma

Precautions: Pregnancy **C**, cardiac disorders, hyperthyroidism, diabetes mellitus, prostatic hypertrophy, elderly (G)

Pharmacokinetics

Absorption	Rapid (INH)
Distribution	Plasma protein binding 61%-64% at concentrations of 0.1-100 ng/mL; 31%-38% at concentrations of 5-500 ng/mL
Metabolism	Liver, lungs, GI tract
Excretion	Urine, feces
Half-life	10 hr mean terminal elimination half-life

Pharmacodynamics

Onset	Unknown
Peak	5 min (INH)
Duration	Unknown

Interactions

Drug classifications

β-blockers: ↓ action of formoterol
Sympathomimetics: ↑ action of both drugs

NURSING CONSIDERATIONS

Assessment

- Assess respiratory function: B/P, pulse, lung sounds
- Assess I&O ratio; check for urinary retention, frequency, hesitancy
- Assess for paresthesias and coldness of extremities; peripheral blood flow may decrease

Nursing diagnoses

- ✓ Airway clearance, ineffective (uses)
- ✓ Impaired gas exchange (uses)
- ✓ Knowledge deficit (teaching)

Implementation

- Store at room temperature, protect from heat, moisture
- Do not use discolored solution

Patient/family education

- Review package insert with patient and inform about all aspects of drug
- Teach correct use of inhaler
- (G) (P) Teach use of spacer device in elderly or children
- Advise patient to avoid getting aerosol in eyes
- Instruct patient to rinse mouth after use
- Advise patient to wash inhaler in warm water and dry qd
- Advise patient to avoid smoking, smoke-filled rooms, persons with respiratory infections

Evaluation

Positive therapeutic outcome

- Absence of dyspnea, wheezing
- Improved airway exchange
- Improved ABGs

Treatment of overdose: Administer β-blocker

frovatriptan (℞)

(froh-vah-trip'tan)
Frova
Func. class.: Antimigraine agent
Chem. class.: 5-HT_1 receptor agonist

Pregnancy category C

Action: Binds selectively to the vascular 5-HT_{1B}, 5-HT_{1D} receptor subtypes, exerts antimigraine effect; binds to benzodiazepine receptor sites

➔ **Therapeutic Outcome:** Absence of migraines

Uses: Acute treatment of migraine with or without aura

Dosage and routes

Adult: PO 2.5 mg, a 2nd dose may be taken after ≥2 hr; max 3 tabs/day (7.5 mg)

Available forms: Tabs 2.5 mg

Adverse effects

CNS: *Hot sensation*, paresthesia, *dizziness*, headache, fatigue, cold sensation

CV: *Flushing*, **MI,** chest pain

GI: Dry mouth, dyspepsia

INTEG: Photosensitivity

MS: Skeletal pain

Contraindications: Angina pectoris, history of MI, documented silent ischemia, Prinzmetal's angina, ischemic heart disease, concurrent ergotamine-containing preparations, uncontrolled hypertension, hypersensitivity, basilar or hemiplegic migraine; ischemic bowel disease; peripheral vascular disease

Precautions: Postmenopausal women, men >40 yr, risk factors for CAD, hypercholesterolemia, obesity, diabetes, impaired hepatic function, P pregnancy **C,** lactation, children, G elderly

Pharmacokinetics

Absorption	Absolute bioavailability of PO dose ~20% in males, 30% in females
Distribution	Protein binding 15%; reversibly bound to blood cells at equilibrium 60%
Metabolism	Liver
Excretion	Urine (32%), feces (62%)
Half-life	25-29 hr

Pharmacodynamics

Onset	10 min-2 hr
Peak	2-4 hr
Duration	Unknown

Interactions

Individual drugs

Ergot: ↑ vasospastic effects
Propranolol: ↑ effects of frovatriptan

Drug classifications

5-HT$_1$ agonists: ↑ vasospastic effects
Ergot derivatives: ↑ vasospastic effects
Oral contraceptives: ↑ effects of frovatriptan
SSRIs: Weakness, incoordination, hyperreflexia

NURSING CONSIDERATIONS

Assessment

- Assess B/P; signs/symptoms of coronary vasospasms
- Assess for stress level, activity, recreation, coping mechanisms
- Assess neurologic status: LOC, paresthesia, hot/cold sensations, dizziness, headache, fatigue
- Assess for ingestion of tyramine-containing foods (pickled products, beer, wine, aged cheese), food additives, preservatives, colorings, artificial sweeteners, chocolate, caffeine, which may precipitate these types of headaches

Nursing diagnoses

✓ Pain (uses)
✓ Knowledge deficit (teaching)

Implementation

- Provide quiet, calm environment with decreased stimulation from noise, bright light, excessive talking

PO route

- ⊘ Ensure that tablets are swallowed whole

Patient/family education

- Instruct patient to report any side effects to prescriber
- Advise patient to use contraception while taking drug
- Advise patient that photosensitivity may occur, to use sunscreen and wear protective clothing when outdoors
- Advise patient to have dark, quiet environment available

Evaluation

Positive therapeutic outcome

- Decrease in frequency, severity of migraine

Treatment of overdose: No specific antidote; monitor patient closely for ≥48 hr, treat any symptoms as necessary

galantamine (℞)
(gah-lan'tah-meen)
Reminyl
Func. class.: Cholinesterase inhibitor

Pregnancy category B

Action: May enhance cholinergic functioning by increasing acetylcholine

Therapeutic Outcome: Decreased signs and symptoms of Alzheimer's dementia

Uses: Alzheimer's dementia

Dosage and routes
Adult: PO 4 mg bid; after 4 wk or more may increase to 8 mg bid; after another 4 wk may increase to 12 mg bid

Available forms: Tabs 4, 8, 12 mg

Adverse effects
CNS: *Tremors, insomnia,* depression, dizziness, headache, somnolence, fatigue
CV: Bradycardia
GI: *Nausea, vomiting, anorexia, abdominal distress, flatulence,* diarrhea
GU: Urinary incontinence
META: Weight decrease
MISC: Anemia, hematuria
MS: Asthenia
RESP: URI, rhinitis

Contraindications: Hypersensitivity to this drug

Precautions: Renal disease, hepatic disease, respiratory disease, seizure disorder, peptic ulcer, pregnancy **B**, asthma, lactation, children, peptic ulcer

Pharmacokinetics

Absorption	Rapidly and completely absorbed
Distribution	Unknown
Metabolism	P450 enzyme
Excretion	Kidneys; clearance ↓ in the elderly, hepatic disease, females (20% lower)
Half-life	Unknown

Pharmacodynamics

Onset	Unknown
Peak	Unknown
Duration	Unknown

Interactions
Individual drugs
Cimetidine: ↑ galantamine bioavailability
Erythromycin: ↑ galantamine bioavailability
Ketoconazole: ↑ galantamine bioavailability
Paroxetine: ↑ galantamine bioavailability
Drug classifications
Cholinesterase inhibitors: Synergistic effect
Cholinomimetics: Synergistic effect

NURSING CONSIDERATIONS
Assessment
- Assess liver function enzymes: AST, ALT, alkaline phosphatase, LDH, bilirubin, CBC
- Assess for severe GI effects: nausea, vomiting, anorexia, weight loss
- Assess B/P, respiration during initial treatment
- Assess mental status: affect, mood, behavioral changes, depression

Nursing diagnoses
- ✓ Knowledge deficit (teaching)
- ✓ Cognitive impairment (uses)

Implementation
- Provide assistance with ambulation during beginning therapy
- Perform complete suicide assessment

PO route

- Give with meals, morning and evening

Patient/family education

- Teach patient or caregiver correct procedure for giving oral solution, using instruction sheet provided
- Instruct patient or caregiver to notify prescriber of severe GI effects
- Instruct patient or caregiver to report hypo/hypertension

Evaluation

Positive therapeutic outcome

- Decreased symptoms of dementia
- Increased coherence
- Improved cognitive performance (memory, orientation, attention, reasoning, language, praxis)

Treatment of overdose:

Administer **IV** atropine titrated to effect at an initial dose of 0.5-1.0 mg, with subsequent doses based on clinical response; provide general supportive measures

imatinib (℞)

(im-ah-tin'ib)

Gleevec

Func. class.: Misc. antineoplastic

Chem. class.: Protein-tyrosine kinase inhibitor

Pregnancy category D

Action: Inhibits Bcr-Abl tyrosine kinase created in chronic myeloid leukemia (CML)

➔ **Therapeutic Outcome:** Decreased tumor size, prevention of spread of cancer

Uses: Treatment of CML

Dosage and routes

Adult: PO 400 mg/day (chronic phase); 600 mg/day (accelerated phase/blast crisis); give with meal and large glass of water, continue as long as response is good, may increase by 200 mg/day as needed

Available forms: Cap 100 mg

Adverse effects

CV: Hemorrhage

CNS: **CNS hemorrhage,** headache

GI: *Nausea,* **hepatotoxicity**, *vomiting, dyspepsia,* **GI hemorrhage**, *anorexia*

HEMA: **Neutropenia, thrombocytopenia**

INTEG: *Rash, pruritus*

META: Edema, fluid retention, hypokalemia, weight increase

MISC: Fatigue, epistaxis, pyrexia, night sweats

MS: Cramps, pain, arthralgia, myalgia

RESP: Cough, dyspnea, nasopharyngitis, pneumonia

Contraindications: Hypersensitivity, pregnancy **D**

P G **Precautions:** Lactation, children, elderly

Pharmacokinetics	
Absorption	Well absorbed; bound to plasma protein (95%)
Distribution	Unknown
Metabolism	Liver (metabolites)
Excretion	Feces, primarily (metabolites)
Half-life	18-40 hr

Pharmacodynamics	
Onset	Unknown
Peak	Unknown
Duration	Unknown

Interactions

Individual drugs

Carbamazepine: ↓ imatinib concentrations

Clarithromycin: ↑ imatinib concentrations

Dexamethasone: ↓ imatinib concentrations

Erythromycin: ↑ imatinib concentrations

Ketoconazole: ↑ imatinib concentrations

Itraconazole: ↑ imatinib concentrations

Phenobarbital: ↓ imatinib concentrations
Phenytoin: ↓ imatinib concentrations
Rifampin: ↓ imatinib concentrations
Simvastatin: ↑ plasma concentrations
Warfarin: ↑ plasma concentration of warfarin; avoid coadministration; use low-molecular weight anticoagulants instead

Drug classifications
Calcium channel blockers, dihydropyridine: ↑ plasma concentrations

Herb/drug
St. John's wort: ↓ imatinib concentration

NURSING CONSIDERATIONS
Assessment
- Assess ANC and platelets; in chronic phase if ANC <1 × 10^9/L and/or platelets <50 × 10^9/L, stop until ANC >1.5 × 10^9/L and platelets >75 × 10^9/L; in accelerated phase/blast crisis if ANC <0.5 × 10^9/L and/or platelets <10 × 10^9/L, determine whether cytopenia is related to biopsy/aspirate, if not, reduce dose by 200 mg, if cytopenia continues, reduce dose by another 100 mg; if cytopenia continues for 4 wks, stop drug until ANC ≥1 × 10^9/L
- Assess for hepatotoxicity: monitor LFTs, before treatment and qmo
- Assess CBC, differential, platelet count weekly; withhold drug if WBC is <3500/mm^3, or platelet count <100,000/mm^3; notify prescriber of these results; drug should be discontinued
- Assess food preferences: list likes, dislikes
- Assess GI symptoms: frequency of stools
- Assess signs of fluid retention, edema: weigh, monitor lung sounds, assess for edema

Nursing diagnoses
✓ Injury, risk for (side effects)
✓ Knowledge deficit (teaching)

Implementation
- Give with meal and large glass of water
- Provide nutritious diet with iron, vit supplement, low fiber, few dairy products
- Store at 25° C (77° F)

Patient/family education
- Instruct patient to report adverse reactions immediately: shortness of breath, swelling of extremities, bleeding

Evaluation
Positive therapeutic outcome
- Decrease in spread of cancer

nesiritide (℞)
(nes-eer'ih-tide)
Natrecor
Func. class.: Vasodilator
Chem. class.: Human B-type natriuretic peptide
Pregnancy category C

Action: Uses DNA technology; human B-type natriuretic peptide binds to the receptor in vascular smooth muscle and endothelial cells, leading to smooth muscle relaxation

Therapeutic Outcome: Improvement in symptoms of congestive heart failure (CHF)

Uses: Acutely decompensated CHF

Dosage and routes
Adult: **IV** 2 μg/kg, then **IV** inf 0.01 μg/kg/min

Available forms: Powder for inj, 1.5 mg single-use vial

Adverse effects
CNS: Headache, insomnia, dizziness, anxiety, confusion, paresthesia, tremor
CV: *Hypotension,* **tachycardia,** dysrhythmias, bradycardia, ventricular tachycardia, ventricular extrasystoles, **atrial fibrillation**
GI: Abdominal pain, vomiting, nausea

INTEG: Rash, sweating, pruritus, inj site reaction
MISC: Back pain
RESP: Increased cough, apnea

Contraindications: Hypersensitivity, cardiogenic shock or B/P <90 mm Hg as primary therapy

Precautions: Pregnancy **C;** mitral stenosis; significant valvular stenosis, restriction, or obstructive cardiomyopathy, or any condition that depends on venous return; renal disease; lactation; P children

Pharmacokinetics

Absorption	Vascular smooth muscle and endothelial cells
Distribution	Unknown
Metabolism	Unknown
Excretion	Bound to cell surfaces, internalized, and proteolyzed; cleaved by endopeptidases on vascular lumenal surface; renal filtration
Half-life	18 min

Pharmacodynamics

Onset	15 min
Peak	1 hr
Duration	Unknown

Interactions

Drug classifications

ACE inhibitors: ↑ symptomatic hypotension

NURSING CONSIDERATIONS

Assessment

- Assess PCWP, RAP, cardiac index, MPAP
- Assess B/P, pulse during treatment until stable

Nursing diagnoses

✓ Tissue perfusion, altered (uses)
✓ Knowledge deficit (teaching)

Implementation

IV **IV route**

- Do not administer nesiritide through a central heparin-coated catheter; heparin should be administered through a separate catheter
- Prime **IV** fluid with inf of 25 ml before connecting to patient's vascular access port and before bolus dose or **IV** inf
- Reconstitute one 1.5 mg vial/5 ml of diluent from prefilled 250 ml plastic **IV** bag with diluent of choice (D_5, 0.9% NaCl, D_5/0.9% NaCl, D_5/0.2% NaCl); do not shake vial, roll gently; use only clear sol
- Withdraw all contents of reconstituted vial and add to the 250 ml plastic **IV** bag (6 μg/ml), invert bag several times
- Use within 24 hr of reconstituting

Evaluation

Positive therapeutic outcome

- Improvement in CHF with improved PCWP, RAP, MPAP

perflutren lipid microsphere

See Appendix F

tenofovir disoproxil fumarate (℞)

(ten-oh-foh'veer dis-oh-prox'il fyoo'mah-rate)

Viread

Func. class.: Antiretroviral
Chem. class.: Nucleoside analog reverse transcriptase inhibitor

Pregnancy category B

Action: Inhibits replication of HIV virus by competing with the natural substrate and then incorporating into cellular DNA by viral reverse transcriptase, thereby terminating cellular DNA chain

➔ **Therapeutic Outcome:** Improved symptoms of HIV infection

Uses: HIV-1 infection with other antiretrovirals

Dosage and routes

Adult: PO 300 mg with meal; if used with didanosine, give tenofovir 2 hr before or 1 hr after didanosine

Available forms: Tabs 300 mg tenofovir disoproxil fumarate (equivalent to 245 mg tenofovir disoproxil)

Adverse effects

CNS: *Headache*

GI: *Nausea, vomiting, diarrhea,* anorexia, *flatulence, abdominal pain*

SYST: Change in body fat distribution

Contraindications: Hypersensitivity

P G **Precautions:** Pregnancy **B,** lactation, children, elderly, renal disease, hepatic insufficiency, pancreatitis

Pharmacokinetics

Absorption	Rapidly absorbed
Distribution	Extravascular space; bound to serum plasma <0.7%; to serum proteins <7.2%
Metabolism	Unknown
Excretion	Urine, unchanged (70%-80%)
Half-life	Unknown

Pharmacodynamics

Onset	Unknown
Peak	0.6-1.4 hr
Duration	Unknown

Interactions

Individual drugs

Acyclovir: ↑ level of tenofovir
Cidofovir: ↑ level of tenofovir
Didanosine: ↑ level of didanosine when coadministered with tenofovir
Ganciclovir: ↑ level of tenofovir
Valacyclovir: ↑ level of tenofovir
Valganciclovir: ↑ level of tenofovir

Drug classifications

↑ levels of tenofovir with any drug that ↓ renal function

NURSING CONSIDERATIONS

Assessment

- Assess liver studies: AST, ALT, bilirubin; amylase, lipase, triglycerides periodically during treatment
- Assess for bone, renal toxicity: if bone abnormalities are suspected, obtain tests: serum phosphorus, creatinine
- Assess for lactic acidosis, severe hepatomegaly with steatosis

Nursing diagnoses

- ✓ Infection, risk for (uses)
- ✓ Injury, risk for (adverse reactions)
- ✓ Knowledge deficit (teaching)

Implementation

- Administer PO qd with meal
- Store at 25° C (77° F)

Patient/family education

- Instruct patient to take this drug 2 hr before or 1 hr after taking didanosine (if used)
- Instruct patient to take drug with meal
- Advise patients that GI complaints resolve after 3-4 wk of treatment
- Caution patient not to breastfeed while taking this drug
- Inform patient that drug must be taken qd even if patient feels better
- Advise patient to continue follow-up visits since serious toxicity may occur; blood counts must be done q2 wk
- Inform patient that drug will control symptoms but is not a cure for HIV; patient is still infectious, may pass HIV virus on to others
- Advise patient that other drugs may be necessary to prevent other infections
- Advise patient that changes in body fat distribution may occur

Evaluation

Positive therapeutic outcome

- Decrease in signs/symptoms of HIV

valdecoxib (℞)
(val-deh-cock'sib)

Bextra

Func. class.: Nonsteroidal antiinflammatory

Chem. class.: COX-2 inhibitor

Pregnancy category
C (1st/2nd trimester),
D (3rd trimester)

Action: Inhibits prostaglandin synthesis by decreasing COX-2 enzyme needed for biosynthesis; analgesic, antiinflammatory, antipyretic properties

→ **Therapeutic Outcome:** Decreased pain, inflammation

Uses: Acute, chronic rheumatoid arthritis, osteoarthritis, primary dysmenorrhea

Dosage and routes

Osteoarthritis/adult rheumatoid arthritis

Adult: PO 10 mg

Primary dysmenorrhea

Adult: PO 20 mg bid, prn

Available forms: Tabs 10, 20 mg

Adverse effects

CNS: *Fatigue, anxiety, depression, nervousness, paresthesia,* dizziness, insomnia

CV: **Tachycardia,** angina, **MI,** palpitations, dysrhythmias, hypertension, fluid retention

EENT: Tinnitus, hearing loss, blurred vision, glaucoma, cataract, conjunctivitis, eye pain

GI: *Nausea, anorexia, vomiting, constipation, dry mouth,* diverticulitis, gastritis, gastroenteritis, hemorrhoids, hiatal hernia, stomatitis, **GI bleeding**

GU: **Nephrotoxicity:** *dysuria,* **hematuria, oliguria, azotemia,** cystitis, UTI

HEMA: *Blood dyscrasias,* epistaxis, bruising, anemia

INTEG: Purpura, rash, pruritus, sweating, erythema, petechiae, photosensitivity, alopecia

RESP: Pharyngitis, shortness of breath, pneumonia, coughing

Contraindications: Hypersensitivity to this drug, aspirin, iodides, other NSAIDs, sulfonamides; asthma triad, asthma, pregnancy 3rd trimester **D**

Precautions: Pregnancy 1st/2nd trimester **C**, lactation; bleeding; GI, cardiac, renal, hepatic disorders; hypersensitivity to other antiinflammatory agents, glucocorticoids, anticoagulants; hypertension, severe dehydration, **G** elderly, **P** children <18 yr

Pharmacokinetics

Absorption	Well absorbed (83%)
Distribution	Plasma protein binding 98%
Metabolism	Liver (P450 and non-P450 systems)
Excretion	Urine (metabolites, 70%)
Half-life	8-11 hr

Pharmacodynamics

Onset	Unknown
Peak	3 hr, delayed 1-2 hr by high-fat meal
Duration	Unknown

Interactions

Individual drugs

Aspirin: ↓ effect of aspirin, ↑ adverse reactions of valdecoxib

Fluconazole: ↑ valdecoxib blood level

Furosemide: ↓ effect of furosemide

Ketoconazole: ↑ valdecoxib blood level

Lithium: ↑ toxicity of lithium

Drug classifications

ACE inhibitors: ↓ effect of ACE inhibitors

Anticoagulants: ↑ effect of anticoagulants

Antineoplastics: ↑ toxicity antineoplastics

Glucocorticoids: ↑ adverse reactions

NSAIDs: ↑ adverse reactions

Thiazide diuretics: ↓ effect of thiazide diuretics

NURSING CONSIDERATIONS

Assessment

- Assess for pain of rheumatoid arthritis, osteoarthritis; check ROM, inflammation of joints, characteristics of pain
- Assess blood counts during therapy; watch for decreasing platelets; if low, therapy may need to be discontinued, restarted after hematologic recovery
- Alert: Assess for blood dyscrasias (thrombocytopenia): bruising, fatigue, bleeding, poor healing

Nursing diagnoses

- ✓ Pain (uses)
- ✓ Mobility, impaired physical (uses)
- ✓ Injury, risk for (side effects)
- ✓ Knowledge deficit (teaching)

Implementation

PO route

- Give with food or milk to decrease gastric symptoms, do not increase dose

Patient/family education

- Instruct patient to check with prescriber to determine when drug should be discontinued before surgery
- Advise patient that drug must be continued for prescribed time to be effective; to avoid other NSAIDs, aspirin, sulfonamides
- Advise patient to notify prescriber if pregnancy is planned or suspected
- Caution patient to notify prescriber of GI symptoms: black, tarry stools; cramping or rash; edema of extremities; weight gain
- Caution patient to report bleeding, bruising, fatigue, malaise since blood dyscrasias do occur
- Instruct patient to take with a full glass of water to enhance absorption

Evaluation

Positive therapeutic outcome

- Decreased pain, inflammation in arthritic conditions
- Decreased dysmenorrhea

Treatment of anaphylaxis: Epinephrine, antihistamines; resuscitate if needed

valganciclovir (℞)

(val-gan-sy'kloh-veer)

Valcyte

Func. class: Antiviral

Chem. class: Synthetic nucleoside analog

Pregnancy category C

Action: Valganciclovir is metabolized to ganciclovir; inhibits replication of human cytomegalovirus in vivo and in vitro by selectively inhibiting viral DNA synthesis

→ **Therapeutic Outcome:** Decreased proliferation of virus responsible for CMV retinitis

Uses: Cytomegalovirus (CMV) retinitis in immunocompromised persons, including those with AIDS, after indirect ophthalmoscopy confirms diagnosis

Dosage and routes

Adult: PO induction 900 mg bid × 21 days with food; maintenance 900 mg qd with food

Renal Dose

Reduce dose; CrCl ≥60 ml/min same dosage as above; CrCl 40-59 ml/min 450 mg bid, then 450 mg qd; CrCl 25-39 ml/min 450 mg qd, then 450 mg q2 days; CrCl 10-24 ml/min 450 mg q2 days, then 450 mg 2×/ week

Available forms: Tab 450 mg

Adverse effects

CNS: *Fever*, chills, **coma**, *confusion*, abnormal thoughts, dizziness, bizarre dreams, *headache*, psychosis, tremors, somnolence, *paresthesia, weakness, seizures*

EENT: Retinal detachment in CMV retinitis

GI: *Abnormal LFTs, nausea, vomit-*

ing, anorexia, diarrhea, abdominal pain, **hemorrhage**
GU: **Hematuria**, increased creatinine, BUN
HEMA: **Granulocytopenia, thrombocytopenia, irreversible neutropenia, anemia, eosinophilia**
INTEG: Rash, alopecia, *pruritus*, urticaria, pain at inj site, phlebitis
MISC: Local and systemic infections and sepsis

Contraindications: Hypersensitivity to acyclovir or ganciclovir, absolute neutrophil count <500/mm^3, platelet count <25,000/mm^3, hemodialysis

Precautions: Preexisting cytopenias, renal function impairment, P pregnancy **C**, lactation, children <6 G mo, elderly

Pharmacokinetics

Absorption	Well absorbed from GI tract
Distribution	Plasma protein binding unknown; crosses blood-brain barrier, CSF
Metabolism	Rapidly metabolized in intestinal wall and liver to ganciclovir
Excretion	Kidneys (ganciclovir)
Half-life	3-4 ½ hr

Pharmacodynamics

Onset	Unknown
Peak	1-3 hr
Duration	Unknown

Interactions
Individual drugs
Adriamycin: ↑ toxicity
Amphotericin B: ↑ toxicity
Cyclosporine: ↑ toxicity
Dapsone: ↑ toxicity
Doxorubicin: ↑ toxicity
Flucytosine: ↑ toxicity
Imipenem/cilastatin: ↑ seizures
Pentamidine: ↑ toxicity
Probenecid: ↓ renal clearance of valganciclovir
Radiation: Severe granulocytopenia; do not coadminister
Trimethoprim-sulfamethoxazole combinations: ↑ toxicity
Vinblastine: ↑ toxicity
Vincristine: ↑ toxicity
Zidovudine: Severe granulocytopenia; do not coadminister

Drug classifications
Nucleoside analogs, other: ↑ toxicity
Antineoplastics: Severe granulocytopenia; do not coadminister

NURSING CONSIDERATIONS
Assessment
- Assess for leukopenia/neutropenia/thrombocytopenia: WBCs, platelets q2d during 2×/d dosing and then qwk
- Assess for leukopenia qd with WBC count in patients with prior leukopenia using other nucleoside analogs or for whom leukopenia counts are <1000 cells/mm^3 at start of treatment
- Assess serum creatinine or CrCl ≥q2 wk

Nursing diagnoses
✓ Infection, risk for (uses)
✓ Injury, risk for (uses, adverse reactions)
✓ Knowledge deficit (teaching)

Implementation
PO route
- Give with food

Patient/family education
- Inform patient that drug does not cure condition, that regular ophthalmologic examinations are necessary
- Caution patient that major toxicities may necessitate discontinuing drug
- Caution patient to use contraception during treatment and that infertility may occur; men should use barrier contraception for 90 days after treatment
- Instruct patient to take with food
- ❗ Instruct patient to report infection: fever, chills, sore throat; blood dyscrasias: bruising, bleeding, petechiae

- Advise patient to avoid crowds, persons with respiratory infections
- Caution patient to use sunscreen to prevent burns

Evaluation

Positive therapeutic outcome

- Decreased symptoms of CMV

Treatment of overdose:

Maintain adequate hydration; dialysis may help reduce serum concentrations; consider use of hematopoietic growth factors

zoledronic acid (℞)

(zoh'leh-drah'nick ass'id))

Zometa

Func. class.: Bone-resorption inhibitor, electrolyte modifier

Chem. class.: Bisphosphonate

Pregnancy category C

Action: Potent inhibitor of osteoclastic bone resorption; inhibits osteoclastic activity, reduces bone resorption and inhibits skeletal calcium release caused by stimulating factors released by tumors; reduction of abnormal bone resorption is responsible for therapeutic effect in hypercalcemia; may directly block dissolution of hydroxyapatite bone crystals; inhibits normal and abnormal bone resorption, apparently without inhibiting bone formation and mineralization

➡ **Therapeutic Outcome:** Serum calcium at normal level

Uses: Moderate to severe hypercalcemia associated with malignancy

Dosage and routes

***Adult:* IV** inf 4 mg, given as a single inf over ≥15 min, may re-treat with 4 mg if serum calcium does not return to normal within 1 wk

Available forms: Powder for inj 4 mg

Adverse effects

CV: Hypertension

GI: Abdominal pain, anorexia, constipation, nausea, diarrhea

GU: UTI, fluid overload, possible reduced renal function

INTEG: Redness, swelling, induration, pain on palpation at site of catheter insertion

META: Anemia, hypokalemia, hypomagnesemia, hypophosphatemia

MISC: ***Fever, chills, arthralgias, myalgias, flu-like symptoms***

MS: Bone pain

Contraindications: Hypersensitivity to bisphosphonates

P **Precautions:** Children, nursing mothers, pregnancy **C,** renal dysfunction, asthma-sensitive asthmatic patients

Pharmacokinetics	
Absorption	Rapidly cleared from circulation
Distribution	Taken up mainly by bones; plasma protein binding ~22%
Metabolism	Not metabolized
Excretion	Kidneys (~50% eliminated in urine within 24 hr)
Half-life	146 hr

Pharmacodynamics	
Onset	Unknown
Peak	15 min
Duration	Unknown

Interactions

Individual drugs

Calcium: ↓ effect of zoledronic acid

Digoxin: Hypomagnesemia, hypokalemia

Infusion solutions, calcium-containing: Do not mix with Ca-containing infusion sol such as Ringer's sol

Vitamin D: ↓ effect of zoledronic acid

NURSING CONSIDERATIONS

Assessment

- Assess renal studies and Ca, P, Mg, K
- Assess for hypercalcemia: paresthesia, twitching, laryngospasm; Chvostek's, Trousseau's signs

Nursing diagnoses

✓ Injury, risk for (uses, adverse reactions)
✓ Fluid excess (side effects)
✓ Knowledge deficit (teaching)

Implementation

- Saline hydration must be performed before administration; urine output should be 2 L/day during treatment, do not overhydrate
- Sol reconstituted with sterile water may be stored under refrigeration for up to 24 hr **IV**
- Administer after reconstituting by adding 5 ml of sterile water for inj to each vial, then add to ≥100 ml of sterile 0.9% NaCl, D_5, run over ≥5 min
- Administer in separate **IV** line from all other drugs

Patient/family education

- Instruct patient to report hypercalcemic relapse: nausea, vomiting, bone pain, thirst
- Advise patient to continue with dietary recommendations including calcium and vit D

Evaluation

Positive therapeutic outcome

- Calcium levels decreased to normal

Treatment of overdose:

Correct clinically relevant reductions in serum calcium by administering **IV** calcium gluconate; in serum phosphorus, with potassium or sodium phosphate; in serum magnesium, with magnesium sulfate

Appendix B

Recent FDA Drug Approvals

GENERIC NAME	TRADE NAME	USE
estradiol	Alora	For the prevention of postmenopausal osteoporosis at all strengths
ibritumomab	Zevalin	For treatment of non-Hodgkin's lymphoma
olmesartan	Benicar	For use in treating hypertension
morphine sulfate	Avinza	For the relief of moderate to severe pain requiring continuous around-the-clock opioid therapy for an extended time
thyrotropin alfa	Thyrogen	For use as an adjunctive tool for serum Tg testing
urofollitropin	Bravelle	Follicle-stimulating hormone for infertility treatment

Tg, Thyroglobulin.

Appendix C

High Alert Drugs

The Joint Commission on Accreditation of Healthcare Organizations recently released a list of medications with the highest risk of injury when misused. Based on a study performed by the Institute for Safe Medication Practices, these high-alert medications have been divided into six groups: insulins, opiates, antineoplastics, injectable potassium chloride or phosphate, intravenous anticoagulants, and sodium chloride solutions stronger than 0.9%. To help nurses identify these drugs, each specific drug monograph has been identified with a "HIGH ALERT" heading throughout the book. A complete list of high-alert drugs located in this book follows.

abciximab
adenosine
aldesleukin
alteplase
amiodarone
anistreplase
antihemophilic factor
antithrombin III
ardeparin
argatroban
arsenic trioxide
asparaginase
atropine
basiliximab
bivalirudin
bleomycin
bretylium
busulfan
calfactant
carboplatin
carmustine
cisplatin
coagulation factor VIIa, recombinant
cyclophosphamide
cytarabine
dacarbazine
daclizumab
dactinomycin
dalteparin
danaparoid
daunorubicin
dezocine
digoxin
diltiazem
dopamine
doxacurium
doxorubicin
droperidol
enoxaparin
ephedrine
epinephrine
epirubicin
eptifibatide
etoposide
factor IX complex/Factor IV
fentanyl
fentanyl/droperidol
fluorouracil
gallamine
gemtuzumab
heparin
hydromorphone
ibutilide
idarubicin
ifosfamide
insulin
irinotecan
ketamine
lepirudin
leuprolide
lidocaine
magnesium sulfate
melphalan
meperidine
methadone
methotrexate
milrinone
mitomycin
mitoxantrone
mivacurium
morphine
nalbuphine
nitroprusside
norepinephrine
oxycodone
oxymorphone
oxytocin
pancuronium

pegaspargase
pentazocine
pentobarbital IV
pentostatin
phenobarbital IV
pipecuronium
plicamycin
poractant alfa
propofol
propoxyphene
remifentanil
rocuronium
secobarbital IV
streptokinase
succinylcholine
sufentanil
tenecteplase
thiopental
tinzaparin
topotecan
trastuzumab
tubocurarine
urokinase
vecuronium
vinblastine
vincristine
vinorelbine
warfarin

1. Cohen MR, Kilo CM: High-alert medications: safeguarding against errors. In Cohen MR, editor: *Medication Errors,* Washington, D.C., 1999, American Pharmaceutical Association.
2. Joint Commission on Accreditation of Healthcare Organizations: High-alert medications and patient safety, *Sentinel Event Alert,* Nov, 1999. Available at www.jcaho.org/edu_pub/sealert/sea11.html [Accessed on 4/30/02].

Appendix D

Ophthalmic, Nasal, Topical, and Otic Products

OPHTHALMIC PRODUCTS

α-ADRENERGIC BLOCKER

dapiprazole (℞)
(da-pip'ra-zole)
Rev-Eyes

ANESTHETICS

proparacaine (℞)
(proe-par'a-kane)
AK-Taine, Alcaine, Diocaine ✤, Ocu-Caine, Ophthaine, Ophthestic, Specto-Caine

tetracaine
(tet'ra-kane)
Minims Tetracaine, Pontocaine Eye, Pontocaine Hcl

ANTIHISTAMINES

emedastine
(ee-med'-a-steen)
Emadine

levocabastine (℞)
(lee-voh-cab'ah-steen)
Livostin

olopatadine (℞)
(oh-loh-pat'ah-deen)
Patanol

ANTIINFECTIVES

bacitracin (℞)
(bass-i-tray'sin)
AK-Tracin, Bacitracin Ophthalmic

brimonidine
(bri-moe'ni-deen)
Alphagan

chloramphenicol (℞)
(klor-am-fen'i-kole)
AK-Chlor, Chloramphenicol, Chloramphenicol Ophthalmic, Chloromycetin Ophthalmic, Chloroptic, Chloroptic S.O.P., Fenicol ✤, Isopto Fenical ✤, Pentamycin ✤

ciprofloxacin (℞)
(sip-ro-floks'a-sin)
Ciloxan

erythromycin (℞)
(er-ith-roe-mye'sin)
AK-Mycin, erythromycin, Ilotycin

gentamicin (℞)
(jen-ta-mye'sin)
Garamycin Ophthalmic, Genoptic Ophthalmic, Genoptic S.O.P., Gentacidin, Gent-AK, gentamicin, Gentamicin Ophthalmic Liquifilm, Gentak

idoxuridine-IDU (℞)
(eye-dox-yoor'i-deen)
Herplex, Stoxil

levofloxacin (℞)
(lee-voh-flock'sah-sin)
Quixin

natamycin (℞)
(nat-a-mye'sin)
Natacyn

norfloxacin (℞)
(nor-floks'a-sin)
Chibroxin

ofloxacin (℞)
(oh-floks'a-sin)
Ocuflox

polymyxin B (℞)
(pol-ee-mix′in)
Aerosporin, polymyxin B sulfate

silver nitrate 1% (℞)

sulfacetamide sodium (℞)
(sul-fa-seet′a-mide)
AK-Sulf, Bleph-10 Liquifilm, Bleph-10 S.O.P., Isopto Cetamide, Ophthacet, Sodium Sulamyd, sodium sulfacetamide 10%, sodium sulfacetamide 15%, sodium sulfacetamide 30%, SOSS-10, Sulfair 15

tetracycline (℞)
(tet-ra-sye′kleen)
Achromycin Ophthalmic

tobramycin (℞)
(toe-bra-mye′sin)
Tobrex

trifluridine (℞)
(trye-floor′i-deen)
Viroptic

vidarabine (℞)
(vye-dare′a-been)
Vira-A

β-ADRENERGIC BLOCKERS

betaxolol (℞)
(beh-tax′oh-lole)
Betoptic, Betoptic S

carteolol (℞)
(kar-tee′oh-lole)
Ocupress

levobetaxolol (℞)
(lee-voh-beh-tax′oh-lohl)
Betaxon

levobunolol (℞)
(lee-voe-byoo′no-lole)
Betagen

metipranolol (℞)
(met-ee-pran′oh-lole)
Optipranolol

timolol (℞)
(tym′-moe-lole)
Apo-Timop ✤, Betimol, Timoptic

CHOLINERGICS (Direct-acting)

carbachol (℞)
(kar′ba-kole)
Isopto Carbachol, Miostat

pilocarpine (℞)
(pye-loe-kar′peen)
Adsorbocarpine, Akarpine, Isopto Carpine, Ocu-Carpine, Ocusert-Pilo, Pilagan, Pilocar, pilocarpine, Pilopine HS, Piloptic-1, Piloptic-2, Pilostat, Pilopto-Carpine

(cholinesterase inhibitors)

demecarium (℞)
(dem-e-kare′ee-um)
Humorsol

ecothiophate (℞)
(ek-oh-thye′eh-fate)
Ecostigmine Iodide, Phospholine Iodide

isoflurophate
(eye-soe-floor′oh-fate)
Floropryl

physostigmine (℞)
(fi-zoe-stig′meen)
Eserine Salicylate, Isopto Eserin

CYCLOPLEGIC MYDRIATICS

atropine (℞)
(a′troe-peen)
Atropine-1, Atropine Care Ophthalmic, Atropine Sulfate Ophthalmic, Atropine Sulfate S.O.P., Atropisol, Isopto Atropine

cyclopentolate (℞)
(sye-kloe-pen′toe-late)
AK-Pentolate, Cyclogyl, I-Pentolate

homatropine (℞)
(home-a′troe-peen)
AK-Homatropine, I-Homatrine, Isopto Homatropine, Minims Homatropine ✤, Spectro-Homatropine

physostigmine (℞)
(fi-zoe-stig′meen)
Fisostin, Isopto Eserine Solution/ Eserine Sulfate Ointment

scopolamine (℞)
(skoe-pol′a-meen)
Isopto-Hyoscine

tropicamide (℞)
(troe-pik′a-mide)
Mydriacyl, Tropicacyl, I-Piramide

GLUCOCORTICOIDS

dexamethasone
(dex-a-meth′a-sone)
AK-Dex, Decadron Phosphate, Dexamethasone Ophthalmic Suspension, Maxidex

fluorometholone (℞)
(flure-oh-meth′oh-lone)
Flarex, Fluor-Op, FML, FML Forte, FML Liquifilm

medrysone (℞)
(me′dri-sone)
HMS

prednisolone (℞)
(pred-niss′oh-lone)
Econopred, Econopred Plus, AK-Pred, Inflamase Forte, Inflamase Mild Ophthalmic, Metreton Ophthalmic, Pred-Forte, Pred-Mild

rimexolone (℞)
(ri-mex′a-lone)
Vexol

NONSTEROIDAL ANTIINFLAMMATORIES

diclofenac (℞)
(dye-kloe′fen-ak)
Voltaran

flurbiprofen (℞)
(flure-bi′-pro-fen)
Ocufen

ketorolac (℞)
(kee-toe′role-ak)
Acular

suprofen
(soo-proe′fen)
Profenal

SYMPATHOMIMETICS

apraclonidine
(a-pra-klon′i-deen)
Iopidine

brimonidine (℞)
(brem-on′-ii-dine)
Alphagan

dipivefrin
(dye-pi′vef-rin)
Propine

epinephrine bitartrate/ epinephrine HCl/ epinephryl borate (℞)
(ep-i-nef′rin)
Epitrate, Mytrate/Epifrin, Glaucon/ Epinal, Eppy ✤

OPHTHALMIC DECONGESTANTS/ VASOCONSTRICTORS

naphazoline (OTC, ℞)
(naf-az′oh-leen)
AK-Con Ophthalmic, Albalon Liquifilm Ophthalmic, Allerest Eye Drops, Clear Eyes, Comfort Eye Drops, Degest 2, Nafazair, naphazoline HCl, Naphcon, Naphcon Forte, Opcon, Vasoclear, Vasocon Regular, Estivin II

oxymetazoline (℞, OTC)
(ox-i-met-ah-zoh′leen)
OcuClear, Visine LR

phenylephrine (OTC)
(fen-ill-ef′rin)
AK-Dilate Ophthalmic, AK-Nefrin Ophthalmic, Isopto Frin, Neo-Synephrine 2.5%, Neo-Synephrine 10% Plain, Neo-Synephrine Viscous, phenylephrine HCl, 2.5% Mydfrin Ophthalmic, Phenoptic Relief, Prefrin

tetrahydrozoline (OTC)
(tet-ra-hye-dro'zoe-leen)
Collyrium Fresh Eye Drops, Eyesine, Murine Plus Eye Drops, Optigene 3 Eye Drops, Soothe Eye Drops, tetrahydrozoline HCl, Tyzine HCl, Tyzine Pediatric, Visine Eye Drops

MISCELLANEOUS OPHTHALMICS

bimatoprost (℞)
(by-mat'oh-prahst)
Lumigan

brinzolamide (℞)
(brin-zole'aa-mide)
Azopt

dorzolamide (℞)
(dor-zol'a-mid)
Trusopt

ketotifen
(ke-toe-tie'fen)
Zaditor

latanoprost (℞)
(la-tan'oh-proest)
Xalatan

lodoxamide
(loe-dox'ah-mide)
Alomide

travoprost (℞)
(trav'oh-prahst)
Travatan

unoprostone (℞)
(yoo-noh-prahs'tohn)
Rescula

Pregnancy category: demecarium, isoflurophate **X;** apraclonidine, cyclopentolate, ecothipate, glucocorticoids, levobunalol, metipranolol, pilocarpine, proparacaine, suprofen, tetracaine **C;** dapiprazole, dipivefrin **B**

β-Adrenergic blockers
Action: Reduces production of aqueous humor by unknown mechanism

Uses: Ocular hypertension, chronic open-angle glaucoma

Anesthetics
Action: Decreases ion permeability by stabilizing neuronal membrane

Uses: Cataract extraction, tonometry, gonioscopy, removal of foreign objects, corneal suture removal, glaucoma surgery (ophth); pruritus, sunburn, toothache, sore throat, cold sores, oral pain, rectal pain and irritation, control of gagging (top)

Antiinfectives
Action: Inhibits folic acid synthesis by preventing PABA use, which is necessary for bacterial growth

Uses: Conjunctivitis, superficial eye infections, corneal ulcers, prophylaxis against infection after removal of foreign matter from the eye

Antiinflammatories
Action: Decreases inflammation, resulting in decreased pain, photophobia, hyperemia, cellular infiltration

Uses: Inflammation of eye, eyelids, conjunctiva, cornea; uveitis, iridocyclitis, allergic conditions, burns, foreign bodies, postoperatively in cataract

Carbonic anhydrase inhibitor
Action: Converted to epinephrine, which decreases aqueous production and increases outflow

Uses: Open-angle glaucoma, ocular hypertension

Direct-acting miotic
Action: Acts directly on cholinergic receptor sites; induces miosis, spasm of accommodation, fall in intraocular pressure, caused by stimulation of ciliary, pupillary sphincter muscles, which leads to pulling away of iris from filtration angle, resulting in increased outflow of aqueous humor

Uses: Primary glaucoma, early stages

of wide-angle glaucoma (less useful in advanced stages), chronic open-angle glaucoma, acute narrow-angle glaucoma before emergency surgery; also neutralizes mydriatics used during eye exam; may be used alternately with mydriatics to break adhesions between iris and lens

---

Adverse effects
CNS: Headache
CV: Hypertension, tachycardia, dysrhythmias
EENT: Burning, stinging
GI: Bitter taste

Contraindications: Hypersensitivity

Precautions: Pregnancy, lactation, P children, aphakia, hypersensitivity to carbonic anhydrase inhibitors, sulfonamides, thiazide diuretics, ocular inhibitors, hepatic and renal insufficiency

NURSING CONSIDERATIONS

Assessment
- Monitor ophth exams and intraocular pressure readings
- Monitor blood counts; liver, renal function tests and serum electrolytes during long-term treatment

Nursing diagnoses
✓ Sensory-perceptual alteration: visual (uses)
✓ Knowledge deficit (teaching)

Implementation
- Storage at room temp away from light

Patient/family education
- Teach how to instill drops
- Advise patient that drug may cause burning, itching, blurring, dryness of eye area

Evaluation
Positive therapeutic outcome
- Absence of increased intraocular pressure

NASAL AGENTS

NASAL DECONGESTANTS

azelastine (℞)
(ay-zell'ah-steen)
Astelin

desoxyephedrine (OTC)
(des-oxy-e-fed'rin)
Vicks Inhaler

ephedrine (OTC)
(e-fed'rin)
Kondon's Nasal Jelly, Pretz-D, Vicks Vatronol

epinephrine (OTC)
(ep-i-neff'rin)
Adrenalin

naphazoline (OTC)
(naff-a-zoe'leen)
Privine

oxymetazoline (OTC)
(ox-i-met-az'oh-leen)
Afrin, Afrin Children's Nose Drops, Allerest 12-Hour Nasal, Chlorphed-LA, Coricidin Nasal Mist, Dristan Long Lasting, Duramist Plus, Duration, Genasal, NTZ Long-Acting Nasal, Nafrine ✤, Neo-Synephrine 12 Hour, Nostrilla, oxymetazoline HCl, Sinarest 12-Hour, Sinex Long-Acting, Twice-A-Day Nasal, 4-Way Long Acting Nasal

phenylephrine (OTC)
(fen-ill-eff'rin)
Alconefrin 12, Children's Nostril, Neo-Synephrine, Sinex

propylhexadrine (OTC)
(proe-pil-hex'a-dreen)
Benzedrex Inhaler

tetrahydrozoline (OTC)
(tet-ra-hye-dro'zoe-leen)
Tyzine

xylometazoline (OTC)
(zye-loh-meh-tazz'oh-leen)
Otrivin, Otrivin Pediatric Nasal Drops, xylometazoline HCl

NASAL STEROIDS

beclomethasone (℞)
(be-kloe-meth′a-sone)
Beconase AQ Nasal, Beconase Inhalation, Vancenase AQ Nasal, Vancenase Nasal

dexamethasone (℞)
(dex-a-meth′a-sone)
Decadron Phosphate Turbinaire

Pregnancy category C

Action: Produces vasoconstriction (rapid, long acting) of arterioles, thereby decreasing fluid exudation, mucosal engorgement by stimulation of α-adrenergic receptors in vascular smooth muscle

➔ **Therapeutic Outcome:** Absence of nasal congestion

Uses: Nasal congestion

Dosage and routes

Desoxyephedrine

P ***Adult and child >6 yr:*** 1-2 INH in each nostril q2h or less

Ephedrine

Adult: Fill dropper to the level marked, then use in each nostril q4h or less

Epinephrine

P ***Adult and child >6 yr:*** Apply with swab, drops, spray prn

Naphazoline

P ***Adult and child >6 yr:*** 1-2 drops/spray q6h or less

Oxymetazoline

P ***Adult and child >6 yr:*** INSTILL 2-3 gtt or sprays to each nostril bid

P ***Child 2-6 yr:*** INSTILL 2-3 gtt or sprays 0.025 sol bid, not to exceed 3 days

Phenylephrine

P ***Adult and child >12 yr:*** 2-3 drops/spray (0.25-0.5) in each nostril: q3-4h or less; or 2-3 drops/spray (1%) in each nostril q4h or less

P ***Child 6-12 yr:*** 2-3 drops/spray (0.25%) in each nostril q3-4h

P ***Infant >6 mo:*** 1-2 drops (0.16%) in each nostril q3h

Propylhexadrine

P ***Adult and child >6 yr:*** 1-2 INH in each nostril q2h or less

Tetrahydrozoline

P ***Adult and child >6 yr:*** 2-4 drops (0.1%) q3-4h prn or 3-4 sprays in each nostril q4h prn

P ***Child 2-6 yr:*** 2-3 drops (0.05%) in each nostril q4-6h prn

Xylometazoline

P ***Adult and child >12 yr:*** 2-3 drops/spray (0.1%) in each nostril q8-10h

P ***Child 2-12yr:*** 2-3 drops (0.05%) in each nostril q8-10h

Available forms: Nasal sol 0.025%, 0.05%

Adverse effects

CNS: Anxiety, restlessness, tremors, weakness, insomnia, dizziness, fever, headache
EENT: Irritation, burning, sneezing, stinging, dryness, rebound congestion
GI: Nausea, vomiting, anorexia
INTEG: Contact dermatitis

Contraindications: Hypersensitivity to sympathomimetic amines

P G **Precautions:** Children <6 yr, elderly, diabetes, cardiovascular disease, hypertension, hyperthyroidism, increased intracranial pressure, prostatic hypertrophy, pregnancy **C**, glaucoma

NURSING CONSIDERATIONS

Assessment

- Assess for redness, swelling, pain in nasal passages before and during treatment
- Assess for syst absorption; hypertension, tachycardia; notify prescriber; syst absorption occurs at high doses or after prolonged use

Nursing diagnoses
- ✓ Airway clearance, ineffective (uses)
- ✓ Knowledge deficit (teaching)
- ✓ Noncompliance (teaching)

Implementation
- Have patient tilt head back, squeeze bulb to create a vacuum, and draw correct amount of sol into dropper; insert 2 gtt of sol into nostril; repeat in other nostril
- Store in light-resistant container; do not expose to high temp or let sol come into contact with aluminum
- Give for <4 consecutive days
- Provide environmental humidification to decrease nasal congestion, dryness

Patient/family education
- Advise patient that stinging may occur for several applications; drying of mucosa may be decreased by environmental humidification
- Caution patient to notify prescriber if irregular pulse, insomnia, dizziness, or tremors occur
- Teach patient proper administration to avoid syst absorption
- Advise patient to rinse dropper with very hot water to prevent contamination

Evaluation
Positive therapeutic outcome
- Decreased nasal congestion

TOPICAL GLUCOCORTICOIDS

alclometasone (℞)
(al-kloe-met′a-sone)
Adovate

amcinonide (℞)
(am-sin′oh-nide)
Cyclocort

betamethasone (℞)
(bay-ta-meth′a-sone)
Alphatrex, Beben ✤, Betacort ✤, Betaderm, Betatrex, Beta-Val, Bethovate ✤, Betmethacort, Celestoderm ✤, Dermabet, Diprolene, Diprosone, Ectosonel ✤, Maxivate, Metaderm ✤, Novobetamet, Psorion, Uticort, Valisone, Valnac

clobetasol (℞)
(kloe-bay′ta-sol)
Dermovate ✤, Temovate

clocortolone (℞)
(kloe-kore′toe-lone)
Cloderm

desonide (℞)
(dess′oh-nide)
Des Owen, Tridesilon

desoximetasone (℞)
(dess-ox-i-met′a-sone)
Topicort

dexamethasone (℞)
(dex-a-meth′a-sone)
Aeroseb-Dex, Decaderm, Decaspray

diflorasone (℞)
(dye-flor′a-sone)
Florone, Maxiflor, Psorcon

fluocinolone (℞)
(floo-oh-sin′oh-lone)
Fluocin, Licon, Lidemol ✤, Lidex, Lyderm ✤, Topsyn ✤, Vasoderm

flurandrenolide (℞)
(flure-an-dren′oh-lide)
Cordran, Cordran SP, Cordran Tape, Drenison 1/4 ✤, Drenison Tape ✤

fluticasone (℞)
(floo-tik′a-sone)
Cutivate

halcinonide (℞)
(hal-sin′oh-nide)
Halog, Halog-E

halobetasol (℞)
(hal-oh-bay′ta-sol)
Ultravate

hydrocortisone (℞)
(hye-droe-kor′ti-sone)
Actiocort, Aeroseb-HC, Ala-Cort, Allercort, Alphaderm, Anusol HC, Bactine, Barriere-HC ✤, Calde-CORT Anti-Itch, Carmol HC, Cetacort, Cortacet ✤, Cortaid, Cortate ✤, Cort-Dome, Cortef ✤, Corticaine, Corticreme ✤, Cortifair, Cortizone, Cortoderm ✤, Cortril, Delcort, Dermacort, DemiCort, Dermtex HC, Emo-Cort, Epifoam, FoilleCort, Gly-Cort, Gynecort, Hi-Cor, Hycort, Hyderm ✤, Hydro-Tex, Hytone, Lacti-Care-HC, Lanacort, Lemoderm, Locoid, My Cort, Novoehydrocort ✤, Nutracort Pharm, Pharmacort, Pentacort, Rederm, Rhulicort S-T Cort, Synacort, Sarna HC ✤, Texa-Cort, Unicort ✤, Westcort

methylprednisolone (℞)
(meth-ill-pred-niss′oh-lone)
Depo-Medrol

mometasone (℞)
(moe-met′a-sone)
Elocon

prednicarbate (℞)
(pred-ni-kar′bate)
Dermatop

triamcinolone (℞)
(trye-am-sin′oh-lone)
Aristocort, Flutex, Kenac, Kenalog, Kenonel, Triaderm ✤, Trianide ✤, Triderm, Trymex

Pregnancy category C

Action: Antipruritic, antiinflammatory

➡ **Therapeutic Outcome:** Decreased itching, inflammation

Uses: Psoriasis, eczema, contact dermatitis, pruritus; usually reserved for severe dermatoses that have not responded to less potent formulation

Dosage and routes

P ***Adult and child:*** Apply to affected area

Adverse effects

INTEG: *Acne, atrophy, epidermal thinning, purpura, striae*

Contraindications: Hypersensitivity, viral infections, fungal infections

Precautions: Pregnancy **C**

NURSING CONSIDERATIONS

Assessment

- Temp; if fever develops, drug should be discontinued
- For systemic absorption, increased temp, inflammation, irritation

Nursing diagnoses

✓ Pain, chronic (uses)
✓ Knowledge deficit (teaching)
✓ Skin integrity, impaired (uses)

Implementation

- Apply only to affected areas; do not get in eyes
- Apply and leave site uncovered or lightly covered; occlusive dressing is not recommended—systemic absorption may occur
- Use only on dermatoses; do not use on weeping, denuded, or infected area
- Cleanse area before application of drug
- Continue treatment for a few days after area has cleared
- Store at room temp

Patient/family education

- Teach patient to avoid sunlight on affected area, burns may occur
- Teach patient to limit treatment to 14 days

Evaluation

Positive therapeutic outcome

- Absence of severe itching, patches on skin, flaking

TOPICAL ANTIFUNGALS

amphotericin B (OTC)
(am-foe-ter′i-sin)
Fungizone

butenafine (℞)
(byoo-tin′a-feen)
Mentex

ciclopirox (OTC)
(sye-kloe-peer′ox)
Loprox

clioquinol (OTC)
(klye-oh-kwin′ole)
Vioforim

clotrimazole (OTC)
(kloe-trye′ma-zole)
Canestew ✤, Clotrimaderm ✤, Lotrimin, Lotrimin AF, Mycelex, Mycelex OTC, Myclo ✤, Neozol ✤

econazole (OTC)
(ee-kon′a-zole)
Spectazole

haloprogin (OTC)
(hal-oh-proe′jin)
Halotex

ketoconazole (OTC)
(kee-toe-kon′a-zole)
Nizoral

miconazole (OTC)
(mye-kon′a-zole)
Micatin, Monistat-Derm

naftifine (OTC)
(naf f′ti-feen)
Naftin

nystatin (OTC)
(nye-stat′in)
Mycostatin, Nodostine ✤, Nilstat, Nyoderm ✤, Nystex

oxiconazole (OTC)
(ox-i-kon′a-zole)
Oxistat

selenium (OTC)
(see-leen′ee-um)
Exsel, Head and Shoulders Intensive Treatment, Selenium Sulfide, Selsun, Selsun Blue

terbinafine (OTC)
(ter-bin′a-feen)
Lamisil

tolnaftate (OTC)
(tole-naf′tate)
Absorbine Antifungal, Absorbine Jock Itch, Absorbine Jr. Antifungal, Aftate For Athlete's Foot, Aftate for Jock Itch, Desenex Spray, Genaspor, NP-27, Quinsana Plus, Tinactin, Ting, tolnaftate, Zeasorb-AF

undecylenic acid (OTC)
(un-deh-sih-len′ik)
Caldesene, Cruex, Decylenes, Desenex, Desenex Maximum Strength, Protectol

Pregnancy category B

Action: Interferes with fungal cell membrane permeability

Therapeutic Outcome: Absence of itching and white patches of the skin

Uses: Tinea cruris, tinea pedis, diaper rash, minor skin irritations; amphotericin B is used for *Candida* infections

Dosage and routes
Massage into affected area, surrounding area qd or bid, continue for 7-14 days, not to exceed 4 wk

Adverse effects
INTEG: Burning, stinging, dryness, itching, local irritation

Contraindications: Hypersensitivity

Precautions: Pregnancy **B**, lactation, children

Interactions: None

NURSING CONSIDERATIONS

Assessment

- Assess skin for fungal infections; peeling, dryness, itching before and throughout treatment
- Assess for continuing infection; increased size, number of lesions

Nursing diagnoses

- ✓ Skin integrity, impaired (uses)
- ✓ Infection, risk for (uses)
- ✓ Knowledge deficit (teaching)

Implementation

- Apply to affected area, surrounding area; do not cover with occlusive dressings
- Store below 30° C (86° F)

Teach patient/family

- Instruct to apply with glove to prevent further infection; not to cover with occlusive dressings
- Teach patient that long-term therapy may be needed to clear infection (2 wk-6 mo depending on organism); compliance is needed even after feeling better
- Teach patient proper hygiene; hand-washing technique, nail care, use of concomitant top agents if prescribed
- Caution patient to avoid use of OTC creams, ointments, lotions unless directed by prescriber
- Instruct patient to use medical asepsis (hand washing) before, after each application; to change socks and shoes once a day during treatment of tinea pedis
- Advise patient to report to health care prescriber if infection persists or recurs; if blisters, burning, oozing, swelling occur
- Caution patient to avoid alcohol because nausea, vomiting, hypertension may occur
- Caution patient to use sunscreen or avoid direct sunlight to prevent photosensitivity
- Advise patient to notify prescriber of sore throat, fever, skin rash, which may indicate overgrowth of organisms

Evaluation

Positive therapeutic outcome

- Decrease in size, number of lesions

TOPICAL ANTIINFECTIVES

bacitracin (OTC)
(bass-i-tray′sin)
Baciguent, Bacitin ♣, Bacitracin

chloramphenicol (℞)
(klor-am-fen′i-kole)
Chloromycetin

erythromycin (OTC)
(er-ith-roe-mye′sin)
A/T/S, Akne-Mycin, C-Solve 2, Erycette, Eryderm, Erygel, Erymax, Erythromycin, E-Solve 2, ETS-2%, Staticin, Theramycin Z, T-Statd

gentamicin (℞)
(jen-ta-mye′sin)
G-Myticin, Garamycin, gentamicin

mafenide (℞)
(ma′fe-nide)
Sulfamylon

mupirocin (℞)
(myoo-peer′oh sin)
Bactroban, Pseudomonic Acid A

neomycin (OTC)
(nee-oh-mye′sin)
Myciguent, Neomycin Sulfate

nitrofurazone (℞)
(nye-troe-fyoor′a-zone)
Furacin, Nitrofurazone

silver sulfadiazine (℞)
(sul-fa-dye′a-zeen)
Flamazine ♣, Silvadene, SSD, SSD AF, Thermazene

sodium sulfacetamide lotion 10% (℞)
(sul-fa-see′ta-mide)
Klaron

tetracycline (℞)
(tet-ra-sye'kleen)
Achromycin, Topicycline
Pregnancy category C

Action: Interferes with bacterial protein synthesis

➔ **Therapeutic Outcome:** Resolution of infection

Uses: Skin infections, minor burns, wounds, skin grafts, primary pyodermas, otitis externa

Adverse effects

INTEG: Rash, urticaria, scaling, redness

Contraindications: Hypersensitivity, large areas, burns, ulcerations

Precautions: Pregnancy **C,** lactation, impaired renal function, external ear or perforated eardrum

NURSING CONSIDERATIONS

Assessment

- Assess for allergic reaction: burning, stinging, swelling, redness
- Assess for signs of nephrotoxicity or ototoxicity

Nursing diagnoses

✓ Infection, risk of (uses)
✓ Skin integrity (uses)
✓ Knowledge deficit (teaching)

Implementation

- Apply enough medication to cover lesions completely
- Apply after cleansing with soap, water before each application; dry well
- Apply to less than 20% of body surface area when patient has impaired renal function
- Store at room temp in dry place

Evaluation

Positive therapeutic outcome

- Decrease in size, number of lesions

TOPICAL ANTIVIRALS

acyclovir (℞)
(ay-sye'kloe-ver)
Zovirax
penciclovir (℞)
(pen-sye'kloe-ver)
Denavir
Pregnancy category C

Action: Interferes with viral DNA replication

➔ **Therapeutic Outcome:** Resolution of infection

Uses: Simple mucocutaneous herpes simplex, in immunocompromised clients with initial herpes genitalis

Adverse effects

INTEG: Rash, urticaria, stinging, burning, pruritus, vulvitis

Contraindications: Hypersensitivity

Precautions: Pregnancy **C,** lactation

NURSING CONSIDERATIONS

Assessment

- Assess for allergic reaction: burning, stinging, swelling, redness, rash, vulvitis, pruritus
- Assess for signs of nephrotoxicity or ototoxicity

Nursing diagnoses

✓ Infection, risk of (uses)
✓ Skin integrity (uses)
✓ Knowledge deficit (teaching)

Implementation

- Apply with finger cot or rubber glove to prevent further infection
- Apply enough medication to cover lesions completely
- Apply after cleansing with soap, water before each application; dry well
- Storage at room temp in dry place

Patient/family education

- Teach patient not to use in eyes or when there is no evidence of infection

- Advise patient to apply with glove to prevent further infection
- Advise patient to avoid use of OTC creams, ointments, lotions unless directed by prescriber
- Advise patient to use medical asepsis (hand washing) before, after each application and avoid contact with eyes
- Advise patient to adhere strictly to prescribed regimen to maximize successful treatment outcome
- Advise patient to begin taking drug when symptoms arise

Evaluation

Positive therapeutic outcome

- Decrease in size, number of lesions

TOPICAL ANESTHETICS

benzocaine (OTC)
(ben'zoe-kane)
Anbesol Maximum Strength, Baby Anbesol, Children's Chloraseptic, Medamint, Orabase Baby, Oracin, Ora-Jel, Oratect, Spec-T Anesthetic, T-Caine, Tyrobenz

dibucaine (OTC)
(dyc'byoo-kane)
dibucaine, Nupercainal

lidocaine (OTC, ℞)
(lye'doe-kane)
Aloe Extra, Anestacon, Burn Relief, Derma Flex, lidocaine HCl topical, lidocaine viscous, Solarcaine, Xylocaine, Xylocaine Viscous, Zilactin-L

pramoxine (OTC)
(pra-mox'een)
Fleet Relief, Prax, ProctoFoam, Tronolane, Tronothane

tetracaine (OTC)
(tet'ra-cane)
Pontocaine

Pregnancy category C

Action: Inhibits conduction of nerve impulses from sensory nerves

Therapeutic Outcome: Decreasing inflammation, itching, pain

Uses: Oral irritation, sore throat, toothache, cold sore, canker sore, sunburn, minor cuts, insect bites, pain, itching

Dosage and routes

P ***Adult and child:*** TOP apply qid as needed; RECT insert tid and after each BM

Adverse effects

INTEG: Rash, irritation, sensitization

Contraindications: Hypersensitivity, infants <1 yr, application to large areas

P **Precautions:** Child <6 yr, sepsis, pregnancy **C**, denuded skin

NURSING CONSIDERATIONS

Assessment

- Assess pain: location, duration, characteristics before and after administration
- Assess for infection: redness, drainage, inflammation; this drug should not be used until infection is treated

Implementation

- Store in tight, light-resistant container; do not freeze, puncture, or incinerate aerosol container

Patient/family education

- Teach patient to avoid contact with eyes
- Teach patient not to use for prolonged periods: use for <1 wk; if condition remains, prescriber should be contacted

Evaluation

Positive therapeutic outcome

- Decreased redness, swelling, pain

docosanol (OTC)
(doh-koh'sah-nohl)
Abreva
pimecrolimus (℞)
(pim-eh-kroh-ly'mus)
Elidel
Pregnancy category C

Action: Docosanol unknown; pimecrolimus may bind with macrophilin and inhibit calcium-dependent phosphatase

Therapeutic Outcome: Decreased redness, swelling, pain

Uses: Docosanol applied to fever blisters to promote more rapid healing; pimecrolimus used to treat mild to moderate atopic dermatitis in nonimmunocompromised patients ≥2 yr who are unresponsive to other treatment

Dosage and routes
Docosanol
Adult: TOP rub into blisters ×5/day until healing occurs
Pimecrolimus
P ***Adult and child ≥2 yr:*** TOP apply thin layer 2×/day and rub in, use as long as needed

Adverse effects
Docosanol
None known
Pimecrolimus
INTEG: Burning

Contraindications: Hypersensitivity

Precautions: Lactation, pregnancy **C**, dermal infections

NURSING CONSIDERATIONS
Assessment
- Assess skin condition (color pain, inflammation) before and after administration
- Assess for signs and symptoms of skin infections (redness, draining lesions); if present, avoid use of product (pimecrolimus)

Nursing diagnoses
- ✓ Skin integrity, impaired (uses)
- ✓ Infection, risk for (uses)
- ✓ Knowledge deficit (teaching)

Implementation
- Apply to skin, rub in gently

Patient/family education
- Advise patient to avoid contact between medication and eyes
- Instruct patient to discontinue use of product when condition clears

Evaluation
Positive therapeutic outcome
- Decreased inflammation, redness

VAGINAL ANTIFUNGALS

butoconazole (OTC)
(byoo-toh-kone'ah-zole)
Femstat
clotrimazole (OTC)
(kloe-trye'ma-zole)
Canesten ♣, Gyne-Lotrimin, Mycelex G, Mycelex Twin Pak, Myclo ♣
miconazole (OTC)
(mye-kon'a-zole)
Monistat, Monistat 3, Monistat 7, Monistat Dual Pak
nystatin (OTC)
(nye-stat'in)
mycostatin, Nadostine ♣, Nilstat, Nyoderm ♣, O-V Statin
terconazole (OTC)
(ter-kone'ah-zole)
Terazol

tioconazole (OTC)
(tye-oh-kone'ah-zole)
Gyne-Trosyd ✤, Vagistat

Pregnancy category:
Nystatin A;
clotrimazole B;
butoconazole, terconazole, tioconazole C

Action: Interferes with fungal DNA replication; binds sterols in fungal cell membranes, which increases permeability, leaking of nutrients

➔ **Therapeutic Outcome:** Fungistatic/fungicidal against susceptible organisms: *Candida* only

Uses: Vaginal, vulval, vulvovaginal candidiasis (moniliasis)

Dosage and routes

Butoconazole
Adult: VAG 5 g (1 applicator) hs × 3-6 days

Clotrimazole
Adult: 100 mg (1 vag tab, 100 mg) hs × 1 wk, or 200 mg (2 vag tab, 100 mg) hs × 3 nights, or 500 mg (1 vag tab, 500 mg); or 5 g (1 applicator) hs × 1-2 wks

Miconazole
Adult: 200 mg supp hs × 3 days or 100 mg supp × 1 wk

Nystatin
Adult: 100,000 U qd × 2 wk

Terconazole
Adult: VAG 5 g (1 applicator) hs × 7 days

Tioconazole
Adult: 1 applicator hs × 1 wk

Adverse effects
GU: Vulvovaginal burning, itching, pelvic cramps
INTEG: Rash, urticaria, stinging, burning
MISC: *Headache,* body pain

Contraindications: Hypersensitivity

P **Precautions:** Children <2 yr, pregnancy, lactation

Interactions: None

NURSING CONSIDERATIONS
Assessment
- Assess for allergic reaction: burning, stinging, itching, discharge, soreness

Nursing diagnoses
✓ Skin integrity, impaired (uses)
✓ Infection, risk for (uses)
✓ Knowledge deficit (teaching)

Implementation
Topical route
- Administer one full applicator every night high into the vagina
- Store at room temp in dry place

Teach patient/family
- Instruct patient in asepsis (hand washing) before, after each application
- Teach patient to apply with applicator only; to avoid use of any other vaginal product unless directed by prescriber; sanitary napkin may prevent soiling of undergarments
- Instruct patient to abstain from sexual intercourse until treatment is completed; reinfection and irritation may occur
- Advise patient to notify prescriber if symptoms persist

Evaluation
Positive therapeutic outcome
- Decrease in itching or white discharge (vaginal)

OTIC STEROIDS

hydrocortisone
(hye-droe-kor'ti-sone)
Cortamed ✤, Otall (℞)

Pregnancy category C

Action: Antiinflammatory, antipruritic

➔ **Therapeutic Outcome:** Decreased otic inflammation

Uses: Ear canal inflammation

Adverse effects

EENT: Itching, irritation in ear
INTEG: Rash, urticaria

Contraindications: Hypersensitivity, perforated eardrum

Precautions: Pregnancy **C**

NURSING CONSIDERATIONS

Assessment

- Assess for redness, swelling, fever, pain in ear, which indicates infection

Nursing diagnoses

- ✓ Pain (uses)
- ✓ Knowledge deficit (teaching)

Implementation

- Administer after removing impacted cerumen by irrigation
- Administer after cleaning stopper with alcohol
- Administer after restraining child if necessary
- Instill after warming sol to body temp

Patient/family education

- Teach patient the correct method of instillation using aseptic technique, including not touching dropper to ear
- Advise patient that dizziness may occur after instillation

Evaluation

Positive therapeutic outcome

- Decreased ear pain, inflammation

OTIC ANTIINFECTIVES

chloramphenicol (℞)
(klor-am-fen'i-kole)
Chloromycetin Otic, Sopamycetin ✤

neomycin (℞)
(nee-oh-mye'sin)
Drotic, Otocort

Pregnancy category C

Action: Inhibits protein synthesis in susceptible microorganisms

➔ **Therapeutic Outcome:** Decreased redness, swelling, fever, and/or pain in ear

Uses: Ear infection (external), short-term use

Adverse effects

EENT: Itching, irritation in ear
INTEG: Rash, urticaria

Contraindications: Hypersensitivity, perforated eardrum

Precautions: Pregnancy **C**

NURSING CONSIDERATIONS

Assessment

- Assess for redness, swelling, fever, pain in ear, which indicates superinfection

Nursing diagnoses

- ✓ Pain (uses)
- ✓ Infection, risk for (uses)
- ✓ Knowledge deficit (teaching)

Implementation

- Administer after removing impacted cerumen by irrigation
- Administer after cleaning stopper with alcohol
- Administer after restraining child if necessary
- Instill after warming sol to body temp

Patient/family education

- Teach patient the correct method of instillation using aseptic technique, including not touching dropper to ear
- Advise patient that dizziness may occur after instillation

Evaluation

Positive therapeutic outcome

- Decreased ear pain

Appendix E

Combination Products

***222:**
aspirin 375 mg
codeine 8 mg
caffeine 30 mg
Uses: Narcotic analgesic
***282 MEP:**
aspirin 375 mg
codeine 15 mg
caffeine 30 mg
Uses: Narcotic analgesic
***292:**
aspirin 375 mg
codeine 30 mg
caffeine 30 mg
Uses: Narcotic analgesic
***692:**
aspirin 375 mg
propoxyphene 65 mg
caffeine 30 mg
Uses: Narcotic analgesic
A-200 Shampoo:
0.33% pyrcthrins
4% piperonyl butoxide
Uses: Scabicide, pediculicide
Aceta w/Codeine:
acetaminophen 300 mg
codeine 30 mg
Uses: Narcotic analgesic
Aceta-Gesic:
325 mg acetaminophen
30 mg phenyltoloxamine
Uses: Nonnarcotic analgesic
Acid-X:
acetaminophen 500 mg
calcium carbonate 250 mg
Uses: Analgesic, antacid
Actifed:
pseudoephedrine 60 mg
triprolidine 2.5 mg
Uses: Decongestant
Actifed, Allergy, Nighttime:
pseudoephedrine 30 mg
diphenhydramine 25 mg
Uses: Decongestant, antihistamine
Actifed Plus:
pseudoephedrine 30 mg
triprolidine 1.25 mg
acetaminophen 500 mg
Uses: Decongestant, antihistamine
Actifed Sinus Daytime:
pseudoephedrine 30 mg
acetaminophen 500 mg
Uses: Decongestant
Actifed Sinus Nighttime:
pseudoephedrine 30 mg
diphenhydramine 25 mg
acetaminophen 500 mg
Uses: Decongestant, antihistamine
Adderall 5 mg:
dextroamphetamine sulfate 1.25 mg
dextroamphetamine saccharate 1.25 mg
amphetamine sulfate 1.25 mg
amphetamine aspartate 1.25 mg
Uses: CNS stimulant
Adderall 10 mg:
dextroamphetamine sulfate 5 mg
dextroamphetamine saccharate 2.5 mg
amphetamine sulfate 2.5 mg
amphetamine aspartate 2.5 mg
Uses: CNS stimulant
Adderall 20 mg:
dextroamphetamine sulfate 5 mg
dextroamphetamine saccharate 5 mg
amphetamine sulfate 5 mg
amphetamine aspartate 5 mg
Uses: CNS stimulant
Adderall 30 mg:
dextroamphetamine sulfate 7.5 mg
dextroamphetamine saccharate 7.5 mg
amphetamine sulfate 7.5 mg
amphetamine aspartate 7.5 mg
Uses: CNS stimulant
Advil Cold & Sinus Caplets:
pseudoephedrine 30 mg
ibuprofen 200 mg
Uses: Decongestant
Aggrenox:
200 mg ext rel dipyridamole
25 mg aspirin
Uses: Antiplatelet
AK-Cide Ophthalmic Suspension/Ointment:
10% sulfacetamide sodium
0.5% prednisolone acetate
Uses: Ophth antiinfective, antiinflammatory

Alamast:
0.005% lauralkonium
glycerin
dibasic/monobasic sodium phosphate
phosphoric acid
Aldactazide 25/25:
spironolactone 25 mg
hydrochlorothiazide 25 mg
Uses: Diuretic
Aldactazide 50/50:
spironolactone 50 mg
hydrochlorothiazide 50 mg
Uses: Diuretic
Aldoclor-150:
methyldopa 250 mg
chlorothiazide 150 mg
Uses: Antihypertensive
Aldoclor-250:
methyldopa 250 mg
chlorothiazide 250 mg
Uses: Antihypertensive
Aldoril-15:
methyldopa 250 mg
hydrochlorothiazide 15 mg
Uses: Antihypertensive
Aldoril-25:
methyldopa 250 mg
hydrochlorothiazide 25 mg
Uses: Antihypertensive
Alka-Seltzer Effervescent, Original:
sodium bicarbonate 1916 mg
citric acid 1000 mg
aspirin 325 mg
Uses: Antacid, adsorbent, antiflatulent
Alka-Seltzer Gold:
sodium bicarbonate 958 mg
citric acid 832 mg
potassium bicarbonate 312 mg
Uses: Antacid, adsorbent
Alka-Seltzer Plus Allergy Liqui-Gels:
pseudoephedrine 30 mg
chlorpheniramine 2 mg
acetaminophen 325 mg
Uses: Decongestant, antihistamine
Alka-Seltzer Plus Night-Time Cold Liqui-Gels:
doxylamine 6.25 mg
dextromethorphan 10 mg
pseudoephedrine 30 mg
acetaminophen 250 mg
Uses: Antitussive, decongestant
Alka-Seltzer Plus Cold & Cough Liqui-Gels:
pseudoephedrine 30 mg
chlorpheniramine 2 mg
dextromethorphan 10 mg
acetaminophen 250 mg
Uses: Antitussive, decongestant
Alka-Seltzer Plus Cold Liqui-Gels:
pseudoephedrine 30 mg
chlorpheniramine 2 mg
acetaminophen 250 mg
Uses: Decongestant, antihistamine
Alka-Seltzer Plus Flu & Body Aches Non-Drowsy Liqui-Gels:
pseudoephedrine 30 mg
dextromethorphan 10 mg
acetaminophen 250 mg
Uses: Decongestant, antitussive, analgesic
Allerest Headache Strength Advanced Formula:
pseudoephedrine 30 mg
chlorpheniramine 2 mg
acetaminophen 325 mg
Uses: Decongestant, antihistamine
Allerest Maximum Strength Tablets:
pseudoephedrine 30 mg
chlorpheniramine 2 mg
Uses: Decongestant, antihistamine
Allerest No-Drowsiness:
pseudoephedrine 30 mg
acetaminophen 325 mg
Uses: Decongestant, analgesic
Allerest Sinus Pain Formula:
pseudoephedrine 30 mg
chlorpheniramine 2 mg
acetaminophen 500 mg
Uses: Decongestant, antihistamine, analgesic
All-Nite Cold Formula Liquid:
Per 5 ml:
pseudoephedrine 10 mg
doxylamine 1.25 mg
dextromethorphan 5 mg
acetaminophen 167 mg
Uses: Decongestant, antihistamine, analgesic
Alor 5/500:
hydrocodone 5 mg
aspirin 500 mg
Uses: Analgesic
Amaphen:
acetaminophen 325 mg
butalbital 50 mg
caffeine 40 mg
Uses: Analgesic, barbiturates
Ambenyl Cough Syrup:
Per 5 ml:
bromodiphenhydramine 12.5 mg
codeine 10 mg
5% alcohol
Uses: Antihistamine, opioid analgesic

Anacin:
aspirin 400 mg
caffeine 32 mg
Uses: Analgesic
Anacin Maximum Strength:
aspirin 500 mg
caffeine 32 mg
Uses: Analgesic
Anacin PM (Aspirin Free):
diphenhydramine 25 mg
acetaminophen 500 mg
Uses: Analgesic
Anacin w/Codeine:
aspirin 325 mg
codeine 8 mg
caffeine 32 mg
Uses: Narcotic analgesic
Anaplex HD Syrup:
Per 5 ml:
hydrocodone 1.7 mg
phenylephrine 5 mg
chlorpheniramine 2 mg
Uses: Analgesic, adrenergic, antihistamine
Anaplex Liquid:
Per 5 ml:
chlorpheniramine 2 mg
pseudoephedrine 30 mg
Uses: Antihistamine, decongestant
Anatuss DM:
guaifenesin 400 mg
pseudoephedrine 60 mg
dextromethorphan 20 mg
Uses: Expectorant, adrenergic, antitussive
Anatuss DM Syrup:
Per 5 ml:
guaifenesin 100 mg
pseudoephedrine 30 mg
dextromethorphan 10 mg
Uses: Expectorant, adrenergic, antitussive
Anatuss LA:
pseudoephedrine 120 mg
guaifenesin 400 mg
Uses: Adrenergic, expectorant
Anexsia 5/500:
hydrocodone 5 mg
acetaminophen 500 mg
Uses: Analgesic
Anexsia 5/500:
hydrocodone 5 mg
acetaminophen 500 mg
Uses: Narcotic analgesic
Anexsia 7.5/650:
hydrocodone 7.5 mg
acetaminophen 650 mg
Uses: Analgesic
Anexsia 10/660:
hydrocodone 10 mg
acetaminophen 660 mg
Uses: Analgesic
Anoquan:
acetaminophen 325 mg
caffeine 40 mg
butalbital 50 mg
Uses: Nonnarcotic analgesic, antipyretic
Antrocol Elixir:
Per 5 ml:
atropine 0.195 mg
phenobarbital 16 mg
alcohol 20%
Uses: Anticholinergic, barbiturate
Apresazide 25/25:
hydralazine 25 mg
hydrochlorothiazide 25 mg
Uses: Antihypertensive
Apresazide 50/50:
hydralazine 50 mg
hydrochlorothiazide 50 mg
Uses: Antihypertensive
Aprodine w/Codeine Syrup:
Per 5 ml:
pseudoephedrine 30 mg
triprolidine 1.25 mg
codeine 10 mg
Uses: Adrenergic, analgesic
Aprodine Syrup:
Per 5 ml:
pseudoephedrine 30 mg
triprolidine 1.25 mg
Uses: Adrenergic, analgesic
Arthritis Pain Formula:
aspirin 500 mg
aluminum hydroxide 27 mg
magnesium hydroxide 100 mg
Uses: Analgesic, antacid
Arthrotec:
diclofenac 50 or 75 mg
misoprostol 200 μg
Uses: NSAID, gastric protectant
Asbron G Elixir:
theophylline 150 mg
guaifenesin 100 mg
alcohol 15%
Uses: Bronchodilator, expectorant
Asbron G Inlay:
theophylline 150 mg
guaifenesin 100 mg
sucrose
Uses: Bronchodilator, expectorant

Ascriptin:
aspirin 325 mg
magnesium hydroxide 50 mg
aluminum hydroxide 50 mg
calcium carbonate 50 mg
Uses: Nonnarcotic analgesic, antipyretic
Ascriptin A/D:
aspirin 325 mg
aluminum hydroxide 75 mg
magnesium hydroxide 75 mg
calcium carbonate 75 mg
Uses: Analgesic
Aspirin-Free Bayer Select Allergy Sinus:
pseudoephedrine 30 mg
chlorpheniramine 2 mg
acetaminophen 500 mg
Uses: Adrenergic, antihistamine, analgesic
Aspirin-Free Bayer Select Head & Chest Cold:
pseudoephedrine 30 mg
guaifenesin 100 mg
dextromethorphan 10 mg
acetaminophen 325 mg
Uses: Adrenergic, antitussive, expectorant, analgesic
Aspirin Free Excedrin:
acetaminophen 500 mg
caffeine 65 mg
Uses: Analgesic
Aspirin Free Excedrin Dual:
acetaminophen 500 mg
calcium carbonate 111 mg
magnesium carbonate 64 mg
magnesium oxide 30 mg
Uses: Analgesic, antacid
Augmentin 250:
amoxicillin 250 mg
clavulanic acid 125 mg
Uses: Antiinfective
Augmentin 500:
amoxicillin 500 mg
clavulanic acid 125 mg
Uses: Antiinfective
Augmentin 875:
amoxicillin 875 mg
clavulanic acid 125 mg
Uses: Antiinfective
Augmentin 125 Chewable:
amoxicillin 125 mg
clavulanic acid 31.25 mg
Uses: Antiinfective
Augmentin 250 Chewable:
amoxicillin 250 mg
clavulanic acid 62.5 mg
Uses: Antiinfective
Augmentin 125 mg/5 ml Suspension:
Per 5 ml:
amoxicillin 125 mg
clavulanic acid 31.25 mg
Uses: Antiinfective
Augmentin 250 mg/5 ml Suspension:
Per 5 ml:
amoxicillin 250 mg
clavulanic acid 62.5 mg
Uses: Antiinfective
Auralgan Otic Solution:
5.4% antipyrine
1.4% benzocaine
Uses: Otic analgesic
Azo-Gantanol:
sulfamethoxazole 500 mg
phenazopyridine 100 mg
Uses: Sulfonamide
Azo-Gantrisin:
sulfisoxazole 500 mg
phenazopyridine 50 mg
Uses: Sulfonamide
Azo-Sulfamethoxazole:
sulfamethoxazole 500 mg
phenazopyridine 100 mg
Uses: Sulfonamide
Azo-Sulfisoxazole:
sulfisoxazole 500 mg
phenazopyridine 50 mg
Uses: Sulfonamide
B&O Supprettes No. 15A Supps:
belladonna extract 15 mg
opium 30 mg
Uses: Anticholinergic, narcotic analgesic
B&O Supprettes No. 16A Supps:
belladonna extract 16.2 mg
opium 60 mg
Uses: Anticholinergic, narcotic analgesic
Bactrim:
trimethoprim 80 mg
sulfamethoxazole 400 mg
Uses: Antiinfective
Bactrim DS:
trimethoprim 160 mg
sulfamethoxazole 800 mg
Uses: Antiinfective
Bactrim I.V.:
trimethoprim 80 mg
sulfamethoxazole 400 mg
Uses: Antiinfective
Bancap HC:
acetaminophen 500 mg
hydrocodone 5 mg
Uses: Analgesic

Bayer Plus, Extra Strength:
aspirin 500 mg
calcium carbonate
magnesium carbonate
magnesium oxide
Uses: Analgesic, antacid

Bayer Select Chest Cold:
dextromethorphan 15 mg
acetaminophen 500 mg
Uses: Antitussive, analgesic

Bayer Select Flu Relief:
acetaminophen 500 mg
pseudoephedrine 30 mg
dextromethorphan 15 mg
chlorpheniramine 2 mg
Uses: Analgesic, adrenergic, antitussive, antihistamine

Bayer Select Head & Chest Cold, Aspirin Free Caplets:
pseudoephedrine 30 mg
dextromethorphan 10 mg
guaifenesin 100 mg
acetaminophen 325 mg
Uses: Adrenergic, antitussive, expectorant, analgesic

Bayer Select Head Cold:
pseudoephedrine 30 mg
acetaminophen 500 mg
Uses: Adrenergic, analgesic

Bayer Select Maximum Strength Headache:
acetaminophen 500 mg
caffeine 65 mg
Uses: Nonnarcotic analgesic

Bayer Select Maximum Strength Menstrual:
acetaminophen 500 mg
pamabrom 25 mg
Uses: Nonnarcotic analgesic

Bayer Select Maximum Strength Night-Time Pain Relief:
acetaminophen 500 mg
diphenhydramine 25 mg
Uses: Analgesic, antihistamine

Bayer Select Maximum Strength Sinus Pain Relief:
acetaminophen 500 mg
pseudoephedrine 30 mg
Uses: Analgesic, adrenergic

Bayer Select Night Time Cold:
acetaminophen 500 mg
pseudoephedrine 30 mg
dextromethorphan 15 mg
triprolidine 1.25 mg
Uses: Analgesic, adrenergic, antitussive, antihistamine

BC Powder Original Formula:
aspirin 650 mg
salicylamide 195 mg
caffeine 33.3 mg
Uses: Nonnarcotic analgesic

BC Powder Arthritis Strength:
aspirin 742 mg
salicylamide 222 mg
caffeine 38 mg
Uses: Nonnarcotic analgesic

Bellatal:
phenobarbital 16.2 mg
hyoscyamine sulfate 0.1037 mg
atropine sulfate 0.0194 mg
scopolamine hydrobromide 0.0065 mg
Uses: Barbiturate, anticholinergic

Bellergal-S:
ergotamine 0.6 mg
belladonna alkaloids 0.2 mg
phenobarbital 40 mg
Uses: α-Adrenergic blocker, anticholinergic, barbiturate

Bel-Phen-Ergot-SR:
phenobarbital 40 mg
ergotamine tartrate 0.6 mg
belladonna alkaloids 0.2 mg
Uses: α-Adrenergic blocker, anticholinergic, barbiturate

Benadryl Allergy Decongestant Liquid:
Per 5 ml:
diphenhydramine 12.5 mg
pseudoephedrine 30 mg
Uses: Antihistamine, adrenergic

Benadryl Allergy/Sinus Headache Caplets:
diphenhydramine 12.5 mg
pseudoephedrine 30 mg
acetaminophen 500 mg
Uses: Antihistamine, adrenergic, analgesic

Benadryl Decongestant Allergy:
pseudoephedrine 60 mg
diphenhydramine 25 mg
Uses: Adrenergic, antihistamine

Benylin Expectorant Liquid:
Per 5 ml:
dextromethorphan 5 mg
guaifenesin 100 mg
5% alcohol
Uses: Expectorant, antitussive

Benylin Multi-Symptom Liquid:
Per 5 ml:
dextromethorphan 5 mg
pseudoephedrine 15 mg
guaifenesin 100 mg
Uses: Antitussive, adrenergic, expectorant

Betoptic-Pilo:
0.25% betaxolol
1.75% pilocarpine
Uses: Ophthalmic
Biohist-LA Tablets:
pseudoephedrine 120 mg
carbinoxamine 8 mg
Uses: Adrenergic
Blephamide Ophthalmic Suspension/Ointment:
0.2% prednisolone
10% sodium sulfacetamide
Uses: Ophthalmic antiinfective, antiinflammatory
Bromfed Capsules:
pseudoephedrine 120 mg
brompheniramine 12 mg
Uses: Antihistamine, adrenergic
Bromfed-PD Capsules:
pseudoephedrine 60 mg
brompheniramine 6 mg
Uses: Adrenergic, antihistamine
Bromfed Tablets:
pseudoephedrine 60 mg
brompheniramine 4 mg
Uses: Antihistamine, adrenergic
Bromfenex:
brompheniramine 12 mg
pseudoephedrine 120 mg
Uses: Antihistamine, adrenergic
Bromfenex PD:
brompheniramine 6 mg
pseudoephedrine 60 mg
Uses: Antihistamine, adrenergic
Bromo-Seltzer:
sodium bicarb 2781 mg
acetaminophen 325 mg
citric acid 2224 mg
Uses: Antacid, analgesic
Brondelate Elixir:
theophylline 192 mg
guaifenesin 150 mg
Uses: Bronchodilator, expectorant
Brontex:
codeine 10 mg
guaifenesin 300 mg
Uses: Analgesic, expectorant
Bufferin:
aspirin 325 mg
calcium carbonate 158 mg
magnesium oxide 63 mg
magnesium carbonate 34 mg
Uses: Analgesic, antacid
Bufferin AF Nite-Time:
acetaminophen 500 mg
diphenhydramine 38 mg
Uses: Analgesic, antihistamine
Butace:
acetaminophen 325 mg
caffeine 40 mg
butalbital 50 mg
Uses: Nonnarcotic analgesic
Butibel:
belladonna extract 15 mg
butabarbital 15 mg
Uses: Anticholinergic, barbiturate
Cafatine PB:
ergotamine 1 mg
caffeine 100 mg
belladonna alkaloids 0.125 mg
pentobarbital 30 mg
Uses: Migraine agent
Cafergot:
ergotamine 1 mg
caffeine 100 mg
Uses: Adrenergic blocker
Cafergot Suppositories:
ergotamine 2 mg
caffeine 100 mg
Uses: Adrenergic blocker
Caladryl:
8% calamine, camphor
2.2% alcohol
1% pramoxine
Uses: Top antihistamine
Caladryl Clear:
1% pramoxine
0.1% zinc acetate
2% alcohol
camphor
Uses: Top antihistamine
Calcet:
calcium 152.8 mg
vitamin D 100 IU
Uses: Supplement
Calcidrine Syrup:
Per 5 ml:
codeine 8.4 mg
calcium iodide 152 mg
Uses: Analgesic
Caltrate 600+D:
vitamin D 200 IU
calcium 600 mg
Uses: Supplement
Cama Arthritis Pain Reliever:
aspirin 500 mg
magnesium oxide 150 mg
aluminum hydroxide 125 mg
Uses: Nonnarcotic analgesic, antacid
Capital w/Codeine:
Per 5 ml:
acetaminophen 120 mg
codeine 12 mg
Uses: Narcotic analgesic

Capozide 25/15:
captopril 25 mg
hydrochlorothiazide 15 mg
Uses: Antihypertensive
Capozide 25/25:
captopril 25 mg
hydrochorothiazide 25 mg
Uses: Antihypertensive
Capozide 50/15:
captopril 50 mg
hydrochlorothiazide 15 mg
Uses: Antihypertensive
Capozide 50/25:
captopril 50 mg
hydrochlorothiazide 25 mg
Uses: Antihypertensive
Cardec DM Syrup:
Per 5 ml:
pseudoephedrine 60 mg
carbinoxamine 4 mg
dextromethorphan 15 mg
Uses: Adrenergic, antitussive
Cetacaine Topical:
14% benzocaine
2% tetracaine
0.5% benzalkonium chloride
0.005% cetyl dimethyl ethyl ammonium bromide
Uses: Local analgesic
Ceta Plus:
hydrocodone 5 mg
acetaminophen 500 mg
Uses: Analgesic
Cetapred Ointment:
0.25% prednisolone
10% sodium sulfacetamide
Uses: Ophthalmic antiinfective, antiinflammatory
Cheracol Syrup:
Per 5 ml:
codeine 10 mg
guaifenesin 100 mg
Uses: Analgesic, expectorant
Children's Cepacol Liquid:
Per 5 ml:
acetaminophen 160 mg
pseudoephedrine 15 mg
Uses: Analgesic, adrenergic
Chlor-Trimeton Allergy 4 Hour Decongestant:
pseudoephedrine 60 mg
chlorpheniramine 4 mg
Uses: Antihistamine, adrenergic
Chlor-Trimeton 12 Hour Relief Tablets:
pseudoephedrine 120 mg
chlorpheniramine 8 mg
Uses: Antihistamine, adrenergic
Chromagen:
ferrous fumarate 66 mg
vitamin B_{12} 10 μg
vitamin C 250 mg
intrinsic factor 100 mg
Uses: Supplement
Claritin-D:
loratidine 5 mg
pseudoephedrine 120 mg
Uses: Antihistamine, adrenergic
Claritin-D 24-Hour:
loratidine 10 mg
pseudoephedrine 240 mg
Uses: Antihistamine, adrenergic
Clindex:
chlordiazepoxide 5 mg
clidinium 2.5 mg
Uses: Antianxiety, anticholinergic
Clomycin Ointment:
bacitracin 500 U
neomycin sulfate 3.5 g
polymyxin B sulfate 500 U
lidocaine 40 mg
Uses: Antiinfective, local anesthetic
Co-Apap:
pseudoephedrine 30 mg
chlorpheniramine 2 mg
dextromethorphan 15 mg
acetaminophen 325 mg
Uses: Adrenergic, antihistamine, antitussive, analgesic
Co-Gesic:
acetaminophen 500 mg
hydrocodone 5 mg
Uses: Analgesic
Codehist DH Elixir:
Per 5 ml:
pseudoephedrine 30 mg
chlorpheniramine 2 mg
codeine 10 mg
Uses: Adrenergic, antihistamine, analgesic
Codiclear DH Syrup:
Per 5 ml:
hydrocodone 5 mg
guaifenesin 100 mg
Uses: Analgesic, expectorant
Codimal:
pseudoephedrine 30 mg
chlorpheniramine 2 mg
acetaminophen 500 mg
Uses: Adrenergic, antihistamine, analgesic

Codimal DH Syrup:
Per 5 ml:
hydrocodone 1.66 mg
phenylephrine 5 mg
pyrilamine 8.33 mg
Uses: Analgesic, adrenergic

Codimal DM Syrup:
Per 5 ml:
phenylephrine 5 mg
pyrilamine 8.33 mg
dextromethorphan 10 mg
Uses: Adrenergic, antitussive

Codimal-LA:
chlorpheniramine 8 mg
pseudoephedrine 120 mg
Uses: Antihistamine, adrenergic

Codimal PII Syrup:
Per 5 ml:
codeine 10 mg
phenylephrine 5 mg
pyrilamine 8.33 mg
Uses: Analgesic, adrenergic

Col-Probenecid:
probenecid 500 mg
colchicine 0.5 mg
Uses: Antigout agent

ColBenemid:
probenecid 500 mg
colchicine 0.5 mg
Uses: Antigout agent

Coldrine:
pseudoephedrine 30 mg
acetaminophen 500 mg
Uses: Decongestant, nonnarcotic analgesic

Coly-Mycin S Otic Suspension:
1% hydrocortisone
neomycin base 3.3 mg/ml
colistin 3 mg/ml
0.05% thonzonium bromide
Uses: Otic antiinfective

Combipres 0.1:
chlorthalidone 15 mg
clonidine 0.1 mg
Uses: Antihypertensive

Combipres 0.2:
chlorthalidone 15 mg
clonidine 0.2 mg
Uses: Antihypertensive

Combipres 0.3:
chlorthalidone 15 mg
clonidine 0.3 mg
Uses: Antihypertensive

Combivent:
ipratropium bromide 18 μg
albuterol 103 μg/actuation
Uses: Bronchodilator

Combivir:
lamivudine 150 mg
zidovudine 300 mg
Uses: Antiviral

Comhist Tablets:
phenylephrine 10 mg
chlorpheniramine 2 mg
phenyltoloxamine 25 mg
Uses: Adrenergic, antihistamine

Comhist LA:
phenylephrine 20 mg
chlorpheniramine 4 mg
phenyltoloxamine 50 mg
Uses: Adrenergic, antihistamine

Comtrex Liquid:
Per 5 ml:
chlorpheniramine 0.67 mg
acetaminophen 108.3 mg
dextromethorphan 3.3 mg
pseudoephedrine 10 mg
Uses: Antihistamine, analgesic, antitussive, decongestant

Comtrex Allergy-Sinus:
chlorpheniramine 2 mg
acetaminophen 500 mg
pseudoephedrine 30 mg
Uses: Antihistamine, analgesic, decongestant

Comtrex Maximum Strength Caplets:
acetaminophen 500 mg
pseudoephedrine 30 mg
chlorpheniramine 2 mg
dextromethorphan 15 mg
Uses: Analgesic, decongestant, antihistamine, antitussive

Comtrex Maximum Strength Multi-Symptoms Cold, Flu Relief:
pseudoephedrine 30 mg
dextromethorphan 15 mg
chlorpheniramine 2 mg
acetaminophen 500 mg
Uses: Analgesic, decongestant, antihistamine, antitussive

Comtrex Maximum Strength Non-Drowsy Caplets:
acetaminophen 500 mg
pseudoephedrine 30 mg
dextromethorphan 15 mg
Uses: Analagesic, decongestant, antitussive

Congess SR:
guaifenesin 250 mg
pseudoephedrine 120 mg
Uses: Expectorant, decongestant

Congestac:
guaifenesin 400 mg
pseudoephedrine 60 mg
Uses: Expectorant, decongestant

Contac Cough & Chest Cold Liquid:
Per 5 ml:
pseudoephedrine 15 mg
dextromethorphan 5 mg
guaifenesin 50 mg
acetaminophen 125 mg
Uses: Decongestant, antitussive, expectorant, analgesic

Contac Cough & Sore Throat Liquid:
Per 5 ml:
dextromethorphan 5 mg
acetaminophen 125 mg
Uses: Antitussive, analgesic

Contac Day Allergy/Sinus:
pseudoephedrine 60 mg
acetaminophen 650 mg
Uses: Decongestant, analgesic

Contac Day Cold and Flu:
pseudoephedrine 60 mg
dextromethorphan 30 mg
acetaminophen 650 mg
Uses: Decongestant, antitussive, analgesic

Contac Night Allergy Sinus:
pseudoephedrine 60 mg
diphenhydramine 50 mg
acetaminophen 650 mg
Uses: Decongestant, antihistamine, analgesic

Contac Night Cold and Flu Caplets:
pseudoephedrine 60 mg
diphenhydramine 50 mg
acetaminophen 650 mg
Uses: Decongestant, antihistamine, antitussive, analgesic

Contac Severe Cold & Flu Nighttime Liquid:
Per 5 ml:
pseudoephedrine 10 mg
chlorpheniramine 0.67 mg
dextromethorphan 5 mg
acetaminophen 167 mg
18.5% alcohol
Uses: Decongestant, antihistamine, antitussive, analgesic

Coricidin:
chlorpheniramine 2 mg
acetaminophen 325 mg
Uses: Antihistamine, analgesic

Coricidin D Tablets:
chlorpheniramine 2 mg
acetaminophen 325 mg
Uses: Antihistamine, analgesic

Coricidin D Cold, Flu & Sinus:
chlorpheniramine 2 mg
acetaminophen 325 mg
pseudoephedrine sulfate 30 mg
Uses: Antihistamine, analgesic, decongestant

Cortisporin Ophthalmic/Otic Suspension:
0.35% neomycin polymyxin B 10,000 U/ml
1% hydrocortisone
Uses: Ophthalmic antiinfective, antiinflammatory

Cortisporin Ophthalmic Ointment:
0.35% neomycin base
bacitracin 400 U
polymyxin B 10,000 U
hydrocortisone 1%
Uses: Ophthalmic antiinfective

Cortisporin Topical Cream:
0.5% neomycin sulfate
polymyxin B 10,000 U
0.5% hydrocortisone
Uses: Topical antiinfective

Cortisporin Topical Ointment:
0.5% neomycin sulfate
bacitracin 400 U
polymyxin B 5,000 U
1% hydrocortisone
Uses: Topical antiinfective

Corzide 40/5:
nadolol 40 mg
bendroflumethiazide 5 mg
Uses: Antihypertensive

Corzide 80/5:
nadolol 80 mg
bendroflumethiazide 5 mg
Uses: Antihypertensive

Cough-X:
dextromethorphan 5 mg
benzocaine 2 mg
Uses: Antitussive, local anesthetic

Creon:
lipase 8,000 U
amylase 30,000 U
protease 13,000 U
pancreatin 300 mg
Uses: Digestive enzyme

Cyclomydril Ophthalmic Solution:
0.2% cyclopentolate
1% phenylephrine
Uses: Mydriatic

Dallergy Caplets:
chlorpheniramine 8 mg
phenylephrine 20 mg
methscopolamine 2.5 mg
Uses: Antihistamine, adrenergic

Dallergy Syrup:
Per 5 ml:
chlorpheniramine 2 mg
phenylephrine 10 mg
methscopolamine 0.625 mg
Uses: Antihistamine, adrenergic

Dallergy Tablets:
chlorpheniramine 4 mg
phenylephrine 10 mg
methscopolamine 1.25 mg
Uses: Antihistamine, adrenergic

Dallergy-D Syrup:
Per 5 ml:
phenylephrine 5 mg
chlorpheniramine 2 mg
Uses: Antihistamine, adrenergic

Damason-P:
hydrocodone 5 mg
aspirin 500 mg
Uses: Analgesic

Darvocet-N50:
acetaminophen 325 mg
propoxyphene 50 mg
Uses: Analgesic

Darvocet-N 100:
propoxyphene-N 100 mg
acetaminophen 650 mg
Uses: Analgesic

Darvon Compound-65:
propoxyphene 65 mg
aspirin 389 mg
caffeine 32.4 mg
Uses: Analgesic

***Darvon-N Compound:**
aspirin 375 mg
propoxyphene 100 mg
caffeine 30 mg
Uses: Analgesic

***Darvon-N w/A.S.A.:**
aspirin 325 mg
propoxyphene 100 mg
Uses: Analgesic

Deconamine:
pseudoephedrine 60 mg
chlorpheniramine 4 mg
Uses: Antihistamine, decongestant

Deconamine CX:
hydrocodone 5 mg
pseudoephedrine 30 mg
guaifenesin 300 mg
Uses: Analgesic, decongestant, expectorant

Deconamine SR:
pseudoephedrine 120 mg
chlorpheniramine 8 mg
Uses: Antihistamine, decongestant

Deconamine Syrup:
Per 5 ml:
pseudoephedrine 30 mg
chlorpheniramine 2 mg
Uses: Antihistamine, decongestant

Defen-LA:
pseudoephedrine 60 mg
guaifenesin 600 mg
Uses: Decongestant, expectorant

Demi-Regroton:
chlorthalidone 25 mg
reserpine 0.125 mg
Uses: Antihypertensive

Demulen 1/50:
ethinyl estradiol 50 μg
ethynodiol diacetate 1 mg
Uses: Oral contraceptive

Dexacidin Ophthalmic Ointment/Suspension:
Per ml:
0.1% dexamethasone
0.35% neomycin
polymyxin B 10,000 U/g
Uses: Ophth, antiinfective/antiinflammatory

Dexasporin Ophthalmic Ointment:
Per gram:
0.1% dexamethasone
0.35% neomycin
polymyxin B 10,000 U
Uses: Ophth, antiinfective/antiinflammatory

DHC Plus:
dihydrocodeine 16 mg
acetaminophen 356.4 mg
caffeine 30 mg
Uses: Analgesic

Dialose Plus:
docusate sodium 100 mg
yellow phenolphthalein 65 mg
Uses: Laxative

Di-Gel Advanced Formula:
magnesium hydroxide 128 mg
calcium carbonate 280 mg
simethicone 20 mg
Uses: Antacid, adsorbent, antiflatulent

Di-Gel Liquid:
Per 5 ml:
aluminum hydroxide 200 mg
magnesium hydroxide 200 mg
simethicone 20 mg
Uses: Antacid, adsorbent, antiflatulent

Dihistine DH Liquid:
Per 5 ml:
pseudoephedrine 30 mg
chlorpheniramine 2 mg
codeine 10 mg
Uses: Decongestant, antihistamine, analgesic

Dilaudid Cough Syrup:
Per 5 ml:
guaifenesin 100 mg
hydromorphone 1 mg
5% alcohol
Uses: Expectorant, analgesic

Dilor-G Liquid:
dyphylline 300 mg
guaifenesin 300 mg
Uses: Bronchodilator, expectorant

Dilor-G Tablets:
dyphylline 200 mg
guaifenesin 200 mg
Uses: Bronchodilator, expectorant

Dimetane Decongestant:
brompheniramine 4 mg
phenylephrine 10 mg
Uses: Antihistamine, adrenergic

Dimetane-DX Cough Syrup:
Per 5 ml:
brompheniramine 2 mg
pseudoephedrine 30 mg
dextromethorphan 10 mg
Uses: Antihistamine, decongestant, antitussive

Dimetapp Sinus:
pseudoephedrine 30 mg
ibuprofen 200 mg
Uses: Decongestant, analgesic

Diurigen w/Reserpine:
chlorothiazide 250 mg
reserpine 0.125 mg
Uses: Antihypertensive

Diutensin-R:
methylclothiazide 2.5 mg
reserpine 0.1 mg
Uses: Antihypertensive

Doan's PM Extra Strength:
magnesium salicylate 500 mg
diphenhydramine 25 mg
Uses: Analgesic, antihistamine

Dolacet:
hydrocodone 5 mg
acetaminophen 500 mg
Uses: Analgesic

Donnatal:
phenobarbital 16.2 mg
hyoscyamine 0.1037 mg
atropine 0.0194 mg
scopolamine 0.0065 mg
Uses: Anticholinergic, barbiturate

Donnatal Elixir:
Per 5 ml:
phenobarbital 16.2 mg
hyoscyamine 0.1037 mg
atropine 0.0194 mg
scopolamine 0.0065 mg
23% alcohol
Uses: Anticholinergic, barbiturate

Donnatal Extentabs:
phenobarbital 48.6 mg
hyoscyamine 0.3111 mg
atropine 0.0582 mg
scopolamine 0.0195 mg
Uses: Anticholinergic, barbiturate

Donnazyme:
pancreatin 500 mg
lipase 1000 U
protease 12,500 U
amylase 12,500 U
Uses: Pancreatic enzymes

Dorcol Children's Cold Formula Liquid:
Per 5 ml:
pseudoephedrine 15 mg
chlorpheniramine 1 mg
Uses: Decongestant, antihistamine

Doxidan:
docusate calcium 60 mg
phenolphthalein 65 mg
Uses: Stool softener

Dristan Cold:
pseudoephedrine 30 mg
acetaminophen 500 mg
Uses: Decongestant, analgesic

Dristan Cold Maximum Strength Caplets:
pseudoephedrine 30 mg
brompheniramine 2 mg
acetaminophen 500 mg
Uses: Decongestant, antihistamine, analgesic

Dristan Cold Multi-Symptom Formula:
acetaminophen 325 mg
phenylephrine 5 mg
chlorpheniramine 2 mg
Uses: Analgesic, adrenergic, antihistamine

Dristan Sinus:
pseudoephedrine 30 mg
ibuprofen 200 mg
Uses: Decongestant, analgesic

Drixoral Allergy Sinus:
pseudoephedrine 60 mg
dexbrompheniramine 3 mg
acetaminophen 500 mg
Uses: Decongestant, antihistamine, analgesic

Drixoral Cold & Allergy:
pseudoephedrine 120 mg
dexbrompheniramine 6 mg
Uses: Decongestant, antihistamine
Drixoral Cold & Flu:
pseudoephedrine 60 mg
dexbrompheniramine 3 mg
acetaminophen 500 mg
Uses: Decongestant, antihistamine, analgesic
Drixoral Cough & Congestion Liquid Caps:
pseudoephedrine 60 mg
dextromethorphan 30 mg
Uses: Decongestant, antitussive
Drixoral Cough & Sore Throat Liquid Caps:
dextromethorphan 15 mg
acetaminophen 325 mg
Uses: Antitussive, analgesic
Drixoral Plus:
pseudoephedrine 60 mg
dexbrompheniramine 3 mg
acetaminophen 500 mg
Uses: Decongestant, antihistamine, analgesic
DT:
Per 5 ml dose:
diphtheria toxoid 2LfU
tetanus toxoid 5LfU
Uses: Vaccine
DTP:
Per 0.5 ml dose:
diphtheria toxoid 6.5LfU
tetanus toxoid 5LfU
pertussis 4LfU
Uses: Vaccine
Dura-Vent/DA:
phenylephrine 20 mg
chlorpheniramine 8 mg
methscopolamine 2.5 mg
Uses: Adrenergic, antihistamine
Dyazide:
hydrochlorothiazide 25 mg
triamterene 37.5 mg
Uses: Diuretic
Dylline-GG Liquid:
dyphylline 300 mg
quaifenesin 300 mg
Uses: Bronchodilator, expectorant
Dynafed Asthma Relief:
ephedrine 25 mg
guaifenesin 200 mg
Uses: Adrenergic, expectorant
Dynafed Plus Maximum Strength:
pseudoephedrine 30 mg
acetaminophen 500 mg
Uses: Decongestant, analgesic
Dyphylline-GG Elixir:
Per 5 ml:
dyphylline 100 mg
guaifenesin 100 mg
Uses: Bronchodilator, expectorant
E-Lor:
acetaminophen 650 mg
propoxyphene 65 mg
Uses: Analgesic
E-Pilo-1 Ophthalmic Solution:
1% epinephrine bitartrate
1% pilocarpine
Uses: Miotic
E-Pilo-2 Ophthalmic Solution:
1% epinephrine bitartrate
2% pilocarpine
Uses: Miotic
E-Pilo-4 Ophthalmic Solution:
1% epinephrine bitartrate
4% pilocarpine
Uses: Miotic
Elase-Chloromycetin Ointment:
Per gram:
fibrinolysin 1 U
desoxyribonuclease 666.6 U
chloramphenicol 10 mg
Uses: Enzyme, antiinfective
Elase Ointment:
Per gram:
fibrinolysin 1 U
desoxyribonuclease 666.6 U
Uses: Enzyme
Elixophyllin GG Liquid:
Per 5 ml:
theophylline 100 mg
guaifenesin 100 mg
Uses: Expectorant, bronchodilator
EMLA Cream:
lidocaine 2.5 mg
prilocaine 2.5 mg
Uses: Local anesthetic
Empirin w/Codeine #3:
aspirin 325 mg
codeine phosphate 30 mg
Uses: Analgesic
Empirin w/Codeine #4:
aspirin 325 mg
codeine phosphate 60 mg
Uses: Analgesic
***Empracet-60:**
acetaminophen 300 mg
codeine 60 mg
Uses: Analgesic
Endocet:
acetaminophen 325 mg
oxycodone 5 mg
Uses: Analgesic

***Endodan:**
aspirin 325 mg
oxycodone 5 mg
Uses: Analgesic
Endolor:
acetaminophen 325 mg
caffeine 40 mg
butalbital 50 mg
Uses: Nonnarcotic analgesic
Enduronyl:
methyclothiazide 5 mg
deserpidine 0.25 mg
Uses: Antihypertensive
Enduronyl Forte:
methyclothiazide 5.0 mg
deserpidine 0.5 mg
Uses: Antihypertensive
Entex PSE:
pseudoephedrine 120 mg
guaifenesin 600 mg
Uses: Adrenergic, expectorant
Epifoam Aerosol Foam:
1% hydrocortisone
1% pramoxine
Uses: Topical corticosteroid
Equagesic:
meprobamate 200 mg
aspirin 325 mg
Uses: Antianxiety
Eryzole:
Per 5 ml:
erythromycin 200 mg
sulfisoxazole 600 mg
Uses: Macrolide antiinfective
Esgic-Plus:
butalbital 50 mg
acetaminophen 500 mg
caffeine 40 mg
Uses: Barbiturate, analgesic
Esimil:
guanethidine 10 mg
hydrochlorothiazide 25 mg
Uses: Antihypertensive
Estratest:
esterified estrogens 1.25 mg
methyltestosterone 2.5 mg
Uses: Androgen, estrogen
Etrafon:
perphenazine 2 mg
amitriptyline 25 mg
Uses: Antipsychotic, antidepressant
Etrafon 2-10:
perphenazine 2 mg
amitriptyline 10 mg
Uses: Antidepressant
Etrafon A:
perphenazine 4 mg
amitriptyline 10 mg
Uses: Antidepressant
Etrafon Forte:
perphenazine 4 mg
amitriptyline 25 mg
Uses: Antipsychotic, antidepressant
Excedrin Aspirin Free Caplets and Geltabs:
500 mg acetaminophen
65 mg caffeine
Uses: Nonnarcotic analgesic
Excedrin Extra Strength:
aspirin 250 mg
acetaminophen 250 mg
caffeine 65 mg
Uses: Nonnarcotic analgesic
Excedrin Migraine:
aspirin 250 mg
acetaminophen 250 mg
caffeine 65 mg
Uses: Migraine agent
Excedrin P.M.:
acetaminophen 500 mg
diphenhydramine citrate 38 mg
Uses: Analgesic, antihistamine
Excedrin P.M. Liquid:
Per 30 ml:
acetaminophen 1000 mg
diphenhydramine 50 mg
Uses: Analgesic, antihistamine
Excedrin P.M. Liquigels:
acetaminophen 500 mg
diphenhydramine 25 mg
Uses: Analgesic, antihistamine
Excedrin Sinus Extra Strength:
pseudoephedrine 30 mg
acetaminophen 500 mg
Uses: Decongestant, analgesic
Fansidar:
sulfidoxine 500 mg
pyrimethamine 25 mg
Uses: Antimalarial
Fedahist:
pseudoephedrine 60 mg
chlorpheniramine 4 mg
Uses: Decongestant, antihistamine
Fedahist Expectorant Syrup:
Per 5 ml:
guaifenesin 200 mg
pseudoephedrine 20 mg
Uses: Expectorant, decongestant
Fedahist Gyrocaps:
pseudoephedrine 65 mg
chlorpheniramine 10 mg
Uses: Decongestant, antihistamine

Fedahist Timecaps:
pseudoephedrine 120 mg
chlorpheniramine 8 mg
Uses: Decongestant, antihistamine

Feen-A-Mint Pills:
docusate sodium 100 mg
phenolphthalein 65 mg
Uses: Laxative

Fem-1:
acetaminophen 500 mg
pamabrom 25 mg
Uses: Nonnarcotic analgesic

FemBack Caplets:
150 mg acetaminophen
150 mg salicylamide
44 mg phenyltoloxamine
Uses: Nonnarcotic analgesic

Femcet:
acetaminophen 325 mg
caffeine 40 mg
butalbital 50 mg
Uses: Nonnarcotic analgesic

Ferro-Sequels:
docusate sodium 100 mg
ferrous fumarate 150 mg
Uses: Laxative, hematinic

Fiorgen:
aspirin 325 mg
caffeine 40 mg
butalbital 50 mg
Uses: Nonnarcotic analgesic

Fioricet:
acetaminophen 325 mg
caffeine 40 mg
butalbital 50 mg
Uses: Analgesic, barbiturate

Fioricet w/Codeine:
acetaminophen 325 mg
caffeine 40 mg
butalbital 50 mg
codeine 30 mg
Uses: Analgesic, barbiturate

Fiorinal:
aspirin 325 mg
caffeine 40 mg
butalbital 50 mg
Uses: Analgesic, barbiturate

Fiorinal w/Codeine:
aspirin 325 mg
caffeine 40 mg
butalbital 50 mg
codeine 30 mg
Uses: Analgesic, barbiturate

FML-S Ophthalmic Suspension:
0.1% flurometholone
10% sulfacetamide
Uses: Ophth, antiinfective/antiinflammatory

Gas-Ban:
calcium carbonate 500 mg
simethicone 40 mg
Uses: Antiflatulent, antacid

Gas-Ban DS Liquid:
Per 5 ml:
aluminum hydroxide 400 mg
magnesium hydroxide 400 mg
simethicone 40 mg
Uses: Antiflatulent, antacid

Gaviscon:
magnesium trisilicate 20 mg
aluminum hydroxide 80 mg
Uses: Antacid, adsorbent, antiflatulent

Gaviscon Liquid:
Per 5 ml:
aluminum hydroxide 31.7 mg
magnesium carbonate 119.3 mg
Uses: Antacid, adsorbent, antiflatulent

Gelprin:
acetaminophen 125 mg
aspirin 240 mg
caffeine 32 mg
Uses: Analgesic

Gelusil:
aluminum hydroxide 200 mg
magnesium hydroxide 200 mg
simethicone 25 mg
Uses: Antacid, adsorbent, antiflatulent

Genatuss DM Syrup:
Per 5 ml:
guaifenesin 100 mg
dextromethorphan 10 mg
Uses: Expectorant, antitussive

Glucovance:
glyburide: 1.25 mg
metformin: 250 mg
Uses: Antidiabetic

Glucovance:
glyburide: 2.5 mg
metformin: 500 mg
Uses: Antidiabetic

Glucovance:
glyburide: 5 mg
metformin: 500 mg
Uses: Antidiabetic

Goody's Extra Strength Headache Powder:
250 mg acetaminophen
520 mg aspirin
32.5 mg caffeine
Uses: Nonopiate analgesic

Goody's Body Pain Powder:
325 mg acetaminophen
500 mg aspirin

Granulex Aerosol:
Per 0.82 ml:
trypsin 0.1 mg
balsam peru 72.5 mg
castor oil 650 mg
Uses: Top enzyme
Guaifenex PSE 60:
pseudoephedrine 60 mg
guaifenesin 600 mg
Uses: Decongestant, expectorant
Guaifenex PSE 120:
pseudoephedrine 120 mg
guaifenesin 600 mg
Uses: Decongestant, expectorant
Haley's M-O Liquid:
Per 15 ml:
magnesium hydroxide 900 mg
mineral oil 3.75 ml
Uses: Laxative
Halotussin-DM Sugar Free Liquid:
Per 5 ml:
guaifenesin 100 mg
dextromethorphan 10 mg
Uses: Expectorant, antitussive
Helidac:
In a compliance package:
bismuth subsalicylate 262.4 mg tabs
metronidazole 250 mg tabs
tetracycline 500 mg caps
Uses: Antiinfective
Ilumibid DM Sprinkle Caps:
dextromethorphan 15 mg
guaifenesin 300 mg
Uses: Expectorant, antitussive
Humibid DM Tablets:
dextromethorphan 30 mg
guaifenesin 600 mg
Uses: Expectorant, antitussive
Hycodan:
hydrocodone 5 mg
homatropine 1.5 mg
Uses: Analgesic, mydriatic
Hycodan Syrup:
Per 5 ml:
hydrocodone 5 mg
homatropine 1.5 mg
Uses: Analgesic, mydriatic
Hycomine Compound:
chlorpheniramine 2 mg
acetaminophen 250 mg
phenylephrine 10 mg
hydrocodone 5 mg
caffeine 30 mg
Uses: Antihistamine, analgesic, adrenergic
Hycotuss Expectorant:
Per 5 ml:
guaifenesin 100 mg
hydrocodone 5 mg
10% alcohol
Uses: Expectorant
Hydergine:
dihydroergocornine 0.167 mg
dihydroergocristine 0.167 mg
dihydroergocryptine 0.167 mg
Uses: Adrenergic blocker
Hydro-Serp:
hydrochlorothiazide 50 mg
reserpine 0.125 mg
Uses: Antihypertensive
Hydrocet:
hydrocodone 5 mg
acetaminophen 500 mg
Uses: Narcotic, opioid analgesic
Hydrogesic:
hydrocodone 5 mg
acetaminophen 500 mg
Uses: Narcotic, opioid analgesic
Hydropres-50:
hydrochlorothiazide 50 mg
reserpine 0.125 mg
Uses: Antihypertensive
Hydroserpine:
hydrochlorothiazide 25 mg
reserpine 0.125 mg
Uses: Antihypertensive
Hydroserpine:
hydrochlorothiazide 50 mg
reserpine 0.125 mg
Uses: Antihypertensive
Hyzaar:
losartan potassium 50 mg
hydrochlorothiazide 12.5 mg
potassium 4.24 mg
Uses: Antihypertensive
Iberet Filmtab:
ferrous sulfate 105 mg
ascorbic acid 150 mg
B-complex vitamins
Uses: Supplement
Iberet Liquid:
Per 5 ml:
ferrous sulfate 78.75 mg
ascorbic acid 112.5 mg
B-complex vitamins
Uses: Supplement
Imodium Advanced:
loperamide 2 mg
simethicone 125 mg
Uses: Antidiarrheal, antiflatulent

Inderide 40/25:
propranolol 40 mg
hydrochlorothiazide 25 mg
Uses: Antihypertensive
Inderide 80/25:
propranolol 80 mg
hydrochlorothiazide 25 mg
Uses: Antihypertensive
Inderide LA 80/50:
propranolol 80 mg
hydrochlorothiazide 50 mg
Uses: Antihypertensive
Inderide LA 120/50:
propranolol 120 mg
hydrochlorothiazide 50 mg
Uses: Antihypertensive
Inderide LA 160/50:
propranolol 160 mg
hydrochlorothiazide 50 mg
Uses: Antihypertensive
Innovar:
Per ml:
droperidol 2.5 mg
fentanyl 0.05 mg
Uses: Narcotic analgesic, general anesthetic
Iofed:
brompheniramine 12 mg
pseudoephedrine 120 mg
Uses: Antihistamine, adrenergic
Iofed PD:
brompheniramine 6 mg
pseudoephedrine 60 mg
Uses: Antihistamine, adrenergic
Iophen-C Liquid:
Per 5 ml:
iodinated glycerol 30 mg
codeine 10 mg
Uses: Expectorant, analgesic
Iophen-DM Liquid:
Per 5 ml:
iodinated glycerol 30 mg
dextromethorphan 10 mg
Uses: Expectorant, antitussive
Isollyl:
aspirin 325 mg
caffeine 40 mg
butalbital 50 mg
Uses: Nonnarcotic analgesic
Isopap:
isometheptene 65 mg
APAP 325 mg
dicloral-phenazone 100 mg
Uses: Migraine agent
Kaletra:
lopinavir 133.3 mg
ritonavir 33.3 mg
Uses: HIV
Kondremul w/Phenolphthalein:
Per 15 ml:
phenolphthalein 150 mg
55% mineral oil
Irish moss
Uses: Laxative
Lactinex:
Mixed culture of:
Lactobacillus acidophilus and
Lactobacillus bulgaricus
Uses: Supplement
Lanorinal:
aspirin 325 mg
caffeine 40 mg
butalbital 50 mg
Uses: Nonnarcotic analgesic
Lenoltec w/Codeine No. 1:
acetaminophen 650 mg
hydrocodone 10 mg
Uses: Analgesic
Levsin PB Drops:
Per ml:
hyoscyamine 0.125 mg
phenobarbital 15 mg
5% alcohol
Uses: Anticholinergic, barbiturate
Levsin w/Phenobarbital:
hyoscyamine 0.125 mg
phenobarbital 15 mg
Uses: Anticholinergic, barbiturate
Lexxel:
enalapril 5 mg
felodipine 5 mg
Uses: Antihypertensive
Librax:
chlordiazepoxide 5 mg
clidinium 2.5 mg
Uses: Antianxiety, anticholinergic
Lida-Mantel-HC-Cream:
0.5% hydrocortisone
3% lidocaine
Uses: Antiinflammatory, analgesic
Limbitrol DS:
chlordiazepoxide 10 mg
amitriptyline 25 mg
Uses: Antidepressant, antianxiety
Lobac:
salicylamide 200 mg
phenyltoloxamine 20 mg
acetaminophen 300 mg
Uses: Skeletal muscle relaxant, analgesic
Loestrin Fe 1.5/30:
norethindrone acetate 1.5 mg
ethinyl estradiol 30 μg
Uses: Oral contraceptive

Lomotil:
diphenoxylate 2.5 mg
atropine 0.025 mg
Uses: Antidiarrheal, anticholinergic
Lomotil Liquid:
Per 5 ml:
diphenoxylate 2.5 mg
atropine 0.025 mg
Uses: Antidiarrheal, anticholinergic
Lo Ovral:
ethinyl estradiol 30 μg
norgestrel 0.3 mg
Uses: Oral contraceptive
Lopressor HCT 50/25:
metoprolol 50 mg
hydrochlorothiazide 25 mg
Uses: Antihypertensive
Lopressor HCT 100/25:
metoprolol 100 mg
hydrochlorothiazide 25 mg
Uses: Antihypertensive
Lopressor HCT 100/50:
metoprolol 100 mg
hydrochlorothiazide 50 mg
Uses: Antihypertensive
Lorcet 10/650:
acetaminophen 650 mg
hydrocodone 10 mg
Uses: Analgesic
Lorcet Plus:
acetaminophen 650 mg
hydrocodone 7.5 mg
Uses: Analgesic
Lortab 2.5/500:
hydrocodone 2.5 mg
acetaminophen 500 mg
Uses: Analgesic
Lortab 5/500:
hydrocodone 5 mg
acetaminophen 500 mg
Uses: Analgesic
Lortab 7.5/500:
hydrocodone 7.5 mg
acetaminophen 500 mg
Uses: Analgesic
Lortab 10/500:
hydrocodone 10 mg
acetaminophen 500 mg
Uses: Analgesic
Lortab ASA:
aspirin 500 mg
hydrocodone 5 mg
Uses: Analgesic
Lortab Elixir:
Per 5 ml:
hydrocodone 2.5 mg
acetaminophen 167 mg
Uses: Analgesic
Lotensin HCT 5/6.25:
benazepril 5 mg
hydrochlorothiazide 6.25 mg
Uses: Antihypertensive
Lotensin HCT 10/12.5:
benazepril 10 mg
hydrochlorothiazide 12.5 mg
Uses: Antihypertensive
Lotensin HCT 20/12.5:
benazepril 20 mg
hydrochlorothiazide 12.5 mg
Uses: Antihypertensive
Lotensin HCT 20/25:
benazepril 20 mg
hydrochlorothiazide 25 mg
Uses: Antihypertensive
Lotrel 2.5/10:
amlopidine 2.5 mg
benazepril 10 mg
Uses: Antihypertensive
Lotrel 5/10:
amlodipine 5 mg
benazepril 10 mg
Uses: Antihypertensive
Lotrel 5/20:
amlodipine 5 mg
benazepril 20 mg
Uses: Antihypertensive
Lotrisone Topical:
0.05% betamethasone
1% clotrimazole
Uses: Local antiinfective, antiinflammatory
Lufyllin-EPG Elixir:
Per 5 ml:
dyphylline 150 mg
ephedrine 24 mg
guaifenesin 300 mg
phenobarbital 24 mg
Uses: Bronchodilator, expectorant
Lufyllin-EPG Tablets:
dyphylline 100 mg
ephedrine 16 mg
guaifenesin 200 mg
phenobarbital 16 mg
Uses: Bronchodilator, adrenergic, expectorant, barbiturate
Lufyllin-GG:
dyphylline 200 mg
guaifenesin 200 mg
Uses: Bronchodilator, expectorant
Lufyllin-GG Elixir:
dyphylline 100 mg
guaifenesin 100 mg
alcohol 17%
Uses: Bronchodilator, expectorant

Lunelle:
25 mg medroxyprogesterone
5 mg estradiol cypionate/0.5 ml
Uses: Contraceptive
M-M-R-II:
measles
mumps
rubella
Uses: Vaccine, toxoid
M-R Vax II:
measles
rubella
Uses: Vaccine, toxoid
Maalox:
aluminum hydroxide 200 mg
magnesium hydroxide 200 mg
Uses: Antacid, adsorbent, antiflatulent
Maalox Plus:
aluminum hydroxide 200 mg
magnesium hydroxide 200 mg
simethicone 25 mg
Uses: Antacid, adsorbent, antiflatulent
Maalox Plus Extra Strength Suspension:
Per 5 ml:
aluminum hydroxide 500 mg
magnesium hydroxide 450 mg
simethicone 40 mg
Uses: Antacid, adsorbent, antiflatulent
Maalox Suspension:
Per 5 ml:
aluminum hydroxide 225 mg
magnesium hydroxide 200 mg
Uses: Antacid, adsorbent, antiflatulent
Macrobid:
nitrofurantoin macrocrystals 25 mg
nitrofurantoin monohydrate 75 mg
Uses: Antiinfective
Magnaprin:
aspirin 325 mg
magnesium hydroxide 50 mg
aluminum hydroxide 50 mg
calcium carbonate 50 mg
Uses: Nonnarcotic analgesic
Magnaprin Arthritis Strength:
aspirin 325 mg
magnesium hydroxide 75 mg
aluminum hydroxide 75 mg
calcium carbonate 75 mg
Uses: Nonnarcotic analgesic
Malarone:
250 mg atovaquone
100 mg proguanil
Uses: Malaria
Malarone Pediatric:
62.5 mg atovaquone
25 mg proguanil
Uses: Malaria
Mapap Cold Formula:
acetaminophen 325 mg
chlorpheniramine 2 mg
pseudoephedrine 30 mg
dextromethorphan 15 mg
Uses: Bronchodilator, expectorant
Marax:
ephedrine 25 mg
theophylline 130 mg
hydroxyzine 10 mg
Uses: Bronchodilator, sedative/ hypnotic
Marnal:
aspirin 325 mg
caffeine 40 mg
butalbital 50 mg
Uses: Nonnarcotic analgesic
Maxzide 1:
polythiazide 0.5 mg
prazosin 1 mg
Uses: Antihypertensive
Maxzide 2:
polythiazide 0.5 mg
prazosin 2 mg
Uses: Antihypertensive
Maxitrol Ophthalmic Suspension/ Ointment:
Per ml:
0.35% neomycin
0.1% dexamethasone
polymyxin B 10,000 U
Uses: Ophthalmic antiinfective, antiinflammatory
Maxzide:
hydrochlorothiazide 50 mg
triamterene 75 mg
Uses: Antihypertensive, diuretic
Maxzide-25 MG:
hydrochlorothiazide 25 mg
triamterene 37.5 mg
Uses: Diuretic
Medi-Flu Liquid:
Per 5 ml:
pseudoephedrine 10 mg
chlorpheniramine 0.67 mg
dextromethorphan 5 mg
acetaminophen 167 mg
18.5% alcohol
Uses: Decongestant, antihistamine, antitussive, analgesic
Medigesic:
acetaminophen 325 mg
caffeine 40 mg
butalbital 50 mg
Uses: Nonnarcotic analgesic
Mepergan Fortis:
meperidine 50 mg
promethazine 25 mg
Uses: Analgesic, antihistamine

Mepergan Injection:
meperidine 25 mg
promethazine 25 mg
Uses: Analgesic
Metimyd Ophthalmic Suspension/ Ointment:
0.5% prednisolone
10% sodium sulfacetamide
Uses: Ophthalmic antiinfective, antiinflammatory
Midol Maximum Strength Multi-Symptom Menstrual Gelcaps:
acetaminophen 500 mg
pyrilamine 15 mg
caffeine 60 mg
Uses: Analgesic
Midol PM:
acetaminophen 500 mg
diphenhydramine 25 mg
Uses: Analgesic, antihistamine
Midol PMS Maximum Strength Caplets:
acetaminophen 500 mg
pyrilamine 15 mg
pamabrom 25 mg
Uses: Analgesic
Midol, Teen:
acetaminophen 400 mg
pamabrom 25 mg
Uses: Analgesic
Midrin:
isometheptene 65 mg
acetaminophen 325 mg
dichloralphenazone 100 mg
Uses: Analgesic
Minizide 1:
prazosin 1 mg
polythiazide 0.5 mg
Uses: Antihypertensive
Minizide 2:
prazosin 2 mg
polythiazide 0.5 mg
Uses: Antihypertensive
Minizide 5:
prazosin 5 mg
polythiazide 0.5 mg
Uses: Antihypertensive
Modane Plus:
docusate sodium 100 mg
phenolphthalein 65 mg
Uses: Laxative
Moduretic:
hydrochlorothiazide 50 mg
amiloride 5 mg
Uses: Diuretic
Motrin IB Sinus:
pseudoephedrine 30 mg
ibuprofen 200 mg
Uses: Adrenergic, analgesic
Murocoll-2 Ophthalmic Drops:
0.3% scopolamine
10% phenylephrine
Uses: Ophth anticholinergic, mydriatic
Mycolog II Topical:
Per gram:
0.1% triamcinolone acetonide
nystatin 100,000 U
Uses: Local antiinfective, antiinflammatory
Mylanta:
aluminum hydroxide 200 mg
magnesium hydroxide 200 mg
simethicone 20 mg
Uses: Antacid, adsorbent, antiflatulent
Mylanta Double Strength Liquid:
Per 5 ml:
aluminum hydroxide 400 mg
magnesium hydroxide 400 mg
simethicone 40 mg
Uses: Antacid, adsorbent, antiflatulent
Mylanta Gelcaps:
calcium carbonate 311 mg
magnesium carbonate 232 mg
Uses: Antacid, adsorbent, antiflatulent
Naldecon Tablets:
phenylpropanolamine 40 mg
phenylephrine 10 mg
phenyltoloxamine 15 mg
chlorpheniramine 5 mg
Uses: Antihistamine, decongestant
Naldecon Senior DX Liquid:
Per 5 ml:
dextromethorphan 10 mg
guaifenesin 200 mg
Uses: Expectorant, antitussive
Naphcon-A Ophthalmic Solution:
0.25% naphazoline
0.3% pheniramine
Uses: Ophth vasoconstrictor
Nasatab LA:
guaifenesin 500 mg
pseudoephedrine 120 mg
Uses: Expectorant, decongestant
NeoDecadron Ophthalmic Ointment:
0.35% neomycin
0.05% dexamethasone
Uses: Ophth antiinfective, antiinflammatory
NeoDecadron Ophthalmic Solution:
0.35% neomycin
0.1% dexamethasone
Uses: Ophth antiinfective, antiinflammatory

NeoDecadron Topical:
neomycin 0.5%
dexamethasone 0.1%
Uses: Top antiinfective, antiinflammatory
Neosporin Cream:
Per gram:
polymyxin B 10,000 U
neomycin 3.5 mg
Uses: Top antiinfective
Neosporin G.U. Irrigant:
Per ml:
neomycin 40 mg
polymyxin B 200,000 U
Uses: Antiinfective
Neosporin Ointment:
Per gram:
polymyxin B 5000 U
bacitracin zinc 400 U
neomycin 3.5 mg
Uses: Top antiinfective
Neosporin Ophthalmic Solution:
Per ml:
neomycin 1.75 mg
polymyxin B 10,000 U
gramicidin 0.025 mg
Uses: Ophthalmic antiinfective
Neosporin Ophthalmic Ointment:
Per gram:
neomycin 3.5 mg
polymyxin B 10,000 U
bacitracin zinc 400 U
Uses: Ophthalmic antiinfective
Neosporin Plus Cream:
polymyxin B 10,000 U
neomycin 3.5 mg
lidocaine 40 mg
Uses: Top antiinfective
Niferex-150 Forte:
ferrous sulfate 150 mg
vitamin B_{12} 25 μg
folic acid 1 mg
Uses: Supplement
Norgesic:
orphenadrine 25 mg
aspirin 385 mg
caffeine 30 mg
Uses: Skeletal muscle relaxant, analgesic
Norgesic Forte:
orphenadrine 50 mg
aspirin 770 mg
caffeine 60 mg
Uses: Skeletal muscle relaxant, analgesic
Novacet Lotion:
sodium sulfacetamine 10%
sulfur 5%
Uses: Acne agent
Novafed A:
pseudoephedrine 120 mg
chlorpheniramine 8 mg
Uses: Adrenergic, antihistamine
Novahistone Elixir:
Per 5 ml:
phenylephrine 5 mg
chlorpheniramine 2 mg
alcohol 5%
Uses: Antihistamine
Novo-Gesic* C8:
acetaminophen 300 mg
codeine 8 mg
caffeine 15 mg
Uses: Analgesic
NuLytely:
PEG 3350/420 g
sodium bicarbonate 5.72 g
sodium chloride 11.2 g
potassium chloride 1.48 g
Uses: Laxative
NyQuil Hot Therapy:
Per packet:
acetaminophen 1000 mg
pseudoephedrine 60 mg
dextromethorphan 30 mg
doxylamine 12.5 mg
Uses: Analgesic, adrenergic, antitussive
NyQuil Nightime Cold/Flu Medicine Liquid:
Per 5 ml:
pseudoephedrine 10 mg
doxylamine 1.25 mg
dextromethorphan 5 mg
acetaminophen 167 mg
25% alcohol
Uses: Adrenergic, antitussive, analgesic
Octicair Otic Suspension:
hydrocortisone 1%
neomycin 5 mg/ml
polymyxin B 10,000 U/ml
Uses: Otic antiinflammatory, antiinfective
Opcon-A Ophthalmic Solution:
0.027% naphazoline
0.315% pheniramine
Uses: Ophth vasoconstrictor
Ornade Spansules:
phenylpropanolamine 75 mg
chlorpheniramine 12 mg
Uses: Antihistamine, decongestant
Ornex:
pseudoephedrine 30 mg
acetaminophen 500 mg
Uses: Adrenergic, analgesic
Ornex No Drowsiness Caplets:
acetaminophen 325 mg
pseudoephedrine 30 mg
Uses: Adrenergic, analgesic

Ortho-cept:
ethinyl estradiol 30 μg
desogestrel 0.15 mg
Uses: Oral contraceptive
Ortho-Novum 7/7/7:
Phase I:
0.5 mg norethindrone
35 μg ethinyl estradiol
Phase II:
0.75 mg norethindrone
35 μg ethinyl estradiol
Phase III:
1 mg norethinidrone
35 μg estradiol
Uses: Oral contraceptive
Otocort Otic Suspension:
hydrocortisone 1%
neomycin 5 mg/ml
polymyxin B 10,000 U
Uses: Otic antiinflammatory, antiinfective
***Oxycocet:**
acetaminophen 325 mg
oxycodone 5 mg
Uses: Analgesic
P-A-C Analgesic:
aspirin 400 mg
caffeine 32 mg
Uses: Nonnarcotic analgesic
Pain-X Topical:
0.05% capsaicin
5% menthol
4% camphor
Uses: Top analgesic
Pamprin Maximum Pain Relief:
acetaminophen 250 mg
pamabrom 25 mg
magnesium salicylate 250 mg
Uses: Analgesic
Pamprin Multi-Symptom:
acetaminophen 500 mg
pamabrom 25 mg
pyrilamine 15 mg
Uses: Analgesic
Panacet 5/500:
hydrocodone 5 mg
acetaminophen 500 mg
Uses: Analgesic
Panasal 5/500:
hydrocodone 5 mg
aspirin 500 mg
Uses: Analgesic
Pancrease Capsules:
amylase 20,000 U
protease 25,000 U
lipase 4500 U (microspheres)
Uses: Digestive enzyme
Pedia Care Cold-Allergy Chewable:
pseudoephedrine 15 mg
chlorpheniramine 1 mg
Uses: Adrenergic, antihistamine
Pedia Care Cough-Cold Liquid:
Per 5 ml:
pseudoephedrine 15 mg
chlorpheniramine 1 mg
dextromethorphan 5 mg
Uses: Adrenergic, antihistamine, antitussive
Pedia Care NightRest Cough-Cold Liquid:
Per 5 ml:
pseudoephedrine 15 mg
chlorpheniramine 1 mg
dextromethorphan 7.5 mg
Uses: Adrenergic, antihistamine, antitussive
Pediacof Syrup:
Per 5 ml:
codeine 5 mg
phenylephrine 2.5 mg
chlorpheniramine 0.75 mg
potassium iodide 75 mg
5% alcohol
Uses: Opioid, narcotic analgesic, antihistamine
Pediazole Suspension:
Per 5 ml:
erythromycin 200 mg
sulfisoxazole 600 mg
Uses: Antiinfective
Percocet:
oxycodone 5 mg
acetaminophen 325 mg
Uses: Analgesic
Percodan:
oxycodone 4.88 mg
aspirin 325 mg
Uses: Analgesic
Percodan-Demi:
aspirin 325 mg
oxycodone HCl 2.25 mg
oxycodone terephthalate 0.19 mg
Uses: Analgesic
***Percodan-Demi:**
aspirin 325 mg
oxycodone 2.5 mg
Uses: Analgesic
Percogesic:
phenyltoloxamine 30 mg
acetaminophen 325 mg
Uses: Analgesic

Perdiem Granules:
Per teaspoon:
senna 0.74 g
psyllium 3.25 g
sodium 1.8 mg
potassium 35.5 mg
Uses: Laxative
Peri-Colace Capsules:
docusate sodium 100 mg
casanthranol 30 mg
Uses: Laxative
Peri-Colace Syrup:
Per 15 ml:
docusate sodium 60 mg
casanthranol 30 mg
Uses: Laxative
Phenaphen w/Codeine No. 3:
aspirin 325 mg
codeine 30 mg
Uses: Analgesic
Phenaphen w/Codeine No. 4:
aspirin 325 mg
codeine 60 mg
Uses: Analgesic
Phenerbel-S:
ergotamine tartrate 0.6 mg
belladonna alkaloids 0.2 mg
phenobarbital 40 mg
Uses: α-Adrenergic blocker, anticholinergic
Phenergan VC Syrup:
Per 5 ml:
phenylephrine 5 mg
promethazine 6.25 mg
Uses: Adrenergic, antihistamine
Phenergan VC w/Codeine Syrup:
Per 5 ml:
phenylephrine 5 mg
promethazine 6.25 mg
codeine 10 mg
Uses: Adrenergic, antihistamine, opioid analgesic
Phenergan w/Codeine Syrup:
Per 5 ml:
promethazine 6.25 mg
codeine 10 mg
Uses: Antihistamine, analgesic
Pherazine DM Syrup:
Per 5 ml:
dextromethorphan 15 mg
promethazine 6.25 mg
7% alcohol
Uses: Antitussive, antihistamine
Phillips' Laxative Gelcaps:
docusate sodium 83 mg
phenolphthalein 90 mg
Uses: Laxative
Phrenilin:
acetaminophen 325 mg
butalbital 50 mg
Uses: Nonnarcotic analgesic
Phrenilin Forte:
acetaminophen 650 mg
butalbital 50 mg
Uses: Nonnarcotic analgesic
PMB-400:
conjugated estrogens 0.45 mg
meprobamate 400 mg
Uses: Oral contraceptive
Polaramine Expectorant Liquid:
Per 5 ml:
guaifenesin 100 mg
dexchlorpheniramine 2 mg
pseudoephedrine 20 mg
7.5% alcohol
Uses: Expectorant
Polycillin-PRB Oral Suspension:
Per single dose:
ampicillin 3.5 g
probenecid 1 g
Uses: Antiinfective
Polycitra Syrup:
Per 5 ml:
potassium citrate 550 mg
sodium citrate 500 mg
citric acid 334 mg
Uses: Laxative
Poly-Histine Elixir:
Per 5 ml:
pheniramine 4 mg
pyrilamine 4 mg
phenyltoloxamine 4 mg
4% alcohol
Uses: Antihistamine
Poly-Pred Ophthalmic Suspension:
Per ml:
0.5% prednisolone acetate
0.35% neomycin
polymyxin B 10,000 U
Uses: Ophth antiinflammatory, antiinfective
Polysporin Ointment:
Per gram:
polymyxin B 10,000 U
bacitracin zinc 500 U
Uses: Top antiinfective
Polysporin Ophthalmic Ointment:
Per gram:
polymyxin B 10,000 U
bacitracin zinc 500 U
Uses: Ophthalmic antiinfective

Polytrim Ophthalmic:
Per ml:
trimethoprim 1 mg
polymyxin B 10,000 U
Uses: Ophthalmic antiinfective
Premphase:
In a compliance package:
conjugated estrogens 0.625 mg
medroxyprogesterone 5 mg
Uses: Oral contraceptive
Prempro:
In a compliance package:
conjugated estrogens 0.625 mg
medroxyprogesterone 2.5 mg
Uses: Oral contraceptive
Premsyn PMS:
acetaminophen 500 mg
pamabrom 25 mg
pyrilamine 15 mg
Uses: Analgesic
Prevpac:
In a compliance package:
amoxicillin 500 mg caps
clarithromycin 500 mg tabs
lansoprazole 30 mg caps
Uses: Antiinfective
Primatene:
theophylline 130 mg
ephedrine 24 mg
phenobarbital 7.5 mg
Uses: Bronchodilator, barbiturate
Primatene Dual Action:
theophylline 60 mg
ephedrine 12.5 mg
guaifenesin 100 mg
Uses: Bronchodilator, expectorant, adrenergic
Primaxin 250 mg
IV for Injection:
imipenem 250 mg
cilastatin sodium 250 mg
Uses: Antiinfective
Primaxin 500 mg
IV for Injection:
imipenem 500 mg
cilastatin sodium 500 mg
Uses: Antiinfective
Prinzide 10-12.5:
lisinopril 10 mg
hydrochlorothiazide 12.5 mg
Uses: Antihypertensive
Prinzide 12.5:
lisinopril 20 mg
hydrochlorothiazide 12.5 mg
Uses: Antihypertensive
Prinzide 25:
lisinopril 20 mg
hydrochlorothiazide 25 mg
Uses: Antihypertensive
Probampacin Oral Suspension:
Per single dose:
ampicillin 3.5 g
probenecid 1 g
Uses: Antiinfective
Proben-C:
colchicine 0.5 mg
probenecid 500 mg
Uses: Antigout agent
Proctofoam-HC Aerosol Foam:
1% hydrocortisone
1% pramoxine
Uses: Topical corticosteroid
Propacet 100:
propoxyphene-N 100 mg
acetaminophen 650 mg
Uses: Analgesic
Pseudo-Chlor:
pseudoephedrine 120 mg
chlorpheniramine 8 mg
Uses: Antihistamine
Pseudo-Gest Plus:
pseudoephedrine 60 mg
chlorpheniramine 4 mg
Uses: Antihistamine
P-V-Tussin:
phenindamine 25 mg
guaifenesin 200 mg
hydrocodone 5 mg
Uses: Antihistamine, analgesic
P-V-Tussin Syrup:
Per 5 ml:
chlorpheniramine 2 mg
phenindamine 5 mg
phenylephrine 5 mg
pyrilamine 6 mg
Uses: Antihistamine, decongestant
Quadrinal:
ephedrine 24 mg
theophylline 65 mg
potassium iodide 320 mg
phenobarbital 24 mg
Uses: Adrenergic, bronchodilator, barbiturate
Quelidrine Cough Syrup:
Per 5 ml:
dextromethorphan 10 mg
phenylephrine 5 mg
ephedrine 5 mg
chlorpheniramine 2 mg
ammonium chloride 40 mg
ipecac 0.005 ml
Uses: Expectorant, adrenergic, antihistamine

Quibron-300:
theophylline 300 mg
guaifenesin 180 mg
Uses: Bronchodilator, expectorant
Quibron:
theophylline, 150 mg
guaifenesin 90 mg
Uses: Bronchodilator, expectorant
R&C Shampoo:
0.3% pyrethrins
3% piperonyl butoxide
Uses: Scabicide, pediculicide
Rauzide:
bendroflumethiazide 4 mg
powdered Rauwolfia serpentina 50 mg
Uses: Diuretic, antihypertensive
Regroton:
chlorthalidone 50 mg
reserpine 0.25 mg
Uses: Diuretic, antihypertensive
Regulace:
docusate sodium 100 mg
casanthranol 30 mg
Uses: Laxative
Renese-R:
polythiazide 2 mg
reserpine 0.25 mg
Uses: Diuretic, antihypertensive
Repan:
acetaminophen 325 mg
caffeine 40 mg
butalbital 50 mg
Uses: Nonnarcotic analgesic
Respahist:
pseudoephedrine 60 mg
brompheniramine 6 mg
Uses: Adrenergic, antihistamine
Respaire-60:
guaifenesin 200 mg
pseudoephedrine 60 mg
Uses: Expectorant, adrenergic
RID Shampoo:
0.3% pyrethrins
3% piperonyl butoxide
Uses: Scabicide, pediculicide
Rifamate:
isoniazid 150 mg
rifampin 300 mg
Uses: Antitubercular, antileprotic
Rifater:
rifampin 120 mg
isoniazid 50 mg
pyrazinamide 300 mg
Uses: Antitubercular
Rimactane/INH Dual Pack:
isoniazid 300 mg (30 tabs)
rifampin 300 mg (60 caps)
Uses: Antitubercular
Riopan Plus Suspension:
Per 5 ml:
magaldrate 540 mg
simethicone 40 mg
Uses: Antacid, adsorbent, antiflatulent
Robaxisal:
methocarbamol 400 mg
aspirin 325 mg
Uses: Skeletal muscle relaxant, analgesic
Robitussin A-C Syrup:
Per 5 ml:
codeine 10 mg
guaifenesin 100 mg
3.5% alcohol
Uses: Analgesic, expectorant
Robitussin Cold & Cough Liqui-Gels:
pseudoephedrine 30 mg
guaifenesin 200 mg
dextromethorphan 10 mg
Uses: Antitussive, expectorant
Robitussin-DAC Syrup:
Per 5 ml:
codeine 10 mg
guaifenesin 100 mg
pseudoephedrine 30 mg
1.4% alcohol
Uses: Analgesic, expectorant, adrenergic
Robitussin-DM Liquid:
Per 5 ml:
guaifenesin 100 mg
dextromethorphan 10 mg
Uses: Expectorant, antitussive
Robitussin Maximum Strength Cough and Cold Liquid:
dextromethorphan 15 mg
pseudoephedrine 30 mg
Uses: Antitussive, adrenergic
Robitussin Night Relief Liquid:
dextromethorphan 5 mg
pyrilamine 8.3 mg
pseudoephedrine 10 mg
acetaminophen 108.3 mg
Uses: Antitussive, adrenergic
Robitussin Pediatric Cough & Cold Liquid:
Per 5 ml:
pseudoephedrine 15 mg
dextromethorphan 7.5 mg
Uses: Antitussive, adrenergic
Robitussin-PE Syrup:
guaifenesin 100 mg
pseudoephedrine 30 mg
1.4% alcohol
Uses: Expectorant, adrenergic

Robitussin Severe Congestion Liqui-Gels:
guaifenesin 200 mg
pseudoephedrine 30 mg
Uses: Expectorant, adrenergic
Rolaids Calcium Rich:
magnesium hydroxide 80 mg
calcium carbonate 412 mg
Uses: Antacid, adsorbent, antiflatulent
Rondec:
pseudoephedrine 60 mg
carbinoxamine 4 mg
Uses: Adrenergic
Rondec DM Drops:
Per ml:
pseudoephedrine 25 mg
carbinoxamine 2 mg
dextromethorphan 4 mg
Uses: Adrenergic, antitussive
Rondec DM Syrup:
Per 5 ml:
pseudoephedrine 60 mg
carbinoxamine 4 mg
dextromethorphan 15 mg
Uses: Adrenergic, antitussive
Rondec Oral Drops:
Per 5 ml:
pseudoephedrine 25 mg
carbinoxamine 2 mg
Uses: Adrenergic
Roxicet:
Per 5 ml:
acetaminophen 325 mg
oxycodone 5 mg
Uses: Opioid analgesic
Roxicet 5/500:
oxycodone 5 mg
acetaminophen 500 mg
Uses: Opioid analgesic
Roxiprin:
aspirin 325 mg
oxycodone HCl 4.5 mg
oxycodone terephthalate 0.38 mg
Uses: Analgesic
Roxicet Oral Solution:
Per 5 ml:
acetaminophen 325 mg
oxycodone 5 mg
Uses: Analgesic
Ru-Tuss DE:
pseudoephedrine 120 mg
guaifenesin 600 mg
Uses: Adrenergic, expectorant
Ru-Tuss Expectorant Liquid:
Per 5 ml:
guaifenesin 100 mg
pseudoephedrine 30 mg
dextromethorphan 10 mg
10% alcohol
Uses: Adrenergic, expectorant, antitussive
Ryna-C Liquid:
Per 5 ml:
pseudoephedrine 30 mg
chlorpheniramine 2 mg
codeine 10 mg
Uses: Adrenergic, antihistamine, analgesic
Ryna Liquid:
Per 5 ml:
pseudoephedrine 30 mg
chlorpheniramine 2 mg
Uses: Adrenergic, antihistamine
Rynatan:
phenylephrine 25 mg
chlorpheniramine 8 mg
pyrilamine 25 mg
Uses: Adrenergic, antihistamine
Rynatan Pediatric Suspension:
Per 5 ml:
phenylephrine 5 mg
chlorpheniramine 2 mg
pyrilamine 12.5 mg
Uses: Adrenergic, antihistamine
Rynatuss:
ephedrine 10 mg
carbetapentane 60 mg
chlorpheniramine 5 mg
phenylephrine 10 mg
Uses: Adrenergic, antihistamine
Saleto Tablets:
115 mg acetaminophen
210 mg aspirin
65 mg salicylamide
16 mg caffeine
Uses: Nonnarcotic analgesic
Salutensin:
hydroflumethiazide 50 mg
reserpine 0.125 mg
Uses: Antihypertensive
Salutensin Demi:
hydroflumethiazide 25 mg
reserpine 0.125 mg
Uses: Antihypertensive
Scot-Tussin DM Liquid:
Per 5 ml:
chlorpheniramine 2 mg
dextromethorphan 15 mg
Uses: Antihistamine, antitussive

Scot-Tussin Original 5-Action Liquid:
phenylephrine 4.2 mg
pheniramine 13.3 mg
sodium citrate 83.3 mg
sodium salicylate 83.3 mg
caffeine citrate 25 mg
Uses: Adrenergic, analgesic
Scot-Tussin Senior Clear Liquid:
Per 5 ml:
guaifenesin 200 mg
dextromethorphan 15 mg
Uses: Antitussive, expectorant
Sedapap-10:
acetaminophen 650 mg
butalbital 50 mg
Uses: Analgesic, barbiturate
Semprex-D:
acrivastine 8 mg
pseudoephedrine 60 mg
Uses: Adrenergic, bronchodilator
Senokot-S:
docusate 50 mg
senna concentrate 187 mg
Uses: Laxative
Septra:
sulfamethoxazole 400 mg
trimethroprim 80 mg
Uses: Antiinfective
Septra DS:
sulfamethoxazole 800 mg
trimethroprim 160 mg
Uses: Antiinfective
Septra I.V. for Injection:
Per 5 ml:
trimethoprim 80 mg
sulfamethoxazole 400 mg
Uses: Antiinfective
Septra Suspension:
Per 5 ml:
trimethoprim 40 mg
sulfamethoxazole 200 mg
Uses: Antiinfective
Ser-A-Gen:
hydrochlorothiazide 15 mg
hydralazine 25 mg
reserpine 0.1 mg
Uses: Antihypertensive
Ser-Ap-Es:
hydrochlorothiazide 15 mg
reserpine 0.1 mg
hydralazine 25 mg
Uses: Diuretic, antihypertensive
Seralazide:
hydrochlorothiazide 15 mg
hydralazine 25 mg
reserpine 0.1 mg
Uses: Antihypertensive
Serpazide:
hydrochlorothiazide 15 mg
hydralazine 25 mg
reserpine 0.1 mg
Uses: Antihypertensive
Silafed Syrup:
Per 5 ml:
pseudoephedrine 30 mg
triprolidine 1.25 mg
Uses: Adrenergic, antihistamine
Sinarest Extra Strength:
pseudoephedrine 30 mg
chlorpheniramine 2 mg
acetaminophen 500 mg
Uses: Adrenergic, antihistamine, analgesic
Sinarest No Drowsiness:
pseudoephedrine 30 mg
acetaminophen 500 mg
Uses: Adrenergic, analgesic
Sinarest Sinus:
pseudoephedrine 30 mg
chlorpheniramine 2 mg
acetaminophen 325 mg
Uses: Adrenergic, antihistamine, analgesic
Sine-Aid IB:
pseudoephedrine 30 mg
ibuprofen 200 mg
Uses: Adrenergic, analgesic
Sine-Aid Maximum Strength:
pseudoephedrine 30 mg
acetaminophen 500 mg
Uses: Adrenergic, analgesic
Sinemet 10/100:
carbidopa 10 mg
levodopa 100 mg
Uses: Antiparkinsonian
Sinemet 25/100:
carbidopa 25 mg
levodopa 100 mg
Uses: Antiparkinsonian
Sinemet 25/250:
carbidopa 25 mg
levodopa 250 mg
Uses: Antiparkinsonian
Sinemet CR 25-100:
carbidopa 25 mg
levodopa 100 mg
Uses: Antiparkinsonian
Sinemet CR 50-200:
carbidopa 50 mg
levodopa 200 mg
Uses: Antiparkinsonian

Sine-Off Maximum Strength No Drowsiness Formula Caplets:
pseudoephedrine 30 mg
acetaminophen 500 mg
Uses: Adrenergic, analgesic

Sine-Off Sinus Medicine:
pseudoephedrine 30 mg
chlorpheniramine 2 mg
acetaminophen 500 mg
Uses: Adrenergic, antihistamine, analgesic

Sinus Excedrin Extra Strength:
acetaminophen 500 mg
pseudoephedrine 30 mg
Uses: Nonnarcotic analgesic

Sinus-Relief:
acetaminophen 325 mg
pseudoephedrine 30 mg
Uses: Nonnarcotic analgesic

Sinutab:
acetaminophen 325 mg
chlorpheniramine 2 mg
pseudoephedrine 30 mg
Uses: Nonnarcotic analgesic

Sinutab without Drowsiness:
acetaminophen 325 mg
pseudoephedrine 30 mg
Uses: Nonnarcotic analgesic

Sinutab Maximum Strength Sinus Allergy:
acetaminophen 500 mg
pseudoephedrine 30 mg
chlorpheniramine 2 mg
Uses: Analgesic, adrenergic, antihistamine

Sinutab Maximum Strength Without Drowsiness:
acetaminophen 500 mg
pseudoephedrine 30 mg
Uses: Analgesic, adrenergic

Sinutab Non-Drying:
pseudoepedrine 30 mg
guaifenesin 200 mg
Uses: Adrenergic, expectorant

Slo-Phyllin GG Syrup:
theophylline 150 mg
guaifenesin 90 mg
Uses: Bronchodilator, expectorant

Soma Compound w/Codeine:
carisoprodol 200 mg
aspirin 325 mg
codeine 16 mg
Uses: Skeletal muscle relaxant

Synophylate-GG Syrup:
theophylline 150 mg
guaifenesin 100 mg
alcohol 15%
Uses: Bronchodilator, expectorant

Soma Compound:
carisoprodol 200 mg
aspirin 325 mg
Uses: Skeletal muscle relaxant, analgesic

Spec-T Lozenge:
dextromethorphan 10 mg
benzocaine 10 mg
Uses: Antitussive, topical anesthetic

Sudafed Cold & Cough Liquicaps:
pseudoephedrine 30 mg
dextromethorphan 10 mg
guaifenesin 100 mg
acetaminophen 250 mg
Uses: Adrenergic, antitussive, expectorant, analgesic

Sudafed Plus:
pseudoephedrine 60 mg
chlorpheniramine 4 mg
Uses: Adrenergic, antihistamine

Sudafed Severe Cold:
pseudoephedrine 30 mg
dextromethorphan 15 mg
Uses: Adrenergic, antitussive

Sudafed Sinus Maximum Strength:
pseudoephedrine 30 mg
acetaminophen 500 mg
Uses: Adrenergic, analgesic

Sudal 60/500:
pseudoephedrine 60 mg
guaifenesin 500 mg
Uses: Adrenergic, expectorant

Sudal 120/600:
pseudoephedrine 120 mg
guaifenesin 600 mg
Uses: Adrenergic, expectorant

Sulfimycin:
Per 5 ml:
erythromycin 200 mg
sulfisoxazole 600 mg
Uses: Macrolide antiinfective

Sultrin Triple Sulfa Vaginal Cream:
3.42% sulfathiazole
2.86% sulfacetamine
3.7% sulfabenzamide
Uses: Antiinfective

Sultrin Triple Sulfa Vaginal Tablets:
sulfathiazolc 172.5 mg
sulfacetamide 143.75
sulfabenzamide 184 mg
Uses: Antiinfective

Synalgos-DC:
aspirin 356.4 mg
caffeine 30 mg
dihydrocodeine 16 mg
Uses: Analgesic

Synercid:
quinupristin 150 mg
dalfopristin 350 mg
Uses: Antiinfective

Talacen:
acetaminophen 650 mg
pentazocine 25 mg
Uses: Analgesic

Talwin Compound:
aspirin 325 mg
pentazocine 12.5 mg
Uses: Analgesic

Talwin NX:
pentazocine 50 mg
naloxone 0.5 mg
Uses: Analgesic, opioid antagonist

Tarka 182:
trandolapril 2 mg (immed rel)
verapamil 180 mg (sus rel)
Uses: Antihypertensive, calcium channel blocker

Tarka 241:
trandolapril 1 mg (immed rel)
verapamil 240 mg (sus rel)
Uses: Antihypertensive, calcium channel blocker

Tarka 242:
trandolapril 2 mg (immed rel)
verapamil 240 mg (sus rel)
Uses: Antihypertensive, calcium channel blocker

Tarka 244:
trandolapril 4 mg (immed rel)
verapamil 240 mg (sus rel)
Uses: Antihypertensive, calcium channel blocker

Tavist Sinus:
acetaminophen 500 mg
pseudoephedrine 30 mg
Uses: Analgesic, adrenergic

***Tecnal:**
aspirin 330 mg
caffeine 40 mg
butalbital 50 mg
Uses: Nonnarcotic analgesic

Teczem:
enalapril 5 mg (extended release)
diltiazem 180 mg (extended release)
Uses: Antihypertensive, calcium channel blocker

Tedrigen:
ephedrine 22.5 mg
theophylline 120 mg
phenobarbital 7.5 mg
Uses: Adrenergic, bronchodilator, barbiturate

Tegrin-LT Shampoo:
0.33% pyrethrins
3.15% piperonyl butoxide
Uses: Scabicide, pediculicide

Tencet:
acetaminophen 325 mg
caffeine 40 mg
butalbital 50 mg
Uses: Nonnarcotic analgesic

Tenoretic 50:
atenolol 50 mg
chlorthalidone 25 mg
Uses: Antihypertensive

Tenoretic 100:
atenolol 100 mg
chlorthalidone 25 mg
Uses: Antihypertensive

Terra-Cortril Ophthalmic Suspension:
1.5% hydrocortisone acetate
0.5% oxytetracycline
Uses: Ophth antiinflammatory, antiinfective

Terramycin w/Polymycin B Sulfate Ophthalmic Ointment:
Per gram:
polymyxin B 10,000 units
oxytetracycline 5 mg
Uses: Ophth antiinfective

T-Gesic:
hydrocodone 5 mg
acetaminophen 500 mg
Uses: Analgesic

Theodrine:
ephedrine 22.5 mg
theophylline 120 mg
Uses: Adrenergic, bronchodilator

Theolate Liquid:
theophylline 150 mg
guaifenesin 90 mg
Uses: Bronchodilator, expectorant

Theophylline KI Elixir:
theophylline 80 mg
potassium iodide 130 mg
Uses: Bronchodilator, expectorant

Thera-Flu, Flu & Cold Medicine Powder:
Per packet:
pseudoephedrine 60 mg
chlorpheniramine 4 mg
acetaminophen 650 mg
Uses: Adrenergic, antihistamine, analgesic

Thera-Flu, Flu, Cold & Cough Powder:
Per packet:
pseudoephedrine 60 mg
chlorpheniramine 4 mg
dextromethorphan 20 mg
acetaminophen 650 mg
Uses: Adrenergic, antihistamine, antitussive, analgesic

Thera-Flu NightTime Powder:
Per packet:
pseudoephedrine 60 mg
chlorpheniramine 4 mg
dextromethorphan 30 mg
acetaminophen 1000 mg
Uses: Adrenergic, antihistamine, antitussive, analgesic

Thera-Flu Non-Drowsy Flu, Cold & Cough Maximum Strength Powder
Per packet:
pseudoephedrine 60 mg
dextromethorphan 30 mg
acetaminophen 1000 mg
Uses: Adrenergic, antitussive, analgesic

Thera-Flu Non-Drowsy Formula Maximum Strength Caplets:
pseudoephedrine 30 mg
dextromethorphan 15 mg
acetaminophen 500 mg
Uses: Adrenergic, antitussive, analgesic

Timentin for Injection:
Per 3.1-g vial:
ticarcillin 3 g
clavulanic acid 0.1 g
Uses: Antiinfective

Timolide 10/25:
timolol 10 mg
hydrochlorothiazide 25 mg
Uses: Antihypertensive

Titralac Plus:
calcium carbonate 420 mg
simethicone 21 mg
Uses: Antacid, adsorbent, antiflatulent

Tobra Dex Ophthalmic Suspension/Ointment:
tobramycin 0.3%
dexamethasone 0.1%
Uses: Ophth antiinfective, antiinflammatory

Triacin-C Cough Syrup:
Per 5 ml:
codeine 10 mg
pseudoephedrine 30 mg
triprolidine 1.25 mg
Uses: Analgesic, adrenergic, antihistamine

Triad:
acetaminophen 325 mg
caffeine 40 mg
butalbital 50 mg
Uses: Nonnarcotic analgesic

Triaminic-12:
phenylpropanolamine 75 mg
chlorpheniramine 12 mg
Uses: Antihistamine

Tri-Hydroserpine:
hydralazine 25 mg
hydrochlorothiazide 15 mg
reserpine 0.1 mg
Uses: Antihypertensive

Tri-Levlen:
Phase I:
levonorgestrel 0.05 mg
ethinyl estradiol 30 μg
Phase II:
levonorgestrel 0.075 mg
ethinyl estradiol 40 μg;
Phase III:
levonorgestrel 0.125 mg
ethinyl estradiol 30 μg
Uses: Oral contraceptive

Triaminic AM Cough & Decongestant Formula Liquid:
Per 5 ml:
pseudoephedrine 15 mg
dextromethorphan 7.5 mg
Uses: Adrenergic, antitussive

Triaminic Nite Light Liquid:
Per 5 ml:
pseudoephedrine 15 mg
chlorpheniramine 1 mg
dextromethorphan 7.5 mg
Uses: Adrenergic, antihistamine, antitussive

Triaminic Sore Throat Formula Liquid:
Per 5 ml:
pseudoephedrine 15 mg
dextromethorphan 7.5 mg
acetaminophen 160 mg
Uses: Adrenergic, antitussive

Triavil 2-10:
perphenazine 2 mg
amitriptyline 10 mg
Uses: Antidepressant, antipsychotic

Triavil 4-10:
perphenazine 4 mg
amitriptyline 10 mg
Uses: Antidepressant, antipsychotic

Triavil 2-25:
perphenazine 2 mg
amitriptyline 25 mg
Uses: Antidepressant, antipsychotic

Trinalin Repetabs:
azatadine maleate 1 mg
pseudoephedrine 120 mg
Uses: Antihistamine
Triphasil:
Phase I:
levonorgestrel 0.05 mg
ethinyl estradiol 30 μg
Phase II:
levonorgestrel 0.075 mg
ethinyl estradiol 40 μg
Phase III:
levonorgestrel 0.125 mg
ethinyl estradiol 30 μg
Uses: Oral contraceptive
Triple Antibiotic Ophthalmic Ointment:
Per gram:
polymyxin B 10,000 U
neomycin 3.5 mg
bacitracin 400 U
Uses: Antiinfective
Trizivir:
300 mg abacavir
150 mg lamivudine
300 mg zidovudine
Uses: HIV
Tuinal 100 mg:
amobarbital 50 mg
secobarbital 50 mg
Uses: Sedative-hypnotic
Tuinal 200 mg:
amobarbital 100 mg
secobarbital 100 mg
Uses: Sedative-hypnotic
Tusibron-DM Syrup:
Per 5 ml:
guaifenesin 100 mg
dextromethorphan 15 mg
Uses: Expectorant, antitussive
Tussionex Pennkinetic Suspension:
Per 5 ml:
chlorpheniramine 8 mg
hydrocodone 10 mg
Uses: Antihistamine, analgesic
Tussi-Organidin NR Liquid:
Per 5 ml:
codeine 10 mg
guaifenesin 100 mg
Uses: Analgesic, expectorant
Tussi-Organidin DM NR Liquid:
Per 5 ml:
guaifenesin 100 mg
dextromethorphan 10 mg
Uses: Expectorant, antitussive
Two-Dyne:
acetaminophen 325 mg
caffeine 40 mg
butalbital 50 mg
Uses: Nonnarcotic analgesic
Tylenol Allergy Sinus, Maximum Strength Gelcaps:
acetaminophen 500 mg
chlorpheniramine 2 mg
pseudoephedrine 30 mg
Uses: Antihistamine, adrenergic, analgesic
Tylenol Children's Cold:
acetaminophen 80 mg
chlorpheniramine 0.5 mg
pseudoephedrine 7.5 mg
Uses: Antihistaminc, adrenergic, analgesic
Tylenol Children's Cold Liquid:
Per 5 ml:
acetaminophen 160 mg
chlorpheniramine 1 mg
pseudoephedrine 15 mg
Uses: Antihistamine, adrenergic, analgesic
Tylenol Children's Cold Multi-Symptom Plus Cough Liquid:
Per 5 ml:
acetaminophen 160 mg
dextromethorphan 5 mg
chlorpheniramine 1 mg
pseudoephedrine 15 mg
Uses: Antihistamine, adrenergic, analgesic
Tylenol Children's Cold Plus Cough Chewable:
acetaminophen 80 mg
pseudoephedrine 7.5 mg
dextromethorphan 2.5 mg
chlorpheniramine 0.5 mg
Uses: Antihistamine, adrenergic, analgesic
Tylenol Cold Multi-Symptom:
acetaminophen 325 mg
chlorpheniramine 2 mg
pseudoephedrine 30 mg
dextromethorphan 15 mg
Uses: Antihistamine, adrenergic, analgesic
Tylenol Cold No Drowsiness:
acetaminophen 325 mg
pseudoephedrine 30 mg
dextromethorphan 15 mg
Uses: Analgesic, adrenergic, antitussive

Tylenol Flu Maximum Strength Gelcaps:
dextromethorphan 15 mg
pseudoephedrine 30 mg
acetaminophen 500 mg
Uses: Analgesic, adrenergic, antitussive

Tylenol Flu NightTime Maximum Strength Gelcaps:
pseudoephedrine 30 mg
chlorpheniramine 2 mg
acetaminophen 500 mg
Uses: Adrenergic, antihistamine, analgesic

Tylenol Flu NightTime Maximum Strength Powder:
pseudoephedrine 60 mg
diphenhydramine 50 mg
acetaminophen 1000 mg
Uses: Adrenergic, antihistamine, analgesic

Tylenol Headache Plus, Extra Strength:
acetaminophen 500 mg
calcium carbonate 250 mg
Uses: Analgesic, antacid

Tylenol Multi-Symptom Cough Liquid:
Per 5 ml:
dextromethorphan 10 mg
acetaminophen 216.7 mg
5% alcohol
Uses: Antitussive, analgesic

Tylenol Multi-Symptom Cough w/Decongestant Liquid:
Per 5 ml:
dextromethorphan 10 mg
acetaminophen 200 mg
pseudoephedrine 20 mg
Uses: Antitussive, analgesic, adrenergic

Tylenol Multi-Symptom Hot Medication:
Per packet:
acetaminophen 650 mg
chlorpheniramine 4 mg
pseudoephedrine 60 mg
dextromethorphan 30 mg
Uses: Analgesic, antihistamine, adrenergic, antitussive

Tylenol PM, Extra Strength:
acetaminophen 500 mg
diphenhydramine 25 mg
Uses: Analgesic, antihistamine

Tylenol Severe Allergy:
diphenhydramine 12.5 mg
acetaminophen 500 mg
Uses: Analgesic, antihistamine

Tylenol Sinus Maximum Strength:
pseudoephedrine 30 mg
acetaminophen 500 mg
Uses: Adrenergic, analgesic

Tylenol w/Codeine Elixir:
Per 5 ml:
acetaminophen 120 mg
codeine 12 mg
Uses: Analgesic

Tylenol w/Codeine No. 1:
acetaminophen 300 mg
codeine 7.5 mg
Uses: Analgesic

Tylenol w/Codeine No. 2:
acetaminophen 300 mg
codeine 15 mg
Uses: Analgesic

Tylenol w/Codeine No. 3:
acetaminophen 300 mg
codeine 30 mg
Uses: Analgesic

Tylenol w/Codeine No. 4:
acetaminophen 300 mg
codeine 60 mg
Uses: Analgesic

Tylox:
oxycodone 5 mg
acetaminophen 500 mg
Uses: Analgesic

Tyrodone Liquid:
Per 5 ml:
hydrocodone 5 mg
pseudoephedrine 60 mg
5% alcohol
Uses: Analgesic, adrenergic

Unasyn for Injection 1.5 g:
ampicillin 1 g
sulbactam 0.5 g
Uses: Antiinfective

Unasyn for Injection 3 g:
ampicillin 2 g
sulbactam 1 g
Uses: Antiinfective

Uniretic:
moexipril 7.5 mg
hydrochlorothiazide 12.5 mg
or moexipril 15 mg
hydrochlorothiazide 25 mg
Uses: Antihypertensive, diuretic

Unituss HC Syrup:
hydrocodone 2.5 mg
phenylephrine 5 mg
chlorpheniramine 2 mg
Uses: Analgesic, adrenergic, antihistamine

Urised:
methenamine 40.8 mg
phenylsalicylate 18.1 mg
atropine 0.03 mg
hyoscyamine 0.03 mg
benzoic acid 4.5 mg
methylene blue 5.4 mg
Uses: Antiinfective

Urobiotic 250:
oxytetracycline 250 mg
sulfamethizole 250 mg
phenazopyridine 50 mg
Uses: Antiinfective

Ursinus Inlay:
pseudoephedrine 30 mg
aspirin 325 mg
Uses: Adrenergic, analgesic

Vanquish:
aspirin 227 mg
acetaminophen 194 mg
caffeine 33 mg
aluminum hydroxide 25 mg
magnesium hydroxide 50 mg
Uses: Nonnarcotic analgesic

Vaseretic 10-25:
enalapril 10 mg
hydrochlorothiazide 25 mg
Uses: Antihypertensive, diuretic

Vasocidin Ophthalmic Ointment:
sulfacetamide 10%
prednisolone 0.5%
Uses: Ophthalmic antiinfective, antiinflammatory

Vasocidin Ophthalmic Solution:
sulfacetamide 10%
prednisolone 0.25%
Uses: Ophthalmic antiinfective, antiinflammatory

Vasocon-A Ophthalmic Solution:
naphazoline 0.05%
antazoline 0.5%
Uses: Ophthalmic vasoconstrictor

Vicks 44D Cough & Head Congestion Liquid:
Per 5 ml:
dextromethorphan 10 mg
pseudoephedrine 20 mg
Uses: Antitussive, adrenergic

Vicks 44E Liquid:
Per 5 ml:
dextromethorphan 6.7 mg
guaifenesin 66.7 mg
Uses: Antitussive, expectorant

Vicks 44M Cold, Flu, & Cough LiquiCaps:
dextromethorphan 10 mg
pseudoephedrine 30 mg
chlorpheniramine 2 mg
acetaminophen 250 mg
Uses: Antitussive, adrenergic, antihistamine, analgesic

Vicks 44 Non-Drowsy Cold & Cough LiquiCaps:
dextromethorphan 30 mg
pseudoephedrine 60 mg
Uses: Antitussive, adrenergic

Vicks Children's NyQuil Nighttime Cough/Cold Liquid:
Per 5 ml:
pseudoephedrine 10 mg
chlorpheniramine 0.67 mg
dextromethorphan 5 mg
Uses: Adrenergic, antihistamine, antitussive

Vicks Cough Silencers:
dextromethorphan 2.5 mg
benzocaine 1 mg
Uses: Antitussive, top anesthetic

Vicks DayQuil Liquid:
Per 5 ml:
dextromethorphan 3.3 mg
pseudoephedrine 10 mg
acetaminophen 108.3 mg
guaifenesin 33.3 mg
Uses: Antitussive, adrenergic, analgesic, expectorant

Vicks DayQuil Sinus Pressure & Pain Relief:
pseudoephedrine 30 mg
acetaminophen 500 mg
Uses: Adrenergic, analgesic

Vicks NyQuil Liquicaps:
pseudoephedrine 30 mg
doxylamine 6.25 mg
dextromethorphan 10 mg
acetaminophen 250 mg
Uses: Adrenergic, antihistamine, antitussive, analgesic

Vicks NyQuil Multi-Symptom Cold Flu Relief Liquid:
pseudoephedrine 10 mg
doxylamine 2.1 mg
dextromethorphan 5 mg
acetaminophen 167 mg
Uses: Adrenergic, antihistamine, antitussive, analgesic

Vicks Pediatric Formula 44e Liquid:
Per 5 ml:
dextromethorphan 3.3 mg
guaifenesin 33.3 mg
Uses: Expectorant, antitussive

Vicks Pediatric Formula 44 m Multi-Symptom Cough & Cold Liquid
pseudoephedrine 10 mg
chlorpheniramine 0.67 mg
dextromethorphan 5 mg
Uses: Adrenergic, antihistamine, antitussive

Vicodin:
acetaminophen 500 mg
hydrocodone 5 mg
Uses: Analgesic

Vicodin ES:
acetaminophen 750 mg
hydrocodone 7.5 mg
Uses: Analgesic

Vicodin HP:
hydrocodone 10 mg
acetaminophen 660 mg
Uses: Analgesic

VicodinTuss:
Per 5 ml:
hydrocodone 5 mg
guaifenesin 100 mg
Uses: Analgesic, expectorant

Vicoprofen:
hydrocodone 7.5 mg
ibuprofen 200 mg
Uses: Analgesic

Wigraine Suppositories:
ergotamine 2 mg
caffeine 100 mg
Uses: α-Adrenergic blocker

Yasmin:
ethinylestadiol 30 μg
dropirenone 3 mg
Uses: Oral contraceptive

Zestoretic 10/12.5:
lisinopril 10 mg
hydrochlorothiazide 12.5 mg
Uses: Antihypertensive

Zestoretic 20/12.5:
lisinopril 20 mg
hydrochlorothiazide 12.5 mg
Uses: Antihypertensive

Zestoretic 20/25:
lisinopril 20 mg
hydrochlorothiazide 25 mg
Uses: Antihypertensive

Ziac 2.5:
bisoprolol 2.5 mg
hydrochlorothiazide 6.25 mg
Uses: Antihypertensive

Ziac 5:
bisoprolol 5 mg
hydrochlorothiazide 6.25 mg
Uses: Antihypertensive

Ziac 10:
bisoprolol 10 mg
hydrochlorothiazide 6.25 mg
Uses: Antihypertensive

Zydone:
hydrocodone 5 mg
acetaminophen 500 mg
Uses: Analgesic

Appendix F

Rarely Used Drugs

HIGH ALERT

abciximab (℞)

Func. class.: Platelet aggregation inhibitor

Dosage and routes

Adult: **IV** 250 μg (0.25 mg)/kg bolus 10-60 min before percutaneous transluminal angioplasty (PTCA), followed by 10 μg/min cont inf for 12 hr

Uses: Used with heparin and aspirin to prevent acute cardiac ischemia following PTCA in patients at high risk for reclosure of affected arteries

Contraindications: Hypersensitivity to this drug or murine protein; GI, GU bleeding; CVA within 2 yr, bleeding disorders, intracranial neoplasm, intracranial arteriovenous malformations, intracranial aneurysm, platelet count <100,000 cells/mm^3, recent surgery, aneurysm, uncontrolled severe hypertension, vasculitis

alfentanil (℞)

Func. class.: Opioid analgesic

Controlled Substance Schedule II

Dosage and routes

Anesthesia <30 min

Combination

Adult: **IV** 8-50 μg/kg, may increase by 3-15 μg/kg

Anesthetic induction

Adult: **IV** 3-5 μg/kg, then 0.5-1.5 μg/kg/min; total dose is 8-40 μg/kg

Anesthesia 30-60 min

Induction

Adult: **IV** 20-50 μg/kg

Maintenance

Adult: **IV** 5-15 μg/kg; may give up to 75 μg/kg total dose

Continuous anesthesia >45 min

Induction

Adult: **IV** 50-75 μg/kg

Maintenance

Adult: **IV** 0.5-3.0 μg/kg/min; rate should be decreased by 30%-50% after 1 hr maintenance inf; may be increased to 4 μg/kg/min or bol doses of 7 μg/kg

Induction of anesthesia >45 min

Adult: **IV** 130-245 μg/kg, then 0.5-1.5 μg/kg/min

MAC

Induction

Adult: **IV** duration ≤½ hr 3-8 μg/kg

Maintenance

Adult: 3-5 μg/kg q5-20min to 1 μg/kg/min, total dose 3-40 μg/kg

Uses: In combination with other drugs in general anesthesia, as a primary anesthetic in general surgery, monitored anesthesia care (MAC)

Contraindications: Child <12 yr, hypersensitivity

alprostadil (℞)

Func. class.: Hormone

Dosage and routes

Patent ductus arteriosus

Infants: **IV** INF 0.1 μg/kg/min, until desired response, then reduce to lowest effective amount, 0.4 μg/kg/min not likely to produce greater beneficial effects

Erectile dysfunction of vasculogenic or mixed etiology, psychogenic

Men: Intracavernosal 2.5 μg may increase by 2.5 μg; may then increase by 5-10 μg until adequate response occurs; intraurethral administer as needed to achieve erection

Uses: To maintain patent ductus arteriosus (temporary treatment), erectile dysfunction

Contraindications: Hypersensitivity, respiratory distress syndrome (RDS)

amantadine (℞)

Func. class.: Antiviral, antiparkinsonian agent

Dosage and routes

Influenza type A

Adult and child >12 yr: PO 200 mg/day in single dose or divided bid

Child 9-12 yr: PO 100 mg bid

Child 1-9 yr: PO 4.4-8.8 mg/kg/day divided bid-tid, not to exceed 200 mg/day

Extrapyramidal reaction/ parkinsonism

Adult: PO 100 mg bid, up to 400 mg/day in EPS; give for 1 wk, then 100 mg as needed up to 400 mg in parkinsonism; CrCl 40-50 ml/min 100 mg/day; CrCl 30 ml/min 200 mg 2×/wk; CrCl 20 ml/min 100 mg 3×/wk; CrCl <10 ml/min 100 mg alternating with 200 mg q7days

Uses: Prophylaxis or treatment of influenza type A, extrapyramidal reactions, parkinsonism, respiratory tract infections

Contraindications: Hypersensitivity, lactation, child <1 yr , eczematic rash

Do not confuse

amantadine/ranitidine, amantadine/rimantidine, Symmetrel/Synthroid

aminocaproic acid (℞)

Func. class.: Hemostatic

Dosage and routes

Adult: PO/**IV** 5-g loading dose, then 1-1.25 g qh if needed, not to exceed 30 g/day

Uses: Hemorrhage from hyperfibrinolysis; adjunctive therapy in hemophilia, amega- karyocytic thrombocytopenia, hereditary angioneurotic edema

Investigational uses: Prevention of recurrent subarachnoid hemorrhage

Contraindications: Hypersensitivity, abnormal bleeding, postpartum bleeding, DIC, upper urinary tract bleeding, new burns

aminoglutethimide (℞)

Func. class.: Antineoplastic, adrenal steroid inhibitor

Dosage and routes

Adult: PO 250 mg qid at 6 hr intervals, may increase by 250 mg/day q1-2wk, not to exceed 2 g/day

Uses: Suppression of adrenal function in Cushing's syndrome, adrenal cancer

Contraindications: Hypersensitivity, hypothyroidism, pregnancy **D**

aminolevulinic acid (℞)

Func. class.: Photochemotherapy

Dosage and routes

Adult: Top 1 application of solution and 1 dose of illumination/treatment site × 8wk

Uses: Face/scalp nonhyperkeratotic actinic keratoses

Contraindications: Hypersensitivity to porphyrins

ammonium chloride (PO-OTC, IV-℞)

Func. class.: Acidifier

Dosage and routes

Alkalosis

Adult and child: **IV** Inf 0.9-1.3 ml/min of a 2.14% sol, not to exceed 5 ml/min

Acidifier

Adult: PO 4-12 g/day in divided doses

Child: PO 75 mg/kg/day in divided doses

Expectorant

Adult: PO 250-500 mg q2-4h as needed

Uses: Alkalosis (metabolic), systemic and urinary acidifier, expectorant, diuretic

Contraindications: Hypersensitivity, severe hepatic disease, severe renal disease

amyl nitrite (℞)

Func. class.: Coronary vasodilator (antianginal, antidote for cyanide)

Dosage and routes

Angina

Adult: INH 0.18-0.3 ml as needed, 1-6 puffs from 1 cap; may repeat in 3-5 min

Cyanide poisoning

Adult: INH 0.3-ml ampule 15 sec until preparation of sodium nitrite infusion is ready

Uses: Acute angina pectoris

Contraindications: Hypersensitivity to nitrites, severe anemia, increased intracranial pressure, hypertension, pregnancy **X**

atracurium (℞)

Func. class.: Neuromuscular blocker (nondepolarizing)

Dosage and routes

Adult and child >2 yr: **IV** bol 0.3-0.5 mg/kg, then 0.08-0.10 mg/kg 20-45 min after first dose if needed for prolonged procedures

Child, 1 mo-2 yr: **IV** bol 0.3-0.4 mg/kg

Uses: Facilitation of endotracheal intubation, skeletal muscle relaxation during mechanical ventilation, surgery, or general anesthesia

Contraindications: Hypersensitivity

auranofin (℞)

Func. class.: Antiinflammatory

Dosage and routes

Adult: PO 6 mg qd or 3 mg bid; may increase to 9 mg/day after 3 mo

Uses: Rheumatoid arthritis; not for first-line therapy

Investigational uses: SLE, psoriatic arthritis, pemphigus

Contraindications: Hypersensitivity to gold, necrotizing enterocolitis, bone marrow aplasia, child <6 yr, lactation, pulmonary fibrosis, exfoliative dermatitis, blood dyscrasias, recent radiation therapy, renal/hepatic disease, marked hypertension, uncontrolled CHF

Do not confuse
Ridaura/Cardura

aurothioglucose/gold sodium thiomalate (℞)

Func. class.: Antiinflammatory (gold)

Dosage and routes

Adult: IM 10 mg; then 25 mg weekly × 2-3 wk; then 50 mg/wk until total of 1 g is administered; then 25-50 mg q3-4 wk if there is improvement without toxicity (aurothioglucose); total of 800 mg-1 g

Adult: IM 10 mg, then 25 mg after 1 wk, then 50 mg weekly for total of 14-20 doses; then 50 mg q2 wk × 4; then 50 mg q3 wk × 4; then 50 mg monthly for maintenance (gold sodium thiomalate)

P ***Child 6-12 yr:*** IM 1 mg/kg/wk × 20 wk, or ¼ of adult dosage (aurothioglucose)

P ***Child <6 yr:*** IM 1 mg/kg/wk × 20 wk, then q3-4 wk if improvement without toxicity (gold sodium thiomalate), not to exceed 2.5 mg

Uses: Rheumatoid arthritis resistant to other treatment, psoriatic arthritis

Contraindications: Hypersensitivity to gold, SLE, uncontrolled diabetes mellitus, marked hypertension, recent radiation therapy, CHF, lactation, renal disease, liver disease

bacitracin (℞)

Func. class.: Antiinfective, misc.

Dosage and routes

Infant >2.5 kg: IM 1000 U/kg/day in divided doses q8-12h

Infant ≤2.5 kg: IM 900 U/kg/day in divided doses q8-12h

Uses: Staphylococcal pneumonia, empyema

Contraindications: Hypersensitivity, severe renal disease (IM use)

benzonatate (℞)

Func. class.: Antitussive, nonnarcotic

Dosage and routes

Adult and child: PO 100 mg tid, not to exceed 600 mg/day

Child <10 yr: PO 8 mg/kg in 3-6 divided doses

Uses: Nonproductive cough

Contraindications: Hypersensitivity

benzoyl peroxide (OTC)

Func. class.: Antiacne medication

Dosage and routes

Adult and child: Top apply to affected area qd or bid

Uses: Mild to moderate acne

Contraindications: Hypersensitivity to benzoic acid derivatives

benzquinamide (℞)

Func. class.: Antiemetic

Dosage and routes

Adult: IM 50 mg or 0.5-1 mg/kg; may be repeated in 1 hr, then q3-4h prn; **IV** 25 mg or 0.2-0.4 mg/kg as a one-time dose

Uses: To inhibit nausea, vomiting associated with anesthetic

Contraindications: Hypersensitivity, hypertension

P **beractant** (℞)
Func. class.: Natural lung surfactant

Dosage and routes
Intratracheal instill: 4 doses can
P be administered in the 1st 48 hr of life; give doses no more frequently than q6h; each dose is 100 mg of phospholipids/kg birth weight (4 ml/kg)

Uses: Prevention and treatment (rescue) of respiratory distress
P syndrome in premature infants

bitolterol (℞)
Func. class.: Bronchodilator, adrenergic β_2-agonist

Dosage and routes
Inhaler
Adult and child >12 yr: INH 2 puffs, wait 1-3 min before 3rd puff if needed, not to exceed 3 INH q6h or 2 INH q4h
Nebulization
Adult and child >12 yr: INH 0.5 ml (1 mg) tid by intermittent flow or 1.25 mg tid by cont flow, max 8 mg (intermittent), 14 mg (cont)

Uses: Asthma, bronchospasm

Contraindications: Hypersensitivity to sympathomimetics

cabergoline (℞)
Func. class.: Dopamine receptor/ agonist

Dosage and routes
Hyperprolactinemic indications
Adult: PO 0.25 mg 2×/wk, may increase by 0.25 mg 2×/wk at 4 wk intervals, max 1 mg 2×/wk; maintenance therapy may be needed for 6 mo

Uses: Reduced prolactin/secretion in postpartum lactation

Investigational uses: Parkinson's disease, normalization of androgen levels and improved menstrual cycles in polycystic ovarian syndrome

Contraindications: Hypersensitivity to uncontrolled hypertension

chlorpropamide (℞)
Func. class.: Antidiabetic, oral

Dosage and routes
Adult: PO 100-250 mg qd initially, then 100-500 mg maintenance according to response; not to exceed 750 mg/day

Uses: Stable adult-onset diabetes mellitus (type II; NIDDM)

Contraindications: Hypersensi-
P tivity to sulfonylureas, juvenile or brittle diabetes, pregnancy **C**, renal failure

cladribine (CdA) (℞)
Func. class.: Antineoplastic antiinfective

Dosage and routes
Adult: **IV** 0.09 mg/kg diluted with 0.9% NaCl qs to 100 ml; pass through 0.22 μm microfilter, given for 1 wk

Uses: Treatment of active hairy cell leukemia; may be useful in chronic lymphocytic leukemia, non-Hodgkin's lymphomas, acute myeloid leukemia, autoimmune hemolytic anemia

Contraindications: Hypersensitivity, lactation

clioquinol (OTC)
Func. class.: Local antiinfective

Dosage and routes
Top apply to affected area bid-tid × 7 days only

Uses: Cutaneous infections: athlete's foot, eczema, and other fungal infections

Contraindications: Hypersensitivity to iodine, chloroxine

clobetasol (℞)
Func. class.: Topical corticosteroid

Dosage and routes
P ***Adult and child:*** Top apply to affected area bid

Uses: Psoriasis, eczema, contact dermatitis, pruritus; usually reserved for severe dermatoses that have not responded to less potent formulation

Contraindications: Hypersensitivity to corticosteroids, fungal infections

clocortolone (℞)
Func. class.: Topical corticosteroid

Dosage and routes
P ***Adult and child:*** Top apply to affected area tid-qid

Uses: Psoriasis, eczema, contact dermatitis, pruritus

Contraindications: Hypersensitivity to corticosteroids, fungal infections

clofazimine (℞)
Func. class.: Leprostatic

Dosage and routes
Erythema nodosum leprosum
Adult: PO 100-200 mg qd × 3 mo, then taper dosage to 100 mg when disease is controlled; do not exceed 200 mg/day

Dapsone-resistant leprosy
Adult: PO 100 mg/day in combination with at least one other antileprosy drug × 3 yr, then 100 mg qd clofazimine (only)

Uses: Lepromatous leprosy, dapsone-resistant leprosy, lepromatous leprosy complicated by erythema nodosum leprosum

Contraindications: Hypersensitivity to this drug

clotrimazole (℞) (OTC)
Func. class.: Local antiinfective

Dosage and routes
P ***Adult and child:*** Top rub into affected area bid × 1-4 wk; loz dissolve in mouth 5 times/day × 2 wk; intravag 1 applicator/1 tab × 1-2 wk hs; oral troches 10 mg 5 times/day × 14 days

Uses: Tinea pedis, tinea cruris, tinea corporis, tinea versicolor, *C. albicans* infection of the vagina, vulva, throat, mouth

Contraindications: Hypersensitivity

colfosceril (℞)
Func. class.: Synthetic lung surfactant

Dosage and routes
Prophylactic treatment
Endotracheally: 5 ml/kg as soon as possible after birth and repeat
P doses 12 and 24 hr later to infants remaining on mechanical ventilation

Rescue treatment
Endotracheally: Administer in two half doses of 5 ml/kg doses; give

initial dose after treatment of RDS, then second dose in 12 hr

Uses: Treatment of RDS in premature infants

corticotropin (ACTH) (℞)

Func. class.: Pituitary hormone

Dosage and routes

Testing of adrenocortical function

Adult: IM/SC up to 80 U in divided doses; **IV** 10-25 U in 500 ml D_5W given over 8 hr

Inflammation

Adult: SC/IM 40 U in 4 divided doses (aqueous) or 40 U q12-24h (gel/repository form)

Infantile spasms

Infant: IM Gel 20 U/day × 2 wks, increase if needed

Uses: Testing adrenocortical function, treatment of adrenal insufficiency caused by administration of corticosteroids (long term), multiple sclerosis, infantile spasms

Contraindications: Hypersensitivity, scleroderma, osteoporosis, CHF, peptic ulcer disease, hypertension, systemic fungal infections, smallpox vaccination, recent surgery, ocular herpes simplex, primary adrenocortical insufficiency/hyperfunction

cosyntropin (℞)

Func. class.: Pituitary hormone

Dosage and routes

Adult and child >2 yr: IM/ **IV** 0.25-1 mg between blood sampling

Child <2 yr: IM/**IV** 0.125 mg

Uses: Testing adrenocortical function

Contraindications: Hypersensitivity

crotamiton (℞)

Func. class.: Scabicide

Dosage and routes

Scabies

Adult and child: Cream wash area with soap, water; remove visible crusts, apply cream, apply another coat in 24 hr, remove with soap, water in 48 hr

Pruritus: Massage into affected area, repeat as necessary

Uses: Scabies, pruritus

Contraindications: Hypersensitivity, skin inflammation, abrasions, breaks in skin, mucous membranes

dapsone (DDS) (℞)

Func. class.: Leprostatic

Dosage and routes

Hansen's disease

Adult: PO 100 mg qd with rifampin 600 mg qd × 6 mo, then dapsone alone for 3-10 yr

Child: PO 1-2 mg/kg/day

PCP

Adult: PO 50-100 mg/day usually given with trimethoprim 20 mg/kg/day in 4 divided doses for 3 wk

Child: PO 2 mg/kg/day

Uses: Hansen's disease, PCP (*Pneumocystis carinii* pneumonia), malaria, dermatitis herpetiformis

Contraindications: Hypersensitivity to sulfones, severe anemia

deferoxamine (℞)

Func. class.: Heavy metal antagonist

Dosage and routes

Acute iron toxicity

Adult and child: IM/**IV** 1 g; then 500 mg q4h × 2 doses; then 500 mg q4-12h × 2 doses, not to exceed 15 mg/kg/hr or 6 g/24 hr

Chronic iron toxicity

P ***Adult and child:*** IM 500 mg-1 g/day plus **IV** inf 2 g given by separate line with each blood transfusion, not to exceed 15 mg/kg/hr or 6 g/24 hr; SC 1-2 g over 8-24 hr by SC infusion pump

Uses: Acute, chronic iron intoxication, hemochromatosis, hemosiderosis

Contraindications: Hypersensitivity, anuria, severe renal disease

demeclocycline (℞)

Func. class.: Antiinfective
Chem. class.: Tetracycline

Dosage and routes

Adult: PO 150 mg q6h or 300 mg q12h

Child >8 yr: PO 6-12 mg/kg/day in divided doses q6-12h

Gonorrhea

Adult: PO 600 mg, then 300 mg q12h × 4 days, total 3 g

Uses: Uncommon gram-positive/gram-negative bacteria, protozoa, *Rickettsia, Mycoplasma, Haemophilus ducreyi, Yersinia pestis, Campylobacter fetus, Chlamydia trachomatis,* psittacosis, granuloma inguinale

Contraindications: Hypersensitivity to tetracyclines, children <8 yr, pregnancy **D**

desipramine

Func. class.: Antidepressant, tricyclic

Dosage and routes

Adult: PO 75-150 mg/day in divided doses; may increase to 300 mg/day or may give daily dose hs

P G ***Adolescent and elderly:*** PO 25-50 mg/day, may increase to 100 mg/day

Uses: Depression

Contraindications: Hypersensitivity to tricyclics, recovery phase of myocardial infarction, narrow-angle glaucoma, convulsive disorders, prostatic hypertrophy, child <12 yr

dicyclomine (℞)

Func. class.: Gastrointestinal anticholinergic

Dosage and routes

Adult: PO 10-20 mg tid-qid; IM 20 mg q4-6h

Child >2 yr: PO 10 mg tid-qid

Child 6 mo-2 yr: PO 5 mg tid-qid

Uses: Treatment of peptic ulcer disease in combination with other drugs; infant colic, urinary incontinence

Contraindications: Hypersensitivity to anticholinergics, narrow-angle glaucoma, GI obstruction, myasthenia gravis, paralytic ileus, GI atony, toxic megacolon

dienestrol (℞)

Func. class.: Estrogen

Dosage and routes

Adult: Vag cream 1-2 applications qd × 2 wk, then ½ dose × 2 wk, then 1 application

Uses: Atrophic vaginitis, kraurosis vulvae

Contraindications: Breast cancer, thromboembolic disorders, reproductive cancer, genital bleeding (abnormal, undiagnosed), pregnancy **X**

diflunisal (℞)

Func. class.: Nonsteroidal anti-inflammatory/analgesic (nonopioid)

Dosage and routes
Adult: PO loading dose 1 g; then 500-1000 mg/day in 2 divided doses, q12h, not to exceed 1500 mg/day

Geriatric: PO ½ adult dose

Uses: Mild to moderate pain or fever including arthritis; 3-4 × more potent than aspirin

Contraindications: Hypersensitivity to salicylates, GI bleeding, bleeding disorders, children <12 yr, vit K deficiency

dimercaprol (℞)

Func. class.: Heavy metal antagonist

Dosage and routes
Severe gold/arsenic poisoning
Adult: IM 3 mg/kg q4h × 2 days; then qid × 1 day; then bid × 10 days

Mild gold/arsenic poisoning
Adult: IM 2.5 mg/kg qid × 2 days; then bid × 1 day; then qd × 10 days

Acute lead poisoning
Adult: IM 4 mg/kg; then q4h with edetate calcium disodium 12.5 mg/kg IM; not to exceed 5 mg/kg/dose

Mercury poisoning
Adult: IM 5 mg/kg; then 2.5 mg/kg/day or bid × 10 days

Uses: Arsenic, gold, mercury, lead poisoning; adjunct in severe lead poisoning with encephalopathy

Contraindications: Hypersensitivity, anuria, hepatic insufficiency, poisoning with other metals, severe P renal disease, child <3 yr, pregnancy **D**

disulfiram (℞)

Func. class.: Alcohol deterrent

Dosage and routes
Adult: PO 250-500 mg qd × 1-2 wk, then 125-500 mg qd until fully socially recovered

Uses: Chronic alcoholism (as adjunct)

Contraindications: Hypersensitivity, alcohol intoxication, psychoses, CV disease, pregnancy **X**

D-penicillamine (℞)

Func. class.: Heavy metal antagonist
Chem. class.: Chelating agent

Dosage and routes
Cystinuria
Adult: PO 250 mg qid ac, not to exceed 5 g/day

Child: PO 30 mg/kg/day in divided doses qid ac

Wilson's disease
Adult: PO 250 mg qid ac

Child: PO 20 mg/kg/day in divided doses ac

Rheumatoid arthritis
Adult: PO 125-250 mg/day, then increase 250 mg q2-3mo if needed, not to exceed 1 g/day

Child: PO 3 mg/kg/day × 3 mo, then 6 mg/kg/day in divided doses × 3 mo, then increase to max 10 mg/kg/day

Uses: Wilson's disease, rheumatoid arthritis, cystinuria, heavy metal poisoning (lead, mercury, gold)

Contraindications: Hypersensitivity to penicillins, anuria, agranulocytosis, severe renal disease, pregnancy **D**, lactation

edetate calcium disodium (℞)

Func. class.: Heavy metal antagonist; antidote

Dosage and routes

Acute lead encephalopathy

P ***Adult and child:*** 1.5 g/m^2/day × 3-5 days, with dimercaprol; may be given again after 4 days off drug

Lead poisoning

Adult: **IV** 1 g/250-500 ml D_5W or 0.9% NaCl over 1-2 hr or q12h × 3-5 days; may repeat after 2 days; not to exceed 50 mg/kg/day; may be given as a cont inf over 8-24 hr

Adult: IM 35 mg/kg bid

P ***Child:*** IM 35 mg/kg/day in divided doses q8-12h, not to exceed 50 mg/kg/day; may give for 3-5 days, off 4 days before next course

Uses: Lead poisoning, acute lead encephalopathy

Contraindications: Hypersensitivity, anuria, poisoning of other P metals, severe renal disease, child <3 yr

edetate disodium (℞)

Func. class.: Metal antagonist

Dosage and routes

Adult and child: **IV** inf 15-50 mg/kg/day in 2 divided doses, diluted in 500 ml D_5W or 0.9% NaCl, given over 3-4 hr, not to exceed 3 g/day (adult) or 70 mg/kg/day (child); allow 5 days between courses (child), 2 days (adult)

Uses: Hypercalcemic crisis, control of ventricular dysrhythmias associated with digitalis toxicity

Contraindications: Hypersensitivity, anuria, hepatic insufficiency, poisoning of other metals, severe renal disease, child <3 yr, seizure disorders, active/inactive TB

estramustine

Func. class.: Antineoplastic

Dosage and routes

Adult: PO 10-16 mg/kg in 3-4 divided doses/day; treatment may continue for ≥3 mo or 600 mg/m^2/day in 3 divided doses

Uses: Metastatic prostate cancer

Contraindications: Hypersensitivity to estradiol, thromboembolic disorders, pregnancy **D**

ethosuximide (℞)

Func. class.: Anticonvulsant

Dosage and routes

Adult and child >6 yr: PO 250 mg bid initially; may increase by 250 mg q4-7d, not to exceed 1.5 g/day

Child 3-6 yr: PO 250 mg/day or 125 mg bid; may increase by 250 mg q4-7d, not to exceed 1.5 g/day

Uses: Absence seizures, partial seizures, tonic-clonic seizures

Contraindications: Hypersensitivity to succinimide derivatives

etomidate (℞)

Func. class.: General anesthetic

Dosage and routes

Adult and child >10 yr: **IV** 0.2-0.6 mg/kg over ½-1 min

Uses: Induction of general anesthesia

Contraindications: Hypersensitivity, labor/delivery

felbamate (℞)

Func. class.: Anticonvulsant

Dosage and routes

Adjunctive therapy

Adult: PO add 1.2 g/day in 3-4

divided doses; reduce other anticonvulsants (valproic acid, phenytoin, carbamazepine, and derivatives) by 20% to control plasma concentrations; may increase felbamate in 1.2 g/day increments qwk, up to 3.6 g/day

Monotherapy
Adult: PO 1.2 g/day in 3-4 divided doses; titrate with close supervision; increase dose in 600-mg increments q2 wk to 3.6 g/day if needed

Lennox-Gastaut syndrome
P ***Child (2-14 yr):*** PO add 15 mg/kg/day in 3-4 divided doses; reduce other anticonvulsants (valproic acid, phenytoin, carbamazepine, and derivatives) by 20% to control plasma concentrations; may increase felbamate 15 mg/kg/day qwk up to 45 mg/day

Uses: Partial seizures, with or without generalization in adults; partial and generalized seizures in P children with Lennox-Gastaut syndrome

Contraindications: Hypersensitivity to this drug, other carbamates

fenoprofen (℞)

Func. class.: Nonsteroidal antiinflammatory/nonopioid analgesic

Dosage and routes
Pain
Adult: PO 200 mg q4-6h prn

Arthritis
Adult: PO 300-600 mg qid, not to exceed 3.2 g/day

Uses: Mild to moderate pain, osteoarthritis, rheumatoid arthritis, acute gout, arthritis, ankylosing spondylitis, inflammation, dysmenorrhea

Contraindications: Hypersensitivity, asthma, severe renal disease, severe hepatic disease

flavoxate (℞)

Func. class.: Spasmolytic

Dosage and routes
Adult and child >12 yr: PO 100-200 mg tid-qid

Uses: Relief of nocturia, incontinence, suprapubic pain, dysuria, frequency associated with urologic conditions (symptomatic only)

Contraindications: Hypersensitivity, GI obstruction, GI hemorrhage, GU obstruction

floxuridine (℞)

Func. class.: Antineoplastic, antimetabolite

Dosage and routes
Adult: Intraarterial by cont inf 0.1-0.6 mg/kg/day × 1-6 wk; hepatic artery inj 0.4-0.6 mg/kg/day × 1-6 wk

Uses: GI adenocarcinoma metastatic to liver; cancer of breast, head, neck, liver, brain, gallbladder, bile duct

Contraindications: Hypersensitivity, myelosuppression, pregnancy **D**, poor nutritional status, serious infections

fludarabine (℞)

Func. class.: Antineoplastic, antimetabolite

Dosage and routes
Adult: **IV** 25 mg/m^2 over 30 min qd × 5 days, may repeat q28 days; reconstitute with 2 ml of sterile water for inj; dissolution should occur in <15 sec

Uses: Chronic lymphocytic leukemia; non-Hodgkin's lymphoma

Contraindications: Hypersensitivity, pregnancy **D**

flunisolide (℞)
Func. class.: Steroid, intranasal

Dosage and routes
Adult: Instill 2 sprays in each nostril bid, then increase to tid if needed, not to exceed 8 sprays/day in each nostril

P ***Child 6-14 yr:*** Instill 1 spray in each nostril tid or 2 sprays bid, not to exceed 4 sprays/day in each nostril

P ***Adult and child >6 yr:*** Spray 2 puffs bid, not to exceed 4 puffs bid

Uses: Rhinitis (seasonal or perennial), nasal polyps; chronic steroid-dependent asthma (inh)

Contraindications: Hypersensitivity, P child <12 yr; fungal, bacterial infection of nose

glycerin, anhydrous (℞)
Func. class.: Ophthalmic

Dosage and routes
Adult: Instill 1-2 gtt after local anesthetic

Uses: Reduce corneal edema

Contraindications: Hypersensitivity

guanabenz (℞)
Func. class.: Antihypertensive

Dosage and routes
Adult: PO 4 mg bid, increasing in increments of 4-8 mg/day q1-2wk, not to exceed 32 mg bid

Uses: Hypertension

Contraindications: Hypersensitivity to guanabenz

guanadrel (℞)
Func. class.: Antihypertensive

Dosage and routes
Adult: PO 5 mg bid, adjusted to desired response weekly or monthly; may need 20-75 mg/day in divided doses; higher doses are given tid or qid

G ***Elderly:*** PO 5 mg/day, titrate as needed

Renal dose
- CrCl 10-50 ml/min dose q12-24h; CrCl <10 ml/min dose q24-48h

Uses: Hypertension (moderate to severe as an adjunct)

Contraindications: Hypersensitivity, pheochromocytoma, lactation, CHF, child <18 yr

guanethidine (℞)
Func. class.: Antihypertensive

Dosage and routes
Adult: PO 10-12.5 mg qd, increase by 10 mg qwk; may require 25-50 mg qd

Adult: (hospitalized) 25-50 mg; may increase by 25-50 mg/day or every other day

Child: PO 0.2 mg/kg/day; (6 mg/m^2/day) increase q7-10d, 0.2 mg/kg or 6 mg/m^2/day, not to exceed 3000 µg/kg/24 hr

Uses: Moderate to severe hypertension

Contraindications: Hypersensitivity, pheochromocytoma, recent MI, CHF, cardiac failure, sinus bradycardia

guanfacine (℞)
Func. class.: Antihypertensive

Dosage and routes
Adult: PO 1 mg/day hs; may increase dose in 2-3 wk to 2-3 mg/day

Uses: Hypertension in individual using a thiazide diuretic

Investigational uses: ADHD

Contraindications: Hypersensitivity

halcinonide (℞)
Func. class.: Corticosteroid, synthetic

Dosage and routes
Adult: Top apply to affected area bid-tid (not around eyes)

Uses: Inflammation of corticosteroid-responsive dermatoses

Contraindications: Hypersensitivity, viral infections, fungal infections

halofantrine (℞)
Func. class.: Antimalarial

Dosage and routes
Adult: PO 500 mg q6h × 3 doses; may need to repeat after 1 wk

Uses: Mild to moderate malaria

Contraindications: Hypersensitivity, pregnancy, lactation, QT interval prolongation, AV conduction disorders, thiamine deficiency, ventricular dysrhythmias

hyaluronidase (℞)
Func. class.: Enzyme

Dosage and routes
Adjunct
Adult and child: Inj 150 U with other drug

Urography
Adult and child: SC 75 U over scapula, then contrast medium injected at same site

Hypodermoclysis
Adult and child >3 yr: SC 150 U/L of lysis sol

Uses: Hypodermoclysis, subcutaneous urography; adjunct to dispersion of other drugs

Contraindications: Hypersensitivity to bovine products, CHF, hypoproteinemia, around infected/inflamed or cancerous area

hydroquinone (℞)
Func. class.: Depigmentating agent

Dosage and routes
Adult and child: Top apply to affected area qd-bid

Uses: Bleaching skin, including age spots, freckles, lentigo, chloasma

Contraindications: Hypersensitivity, inflamed skin, prickly heat, sunburn

hydroxychloroquine (℞)
Func. class.: Antimalarial, antiarthritic

Dosage and routes
Malaria
P ***Adult and child:*** PO 5 mg/kg/wk on same day of week, not to exceed 400 mg; treatment should begin 2 wk before entering endemic area; continue 8 wk after leaving; if treatment begins after exposure, 800 mg for P adult, 10 mg/kg for children in 2 divided doses 6 hr apart

Lupus erythematosus
Adult: PO 400 mg qd-bid; length depends on patient response; maintenance 200-400 mg qd

Rheumatoid arthritis
Adult: PO 400-600 mg qd, then 200-300 mg qd after good response

Uses: Malaria caused by *Plasmodium vivax, P. malariae, P. ovale, P. falciparum* (some strains); SLE, rheumatoid arthritis

Contraindications: Hypersensitivity, retinal field changes, porphyria, P children (long-term)

hydroxyprogesterone (℞)

Func. class.: Progestin, hormone

Dosage and routes
Menstrual disorders
Adult: IM 125-375 mg q4 wk; discontinue after 4 cycles
Uterine cancer
Adult: IM 1 g 5-7 times/wk

Uses: Uterine carcinoma, menstrual disorders (abnormal uterine bleeding, amenorrhea)

Contraindications: Breast cancer, hypersensitivity, thromboembolic disorders, reproductive cancer, genital bleeding (abnormal, undiagnosed), pregnancy

idoxuridine-IDU (℞)

Func. class.: Antiviral

Dosage and routes
Adult and child: Instill 1 gtt qh during day and q2h during night

Uses: Herpes simplex keratitis, CMV, varicella-zoster alone or with corticosteroids

Contraindications: Hypersensitivity

indecainide (℞)

Func. class.: Antidysrhythmic (Class IC)

Dosage and routes
Adult: PO 100-200 mg/day in divided dose q12h; 50 mg q12h initially, then increase dose by 25 mg increments q4d, max 400 mg/day

Uses: Life-threatening dysrhythmias, sustained ventricular tachycardia

Contraindications: 2nd- or 3rd-degree AV block, right bundle branch block, cardiogenic shock, hypersensitivity

iodoquinol (℞)

Func. class.: Amebicide

Dosage and routes
Adult: PO 630-650 mg tid × 20 days, not to exceed 2 g/day
Child: PO 30-40 mg/kg/day in 2-3 divided doses × 20 days, not to exceed 1.95 g/24 hr × 20 days; do not repeat treatment before 2-3 wk

Uses: Intestinal amebiasis

Contraindications: Hypersensitivity to this drug or iodine, renal disease, hepatic disease, severe thyroid disease, preexisting optic neuropathy

isotretinoin (℞)

Func. class.: Dermatologic antiacne agent

Dosage and routes
Adult: PO 0.5-2 mg/kg/day in 2 divided doses × 15-20 wk; if relapse occurs, repeat after 8 wk off drug

Uses: Severe recalcitrant cystic acne

Contraindications: Hypersensitivity, inflamed skin, pregnancy **X**

isoxsuprine (℞)
Func. class.: Peripheral vasodilator

Dosage and routes
Adult: PO 10-20 mg tid or qid

Uses: Symptoms of cerebrovascular insufficiency, peripheral vascular disease including arteriosclerosis obliterans, thromboangitis obliterans, Raynaud's disease

Contraindications: Hypersensitivity, postpartum, arterial bleeding

HIGH ALERT

ketamine (℞)
Func. class.: General anesthetic

Dosage and routes
P ***Adult and child:*** **IV** 1-4.5 mg/kg over 1 min
P ***Adult and child:*** IM 6.5-13 mg/kg
Maintenance: ½ to full induction dose may be repeated

Uses: Short anesthesia for diagnostic/surgical procedures; as an adjunct with other anesthetics

Contraindications: Hypersensitivity, CVA, increased intracranial pressure, severe hypertension, cardiac decompensation, P child <2 yr

levobupivacaine (℞)
Func. class.: Local anesthetic

Dosage and routes
Varies with route of anesthesia

Uses: Local, regional anesthesia, surgical anesthesia, pain management, continuous epidural analgesia

Contraindications: Hypersensitivity, children <12 yr, elderly, severe liver disease

levorphanol (℞)
Func. class.: Opioid analgesic (agonist)

Controlled Substance Schedule II

Dosage and routes
Adult: PO/SC/**IV** 2-3 mg q4-5h prn; PCA 0.1 mg/ml

Uses: Moderate to severe pain

Contraindications: Hypersensitivity, addiction (narcotic)

lincomycin (℞)
Func. class.: Antibacterial

Dosage and routes
Adult: PO 500 mg q6-8h, not to exceed 8 g/day; IM 600 mg/day or q12h; **IV** 600 mg-1 g q8-12h; dilute in 100 ml **IV** sol; infuse over 1 hr, not to exceed 8 g/day
Child >1 mo: PO 30-60 mg/kg/day in divided doses q6-8h; IM 10 mg/kg/day q12h; **IV** 10-20 mg/kg/day in divided doses q8-12h; dilute to 100 ml **IV** sol; infuse over 1 hr

Uses: Infections caused by group A β-hemolytic streptococci, pneumococci, staphylococci (respiratory tract, skin, soft tissue, urinary tract infections, osteomyelitis, septicemia)

Contraindications: Hypersensitivity, ulcerative colitis/enteritis, infants <1 mo

masoprocol (℞)
Func. class.: Miscellaneous topical product

Dosage and routes
Adult: Top apply to lesion bid × 2-4 wk

Uses: Actinic keratoses

Contraindications: Hypersensitivity, children

mazindol (℞)
Func. class.: Anorexiant

Dosage and routes
Adult: PO 1 mg/hr ac, or 2 mg 1 hr ac lunch, or 1 mg tid 1 hr ac

Uses: Exogenous obesity

Contraindications: Hypersensitivity to sympathomimetic amine, glaucoma, drug abuse, cardiovascular disease, children <12 yr, hypertension, severe arteriosclerosis, agitated states, hyperthyroidism, concurrent MAOI use or use within 14 days

mefenamic acid (℞)
Func. class.: Nonsteroidal anti-inflammatory

Dosage and routes
Adult and child >14 yr: PO 500 mg, then 250 mg q6h, use not to exceed 1 wk

Uses: Mild to moderate pain, dysmenorrhea, inflammatory disease

Contraindications: Hypersensitivity, asthma, severe renal disease, severe hepatic disease, ulcer disease

mefloquine (℞)
Func. class.: Antimalarial

Dosage and routes
Adult: PO 1250 mg as a single dose (treatment); 250 mg 1 wk before trip, then for 4 wk after returning, then 250 mg q2 wk (prevention)

Uses: Treatment and prevention of *Plasmodium falciparum, P. vivax,* malaria

Contraindications: Hypersensitivity

mepenzolate (℞)
Func. class.: GI anticholinergic

Dosage and routes
Adult: PO 25-50 mg qid with meals, hs; titrate to patient response

Uses: Treatment of peptic ulcer disease, irritable bowel syndrome in combination with other drugs; for other GI disorders

Contraindications: Hypersensitivity to anticholinergics, narrow-angle glaucoma, GI obstruction, myasthenia gravis, paralytic ileus, GI atony, toxic megacolon

methohexital (℞)
Func. class.: General anesthetic

Dosage and routes
Induction
P ***Adult and child:*** **IV** 50-120 mg given 1 ml/5 sec
Maintenance
P ***Adult and child:*** **IV** 20-40 mg q4-7 min of a 0.1% sol

Uses: General anesthesia for electroshock therapy, reduction of fractures, adjunct with other anesthetics, balanced anesthesia

Contraindications: Hypersensitivity, status asthmaticus, hepatic/intermittent porphyrias

methoxsalen (℞)
Func. class.: Pigmentating agent

Dosage and routes
Vitiligo
Adult and child >12 yr: PO 20 mg qd 2-4 hr before exposure to therapeutic ultraviolet rays; administer on alternate days; Top apply 1-2 hr before exposure to UVA light; treatment intervals regulated by erythema response

Psoriasis
Adult: PO dosage individualized to weight; taken 2 hr before exposure to therapeutic ultraviolet rays

Uses: Vitiligo, psoriasis

Contraindications: Hypersensitivity, melanoma, LE, albinism, sunburn, cataracts, squamous cell cancer, child ≤12 yr, diseases associated with photosensitivity

methscopolamine (℞)

Func. class.: GI anticholinergic

Dosage and routes
Adult: PO 2.5-5 mg ½ hr ac, hs

Uses: Peptic ulcer disease, preoperatively

Contraindications: Hypersensitivity to anticholinergics, narrow-angle glaucoma, GI obstruction, myasthenia gravis, paralytic ileus, GI atony, toxic megacolon

methsuximide (℞)

Func. class.: Anticonvulsant

Dosage and routes
Adult and child: PO 300 mg/day; may increase by 300 mg/wk, not to exceed 1.2 g/day in divided doses

Uses: Refractory absence seizures (petit mal)

Contraindications: Hypersensitivity to succinimide derivatives

mitotane (℞)

Func. class.: Antineoplastic

Dosage and routes
Adult: PO 9-10 g/day in divided doses tid or qid; may have to decrease dosage if severe reactions occur

Uses: Adrenocortical carcinoma

Investigational uses: Pituitary disorders with cushingoid symptoms

Contraindications: Hypersensitivity

molindone (℞)

Func. class.: Antipsychotic/neuroleptic

Dosage and routes
Adult: PO 50-75 mg/day increasing to 225 mg/day if needed

Uses: Psychotic disorders

Contraindications: Hypersensitivity, coma, P child

papaverine (℞)

Func. class.: Peripheral vasodilator

Dosage and routes
Adult: PO 100-300 mg 3-5 × day; sus rel cap 150-300 mg q8-12h; IM/**IV** 30-120 mg q3h prn; Intracavernosal (IC) 30 mg/0.5-1 mg phentolamine or 60 mg alone

Uses: Arterial spasm resulting in cerebral and peripheral ischemia, myocardial ischemia associated with vascular spasm or dysrhythmias, angina pectoris, peripheral pulmonary embolism, visceral spasm as in ureteral, biliary, GI colic, peripheral vascular disease

Contraindications: Hypersensitivity, complete AV heart block

paraldehyde (℞)

Func. class.: Anticonvulsant

Dosage and routes
Seizures
Adult: IM 5-10 ml; divide 10 ml into 2 inj; **IV** 0.2-0.4 ml/kg in NS inj

Child: IM 0.15 ml/kg; rect 0.3 ml/kg

q4-6h or 1 ml/yr of age, not to exceed 5 ml; may repeat in 1 hr prn; **IV** 5 ml/90 ml NS inj; begin infusion at 5 ml/hr; titrate to patient response

Alcohol withdrawal

Adult: PO/rect 5-10 ml, not to exceed 60 ml; IM 5 ml q4-6h × 24 hr, then q6h on following days, not to exceed 30 ml

Sedation

Adult: PO/rec 4-10 ml; IM 5 ml; **IV** 3-5 ml in emergency only; Child: PO/rec/IM 0.15 ml/kg

Tetanus

Adult: **IV** 4-5 ml or 12 ml by gastric tube q4h diluted with water; IM 5-10 ml prn

Uses: Refractory seizures, status epilepticus, sedation, insomnia, alcohol withdrawal, tetanus, eclampsia

Contraindications: Hypersensitivity, gastroenteritis with ulceration

paramethadione (℞)

Func. class.: Anticonvulsant

Dosage and routes

Adult: PO 300 mg tid; may increase by 300 mg/wk, not to exceed 600 mg qid

Child >6 yr: PO 0.9 g/day in divided doses tid or qid

Child 2-6 yr: PO 0.6 g/day in divided doses tid or qid

Child <2 yr: PO 0.3 g/day in divided doses tid or qid

Uses: Refractory absence (petit mal) seizures

Contraindications: Hypersensitivity, blood dyscrasias, pregnancy **D**, lactation

paromomycin (℞)

Func. class.: Amebicide

Dosage and routes

Intestinal amebiasis

Adult and child: PO 25-35 mg/kg/day in 3 divided doses × 5-10 day pc

Hepatic coma

Adult: 4 g qd in divided doses × 5-6 day

Uses: Intestinal amebiasis, adjunct in hepatic coma

Contraindications: Hypersensitivity, renal disease, GI obstruction

permethrin (OTC, ℞)

Func. class.: Pediculicide

Dosage and routes

Lice (head)

Adult and child: Wash hair, towel dry; apply liberally to hair, leave on 10 min, rinse with water

Scabies

Adult and child: Top 5% cream applied and massaged into all skin surfaces; leave cream on 8-14 hr, then wash

Uses: Lice, nits, ticks, flea nits

Contraindications: Hypersensitivity

phenacemide (℞)

Func. class.: Anticonvulsant

Dosage and routes

Adult: PO 500 mg tid, may increase by 500 mg/wk, not to exceed 5 g/day

Child 5-10 yr: PO 250 mg tid, may increase by 250 mg/wk, not to exceed 1.5 g/day prn

Uses: Refractory, generalized tonic-clonic (grand mal), complex-partial (psychomotor), absence (petit mal), atypical seizures

Contraindications: Hypersensitivity, psychiatric condition, pregnancy **D**, lactation

phendimetrazine (℞)

Func. class.: Anorexiant

Dosage and routes

Adult: PO 35 mg bid-tid 1 hr ac, not to exceed 70 mg tid; sus rel 105 mg qd ac AM

Uses: Exogenous obesity

Contraindications: Hypersensitivity, hyperthyroidism, hypertension, glaucoma, severe arteriosclerosis, severe cardiovascular disease, children <12 yr, agitated states, drug abuse, MAOI use within 14 days

phenoxybenzamine (℞)

Func. class.: Antihypertensive

Dosage and routes

Adult: PO 10 mg qd; increase by 10 mg qod; usual range 20-40 mg bid-tid

P ***Child:*** PO 0.2 mg/kg or 6 mg/m^2/day, max 10 mg, may increase at 4-day intervals; maintenance dosage 0.4-1.2 mg/kg/day or 12-36 mg/m^2/day given in divided doses tid or qid

Uses: Pheochromocytoma

Contraindications: Hypersensitivity, CHF, angina, cerebral vascular insufficiency, coronary arteriosclerosis

phentermine (℞)

Func. class.: Cerebral stimulant

Dosage and routes

Adult: PO 8 mg tid 30 min before meals or 15-37.5 mg qd before breakfast

Uses: Exogenous obesity

Contraindications: Hypersensitivity, hyperthyroidism, hypertension, glaucoma, severe arteriosclerosis, angina pectoris, cardiovascular disease, pregnancy **C**, child <12 yr

physostigmine (℞)

Func. class.: Antidote, reversible anticholinesterase

Dosage and routes

Overdose of anticholinergics

Adult: IM/**IV** 2 mg; give no more than 1 mg/min; may repeat

Child: IM/**IV** inj 0.02 mg/kg, not more than 0.5 mg/min; may repeat at 5-10 min intervals until max dose of 2 mg

Postanesthesia

Adult: IM/**IV** 0.5-1 mg; give no more than 1 mg/min (**IV**); can repeat at 10 to 30 min intervals

Uses: To reverse CNS effects of diazepam; anticholinergic, tricyclics, Alzheimer's disease, hereditary ataxia

Contraindications: Hypotension, obstruction of intestine or renal system , asthma, gangrene, CV disease, choline esters, depolarizing neuromuscular blocking agents, diabetes

pinacidil (℞)

Func. class.: Antihypertensive

Dosage and routes

Adult: PO 12.5-25 mg bid

Uses: Severe hypertension not responsive to other therapy

Contraindications: Acute MI, dissecting aortic aneurysm, hypersensitivity, pheochromocytoma

pralidoxime (℞)

Func. class.: Cholinesterase reactivator

Dosage and routes

Anticholinesterase overdose

Adult: **IV** 1-2 g, then 250 mg q5 min until desired response

Organophosphate poisoning

Adult: **IV** inf 1-2 g/100 ml 0.9% NaCl over 15-30 min; may repeat in 1 hr; PO 1-3 g q5h

P ***Child:*** **IV** inf 20-40 mg/kg/dose diluted in 100 ml 0.9% NaCl over 15-30 min

Uses: Cholinergic crisis in myasthenia gravis, organophosphate poisoning antidote, early relief of paralysis of respiratory muscles; used as an adjunct to systemic atropine administration

Contraindications: Hypersensitivity, carbamate insecticide poisoning

prazepam (℞)

Func. class.: Sedative/hypnotic; antianxiety agent

Dosage and routes

Adult: PO 10 mg tid; 20-60 mg in divided doses or 20 mg at hs

G ***Elderly:*** PO 10-15 mg/day in divided doses

Uses: Anxiety

Contraindications: Hypersensitivity to benzodiazepines, narrow-angle glaucoma, psychosis, pregnancy **D**,
P child <18 yr

sevelamer (℞)

Func. class.: Polymeric phosphate binder

Dosage and routes

Reduction of serum phosphorus in adults not taking phosphate binders

Adult: PO initially 800-1600 mg tid with meals based on serum phosphorus level (see below); adjust dose gradually at 2-wk intervals until serum phosphorus 6 mg/dl

Adult, serum phosphorus 9 mg/dl: 1600 mg tid with meals

Adult, serum phosphorus 7.5 and <9 mg/dl: 1200-1600 mg tid with meals

Adult, serum phosphorus >6 and <7.5 mg/dl: 800 mg tid with meals

Uses: End-stage renal disease (ESRD)

Contraindications: Hypophosphatemia, bowel obstruction, hypersensitivity

sibutramine (℞)

Func. class.: Appetite suppressant

Controlled Substance Schedule IV

Dosage and routes

Adult: PO 10 mg qd; may be increased to 15 mg qd after 4 wk, or lowered to 5 mg qd depending on response

Uses: Obesity in conjunction with other treatments

Contraindications: Hypersensitivity, hypothyroidism, anorexia nervosa, severe hepatic/renal disease, uncontrolled hypertension, history of CAD, CHF, dysrhythmias, lactation, CVA

streptozocin (℞)

Func. class.: Antineoplastic alkylating agent

Dosage and routes
Adult: **IV** 500 mg/m^2 × 5 days q6 wk until desired response; or 1 g/m^2 qwk × 2 wk, not to exceed 1.5 g/m^2 in 1 dose

Uses: Metastatic islet cell carcinoma of pancreas

Investigational uses: Prevention of spread of Hodgkin's disease, metastatic carcinoid tumor, pancreatic adenocarcinoma, colon malignancies

Contraindications: Hypersensitivity

teniposide (℞)

Func. class.: Antineoplastic

Dosage and routes
P ***Child:*** **IV** inf Combo teniposide 165 mg/m^2 and cytarabine 300 mg/m^2 2 ×/wk × 8-9 doses or combo teniposide 250 mg/m^2 and vincristine 1.5 mg/m^2 qwk × 4-8 wk and prednisone 40 mg/m^2 PO × 28 days

Uses: Childhood acute lymphoblastic leukemia (ALL), refractory childhood acute lymphocytic leukemia

Contraindications: Hypersensitivity, bone marrow depression, severe hepatic disease, severe renal disease, bacterial infection, pregnancy **D**

thioguanine (6-TG) (℞)

Func. class.: Antineoplastic-antimetabolite

Dosage and routes
Adult and child: PO 2 mg/kg/day, then increase slowly to 3 mg/kg/day after 4 wk

Uses: Acute leukemias, chronic granulocytic leukemia, lymphomas, multiple myeloma, solid tumors

Contraindications: Prior drug resistance, leukopenia (<2500/mm^3), thrombocytopenia (<100,000/mm^3), anemia, pregnancy **D**

HIGH ALERT

thiopental (℞)

Func. class.: General anesthetic

Dosage and routes
Induction
Adult: **IV** 210-280 mg or 3-5 ml/kg

General anesthetic
Adult: **IV** 50-75 mg given at 20-40 sec intervals

Narcoanalysis
Adult: **IV** 100 mg/min, not to exceed 50 ml/min

Sedation or narcosis
Adult: Rec 12-20 mg/lb

Increased intracranial pressure
Adult: 1.5-3.5 mg/kg

Uses: Short general anesthesia, narcoanalysis, induction anesthesia before other anesthetics

Investigational uses: Increased intracranial pressure

Contraindications: Hypersensitivity, status asthmaticus, hepatic/intermittent porphyrias

thiotepa (℞)

Func. class.: Antineoplastic

Dosage and routes
Adult: **IV** 0.3-0.4 mg/kg at 1-4 wk intervals

Neoplastic effusions
Adult: Intracavity 0.6-0.8 mg/kg

Bladder cancer
Adult: Instill 60 mg/30-60 ml water for inj instilled in bladder for 2 hr once weekly × 4 wk

Uses: Hodgkin's disease, lymphomas; breast, ovarian, lung, bladder cancer; neoplastic effusions

Contraindications: Hypersensitivity, pregnancy **D**

thiothixene (℞)

Func. class.: Antipsychotic, neuroleptic

Dosage and routes
Adult: PO 2-5 mg bid-qid depending on severity of condition; dose gradually increased to 15-30 mg if needed; IM 4 mg bid-qid; max dose 30 mg qd; administer PO dose as soon as possible

G ***Elderly:*** PO 1-2 mg qd-bid, increase by 1-2 mg q4-7 days to desired dose

Uses: Psychotic disorders, schizophrenia, acute agitation

Contraindications: Hypersensitivity, blood dyscrasias, child <12 yr, bone marrow depression, circulatory collapse, CNS depression, coma, alcoholism, CV disease, hepatic disease, Reye's syndrome, narrow-angle glaucoma

Do not confuse:
Navane/Norvasc

tolazamide (℞)

Func. class.: Antidiabetic, oral

Dosage and routes
Adult: PO 100 mg/day for FBS <200 mg/dl or 250 mg/day for FBS >200 mg/dl; dose should be titrated to patient response (1 g or less/day)

Uses: Type II (NIDDM) diabetes mellitus

Contraindications: Hypersensitivity to sulfonylureas, juvenile or brittle diabetes

tolbutamide 🔑 (℞)

Func. class.: Antidiabetic

Dosage and routes
Adult: PO 1-2 g/day in divided doses, titrated to patient response; **IV** 1 g (Fajan's test)

Uses: Type II (NIDDM) diabetes mellitus

Contraindications: Hypersensitivity to sulfonylureas, juvenile or brittle diabetes

trientine (℞)

Func. class.: Heavy-metal antagonist

Dosage and routes
Adult: PO 750-1250 mg in divided doses bid-qid, max 2000 mg/day

Child: PO 500-1500 mg in divided doses bid-qid

Uses: Wilson's disease, chelating agent if other agents are not tolerated

Contraindications: Hypersensitivity, cystinuria, rheumatoid arthritis, biliary cirrhosis

vasopressin 🔑 (℞)

Func. class.: Pituitary hormone

Dosage and routes
Diabetes insipidus
Adult: IM/SC 5-10 units bid-qid prn; IM/SC 2.5-5 units q2-3 days (Pitressin Tannate) for chronic therapy

P ***Child:*** IM/SC 2.5-10 units bid-qid prn; IM/SC 1.25-2.5 units q2-3 days (Pitressin Tannate) for chronic therapy

Abdominal distention

Adult: IM 5 units, then q3-4h, increasing to 10 units if needed (aqueous)

Uses: Diabetes insipidus (nonnephrogenic/nonpsychogenic), abdominal distention postoperatively, bleeding esophageal varices

Contraindications: Hypersensitivity, chronic nephritis

xylometazoline (OTC)

Func. class.: Nasal decongestant

Dosage and routes

P ***Adult and child >12 yr:*** Instill 2-3 gtt or 2 sprays q8-10h (0.1%)

P ***Child <12 yr:*** Instill 2-3 gtt or 1% spray q8-10h (0.05%)

Uses: Nasal congestion; adjunct in otitis media

Contraindications: Hypersensitivity to sympathomimetic amines

Appendix G Less Frequently Used Antihistamines

GENERIC NAME	TRADE NAME(S)	USES	DOSAGES AND ROUTES	AVAILABLE FORMS	INTERACTIONS	CONTRAINDICATIONS
acrivastine/ pseudoephedrine (℞)	Semprex-D	• Rhinitis • Allergy symptoms • Chronic idiopathic urticaria	• Adult, child >12 yr: PO 8 mg q4-6h	• Caps 8 mg/60 mg	• Increased CNS depression: alcohol, narcotics, sedatives, hypnotics • Hypertensive crisis: MAOIs ▨ May increase CNS depression: kava ▨ May increase anticholinergic effect: henbane leaf	• Hypersensitivity to this drug or triprolidine • Severe hypertension • Cardiac disease
azatadine (℞)	Optimine	• Allergy symptoms • Rhinitis • Chronic urticaria	• Adult: PO 1-2 mg bid, not to exceed 4 mg/day G Elderly: PO 1 mg qd-bid	• Tabs 1 mg	• Increased CNS depression: barbiturates, narcotics, hypnotics, tricyclic antidepressants, alcohol • Decreased effect of: oral anticoagulants ▨ Increased effect of azatadine: MAOIs ▨ Increased CNS depression: kava ▨ Increased anticholinergic effect: henbane leaf	• Hypersensitivity to H_1-receptor antagonists • Acute asthma attack • Lower respiratory tract disease • Child <12 yr
buclizine (℞)	Buclacin-S, Softabs	• Motion sickness • Dizziness • Nausea • Vomiting • Antihistamine	• Adult: PO 25-50 mg prn ½ hr before travel; may be repeated q4-6h prn	• Tabs 50 mg	▨ Increased anticholinergic effect: henbane leaf ▨ Increased CNS depression: kava	• Hypersensitivity to cyclizines • Shock

cyclizine (OTC, ℞)	Marezine	• Motion sickness • Prevention of postoperative vomiting • Antihistamine	*Vomiting* • Adult: IM 25-50 mg ½ hr before termination of surgery, then q4-6h prn (lactate) P Child: IM 3 mg/kg divided in 3 equal doses *Motion sickness* • Adult: PO 50 mg then q4-6h prn, not to exceed 200 mg/day (HCl) P Child: PO 25 mg q4-6h prn	• Tabs (HCl) 50 mg • Inj (lactate) 50 mg/ml	• May increase CNS effect: alcohol, tranquilizers, narcotics ▨ Increased CNS depression: kava	• Hypersensitivity to cyclizines • Shock
dexchlorpheniramine (℞)	Dexchlor, dexclorpheniramine maleate, Poladex, Polaramine	• Allergy symptoms • Rhinitis • Pruritus • Contact dermatitis	• Adult: PO 1-2 mg tid-qid; repeat action 4-6 mg bid-tid P Child 6-11 yr: PO 1 mg q4-6h, or time rel 4 mg hs P Child 2-5 yr: PO 0.5 mg q4-6h; do not use repeat action form	• Tabs 2 mg • Repeat action tabs 4, 6 mg • Syr 2 mg/5 ml	• Increased CNS depression: barbiturates, narcotics, hypnotics, tricyclic antidepressants, alcohol • Decreased effect: oral anticoagulants, heparin • Increased effect of dexchlorpheniramine: MAOIs ▨ Increased anticholinergic effect: henbane leaf	• Hypersensitivity to H_1-receptor antagonists • Acute asthma attack • Lower respiratory tract disease

KEY: ▨ = Herb/drug interaction

Continued

Appendix G Less frequently used antihistamines—cont'd

GENERIC NAME	TRADE NAME(S)	USES	DOSAGES AND ROUTES	AVAILABLE FORMS	INTERACTIONS	CONTRAINDICATIONS
trimeprazine (℞)	Panectyl ✱, Temaril	• Pruritus	• Adult: PO 2.5 mg qid; time-rel 5 mg bid G Elderly: PO 2.5 mg bid P Child 3-12 yr: PO 2.5 mg tid or hs P Child 6 mo-1 yr: PO 1.25 mg tid or hs	• Tabs 2.5 mg • Time rel spanules 5 mg • Syr 2.5 mg/5 ml	• Increased CNS depression: barbiturates, narcotics, hypnotics, tricyclic antidepressants, alcohol • Decreased effect of oral anticoagulants, heparin • Increased effect of trimeprazine: MAOIs ▨ Increased anticholinergic effect: henbane leaf	• Hypersensitivity to H_1-receptor antagonists • Acute asthma attack • Lower respiratory tract disease
tripelennamine (℞)	PBZ, PBZ-SR, Pelamine, tripelennamine HC1	• Rhinitis • Allergy symptoms	• Adults: PO 25-50 mg q4-6h, not to exceed 600 mg/day; time-rel 100 mg bid-tid, not to exceed 600 mg/day P Child >5 yr: PO time-rel 50 mg q8-12h, not to exceed 300 mg/day P Child <5 yr: PO 5 mg/kg/day in 4-6 divided doses, not to exceed 300 mg/day	• Tabs 25, 50 mg • Time-rel tabs 100 mg • Elix 37.5 mg/5 ml	• Increased CNS depression: barbiturates, narcotics, hypnotics, tricyclic antidepressants, alcohol • Decreased effect of oral anticoagulants, heparin • Increased effect of tripelennamine: MAOIs ▨ Increased anticholinergic effect: henbane leaf	• Hypersensitivity to H_1-receptor antagonists • Acute asthma attack • Lower respiratory tract disease

KEY: ✱ = Canada only

Appendix H Vaccines and Toxoids

GENERIC NAME	TRADE NAME	USES	DOSAGES AND ROUTES	CONTRAINDICATIONS
BCG vaccine	TICE BCG	TB exposure	Adult/child >1 mo: 0.2-0.3 ml P Child<1 mo: Reduce dose by 50% using 2 ml of sterile water after reconstituting	Hypersensitivity, hypogammaglobulinemia, positive TB test, burns
cholera vaccine	No trade name	Immunization for cholera in other countries	P Adult/child >10 yr: IM/SC 2× of 0.5 ml, 7-30 days before travelling to areas with cholera. Booster is used q6 mo 0.5 ml prn	Hypersensitivity, acute febrile illness
diphtheria and tetanus toxoids, adsorbed	No trade name	Induces antitoxins to provide immunity to diphtheria & tetanus	P Adult/child ≥7 yr: IM (Adult strength) 0.5 ml q4-8 wk × 2 doses, then 3rd dose 6-12 mo after 2nd dose, booster IM 0.5 ml q10 yr P Child 1-6 yr: IM (Pediatric strength) 0.5 ml q4 wk × 2 doses, booster 6-12 mo after 2nd dose P Infant 6 wk-1 yr: IM (Pediatric strength) 0.5 ml q4 wk × 3 doses, booster 6-12 mo after 3rd dose	Hypersensitivity to mercury, thimerosal, immunocompromised patients, radiation, corticosteroids, acute illness
diphtheria and tetanus toxoids and whole-cell pertussis vaccine (DPT, DTP)	DTwP, Tr-Immunol	Prevention of diphtheria, tetanus, pertussis	Adult: booster dose q10 yr P Child >6 wk-6 yr: IM 0.5 ml at 2, 4, 6 mo, 1-½ yr; booster needed 0.5 ml at age 6	Hypersensitivity, active infection, poliomyelitis outbreak, immunosuppression, febrile illness
diphtheria and tetanus toxoids and acellular pertussis vaccine	Acel-Imune, DTaP, Tripedia			

TB, Tuberculosis; *DPT*, diphtheria-pertussis-tetanus (vaccine); *DTP*, diphtheria and tetanus toxoids and pertussis vaccine.

Continued

GENERIC NAME	TRADE NAME	USES	DOSAGES AND ROUTES	CONTRAINDICATIONS
haemophilus b conjugate vaccine, diphtheria CRM_{197} protein conjugate (HbOC) haemophilus b conjugate vaccine, meningococcal protein conjugate (PRP-OMP)	HibTITER PedvaxHIB	Polysaccharide immunization of children 2-6 yr against *H. influenzae b*, conjugate immunization of child 2, 4, 6 mo	**HibTITER (IM only)** P Child: IM 0.5 ml P Child 2-6 mo: 0.5 ml q2 mo × 3 inj P Child 7-11 mo: Previously unvaccinated 0.5 ml q2 mo inj P Child 12-14 mo: previously unvaccinated 0.5 ml × 1 inj **PEDVAXHIB (IM only)** P Child 2-14 mo: 0.5 ml × 2 inj at 2, 4 mo of age (6 mo dose not needed), then booster at 12-18 mo against invasive disease P Child ≥15 mo: Previously unvaccinated 0.5 ml inj	Hypersensitivity, febrile illness, active infection
hepatitis A vaccine, inactivated	Havrix, Vaqta	Active immunization against hepatitis A virus	Adults: IM 1, 440 EL. U (Havrix) or 50 U (Vagta) as a single dose, booster dose is the same given at 6, 12 mo P Child 2-18 yr: IM 720 EL. U (Havrix) or 25 U (Vagta) as a single dose, booster dose is the same given at 6, 12 mo	Hypersensitivity
hepatitis B vaccine, recombinant	Engerix-B, Recombivax HB	Immunization against all subtypes of hepatitis B virus	Varies widely	Hypersensitivity to this vaccine or yeast

influenza virus vaccine, trivalent A and B (whole virus/split virus)	Fluogen, FluShield, Fluviral ✱, Fluvirin, Fluzone, influenza virus vaccine, trivalent	Prevention of Russian, Chilean, Philippine influenza	P Adult/child >12 yr: IM 0.5 ml in 1 dose P Child 3-12 yr: IM 0.5 ml, repeat in 1 mo (split) unless 1978-1985 vaccine was given P Child 6 mo to 3 yr: IM 0.25 ml, repeat in 1 mo (split) unless 1978-1985 vaccine was given	Hypersensitivity, active infection, chicken egg allergy, Guillain-Barr fe syndrome, active neurologic disorders
Japanese encephalitis virus vaccine, inactivated	JE-VAX	Active immunity against Japanese encephalitis (JE)	P Adult/child ≥3 yr: SC 1 ml, days 0, 7, 30; booster SC 1 ml 2 yr after last dose P Child 1-3 yr: SC 0.5 ml, days 0, 7, 30; booster SC 0.5 ml 2 yr after last dose	Hypersensitivity to murine, thimerosal; allergic reactions to previous dose
Lyme disease vaccine (recombinant OspA)	LYMErix	Immunization against Lyme disease	Adult and adolescent 15-70: IM 30 μg in deltoid, repeat at 1, 12 mo after first dose	Hypersensitivity, antibiotic refractory Lyme arthritis
measles and rubella virus vaccine, live attenuated	M-R-Vax II	Immunity to measles and rubella by antibody production	P Adult/child ≥15 mo: SC 0.5 ml (1000 U)	Hypersensitivity, immunocompromised patients, active untreated TB, cancer, blood dyscrasias, radiation, corticosteroids, pregnancy; allergic reactions to neomycin, eggs
measles, mumps, and rubella vaccine, live	M-M-R-II	Prevention of measles, mumps, rubella	Adult: SC 1 vial; 2 vials separated by 1 mo, in person born after 1957 P Child >15 mo and adult: SC 0.5 ml	Hypersensitivity, blood dyscrasias, anemia, active infection, immunosuppression; egg, chicken allergy; pregnancy, febrile illness, neomycin allergy, neoplasms

✱Canada only.

Continued

GENERIC NAME	TRADE NAME	USES	DOSAGES AND ROUTES	CONTRAINDICATIONS
measles virus vaccine, live attenuated	Attenuvax	Immunity to measles by antibody production	P Adult/child ≥15 mo: SC 0.5 ml (1000 U), one dose 15 mo, 2nd dose age 4-6 or 11, or 12	Hypersensitivity to eggs, neomycin; cancer, radiation, corticosteroids, pregnancy, immunocompromised patients, blood dyscrasias, active untreated TB
meningococcal polysaccharide vaccine	Menomune-A/C/Y/W-135	Prophylaxis to meningococcal meningitis	P Adult/child >2 yr: SC 0.5 ml	Hypersensitivity to thimerosal, pregnancy, acute illness
mumps virus vaccine, live	Mumpsvax	Active immunity to mumps	P Adult/child ≥1 yr: SC 0.5 ml (20,000 U)	Hypersensitivity to eggs, neomycin; cancer, radiation, corticosteroids, pregnancy, immunocompromised patients, blood dyscrasias, active untreated TB
plague vaccine	No trade name	Active immunity to *Yersinia pestis* plague	Adult: IM 1 ml, then 0.2 ml in 4-12 wk, then 0.2 ml 5-6 mo after 2nd dose; booster 0.1-0.2 ml q6 mo when in area where plague is present	Hypersensitivity to phenol, sulfites, formaldehyde, beef, soy, casein; pregnancy, coagulation disorders
pneumococcal 7-valent conjugate vaccine	Prevnar	Immunity against streptococcus pneumoniae	P Child: IM 0.5 ml × 3 doses (7-11 mo); × 2 doses (12-23 mo); × 1 dose >2-9 yr	Hypersensitivity to diphtheria toxoid or this product
pneumococcal vaccine, polyvalent	Pneumovax 23, Pnu-Imune 23	Pneumococcal immunization	P Adult/child >2 yr: IM/SC 0.5 ml	Hypersensitivity, Hodgkin's disease, ARDS
poliovirus vaccine, live, oral, trivalent (TOPV) poliovirus vaccine (IPV)	Orimune, IPOL	Prevention of polio	P Adult/child >2 yr: PO 0.5 ml, given q8 wk × 2 doses, then 0.5 ml ½-1 yr after dose 2 P Infant: PO 0.5 at 2, 4, 18 mo; booster at 4-6 yr; may also be given IPV at 2, 4 mo, then TOPV at 12-18 mo, booster at 4-6 yr	Hypersensitivity, active infection, allergy to neomycin/streptomycin, immunosuppression, vomiting, diarrhea

rabies vaccine, adsorbed	No trade name	Active immunity to rabies	**Preexposure** P Adult/child: IM 1 ml day 0, 7, 21, or 28 days (total 3 doses); booster IM 1 ml PRN q2-5 yr **Postexposure** P Adult/child not vaccinated: IM 20 IU/kg of HRIG and 5 1 ml inj of rabies vaccine on days 0, 7, 14, 28	Severe hypersensitivity to previous inj of vaccine, thimerosal
rabies vaccine, HDCV	IMOVax Rabies, IMOVax Rabies I.D.	Active immunity to rabies	**Preexposure** P Adult/child: IM 1 ml day 0, 7, 21 or 28 **Postexposure** P Adult/child: IM 1 ml on day 0, 3, 7, 14, 28	No contraindications
rubella and mumps virus vaccine, live	Biavax II	Immunity to rubella and mumps by antibody production	P Adult/child ≥1 yr: SC 0.5 ml	Hypersensitivity to eggs, neomycin; cancer, radiation, corticosteroids, pregnancy, immunocompromised patients, blood dyscrasias, active untreated TB
rubella virus vaccine, live attenuated (RA 27/3)	Meruvax II	Immunity to rubella by antibody production	P Adult/child ≥1 yr: SC 0.5 ml (1000 U)	Hypersensitivity to eggs, neomycin; cancer, radiation, corticosteroids
tetanus toxoid, adsorbed/tetanus toxoid	No trade name	Tetanus toxoid: used for prophylactic treatment of wounds	P Adult/child: IM 0.5 ml q4-6 wk × 2 doses, then 0.5 ml 1 yr after dose 2 (adsorbed); SC/IM 0.5 ml q4-8 wk × 3 doses, then 0.5 ml 1/2-1 yr after dose 3, booster dose 0.5 ml q10 yr	Hypersensitivity, active infection, poliomyelitis outbreak, immunosuppression

ARDS, Acute respiratory distress syndrome; *HRIG,* human rabies immune globulin; *HDCV,* human diploid cell vaccine.

Continued

GENERIC NAME	TRADE NAME	USES	DOSAGES AND ROUTES	CONTRAINDICATIONS
typhoid vaccine, parenteral typhoid vaccine, oral	No trade name Vivotif Berna Vaccine	Active immunity to typhoid fever	Adult: PO 1 cap 1 hr before meals × 4 doses, booster q5 yr P Adult/child >10 yr: SC 0.5 ml, repeat in 4 wk, booster q3 yr P Child 6 mo-10 yr: SC 0.25 ml, repeat in 4 wk, booster q3 yr	Parenteral: systemic or allergic reaction, acute respiratory or other acute infection, intensive physical exercise in high temp Oral: hypersensitivity, acute febrile illness, suppressive or antibiotic drugs
typhoid Vi polysaccharide vaccine	Typhim Vi	Active immunity to typhoid fever	P Adult/child ≥2 yr: IM 0.5 ml as a single dose, reimmunize q2 yr 0.5 ml IM, if needed	Hypersensitivity, chronic typhoid carriers
varicella virus vaccine	Varivax	Prevention of varicella-zoster (chickenpox)	P Adult/child ≥13 yr: SC 0.5 ml, 2nd dose SC 0.5 ml 4-8 wk later	Hypersensitivity to neomycin; blood dyscrasias, immunosuppression, active untreated TB, acute illness, pregnancy, diseases of lymphatic system
yellow fever vaccine	YF-Vax	Active immunity to yellow fever	P Adult/child ≥9 mo: SC 0.5 ml deeply, booster q10 yr P Child 6-9 mo: same as above if exposed	Hypersensitivity to egg or chicken embryo protein, pregnancy, child <6 mo, immunodeficiency

Appendix I

Herbal Products

agrimony

Uses: Mild diarrhea, gastroenteritis, intestinal mucous secretion, inflammation of the mouth and throat, cuts and scrapes, amenorrhea

alfalfa

Uses: Poor appetite, hay fever and asthma, high cholesterol, nutrient source

aloe

Uses of aloe vera gel:
External: Minor burns, skin irritations, minor wounds, frostbite, radiation-caused injuries

Internal: To heal intestinal inflammation and ulcers, as a digestive aid to stimulate bile secretion

angelica

Uses: Heartburn, indigestion, gas, colic, poor blood flow to the extremities, bronchitis, poor appetite, psoriasis, vitiligo, as an antiseptic

arnica

Uses: Topical application for muscle and joint inflammation and swelling; in homeopathic preparations as a remedy for shock, injury, pain

astragalus

Uses: Immune stimulant, viral infections, HIV/AIDS, cancer, vascular disorders, improve circulation, lower blood pressure, possible efficacy in myasthenia gravis

bilberry

Uses: Diabetic retinopathy, macular degeneration, glaucoma, cataract, capillary fragility, varicose veins, hemorrhoids, mild diarrhea

black cohosh

Uses:
Menopause: Hot flashes, nervous conditions associated with menopause

Dysmenorrhea: Menstrual cramps, pain, inflammation

black haw (cramp bark)

Uses: Dysmenorrhea, menstrual cramps and pain, menopausal metrorrhagia, hysteria, asthma, lower blood pressure, heart palpitations

blessed thistle

Uses: Loss of appetite, indigestion, intestinal gas

Adapted from: Dubusk, Ruth, and Treadwell, Phillip. *Serious Drug/Herb Interactions.* Skidmore-Roth Publishing, Inc. 1999.

blue cohosh

Uses: Menopausal symptoms, uterine and ovarian pain, improve flow of menstrual blood, antiinflammatory, antirheumatic, popular remedy in black ethnic medicine

borage

Uses: Antiinflammatory for premenstrual syndrome, rheumatoid arthritis, Raynaud's disease, other inflammatory conditions, atopic dermatitis, infant cradle cap, cystic fibrosis, high blood pressure, diabetes

burdock root

Uses: Skin diseases, inflammation, rashes, cold and fever, cancer, gout, arthritis

calendula

Uses:
External: Minor skin ailments

Internal: Inflammation throughout the gastrointestinal tract, toxic liver and gallbladder, menstrual bleeding and pain, yeast infections

capsicum (cayenne)

Uses: Muscle spasms, pain of inflammation, neuromas, psoriasis, dry mouth, as an antioxidant food, as a food seasoning

cascara

Uses: Chronic constipation, hepatitis, gallstones

cat's claw

Uses: Cancer, herpes, HIV/AIDS, rheumatoid arthritis, gastritis, gout, wounds, gastric ulcers

chamomile

Uses:
External: As an antiseptic and soothing agent for inflamed skin and minor wounds

Internal: As an antispasmodic, gas-relieving, and antiinflammatory agent for the treatment of digestive problems; light sleep aid and sedative for adults and children; possible anticancer agent

chaparral

Uses: Not recommended—potentially toxic to the liver and kidneys

chicory

Uses: Coffee substitute, source of fructo-oligosaccharides, mild laxative for children, gout, rheumatism, loss of appetite, digestive distress

comfrey

Uses: Bruises, sprains, broken bones, acne, boils

cranberry

Uses: UTIs; susceptibility to kidney stones

dong quai

Uses: To restore vitality to tired women; for a variety of gynecologic, menstrual, and menopausal symptoms; cirrhosis of the liver

echinacea

Uses: Low immune status, hard-to-heal superficial wounds, sun protection

elder (elderberry)

Uses: Susceptibility to colds, flu, yeast infections; nasal and chest congestion; earache associated with chronic congestion; hay fever

eleuthero (See siberian ginseng)

ephedra *(ma huang)*

Uses: Seasonal and chronic asthma, nasal congestion, cough

evening primrose

Uses: Premenstrual syndrome, arthritis and inflammatory disorders in general, dry skin, eczema, asthma, diabetes, migraines, chronic fatigue syndrome, heart disease and stroke, circulatory disorders, Raynaud's disease, NSAID use, multiple sclerosis

fenugreek

Uses: Loss of appetite, inflamed areas of the skin, water retention, cancer, constipation, diarrhea, high cholesterol, high blood sugar, calcium oxalate stones

feverfew

Uses: Migraines, cluster headaches, fever, psoriasis, inflammation

flaxseed

Uses: Constipation, as a source of omega-3 fatty acids

fo-ti

Uses: Tiredness, constipation, elevated cholesterol

garcinia cambogia

Uses: Appetite control, weight loss, high cholesterol

garlic

Uses: Vascular disease, elevated LDL, elevated triglycerides, low HDL, high blood pressure, poor circulation, risk of cancer, inflammatory disorders, childhood ear infection, yeast infection

ginger

Uses: Nausea, motion sickness, indigestion, inflammation

ginkgo

Uses: Poor circulation; age-related decline in cognition, memory; diabetes; vascular disease; cancer; inflammatory disorders; impotence; degenerative nerve conditions

ginseng

Uses: Physical and mental exhaustion, stress, viral infections, diabetes, sluggishness, fatigue, weak immunity, convalescence

goldenseal

Uses: High blood pressure, poor appetite, infections, menstrual problems, minor sciatic pain, muscle spasms, eye washes

gotu kola

Uses: Chronic wounds, psoriasis

grape seed

Uses: Antioxidant, chronic disease prevention, inflammation

green tea

Uses: Cancer prevention, heart disease prevention, hypercholesterolemia, diarrhea

guggul

Uses: High LDL cholesterol, elevated triglycerides, weight loss

gymnema sylvestre

Uses: High blood sugar levels

hawthorn

Uses: Poor circulation, chest pain, irregular heartbeat, high blood fats, high blood pressure

hops

Uses: Mild sedative, diuretic, weak antibiotic, insomnia, hyperactivity, pain, fever, jaundice, improve appetite

horse chestnut

Uses: Fever, fluid retention, frostbite, hemorrhoids, inflammation, lower extremity swelling, phlebitis, varicose veins, wounds

horsetail

Uses: Diuretic, genitourinary astringent, anti-hemorrhagic, Bell's Palsy, healing broken bones

kava

Uses: Anxiety, restlessness, sleep disturbances, stress

khat

Uses: Obesity, gastric ulcers, stimulant

kombucha

Uses: Numerous claims for a wide variety of ills; none has been substantiated to date

konjac

Uses: Blood sugar control, constipation, high blood fats, high blood pressure, excessive appetite

kudzu

Uses: Alcohol cravings, menopausal symptoms

lapacho (pau d'arco)

Uses: Cancer, inflammation, infection

lemon balm (melissa)

Uses: Abdominal gas and cramping, cold sores

licorice

Uses: Allergies, arthritis, asthma, constipation, esophagitis, gastritis, hepatitis, inflammatory conditions, peptic ulcers, poor adrenal function, poor appetite

maitake

Uses: Immunostimulant activity, diabetes, hypertension, high cholesterol, obesity

maté

Uses: Diuretic, depurative

melatonin

Uses: Jet lag, insomnia, cancer protection, oral contraceptive

milk thistle

Uses: Protection for alcoholic cirrhosis and hepatitis, antiinflammatory

monascus

Uses: Maintaining acceptable cholesterol levels

morinda

Uses: Headache, digestive, heart and liver conditions, arthritis

nettle

Uses: Diuretic, hay fever

octacosanol

Uses: Herpes, inflammation of the skin, physical endurance

passionflower

Uses: Antifungal, hypertension, sedative, group A hemolytic streptococcus

peppermint

Uses: GI disorders

pygeum

Uses: Benign prostate hypertrophy, antiinflammatory

raspberry leaves

Uses: Facilitation of childbirth, dysmenorrhea, uterine tonic, fever, vomiting

red clover

Uses: Antispasmodic, expectorant, sedative, psoriasis, eczema, amenorrhea

rose hips

Uses: Source of vit C, cold, fever, mild infection

st. john's wort

Uses: Depression, antiviral

sarsaparilla

Uses: Antiinflammatory, antiseptic, syphilis, skin diseases, rheumatism, necrosis, mercury poisoning

sassafras

Uses: Banned in the United States

saw palmetto

Uses: Benign prostatic hypertrophy

schisandra

Uses: GI disorders, liver protection, tonic

scull cap

Uses: Antibacterial, sedative

senna

Uses: Laxative

siberian ginseng (eleuthero)

Uses: Improve appetite, memory loss, hypertension, insomnia, rheumatism, circulation, heart ailments, diabetes, headache

tea tree oil

Uses: Topical use for infections; inhaled for respiratory disorders

uva ursi

Uses: Diuretic, urinary tract infections, contact dermatitis, arthritis

valerian

Uses: Sedative

vitex

Uses: Premenstrual and menstrual disorders, spasms, estrogen gestagen imbalance

yarrow

Uses: To decrease bleeding, Gi disorders, hypertension, thrombi, to improve circulation

yohimbine

Uses: Male organic impotence

Appendix J

FDA Pregnancy Categories

A No risk demonstrated to the fetus in any trimester

B No adverse effects in animals, no human studies available

C Only given after risks to the fetus are considered; animal studies have shown adverse reactions, no human studies available

D Definite fetal risks, may be given in spite of risks if needed in life-threatening conditions

X Absolute fetal abnormalities; not to be used anytime during pregnancy

Appendix K

Controlled Substance Chart

DRUGS	UNITED STATES	CANADA
Heroin, LSD, peyote, marijuana, mescaline	Schedule I	Schedule H
Opium (morphine), meperidine, amphetamines, cocaine, short-acting barbiturates (secobarbital)	Schedule II	Schedule G
Glutethimide, paregoric, phendimetrazine	Schedule III	Schedule F
Chloral hydrate, chlordiazepoxide, diazepam, mazindol, meprobamate, phenobarbital (Canada-G)	Schedule IV	Schedule F
Antidiarrheals with opium (Canada-G), antitussives	Schedule V	Schedule F

Appendix L

Commonly Used Abbreviations

abd abdomen
ABG arterial blood gas
ac before meals
ACE angiotensin-converting enzyme
ACT activated clotting time
ADA American Diabetes Association
ADH antidiuretic hormone
ALT alanine aminotransferase
ANA antinuclear antibody
AP anteroposterior
APTT activated partial thromboplastin time
ASA acetylsalicylic acid, aspirin
ASHD arteriosclerotic heart disease
AST aspartate aminotransferase (SGOT)
AV atrioventricular
bid twice a day
BM bowel movement
BMR basal metabolic rate
B/P blood pressure
BPH benign prostatic hypertrophy
BPM beats per minute
BS blood sugar
BUN blood urea nitrogen
C Celsius (centigrade)
Ca cancer
CAD coronary artery disease
cap capsule
Cath catheterization or catheterize
CBC complete blood cell count
CC chief complaint
cc cubic centimeter
CHF congestive heart failure
cm centimeter
CNS central nervous system
CO_2 carbon dioxide
cont continuous
COPD chronic obstructive pulmonary disease
CPAP continuous positive airway pressue
CPK creatinine phosphokinase
CPR cardiopulmonary resuscitation
CrCl creatinine clearance
C&S culture and sensitivity
C sect cesarean section
CSF cerebrospinal fluid
CV cardiovascular
CVA cerebrovascular accident
CVP central venous pressure
D&C dilatation and curettage
dir inf direct infusion
dr dram
D_5W 5% glucose in distilled water
ECG electrocardiogram (EKG)
EDTA ethylenediamine tetraacetic acid
EEG electroencephalogram

EENT ear, eye, nose, and throat
EPS extrapyramidal symptom
ESR erythrocyte sedimentation rate
ext rel extended release
EXTRA STREN extra strength
susp suspension
FBS fasting blood sugar
FHT fetal heart tones
FSH follicle-stimulating hormone
g gram
GABA γ-aminobutyric acid
GI gastrointestinal
gr grain
GTT glucose tolerance test
gtt drops
GU genitourinary
H_2 histamine$_2$
HCG human chorionic gonadotropin
Hct hematocrit
HDCV human diploid cell rabies vaccine
Hgb hemoglobin
H & H hematocrit and hemoglobin
5-HIAA 5-hydroxyindoleacetic acid
HIV human immunodeficiency virus (AIDS)
H_2O water
HOB head of bed
HR heart rate
hr hour
hs at bedtime
IgG immunoglobulin G
IM intramuscular
inf infusion
INH inhalation
inj injection
I&O intake and output
IPPB intermittent positive-pressure breathing
ITP idiopathic thrombocytopenic purpura
IUD intrauterine device
IV intravenous
IVP intravenous pyelogram
K potassium
kg kilogram
L liter
lb pound
LDH lactic dehydrogenase
LE lupus erythematosus
LH luteinizing hormone
LLQ left lower quadrant
LMP last menstrual period
LOC level of consciousness
LR lactated Ringer's solution
LUQ left upper quadrant
M meter
m minim
m^2 square meter
MAOI monoamine oxidase inhibitor
mEq milliequivalent
mg milligram
μg microgram
MI myocardial infarction
min minute
ml milliliter
mm millimeter
mo month
Na sodium
neg negative
NPO nothing by mouth (Lat. *nulla per os*)
NS normal saline
O_2 oxygen
OBS organic brain syndrome
OD right eye
OR operating room
OS left eye
OTC over-the-counter
OU each eye
oz ounce
p̄ after
P56 plasma-lyte 56

$PaCO_2$ arterial carbon dioxide tension (pressure)
PaO_2 arterial oxygen tension (pressure)
PAT paroxysmal atrial tachycardia
PBI protein-bound iodine
PCWP pulmonary capillary wedge pressure
PEEP positive end-expiratory pressure
PERRLA pupils equal, round, react to light and accommodation
pH hydrogen ion concentration
PO by mouth
postop postoperative
PP postprandial
preop preoperative
prn as required
PT prothrombin time
PTT partial thromboplastin time
PVC premature ventricular contraction
q every
qAM every morning
qd every day
qh every hour
q2h every 2 hours
q3h every 3 hours
q4h every 4 hours
q6h every 6 hours
q12h every 12 hours
qid four times daily
qod every other day
qPM every night
qs sufficient quantity
qt quart
R right
RAIU radioactive iodine uptake
RBC red blood count or cell
RLQ right lower quadrant
ROM range of motion
RUQ right upper quadrant
SC subcutaneous
SIMV synchronous intermittent mandatory ventilation
SL sublingual
SLE systemic lupus erythematosus
SOB shortness of breath
sol solution
ss one half
supp suppository
sus rel sustained release
syr syrup
T&A tonsillectomy and adenoidectomy
tab tablet
tbsp tablespoon
temp temperature
tid three times daily
tinc tincture
TPN total parenteral nutrition
top topical
TRANS transdermal
TSH thyroid-stimulating hormone
tsp teaspoon
TT thrombin time
U unit
UA urinalysis
UTI urinary tract infection
UV ultraviolet
vag vaginal
VMA vanillylmandelic acid
vol volume
VS vital sign
WBC white blood cell count
wk week
wt weight
yr year
> greater than
< less than
= equal
° degree
% percent
γ gamma
β beta

Appendix M

IV Drug/Solution Compatibility Chart

	D_5	D_{10}	D_5 ½S	D_5 S	NS	R	LR	OTHER
Acetazolamide	C	C	C	C	C	C	C	
Acyclovir	C							
Alpha$_1$-proteinase inhibitor								Sterile water for inj
Alprostadil	C	C			C			
Alteplase								Sterile water for inj
Amdinocillin	C	C	C	C	C	C	C	D_5 in R
Amikacin	C				C			
Aminocaproic acid			C	C	C	C		D in distilled water
Ammonium Cl					C			May add KCl to solution
Amphotericin B	C							
Ampicillin	C				C			
Amrinone lactate					C			0.45% saline
Antithrombin III	C				C			Sterile water for inj
Ascorbic acid	C				C	C	C	Sodium lactate
Azlocillin	C		C		C			
Atenolol	C				C			0.45% saline
Aztreonam	C	C			C	C	C	Normosol-R
Bretylium tosylate	C				C			
Cefamandole	C				C			
Cefazolin	C				C			
Cefotetan	C				C			
Cefoxitin	C	C			C	C	C	Aminosol
Ceftrazidime	C		C	C	C	C	C	M/G Sodium lactate
Ceftriaxone	C				C			
Cefuroxime	C		C	C		C		M/G Sodium lactate
Cephalothin	C				C	C	C	M/G Sodium lactate

This chart is not inclusive and is based on manufacturers' recommendations.

Key

C = Compatible
D_5 = Dextrose 5%
D_{10} = Dextrose 10%
D_5½S = Dextrose 5% in saline 0.45%
D_5S = Dextrose 5% in saline 0.9%
NS = Sodium chloride 0.9% (normal saline)
R = Ringer's solution
LR = Lactated Ringer's solution

	D_5	D_{10}	D_5 ½S	D_5 S	NS	R	LR	OTHER
Cephapirin	C				C			
Ciprofloxacin	C				C			
Cyclosporine	C				C			Use only glass containers
Dobutamine					C			Sodium lactate
Dopamine	C		C	C	C		C	M/G Sodium lactate
Doxycycline	C				C			Invert sugar 10%
Edetate Na	C	C						Isotonic saline
Ganciclovir	C				C	C	C	
Gentamicin	C				C			Normosol-R
Heparin Na	C	C			C	C		
Ifosfamide	C				C		C	Sterile water for inj
Isoproterenol	C			C	C	C		Invert sugar 5% & 10%
Kanamycin	C				C			
Metaraminol	C			C	C	C	C	Normosol-R
Methicillin	C			C				
Metoclopramide	C			C		C	C	
Mezlocillin	C	C	C	C	C	C	C	Fructose 5%
Moxalactam	C	C	C	C	C	C	C	M/G Sodium lactate
Netilmicin	C	C		C	C	C	C	Normosol-R
Norepinephrine	C	C		C			C	
Nitroglycerin	C	C			C			
Piperacillin	C			C	C		C	
Ritodrine	C							
Ticarcillin	C				C		C	
Tobramycin	C				C			
Vidarabine	C	C			C			

Appendix N

Nomogram for Calculation of Body Surface Area

Place a straight edge from the patient's height in the left column to his or her weight in the right column. The point of intersection on the body surface area column indicates the body surface area (BSA). Reproduced from Behrman RE, and Vaughn VC (editors): Nelson's textbook of pediatrics, ed 12, Philadelphia, 1983, WB Saunders.

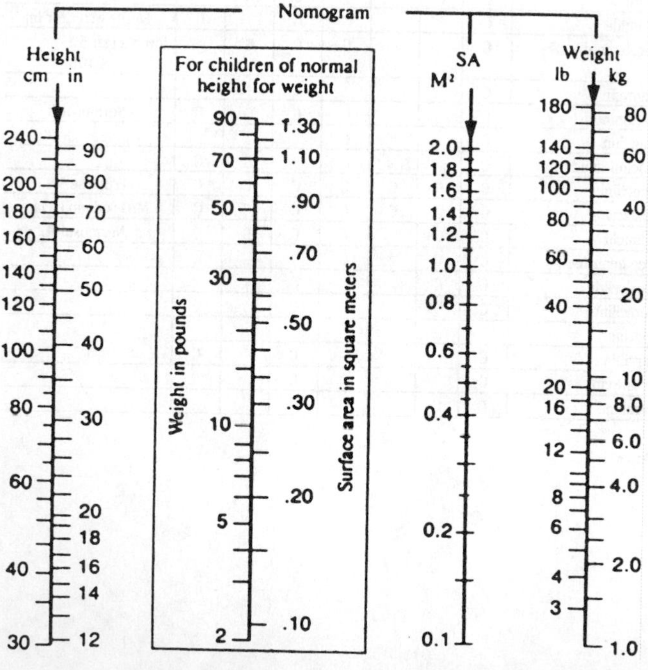

Disorders Index

S

T

V

Z

Index

Entries can be identified as follows: generic name, Trade Name, DRUG CATEGORY, *Combination Product.*

Entries can be identified as follows: generic name, Trade Name, DRUG CATEGORY, *Combination Product.*

B

Entries can be identified as follows: generic name, Trade Name, DRUG CATEGORY, *Combination Product.*

Entries can be identified as follows: generic name, Trade Name, DRUG CATEGORY, *Combination Product.*

Entries can be identified as follows: generic name, Trade Name, DRUG CATEGORY, *Combination Product.*

F

Entries can be identified as follows: generic name, Trade Name, DRUG CATEGORY, *Combination Product.*

H

I

J

K

L

Entries can be identified as follows: generic name, Trade Name, DRUG CATEGORY, *Combination Product.*

N

P

Q

R

S

T

Entries can be identified as follows: generic name, Trade Name, DRUG CATEGORY, *Combination Product.*

W

X

Y

Z

Mosby's DrugSmart CD-ROM to accompany Mosby's Drug Guide for Nurses

Fifth Edition

Learn to administer drugs with ease and confidence using *Mosby's DrugSmart to Accompany Mosby's Drug Guide for Nurses, Fifth Edition*. This three-in-one CD-ROM provides you with interactive information and exercises on dosages and solutions, alternative remedies and pharmacology principles.

Mosby's DrugSmart includes:

- **Dosages and Solutions** by Virginia Daugherty, RN, MSN & Diana Romans, RN, BSN
  Use this tutorial to master dug calculations. First, review drug dosage calculations with key examples. Then, test your knowledge with abundant practice problems and answers.
- **Herbal Remedies** by Steve Blake, ND, MH, DSc, MT
  Use this electronic encyclopedia to search for reliable, up-to-date information and photos on more than 30 of the most commonly used herbal remedies. *Herbal Remedies* allows you to search by alternative names, actions, constituents, body systems and health conditions.
- **Pharmacology Principles** by Linda Skidmore-Roth, RN, MSN, NP
  Use this information to refresh your memory of calculation methods and formulas for all drug forms, as well as brush up on life span considerations – including pediatric, geriatric, and pregnancy dosing recommendations.

Contact Us
For further information, visit us at www.mosby.com or call us at (800) 545-2522.

Mini CD-ROM
This mini CD-ROM will work in your CD-ROM drive. Place it on the inner ring of the tray, as shown, and follow the on-screen installation instructions.

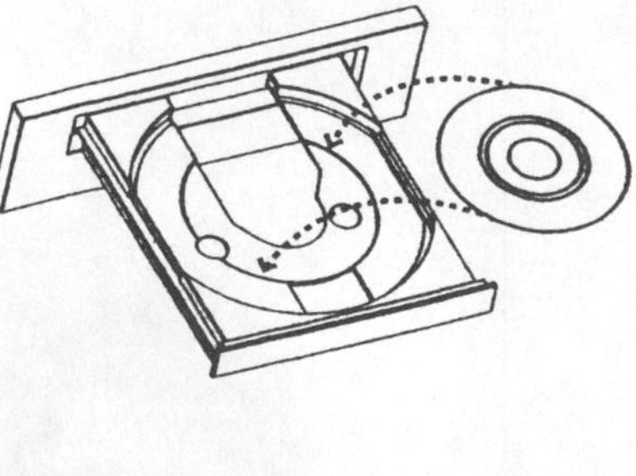

This mini-CD does not work in:
- Floppy Drives
- Slot Drives
- Zip Drives
- Stereos

Insert this mini-CD into your CD-ROM drive as shown at left.

Important
No credit or refund will be issued on this book if the CD envelope has been opened, torn, or otherwise tampered with.

Mosby's DrugSmart

SYSTEM REQUIREMENTS

Windows®
486, Pentium®, or faster processor
Windows® 95, 98, NT 4.0, or newer
16 MB or available RAM
35 MB or available hard-disk space
2× or faster CD-ROM drive
640 × 480 minimum resolution monitor supporting 256 colors (thousands recommended)

CD INSTALLATION INSTRUCTIONS
Windows® 95, 98, NT 4.0, or newer

1. Start Microsoft Windows® and insert CD-ROM.
2. Follow the on-screen instructions for installation.

TECHNICAL SUPPORT
Technical support for this product is available at no charge by calling the Technical Support Hotline between 9 a.m. and 5 p.m. CST, Monday through Friday. Inside the United States, call 1-800-692-9010. Outside the United States, call 314-872-8370. You may also contact Technical Support through e-mail: technical.support@elsevier.com